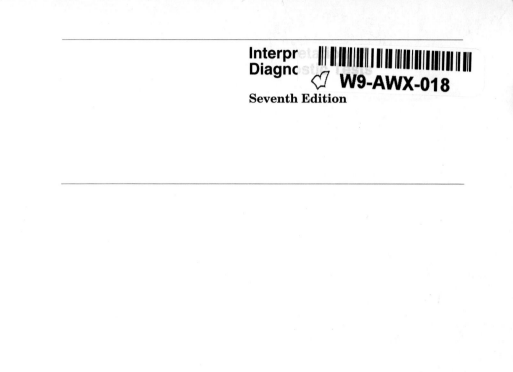

Interpretation of
Diagnostic Tests

Seventh Edition

Seventh Edition

Interpretation of Diagnostic Tests

Jacques Wallach, M.D.
Clinical Professor of Pathology,
State University of New York
Health Science Center at Brooklyn;
Attending Pathologist,
Kings County Hospital Center,
Brooklyn, New York

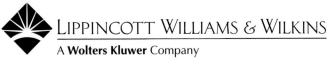

LIPPINCOTT WILLIAMS & WILKINS
A **Wolters Kluwer** Company
Philadelphia · Baltimore · New York · London
Buenos Aires · Hong Kong · Sydney · Tokyo

Acquisitions Editor: Richard Winters
Developmental Editor: Michelle LaPlante
Supervising Editor: Mary Ann McLaughlin
Production Editor: Shannon Garza, Silverchair Science + Communications
Manufacturing Manager: Kevin Watt
Cover Designer: Tik Chuaviriya
Compositor: Silverchair Science + Communications
Printer: RR Donnelly, Crawfordsville

© 2000 by LIPPINCOTT WILLIAMS & WILKINS
530 Walnut Street
Philadelphia, PA 19106 USA
LWW.com

Library of Congress Cataloging-in-Publication Data

Wallach, Jacques B. (Jacques Burton), 1926-
    Interpretation of diagnostic tests / Jacques Wallach.-- 7th ed.
        p. ; cm.
    Includes bibliographical references and index.
    ISBN 0-7817-1659-4
    1. Diagnosis, Laboratory--Handbooks, manuals, etc. I. Title.
    [DNLM: 1. Laboratory Techniques and Procedures. QY 25 W195i 2000]
    RB38.2 .W35 2000
    616.07'56--dc21

                                                      99-055267

10 9 8 7 6 5 4 3 2

To Doris
and
To Kim, Lisa, and Tracy
and
To Gabriel, Jonah, Zachary, and Ariel

Translations

INTERPRETATION OF DIAGNOSTIC TESTS is published in the following translations:

First Edition

INTERPRETACIÓN DE LOS DIAGNÓSTICOS DE LABORATORIO

Ἑρμηνεία τῶμ Διαγνωστικῶν Ἐξετάσεων καὶ Δοκιμασιῶν

INTERPRETAÇOÄ DOŚ DIAGNÓSTICOS DE LABORATÓRIO

Second Edition

INTERPRETAZIONE DEI TESTS DI LABORATORIO IN MEDICINA

如何解释临床检验: 实验室医学手册

Third Edition

INTERPRETAÇOÄ DOŚ DIAGNÓSTICOS DE LABORATÓRIO

INTERPRETAZIONE DEI TESTS DI LABORATORIO IN MEDICINA

INTERPRETACIÓN DE LOS DIAGNÓSTICOS DE LABORATORIO

Fourth Edition

INTERPRETAÇOÄ DOŚ DIAGNÓSTICOS DE LABORATÓRIO

Fifth Edition

Teşhiste Laboratuvar Testleri: Özet Laboratuvar Bilgileri

Ἑρμηνεία τῶμ Διαγνωστικῶν Ἐξετάσεων καὶ Δοκιμασιῶν

INTERPRETAÇOÄ DOŚ DIAGNÓSTICOS DE LABORATÓRIO

Sixth Edition

INTERPRETACIÓN DE LOS DIAGNÓSTICOS DE LABORATORIO

Ἑρμηνεία τῶμ Διαγνωστικῶν Ἐξετάσεων καὶ Δοκιμασιῶν

INTERPRETAÇOÄ DOŚ DIAGNÓSTICOS DE LABORATÓRIO

ワラック
検査値ハンドブック

Contents

Preface

The history is important in the selection of appropriate diagnostic tests and for an estimate of prior prevalence for interpreting the test sensitivity and specificity. Laboratory tests have greater specificity and sensitivity than the physical examination for many disorders.

Test selection depends largely on the clinical purpose for testing (e.g., screening, case finding, monitoring the course of disease, following the effects of therapy, determining drug levels or drug effects) and on the patient population being evaluated. Whereas formerly it was common to order a multiphasic panel of blood chemistry and hematology tests, this practice is now discouraged to decrease costs and to avoid the "Ulysses syndrome."

Appropriate diseases for screening should be sufficiently prevalent, life threatening, disabling, or financially burdensome; detectable by tests of sufficient sensitivity and specificity with high predictive value; and susceptible to available therapy that can prevent, ameliorate, or delay the onset of disease or prolong useful life. Common examples of conditions for screening and case finding in asymptomatic persons include cytology for cervical cancer, testing for HIV and other transmissible diseases in blood donors, and for phenylketonuria (PKU) and hypothyroidism in newborns.

Laboratory tests are an increasing part of most patient-physician relationships and contribute greatly to the selection of additional diagnostic procedures and, ultimately to diagnosis and treatment. They often precede the history and physical examination. The use of physician office laboratories and increased consolidation of distant reference laboratories diminishes the opportunity for clinicians to consult with local laboratory directors even as there are greater economic constraints and criticisms regarding inappropriate utilization of health resources.

Many remarkable advances have occurred in laboratory medicine since the first edition of *Interpretation of Diagnostic Tests* was published in 1970. A wealth of new laboratory tests has become essential to the modern practice of medicine, and each edition has paralleled these changes by including more recently described disorders and newer tests, which accounts for the increased size of each edition. The number, cost, complexity, sophistication, variety, utility, and availability of laboratory tests continues to grow along with clinicians' dependence on them.

Many diagnoses can only be established, or etiologies confirmed or appropriate therapy selected, by such tests. The size of this medical knowledge database defies and challenges the ability of any individual to use it to its greatest advantage.

I have attempted to address these issues in the following ways:

1. Maintaining the organization, format, style, ease of use, nominal cost, thoroughness, and practical utility.
2. Making significant improvements through extensive editing, remodeling, cross-referencing, and book design (e.g., edge tabs) to make the data more readable and more useful.
3. Information about tests and diseases has been extensively updated, including newer technologies such as monoclonal antibodies, DNA probes, polymerase chain reaction, specific hormone assays, immunochemical and cytochemical staining, flow cytometry, cytogenics, and chromosomal studies that have markedly improved our accuracy and diagnostic ability. Outmoded or rarely used tests have been deleted.
4. Additional algorithms and tables may clarify and expedite the patient's workup.
5. More data on test sensitivity, specificity, and predictive value and more current references have been included.

6. Reorganization includes improved alphabetizing and organizing of the tests and diseases within each chapter and deleting redundancies and repetitions that may have crept in during the previous 25 years, thereby simplifying the reader's search as well as reducing the size of the extensive index that characterized previous editions. The reader can now find answers more quickly and expeditiously.

7. A symbol is used to mark tests that are diagnostic for a disease (♦), and a different icon (○) is used for those tests that are suggestive or supportive or should arouse suspicion of, but are not diagnostic for, that disease, thus encouraging more cost-effective and immediate diagnosis. Unmarked tests simply let the reader know that such test results may occur and are nonspecific, although they may occasionally provide useful collateral information in the differential diagnosis of an individual problem.

8. The effect of drugs on laboratory tests that appeared in a separate chapter in previous editions has been included with the tests themselves, diminishing the need for the reader to cross-check between chapters and possible redundancy.

9. Electronic versions are available for easier pursuit of information and cross-referencing and ultimately for integration with computerized laboratory test reporting.

10. A more concise pocket version (*Handbook of Interpretation of Diagnostic Tests*) has been published for those who may need less detail and more portability.

11. This edition continues to mostly use conventional rather than Système International (SI) units because many journals do so and especially because most physicians are more familiar with them; a table for converting units is included in Appendix B.

12. Computerized consolidation of laboratory results brings clinicians closer to the goal of integrating these results and clinical findings with their interpretation and constitutes an increasing unique opportunity in medicine.

These modifications should permit this book to continue to meet the needs of students in medicine, dentistry, nursing, laboratory technology, and veterinary medicine, as well as a wide range of health care providers from novices and house officers to seasoned clinicians, laboratorians, and pathologists. Its success is indicated in the use of hundreds of thousands of copies of earlier editions in various languages and countries for 30 years, the many favorable comments received, and the number of authors who have tried to emulate it. Readers are encouraged to continue their suggestions and criticisms.

The author's perspective as a practicing pathologist, laboratory director, clinician, and teacher who personally needs current, concise, and practical diagnostic data without the distraction of other material, such as methodology, technology, physiologic mechanisms, and Medicare code numbers, has informed the preparation of this edition and continues to distinguish it from other laboratory books.

J.W.

Preface to the First Edition

Results of laboratory tests may aid in
  Discovering occult disease
  Preventing irreparable damage (e.g., phenylketonuria)
  Early diagnosis after onset of signs or symptoms
  Differential diagnosis of various possible diseases
  Determining the stage of the disease
  Estimating the activity of the disease
  Detecting the recurrence of disease
  Monitoring the effect of therapy
  Genetic counseling in familial conditions
  Medicolegal problems, such as paternity suits
This book is written to help the physician achieve these purposes with the least amount of
  Duplication of tests
  Waste of patient's money
  Overtaxing of laboratory facilities and personnel
  Loss of physician's time
  Confusion caused by the increasing number, variety, and complexity of tests currently available. Some of these tests may be unrequested but performed as part of routine surveys or hospital admission multitest screening.
In order to provide quick reference and maximum availability and usefulness, this handy-sized book features
  Tabular and graphic style of concise presentation
  Emphasis on serial time changes in laboratory findings in various stages of disease
  Omission of rarely performed, irrelevant, esoteric, and outmoded laboratory tests
  Exclusion of discussion of physiologic mechanisms, metabolic pathways, clinical features, and nonlaboratory aspects of disease
  Discussion of only the more important diseases that the physician encounters and should be able to diagnose
This book is not
  An encyclopedic compendium of clinical pathology
  A technical manual
  A substitute for good clinical judgment and basic knowledge of medicine
Deliberately omitted are
  Technical procedures and directions
  Photographs and illustrations of anatomic changes (e.g., blood cells, karyo-types, isotope scans)
  Discussions of quality control
  Selection of a referral laboratory
  Performance of laboratory tests in the clinician's own office
  Bibliographic references, except for the most general reference texts in medicine, hematology, and clinical pathology and for some recent references to specific conditions
The usefulness and need for a book of this style, organization, and contents have been increased by such current trends as
  The frequent lack of personal assistance, advice, and consultation in large commercial laboratories and hospital departments of clinical pathology, which are often specialized and fragmented as well as impersonal
  Greater demand for the physician's time

The development of many new tests

Faculty and administrators still assume that this essential area of medicine can be learned "intuitively" as it was 20 years ago and that it therefore requires little formal training. This attitude ignores changes in the number and variety of tests now available as well as their increased sophistication and basic value in establishing a diagnosis.

The contents of this book are organized to answer the questions most often posed by physicians when they require assistance from the pathologist. There is no other single adequate source of information presented in this fashion. It appears from numerous comments I have received that this book has succeeded in meeting the needs not only of practicing physicians and medical students but also of pathologists, technologists, and other medical personnel. It has been adopted by many schools of nursing and of medical technology, physicians assistant training programs, and medical schools. Such widespread acceptance confirms my original premise in writing this book and is most gratifying.

A perusal of the table of contents and index will quickly show the general organization of the material by type of laboratory test or organ system or certain other categories. In order to maintain a concise format, separate chapters have not been organized for such categories as newborn, pediatric, and geriatric periods or for primary psychiatric or dermatologic diseases. A complete index provides maximum access to this information.

Obviously these data are not original but have been adapted from many sources over the years. Only the selection, organization, manner of presentation, and emphasis are original. I have formulated this point of view during 40 years as a clinician and pathologist, viewing with pride the important and growing role of the laboratory but deeply regretting its inappropriate utilization.

This book was written to improve laboratory utilization by making it simpler for the physician to select and interpret the most useful laboratory tests for his clinical problems.

J.W.

Acknowledgments

I thank colleagues in various parts of the world who have shared their clinical and laboratory problems with me and encouraged the continuation of this book. The universal need to convert an ever-expanding mass of raw laboratory data into accessible, cost-effective, clinically usable information continues to be a matter of increasing significance throughout the medical community and a chief concern of mine in producing this book and in other teaching and research efforts. The need for expeditious, unencumbered information has been repeatedly confirmed during teaching of medical students and house officers, in the daily practice of pathology, by discussions with physicians in many countries that I have visited or in which I have worked or taught, and by the translation of this volume into various other languages. I am rewarded by numerous instances of friendship, criticism, kindness, and help and by learning far more than I could include in this small volume. I continue to be gratified and stimulated beyond expectation.

My thanks to Executive Editor Rich Winters for his sensible advice and support, to Developmental Editor Michelle LaPlante, to Supervising Editor Mary Ann McLaughlin, and to the other people behind the scenes at Lippincott Williams & Wilkins who were so uniformly helpful; to Production Editor Shannon Garza and staff at Silverchair Science + Communications for their tireless, diligent, and meticulous work on this project; and to Linda Hallinger for her careful indexing.

The friendship, love, care, and generosity of my wife, Doris, can never be sufficiently acknowledged.

Acknowledgments

Normal Values

1 Introduction to Normal Values (Reference Ranges)

General Principles

The purpose of all testing (laboratory, radiologic, electrocardiographic [ECG], etc.) is to reduce clinical uncertainty. The degree of reduction varies with the test characteristics and clinical situation. Modern medicine has superseded Voltaire's dictum that "the art of medicine consists of amusing the patient while nature cures the disease."

Many clinicians are still largely unaware of the reasoning process that they pursue in seeking a diagnosis and tend to follow an empirical path that was previously successful or was learned during early training periods by observing their mentors during clinical rounds without appreciating the rationale for selecting, ordering, and interpreting laboratory tests; this is often absorbed in a subliminal, informal, or rote fashion. The need to control health care costs and many recent studies on laboratory test utilization have emphasized the need for a selective approach.

Some important principles in utilizing laboratory (and all other) tests are as follows:

1. Under the best of circumstances, no test is perfect (e.g., 100% sensitivity, specificity, predictive value). In any specific case, the results may be misleading. The most sensitive tests are best used to rule out a suspected disease so that the number of false-negative tests is minimal; thus a negative test tends to exclude the disease. The most specific tests are best used to confirm or exclude a suspected disease and minimize the number of false-positive results. Sensitivity and specificity may be markedly altered by the coexistence of other disorders or by complications or sequelae of the primary disease.

2. Choice of tests should be based on the prior probability of the diagnosis being sought, which affects the predictive value of the test. This prior probability is determined by the history, physical examination, and prevalence of the suspected disorder (in that community at that time), which is why history and physical examination should precede ordering of tests. The clinician need not know the exact prior probability of the disease. Estimating this as high, intermediate, or low is usually sufficient. Moderate errors in estimating prior probability have only relatively limited effects on interpretation of the tests. If the prior prevalence is high, a positive result tends to confirm the presence of the disease, but an unexpected negative result is not very useful in ruling out the disease. Conversely, when the prior prevalence is low, a normal result tends to rule out the disease, but an unexpected positive result is not very useful in confirming the disease. (See Tables 1-1 and 1-2.)

3. In the majority of laboratory measurements, the combination of short-term physiologic variation and analytic error is sufficient to render the interpretation of single determinations difficult when the concentrations are in the borderline range. Any particular laboratory result may be incorrect for a large variety of reasons, regardless of the high quality of the laboratory; such results should be rechecked. If indicated, a new specimen sample should be submitted with careful confirmation of patient identification, prompt delivery to the laboratory, and immediate processing; in some circumstances, confirmation of test results at another laboratory may be appropriate.

4. Reference ranges vary from one laboratory to another; the user should know what these ranges are for each laboratory used and should also be aware of variations due to age, sex, race, size, physiologic status (e.g., pregnancy, lactation) that apply

Table 1-1. Assuming a Low Prior Probability (10%) (in 1000 Tests, Disease is Present in 100 and Absent in 900)

[Prevalence = (90 + 10)/(90 + 180 + 10 + 720) or (100/1000) = 10%]

Test Result	Disease Present	Disease Absent
Positive	90	180
Negative`	10	720
Total	100	900

Even with a test of high sensitivity (e.g., 90%), the positive predictive value (probability that those with a positive test have the disease) is only 33% [90/(90 + 180)].
In contrast, the negative predictive value (percentage of those with a negative result who do not have the disease) is [720/(10 + 720)] = 99%. Thus, a negative test indicates 99% probability of no disease.
The specificity = 720/(180 + 720) = 80%.

Table 1-2. Assuming a High Prior Probability (90%) (in 1000 Cases Tested, Disease is Present in 900 and Absent in 100)

[Prevalence = (810 + 90)/(810 + 20 + 90 + 80) or (900/1000) = 90%]

Test Result	Disease Present	Disease Absent
Positive	810	20
Negative	90	80
Total	900	100

With a test of high sensitivity (e.g., 90%), the positive predictive value (probability that those with a positive test have the disease) is 98% [810/(810 + 20)], indicating near certainty that disease is present is confirmatory.
In contrast, the negative predictive value (percentage of those with a negative result who do not have the disease) is [80/(90 + 80)] = 47%. Thus, a negative test (probability of no disease) indicates that the patient still has a fairly high likelihood of having the disease (47%).
The specificity = 80/(20 + 80) = 80%.

to the particular patient. These "normal" ranges represent collected statistical data rather than classification of patients as having disease or being healthy and are based on the statistical definition of normal as 95% range of values, whereby 5% of independent tests will be outside this normal range in the absence of disease. This is best illustrated in the use of multitest chemical profiles for screening persons known to be free of disease. The probability of any given test being abnormal is approximately 2% to 5% and the probability of disease if a screening test is abnormal is generally low (0% to 15%). The frequency of abnormal single tests is 1.5% (albumin) to 5.9% (glucose) and up to 16.6% for sodium. Based on statistical expectations, when a panel of 8 tests is performed in a multiphasic health program, 25% of the patients have one or more abnormal results and when the panel includes 20 tests, 55% have one or more test abnormalities.[1]
5. Tables of reference values represent statistical data for 95% of the population; values outside of these ranges do not necessarily represent disease. Results may still be within the reference range but be elevated above the patient's baseline, which is why serial testing is important in a number of conditions. For example, in acute myocardial infarction, the increase in serum total creatine kinase (CK) may be abnormal for that patient although the value may be within "normal" range.
6. An individual's test values when measured by a good laboratory tend to remain fairly consistent over a period of years when performed with comparable technology; comparison of results with previous values obtained when the patient was not ill (if available) are often a better reference value than "normal" ranges.

[1]Friedman GD, Golberg M, Ahuja JN, Siegelaub AB, Bassis ML, Collen MI. Biochemical screening tests: effect of panel size on medical care. *Arch Int Med* 1972;129:91.

7. Multiple test abnormalities are more likely to be significant than single test abnormalities. When two or more tests for the same disorder are positive, the results reinforce the diagnosis, but when only one test is positive and the other is not positive, the strength of the interpretation is diluted.

8. The greater the degree of abnormality of a test result, the more likely that a confirmed value is clinically significant or represents a real disorder. Thus, an increase ten times the upper reference range is much more likely to be significant compared to a result that is only slightly increased. Most slightly abnormal results are due to preanalytic factors.

9. Characteristic laboratory test profiles that are described in the literature and in this book represent the full-blown picture of the well-developed or far-advanced case, but all abnormal tests may be present simultaneously in only a small fraction (e.g., one-third) of patients with that condition. Even when a test profile (combination of tests) is characteristic of a particular disorder, other disorders or groups of conditions may produce exactly the same combination of laboratory test changes.

10. Excessive repetition of tests is wasteful, and the excess burden increases the possibility of laboratory errors. Appropriate intervals between tests should be dictated by the patient's clinical condition.

11. Tests should be performed only if they will alter the patient's diagnosis, prognosis, treatment, or management. Incorrect test values or isolated individual variation in results may cause "Ulysses syndrome" and result in loss of time, money, and peace of mind.

12. Clerical errors are far more likely than technical errors to cause incorrect results. Greatest care should be taken to completely and properly label and identify every specimen, which should *always* be accompanied by a test requisition form. Busy hospital laboratories receive inordinate numbers of unlabeled, unidentified specimens each day, which are useless, burdensome, and sometimes dangerous.

13. The effect of drugs on laboratory test values must never be overlooked. Test abnormalities may be due to drugs as often as to disease. The clinician should always be aware of what drugs the patient has been taking, including over-the-counter medications, vitamins, iron, and such. Patients often do not tell their physicians about medications they are taking (prescribed by other doctors or by the patients themselves) which may produce false-negative as well as false-positive results. In addition, there is environmental exposure to many drugs and chemicals. The classes of drugs most often involved include the anticoagulants, anticonvulsants, antihypertensives, antiinfectives, oral hypoglycemics, hormones, and psychoactive agents. A number of causative mechanisms may operate, sometimes simultaneously (e.g., interference with the chemical reaction in the testing procedure, damage to a specific organ such as liver or kidney, competition for binding sites, accelerated or retarded formation or excretion of a specific chemical, and such). Often the mechanism of these altered laboratory test values is not known.

14. Laboratory values in the elderly must be interpreted in light of the many factors that affect "normal" values in this group:
    - Altered function due to aging (e.g., diminished renal function).
    - Presence of chronic disease that is more prevalent in older populations and may be asymptomatic or occult.
    - Occurrence of multiple concurrent conditions or diseases, some of which may have additive effects on laboratory results.
    - Use of medications that affect laboratory analytes (e.g., 10% to 30% of elderly persons may be taking diuretics).
    - Homeostasis is not compromised by age alone.
    - Biological variability does not increase simply with age.
    - Values given for age are always in comparison to young adults of the same sex unless otherwise stated. Values given for sex are always in comparison to opposite sex of comparable age. When sex is not specified, it refers to both sexes.

15. The reader must be aware of the effect of artifacts causing spurious values and of factitious disorders *especially in the face of discrepant laboratory results*.

16. Negative laboratory (or any other type of tests) do not necessarily rule out a clinical diagnosis.

Table 1-3. Reference Ranges for Complete Blood Cell Count at Various Ages

Age	RBC (× 10⁶/cu mm)	Hb (g/dL)	Hct (%)	MCV (fL)	MCH (pg)	RDW (%)
Newborn	4.1–6.7	15.0–24.0	44–70	102–115	33–39	13.0–18.0
1–23 mos	3.8–5.4	10.5–14.0	32–42	72–88	24–30	11.5–16.0
2–9 yrs	4.0–5.3	11.5–14.5	33–43	76–90	25–31	11.5–15.0
10–17 yrs						
Males	4.2–5.6	12.5–16.1	36–47	78–95	26–32	11.5–14.0
Females	4.1–5.3	12.0–15.0	35–45	78–95	26–32	11.5–14.0
>18 yrs						
Males	4.7–6.0	13.5–18.0	42–52	78–100	27–31	11.5–14.0
Females	4.2–5.4	12.5–16.0	37–47	78–100	27–31	11.5–14.0

Mean platelet volume = 6.0–9.5 fL for all age groups. Platelets = 150,000–450,000/cu mm for all age groups. Mean corpuscular hemoglobin concentration = 32–36 gm/dL for all age groups.
Source: Clinical Laboratories of Children's Hospital of Buffalo.

References Values[2]

Hematology Reference Values

Complete blood cell count (CBC)	See Tables 1-3, 1-4, 1-5, and 1-6
Carboxyhemoglobin	<5% of total
Delta-aminolevulinic acid	1.5–7.5 mg/24-hr urine
Erythrocyte sedimentation rate (ESR)	
Westergren	
Males	0–13 mm in 1 hr
Females	0–20 mm in 1 hr
Wintrobe	
Males	0–10 mm in 1 hr
Females	0–15 mm in 1 hr
Children	0–13 mm in 1 hr
Newborns	0–2 mm in 1 hr
Erythropoietin (radioimmunoassay [RIA])	
Males	17.2 mU/mL (mean)
Females	18.8 mU/mL (mean)
Ferritin	
Newborns	25–200 ng/mL
1 mo	200–600 ng/mL
2–5 mos	50–200 ng/mL
6 mos–15 yrs	7–142 ng/mL
Adult males	20–300 ng/mL
Adult females	15–120 ng/mL
Borderline (males or females)	10–20 ng/mL
Iron excess	>400 ng/mL

[2]Burritt ME, Slockbower JM, Forsman RW, Offord KP, Bergstralh EJ, Smithson WA. Pediatric reference intervals for 19 biologic variables in healthy children. *Mayo Clin Proc* 1990;65:329.
Leavelle DE, ed. *Mayo Medical Laboratories 1995 test catalog*. Rochester, MN: Mayo Medical Laboratories, 1995.
Lockitch G, Halstead AC, Quigley G, MacCallum C. Age- and sex-specific pediatric reference intervals—various analytes. *Clin Chem* 1988;34:1618.
Kratz A, Lewandrowski KB. Case records of the Massachusetts General Hospital. Normal reference laboratory values. *N Engl J Med* 1998;339:1063.
Soldin SJ, Hicks JM, eds. *Pediatric reference ranges*. Washington: AACC Press, 1995.
Tietz NW, Shuey DF, Wekstein DR. Laboratory values in fit aging individuals—sexagenarians through centenarians. *Clin Chem* 1992;38:1167.
Green A, Morgan I. *Neonatology and clinical biochemistry*. London: CB Venture Publications, 1993.

Table 1-4. Reference Ranges for White Blood Cell Count (WBC) at Various Ages (Differential Count in Absolute Numbers)

Age	WBC (× 1000/cu mm)	Total Neutrophils*	Segs	Bands	Lymphs	Monos	Eos	Baso
Newborn	9.1–34.0	6.0–23.5	6.0–20.0	<3.5	2.5–10.5	<3.5	<2.0	<0.4
1–23 mos	6.0–14.0	1.1–6.6	1.0–6.0	<1.0	1.8–9.0	<1.0	<0.7	<0.1
2–9 yrs	4.0–12.0	1.4–6.6	1.2–6.0	<1.0	1.0–5.5	<1.0	<0.7	<0.1
10–17 yrs	4.0–10.5	1.5–6.6	1.3–6.0	<1.0	1.0–3.5	<1.0	<0.7	<0.1
>18 yrs	4.0–10.5	1.5–6.6	1.3–6.0	<1.0	1.5–3.5	<1.0	<0.7	<0.1

Segs = segmented neutrophils; Bands = band neutrophils; Lymphs = lymphocytes; Monos = monocytes; Eos = eosinophils; Baso = basophils.
*Total Neutrophils = Segs + Bands.
Source: Clinical Laboratories of Children's Hospital of Buffalo.

Table 1-5. Reference Ranges for Blood Cell Count at Various Fetal Ages

	Age (wks)			
	18–20	21–22	23–25	25–30
RBC ($\times 10^6$/cu mm)	2.35–2.95	2.70–3.22	2.80–3.32	3.20–3.84
Hb (gm/dL)	10.7–12.3	11.4–13.2	12.1–12.7	12.2–14.5
Hct (%)	33–39	35–41	36–41	38–45
MCV (fL)	125–142	123–136	119–132	112–124
WBC ($\times$ 1000/cu mm)	3.6–5.0	3.4–5.0	3.3–4.6	3.5–5.2
Platelets ($\times$ 1000/cu mm)	208–277	203–312	217–301	216–290

RBC = red blood cell count; Hb = hemoglobin; Hct= hematocrit; MCV = mean corpuscular volume;
WBC = white blood cell count.
Source: Daffos F. Fetal blood sampling. In: Harrison WR, Globus MS, Filly RA, eds. *The unborn patient*,
2nd ed. Philadelphia: WB Saunders, 1991:79.

Folate, erythrocyte	
<1 yr	74–995 ng/mL
1–11 yrs	96–362 ng/mL
≥ 12 yrs	180–600 ng/mL
Folate, serum	≥ 3.5 μg/L
Free erythrocyte protoporphyrin	<100 μg/dL packed red blood cells
(FEP)	(RBCs)
Glucose-6-phosphate dehydrogenase	
(G-6-PD) erythrocyte	
2–17 yrs	6.4–15.6 U/gm hemoglobin (Hb)
≥ 18 yrs	8.6–18.6 U/gm Hb
Haptoglobins	Genetic absence in 1% of population
Newborns	Absent in 90%; 10 mg/dL in 10%
Age 1–6 mos	Gradual increase to 30 mg/dL
6 mos–17 yrs	40–180 mg/dL
Adults	40–270 mg/dL
Hemoglobin, plasma	
≥ 18 yrs old	<15 mg/dL
Infants and newborns	May be higher
Hemoglobin electrophoresis	
HbA	
0–30 days	10–40%
6 mos to adult	>95%
HbA_2	
0–30 days	<1%
1 yr to adult	1.5–3.0%
	3–3.5% (borderline)
HbF	<2%
No abnormal Hb variants	
Hemoglobin F, RBC	HbF remaining in <1% of RBCs
Hemosiderin, urine	Negative
Iron, liver tissue	530–900 μg/gm dry weight
Iron, serum	
Newborns	100–250 μg/dL
Infants	40–100 μg/dL
Children	50–120 μg/dL
Adults	
Males	65–175 μg/dL
Females	50–170 μg/dL
Iron, urine	100–300 ng/24 hrs
Iron-binding capacity	250–450 μg/dL
% saturation	14–50%
Leukocyte alkaline phosphatase score	40–100

Table 1-6. Pediatric Reference Ranges for Lymphocyte Counts

Lymphocytes	0–6	6–12	12–18	18–24	24–30	30–36	>36
				Age (mos)			
Total %	62–72	60–69	56–63	52–29	45–57	38–53	22–69
Total absolute	5395–7211	5284–6714	4943–5943	4431–5508	3855–5248	3315–5058	1622–5370
CD4 %	5057	4955	4651	4248	3846	3344	2757
CD4 absolute	2780–3908	2630–3499	2307–2864	1919–2472	1538–2213	1216–2009	562–2692
CD8 %				8–31			14–34
CD8 absolute				351–2479			331–1445
CD2 %				55–88			65–84
CD2 absolute	3929–5275	3806–4881	3516–3868	3101–3868	2640–3639	2236–3463	1230–4074
CD3 %				55–82			55–82
CD3 absolute	3505–5009	3409–4575	3156–3899	2766–3508	2324–3295	1923–3141	1072–3890
CD19 %				11–45			9–29
CD19 absolute				432–3345			200–1259
Helper-suppressor ratio				1.2–6.2			0.98–3.24

Source: Riley Hospital for Children, Indiana University Medical Center, 1992.

Lysozyme (muramidase), plasma	0.2–15.8 μg/mL
Lysozyme (muramidase), urine	<3 mg/24 hrs
Marrow sideroblasts	≥ 30% of normoblasts
Methemoglobin	<3% of total
Myoglobin, serum	≤ 90 ng/mL
Myoglobin, urine	0–2 mg/mL
Osmotic fragility of RBC	Increased if hemolysis occurs in >0.5% NaCl
	Decreased if incomplete in 0.30% NaCl
Phosphofructokinase, erythrocyte	3.0–6.0 U/gm Hb
Plasma iron turnover rate	38 mg/24 hrs (0.47 mg/kg)
Pyruvate kinase, erythrocyte	2.0–8.8 U/gm Hb
Red blood cell survival time (sodium chromate [^{51}Cr])	Half-life: 25–35 days
Reticulocyte count	
%	0.5–1.85% of erythrocytes
Absolute	29–87 × 10^9/L
Ringed sideroblasts	None
Transferrin	240–480 mg/dL
Unsaturated vitamin B$_{12}$–binding capacity	870–1800 pg/mL
Urobilinogen, stool	50–300 mg/24 hrs
Urobilinogen, urine	<4 mg/24 hrs
Vitamin B$_{12}$, serum	190–900 ng/L
By seventh decade	Decrease to 60–80%
Higher in black than in white populations	

Volume (mL/kg body weight)	**Males**	**Females**
Blood	75	67
RBC	30	24
Plasma	44	43

Blood Coagulation Tests—Reference Values

Antithrombin III, plasma	
Immunologic	17–30 mg/dL
Functional	80–120%
Bleeding time (Simplate)	3–9.5 mins
Clot retraction, qualitative	Begins in 30–60 mins; complete within 24 hrs, usually within 6 hrs

Coagulation factor assay[3]	**Activity**	**Plasma Levels**
I (fibrinogen)		
Males		180–340 mg/dL
Females		190–420 mg/dL
II (prothrombin)	70–140%*	100 μg/mL
V (accelerator globulin)	70–160%*†	10 μg/mL
VII (proconvertin-Stuart)	65–170%*†	0.5 μg/mL
VIII (anti-hemophilic globulin)	55–145%*	0.1 μg/mL
IX	70–140%*†	5 μg/mL
X (Stuart factor)	70–140%*†	10 μg/mL
XI	65–145%*	5 μg/mL
XII (Hageman factor)	60–160%*	30 μg/mL
XIII	50–200%*	10 μg/mL
Factor VIII–related antigen	45–185%	
Coagulation factor VIII inhibitor	Negative	

*Infants may not reach adult level until age 6 mos.
†Increased with age in elderly.

[3]Roberts HR, Lozier J. New perspectives on the coagulation cascade. *Hosp Pract* 1992;27:99.

Coagulation time (Lee-White)	6–17 mins (glass tubes)
	19–60 mins (siliconized tubes)
Euglobulin lysis	No lysis in 2 hrs
Fibrinogen	
Males	180–340 mg/dL
Females	190–420 mg/dL
Fibrinogen split products	Negative at >1:4 dilution
	Positive at >1:8 dilution
Fibrinolysins	No clot lysis in 24 hrs
Lupus anticoagulant (dilute Russell viper venom time [dRVVT]) (plasma [P])	Negative
Partial thromboplastin time, activated (aPTT)	25–38 secs
Platelet aggregation	Full response to adenosine diphosphate, epinephrine, and collagen
Platelet antibody, serum	Negative
Platelet count	140,000–340,000/cu mm (Rees-Ecker)
	150,000–350,000/cu mm (Coulter counter)
Protein C activity (P)	70–130%
Protein C antigen (P)	60–125%
Protein S activity, total or free (P)	
Males	60–130%
Females	50–120%
Prothrombin time (PT), one stage	±2 secs of control (control should be 11–16 secs)
Ristocetin cofactor (P)	45–140%
Ristocetin-von Willebrand's factor (vWF)	45–140%
Thrombin time (TT)	±5 secs of control
vWF antigen, plasma	45–165%
Whole blood clot lysis	No clot lysis in 24 hrs

Blood Chemistries—Reference Values

These values will vary, depending on the individual laboratory as well as the methods and instruments used. Each clinician should compare the applicability of these data to his or her own situation.

Acetone	0.3–2.0 mg/dL
Aldolase	
0–2 yrs	3.4–11.8 U/L
2–16 yrs	1.2–8.8 U/L
Adults (≥ 17 yrs)	1.7–4.9 U/L
Ammonia	9–33 U/L
Newborns at term or premature	<50 U/L
Amylase (total)	
<18 yrs	0–260 U/L
Adults (≥ 18 yrs)	35–115 U/L
Apolipoprotein A-I	
Males	90–155 mg/dL
Females	94–172 mg/dL
Apolipoprotein B	
Males	55–100 mg/dL
Females	45–110 mg/dL
Base, excess	
Newborns	–10 to –2 mEq/L
Infants	–7 to –1 mEq/L
Children	–4 to +2 mEq/L
Adults	–3 to +3 mEq/L

Bicarbonate

Males	**Females**	
1–2 yrs	1–3 yrs	17–25 mEq/L
3–4 yrs	4–5 yrs	18–26 mEq/L
4–5 yrs	6–7 yrs	19–27 mEq/L
6–7 yrs	8–9 yrs	20–28 mEq/L
≥ 8* yrs	≥ 10* yrs	21–29 mEq/L

*Adult value.

Bilirubin
  Total

<1 day	<5.8 mg/dL
1–2 days	<8.2 mg/dL
3–5 days	<11.7 mg/dL
>1 mo	<1.0 mg/dL

  Direct

1 mo to adult	<0.6 mg/dL

Calcium
  Total

1–3 yrs	8.7–9.8 mg/dL
4–11 yrs	8.8–10.1 mg/dL
12–13 yrs	8.8–10.6 mg/dL
14–15 yrs	9.2–10.7 mg/dL
>16 yrs	8.9–10.7 mg/dL

Males	**Females**	*Ionized*
1–19 yrs	1–17 yrs	4.9–5.5 mg/dL
≥ 20 yrs	≥ 18 yrs	4.75–5.3 mg/dL

Carbon dioxide

CO_2	17–31 mEq/L
Partial pressure of carbon dioxide (pCO_2) (whole blood)	
Adults	32–48 mm Hg
Infants	27–41 mm Hg

Ceruloplasmin

1–3 yrs	24–46 mg/dL
4–6 yrs	24–42 mg/dL
7–9 yrs	24–40 mg/dL
10–13 yrs	22–36 mg/dL
14–19 yrs	14–34 mg/dL
Chloride	96–109 (mEq/L)
Cholesterol (Table 1-7)	See Lipid Fractionation, p. 15

Cholinesterase

Plasma	7–25 U/mL
RBC	0.65–1.3 pH units

Complement

Total complement	25–110 U
C1 esterase inhibitor	8–24 mg/dL
C1q complement component	7–15 mg/dL
C2 (second component of complement)	50–250% of normal
C3 (third component of complement)	70–150 mg/dL
C4 (fourth component of complement)	10–30 mg/dL
C5 (fifth component of complement)	9–18 mg/dL
Copper	75–145 μg/dL

Table 1-7. Lipid Fractionation: Desirable Levels for Cholesterol and Triglycerides[a]

	Cholesterol (mg/dL)						Triglycerides (mg/dL)			
	Males (percentile)			Females (percentile)			Males (percentile)		Females (percentile)	
Age (yrs)	5 95	75[b]		5 95	75[b]		5 95		5 95	
5–9	126–191	172		122–209	173		27–102		34–76	
10–14	130–204	179		124–217	174		30–103		33–121	
15–19	114–198	167		125–212	175		31–124		32–122	
20–24	128–216	185		128–209	181		34–137		32–97	
25–29	140–236	202		134–218	190		40–157		33–100	
30–34	150–250	216		141–229	199		43–171		35–106	
35–39	156–264	226		147–240	209		45–182		38–110	
40–44	162–274	235		155–253	219		48–189		40–117	
45–49	166–280	242		162–265	229		50–193		41–122	
50–54	170–286	246		171–278	241		50–195		43–128	
55–59	173–291	250		179–291	253		51–197		45–134	
60–64	175–295	253		188–306	265		51–198		47–140	
65–69	176–298	255		197–320	278		51–199		50–147	
70–74	177–299	256		207–336	291		51–199		52–154	
>74	178–300	257		217–352	306		51–199		54–162	

[a]Recently, data have been presented as "desirable levels" rather than "reference ranges" or "normal values." See Chapter 12.
[b]Seventy-fifth percentile has been recommended as upper limit for serum cholesterol and low-density lipoprotein (LDL) cholesterol.

Creatine kinase
    Males   55–170 U/L
    Females   45–135 U/L
Creatine kinase isoenzyme MB   <5%
    (CK-MB)   <10 ng/mL (mass)
Creatinine
    <1 wk   0.6–1.1 mg/dL
    1–4 wks   0.3–0.7 mg/dL
    1–12 mos   0.2–0.4 mg/dL
    >1 yr   0.2–0.7 mg/dL

Males	**Females**	
1–2 yrs	1–3 yrs	0.2–0.6 mg/dL
3–4 yrs	4–5 yrs	0.3–0.7 mg/dL
5–9 yrs	6–8 yrs	0.5–0.8 mg/dL
10–11 yrs	≥ 9 yrs	0.6–0.9 mg/dL
12–13 yrs		0.6–1.0 mg/dL
14–15 yrs		0.7–1.1 mg/dL
≥ 16 yrs (adult values)		0.8–1.2 mg/dL

Cryoglobulins   0
Gamma-glutamyl transferase (GGT)
    1–3 yrs   6–19 U/L
    4–6 yrs   10–22 U/L
    7–9 yrs   13–25 U/L

	Males	**Females**
10–11 yrs	17–30 U/L	17–28 U/L
12–13 yrs	17–44 U/L	14–25 U/L
14–15 yrs	12–33 U/L	14–26 U/L
16–19 yrs	11–34 U/L	11–28 U/L

Glucose (fasting)	60–100 mg/dL (depends on method)
Homocysteine, total	5–15 μmol/L
Desirable	<10 μmol/L
Optimal	<12 μmol/L
Borderline	12–15 μmol/L
Moderate hyperhomocystinemia	>15–30 μmol/L
Intermediate hyperhomocystinemia	>30–100 μmol/L
Severe hyperhomocystinemia	>100 μmol/L
Isocitrate dehydrogenase (ICD)	3–85 U/L
Lactate	6.3–18.9 mg/dL
Lactate dehydrogenase (LD)	
Newborn	160–1500 U/L
Infant	150–360 U/L
Child	150–300 U/L
Adult	100–250 U/L
LD isoenzymes	
LD-1	17–28%
LD-2	30–36%
LD-3	19–25%
LD-4	10–16%
LD-5	6–13%
Lead	
Adults	<20 μg/dL
≤ 15 yrs	<10 μg/dL
Leptin	
<15% body fat in men and	1–16 μg/L
<25% in women	
Leucine aminopeptidase (LAP)	Depends on method
Lipase	56–239 U/L
Lipid fractionation (see Tables 1-7 and 1-8)	
Cholesterol esters	60–75% of total
Phospholipids	180–320 mg/dL
Magnesium	1.7–2.3 mg/dL
Myoglobin (serum [S])	≤ 90 ng/mL
Osmolality	275–295 mOsm/kg
Oxygen	
Saturation, arterial	96–100% of capacity
Tension, partial pressure of oxygen (pO_2), arterial while breathing room air	
Newborns	60–75 mm Hg
<60 yrs	>85 mm Hg
60 yrs	>80 mm Hg
70 yrs	>70 mm Hg
80 yrs	>60 mm Hg
90 yrs	>50 mm Hg
While breathing 100% oxygen	>500 mm Hg
Oxygen dissociation, P^{50} (RBCs)	26–30 mm Hg
pH, arterial	7.36–7.44
pH, venous	7.32–7.38
Phenylalanine	
≤ 1 wk	42–124 μmol/L
<16 yrs	26–86 μmol/L
≥ 16 yrs	41–68 μmol/L

Table 1-8. Lipid Fractionation: Desirable Levels for HDL Cholesterol and LDL Cholesterol[a]

	HDL Cholesterol (mg/dL)						LDL Cholesterol (mg/dL)					
	Males (percentile)			Females (percentile)			Males (percentile)			Females (percentile)		
Age (yrs)	5	95	75[b]	5	95	75[b]	5	95	75[b]	5	95	75[b]
6–11	30–70		55	34–65		59	60–140		114	60–150		114
12–14	30–65		50	30–65		49	60–140		111	60–150		114
15–19	30–60		53	33–65		47	60–140		113	60–150		118
20–29	30–65		55	34–75		47	60–175		131	60–160		128
30–39	30–70		60	35–80		47	70–190		147	70–170		140
40–49	30–70		63	35–80		47	70–205		160	80–190		150
>50	30–70		65	35–80		47	80–220		170	80–200		164

HDL = high-density lipoprotein; LDL = low-density lipoprotein.
[a]Recently, data have been presented as "desirable levels" rather than "reference ranges" or "normal values." See Chapter 12.
[b]Seventy-fifth percentile has been recommended as upper limit for serum cholesterol and LDL cholesterol.

Phosphatase, prostatic acid (PAP)	<3.7 ng/mL	
Phosphatase, alkaline (ALP)		
1–3 yrs	145–320 U/L	
4–6 yrs	150–380 U/L	
7–9 yrs	175–420 U/L	
	Males	**Females**
10–11 yrs	135–530 U/L	130–560 U/L
12–13 yrs	200–495 U/L	105–420 U/L
14–15 yrs	130–525 U/L	70–230 U/L
16–19 yrs	65–260 U/L	50–130 U/L
Phosphate		
<5 days	4.6–8.0 mg/dL	
1–3 yrs	3.9–6.5 mg/dL	
4–6 yrs	3.7–5.4 mg/dL	
7–11 yrs	3.7–5.6 mg/dL	
12–13 yrs	3.3–5.4 mg/dL	
14–15 yrs	2.9–5.4 mg/dL	
16–19 yrs	2.8–4.6 mg/dL	
Potassium		
1–15 yrs	3.7–5.0 mEq/L	
16–59 yrs	3.6–4.8 mEq/L	
≥ 60 yrs	3.9–5.3 mEq/L	
Prostate-specific antigen (PSA)		
(S), males[4]		
Normal	<4.0 ng/mL	
Borderline	4–10 ng/mL	
Values higher in black than in white men; increase with age		
40–49 yrs	1.5 ng/mL	
50–59 yrs	2.5 ng/mL	
60–69 yrs	4.5 ng/mL	
70–79 yrs	7.5 ng/mL	

[4]Anderson JR, et al. Age-specific reference ranges for serum prostate-specific antigen. *Urology* 1995;46:54.

Proteins, serum	Total (gm/dL)	Albumin (gm/dL)
<5 days	5.4–7.0	2.6–3.6
1–3 yrs	5.9–7.0	3.4–4.2
4–6 yrs	5.9–7.8	3.5–5.2
7–9 yrs	6.2–8.1	3.7–5.6
10–19 yrs	6.3–8.6	3.7–5.6

	Globulin (gm/dL)
<1 yr	0.4–3.7
1–3 yrs	1.6–3.5
4–9 yrs	1.9–3.4
10–49 yrs	1.9–3.5

Prealbumin (transthyretin) (mg/dL)

<5 days	6.0–21.0
1–5 yrs	14.0–30.0
6–9 yrs	15.0–33.0
10–13 yrs	20.0–36.0
14–19 yrs	22.0–45.0

Electrophoresis

Albumin	3.1–4.3 gm/dL
Globulin	
Alpha$_1$	0.1–0.3 gm/dL
Alpha$_2$	0.6–1.0 gm/dL
Beta	0.7–1.4 gm/dL
Gamma	0.0–1.6 gm/dL
Alpha$_1$-antitrypsin	>180 mg/dL
Z heterozygotes	79–171 mg/dL
Z homozygotes	19–31 mg/dL

Immunoglobulins (Ig)	IgG (mg/dL)	IgA (mg/dL)	IgM (mg/dL)
0–4 mos	141–930	5–64	14–142
5–8 mos	250–1190	10–87	24–167
9–11 mos	320–1250	17–94	
1–3 yrs	400–1250		
1–2 yrs			35–242 (females)
			35–200 (males)
2–3 yrs		24–192	41–242 (females)
			41–200 (males)
4–6 yrs	560–1307	26–232	
7–9 yrs	598–1379	33–258	
10–12 yrs	638–1453	45–285	
13–15 yrs	680–1531	47–317	
16–17 yrs	724–1611	55–377	
4–17 yrs			56–242 (females)
			47–200 (males)
≥ 18 yrs	700–1500	60–400	60–300
IgE			
<1 yr		0.0–6.6 U/mL	
1–2 yrs		0.0–20.0 U/mL	
2–3 yrs		0.1–15.8 U/mL	
3–4 yrs		0.0–29.2 U/mL	
4–5 yrs		0.3–25.0 U/mL	
5–6 yrs		0.2–17.6 U/mL	
6–7 yrs		0.2–13.1 U/mL	
7–8 yrs		0.3–46.1 U/mL	
8–9 yrs		1.8–60.1 U/mL	
9–10 yrs		3.6–81.0 U/mL	
10–11 yrs		8.0–95.0 U/mL	
11–12 yrs		1.5–99.7 U/mL	
12–13 yrs		3.9–83.5 U/mL	

13–16 yrs	3.3–188.0 U/mL	
IgD	0–14 mg/dL	
Sodium	135–145 mEq/L	

Transaminase
  Aspartate aminotransferase
    (AST; serum glutamic oxalo-
    acetic transaminase [SGOT])

1–3 yrs	20–60 U/L	
4–6 yrs	15–50 U/L	
7–9 yrs	15–40 U/L	
10–11 yrs	10–60 U/L	

	Males	**Females**
12–15 yrs	15–40 U/L	10–30 U/L
16–19 yrs	15–45 U/L	5–30 U/L

Alanine aminotransferase (ALT;
  serum glutamic pyruvic transaminase [SGPT])

1–3 yrs	5–45 U/L	
4–6 yrs	10–25 U/L	
7–9 yrs	10–35 U/L	

	Males	**Females**
10–11 yrs	10–35 U/L	10–30 U/L
12–13 yrs	10–55 U/L	10–30 U/L
14–15 yrs	10–45 U/L	5–30 U/L
16–19 yrs	10–40 U/L	5–35 U/L

Troponin I	<1.6 ng/mL	
Troponin T	<0.1 ng/mL	

Urea nitrogen, blood (BUN)

1–3 yrs	5–17 mg/dL	
4–13 yrs	7–17 mg/dL	
14–19 yrs	8–21 mg/dL	

Uric acid

1–3 yrs	1.8–5.0 mg/dL	
4–6 yrs	2.2–4.7 mg/dL	
7–9 yrs	2.0–5.0 mg/dL	

	Males	**Females**
10–11 yrs	2.3–5.4 mg/dL	3.0–4.7 mg/dL
12–13 yrs	2.7–6.7 mg/dL	3.0–5.8 mg/dL
14–15 yrs	2.4–7.8 mg/dL	3.0–5.8 mg/dL
16–19 yrs	4.0–8.6 mg/dL	3.0–5.9 mg/dL

Viscosity (correlates with fibrinogen, high-density lipoprotein [HDL] cholesterol)
  (viscosimeter)

Plasma	1.38±0.08 relative units
Serum	1.26±0.08 relative units

See Table 1-9.

Normal Blood and Urine Hormone Levels

Adrenocorticotropic hormone (ACTH), plasma	≤ 60 pg/mL

Aldosterone, serum

0–3 wks	16.5–154 ng/dL	
1–11 mos	6.5–86 ng/dL	
1–10 yrs (supine)	3.0–39.5 ng/dL	
1–10 yrs (upright)	3.5–124 ng/dL	
≥ 11 yrs (morning specimen, peripheral vein)		1–21 ng/dL

Aldosterone, urine

0–30 days	0.7–11 μg/24 hrs
1–11 mos	0.7–22 μg/24 hrs

Table 1-9. Reference Blood Values for Fetal Umbilical Blood at 18–40 Wks of Pregnancy (Hitachi 717 Analyzer)

	Fetal	Infant		Adult
Bilirubin, total (mg/dL)	0.9–2.5	1.0–10.0		0.3–1.2
Bilirubin, direct (mg/dL)	0.3–0.8			0.1–0.35
Calcium (mg/dL)	7.6–10			8.5–10.5
Chloride (mEq/L)	97–122			98–108
Cholesterol (mg/dL)	32–76			130–200
Creatinine (mg/dL)	0.4–0.9	0.3–0.7	Male	0.7–1.4
			Female	0.6–1.1
GGT (U/L)	22–146	5–120		5–45
Glucose (mg/dL)	54–103			65–110
Phosphorus, inorganic (mg/dL)	4.0–8.8	4.0–7.0		2.5–4.5
Potassium (mEq/L)	3.2–4.6			3.5–5.0
LD (U/L)	259–552			230–460
Magnesium (mg/dL)	1.4–1.9	1.2–1.8		1.8–2.4
Sodium (mEq/L)	128–147			135–145
Transaminase				
AST (U/L)	9–31			7–45
ALT (U/L)	1–15			7–45
Triglycerides (mg/dL)	2–62			20–170
BUN (mg/dL)	5–16	5–18		10–23
Uric acid (mg/dL)	1.0–5.5		Male	3.5–7.0
			Female	2.4–5.7

Analytes that change with fetal age (approximate numbers taken from figure)

ALP (U/L)	From 525 to 400
CK (U/L)	From ~2 to 20
Total protein (mg/dL)	From 2.5 to 5.0
Albumin (mg/dL)	From 2.0 to 3.2

Source: Guzzo ML, et al. Reference intervals for 18 clinical chemistry analytes in fetal plasma samples between 18 and 40 weeks of pregnancy. *Clin Chem* 1998;44:683.

≥ 1 yr	2–16 μg/24 hrs	
Androstenedione, serum	**Males**	**Females**
0–7 yrs	0.1–0.2 ng/mL	0.1–0.3 ng/mL
8–9 yrs	0.1–0.3 ng/mL	0.2–0.5 ng/mL
10–11 yrs	0.3–0.7 ng/mL	0.4–1.0 ng/mL
12–13 yrs	0.4–1.0 ng/mL	0.8–1.9 ng/mL
14–17 yrs	0.5–1.4 ng/mL	0.7–2.2 ng/mL
≥ 18 yrs	0.3–3.1 ng/mL	0.2–3.1 ng/mL
Angiotensin-converting enzyme (ACE), serum		
≤ 1 yr	10.9–42.1 U/L	
1–2 yrs	9.4–36 U/L	
3–4 yrs	7.9–29.8 U/L	
5–9 yrs	9.6–35.4 U/L	
10–12 yrs	10.0–37.0 U/L	
13–16 yrs	9.0–33.4 U/L	
17–19 yrs	7.2–26.6 U/L	

NORMAL

≥ 20 yrs	6.1–21.1 U/L	
Calcitonin, plasma	**Males**	**Females**
Basal	≤ 19 pg/mL	<14 pg/mL
Calcium infusion (2.4 mg calcium/kg)	≤ 190 pg/mL	≤ 130 pg/mL
Pentagastrin infusion (0.5 μg/kg)	≤ 110 pg/mL	≤ 30 pg/mL
Catecholamine fractionation (free), plasma		
	Supine	**Standing**
Norepinephrine	70–750 pg/mL	200–1700 pg/mL
Epinephrine	≤ 110 pg/mL	≤ 140 pg/mL
Dopamine	<30 pg/mL (any posture)	

Catecholamine fractionation, urine

Epinephrine
<1 yr	<2.5 μg/24 hrs
1–2 yrs	<3.5 μg/24 hrs
2–3 yrs	<6.0 μg/24 hrs
4–9 yrs	0.2–10 μg/24 hrs
10–15 yrs	0.5–20 μg/24 hrs
≥ 16 yrs	0–20 μg/24 hrs

Norepinephrine
<1 yr	0–10 μg/24 hrs
1 yr	1–17 μg/24 hrs
2–3 yrs	4–29 μg/24 hrs
4–6 yrs	8–45 μg/24 hrs
7–9 yrs	13–65 μg/24 hrs
≥ 10 yrs	15–80 μg/24 hrs

Dopamine
<1 yr	<85 μg/24 hrs
1 yr	10–140 μg/24 hrs
2–3 yrs	40–260 μg/24 hrs
≥ 4 yrs	65–400 μg/24 hrs

Catecholamine metabolites fractionation, urine

Homovanillic acid (HVA), urine
<1 yr	<35 μg/mg creatinine
>1 yr	<23 μg/mg creatinine
2–4 yrs	<13.5 μg/mg creatinine
5–9 yrs	<9 μg/mg creatinine
10–14 yrs	<12 μg/mg creatinine
Adults	<8 mg/24 hrs
Metanephrines, urine	<1.3 mg/24 hrs

Vanillylmandelic acid (VMA), urine
<1 yr	<27 μg/mg creatinine
1 yr	<18 μg/mg creatinine
2–4 yrs	<13 μg/mg creatinine
5–9 yrs	<8.5 μg/mg creatinine
10–14 yrs	<7 μg/mg creatinine
15–18 yrs	<5 μg/mg creatinine
Adults	<9 mg/24 hrs

Chorionic gonadotropins, beta-subunit, serum
Females	<5 U/L
Postmenopausal females	<9 U/L
Males	<2.5 U/L
Cerebrospinal fluid (CSF)	≤ 1.5 U/L
Cortisol (for general screening), plasma	a.m.: 7–25 μg/dL p.m.: 2–14 μg/dL
Cortisol, free, urine	24–108 μg/24 hrs

	Males	Females
Deoxycorticosteroids (for metyrapone test), plasma	a.m.: 0–5 µg/dL p.m.: 0–3 µg/dL	
Dehydroepiandrosterone sulfate (DHEA-S), serum	**Males**	**Females**
0–30 days (premature)	0.25–10.0 µg/mL	0.25–10.0 µg/mL
(full-term)	0.25–2.0 µg/mL	0.25–2.0 µg/mL
1–16 yrs	<0.5 µg/mL	<0.5 µg/mL
≥ 17 yrs	<6.0 µg/mL	<3.0 µg/mL
Estradiol, serum		
Children	<10 pg/mL	
Adult males	10–50 pg/mL	
Premenopausal adult females	30–400 pg/mL	
Postmenopausal females	<30 pg/mL	
Estrogen and progesterone receptor assays, tissue		
Negative	<3 fmol/mg cytosol protein	
Borderline	3–9 fmol/mg cytosol protein	
Positive	≥ 10 fmol/mg cytosol protein	
Follicle-stimulating hormone (FSH), serum	**Males**	**Females**
Prepuberty	<2 U/L	<2 U/L
Adult	1–10 U/L	
Follicular		1–10 U/L
Midcycle		6–30 U/L
Luteal		1–8 U/L
Postmenopausal		20–100 U/L
Follicle-stimulating hormone, urine	**Males**	**Females**
Prepuberty	<0.5 U/24 hrs	<0.7 U/24 hrs
Adult	7–10 U/24 hrs	
Not midcycle		0.7–10 U/24 hrs
Postmenopausal		>10 U/24 hrs
Gastrin, serum	≤ 200 pg/mL	
Growth hormone, serum	**Males**	**Females**
	≤ 5 ng/mL	≤ 10 ng/mL
5-Hydroxyindole acetic acid (5-HIAA), urine	≤ 6 mg/24 hrs	
17-Hydroxyprogesterone, serum		
Males	<220 ng/dL	
Prepubertal	<110 ng/dL	
Females		
Follicular phase	<80 ng/dL	
Luteal phase	<285 ng/dL	
Postmenopausal	<51 ng/dL	
Prepubertal	<100 ng/dL	
Newborns	<630 ng/dL	
Insulin, serum	<20 µU/mL	
Borderline	21–25 µU/mL	
17-Ketogenic steroids (17-KGS), urine		
Adult males	4–14 mg/24 hrs	
Adult females	2–12 mg/24 hrs	
Children, 0–10 yrs	0.1–4 mg/24 hrs	
11–14 yrs	2–9 mg/24 hrs	
17-Ketosteroids (17-KS), urine		
Adult males	6–21 mg/24 hrs	
Adult females	4–17 mg/24 hrs	
Children, 0–10 yrs	0.1–3 mg/24 hrs	
11–14 yrs	2–7 mg/24 hrs	
17-KS, fractionation, urine	See Table 1-10	
Luteinizing hormone (LH), serum		
Prepuberty males	<0.5 U/L	
Adult males	1–10 U/L	

Table 1-10. 17-Ketosteroids (Fractionation), Urine (mg/24 hrs)

	Adult Females	Adult Males	Males 10–15 yrs	Females 10–15 yrs	6–9 yrs	3–5 yrs	1–2 yrs	0–1 yr
Pregnanediol	0–4.5	0–1.9	0.1–1.2	0.1–0.7	<0.5	<0.3	<0.1	<0.1
Androsterone	0–3.1	0.9–6.1	0.2–2.0	0.5–2.5	0.1–1.0	<0.3	<0.3	<0.1
Etiocholanolone	0.1–3.5	0.9–5.2	0.1–1.6	0.7–3.1	0.3–1.0	<0.7	<0.4	<0.1
Dehydroepiandrosterone	0–1.5	0–3.1	<0.4	<0.4	<0.2	<0.1	<0.1	<0.1
Pregnanetriol	0–1.4	0.2–2.0	0.2–0.6	0.1–0.6	<0.3	<0.1	<0.1	<0.1
Δ5-Pregnanetriol	0–0.4	0–0.4	<0.3	<0.3	<0.2	<0.2	<0.1	<0.1
11-Ketoandrosterone	0–0.3	0–0.5	<0.1	<0.1	<0.1	<0.1	<0.1	<0.1
11-Ketoetiocholanolone	0–1.0	0–1.6	<0.3	0.1–0.5	0.1–0.5	<0.4	<0.1	<0.1
11-Hydroxyandrosterone	0–1.1	0.2–1.6	0.1–1.1	0.2–1.0	0.4–1.0	<0.4	<0.3	<0.3
11-Hydroxyetiocholanolone	0.1–0.8	0.1–0.9	<0.3	0.1–0.5	0.1–0.5	<0.4	<0.1	<0.1
11-Ketopregnanetriol	0–0.5	0–0.5	<0.3	<0.2	<0.2	<0.2	<0.2	<0.2

Source: Leavelle DE, ed. *Mayo Medical Laboratories Handbook*. Rochester, MN: Mayo Medical Laboratories, 1995.

	Prepuberty females	<0.2 U/L	
	Adult females, follicular	1–20 U/L	
	Adult females, midcycle	25–100 U/L	
	Postmenopausal females	20–100 U/L	

Luteinizing hormone, urine
    Prepuberty males   <0.8 U/24 hrs
    Adult males   0.2–5.0 U/24 hrs
    Prepuberty females   <0.8 U/24 hrs
    Adult females, nonmidcycle 0.5–5.0 U/24 hrs
    Postmenopausal females   >5.0 U/24 hrs

Parathyroid hormone (PTH), serum   1.0–5.0 pmol/L
    (intact + N-terminal PTH)

Pregnanetriol, urine	**Males**	**Females**
0–5 yrs	<0.1 mg/24 hrs	<0.1 mg/24 hrs
6–9 yrs	<0.3 mg/24 hrs	<0.3 mg/24 hrs
10–15 yrs	0.2–0.6 mg/24 hrs	0.1–0.6 mg/24 hrs
>16 yrs	0.2–2.0 mg/24 hrs	0.0–1.4 mg/24 hrs
Progesterone, serum	**Males**	**Females**
0–1 yr	0.87–3.37 ng/mL	0.87–3.37 ng/mL
2–9 yrs	0.12–0.14 ng/mL	0.20–0.24 ng/mL
Postpuberty	<1.0 ng/mL	Increasing values
Follicular phase		≤ 0.7 ng/mL
Luteal phase		2.0–20.0 ng/mL

Prolactin, serum
    Males   0–20 ng/mL
    Females   0–23 ng/mL

Renin activity (peripheral vein),
    plasma (PRA)
    Na-depleted, upright
        18–39 yrs   2.9–24.0 ng/mL/hr
        >40 yrs   2.9–10.8 ng/mL/hr
    Na-replete, upright
        18–39 yrs   ≤ 0.6–4.3 ng/mL/hr
        ≥ 40 yrs   ≤ 0.6–3.0 ng/mL/hr

Sex hormone–binding globulin, serum
    Adult males   10–80 nmol/L
    Adult nonpregnant females 20–130 nmol/L

Somatomedin-C, plasma

Age (yrs)	**Males**	**Females**
0–5	0–103 ng/mL	0–112 ng/mL
6–8	2–118 ng/mL	5–128 ng/mL
9–10	15–148 ng/mL	24–158 ng/mL
11–13	55–216 ng/mL	65–226 ng/mL
14–15	114–232 ng/mL	124–242 ng/mL
16–17	84–221 ng/mL	94–231 ng/mL
18–19	56–177 ng/mL	66–186 ng/mL
20–24	75–142 ng/mL	64–131 ng/mL
25–29	65–131 ng/mL	55–121 ng/mL
30–34	58–122 ng/mL	47–112 ng/mL
35–39	51–115 ng/mL	40–104 ng/mL
40–44	46–109 ng/mL	35–98 ng/mL
45–49	43–104 ng/mL	32–93 ng/mL
≥ 50	40–100 ng/mL	29–90 ng/mL

Testosterone, serum	**Total**	**Free**	**%**
Males	300–1200 ng/dL	9–30 ng/dL	2.0–4.8%
Females	20–80 ng/dL	0.3–1.9 ng/dL	0.9–3.8%

Thyroid function indicators   See Table 1-11
Thyroid microsomal and thyro-
    globulin antibodies   <1:100
Vasoactive intestinal polypeptide
    (VIP), plasma   <75 μg/mL

Table 1-11. Thyroid Function Indicators by Age (Serum Concentration)[a]

Age	T_4 (nmol/L)	FT_4 (pmol/L)	TSH[b] (mIU/L)	TBG (mg/L)	T_3 (nmol/L)	rT_3 (nmol/L)	Thyroglob-ulin (μg/L)
1–4 days	142–277	28–68	1–39	22–42	1.5–11.4		2–110
1–4 wks	106–221	12–30	1.7–9.1		1.6–5.3	0.4–4.5	
1–12 mos	76–210	10–23	0.8–8.2	16–36	1.6–3.8	0.17–2.0	
1–5 yrs	94–193	10–27	0.7–5.7	12–28	1.6–4.1	0.23–1.1	2–65
6–10 yrs	82–171	13–27	0.7–5.7	12–28	1.4–3.7	0.26–1.2	2–65
11–15 yrs	71–151	10–26	0.7–5.7	14–30	1.3–3.3	0.29–1.3	2–36
16–20 yrs	54–152	10–26	0.7–5.7	14–30	1.2–3.2	0.39–1.2	2–36
21–80 yrs	55–160	12–32	0.4–4.2	17–36		0.46–1.2	2–25
21–50 yrs					1.1–3.1		
51–80 yrs					0.6–2.8		

FT_4 = free T_4; rT_3 = reverse triiodothyronine; T_3 = triiodothyronine; T_4 = thyroxine; TBG = thyroxine-binding globulin; TSH = thyrotropin.
[a]No clinically significant difference by gender or race.
[b]Diurnal variation of TSH ~50% between nadir (1500–1700 hrs) and peak (2300–2400 hrs).

Normal Values for Serologic Tests for Infectious Agents

Amebiasis (*Entamoeba histolytica*)	
No invasive disease	<1:32
Borderline	<1:32–1:64
Active or recent infection	≥ 128
Current infection	>1:256
Aspergillosis	Negative
Blastomycosis	Negative (positive in <50% of cases)
Brucellosis	<1:80
Candidosis	Negative (positive in 25% of normal persons)
Chlamydia IgG	<1:10
Chlamydia antigen (endocervix, male urine, male urethra)	Negative
Cold agglutinin titer	<1:16
Cryptococcosis antigen, serum or CSF	Negative
Cryptosporidium antigen, feces	Negative
Cysticercosis, serum	Negative
Cytomegalovirus (CMV)*	
IgG	Negative (<15 U/mL)
IgM	Negative
Echinococcosis	Negative at 1:128
Epstein-Barr virus	See p. 842
Heterophil	See p. 844
Hepatitis	See p. 223
Herpes simplex, serum or CSF	
IgG	<1:5
IgM	<1:10
Polymerase chain reaction (PCR), CSF	Negative
Histoplasmosis, serum or CSF	Negative
Influenza A or B*	<1:10
IgG or IgM	
Lyme disease (*Borrelia burgdorferi*)	See p. 808
Monospot screen	Negative

Mumps*
    IgG   <1:5
    IgM   <1:10

Mumps*		
IgG	<1:5	
IgM	<1:10	
Murine typhus IgG	≤ 1:32	
Mycoplasma pneumoniae IgG or IgM	<1:10	
Respiratory syncytial virus (RSV)		
IgG	<1:10	
IgM	<1:10	
RSV antigen, nasopharynx	Negative	
Q fever*		
Not infected	<1:10	
Previous infection	≥ 1:10	
Recent or active infection	≥ 1:160	
Rocky Mountain spotted fever*	IgG ≤ 1:32	
Rubella		
IgG	>1:10 confirms immunity	
IgM	Negative	
Rubeola, serum or CSF		
IgG	<1:5	
IgM	<1:10	
Scrub typhus	≤ 1:40	
St. Louis encephalitis*	<1:10	
Sporotrichosis	<1:80	
Streptococcal	**ASO**	**Anti-DNase-B**
Preschool children	≤ 85 U	≤ 60 U
School-age children	≤ 170 U	≤ 170 U
Adults	≤ 85 U	≤ 85 U
Syphilis serology	See p. 816	
Toxocara canis antibody	Negative	
Toxoplasmosis		
IgG		
No previous infection (except eye)	<1:16	
Prevalent in general population	1:16–1:256	
Suggests recent infection	>1:256	
Active infection	≥ 1:1024	
IgM		
Adults	≥ 1:64 = active infection	
Children	Any titer is significant	
Trichinosis	Negative	
Tularemia	<1:40	
Varicella		
IgG	<1:10	
IgM	<1:10 nonimmune	
	1:10 borderline immunity	
	1:40 immune	

*Presence of IgM antibodies or ≥ fourfold rise in IgG titer between acute- and convalescent-phase sera drawn within 30 days of each other indicates recent infection. Generally, presence of IgG indicates past exposure and possible immunity. Congenital infections require serial sera from both mother and infant. Passively acquired antibodies in infant will decay in 2–3 mos. Antibody levels that are unchanged or increased in 2–3 mos indicate active infection. Absence of antibody in mother rules out congenital infection in infant.

Normal Blood Antibody Levels

Acetylcholine (ACh)	
Receptor-binding antibodies	≤ 0.02 nmol/L
Receptor-blocking antibodies	<25% blockade of ACh receptors
Receptor-modulating antibodies	<20% loss of ACh receptors
Antiglomerular basement membrane antibody	Negative
Antinuclear antibodies (ANA)	Negative

Antimitochondrial antibodies	Negative
Antibodies to Scl 70 antigen	Negative
Antibodies to Jo 1 antigen	Negative
Anti–double-stranded DNA (dsDNA) antibodies	
Negative	<70 U
Borderline	70–200 U
Positive	>200 U
Antiextractable nuclear antigens (anti-RNP, anti-Sm, anti-SSB, anti-SSA)	Negative
Antineutrophil cytoplasmic antibodies (ANCA) (c-ANCA and p-ANCA)	Negative
Granulocyte antibodies	Negative
Human leukocyte antigen (HLA) B27	
Present in	Whites: 6–8%
	Blacks: 3–4%
	Asians: 1%
Intrinsic factor blocking antibody	Negative
Parietal cell antibodies	Negative
Rheumatoid factor (RF)	
Latex agglutination	Negative
Rate nephelometry	
Nonreactive	0–39 U/mL
Weakly reactive	40–79 U/mL
Reactive	≥ 80 U/mL
Smooth muscle antibody	Negative
Striated muscle antibodies	<1:60

Normal Blood Levels for Metabolic Diseases

U = urine
S = serum
P = plasma
B = whole blood
F = skin fibroblasts
L = leukocytes
RBC = erythrocytes
St = stool

Acid mucopolysaccharides	(U)	
<14 yrs old		Age dependent
Adult		≤ 13.3 μg glucuronic acid/mg creatinine
Alpha$_1$-antitrypsin	(S)	126–226 mg/dL
Alpha-fucosidase	(F)	Compare with controls
	(L)	0.49–1.76 U/gm cellular protein
Alpha-galactosidase	(S)	0.016–0.2 U/L
(Fabry's disease)	(F)	0.24–1.10 U/gm cellular protein
	(L)	0.60–3.63 U/10^{10} cells
Alpha-glucosidase	(F)	0.13–1.84 U/gm protein
Alpha-L-iduronidase	(F)	0.44–1.04 U/gm cellular protein
(Hurler's, Scheie's syndromes)	(L)	0.17–0.54 U/10^{10} cells
Alpha-mannosidase	(F)	0.71–5.92 U/gm cellular protein
(mannosidosis)	(L)	1.50–3.33 U/10^{10} cells
Alpha-N-acetylglucosaminidase	(S)	0.09–0.58 U/L
(Sanfilippo type B)	(F)	0.076–0.291 U/gm cellular protein
Arylsulfatase A (mucolipidosis,	(F)	2.28–15.74 U/gm cellular protein
types II and III)	(L)	≥ 2.5 U/10^{10} cells
	(U)	>1 U/L

Arylsulfatase B	(F)	1.6–14.9 U/gm cellular protein
Beta-galactosidase (Gm$_1$	(F)	4.7–19.1 U/gm cellular protein
gangliosidosis, Morquio's	(L)	1.01–6.52 U/10^{10} cells
syndrome)		
Beta-glucosidase (Gaucher's	(F)	3.80–8.70 U/gm cellular protein
disease)	(L)	0.08–0.35 U/10^{10} cells
Beta-glucuronidase (mucopoly-	(F)	0.34–1.24 U/gm cellular protein
saccharidosis VII)		
Carbohydrate	(U)	Negative
Cystine	(U)	
<1 mo		64–451 μmol/gm creatine
1–5 mos		66–375 μmol/gm creatine
6–11 mos		70–316 μmol/gm creatine
1–2 yrs		53–244 μmol/gm creatine
3–15 yrs		11–53 μmol/gm creatine
≥ 16 yrs		28–115 μmol/gm creatine
Fatty acid profile of serum lipids		
Linoleate		≥ 25% of fatty acids in serum lipids
Arachidonate		≥ 6% of fatty acids in serum lipids
Palmitate		18–26% of fatty acids in serum lipids
Phytanate		≤ 0.3% of fatty acids in serum lipids
		(>0.5% suggests Refsum's disease;
		0.3–0.5% borderline)
Free fatty acids	(S)	239–843 μEq/L
Galactose	(U)	Not detectable
Galactose 1-phosphate	(RBC)	
Nongalactosemic		5–49 μg/gm Hb
Galactosemic (galactose-		80–125 μg/gm Hb
restricted diet)		
Galactosemic (unrestricted diet)		>125 μg/gm Hb
Galactose 1-phosphate uridyl-	(B)	18.5–28.5 U/gm Hb
transferase (galactosemia)		
Galactokinase	(B)	
<2 yrs old		20–80 mU/gm Hb
≥ 2 yrs old		12–40 mU/gm Hb
Galactosylceramide-beta-galactosi-	(F)	10.3–89.7 mU/gm cellular protein
dase (Krabbe's disease,	(L)	>21.5 mU/gm cellular protein
globoid cell leukodystrophy)		
Glucose-6-phosphate dehydro-	(B)	
genase		
2–17 yrs old		6.4–15.6 U/gm Hb
>18 yrs old		8.6–18.6 U/gm Hb
Glucose phosphate isomerase	(B)	49–81 U/gm Hb
Hexosaminidase (≥ 5 yrs old)		
(Tay-Sachs disease, GM$_2$		
gangliosidosis)		
Total	(S)	10.4–23.8 U/L
Hexosaminidase A		
Normal		1.23–2.59 U/L; 56–80% of total
Indeterminate		1.16–1.22 U/L; 50–55% of total
Carrier		0.58–1.15 U/L; <50% of total
Total	(L)	16.4–36.2 U/gm cellular protein
Hexosaminidase A		63–75% of total
Total	(F)	92–184.5 U/gm cellular protein
Hexosaminidase A		41–65% of total
Homogentisic acid	(U)	Negative
Hydroxyproline, free	(24 hr U)	<1.3 mg/24 hrs
Hydroxyproline, total	(24 hr U)	
<5 yrs old		100–400 μg/mg creatinine
5–12 yrs		100–150 μg/mg creatinine

Females ≥ 19 yrs		0.4–2.9 mg/2 hr specimen
Males ≥ 19 yrs		0.4–5.0 mg/2 hr specimen
^{35}S Mucopolysaccharide (I, II, III, VI, VII)	(F)	Normal or abnormal turnover
Phenylalanine	(P)	
≤ 1 wk of age		0.69–2.0 mg/dL (42–124 μmol/L)
<16 yrs old		0.43–1.4 mg/dL (26–86 μmol/L)
>16 yrs old		0.68–1.1 mg/dL (41–68 μmol/L)
Phytanate (phytanic acid)	(S)	<0.3% = normal
		0.3–0.5% = borderline
		>0.5% suggests Refsum's disease
Porphyrins, total	(RBC)	16–60 μg/dL packed cells
Uro (octacarboxylic)		≤ 2 μg/dL
Hepatocarboxylic		≤ 1 μg/dL
Hexacarboxylic		≤ 1 μg/dL
Pentacarboxylic		≤ 1 μg/dL
Copro (tetracarboxylic)		≤ 2 μg/dL
Porphyrins, total	(P)	≤ 1 μg/dL
Fractionation		≤ 1 μg/dL for any fraction
Porphyrins	(St)	
Coproporphyrin		≤ 200 μg/24 hrs
Protoporphyrin		≤ 1500 μg/24 hrs
Uroporphyrin		≤ 1000 μg/24 hrs
Porphyrins, fractionation	(U)	
Uro (octacarboxylic)		
Males		≤ 46 μg/24 hrs
Females		≤ 22 μg/24 hrs
Hepatocarboxylic		
Males		≤ 13 μg/24 hrs
Females		≤ 9 μg/24 hrs
Hexacarboxylic		
Males		≤ 5 μg/24 hrs
Females		≤ 4 μg/24 hrs
Pentacarboxylic		
Males		≤ 4 μg/24 hrs
Females		≤ 3 μg/24 hrs
Copro (tetracarboxylic)		
Males		≤ 96 μg/24 hrs
Females		≤ 60 μg/24 hrs
Porphobilinogen		Normal: ≤ 1.5 mg/24 hrs
		Marginal: 1.5–2.0 mg/24 hrs
		Excess: >2.0 mg/24 hrs
Protoporphyrins	(RBC)	
Free		1–10 μg/dL packed RBCs
Zinc-protoporphyrin		10–38 μg/dL packed RBCs
Sphingomyelinase (Niemann-Pick disease)	(F)	1.53–7.18 U/gm cellular protein
Tyrosine	(P)	
≤ 1 wk		0.6–2.2 mg/dL (33–122 μmol/L)
<16 yrs		0.47–2.0 mg/dL (26–110 μmol/L)
>16 yrs		0.8–1.3 mg/dL (45–74 μmol/L)
Uroporphyrinogen synthase	(RBC)	
Males		7.9–14.7 nM/sec/L
Females		8.0–16.8 nM/sec/L
		Marginal values 6.0–8.0 nM/sec/L are suggestive but indeterminate
		Values <6.0 nM/sec/L are definite for acute, intermittent porphyria
Vitamins		See Chapter 12, pp. 501–502

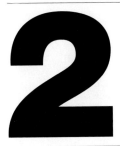

Critical Values

These values may indicate the need for prompt clinical intervention. Any *sudden changes* may also be critical. Also called *action values* or *automatic call back values*. Values will vary according to the laboratory performing the tests as well as patient age and other factors.

Hematology

	Low	High
Hct (packed cell volume)	<20 vol%	>60 vol%
Hb	<7 gm/dL	>20 gm/dL
Platelet count (adult)	<40,000/cu mm	>1,000,000/cu mm
Platelet count (pediatric)	<20,000/cu mm	>1,000,000/cu mm
aPTT	None	>78 secs
PT	None	>30 secs or >3× control level
Positive test for fibrin split products, protamine sulfate, high heparin level		
Fibrinogen	<100 mg/dL	>700 mg/dL
WBC	<2000/cu mm	>30,000/cu mm
Presence of blast cells, sickle cells		
New diagnosis of leukemia, sickle cell anemia, aplastic crisis		

Blood Chemistry

	Low	High
Ammonia	None	>40 μmol/L
Amylase	None	>200 U/L
Arterial pCO$_2$	<20 mm Hg	>70 mm Hg
Arterial pH	<7.2 U	>7.6 U
Arterial pO$_2$ (adults)	<40 mm Hg	None
Arterial pO$_2$ (newborns)	<37 mm Hg (standard deviation [SD] = 7)	92 mm Hg (SD = 12)
Bicarbonate	<10 mEq/L	>40 mEq/L
Bilirubin, total (newborns)	None	>15 mg/dL
Calcium	<6 mg/dL	>13 mg/dL
Carbon dioxide	<10 mEq/L	>40 mEq/L
Cardiac troponin (cTn)		
Cardiac troponin T (cTnT)	None	>0.1 μg/L
Cardiac troponin I (cTnI)	None	>1.6 μg/L
Chloride	<80 mEq/L	>115 mEq/L
CK	None	>3–5× upper limit of normal (ULN)

CK-MB	None	>5% or ≥ 10 μg/L
Creatinine (except dialysis patients)	None	>5.0 mg/dL
Glucose	<40 mg/dL	>450 mg/dL
Glucose (newborns)	<30 mg/dL	>300 mg/dL
Magnesium	<1.0 mg/dL	>4.7 mg/dL
Phosphorus	<1 mg/dL	None
Potassium	<2.8 mEq/L	>6.2 mEq/L
Potassium (newborns)	<2.5 mEq/L	>8.0 mEq/L
Sodium	<120 mEq/L	>160 mEq/L
BUN (except dialysis patients)	2 mg/dL	>80 mg/dL

Cerebrospinal Fluid

	Low	**High**
Glucose	<80% of blood level	
Protein, total	None	>45 mg/dL
Positive bacterial stain (e.g., Gram, acid-fast), antigen detection, culture, or India ink preparation		
WBC in CSF	None	>10/cu mm
Presence of malignant cells or blasts or any other body fluid		

Microbiology

Positive blood culture
Positive Gram stain or culture from any body fluid (e.g., pleural, peritoneal, joint)
Positive acid-fast stain or culture from any site
Positive culture or isolate for *Corynebacterium diphtheriae, Cryptococcus neoformans, Bordetella pertussis, Neisseria gonorrhoeae* (only nongenital sites), dimorphic fungi (*Histoplasma, Coccidioides, Blastomyces, Paracoccidioides*)
Presence of blood parasites (e.g., malaria organisms, *Babesia*, microfilaria)
Positive antigen detection (e.g., *Cryptococcus*, group B streptococci, *Haemophilus influenzae* type B, *Neisseria meningitidis, Streptococcus pneumoniae*)
Stool culture positive for *Salmonella, Shigella, Campylobacter, Vibrio*, or *Yersinia*

Urinalysis

Strongly positive test for glucose and ketone
Presence of reducing sugars in infants
Presence of pathological crystals (urate, cysteine, leucine, tyrosine)

Serology

Incompatible cross match
Positive direct and indirect antiglobulin (Coombs') test on routine specimens
Positive direct antiglobulin (Coombs') test on cord blood
Titers of significant RBC alloantibodies during pregnancy
Transfusion reaction workup showing incompatible unit of transfused blood
Failure to call within 72 hrs for Rh Ig after possible or known exposure to Rh-positive RBCs
Positive confirmed test for hepatitis, syphilis, acquired immunodeficiency syndrome (AIDS)
Increased blood antibody levels for infectious agents (see pp. 23–24)

Therapeutic Drugs

	Blood Levels
Acetaminophen	>150 μg/mL
Carbamazepine	>20 μg/mL
Chloramphenicol	>50 μg/mL (peak)
Digitoxin	>35 ng/mL
Digoxin	>2.5 ng/mL
Ethosuximide	>200 μg/mL
Gentamicin	>12 μg/mL
Imipramine	>400 ng/mL
Lidocaine	>9 μg/mL
Lithium	>2 mEq/L
Phenobarbital	>60 μg/mL
Phenytoin	>40 μg/mL
Primidone	>24 μg/mL
Quinidine	>10 μg/mL
Salicylate	>700 μg/mL
Theophylline	>25 μg/mL
Tobramycin	>12 μg/mL (peak)

See Chapter 18, Therapeutic Drug Monitoring and Toxicology, for toxic levels of various therapeutic drugs and toxic substances.

In addition, the physician is promptly notified of any of the following:

Serum glucose, fasting	>130 mg/dL
Serum glucose, random	>250 mg/dL
Serum cholesterol	>300 mg/dL
Serum total protein	>9.0 mg/dL
Blood lead	Increased
Urinalysis	Pus, blood, or protein ≥ 2+
Urine colony count/culture	>50,000 colonies/mL of single organism
Respiratory culture	Heavy growth of pathogen
Peripheral blood smear	Atypical lymphocytes, plasma cells

Some data from Emmancipator K. Critical values. ASCP practice parameter. *Am J Clin Pathol* 1997;108:247.

CRIT. VALUES

Specific Laboratory Examinations

Core Blood Analytes: Alterations by Diseases

Alanine Aminotransferase (ALT; Serum Glutamic-Pyruvic Transaminase [SGPT])

Use

Differential diagnosis of diseases of hepatobiliary system and pancreas
Repeat testing to establish chronicity of viral hepatitis
Generally parallels but lower than AST in alcohol-related diseases

Increased In

See serum AST (see pp. 41–42)
Obesity (not AST; modest increase to 1–3× ULN)
Severe preeclampsia (both)
Rapidly progressing acute lymphoblastic leukemia (both)
Levels in females ~75% of those in males

Decreased In

GU tract infection
Malignancy
Pyridoxal phosphate deficiency states (e.g., malnutrition, pregnancy, alcoholic liver disease)
Others

Albumin

(Generally parallels total protein except when total protein changes are due to gamma globulins)

Use

Marker of disorders of protein metabolism (e.g., nutritional, decreased synthesis, increased loss)

Increased In

Dehydration (relative increase)
Intravenous (IV) albumin infusions

Decreased In

Inadequate intake (e.g., malnutrition)
Decreased absorption (e.g., malabsorption syndromes)
Increased need (e.g., hyperthyroidism, pregnancy)
Impaired synthesis (e.g., liver diseases, chronic infection, hereditary analbuminemia)
Increased breakdown (e.g., neoplasms, infection, trauma)
Increased loss (e.g., edema, ascites, burns, hemorrhage, nephrotic syndrome, protein-losing enteropathy)
Dilutional states (e.g., IV fluids, SIADH, psychogenic diabetes/water intoxication)
Congenital deficiency

Alkaline Phosphatase (ALP)

(See also Table 13-7.)

Use

Diagnosis of causes and monitoring of course of cholestasis (e.g., neoplasm, drugs)
Diagnosis of various bone disorders (e.g., Paget's disease, osteogenic sarcoma)

Interferences

Intravenous injection of albumin; sometimes marked increase (e.g., 10× normal level)
   lasting for several days (placental origin); total parenteral nutrition (TPN)
Decreased by collection of blood in EDTA, fluoride, or oxalate anticoagulant
Increased (≤ 30%) by standing at room or refrigerator temperature

Increased In

Bone origin—increased deposition of calcium
   • Hyperparathyroidism.
   • Paget's disease (osteitis deformans) (highest reported values 10–20× normal).
     *Marked elevation in absence of liver disease is most suggestive of Paget's disease
     of bone or metastatic carcinoma from prostate.*
   • *Increase in cases of metastases to bone is marked only in prostate carcinoma.*
   • Osteoblastic bone tumors (osteogenic sarcoma, metastatic carcinoma).
   • Osteogenesis imperfecta (due to healing fractures).
   • Familial osteoectasia.
   • Osteomalacia, rickets.
   • Polyostotic fibrous dysplasia.
   • Osteomyelitis.
   • Late pregnancy; reverts to normal level by 20th day postpartum.
   • Children.
   • Administration of ergosterol.
   • Hyperthyroidism.
   • Transient hyperphosphatasemia of infancy.
   • Hodgkin's disease.
   • Healing of extensive fractures (slightly).
Liver disease—any obstruction of biliary system (e.g., stone, carcinoma, primary bil-
   iary cirrhosis); is a sensitive indicator of intra- or extrahepatic cholestasis. Whenever
   the ALP is elevated, a simultaneous elevation of 5'-NT establishes biliary disease as
   the cause of the elevated ALP. If the 5'-NT is not increased, the cause of the elevated
   ALP must be found elsewhere, e.g., bone disease.
   • Nodules in liver (metastatic or primary tumor, abscess, cyst, parasite, tuberculo-
     sis [TB], sarcoid); is a sensitive indicator of a hepatic infiltrate. *Increase >2× upper
     limit of normal in patients with primary breast or lung tumor with osteolytic metas-
     tases is more likely due to liver than bone metastases.*
   • Liver infiltrates (e.g., amyloid or leukemia).
   • Cholangiolar obstruction in hepatitis (e.g., infectious, toxic).
   • Hepatic congestion due to heart disease.
   • Adverse reaction to therapeutic drug (e.g., chlorpropamide) (progressive elevation
     of serum ALP may be first indication that drug therapy should be halted); may be
     2–20× normal.
   • Increased synthesis of ALP in liver.
       Diabetes mellitus—44% of diabetic patients have 40% increase of ALP.
       Parenteral hyperalimentation of glucose.
   • Liver diseases with increased ALP.
       <3–4× increase lacks specificity and may be present in all forms of liver disease.
       2× increase: acute hepatitis (viral, toxic, alcoholic), acute fatty liver, cirrhosis.
       5× increase: infectious mononucleosis, postnecrotic cirrhosis.
       10× increase: carcinoma of head of pancreas, choledocholithiasis, drug chole-
          static hepatitis.
       15–20× increase: primary biliary cirrhosis, primary or metastatic carcinoma.
       Chronic therapeutic use of anticonvulsant drugs (e.g., phenobarbital, phenytoin)
   • Hodgkin's disease.

Placental origin—appears 16th–20th wk of normal pregnancy, increases progressively to 2× normal up to onset of labor, disappears 3–6 days after delivery of placenta. May be increased during complications of pregnancy (e.g., hypertension, preeclampsia, eclampsia, threatened abortion) but difficult to interpret without serial determinations. Lower in diabetic than in nondiabetic pregnancy.

Intestinal origin—is a component in ~25% of normal sera; increases 2 hrs after eating in persons with blood type B or O who are secretors of H blood group. Has been reported to be increased in cirrhosis, various ulcerative diseases of GI tract, severe malabsorption, chronic hemodialysis, acute infarction of intestine.

Benign familial hyperphosphatasemia (see p. 604).

Ectopic production by neoplasm (Regan isoenzyme) without involvement of liver or bone (e.g., Hodgkin's disease, cancer of lung, breast, colon, or pancreas; highest incidence in ovary and cervical cancer)

Vascular endothelium origin—some patients with myocardial, pulmonary, renal (one-third of cases), or splenic infarction, usually after 7 days during phase of organization

Hyperphosphatasia (liver and bone isoenzymes)

Hyperthyroidism (liver and bone isoenzymes). *Increased ALP alone in a chemistry profile, especially with a decreased serum cholesterol and lymphocytosis, should suggest excess thyroid medication or hyperthyroidism.*

Primary hypophosphatemia (often increased)

ALP isoenzyme determinations are not widely used clinically; heat inactivation may be more useful to distinguish bone from liver source of increased ALP. Extremely (90%) heat labile: bone, vascular endothelium, reticuloendothelial system. Extremely (90%) heat stable: placenta, neoplasms. Intermediate (60–80%) heat stable: liver, intestine. Also differentiate by chemical inhibition (e.g., L-phenylalanine) or use serum LAP.

Children—mostly bone; little or no liver or intestine.

Adults—liver with little or no bone or intestine; after age 50, increasing amounts of bone.

Normal In

Inherited metabolic diseases (Dubin-Johnson, Rotor's, Gilbert, Crigler-Najjar syndromes; types I to V glycogenoses, mucopolysaccharidoses; increase in Wilson's disease and hemochromatosis related to hepatic fibrosis)

Consumption of alcohol by healthy persons (in contrast to GGT); may be normal even in alcoholic hepatitis.

In acute icteric viral hepatitis, increase is <2× normal in 90% of cases, but when ALP is high and serum bilirubin is normal, infectious mononucleosis should be ruled out as cause of hepatitis.

Decreased In

Excess vitamin D ingestion
Milk-alkali (Burnett's) syndrome
Congenital hypophosphatasia
Achondroplasia
Hypothyroidism, cretinism
Pernicious anemia (PA) in one-third of patients
Celiac disease
Malnutrition
Scurvy
Zinc deficiency
Magnesium deficiency
Postmenopausal women with osteoporosis taking estrogen replacement therapy
Therapeutic agents (e.g., corticosteroids, trifluoperazine, antilipemic agents, some hyperalimentation)
Cardiac surgery with cardiopulmonary bypass pump

Ammonia

Use

Increased in some inherited metabolic disorders, especially ornithine carbamoyltransferase deficiency, citrullinemia, argininosuccinic aciduria.

BLOOD ANALYT

*Should be measured in cases of unexplained lethargy and vomiting, encephalopathy, or
in any newborn with unexplained neurological deterioration.*
Not useful to assess degree of dysfunction; e.g., in Reye's syndrome, hepatic function
improves and ammonia level falls even in patients who finally die of this.

Increased In

Certain inborn errors of metabolism (see Chapter 12)
Transient hyperammonemia in newborn; unknown etiology; may be life-threatening
in first 48 hrs.
Moribund children—moderate increases ($\leq$ 300 μmol/L) without being diagnostic of a
specific disease.
May occur in any patient with severe liver disease (e.g., acute hepatic necrosis, terminal cirrhosis, hepatectomy). Increased in most cases of hepatic coma but correlates
poorly with degree of encephalopathy. *In cirrhosis, blood ammonia may be increased
after portacaval anastomosis.*
GU tract infection with distention and stasis
Sodium valproate therapy

Decreased In

Hyperornithinemia (deficiency of ornithine aminotransaminase activity) with gyrate
atrophy of choroid and retina

Antistreptococcal Antibody Titers (ASOT)
Use

Individual determinations depend on various factors (e.g., duration and severity of infec-
tion, antigenicity) and are of limited clinical value. Serial determinations are most desir-
able; a 4× increase in ASOT confirms immunologic response to streptococcal organisms.
A high or rising titer is indicative only of current or recent streptococcal infection.
  • Direct diagnostic value in
      Scarlet fever
      Erysipelas
    Streptococcal pharyngitis and tonsillitis
  • Indirect diagnostic value in
      Rheumatic fever (see p. 128)
      Glomerulonephritis (see p. 718)
Detection of subclinical streptococcal infection
Differential diagnosis of joint pains of rheumatic fever and rheumatoid arthritis (RA)

Increased In

Antibody appears as early as 1 wk after infection; titer rises rapidly by 3–4 wks and
then declines quickly; may remain elevated for months.
Even in severe streptococcal infection, ASOT will be increased in only 70–80% of patients.

Conditions	Usual ASO Titer (Todd Units)
Normal persons	12–166
Active rheumatic fever	500–5000
Inactive rheumatic fever	12–250
RA	12–250
Acute GN	500–5000
Streptococcal URI	100–333
Collagen diseases	12–250

False positives are associated with TB, liver disease (e.g., active viral hepatitis), bacterial contamination.
ASOT is increased in only 30–40% of patients with streptococcal pyoderma and 50%
of patients with poststreptococcal GN; DNase antibodies are the most sensitive indicators of these conditions. DNase B titers may also be helpful in diagnosis of delayed
sequelae of Sydenham's chorea because they are detectable for several months.
Other streptococcal antigens may be tested
    Antistreptococcal hyaluronidase (significant titer >128)
    Antideoxyribonuclease (DNase B) (significant titer >10)

Interferences

Latex agglutination method may give false positive in markedly lipemic or contaminated specimens.

Apolipoproteins

Apolipoprotein A-I

Use
Decreased level is associated with increased risk of coronary heart disease (CHD).

Increased In
Familial hyperalphalipoproteinemia
Pregnancy
Estrogen therapy
Alcohol consumption
Exercise

Decreased In
Tangier disease
"Fish-eye" disease
Familial hypoalphalipoproteinemia
Familial lecithin-cholesterol acyltransferase deficiency
Type I and type V hyperlipoproteinemia
Diabetes mellitus
Cholestasis
Hemodialysis
Infection
Drugs (e.g., diuretics, beta-blockers, androgenic steroids, glucocorticoids, cyclosporine)

Apolipoprotein A-II

Increased In
Alcohol consumption

Decreased In
Tangier disease
Cholestasis
Cigarette smoking

Apolipoprotein A-IV

Increased In
Postprandial lipemia

Decreased In
Abetalipoproteinemia
Chronic pancreatitis
Malabsorption
Obstructive jaundice
Acute hepatitis
Total parenteral nutrition

Apolipoprotein (a)

Use
Increased risk of CHD with serum levels >0.03 gm/L

Increased In
Pregnancy
Patients who have had acute myocardial infarction (AMI)

Decreased In
Drugs (e.g., nicotinic acid, neomycin, anabolic steroids)

Apolipoprotein B-48

Normally absent during fasting

Increased In
Hyperlipoproteinemia (types I, V)
Apoprotein (apo) E deficiency

Decreased In
Liver disease
Hypo- and abetalipoproteinemia
Malabsorption

Apolipoprotein B-100

Use
Increased levels are associated with increased risk of CHD.

Increased In
Hyperlipoproteinemia (types IIa, IIb, IV, V)
Familial hyperapobetalipoproteinemia
Nephrotic syndrome
Pregnancy
Biliary obstruction
Hemodialysis
Cigarette smoking
Drugs (e.g., diuretics, beta-blockers, cyclosporine, glucocorticoids)

Decreased In
Hypo- and abetalipoproteinemia
Type I hyperlipoproteinemia (hyperchylomicronemia)
Liver disease
Exercise
Infections
Drugs (e.g., cholesterol-lowering drugs, estrogens)

Apolipoprotein C-1

Increased In
Hyperlipoproteinemia (types I, III, IV, V)

Decreased In
Tangier disease

Apolipoprotein C-II

Increased In
Hyperlipoproteinemia (types I, III, IV, V)

Decreased In
Tangier disease
Hypoalphalipoproteinemia
Apo C-II deficiency
Nephrotic syndrome

Apolipoprotein C-III

Use
With combined hereditary apo A-I and apo C-III deficiency increased risk of premature CHD.

Increased In
Hyperlipoproteinemia (types III, IV, V)

Decreased In
Tangier disease
Combined with hereditary deficiency apo A-I

Apolipoprotein E

Increased In
Hyperlipoproteinemia (types I, III, IV, V)
Pregnancy
Cholestasis
Multiple sclerosis in remission
Drugs (e.g., dexamethasone)

Decreased In
Drugs (e.g., ACTH)

Aspartate Aminotransferase (AST; Serum Glutamic-Oxaloacetic Transaminase [SGOT])

Use

Differential diagnosis of diseases of hepatobiliary system and pancreas
Formerly surrogate test for screening blood donors for hepatitis

Interferences

Increase due to hemolysis, lipemia
Increase due to calcium dust in air (e.g., due to construction in laboratory)
Increased due to enzyme activation during test
  • Therapy with oxacillin, ampicillin, opiates, erythromycin
Decreased (because of increased serum lactate–consuming enzyme during test)
  • Diabetic ketoacidosis
  • Beriberi
  • Severe liver disease
  • Chronic hemodialysis (reason unknown)
  • Uremia—proportional to BUN level (reason unknown)

Increased In

Liver diseases (see Chapter 8)
  • Active necrosis of parenchymal cells is suggested by extremely high levels. Acute viral hepatitis shows greatest increases; may be 20× to 100×.
  • Rapid rise and decline suggests extrahepatic biliary disease.
  • Administration of opiates to patients with diseased biliary tract or previous cholecystectomy causes increase in LD and especially AST. AST increases by 2–4 hrs, peaks in 5–8 hrs; increase may persist for 24 hrs; elevation may be 2.5–65× normal.
  • Congestion, e.g., heart failure, cirrhosis, biliary obstruction, primary or metastatic cancer, granulomas, hepatic ischemia.
  • Eclampsia.
  • Hepatotoxic drugs and chemicals (e.g., carbon tetrachloride).
Musculoskeletal disorders (see Chapter 10), including trauma, surgery, and IM injections
  • Myoglobinuria
Acute myocardial infarction
Others
  • Acute pancreatitis
  • Intestinal injury (e.g., surgery, infarction)
  • Local irradiation injury
  • Pulmonary infarction (relatively slight increase)
  • Cerebral infarction (increased in following week in 50% of patients)
  • Cerebral neoplasms (occasionally)
  • Renal infarction (occasionally)
  • Drugs (e.g., heparin therapy, salicylates, opiates, tetracycline, chlorpromazine [Thorazine], isoniazid)
  • Burns
  • Heat exhaustion
  • Mushroom poisoning

- Lead poisoning (not useful for screening)
- Hemolytic anemia

Marked Increase (>3000 U/L) In

Acute hypotension (e.g., AMI, sepsis, post–cardiac surgery)
Toxic liver injury (e.g., drugs)
Viral hepatitis
Liver trauma
Liver metastases
Rhabdomyolysis

Decreased In

Azotemia
Chronic renal dialysis
Pyridoxal phosphate deficiency states (e.g., malnutrition, pregnancy, alcoholic liver disease)

Normal In

Angina pectoris
Coronary insufficiency
Pericarditis
Congestive heart failure without liver damage
Varies <10 U/day in the same person.

AST/ALT (SGOT/SGPT) Ratio

(Normal = 0.7–1.4 depending on methodology.)

Use

Differential diagnosis of diseases of hepatobiliary system and pancreas

Increased In

Drug hepatotoxicity (>2.0)
Alcoholic hepatitis (>2.0 is highly suggestive; may be ≤ 6.0)
Cirrhosis (1.4–2.0)
Intrahepatic cholestasis (>1.5)
Hepatocellular carcinoma
Chronic hepatitis (slightly increased; 1.3)

Decreased In

Acute hepatitis due to virus, drugs, toxins (with AST increased 3–10× upper limit of
    normal) (usually ≤ 0.65; ratio 0.3–0.6 is said to be a good prognostic sign but higher
    ratio of 1.2–1.6 is a poor prognostic sign)
Extrahepatic cholestasis (normal or slightly decreased; 0.8)[1]

Autohemagglutination, Cold

Use

Primary atypical (*Mycoplasma*) pneumonia (30–90% of patients): titer ≥ 1:14–1:224.
    Not ruled out by negative titer (see p. 810).

Increased In

Atypical hemolytic anemia
Paroxysmal hemoglobinuria
Raynaud's disease
Cirrhosis of the liver
Trypanosomiasis

---

[1]Reg R. Aminotransferases in disease. *Clin Lab Med* 1989;9:667.

Malaria
Infectious mononucleosis
Adenovirus infections
Influenza
Psittacosis
Mumps
Measles
Scarlet fever
Rheumatic fever
Some cases of lymphoma

Bilirubin

See Chapter 8, Hepatobiliary Diseases and Diseases of the Pancreas.

Use

Differential diagnosis of diseases of hepatobiliary system and pancreas and other causes
of jaundice.
- Jaundice becomes apparent clinically at $\geq$ 2.5 mg/dL.

Interferences

Exposure to either white or ultraviolet light decreases total and indirect bilirubin 2% to >20%.
Fasting for 48 hrs produces a mean increase of 240% in healthy persons and 194% in
those with hepatic dysfunction.

Increased Direct (Conjugated) Bilirubin In

Hereditary disorders (e.g., Dubin-Johnson syndrome, Rotor's syndrome)
Hepatic cellular damage. *Increased conjugated bilirubin may be associated with nor-
mal total bilirubin in up to one-third of patients with liver diseases.*
    Viral
    Toxic
    Alcohol related
    Drug related
Methodologic interference
    - Evelyn-Malloy (dextran, novobiocin)
    - Diazo reaction (ethoxazene, histidine, indican, phenazopyridine, rifampin, theo-
      phylline, tyrosine)
    - SMA 12/60 (aminophenol, ascorbic acid, epinephrine, isoproterenol, levodopa,
      methyldopa, phenelzine)
    - Spectrophotometric methods (drugs that cause lipemia)
Other effects (e.g., toxic, cholestasis)
Biliary duct obstruction
    Extrahepatic
    Intrahepatic
Infiltrations, space-occupying lesions, e.g.,
    Metastatic tumor
    Abscess
    Granulomas
    Amyloidosis
Direct bilirubin
    - 20–40% of total: more suggestive of hepatic than posthepatic jaundice
    - 40–60% of total: occurs in either hepatic or posthepatic jaundice
    - >50% of total: more suggestive of posthepatic than hepatic jaundice
Total serum bilirubin >40 mg/dL indicates hepatocellular rather than extrahepatic
obstruction.

Increased Unconjugated (Indirect) Bilirubin (Conjugated <20% of Total)

Increased bilirubin production
    Hemolytic diseases (e.g., hemoglobinopathies, RBC enzyme deficiencies, dissemi-
    nated intravascular coagulation [DIC], autoimmune hemolysis)

BLOOD ANALYT

Ineffective erythropoiesis (e.g., PA)
Blood transfusions
Hematomas
Hereditary disorders (e.g., Gilbert's disease, Crigler-Najjar syndrome)
Drugs (e.g., causing hemolysis)

Decreased In

Drugs (e.g., barbiturates)

Interferences

Presence of hemoglobin
Exposure to sunlight or fluorescent light

Decreased In

Ingestion of certain drugs (e.g., barbiturates)

Blood Urea Nitrogen (BUN)/Creatinine Ratio

(See also Table 15-3.)
Normal range for healthy person on normal diet = 12–20; ratio for most individuals is
12–16. Because of considerable variability, should be used only as a rough guide.

Use

Differentiate pre- and postrenal azotemia from renal azotemia

Increased Ratio (>20:1) with Normal Creatinine In

Prerenal azotemia (BUN rises without increase in creatinine) (e.g., heart failure, salt
depletion, dehydration, blood loss) due to decreased glomerular filtration rate
Catabolic states with increased tissue breakdown
GI hemorrhage. It has been reported that ratio ≥ 36 distinguishes upper from lower GI
hemorrhage in patients with negative gastric aspirate.
High protein intake
Impaired renal function plus
  • Excess protein intake or production or tissue breakdown (e.g., GI bleeding, thy-
    rotoxicosis, infection, Cushing's syndrome, high-protein diet, surgery, burns,
    cachexia, high fever)
  • Urine reabsorption (e.g., ureterocolostomy)
  • Reduced muscle mass (subnormal creatinine production)
Certain drugs (e.g., tetracycline, glucocorticoids)

Increased Ratio (>20:1) with Elevated Creatinine In

Postrenal azotemia (BUN rises disproportionately more than creatinine) (e.g., obstructive uropathy)
Prerenal azotemia superimposed on renal disease

Decreased Ratio (<10:1) with Decreased BUN In

Acute tubular necrosis
Low protein diet, starvation, severe liver disease, and other causes of decreased urea
synthesis
Repeated dialysis (urea rather than creatinine diffuses out of extracellular fluid)
Inherited hyperammonemias (urea is virtually absent in blood)
SIADH (due to tubular secretion of urea)
Pregnancy

Decreased Ratio (<10:1) with Increased Creatinine In

Phenacemide therapy (accelerates conversion of creatine to creatinine)
Rhabdomyolysis (releases muscle creatinine)
Muscular patients who develop renal failure

Inappropriate Ratio

Diabetic ketoacidosis (acetoacetate causes false increase in creatinine with certain methodologies, resulting in normal ratio when dehydration should produce an increased BUN/creatinine ratio)
Cephalosporin therapy (interferes with creatinine measurement)

Calcium, Ionized

See Calcium, Total, p. 46.

Use

In patients with hypo- or hypercalcemia with borderline serum calcium and altered serum proteins
~50% of calcium is ionized; 40–45% is bound to albumin; 5–10% is bound to other anions (e.g., sulfate, phosphate, lactate, citrate); only ionized fraction is physiologically active. Total calcium values may be deceiving because they may be unchanged even if ionized calcium values are changed; e.g., increased blood pH increases protein-bound calcium and decreases ionized calcium, and parathyroid hormone has opposite effect (*blood pH should always be performed with ionized calcium, which is increased in acidosis and decreased in alkalosis*). However, in critically ill patients, elevated total serum calcium usually indicates ionized hypercalcemia, and a normal total serum calcium is evidence against ionized hypocalcemia.
Ionized calcium is the preferred measurement rather than total calcium because it is physiologically active and can be rapidly measured, which may be essential in certain situations (e.g., liver transplantation, rapid or large transfusion of citrated blood that makes interpretation of total calcium nearly impossible).
Life-threatening complications are frequent when serum ionized calcium is <2 mg/dL (<0.50 mmol/L).
With multiple blood transfusions, ionized calcium <3 mg/dL (<0.95 mmol/L) may be an indication to administer calcium.
Reference ranges for ionized calcium vary with method and type of sample preparation (e.g., brand of heparin used) and should be determined by each laboratory. Sample ranges (mmol/L) are:

Age	Values
Adult	1.15–1.35
1 yr to adult	1.29–1.31
5 days	1.24–1.44
3 days	1.16–1.36
1 day	1.11–1.31

Interferences

Hypo- or hypermagnesemia (see p. 66); patients respond to serum magnesium that becomes normal but not to calcium therapy. *Serum magnesium should always be measured in any patient with hypocalcemia.*
Increase of ions to which calcium is bound
  • Phosphate (e.g., phosphorus administration in treatment of diabetic ketoacidosis, chemotherapy causing tumor lysis syndrome, rhabdomyolysis)
  • Bicarbonate
  • Citrate (e.g., during blood transfusion)
  • Radiographic contrast media containing calcium chelators (edetate, citrate)

Increased In

Normal total serum calcium associated with hypoalbuminemia may indicate ionized hypercalcemia.
~25% of patients with hyperparathyroidism have normal total but increased ionized calcium levels.

Decreased In

Hyperventilation (e.g., to control increased intracranial pressure) (total serum calcium may be normal)

Administration of bicarbonate to control metabolic acidosis
Increased serum free fatty acids (increase calcium binding to albumin) due to
  • Certain drugs (e.g., heparin, intravenous lipids, epinephrine, norepinephrine, iso-proterenol, alcohol)
  • Severe stress (e.g., acute pancreatitis, diabetic ketoacidosis, sepsis, AMI)
  • Hemodialysis
Hypoparathyroidism (primary, secondary)
Vitamin D deficiency
Toxic shock syndrome
Fat embolism
Hypokalemia protects patient from hypocalcemic tetany; correction of hypokalemia without correction of hypocalcemia may provoke tetany.

Calcium, Total

See Fig. 13-6 and Table 13-8.

Use

Diagnosis of parathyroid dysfunction, hypercalcemia of malignancy. *90% of cases of hypercalcemia are due to hyperparathyroidism, neoplasms, or granulomatous diseases. Hypercalcemia of sarcoidosis, adrenal insufficiency, and hyperthyroidism tend to be found in clinically evident disease.*
Blood calcium should be monitored in renal failure, effects of various drugs, acute pancreatitis, postoperative thyroidectomy, and parathyroidectomy.

Interferences

Increased by
  • Elevated serum protein
  • Dehydration
  • Venous stasis during blood collection by prolonged application of tourniquet
  • Use of cork-stoppered test tubes
  • Hyponatremia (<120 mEq/L), which increases protein-bound fraction of calcium thereby slightly increasing the total calcium (opposite effect in hypernatremia)
Decreased by
  • Hypomagnesemia (e.g., due to cisplatin chemotherapy)
  • Hyperphosphatemia (e.g., due to laxatives, phosphate enemas, chemotherapy for leukemia or lymphoma, rhabdomyolysis).
  • Hypoalbuminemia
  • Hemodilution
Total serum protein and albumin should always be measured simultaneously for proper interpretation of serum calcium levels, because 0.8 mg of calcium is bound to 1.0 gm of albumin in serum; to correct, add 0.8 mg/dL for every 1.0 g/dL that serum albumin falls below 4.0 g/dL; binding to globulin affects total calcium only if globulin is >6 gm/dL.

Increased In

Hyperparathyroidism
  • Primary
  • Secondary
      Acute and chronic renal failure
      Post–renal transplant
      Osteomalacia with malabsorption
      Aluminum-associated osteomalacia
Malignant tumors (especially breast, lung, kidney; 2% of patients with Hodgkin's or non-Hodgkin's lymphoma)
  • Direct bone metastases (up to 30% of these patients) (e.g., breast cancer, Hodgkin's and non-Hodgkin's lymphoma, leukemia, pancreatic cancer, lung cancer)
  • Osteoclastic activating factor (e.g., multiple myeloma, Burkitt's lymphoma; may be markedly increased in adult T-cell [HTLV] lymphoma)
  • Humoral hypercalcemia of malignancy (parathyroid hormone–related protein [PTHrP])

- Ectopic production of 1,25-dihydroxyvitamin D_3 (e.g., Hodgkin's and non-Hodgkin's lymphoma)

Effect of drugs
- Vitamin D intoxication
- Milk-alkali (Burnett's) syndrome
- Diuretic use (thiazide and chlorthalidone rarely increase serum calcium >1.0 mg/dL)
- Use of therapeutic agents (estrogens, androgens, progestins, tamoxifen, lithium)
- Others (e.g., vitamin A intoxication, thyroid hormone use, parenteral nutrition)

Chronic renal failure
Other endocrine conditions
- Hyperthyroidism (in 20–40% of patients; usually <14 mg/dL)
- Hypothyroidism in some patients, Cushing's syndrome, adrenal insufficiency acromegaly, pheochromocytoma, vasoactive intestinal polypeptide hormone–producing tumor
- Multiple endocrine neoplasia (MEN) syndrome

Granulomatous disease (1,25-dihydroxyvitamin D excess) (e.g., sarcoidosis, TB, leprosy, mycoses, berylliosis, silicone granulomas)
Acute osteoporosis (e.g., immobilization of young patients or in Paget's disease)
Polyuric phase of acute renal failure
Miscellaneous
- Familial hypocalciuric hypercalcemia
- Rhabdomyolysis causing acute renal failure
- Porphyria
- Dehydration with hyperproteinemia
- Hypophosphatasia
- Idiopathic hypercalcemia of infancy

Decreased In

Hypoparathyroidism
- Surgical
- Idiopathic
- Infiltration of parathyroids (e.g., sarcoidosis, amyloidosis, hemochromatosis, tumor)
- Congenital (DiGeorge syndrome)

Pseudohypoparathyroidism
Malabsorption of calcium and vitamin D
Obstructive jaundice
Chronic renal disease with uremia and phosphate retention; Fanconi's syndrome; renal tubular acidosis
Acute pancreatitis with extensive fat necrosis
Insufficient calcium, phosphorus, and vitamin D ingestion
- Bone disease (osteomalacia, rickets)
- Starvation
- Late pregnancy

Use of certain drugs
- Cancer chemotherapy drugs (e.g., cisplatin, mithramycin, cytosine arabinoside)
- Fluoride intoxication
- Antibiotics (e.g., gentamicin, pentamidine, ketoconazole)
- Chronic therapeutic use of anticonvulsant drugs (e.g., phenobarbital, phenytoin)
- Loop-active diuretics
- Calcitonin
- Multiple citrated blood transfusions

Neonates born of complicated pregnancies
- Hyperbilirubinemia
- Respiratory distress, asphyxia
- Cerebral injuries
- Infants of diabetic mothers
- Prematurity
- Maternal hypoparathyroidism

Hypomagnesemia
Malignant disease
Toxic shock syndrome

BLOOD ANALYT

Rhabdomyolysis

Tumor lysis syndrome

Temporary hypocalcemia after subtotal thyroidectomy in >40% of patients; >20% are symptomatic.

Concomitant hypokalemia is not infrequent in hypercalcemia. Concomitant dehydration is almost always present because hypercalcemia causes nephrogenic diabetes insipidus.

Chloride

Use

With sodium, potassium, and carbon dioxide to assess electrolyte, acid-base, and water balance. Usually changes in same direction as sodium except in metabolic acidosis with bicarbonate depletion and metabolic alkalosis with bicarbonate excess when serum sodium levels may be normal.

Interferences

Hyperlipidemia (artifactual change; see Sodium, p. 693)

Increased In

Metabolic acidosis associated with prolonged diarrhea with loss of $NaHCO_3$

Renal tubular diseases with decreased excretion of H^+ and decreased reabsorption of HCO_3^- ("hyperchloremic metabolic acidosis")

Respiratory alkalosis (e.g., hyperventilation, severe central nervous system [CNS] damage)

Drugs

    Excessive administration of certain drugs (e.g., NH_4Cl, IV saline, salicylate intoxication; acetazolamide therapy)

    False (methodological) increase due to bromides or other halogens

    Retention of salt and water (e.g., corticosteroids, guanethidine, phenylbutazone)

Some cases of hyperparathyroidism

Diabetes insipidus, dehydration

Sodium loss > chloride loss (e.g., diarrhea, intestinal fistulas)

Ureterosigmoidostomy

Decreased In

Prolonged vomiting or suction (loss of HCl)

Metabolic acidoses with accumulation of organic anions (see Anion Gap Classification, p. 331)

Chronic respiratory acidosis

Salt-losing renal diseases

Adrenocortical insufficiency

Primary aldosteronism

Expansion of extracellular fluid (e.g., SIADH, hyponatremia, water intoxication, congestive heart failure)

Burns

Drugs

    Alkalosis (e.g., bicarbonates, aldosterone, corticosteroids)

    Diuretic effect (e.g., ethacrynic acid, furosemide, thiazides)

    Other loss (e.g., chronic laxative abuse)

Cholesterol, High-Density Lipoprotein (HDL) Cholesterol, Low-Density Lipoprotein (LDL) Cholesterol, Triglycerides

See Disorders of Lipid Metabolism, see pp. 525.

Complement

Use

Evaluate role of complement in immune disorders.

Determine if deficiency is acquired or genetic.

Normal In

Renal diseases
- IgG-IgA nephropathy (Berger's disease)
- Idiopathic rapidly progressive GN
- Anti–glomerular basement membrane disease
- Immune-complex disease
- Negative immunofluorescence findings

Systemic diseases
- Polyarteritis nodosa
- Hypersensitivity vasculitis
- Wegener's granulomatosis
- Schönlein-Henoch purpura
- Goodpasture's syndrome
- Visceral abscess

Decreased In (Acquired)

Common diseases associated with **arthritis**
- Active SLE, particularly associated with renal disease
- Prodromal hepatitis B virus (HBV) hepatitis
- Essential mixed cryoglobulinemia
- Sjögren's syndrome
- Serum sickness
- Short bowel syndrome

Common diseases associated with **vasculitis**
- Rheumatoid vasculitis
- Essential mixed cryoglobulinemia
- Sjögren's syndrome
- Hypocomplementemic vasculitis
- Wegener's granulomatosis

Common diseases associated with **nephritis**

	% of Cases in Which Occurs
Acute poststreptococcal GN	Transient (3–8 wks) decline in C3
Membranoproliferative GN	
Type I ("classic" membranopro-liferative GN)	50–80%
Type II ("dense deposit disease")	80–90%; C3 often remains depressed
SLE	
Focal	75%
Diffuse	90%
Subacute bacterial endocarditis (SBE)	90%
Cryoglobulinemia	85%
"Shunt" nephritis	90%
Serum sickness	
Atheromatous emboli	

Decreased In (Inherited)

	Deficient Complement
SLE	C1qINH, C1q, C1r, C1s, C2, C4, C5, C8
Hereditary angioedema	C1qINH
Familial Mediterranean fever	C5aINH
Urticarial vasculitis	C3
GN	C1r, C2
Severe combined immunodeficiency	C1q
X-linked hypogammaglobulinemia	C1q
Recurrent infections	C3, C3bINH
Recurrent neisserial infections	C5, C6, C7, C8

Increased In

Inflammatory conditions that increase acute-phase reactants

Use of Individual Complement Levels

CH50 detects activation of classic pathway; measures functional activity of C1 through C9; is useful for screening because a normal result indicates classic complement pathway is functionally intact. Decrease indicates 50–80% of normal amounts have been depleted. Detects all inborn and most acquired complement deficiencies.

AH50 measures only activity of alternative pathway.

C3 is useful for screening for activation of classic and alternate complement pathways. May be increased in subacute inflammation, biliary obstruction, nephrotic syndrome, corticosteroid therapy. May be decreased in immune complex disease (especially lupus nephritis), acute poststreptococcal GN, hypercatabolism (especially C3b inactivator deficiency), massive necrosis and tissue injury, sepsis, viremia, hereditary deficiency, infancy.

C3 or CH50 may be useful for monitoring disease activity in SLE but usefulness may vary from case to case.

C4 may be decreased in immune complex disease (especially lupus nephritis), hereditary angioneurotic edema, hereditary deficiency, acute GN, infancy, or when classic pathway is activated.

Decreased C3 and C4 indicate initiation of classic activation pathway and activation of functional unit (e.g., active viral hepatitis, immune complex formation).

Normal C3 with decreased C4 suggests C4 deficiency (e.g., hereditary angioedema, malaria, some SLE patients).

Normal C4 and decreased C3 suggests congenital C3 deficiency or deficiency of C3b inactivator, or activation of functional unit by alternate pathway (e.g., gram-negative toxemia).

Normal C3 and C4 with decreased C50 indicates isolated deficiency of another complement component and further testing is indicated.

C2 may be decreased in immune complex disease (especially lupus nephritis), hereditary angioedema, hereditary deficiency, infancy.

C1 esterase inhibitor deficiency is characteristic of hereditary angioedema. In heterozygote, C1 inhibitor is substantially decreased. Patients have low CH100, C4, and C2 during attacks.

C1q can be very low in acquired angioedema, severe combined immunodeficiency, and X-linked hypogammaglobulinemia. May be decreased in SLE, infancy.

Absence of or marked decrease in any of the components of complement will cause absence of or marked decrease in the total hemolytic complement assay, but mild to moderate decrease of an individual component may not alter this total.

Deficiency of early classic pathway components (C1q, C1r, C1s, C2, C4)
- Serum shows absence of hemolytic complement activity.
- The affected component is absent or decreased on immunochemical testing.
- Opsonic activity and generation of chemotactic activity are defective.
- Infections are not a problem (because alternative pathway is intact).
- Symptoms due to collagen vascular disorders (e.g., nephritis, arthritis).

Deficiency of C3 and C5
- Serum shows absence of hemolytic complement activity.
- C3 or C5 is absent or decreased in serum.
- Defective opsonic capacity and chemotactic activity.
- Severe recurrent infections (e.g., pneumonia, sepsis, otitis media, chronic diarrhea).
- Often responds to fresh plasma.

Deficiency of late classic pathway components (C6, C7, C8)
- Serum shows absence of hemolytic complement activity.
- Normal opsonization and generation of chemotactic factor.
- Total absence of individual component.
- Recurrent systemic infection due to *Neisseria gonorrhoeae* or *Neisseria meningitidis*.

C-Reactive Protein (CRP)

(An acute-phase reactant; quantitative test is superior; normal value <8 mg/dL)

Use

Inflammatory disorders for monitoring course and effect of therapy:
- In any acute inflammatory change, CRP shows an earlier (begins in 4–6 hrs), more intense increase rise than ESR; with recovery, disappearance of CRP precedes the return to normal of ESR. CRP disappears when inflammatory process is sup-

pressed by steroids or salicylates. Generally parallels ESR but is not influenced by anemia, polycythemia, spherocytosis, macrocytosis, congestive heart failure, hypergammaglobulinemia in which ESR is increased.

Most useful as indicator of activity in a rheumatic disease (e.g., RA, rheumatic fever).

Infection:
- Indicate presence of infection (30–35 mg/dL in 80–85% of acute bacterial infections and <20 mg/dL in viral infections, but not useful to differentiate bacterial from viral infections).
- Normal value is useful to exclude infection.
- Monitor recovery from infection (spontaneous or due to therapy).
- Diagnose postoperative and intercurrent infection: After surgery, CRP begins to increase in 4–6 hrs to peak in 48–72 hrs (usually 25–35 mg/dL), begins to decrease after third day to normal by fifth to seventh day. Should have baseline preoperative value; serial pattern is different with complicating infection or tissue necrosis.

Leukemia: Fever, blast crisis, or cytotoxic drugs cause only modest elevation of CRP, but intercurrent infection stimulates significantly higher CRP levels and measurement is particularly useful to monitor response to antibiotic therapy. Not useful to differentiate graft-versus-host disease from infection after marrow transplant.

Increased In

Inflammatory disorders:
- RA, rheumatic fever, seronegative arthritides (e.g., Reiter's syndrome), vasculitis syndromes (e.g., hypersensitivity vasculitis).
- Inflammatory bowel disease: Significantly higher in Crohn's disease than in ulcerative colitis and corresponds to relapse, remission, and response to therapy in Crohn's disease.
- Chronic inflammatory diseases: Usually <8.0 mg/dL; if >10.0 mg/dL, superimposed infection should be ruled out.

Tissue injury or necrosis:
- AMI: CRP appears within 24–48 hrs, peaks at 72 hrs, and becomes negative after 7 days; correlates with peak CK-MB levels, but CRP peak occurs 1–3 days later. Failure of CRP to return to normal indicates tissue damage in heart or elsewhere. Absent CRP increase raises question of a significant infarct in prior 2–10 days. May be increased in unstable angina but not by angina in absence of tissue necrosis.
- Ischemia or infarction of other tissues.
- Rejection of kidney or marrow transplant but not of heart transplant.
- Malignant (but not benign) tumors, especially breast, lung, GI tract; >10 mg/dL in one-third of cases. May be a useful tumor marker because a high CRP is often present when CEA and other tumor markers are not increased.
- After surgery: CRP increases within 4–6 hrs to peak at 48–72 hrs (usually at 25–35 mg/dL). Begins to decrease after third postoperative day and returns to normal by fifth to seventh day; failure to fall is more sensitive indicator of complications (e.g., infection, pulmonary infarction) than WBC, ESR, temperature, pulse rate.
- Burns, trauma.

Infections:
- Highest levels are found in acute bacterial infections (>30 mg/dL) but <20 mg/dL in acute viral infections.
- Lower in viral compared to bacterial infection but may be very high in both. CSF CRP has been reported specific to differentiate bacterial from viral meningitis.
- Infections in various sites (e.g., newborns; GU, GI, and biliary tracts, pelvic inflammatory disease [PID], CNS) or due to other organisms (e.g., parasites, fungi).
  In premature rupture of membranes, CRP >12.5 mg/dL in cord blood strongly suggests chorioamnionitis.
  Increased CRP in seriously ill neonate is indication for immediate vigorous antibiotic therapy.
  In children younger than 6 yrs with meningitis, CRP >20 mg/dL after 12 hrs (50 mg/dL in older patients) suggests bacterial rather than viral cause.

Not Increased In

Autoimmune diseases (e.g., SLE, mixed connective tissue disease, dermatomyositis, scleroderma): Little or no increase unless infection is present.

BLOOD ANALYT

Pregnancy
Strenuous exercise
Angina
Cerebrovascular accident
Seizures
Asthma
Common cold
Rejection of heart transplant

Creatine

Use

Is rarely used clinically.

Increased In

High dietary intake (meat)
Destruction of muscle
Hyperthyroidism (this diagnosis almost excluded by normal serum creatine)
Active RA
Testosterone therapy

Decreased In

Not clinically significant
Drugs (e.g., TMP/SMX, cimetidine, cefoxitin)

Interferences

Artifactual decrease in diabetic ketoacidosis

Creatine Kinase (CK), Total

Use

Marker for injury or diseases of cardiac with good specificity (see pp. 516–529)
Measurement of choice for striated muscle disorders (see Chapter 10)

Increased In

Necrosis or inflammation of cardiac muscle (see p. 119)
  • Disorders listed under CK-MB (CK index usually >2.5%)
Necrosis, inflammation or acute atrophy of striated muscle (see Chapter 10)
  • Disorders listed under CK-MB (CK index usually <2.5%)
  • Muscular dystrophy (see p. 295)
  • Myotonic dystrophy (see p. 298)
  • Amyotrophic lateral sclerosis (>40% of cases)
  • Polymyositis (70% of cases; average 20× ULN) (see p. 301)
  • Thermal and electrical burns (values usually higher than in AMI)
  • Rhabdomyolysis (especially with trauma and severe exertion); marked increase
    may be 1000× ULN
  • Severe or prolonged exercise as in marathon running (begins 3 hrs after start of
    exercise; peaks after 8–16 hrs; usually normal by 48 hrs); smaller increases in well-
    conditioned athletes
  • Status epilepticus
  • Parturition and frequently the last few weeks of pregnancy
  • Malignant hyperthermia (see p. 299)
  • Hypothermia
  • Familial hypokalemic periodic paralysis
  • McArdle's disease (see p. 546)
Drugs and chemicals
  • Cocaine
  • Alcohol
  • Emetine (ipecac) (e.g., bulimia)

- Toxic chemicals (benzene ring compounds [e.g., xylene] depolarize surface membrane and leach out low-molecular-weight enzymes, producing very high levels of total CK [100% MM] with increased LD 3–5× normal)

Half of patients with extensive brain infarction. Maximum levels in 3 days; increase may not appear before 2 days; levels usually less than in AMI and remain increased for longer time; return to normal within 14 days; high mortality associated with levels >300 IU. Elevated serum CK in brain infarction may obscure diagnosis of concomitant AMI.

Some persons with large muscle mass (≤ 2× normal) (e.g., football players)

Slight Increase Occasionally In

IM injections. Variable increase after IM injection to 2–6× normal level. Returns to normal 48 hrs after cessation of injections. Rarely affects CK-MB, LD-1, AST.

Muscle spasms or convulsions in children
Moderate hemolysis

Normal In

Pulmonary infarction
Renal infarction
Liver disease
Biliary obstruction
Some muscle disorders
- Thyrotoxicosis myopathy
- Steroid myopathy
- Muscle atrophy of neurologic origin (e.g., old poliomyelitis, polyneuritis)

PA
Most malignancies
Scleroderma
Acrosclerosis
Discoid lupus erythematosus

Decreased In

Decreased muscle mass (e.g., old age, malnutrition, alcoholism)
RA (approximately two-thirds of patients)
Untreated hyperthyroidism
Cushing's disease
Connective tissue disease not associated with decreased physical activity
Pregnancy level (8th to 12th wk) is said to be ~75% of nonpregnancy level
Various drugs (e.g., phenothiazine, prednisone, estrogens, tamoxifen, ethanol), toxins, and insecticides (e.g., aldrin, dieldrin)
Metastatic tumor in liver
Multiple organ failure
Intensive care unit patients with severe infection or septicemia

Creatine Kinase (CK) Isoenzymes

Use

CK-MB is the most widely used early marker for myocardial injury (see p. 121).

CK-MB Increased In

Necrosis of cardiac muscle (*CK index >2.5%; in all other causes, CK index usually <2.5%*)
- AMI (see p. 121).
- Cardiac contusion.
- After thoracic/open heart surgery, values return to baseline in 24–48 hrs. AMI is difficult to diagnose in first 24 postoperative hrs.
- Resuscitation for cardiac arrest may increase CK and CK-MB in ~50% of patients with peak at 24 hrs due to defibrillation (>400 J) and chest compression but CK-MB/CK total ratio may not be increased even with AMI.
- Percutaneous transluminal coronary angioplasty.

- Myocarditis.
- Prolonged supraventricular tachycardia.
- Cardiomyopathies (e.g., hypothyroid, alcohol).
- Collagen diseases involving the myocardium.
- Coronary angiography (transient).

Necrosis, inflammation, or acute atrophy of striated muscle (see p. 295)
- Exercise myopathy; slight to significant increases in 14–100% of persons after extreme exercise (e.g., marathons); smaller increases in well-conditioned athletes
- Skeletal muscle trauma with rhabdomyolysis, myoglobinuria
- Skeletal muscle diseases (e.g., myositis, muscular dystrophies, polymyositis, collagen vascular diseases [especially SLE])
- Familial hypokalemic periodic paralysis
- Electrical and thermal burns and trauma (~50% of patients; but not supported by LD-1 > LD-2)
- Drugs (e.g., alcohol, cocaine, halothane [malignant hyperthermia], ipecac)

Endocrine disorders (e.g., hypoparathyroidism, acromegaly, diabetic ketoacidosis; hypothyroidism—total CK 4–8× ULN in 60–80% of cases; becomes normal within 6 wks of initiating replacement therapy)

Some infections
- Viral (e.g., HIV, Epstein-Barr virus [EBV], influenza, picornaviruses, coxsackievirus, echoviruses, adenoviruses)
- Bacterial (e.g., *Staphylococcus, Streptococcus, Clostridium, Borrelia*)
- Rocky Mountain spotted fever
- Fungal
- Parasitic (e.g., trichinosis, toxoplasmosis, schistosomiasis, cysticercosis)

Other conditions
- Malignant hyperthermia; hypothermia
- Reye's syndrome
- Peripartum period for first day beginning within 30 mins
- Acute cholecystitis
- Hyperthyroidism and chronic renal failure may cause persistent increase, although the proportion of CK-MB remains low
- Acute exacerbation of obstructive lung disease
- Drugs (e.g., aspirin, tranquilizers)
- Carbon monoxide poisoning

Some neoplasms (see Tumor Markers, p. 901)
- For example, prostate, breast.
- Increase in 90% of patients after cryotherapy for prostate carcinoma with peak at 16 hrs to ~5× upper limit of normal value; similar increase in total CK.

% Activity Distribution of CK Isoenzymes in Tissue		
CK-MM	**CK-MB**	**CK-BB**
Skeletal muscle	99	1	0
Myocardium	77	22	1
Brain	4	0	96

CK-MB >15–20% should raise the possibility of an atypical macro CK-MB.

CK-MB Not Increased In

Angina pectoris, coronary insufficiency, exercise testing for coronary artery disease, or pericarditis; an increase implies some necrosis of cardiac muscle even if a discrete infarct is not identified.

After cardiopulmonary bypass, cardiac catheterization (including Swan-Ganz), cardiac pacemaker implantation, and coronary arteriography unless myocardium has been injured by catheter

IM injections (total CK may be slightly increased)

Seizures (total CK may be markedly increased)

Brain infarction or injury (total CK may be increased)

CK-BB Isoenzyme

Use

Is rarely encountered clinically.

CK-BB May Be Increased In

Malignant hyperthermia, uremia, brain infarction or anoxia, Reye's syndrome, necrosis of intestine, various metastatic neoplasms (especially prostate), biliary atresia

Atypical Macro Isoenzyme

(High-molecular-mass complex of a CK isoenzyme and immunoglobulin, most often CK-BB and monoclonal IgG and a kappa light chain)
May cause falsely high or low CK-MB results (depending on type of assay), resulting in an incorrect diagnosis of myocardial infarction or delayed recognition of a real myocardial infarction.
Discovered in <2% of all CK isoenzyme electrophoresis studies.

	Type 1	Type 2
Electrophoretic location	Between CK-MM and CK-MB	Cathode side of CK-MM
Prevalence (%)	0.43	1.30
Associated disorders	Myositis	Malignancy
	Autoimmune disease	

Creatinine

Use

Diagnosis of renal insufficiency. *Serum creatinine is a more specific and sensitive indicator of renal disease than BUN. Use of simultaneous BUN and creatinine determinations provides more information in conditions listed in next section.*

Increased In

Diet
  • Ingestion of creatinine (roast meat)
Muscle disease
  • Gigantism
  • Acromegaly
Prerenal azotemia (see BUN, p. 44)
Postrenal azotemia (see BUN, p. 44)
Impaired kidney function; 50% loss of renal function is needed to increase serum creatinine from 1.0 to 2.0 mg/dL; therefore not sensitive to mild to moderate renal injury.

Decreased In

Pregnancy—normal value is 0.4–0.6 mg/dL. *>0.8 mg/dL is abnormal and should alert clinician to further diagnostic evaluation.*

Interferences

(Depending on methodology)
Artifactual decrease by
  • Marked increase of serum bilirubin
  • Enzymatic reaction (glucose >100 mg/dL)
Artifactual increase due to
  • Reducing alkaline picrate (e.g., glucose, ascorbate, uric acid). *Ketoacidosis may substantially increase serum creatinine results with alkaline picrate reaction.*
  • Formation of colored complexes (e.g., acetoacetate, pyruvate, other ketoacids, certain cephalosporins).
  • Enzymatic reaction (flucytosine [5-fluorocytosine] may increase serum creatinine ≤ 0.6 mg/dL).
  • Other methodologic interference (e.g., ascorbic acid, PSP, L-dopa, para-aminohippurate).

Erythrocyte Sedimentation Rate (ESR)

See Table 3-1.

BLOOD ANALYT

Table 3-1. Changes in Erythrocyte Sedimentation Rate

Disease	Increased In	Not Increased In
Infectious	Tuberculosis (especially) Acute hepatitis Many bacterial infections	Typhoid fever Undulant fever Malarial paroxysm Infectious mononucleosis Uncomplicated viral diseases
Cardiac	Acute myocardial infraction Active rheumatic fever After open heart surgery	Angina pectoris Active renal failure with heart failure
Abdominal	Acute pelvic inflammatory disease Ruptured ectopic pregnancy Pregnancy—third month to ~3 wks postpartum Menstruation	Acute appendicitis (first 24 hrs) Unruptured ectopic pregnancy Early pregnancy
Joint	Rheumatoid arthritis Pyogenic arthritis	Degenerative arthritis

Miscellaneous	Significant tissue necrosis, especially
	  neoplasms (most frequently malig-
	  nant lymphoma, cancer of colon
	  and breast)
	Increased serum globulins (e.g., mye-
	  loma, cryoglobulinemia, macro-
	  globulinuria)
	Decreased serum albumin
	Hypothyroidism
	Hyperthyroidism
	Acute hemorrhage
	Nephrosis, renal disease with azotemia
	Arsenic and lead intoxification
	Dextran and polyvinyl compounds
	  in blood
	Temporal arteritis
	Polymyalgia rheumatica
		Peptic ulcer
		Acute allergy

Use

○*Indicates presence and intensity of an inflammatory process; never diagnostic of a specific disease. Changes are more significant than a single abnormal occurrence.*

Detect occult disease (e.g., screening program), but a normal ESR does not exclude malignancy or other serious disease.

Monitor the course of or response to treatment of certain diseases (e.g., temporal arteritis, polymyalgia rheumatica, acute rheumatic fever, RA, SLE, Hodgkin's disease, TB, bacterial endocarditis). *ESR is normal in 5% of patients with RA or SLE.*

♦Confirm or exclude a diagnosis (a normal ESR virtually excludes diagnosis of temporal arteritis or polymyalgia rheumatica; >50 mm/hr in 90% of these patients).

Rarely may assist in differential diagnosis (e.g., acute myocardial infarction versus angina pectoris; early acute appendicitis versus ruptured ectopic pregnancy or acute pelvic inflammatory disease; RA versus osteoarthritis; acute versus quiescent gout).

ESR is said to be useful to differentiate iron deficiency anemia (ESR normal) from anemia of acute or chronic disease alone or combined with iron deficiency, in which ESR is almost always increased.

Rarely (6 in 10,000) useful for screening of asymptomatic persons after history and physical examination. Unexplained increase with no detectable disease occurs in <3% of cases.

○*Hyperviscosity syndrome should be suspected in patients with hyperproteinemia (e.g., multiple myeloma, Waldenström's macroglobulinemia) with rouleaux formation but no increase of ESR.*

○Extreme elevation of ESR is found particularly in association with malignancy (most frequently malignant lymphoma, carcinomas of colon and breast), hematologic diseases (most frequently myeloma), collagen diseases (e.g., RA, SLE), renal diseases (especially with azotemia), drug fever, and other conditions (e.g., cirrhosis). In patients with cancer, ESR >100 mm/hr indicates metastases. Other causes of ESR >100 mm/hr are severe infections (osteomyelitis, SBE), giant cell arteritis, polymyalgia rheumatica, renal diseases.

Interferences That Increase ESR

Macrocytosis
Hypercholesterolemia
Increased fibrinogen, gamma or beta globulins
Technical factors (e.g., tilted ESR tube, high room temperature)
Drugs (e.g., dextran, methyldopa, methysergide, penicillamine, theophylline, trifluperidol, vitamin A)

Interferences That Decrease ESR

Polycythemia, vera or secondary
Abnormal RBCs, especially sickle cells; hereditary spherocytosis; acanthocytosis
Microcytosis (e.g., HbC disease)
Hypofibrinogenemia (e.g., DIC, massive hepatic necrosis)
High WBC count
Technical factors (e.g., short ESR tube, low room temperature, delay in test performance >2 hrs, clotted blood sample, excess anticoagulation)
Drugs (e.g., quinine [therapeutic], salicylates [therapeutic], drugs that cause a high glucose level, high doses of adrenal steroids)

Increased In

Chronic inflammatory diseases, especially collagen and vascular diseases
Postoperative (may be increased for up to 1 mo), postpartum

Decreased In

Congestive heart failure
Cachexia
High doses of adrenal steroids

Factors That Do Not Affect ESR

Body temperature
Recent meal
Aspirin
Nonsteroidal anti-inflammatory drugs
Formula for normal range Westergren ESR:

$$\text{Men:} \quad ESR = \frac{age\ (yrs)}{2}$$

$$\text{Women:} \quad ESR = \frac{[age\ (yrs) + 10]}{2}$$

5'-Nucleotidase (5'-N)

Use

Is rarely used.
May aid in differential diagnosis of hepatobiliary disease during pregnancy.

Increased Only In

Obstructive type os hepatobiliary disease.
May be an early indication of liver metastases in the cancer patient, especially if jaundice is absent.

Normal In

Pregnancy and postpartum period (in contrast to serum LAP and ALP).

BLOOD ANALYT

Gamma-Glutamyl Transferase (GGT)

Use

In liver disease, generally parallels changes in serum ALP.
Sensitive indicator of occult alcoholism
Diagnosis of liver disease in presence of bone disease or pregnancy, or in childhood;
serum ALP and LAP increased but not GGT.

Increased In

Liver disease—generally parallels changes in serum ALP, LAP, and 5'-nucleotidase but
is more sensitive.
* Acute hepatitis. Elevation is less marked than that of other liver enzymes, but it
is the last to return to normal and therefore is useful to indicate recovery.
* Chronic active hepatitis. Increased (average >7× ULN) more than in acute hepatitis.
More elevated than AST and ALT. In dormant stage, may be the only enzyme elevated.
* In alcoholic hepatitis, average increase is >3.5× ULN.
* Cirrhosis. In inactive cases, average values are lower (4× ULN) than in chronic
hepatitis. Increase >10–20 times in cirrhotic patients suggests superimposed pri-
mary carcinoma of the liver (average increase >21× ULN).
* Primary biliary cirrhosis. Elevation is marked: average >13× ULN.
* Fatty liver. Elevation parallels that of AST and ALT but is greater.
* Obstructive jaundice. Increase is faster and greater than that of serum ALP and
LAP. Average increase >5× ULN.
* Liver metastases. Parallels ALP; elevation precedes positive liver scans. Average
increase >14× ULN.
* Cholestasis. In mechanical and viral cholestasis, GGT and LAP are about equally
increased, but in drug-induced cholestasis, GGT is much more increased than LAP.
Average increase >6× ULN.
* Children. Much more increased in biliary atresia than in neonatal hepatitis (300
U/L is useful differentiating level). Children with alpha$_1$-antitrypsin deficiency
have higher levels than other patients with biliary atresia.
Pancreatitis: Always elevated in acute pancreatitis. In chronic pancreatitis is increased
when involvement of the biliary tract or active inflammation is present.
Acute myocardial infarction. Increased in 50% of patients. Elevation begins on fourth
to fifth day, reaches maximum at 8–12 days. With shock or acute right heart failure,
may have early peak within 48 hrs, with rapid decline followed by later rise.
Heavy use of alcohol: *Is the most sensitive indicator and a good screening test for alcoholism*, because elevation exceeds that of other commonly assayed liver enzymes.
Various drugs (e.g., barbiturates, phenytoin, tricyclic antidepressants, acetaminophen)
Some cases of carcinoma of prostate
Neoplasms, even in absence of liver metastases; especially malignant melanoma, car-
cinoma of breast and lung; highest levels in hypernephroma
Other conditions (e.g., gross obesity [slight increase], renal disease, cardiac disease,
postoperative state)

Normal In

Pregnancy (in contrast to serum ALP, LAP) and children older than 3 mos; therefore may
aid in differential diagnosis of hepatobiliary disease occurring during pregnancy and
childhood.
Patients with bone disease or with increased bone growth (children and adolescents);
therefore useful in distinguishing bone disease from liver disease as a cause of
increased serum ALP.
Renal failure
Strenuous exercise

Glucose

Use

Diagnosis of diabetes mellitus (defined by World Health Organization as unequivocal
increase of fasting serum [or plasma] glucose ≥ 126 mg/dL on more than one occasion or any glucose level ≥ 200 mg/dL)

Control of diabetes mellitus
Diagnosis of hypoglycemia

May Be Increased In

Diabetes mellitus, including
- Hemochromatosis
- Cushing's syndrome (with insulin-resistant diabetes)
- Acromegaly and gigantism (with insulin-resistant diabetes in early stages; hypopituitarism later)

Increased circulating epinephrine
- Adrenalin injection
- Pheochromocytoma
- Stress (e.g., emotion, burns, shock, anesthesia)

Acute pancreatitis
Chronic pancreatitis (some patients)
Wernicke's encephalopathy (vitamin B_1 deficiency)
Some CNS lesions (subarachnoid hemorrhage, convulsive states)
Effect of drugs (e.g., corticosteroids, estrogens, alcohol, phenytoin, thiazides, propranolol, vitamin A [chronic hypervitaminosis])

May Be Decreased In

Pancreatic disorders
- Islet cell tumor, hyperplasia
- Pancreatitis
- Glucagon deficiency

Extrapancreatic tumors
- Carcinoma of adrenal gland
- Carcinoma of stomach
- Fibrosarcoma
- Other

Hepatic disease
- Diffuse severe disease (e.g., poisoning, hepatitis, cirrhosis, primary or metastatic tumor)

Endocrine disorders
- Hypopituitarism*
- Addison's disease
- Hypothyroidism
- Adrenal medulla unresponsiveness
- Early diabetes mellitus

Functional disturbances
- Postgastrectomy
- Gastroenterostomy
- Autonomic nervous system disorders

Pediatric anomalies
- Prematurity*
- Infant of diabetic mother*
- Ketotic hypoglycemia
- Zetterstrom's syndrome
- Idiopathic leucine sensitivity
- Spontaneous hypoglycemia in infants

Enzyme diseases
- von Gierke's disease*
- Galactosemia*
- Fructose intolerance*
- Amino acid and organic acid defects*
  Methylmalonic acidemia*
  Glutaric acidemia, type II*
  Maple syrup urine disease*
  3-hydroxy, 3-methyl glutaric acidemia*
- Fatty acid metabolism defects*
  Acyl coenzyme A dehydrogenase defects*
  Carnitine deficiencies*

BLOOD ANALYT

Other
- Exogenous insulin (factitious)
- Oral hypoglycemic medications (factitious)
- Leucine sensitivity
- Malnutrition
- Hypothalamic lesions
- Alcoholism

*May cause neonatal hypoglycemia.

Interferences

Blood samples in which serum is not separated from blood cells will show glucose values decreasing at rate of 3–5%/hr at room temperature.

Most glucose strips and meters quantify whole blood glucose, whereas most laboratories use plasma or serum, which reads 10–15% higher.

Postprandial capillary glucose is ≤ 36 mg/dL higher than venous glucose at peak of 1 hr postprandial; usually returns to negligible difference with fasting level within 4 hrs but in ~15% of patients may still be >20 mg/dL difference.

Considerable imprecision is found between glucose meters from the same manufacturer and between different types of meters.

Only fresh capillary blood should be used with some reflectance meters; low oxygen content (e.g., venous blood, altitudes >3000 m) gives falsely increased values.

Reflectance meter value of ~160 mg/dL on capillary blood corresponds to venous plasma level of ~135 mg/dL in most cases.

Whole blood glucose value multiplied by 0.94 = plasma concentration.

Immunoglobulin A (IgA)

Increased In (in relation to other immunoglobulins)
Gamma-A myeloma (M component)
Cirrhosis of liver
Chronic infections
RA with high titers of RF
SLE (some patients)
Sarcoidosis (some patients)
Wiskott-Aldrich syndrome
Other

Decreased In (Alone)

Healthy persons (1 in 700)
Hereditary telangiectasia (80% of patients)
Type III dysgammaglobulinemia
Malabsorption (some patients)
SLE (occasionally)
Cirrhosis of liver (occasionally)
Still's disease (occasionally)
Recurrent otitis media (occasionally)
Non-IgA myeloma
Waldenström's macroglobulinemia
Acquired immunodeficiency

Decreased In (Combined with Other Immunoglobulin Decreases)

Agammaglobulinemia

- Acquired
   Primary
   Secondary (e.g., multiple myeloma, leukemia, nephrotic syndrome, protein-losing enteropathy)
- Congenital

Hereditary thymic aplasia
Type I dysgammaglobulinemia (decreased IgG and IgA and increased IgM)

Type II dysgammaglobulinemia (absent IgA and IgM and normal levels of IgG)
Infancy, early childhood

Immunoglobulin D (IgD)

Use

Diagnosis of rare IgD myelomas (greatly increased)

Increased In

Chronic infection (moderately)
Autoimmune disease

Decreased In

Hereditary deficiencies
Acquired immunodeficiency
Non-IgD myeloma
Infancy, early childhood

Immunoglobulin E (IgE)

Use

Diagnosis of E-myeloma
Indicates various parasitic or allergic diseases.
A normal serum IgE level excludes the diagnosis of bronchopulmonary aspergillosis.

Increased In

Atopic diseases
  • Exogenous asthma in ~60% of patients
  • Hay fever in ~30% of patients
  • Atopic eczema
      Influenced by type of allergen, duration of stimulation, presence of symptoms, hyposensitization treatment.
Parasitic diseases (e.g., ascariasis, visceral larva migrans, hookworm disease, schistosomiasis, *Echinococcus* infection)

Normal or Low In

Asthma

Decreased In

Hereditary deficiencies
Acquired immunodeficiency
Ataxia-telangiectasia
Non-IgE myeloma

Immunoglobulin G (IgG)

Use

Diagnosis of IgG myeloma
Diagnosis of hereditary and acquired IgG immunodeficiencies

Increased In

Sarcoidosis
Chronic liver disease (e.g., cirrhosis)
Autoimmune diseases
Parasitic diseases
Chronic infection

Decreased In

Protein-losing syndromes
Pregnancy

Non-IgG myeloma
Waldenström's macroglobulinemia

Immunoglobulin M (IgM)

Use

Diagnosis of hereditary and acquired IgM immunodeficiencies
Diagnosis of Waldenström's macroglobulinemia

Increased In

Liver disease
Chronic infections

Decreased In

Protein-losing syndromes
Non-IgM myeloma
Infancy, early childhood

Immunologic Tests

See Table 3-2.

Inflammatory Reactants, Acute

Acute-phase reactants in serum (except CRP) are not used to detect inflammation, but
recognizing this cause of increase is important when they are used in testing for other
conditions (e.g., ceruloplasmin).
- CRP (see p. 50) can increase up to 1000% in severe tissue injury.
- Fibrinogen usually increases by 200–400%.
- Alpha$_1$-antitrypsin increases by 200–400%.
- Haptoglobin increases by 200–400%.
- Ferritin usually increases by 50%.
- Ceruloplasmin.
- Alpha$_1$-acid glycoprotein.

Serum complement (see pp. 48–50) usually increases by 50%.
Total WBC, neutrophils, and bands
ESR (see pp. 55–57)

Lactate Dehydrogenase (LD)

Use

Replaced by cardiac troponins as late marker for AMI.
May be a useful marker of disease activity in cryptogenic fibrosing alveolitis and extrin-
sic allergic alveolitis.
Marker for hemolysis, in vivo (e.g., hemolytic anemias) or in vitro (artifactual)
LD is a very nonspecific test.

Interferences

Artifactual hemolysis (e.g., poor venipuncture, failure to separate clot from serum, heating of blood)

Increased In

Cardiac diseases
- AMI (see p. 121).
- AMI with congestive heart failure. May show increase of LD-1 and LD-5.
- Congestive heart failure alone. LD isoenzymes are normal or LD-5 is increased
due to liver congestion.
- Coronary insufficiency may show mild elevation; flipped LD is less likely.

Table 3-2. Immunologic Tests

Antibody Test	Interpretation
Anti–acetylcholine receptor	Result <1 U makes the diagnosis of myasthenia gravis. May be negative in ocular myasthenia, Eaton-Lambert syndrome, and treated or inactive generalized myasthenia gravis.
Antistriational	Found in >80% of cases of myasthenia gravis with thymoma; ≤ 25% of cases of thymoma without myasthenia gravis; 30% of patients with myasthenia gravis alone. In 25% of drug reactions due to penicillamine.
Antiadrenal	High titers are characteristic of autoimmune hypoadrenalism (70%); rarely found in Addison's disease due to tuberculosis.
Anti–glomerular basement membrane	See Rapidly Progressive Nonstreptococcal GN, Chapter 14.
Anti-intrinsic factor	Antibodies indicate overt or latent pernicious anemia; present in ~75% of cases.
Parietal cell antibodies	See Chapter 11.
Antimitochondrial	Strongly positive in >90% of patients with primary biliary cirrhosis but almost never in extrahepatic biliary obstruction; therefore are useful in differentiating these two conditions. May also be found in 5% of chronic hepatitis cases.
Antireticulin	Presence supports the diagnosis of gluten-sensitive enteropathy. Especially useful in childhood, in which positive in 80% of cases.
Anti-skin, interepithelial	Positive test confirms diagnosis of pemphigus and is helpful in evaluating bullous disease. Positive in >90% of pemphigus cases; absence largely excludes that diagnosis. Rise and fall of titer may indicate impending relapse or effective control of disease. High sensitivity; lower specificity.
Anti-skin, dermal-epidermal	Positive in >80% of bullous pemphigus cases. Absence does not exclude that diagnosis. Some correlation of titer and severity. Low sensitivity; high specificity.
Anti–smooth muscle (antiactin)	Titer ≥ 1:160 in 95% of patients with autoimmune chronic active hepatitis. Less often in other liver and viral diseases.
Antithyroglobulin and antithyroid microsome antibodies	Absence of both antibodies is strong evidence against autoimmune thyroiditis (see Chapter 13).
Thyroid-stimulating immunoglobulin (TSI)	Elevated TSI occurs only in Graves' disease (see p. 585). Failure of TSI to fall after antithyroid therapy predicts relapse. Elevated TSI in a patient who is HLA-DR3 positive predicts poor response to antithyroid therapy and suggests need for alternate mode of treatment.
Rheumatoid factor	See Rheumatoid Arthritis, Chapter 10, and Table 10-7.
Neutrophil antibodies	
Cytoplasmic (c-ANCA)	Wegener's granulomatosis
Perinuclear (p-ANCA)	Vasculitis, Churg-Strauss syndrome, microscopic polyarteritis nodosa, ulcerative colitis

ANCA = antineutrophil cytoplasmic antibodies.
Source: Peter JP. *The use and interpretation of tests in clinical immunology,* 8th ed. Santa Monica, CA: Clinical Immunology Laboratories, 1991.

BLOOD ANALYT

- Insertion of intracardiac prosthetic valves consistently causes chronic hemolysis with increase of total LD and of LD-1 and LD-2. This is also often present before surgery in patients with severe hemodynamic abnormalities of cardiac valves.
- Cardiovascular surgery. LD is increased to ≤ 2 times normal without cardiopulmonary bypass and returns to normal in 3–4 days; with extracorporeal circulation, it may increase to ≤ 4–6 times normal; increase is more marked when transfused blood is older.
- Increases have been described in acute myocarditis and rheumatic fever.

Liver diseases
- Cirrhosis, obstructive jaundice, acute viral hepatitis show moderate increases.
- Hepatitis. Most marked increase is of LD-5, which occurs during prodromal stage and is greatest at time of onset of jaundice; total LD is also increased in 50% of the cases. LD increase is isomorphic in infectious mononucleosis ALT/LD or AST/LD ratio ≥ 1.5 within 24 hrs of admission favors acute hepatitis over acetaminophen or ischemic injury.
- Acute and subacute hepatic necrosis. LD-5 is also increased with other causes of liver damage (e.g., chlorpromazine hepatitis, carbon tetrachloride poisoning, exacerbation of cirrhosis, biliary obstruction) even when total LD is normal.
- Metastatic carcinoma to liver may show marked increases. LD-4/LD-5 ratio <1.05 has been reported to favor diagnosis of hepatocellular carcinoma, whereas ratio >1.05 favors liver metastases in >90% of cases.[2]
- *If liver disease is suspected but total LD is very high and isoenzyme pattern is isomorphic, rule out cancer.*
- Liver disease, per se, does not produce marked increase of total LD or LD-5.
- Various inborn metabolic disorders affecting liver (e.g., hemochromatosis, Dubin-Johnson syndrome, hepatolenticular degeneration, Gaucher's disease, McArdle's disease).

Hematologic diseases
- Untreated PA and folic acid deficiency show some of the greatest increases, chiefly in LD-1, which is >LD-2 (flipped), especially with Hb <8 gm/dL.
- Increased in all hemolytic anemias, which can probably be ruled out if LD-1 and LD-2 are not increased in an anemic patient. Normal in aplastic anemia and iron-deficiency anemia, even when anemia is very severe.

Diseases of lung
- Pulmonary embolus and infarction—*pattern of moderately increased LD with increased LD-3 and normal AST 24–48 hrs after onset of chest pain* (see Lactate Dehydrogenase Isoenzymes section).
- Sarcoidosis.

Malignant tumors
- Increased in ~50% of patients with various solid carcinomas, especially in advanced stages.
- In patients with cancer, a higher LD level generally indicates a poorer prognosis. Whenever the total LD is increased and the isoenzyme pattern is nonspecific or cannot be explained by obvious clinical findings (e.g., myocardial infarction, hemolytic anemia), cancer should always be ruled out. Moderately increased in ~60% of patients with lymphomas and lymphocytic leukemias and ~90% of patients with acute leukemia; degree of increase is not correlated with level of WBC; relatively low levels in lymphatic type of leukemia. Increased in 95% of patients with chronic myelogenous leukemia, especially LD-3. (See also Chapter 11, Hematologic Diseases.)

Diseases of muscle (see p. 295)
- Marked increase of LD-5 is likely due to anoxic injury of striated muscle.
- Electrical and thermal burns and trauma. Marked increase of total LD (about the same as in myocardial infarction) and LD-5.

Renal diseases
- Renal cortical infarction may mimic pattern of AMI. *Rule out renal infarction if LD-1 (>LD-2) is increased in the absence of AMI or anemia; increased LD is out of proportion to AST and ALP levels.*
- May be slightly increased (LD-4 and LD-5) in nephrotic syndrome. LD-1 and LD-2 may be increased in nephritis.

Miscellaneous conditions (may be related to hemolysis, involvement of liver, striated muscle, heart, etc.)

[2]Castaldo G, et al. Serum LD isoenzyme 4/5 ratio discriminates between hepatocellular and secondary liver neoplasms. *Clin Chem* 1991;37:1419.

- Various infectious and parasitic diseases
- Hypothyroidism, subacute thyroiditis
- Collagen vascular diseases
- Acute pancreatitis
- Intestinal obstruction
- Sarcoidosis
- Various CNS conditions (e.g., bacterial meningitis, cerebral hemorrhage or thrombosis)
- Drugs

Decreased In

X-ray irradiation

Lactate Dehydrogenase Isoenzymes

	% Activity Distribution of LD Isoenzymes in Tissue				
	LD-1	**LD-2**	**LD-3**	**LD-4**	**LD-5**
Heart	60	30	5	3	2
Liver	0.2	0.8	1	4	94
Kidney	28	34	21	11	6
Cerebrum	28	32	19	16	5
Skeletal muscle	3	4	8	9	76
Lung	10	18	28	23	21
Spleen	5	15	31	31	18
RBCs	40	30	15	10	5
Skin	0	0	4	17	79

Use

To delineate tissue source of elevated serum total LD.
Interpretation of this test must be correlated with clinical status of the patient. Do serial determinations to obtain maximum information.

Condition	LD Isoenzyme Increased
AMI	LD-1 > LD-2
Acute renal cortical infarction	LD-1 > LD-2
PA	LD-1
Sickle cell crisis	LD-1 and LD-2
Electrical and thermal burn, trauma	LD-5
Mother carrying erythroblastotic child	LD-4 and LD-5
AMI with acute congestion of liver	LD-1 and LD-5
Early hepatitis	LD-5 (may become normal even when ALT is still rising)
Malignant lymphoma	LD-3 and LD-4 (may even increase LD-2) (reflects effect of chemo-therapy)
Active chronic granulocytic leukemia	LD-3 increased in >90% of cases but normal during remission
Carcinoma of prostate	LD-5; LD-5:LD-1 ratio >1
Dermatomyositis	LD-5
SLE	LD-3 and LD-4
Collagen disorders	LD-2, LD-3, and LD-4
Pulmonary embolus and infarction	LD-2, LD-3, and LD-4
Pulmonary embolus with acute cor pulmonale causing acute congestion of liver	LD-3 and LD-5
Congestive heart failure	LD-2, LD-3, and LD-4
Viral infections	LD-2, LD-3, and LD-4
Various neoplasms	LD-2, LD-3, and LD-4
Strenuous physical activity	LD-4 and LD-5
CNS malignant neoplasms	LD-5

Abnormally migrating macroenzymes (circulating complexes of LD with IgA or IgG immunoglobulins) may be found in some autoimmune conditions, cancer, and some miscellaneous conditions but not useful for diagnosis.

Increased total LD with normal distribution of isoenzymes may be seen in AMI, arteriosclerotic heart disease with chronic heart failure, and various combinations of acute and chronic diseases (this may represent a general stress reaction).

Approximately 50% of patients with malignant tumors have altered LD patterns. This change often is nonspecific and of no diagnostic value. Solid tumors, especially of germ cell origin, may increase LD-1.

In megaloblastic anemia, hemolysis, renal cortical infarction, and cancer in some patients the isoenzyme pattern may mimic that of AMI, but the time to peak value and the increase help to differentiate.

Leucine Aminopeptidase (LAP)

Use

Is rarely used.
Parallels serum ALP except that
- LAP is usually normal in the presence of bone disease or malabsorption syndrome.
- LAP is a more sensitive indicator of choledocholithiasis and of liver metastases in anicteric patients.

When serum LAP is increased, urine LAP is almost always increased; but when urine LAP is increased, serum LAP may have already returned to normal.

Magnesium (Mg)

Use

Diagnose and monitor hypo- and hypermagnesemia, especially in renal failure or GI disorders

Increased In

Iatrogenic (usual cause, most often with acute or chronic renal failure)
- Antacids containing magnesium
- Enemas containing magnesium
- Laxative and cathartic abuse
- Parenteral nutrition
- Magnesium for eclampsia or premature labor
- Lithium carbonate intoxication

Renal failure (when glomerular filtration rate [GFR] approaches 30 mL/min); in chronic renal failure, hypermagnesemia is inversely related to residual renal function. Increase is rarely observed with normal renal function.
Diabetic coma before treatment
Hypothyroidism
Addison's disease and after adrenalectomy
Controlled diabetes mellitus in older patients
Accidental ingestion of large amount of sea water

Signs	Approximate Serum Levels in Adults
Neuromuscular depression, hypotension	>4–6 mg/dL
Difficulty in urination	>5 mg/dL
CNS depression	6–8 mg/dL
Nausea, vomiting, cutaneous flushing	6 mg/dL
Hyporeflexia, drowsiness	8 mg/dL
Coma	12–17 mg/dL
ECG changes	>10 mg/dL
Complete heart block	30 mg/dL
Cardiac arrest	34–40 mg/dL

Decreased In

(Almost always due to GI or renal disturbance)
GI disease

- Malabsorption (e.g., sprue, small bowel resection, biliary and intestinal fistulas, abdominal irradiation, celiac disease and other causes of steatorrhea; familial magnesium malabsorption)
- Abnormal loss of GI fluids (chronic ulcerative colitis, Crohn's disease, villous adenoma, carcinoma of colon, laxative abuse, prolonged aspiration of GI tract contents, vomiting, etc.)

Renal disease (>2 mEq/day in urine during hypomagnesemia indicates excessive renal loss)
- Chronic GN
- Chronic pyelonephritis
- Renal tubular acidosis
- Diuretic phase of acute tubular necrosis
- Postobstructive diuresis
- Drug injury
    Diuretics (e.g., furosemide, thiazides, ethacrynic acid)
    Antibiotics (e.g., gentamicin, tobramycin, carbenicillin, ticarcillin, amphotericin B, aminoglycosides)
    Digitalis (in 20% of patients taking digitalis)
    Antineoplastic (e.g., cisplatin)
    Cyclosporine
- Tubular losses due to ions or nutrients
    Hypercalcemia
    Diuresis due to glucose, urea, or mannitol
    Phosphate depletion
    Extracellular fluid volume expansion
    Primary renal magnesium wasting

Nutritional
- Prolonged parenteral fluid administration without magnesium (usually >3 wks)
- Acute alcoholism and alcoholic cirrhosis
- Starvation with metabolic acidosis
- Kwashiorkor, protein-calorie malnutrition

Endocrine
- Hyperthyroidism
- Aldosteronism (primary and secondary)
- Hyperparathyroidism and other causes of hypercalcemia
- Hypoparathyroidism
- Diabetes mellitus (in 25–75% of patients)

Metabolic
- Excessive lactation
- Third trimester of pregnancy
- Insulin treatment of diabetic coma

Other
- Toxemia of pregnancy or eclampsia
- Lytic tumors of bone
- Active Paget's disease of bone due to increased uptake by bone
- Acute pancreatitis
- Transfusion of citrated blood
- Severe burns
- Sweating
- Sepsis
- Hypothermia

Magnesium deficiency frequently coexists with other electrolyte abnormalities. Magnesium deficiency may cause apparently unexplained hypocalcemia and hypokalemia; the patients may have neurologic and GI symptoms (see Calcium, Total, p. 46).

In ~90% of patients, high or low serum magnesium levels are not clinically recognized; therefore routine inclusion of magnesium with electrolyte measurements has been suggested.

Digitalis sensitivity and toxicity frequently occur with hypomagnesemia.

Ionized magnesium may be decreased despite increased or normal total magnesium.

Because deficiency can exist with normal or borderline serum magnesium levels, 24-hr urine testing may be indicated by frequent concomitant disorders.

24-hr urine level <25 mg suggests magnesium deficiency (in absence of conditions or agents that promote magnesium excretion). If due to renal loss, urine magnesium should be >3.65–6.00/day.

If <2.4 mg/day, collect 24-hr urine during IV of 72 mg of MgCl. 60–80% of load is excreted by patients with normal magnesium stores. <50% suggests nonrenal magnesium depletion.

Osmolality

Use

Diagnosis of nonketotic hyperglycemic coma
Monitoring of fluid and electrolyte balance
  • Determine serum water deviation from normal for evaluation of hyponatremia (see Causes of Hyponatremia, p. 693, Fig. 13-27).
  • *Urine and plasma osmolality are more useful to diagnose state of hydration than changes in Hct, serum proteins, and BUN, which are more dependent on other factors than hydration.*

Increased In

Hyperglycemia
Diabetic ketoacidosis. (*Osmolality should be determined routinely in grossly unbalanced diabetic patients.*)
Nonketotic hyperglycemic coma (see p. 617)
Hypernatremia with dehydration
  • Diarrhea, vomiting, fever, hyperventilation, inadequate water intake
  • Diabetes insipidus—central
  • Nephrogenic diabetes insipidus—congenital or acquired (e.g., hypercalcemia, hypokalemia, chronic renal disease, sickle cell disease, effect of some drugs)
  • Osmotic diuresis—hyperglycemia, administration of urea or mannitol
Hypernatremia with normal hydration—due to hypothalamic disorders
  • Insensitivity of osmoreceptors (essential hypernatremia)—water loading does not return serum osmolality to normal; chlorpropamide may lower serum sodium toward normal
  • Defect in thirst (hypodipsia)—forced water intake returns serum osmolality to normal
Hypernatremia with overhydration—iatrogenic or accidental (e.g., infants given feedings with high sodium concentrations or given $NaHCO_3$ for respiratory distress or cardiopulmonary arrest)
Alcohol ingestion is the most common cause of hyperosmolar state and of coexisting coma and hyperosmolar state.

Decreased In (Equivalent to Hyponatremia)

Hyponatremia with hypovolemia (urine sodium is usually >20 mEq/L)
  • Adrenal insufficiency (e.g., salt-losing form of congenital adrenal hyperplasia, congenital adrenal hypoplasia, hemorrhage into adrenals, inadequate replacement of corticosteroids, inappropriate tapering of steroids)
  • Renal losses (e.g., osmotic diuresis, proximal renal tubular acidosis, salt-losing nephropathies, usually tubulointerstitial diseases such as GU tract obstruction, pyelonephritis, medullary cystic disease, polycystic kidneys)
  • GI tract loss (e.g., vomiting, diarrhea)
  • Other losses (e.g., burns, peritonitis, pancreatitis)
Hyponatremia with normal volume or hypervolemia (dilutional syndromes)
  • Congestive heart failure, cirrhosis, nephrotic syndrome
  • SIADH
Formulas for *calculation* or *prediction* of serum osmolality:

$$mOsm/L = (1.86 \times \text{serum NA}) + \left(\frac{\text{serum glucose}}{18} \right) + \left(\frac{BUN}{2.8} \right) + 9 \text{ (in mg/dL) or}$$

in SI units $= (1.86 \times \text{serum Na}) + \text{serum glucose (mmol/L)} + BUN \text{ (mmol/L)} + 9$

Osmolal Gap

Difference between measured and calculated values; <10 in healthy persons.

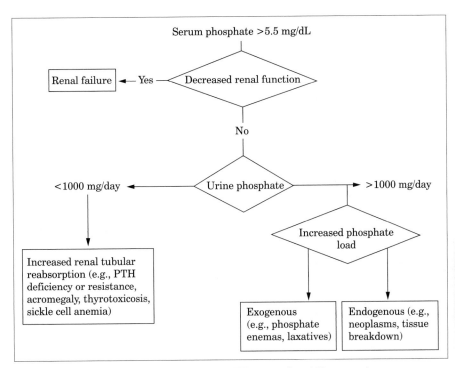

Fig. 3-1. Algorithm for hyperphosphatemia. (PTH = parathyroid hormone.)

Use

Osmolal gap has been used to estimate the blood alcohol. Because serum osmolality increases 22 mOsm/kg for every 100 mg/dL of ethanol:

$$\text{Estimated blood alcohol (mg / dL)} = \text{osmolal gap} \times \frac{100}{22}$$

Osmolal Gap >10 Due To

Decreased serum water content
- Hyperlipidemia (serum will appear lipemic)
- Hyperproteinemia (total protein >10 gm/dL)

Additional low-molecular-weight substances are in serum (measured osmolality will be >300 mOsm/kg water):
- Ethanol. (An especially large osmolal gap with a low or only moderately elevated ethanol level should raise the possibility of another low-molecular-weight toxin [e.g., methanol].)
- Methanol.
- Isopropyl alcohol.
- Mannitol. (Osmolal gap can be used to detect accumulation of infused mannitol in serum.)
- Ethylene glycol, acetone, paraldehyde result in relatively small osmolal gaps even at lethal levels.

Severe illness, especially shock, acidosis (lactic, diabetic, alcoholic), renal failure
Laboratory analytic error
- Random error from all measurements could add or subtract ≤ 15 mOsm/kg.
- Use of incorrect blood collection tubes.

Phosphorus

See Fig. 3-1.

Use

Monitor blood phosphorus level in renal and GI disorders, effect of drugs

Increased In

Most causes of hypocalcemia except vitamin D deficiency, in which it is usually decreased.
Acute or chronic renal failure (most common cause) with decreased GFR
Increased tubular reabsorption of phosphate
- Hypoparathyroidism
   Idiopathic
   Surgical
   Radiation induced
- Secondary hyperparathyroidism (renal rickets)
- Pseudohypoparathyroidism
- Other endocrine disorders
   Addison's disease
   Acromegaly
   Hyperthyroidism
- Sickle cell anemia
Increased cellular release of phosphate
- Neoplasms (e.g., myelogenous leukemia)
- Excessive breakdown of tissue (e.g., chemotherapy for neoplasms, rhabdomyolysis, malignant hyperthermia, lactic acidosis, acute yellow atrophy)
- Bone disease
   Healing fractures
   Multiple myeloma (some patients)
   Paget's disease (some patients)
   Osteolytic metastatic tumor in bone (some patients)
- Childhood
Increased phosphate load
- Exogenous phosphate (e.g., oral or IV)
   Phosphate enemas, laxatives, or infusions
   Excess vitamin D intake
   IV therapy for hypophosphatemia or hypercalcemia
   Milk-alkali (Burnett's) syndrome (some patients)
   Massive blood transfusions
   Hemolysis of blood
Miscellaneous
- High intestinal obstruction
- Sarcoidosis (some patients)

Decreased In

Renal or intestinal loss (>100 mg/day in urine during hypophosphatemia indicates excessive renal loss)
- Administration of diuretics
- Renal tubular defects (Fanconi syndrome; isolated hypophosphatemia due to drugs, neoplasia, X-linked, etc.)
- Primary hyperparathyroidism
- Idiopathic hypercalciuria
- Hypokalemia
- Hypomagnesemia
- Dialysis
- Primary hypophosphatemia
- Idiopathic hypercalciuria
- Acute gout
Decreased intestinal absorption
- Malabsorption
- Vitamin D deficiency and/or resistance, osteomalacia
- Malnutrition, vomiting, diarrhea
- Administration of phosphate-binding antacids*

Intracellular shift of phosphate
- Alcoholism*
- Diabetes mellitus*
- Acidosis (especially diabetic ketoacidosis)
- Hyperalimentation*
- Nutritional recovery syndrome* (rapid refeeding after prolonged starvation)
- Administration of IV glucose (e.g., recovery after severe burns, hyperalimentation)
- Alkalosis, respiratory (e.g., gram-negative bacteremia) or metabolic
- Salicylate poisoning
- Administration of anabolic steroids, androgens, epinephrine, glucagon, insulin
- Cushing's syndrome (some patients)
- Prolonged hypothermia (e.g., open heart surgery)

Sepsis

Often more than one mechanism is operative, usually associated with prior phosphorus depletion.

*Indicates conditions that may be associated with severe hypophosphatemia (<1 mg/dL).

Plasma, Discolored

(Differentiated by spectrophotometric analysis of plasma)

Due To

Total bilirubin (causes of jaundice)
Lipemia
Free hemoglobin (hemolysis)
Ceruloplasmin (green color; see p. 251)
Excess drugs, medications, diet, e.g.:
　Suntanning agents (orange-pink color due to canthaxanthin)
　Carotenoids
Bacterial contamination
Diseases

Potassium

See Table 3-3 and Figs. 3-2 and 3-3.

Use

Diagnosis and monitoring of hyper- and hypokalemia in various conditions (e.g., treatment of diabetic coma, renal failure, severe fluid and electrolyte loss, effect of certain drugs)
Diagnosis of familial hyperkalemic periodic paralysis and hypokalemic paralysis

Increased In

Potassium Retention

Glomerular filtration rate <3–5 mL/min
- Oliguria due to any condition (e.g., renal failure)
- Chronic nonoliguric renal failure associated with dehydration, obstruction, trauma, or excess potassium
- Drugs
　Renal toxicity (e.g., amphotericin B, methicillin, tetracycline)

Glomerular filtration rate >20 mL/min
- Decreased (aldosterone) mineralocorticoid activity
　Addison's disease
　Hypofunction of renin-angiotensin-aldosterone system
　Hyporeninemic hypoaldosteronism with renal insufficiency (GFR 25–75 mL/minute) (see p. 657)
　Various drugs (e.g., nonsteroidal anti-inflammatory drugs [NSAIDs], angiotensin-converting enzyme inhibitors, cyclosporine, pentamidine)

BLOOD ANALYT

Table 3-3. Urine and Blood Changes in Electrolytes, pH, and Volume in Various Conditions

Measurement	Pulmonary Emphysema	Congestive Heart Failure	Excessive Sweating	Diarrhea	Pyloric Obstruction	Dehydration	Starvation	Malabsorption	Salicylate Intoxication	Primary Aldosteronism
Blood										
Sodium	N	N or D	D	D	D	I	N	D	N	I
Potassium	N	N	N	D	D	N	D	D	N or D	D
Bicarbonate	I	N	N	D	I	N or D	D	N or D	D	I
Chloride	D	D	D	D	D	I	N	N	I	D
Volume	N or I	I	N	D	D	D	N or D	D	N	N
Urine										
Sodium	D	D	D	D	D	I	N or I	D	I	D
Potassium	N	N	N	N or D	N	I	I or N	D	N or I	I
pH	D	N	N	D	I	D	D	N or D	I	N or D
Volume	N	D	N	D	D	D	I	N	N	I

Measurement	Adrenal Cortical Insufficiency	Diabetes Insipidus	Diabetic Acidosis	Mercurial Diuretic Administration	Thiazide Diuretic Administration	Ammonium Chloride Administration	Acetazolamide (Diamox) Administration	Renal Tubular Acidosis	Chronic Renal Failure	Acute Renal Failure
Blood										
Sodium	D	N or I	D	D	D	D	D	D	D	D
Potassium	I	N	N or I	D	D	D	D	D	N or D	I
Bicarbonate	N or D	N	D	I	D	D	D	D	D	D
Chloride	D	I	D	D	D	I	I	I	D or N	I
Volume	D	D	D	D	D	D	D	D	V	I
Urine										
Sodium	I	N	I	I	I	I	I	I	I	D
Potassium	N or D	N	I	I	I	I	I	I	I	D
pH	N or I	N	D	D	N or I	I	I	I	I	N or I
Volume	N or D	I	I	I	I	I	I	I	V*	D

N = normal; D = decreased; I = increased; V = variable.
*Usually increased.

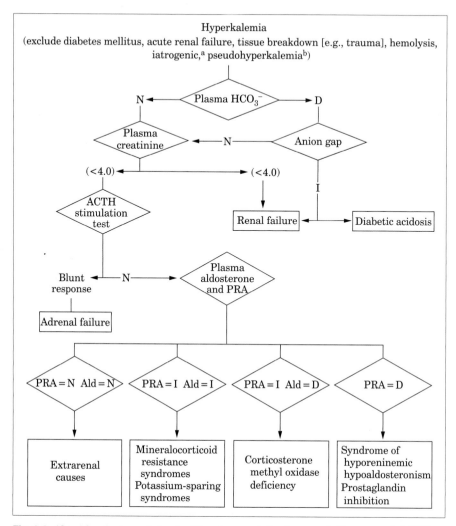

Fig. 3-2. Algorithm for hyperkalemia. (D = decreased; I = increased; N = normal; ACTH = adrenocorticotropic hormone; Ald = aldosterone; PRA = plasma renin activity.)
[a]Potassium-sparing diuretics, administration of potassium (e.g. blood transfusions, salt substitutes, potassium penicillin).
[b]Pseudohyperkalemia = WBC > 100,000/cu mm or platelet count > 1,000,000/cu mm (serum potassium > plasma potassium).

      Decreased aldosterone production
       Pseudohypoaldosteronism
       Aldosterone antagonist drugs (e.g., spironolactone, captopril, heparin)
    • Inhibition of tubular secretion of potassium
       Drugs (e.g., spironolactone, triamterene, amiloride)
       Hyperkalemic type of distal renal tubular acidosis (e.g., sickle cell disease, obstrutive uropathy)

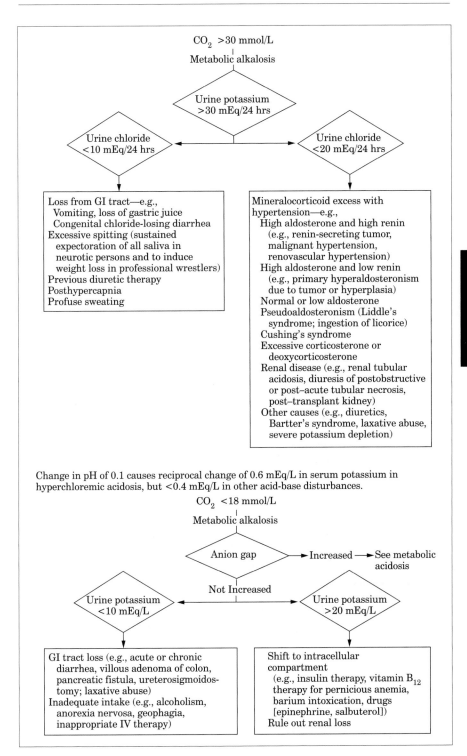

Change in pH of 0.1 causes reciprocal change of 0.6 mEq/L in serum potassium in hyperchloremic acidosis, but <0.4 mEq/L in other acid-base disturbances.

Fig. 3-3. Algorithm for hypokalemia.

- Mineralocorticoid-resistant syndromes (increased renin and aldosterone may be low in those marked with *)
  Primary tubular disorders
    Hereditary
    Acquired (e.g., SLE, amyloidosis, sickle cell nephropathy,* obstructive uropathy,* renal allograft transplant, chloride shift)

Potassium Redistribution

Familial hyperkalemic periodic paralysis (Gamstorp's disease, adynamia episodica hereditaria)
Acute acidosis (especially hyperchloremic metabolic acidosis; less with respiratory acidosis; little with metabolic acidosis due to organic acids) (e.g., diabetic ketoacidosis, lactic acidosis, acute renal failure, acute respiratory acidosis)
- Decreased insulin
- Beta-adrenergic blockade
- Drugs (e.g., succinylcholine, great excess of digitalis, arginine infusion)
- Use of hypertonic solutions (e.g., saline, mannitol)
- Intravascular hemolysis (e.g., transfusion reaction, hemolytic anemia), rhabdomyolysis
- Rapid cellular release (e.g., crush injury, chemotherapy for leukemia or lymphoma, burns, major surgery)

Increased Supply of Potassium

Laboratory artifacts (e.g., hemolysis during venipuncture, conditions associated with thrombocytosis [>1,000,000/cu mm] or leukocytosis [>100,000/cu mm], incomplete separation of serum and clot)
Potassium value can be elevated ~15% in slight hemolysis (Hb ≤ 50 mg/dL); elevated ~30–50% in moderate hemolysis (Hb >100 mg/dL). Thus potassium status can be assessed with slight hemolysis but not with moderate hemolysis.
Prolonged tourniquet use and hand exercise when drawing blood
Excess dietary intake or rapid potassium infusion
Drugs (e.g., those with high potassium content [1 million U of penicillin G potassium contains 1.7 mEq of potassium])

Urinary Diversion

Ureteral implants into jejunum
In neonates—dehydration, hemolysis (e.g., cephalohematoma, intracranial hemorrhage, bruising, exchange transfusion), acute renal failure, congenital adrenal hyperplasia, adrenocortical insufficiency

Decreased In

See Table 12-3 and Fig. 3-3.
(Each 1 mEq/L decrease of serum potassium reflects a total deficit of <200–400 mEq; serum potassium <2 mEq/L may reflect total deficit >1000 mEq.)

Excess Renal Excretion

Osmotic diuresis of hyperglycemia (e.g., uncontrolled diabetes)
Nephropathies
- Renal tubular acidosis (proximal and especially distal) (see p. 709)
- Bartter's syndrome (see p. 654)
- Liddle's syndrome (see p. 663)
- Magnesium depletion due to any cause
- Renal vascular disease, malignant hypertension, vasculitis
- Renin-secreting tumors
Endocrine
- Hyperaldosteronism (primary, secondary)
- Cushing's syndrome, especially due to ectopic ACTH production
- Congenital adrenal hyperplasia
- Hyperthyroidism (especially in Asian persons)
Drugs
- Diuretics (e.g., thiazides, ethacrynic acid, furosemide)
- Mineralocorticoids (e.g., fludrocortisone)

- High-dose glucocorticoids
- High-dose antibiotics (e.g., penicillin, nafcillin, ampicillin, carbenicillin)
- Substances with mineralocorticoid effect (e.g., glycyrrhizic acid [licorice; see p. 663], carbenoxolone, gossypol)
- Drugs associated with magnesium depletion (e.g., aminoglycosides, cisplatin, amphotericin B, foscarnet)

Acute myelogenous, monomyeloblastic or lymphoblastic leukemia

Nonrenal Causes of Excess Potassium Loss

Gastrointestinal

- Vomiting
- Diarrhea (e.g., infections, malabsorption, radiation)
- Drugs (e.g., laxatives [phenolphthalein], enemas, cancer therapy)
- Neoplasms (e.g., villous adenoma of colon, pancreatic vipoma that produces vasoactive intestinal polypeptide >200 pg/mL, Zollinger-Ellison [Z-E] syndrome)
- Excessive spitting (sustained expectoration of all saliva in neurotic persons and to induce weight loss in professional wrestlers)

Skin

- Excessive sweating
- Cystic fibrosis
- Extensive burns
- Draining wounds

Cellular shifts

- Respiratory alkalosis
- Classic periodic paralysis
- Insulin use
- Use of certain drugs (e.g., bronchodilators, decongestants)
- Accidental ingestion of barium compounds
- Treatment of severe megaloblastic anemia with vitamin B_{12} or folic acid
- Physiologic causes (e.g., in highly trained athletes)

Diet

- Severe eating disorders (e.g., anorexia nervosa, bulimia)
- Dietary deficiency

Delirium tremens

In neonates—asphyxia, alkalosis, renal tubular acidosis, iatrogenic causes (glucose and insulin administration), diuretic use

Major causes of hypokalemia with hypertension:

- Diuretic drugs (e.g., thiazides)
- Primary aldosteronism
- Secondary aldosteronism (renovascular disease, renin-producing tumors)
- Cushing's syndrome
- Malignant hypertension
- Renal tubular acidosis

Pregnancy Test

(Immunoassay detection of human chorionic gonadotropin [hCG] in blood)

(See also Urinary Chorionic Gonadotropins, p. 94, Serum Human Chorionic Gonadotropin, pp. 761–763)

Use (Positive In)

Pregnancy. Test becomes positive as early as 4 days after expected date of menstruation; it is >95% reliable by 10th–14th day.

Ectopic pregnancy. See pp. 761–763.

Hydatidiform mole, choriocarcinoma. Test negative one or more times in >60% of these patients and negative at all times in >20% of patients, for whom more sensitive methods (e.g., radioimmunoassay) should be used. Quantitative titers should be performed for diagnosis and for following the clinical course of patients with these conditions. (See p. 766.)

Interferences

False-negative results may occur with dilute urine or in cases of missed abortion, dead fetus syndrome, ectopic pregnancy.

Table 3-4. Changes in Serum Immunoproteins in Various Conditions

Condition	Albumin	Alpha$_1$-Antitrypsin	Haptoglobin	Transferrin	C3
Acute inflammation	D	I	I	D	Slight I
Chronic inflammation	D	V–I	V–I	D	Slight I
Chronic liver disease	D	V–I	V	D	V–D
Obstructive jaundice	N	N	V–I	N	I
Hemolytic anemia	N	N	D	N	N
Iron deficiency	N	N	N	I	N
Acute GN	N	N	N	N	D
SLE	D	I	D[a]	D	V–D[b]
Alpha$_1$-antitrypsin deficiency	N	D	N	N	N
Analbuminemia	D	N	N	N	N
Agammaglobulinemia	N	N	N	N	N
IgG myeloma	D	N	N	N	N
IgA myeloma	D	N	N	N	N
Waldenström's macroglobulinemia	D	N	N	N	N

N = normal; D = decreased; I = increased; V = variable.
[a]D with associated hemolytic anemia.
[b]N if immunosuppressive treatment is effective.

False-positive results may occur in
- Bacterial contamination or protein or blood in urine or in patients on methadone therapy
- Marijuana smokers
- Postorchiectomy patients (secondary to decreased testosterone)

With the latex agglutination type of test, only urine should be used if patient has RA.
Leukocyte alkaline phosphatase scoring has also been used as a pregnancy test (see p. 334).

Protein Gammopathies

Use

Identify hereditary and acquired immunodeficiencies (see p. 398)
Identify monoclonal gammopathies (increases) and associated disorders (concomitant hyperproteinemia is very frequent; see Tables 3-4, 3-5)

Monoclonal Increase In

Classification of monoclonal gammopathies (see p. 417)

Polyclonal Gammopathy with Hyperproteinemia

Collagen diseases (e.g., SLE, RA, scleroderma)
Liver disease (e.g., chronic hepatitis, cirrhosis)
Chronic infection (e.g., chronic bronchitis and bronchiectasis, lung abscess, TB, osteomyelitis, SBE, infectious mononucleosis, malaria, leishmaniasis, trypanosomiasis)
Miscellaneous (e.g., sarcoidosis, malignant lymphoma, acute myeloid and monocytic leukemia, diabetes mellitus)
Idiopathic (family of patients with SLE)

Protein, Total

See Table 3-6.

Use

Screening for nutritional deficiencies and gammopathies

Table 3-5. Serum Immunoglobulin Changes in Various Diseases

Disease	IgG	IgA	IgM
Immunoglobulin disorders (see Tables 11-8 and 11-9, pp. 357 and 362)			
Lymphoid aplasia	D	D	D
Agammaglobulinemia	D	D	D
Type I dysgammaglobulinemia (selective IgG and IgA deficiency)	D	D	N or I
Type II dysgammaglobulinemia (absent IgA and IgM)	N	D	D
IgA globulinemia	N	D	N
Ataxia-telangiectasia	N	D	N
Multiple myeloma, macroglobulinemia, lymphomas (see p. 414)			
Heavy-chain disease	D	D	D
IgG myeloma	I	D	D
IgA myeloma	D	I	D
Macroglobulinemia	D	D	I
Acute lymphocytic leukemia	N	D	N
Chronic lymphocytic leukemia	D	D	D
Acute myelogenous leukemia	N	N	N
Chronic myelogenous leukemia	N	D	N
Hodgkin's disease	N	N	N
Liver diseases			
Hepatitis	I	I	I
Laënnec's cirrhosis	I	I	N
Biliary cirrhosis	N	N	I
Hepatoma	N	N	D
Miscellaneous			
Rheumatoid arthritis	I	I	I
SLE	I	I	I
Nephrotic syndrome	D	D	N
Trypanosomiasis	N	N	I
Pulmonary tuberculosis	I	N	N

N = normal; I = increased; D = decreased.

Increased In

Hypergammaglobulinemias (mono- or polyclonal; see following sections)
Hypovolemic states

Decreased In

Nutritional deficiency, e.g.,
  • Malabsorption
  • Kwashiorkor
  • Marasmus
Decreased or ineffective protein synthesis, e.g.,
  • Severe liver disease
  • Agammaglobulinemia
Increased loss
  • Renal (e.g., nephrotic syndrome)
  • GI disease (e.g., protein-losing enteropathies, surgical resection)
  • Severe skin disease (e.g., burns, pemphigus vulgaris, eczema)
  • Blood loss, plasmapheresis
Increased catabolism, e.g.,
  • Fever
  • Inflammation

Table 3-6. Serum Protein Electrophoretic Patterns in Various Diseases*

Condition	Total Protein	Albumin	Alpha$_1$ Globulin	Alpha$_2$ Globulin	Beta Globulin	Gamma Globulin	Comment
Multiple myeloma	I	D		Dyscrasia of beta$_{2A}$ or gamma$_2$ Ig			Total globulin, marked I; Variable location of M globulin
Macroglobulinemia	I	D		Dyscrasia of beta$_{2M}$		Marked I	Electrophoresis same as multiple myeloma
Hodgkin's disease	D	D	I	I		V	
Lymphatic leukemia and lymphoma	D	D			D	D	
Myelogenous and monocytic leukemia	D	D			D	I	Gamma globulin to differentiate types of acute leukemias
Hypogamma-globulinemia	D	N	N	N	N	D	
Analbuminemia	Marked D	Marked D	N	I	I	I	
GI diseases							
Peptic ulcer	D	D	May be I	May be I			
Ulcerative colitis	D	D	May be I	May be I	D		
Protein-losing enteropathy		Marked D	I	I		D	
Acute cholecystitis	D	D				N	
Nephrosis	D	D		D	D, I (N)	D (N, I)	
Chronic GN	D	D	N	I	N	N	
Laënnec's cirrhosis	D, N, I	D	N	D	Characteristic pattern of beta-gamma "bridging"		Typical pattern
Acute viral hepatitis	D, N	D	D	D	D	V, I	

(indicates acute

Condition						Remarks
				(evidence of hepatocellular damage)		
Stress	D	I	I			"Three-fingered" pattern
Hypersensitivity — Sarcoidosis	D			I	I	"Sarcoid steps" help differentiate from other lung disease
Collagen disease					Stepwise increase of alpha$_2$, beta, and gamma	Gamma globulin levels of prognostic value
SLE	D		I	I	I	
Polyarteritis nodosa	D		I	I	N	
Rheumatoid arthritis	D		I	I	I	No significant changes
Scleroderma	D			I	V	
Acute rheumatic fever	D		I	I	No significant changes	Albumin D due to hemodilution
Essential hypertension ⎰ Congestive heart failure ⎱	D	No significant changes				(Hemodilution, diminished hepatic synthesis, and possible excessive enteric loss)
Metastatic carcinomatosis	D	I	I		D	Nonspecific patterns

(continued)

Table 3-6. * (continued)

Condition	Total Protein	Albumin	Alpha$_1$ Globulin	Alpha$_2$ Globulin	Beta Globulin	Gamma Globulin	Comment
Certain infections (meningitis, pneumonia, osteomyelitis)				D		I	
Myxedema							Changes due to hemodilution
Hyperthyroidism		D	N	N	N	N	
Diabetes mellitus		D		I	I		

I = increased or elevated; D = decreased or diminished; V = variable; N = normal; blank = no significant change.

*Nonspecific changes of decreased albumin and increased globulin occur in many conditions (e.g., infections, neoplasms, metabolic diseases).

Source: Sunderman FW Jr. Recent advances in clinical interpretation of electrophoretic fractionations of the serum proteins. In Sunderman FW, Sunderman JC, eds. *Serum proteins and the dysproteinemias.* Philadelphia: Lippincott, 1964. Harrison HH, Levitt MH. Serum protein electrophoresis: basic principles, interpretations, and practical considerations. *ASCP Check Sample.* Core Chemistry NO. PTS 87-7 (PTS-25). Chicago: ASCP; 1987.

- Hyperthyroidism
- Malignancy
- Chronic diseases

Dilutional, e.g.,

- IV fluid administration
- SIADH
- Water intoxication

Protein Separation (Immunodiffusion, Immunofixation, Electrophoresis)

Use

Diagnosis of Specific Diseases
- Multiple myeloma
- Waldenström's macroglobulinemia
- Hypogammaglobulinemia
- Agammaglobulinemia
- Agamma-A-globulinemia
- Analbuminemia
- Bisalbuminemia
- Afibrinogenemia
- Atransferrinemia
- Alpha$_1$-antitrypsin variant
- Cirrhosis
- Acute-phase reactant

Other Changes

Nonspecific changes in serum proteins
Protein pattern changes in urine, cerebrospinal fluid, peritoneal fluid, etc.

Sodium

See Figs. 13-27 and 13-28, pp. 693–696; Table 3-3.

Use

Diagnosis and treatment of dehydration and overhydration. *Changes in serum sodium most often reflect changes in water balance rather than sodium balance. If patient has not received large load of sodium, hypernatremia suggests need for water and values <130 mEq/L suggest overhydration.* Determinations of blood sodium and potassium levels are not useful in diagnosis or in estimating net ion losses but are performed to monitor changes in sodium and potassium during therapy.

Interference

Hyperglycemia—serum sodium decreases 1.7 mEq/L for every increase of serum glucose of 100 mg/dL).
Hyperlipidemia and hyperproteinemia cause spurious results only with flame photometric technique but not with specific ion electrode techniques for measuring sodium.

Urea Nitrogen (BUN)

Use

Diagnosis of renal insufficiency
Correlates with uremic symptoms better than serum creatinine.
A low BUN of 6–8 mg/dL is frequently associated with states of overhydration.
A BUN of 10–20 mg/dL almost always indicates normal glomerular function.
A BUN of 50–150 mg/dL implies serious impairment of renal function.
Markedly increased BUN (150–250 mg/dL) is virtually conclusive evidence of severely impaired glomerular function.
In chronic renal disease, BUN correlates better with symptoms of uremia than does the serum creatinine.
Evidence of hemorrhage into GI tract
Assessment of patients requiring nutritional support for excess catabolism (e.g., burns, cancer)

Increased In

Impaired kidney function (see Creatinine, p. 55)
Prerenal azotemia—any cause of reduced renal blood flow
  • Congestive heart failure
  • Salt and water depletion (vomiting, diarrhea, diuresis, sweating)
  • Shock
Postrenal azotemia—any obstruction of urinary tract (increased BUN/creatinine ratio)
Increased protein catabolism (serum creatinine remains normal)
  • Hemorrhage into GI tract
  • Acute myocardial infarction
  • Stress
Methodologic interference
  • Nesslerization (chloral hydrate, chloramphenicol, ammonium salts)
  • Berthelot (aminophenol, asparagine, ammonium salts)
  • Fearon (acetohexamide, sulfonylureas)

Decreased In

Diuresis (e.g., with overhydration, often associated with low protein catabolism)
Severe liver damage (liver failure)
  • Drugs
  • Poisoning
  • Hepatitis
  • Other
Increased utilization of protein for synthesis
  • Late pregnancy
  • Infancy
  • Acromegaly
  • Malnutrition
  • Anabolic hormones
Diet
  • Low protein and high carbohydrate
  • IV feedings only
  • Impaired absorption (celiac disease)
  • Malnutrition
Nephrotic syndrome (some patients)
SIADH
Inherited hyperammonemias (urea is virtually absent in blood)
Methodologic interference
  • Berthelot (chloramphenicol, streptomycin)

Uric Acid

Levels are very labile and show day-to-day and seasonal variation in same person; also increased by emotional stress, total fasting, increased body weight.

Use

Monitor treatment of gout.
Monitor chemotherapeutic treatment of neoplasms to avoid renal urate deposition with possible renal failure.

Increased In

Renal failure (does not correlate with severity of kidney damage; urea and creatinine should be used)
Gout (see p. 316)
25% of relatives of patients with gout
Asymptomatic hyperuricemia (e.g., incidental finding with no evidence of gout; clinical significance is not known but people so afflicted should be rechecked periodically for gout). The higher the level of serum uric acid, the greater the likelihood of an attack of acute gouty arthritis.
Increased destruction of nucleoproteins

- Leukemia, multiple myeloma
- Polycythemia
- Lymphoma, especially postirradiation
- Other disseminated neoplasms
- Cancer chemotherapy (e.g., nitrogen mustards, vincristine, mercaptopurine, prednisone)
- Hemolytic anemia
- Sickle cell anemia
- Resolving pneumonia
- Toxemia of pregnancy (serial determinations to follow therapeutic response and estimate prognosis)
- Psoriasis (one-third of patients)

Drugs
- Small doses of salicylates (<4 gm/day)
- Intoxications (e.g., barbiturates, methyl alcohol, ammonia, carbon monoxide); some patients with alcoholism
- Decreased renal clearance or tubular secretion (e.g., various diuretics: thiazides, furosemide, ethacrynic acid)
- Nephrotoxic effect (e.g., mitomycin C)
- Other effects (e.g., levodopa, phenytoin sodium)
- Methodologic interference (e.g., ascorbic acid, levodopa, methyldopa)

Metabolic acidosis

Diet
- High-protein weight reduction diet
- Excess nucleoprotein (e.g., sweetbreads, liver) may increase level ≤ 1 mg/dL.
- Alcohol consumption

Miscellaneous
- von Gierke's disease
- Lead poisoning
- Lesch-Nyhan syndrome
- Maple syrup urine disease
- Down syndrome
- Polycystic kidney disease
- Calcinosis universalis and circumscripta
- Hypoparathyroidism
- Primary hyperparathyroidism
- Hypothyroidism
- Sarcoidosis
- Chronic berylliosis
- Arteriosclerosis and hypertension *(serum uric acid is increased in 80% of patients with elevated serum triglycerides)*
- Certain population groups (e.g., Blackfoot and Pima, Filipinos, New Zealand Maoris)

Most common causes in hospitalized men are azotemia, metabolic acidosis, diuretics, gout, myelolymphoproliferative disorders, other drugs, unknown causes.

("It is difficult to justify therapy in asymptomatic persons with hyperuricemia to prevent gouty arthritis, uric acid stones, urate nephropathy or risk of cardiovascular disease."[3])

Decreased In

Drugs
- ACTH
- Uricosuric drugs (e.g., high doses of salicylates, probenecid, cortisone, allopurinol, coumarins)
- Various other drugs (radiographic contrast agents, glyceryl guaiacolate, estrogens, phenothiazines, indomethacin)

Wilson's disease
Fanconi's syndrome
Acromegaly (some patients)
Celiac disease (slightly)

[3]Duffy WB, et al. Management of asymptomatic hyperuricemia. *JAMA* 1981;246:2215–2216.

PA in relapse (some patients)

Xanthinuria

Neoplasms (occasional cases) (e.g., carcinomas, Hodgkin's disease)

Healthy adults with isolated defect in tubular transport of uric acid (Dalmatian dog mutation)

Decreased in ~5% of hospitalized patients; most common causes are postoperative state (GI surgery, coronary artery bypass), diabetes mellitus, various drugs, SIADH in association with hyponatremia.

Unchanged In

Colchicine administration

Vitamin D

Use

Diagnosis of rickets and vitamin D toxicity

Differential diagnosis of hypercalcemias

Serum/Urine Calcium Increased	1,25-dihydroxy-vitamin D	25-hydroxy-vitamin D
Hyperparathyroidism	N	N, I
Conditions associated with parathyroid hormone–related protein (PTHrP)	N	D
Lymphoma	N	D, I
Granulomatous conditions (e.g., sarcoidosis)	N	I
Idiopathic hypercalciuria	N	N, I
Osteoporosis	N	N, I
Vitamin D and 25-hydroxy-vitamin D intoxication	I	N
1,25-dihydroxy-vitamin D and dihydrotachysterol intoxication	N	I

Serum Calcium Decreased	1,25-dihydroxy-vitamin D	25-hydroxy-vitamin D
Hypoparathyroidism	N	D, N
Pseudohypoparathyroidism	N	D, N
Vitamin D deficiency	D	D, N, I
Vitamin D-dependent rickets		
Type I	N	D
Type II	N	I
Severe liver disease	D	D, N
Nephrotic syndrome	D	D, N
Renal failure	N	D
Hyperphosphatemia	N	D
Hypomagnesemia	N	D, N

Serum Calcium Normal	1,25-dihydroxy-vitamin D	25-hydroxy-vitamin D
Pregnancy, lactation	N	I
Growing children	N	I
Elderly	D, N	D, N, I
Summertime	N	N
Wintertime	D	N
Increased latitude	D	N

I = increased; D = decreased; N = normal.

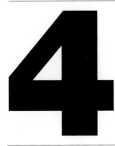

Urine

Normal Values

Addis count (no longer performed)	
RBC	≤ 1,000,000/24 hrs
Casts	≤ 100,000/24 hrs
WBC + epithelial cells	≤ 2,000,000/24 hrs
Calcium	<150 mg/24 hrs on low-calcium (Bauer-Aub) diet
Chloride	140–250 mEq/L
Coproporphyrin	50–300 μg/24 hrs; 0–75 μg/24 hrs in children weighing <80 lb
Creatine	<100 mg/24 hrs (<6% of creatinine); higher in children (<1 yr: may = creatinine; older children: ≤ 30% of creatine) and during pregnancy (≤ 12% of creatinine)
Creatinine	
Males	19–26 mg/kg of body weight/24 hrs
Females	14–21 mg/kg of body weight/24 hrs
Cystine or cysteine	0
Delta-aminolevulinic acid	1.5–7.5 mg/24 hrs
Glucose	Qualitative = 0≤ 0.3 gm/24 hrs
Hemoglobin and myoglobin	0
Homogentisic acid	0
Ketones	Qualitative = 0
Lead	<0.08 μg/mL or 120 μg/24 hrs
Microscopic examination	≤ 1–2 RBC, WBC, epithelial cells/high-power field (HPF); occasional hyaline cast/low-power field (LPF)
Osmolality	500–1200 mOsm/L
Oxalate	
Males	≤ 55 mg/24 hrs
Females	≤ 50 mg/24 hrs
pH	4.6–8.0 (average = 6.0), depending on diet; >9 indicates old specimen
Phenylpyruvic acid	0
Phosphorus	1 gm/24 hrs (average), depending on diet
Porphobilinogen	0–2 mg/24 hrs
Protein	Qualitative = 0
	0–0.1 gm/24 hrs
Specific gravity	1.003–1.030
Total solids	30–70 gm/L (average = 50). To estimate, multiply last two figures of specific gravity by 2.66 (Long's coefficient).
Uric acid	≤ 750 mg/24 hrs
Urobilinogen	0–4 mg/24 hrs
Uroporphyrin	0

Volume
    Adults   600–2500 mL/24 hrs (average = 1200)
                                   Night volume usually <700 mL with specific
                                       gravity <1.018 or osmolality >825 mOsm/kg
                                       of body weight in children
                                   Ratio of night to day volume 1:2–1:4
    Infants
        Premature   1–3 mL/kg/hr
        Full-term   15–60 mL/24 hrs
        2 wks   250–400 mL/24 hrs
        8 wks   250–400 mL/24 hrs
        1 yr   500–600 mL/24 hrs

Bacteriuria

See Chapter 14.

Bilirubinuria

See Chapter 8.

Calciuria

Use

Diagnosis of hypercalciuria causing renal calculi.

Increased In

Hyperparathyroidism
Idiopathic hypercalciuria
High-calcium diet
Excess milk intake
Immobilization (especially in children)
Lytic bone lesions
  • Metastatic tumor
  • Multiple myeloma
  • Osteoporosis (primary or secondary to hyperthyroidism, Cushing's syndrome, acromegaly)
Drugs
  • Diuretics (e.g., ammonium chloride, mercurials)
  • Androgens, anabolic steroids
  • Cholestyramine
  • Dihydrotachysterol, vitamin D, parathyroid injections
  • Viomycin
Fanconi's syndrome
Glucocorticoid excess due to any cause
Paget's disease
Renal tubular acidosis
Rapidly progressive osteoporosis
Sarcoidosis

Decreased In

Hypoparathyroidism
Rickets, osteomalacia
Familial hypocalciuric (benign) hypercalcemia
Steatorrhea
Renal failure
Metastatic carcinoma of prostate
Drugs (e.g., sodium phytate, thiazides)

Hypercalciuria without Hypercalcemia

Due To
Idiopathic hypercalciuria

Sarcoidosis
Glucocorticoid excess due to any cause
Hyperthyroidism
Rapidly progressive bone diseases (Paget's disease, immobilization, malignant tumors)
Renal tubular acidosis
Medullary sponge kidney
Furosemide administration

Chyluria

Use

Diagnosis of injury or obstruction of lymphochylous system of chest or abdomen

Due To

Obstruction of the lymphochylous system, usually filariasis. Microfilariae appear in the urine for 6 wks after acute infection then disappear, unless endemic.
Trauma to chest or abdomen
Abdominal tumors or lymph node enlargement
Milky urine is due to chylomicrons recognized as fat globules by microscopy (this is almost entirely neutral fat). Protein is normal or low. Hematuria is common. Specific gravity is low, and reaction is acid.
A test meal of milk and cream may cause chyluria in 1–4 hrs.
Laboratory findings due to pyelonephritis that is often present.

Color, Abnormal[1]

Red ("red" often includes colors from pink to red-brown)
- No specific test (chlorzoxazone, ethoxazene, oxamniquine, phenothiazines, rifampin)
- Acid urine only (phenolphthalein)

Red-orange
- No specific test (butazopyridine, chlorzoxazone, ethoxazene, mannose, oxamniquine, phenothiazines, rifampin)
- Alkaline urine only (phenindione)
- Acid urine only (phenolphthalein)

Red or pink
- No specific test (aminopyrine, aniline dyes, antipyrine, doxorubicin, fuscin, ibuprofen, phenacetin, phenothiazines, phensuximide, phenytoin)
- Acid urine only (beets, blackberries, anisindione)
- Alkaline urine only (anthraquinone laxatives, rhubarb, santonin, phenolsulfonphthalein, sulfobromophthalein sodium [Bromsulphalein]; eosin produces green fluorescence)
- Darkens on standing (porphyrins)
- Presence of urates and bile
- On contact with hypochlorite bleach (toilet bowl cleaner) (aminosalicylic acid)
- Centrifuged specimen shows RBC in base (blood)

Purple
- Alkaline urine only (phenolphthalein)
- Darkens on standing (porphyrins; fluoresces with ultraviolet light)
- No specific test (chlorzoxazone)

Red-brown
- Acid urine only (methemoglobin, metronidazole, anisindione) (Fig. 4-1)
- Alkaline urine only (anthraquinone laxatives, levodopa, methyldopa, parahydroxyphenylpyruvic acid, phenazopyridine)
- Positive *o*-toludine test for blood
  Centrifuged urine shows RBC in base if blood; centrifuged blood shows pink supernatant plasma if Hb but clear plasma if myoglobin.
- Green in reflected light (antipyrine)
- Orange with addition of HCl (phenazopyridine)
- No specific test (chloroquine, deferoxamine, ethoxazene, ibuprofen, iron sorbitex, pamaquine, phenacetin, phenothiazines, phensuximide, phenytoin, trinitrophenol)

[1]Raymond JR, Yarger WE. Abnormal urine color: differential diagnosis. *South Med J* 1988;81:837.

URINE

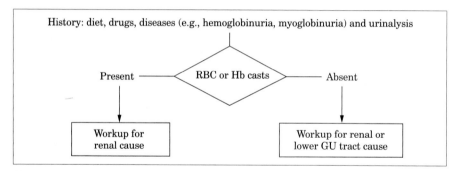

Fig. 4-1. Algorithm for red or brown urine. (GU = genitourinary; Hb = hemoglobin; RBC = red blood cell.)

Brown-black
- Darkens on standing (homogentisic acid, melanin, melanogen, nitrobenzene, parahydroxyphenylpyruvic acid [alkaline urine only], phenol, cresol, naphthol)
- Does not darken on standing
     Ferric chloride test
     Color fades (Argyrol)
     Blue-green (homogentisic acid)
     Black (melanin or melanogen)
        Nitroprusside test is red with melanin, black with melanogen.
Yellow-brown
- Darkens on standing in acid urine (anthraquinone laxatives, rhubarb)
- Positive test for bile (bilirubin, urobilin)
- No specific test (niridazole, nitrofurantoin, pamaquine, primaquine, sulfa-methoxazole)
Yellow
- Acid urine only (quinacrine, santonin)
- Alkaline urine only (beets)
- Positive test for bile (bilirubin, urobilin)
- No specific test (fluorescein dye, phenacetin, riboflavin, trinitrophenol)
Yellow-orange
- Alkaline urine only (anisindione, sulfasalazine)
- Positive test for bile (bilirubin, urobilin)
- Color increases with HCl (phenazopyridine)
- Ether soluble (carrots, vitamin A)
- High specific gravity (dehydration)
- No specific test (aminopyrine, warfarin)
Yellow-green or brown-green
- Darkens on standing (cresol, phenol [Chloraseptic], methocarbamol [Robaxin], resorcinol)
- Positive test for bile (biliverdin)
Blue-green
- Darkens on standing (methocarbamol, resorcinol)
- Blue fluorescence in acid urine (triamterene)
- Bacteriuria, pyuria (*Pseudomonas* infection [rare])
- Decolorizes with alkali (indigo-carmine dye)
- Positive Obermayer's test (indican)
- No specific test (chlorophyll breath mints [Clorets], Evans blue dye, guaiacol, magnesium salicylate [Doan's Pills], methylene blue, thymol [Listerine])
- Biliverdin due to oxidation of bilirubin in poorly preserved specimens.
     Gives negative diazo tests for bilirubin (Ictotest), but oxidative tests (Harrison spot test) may still be positive.

Milky
- Lipuria, chyluria (ether soluble)
- Many polymorphonuclear neutrophils (PMNs) (microscopic examination)

White cloud is due to excessive oxalic acid and glycolic acid in urine; occurs in oxalosis (primary hyperoxaluria).

Colorless
  Specific gravity
    High (diabetes mellitus with glycosuria; positive test for glucose)
    Low (diabetes insipidus, recent fluid intake)
    Variable (diuretics, ethyl alcohol, hypercalcemia)

Clear to deep yellow
- Normal (due to urochrome pigment)

Blue diaper syndrome results from indigo blue in urine due to familial metabolic defect in tryptophan absorption associated with idiopathic hypercalcemia and nephrocalcinosis.

Red diaper syndrome is due to a nonpathogenic chromobacterium (*Serratia marcescens*) that produces a red pigment when grown aerobically at 25–30°C.

Darkening of urine on standing, alkalinization, or oxygenation is nonspecific and may be due to
- Melanogen, Hb, indican, urobilinogen, porphyrins, phenols, salicylate metabolites (e.g., gentisic acid), homogentisic acid (due to alkaptonuria), administration of metronidazole hydrochloride (Flagyl). In acid pH, urine may not darken for hours (e.g., tyrosinosis).
- Sickle cell crises produce a characteristic dark-brown color independent of volume or specific gravity that becomes darker on standing or on exposure to sunlight due to increase in porphyrins.

URINE

Creatine

Increased In

Physiologic states
- Childhood growth
- Pregnancy
- Puerperium (2 wks)
- Starvation
- Raw meat diet

Increased formation
- Myopathy
    Amyotonia congenita
    Muscular dystrophy
    Poliomyelitis
    Myasthenia gravis
    Crush injury
    Acute paroxysmal myoglobinuria
- Endocrine diseases
    Hyperthyroidism
    Addison's disease
    Cushing's syndrome
    Acromegaly
    Diabetes mellitus
    Eunuchoidism
    Therapy with ACTH, cortisone, or desoxycorticosterone acetate

Increased breakdown
- Infections
- Burns
- Fractures
- Leukemia
- SLE

Decreased In

Hypothyroidism

Creatinine

Use

Determine urine concentration of various substances when 24-hr urine cannot be obtained.
Detect artifactual dilution of urine in drug abuse testing.
In healthy young men on meat-free diet, can be used to calculate muscle mass[2]:

Total muscle mass (kg) = creatinine (gm) excreted/24 hrs × 21.8

Crystalluria

Disorder	Substance
Massive hepatic necrosis (acute yellow atrophy), tyrosinemia, tyrosinosis	Tyrosine
Cystinuria, cystinosis	Cystine
Fanconi's syndrome	Leucine
Hyperoxaluria, oxalosis	Calcium oxalate
Lesch-Nyhan syndrome	Uric acid
Orotic aciduria	Orotic acid
Xanthinuria	Xanthine

Cytology

Use

Screen persons exposed to urothelial or bladder carcinogens
Detect urothelial dysplasia and carcinomas (see Chapter 14, p. 750)
Monitor effects of radiation or chemotherapy
Detect nonbacterial infections (parasitic, fungal, viral)
Characterize cells with inclusions
Characterize inflammatory conditions
Confirm abnormal routine urinalysis microscopy findings
Flow cytometry and DNA analysis are used for diagnosis, prognosis, and monitoring of therapy but not for screening.

Diagnostic Indices

See Table 14-12.

Electrolytes

Use

Diagnosis of causes of hyponatremia (see p. 693 and Table 13-27) and hypokalemia
Identify suspected disorders of adrenal cortex
Aid diagnosis of causes of acute renal failure (Table 14-12 and Table 4-1)

Interferences

Value may be limited due to failure to obtain 24-hr excretion levels rather than random samples or administration of diuretics.

Eosinophiluria[3]

(Refers to >1% of urinary leukocytes as eosinophils; should be performed using Hansel's rather than Wright's stain)

---

[2]Wang Z-M, Gallagher D, Nelson ME, et al. Total-body skeletal muscle mass: evaluation of 24-h urinary creatinine excretion by computerized axial tomography. *Am J Clin Nutr* 1996;63:863.
[3]Corwin HL, Bray BA, Haber MH. The detection and interpretation of urinary eosinophils. *Arch Pathol Lab Med* 1989;113:1256.

Table 4-1. Urine Electrolytes in Various Metabolic Conditions

Metabolic Problem	Cause	Urine Electrolytes*
Volume depletion	Extrarenal sodium loss Adrenal insufficiency or renal salt wasting	Sodium <10 mEq/L Sodium >10 mEq/L
Acute oliguria	Prerenal azotemia Acute tubular necrosis	Sodium <10 mEq/L Sodium >30 mEq/L

Hyponatremia	Severe volume depletion: edematous states
	SIADH; adrenal insufficiency; salt-wasting
	  nephropathies
		Sodium <10 mEq/L
		Sodium ≥ dietary
		  intake

Hypokalemia	Extrarenal potassium loss Renal potassium loss (often associated with diuretic therapy)	Potassium <10 mEq/L Potassium >10 mEq/L
Metabolic alkalosis	Chloride-responsive alkalosis Chloride-resistant alkalosis	Chloride <10 mEq/L Chloride parallels dietary intake

*Values based on patient not receiving diuretics.

Use

May be useful to distinguish acute interstitial nephritis from acute tubular necrosis, in
which it is absent.

Due To

Acute interstitial nephritis (drug induced); sensitivity = 60–90%, specificity >85%, positive predictive value ~50%, negative predictive value 98%.
Acute GN (rapidly progressive; acute including poststreptococcal)
IgA nephropathy (Henoch-Schönlein purpura)
Chronic pyelonephritis
Acute rejection of renal allograft
Obstructive uropathy
Prostatitis
Eosinophilic cystitis
Schistosoma hematobium infestation
Bladder cancer
Cholesterol embolization to kidney

Ferric Chloride Test

(Primarily used as screening test for phenylketonuria)

Positive In	Phenistix color
Phenylketonuria (unreliable for diagnosis)	Gray-green
Tyrosinuria (transient elevation in newborns)	Green
Maple syrup urine disease	Negative
Alkaptonuria	Negative
Histidinemia	Blue-gray to green
Tyrosinosis	Green (fades quickly)
Oasthouse urine disease	—
Bilirubin	—
Lactic acidosis	Gray
Melanin	—
Methionine malabsorption	—
Pyruvic acid	Yellow
Xanthurenic acid	Negative
Acetoacetic acid	Negative

URINE

Drugs
      Para–aminosalicylic acid   Purple
      Phenothiazines   Purple
      Salicylates   Purple
A positive test should always be followed by other tests (e.g., chromatography of blood and urine) to rule out genetic metabolic disorders.

Gonadotropins, Chorionic

(See also Pregnancy Test, p. 77; Human Chorionic Gonadotropin, Serum, p. 77.)

Increased In

Normal pregnancy (secreted first by trophoblastic cells of conceptus and later by placenta). Becomes positive as early as 4 days after expected date of menstruation; it is >95% reliable by 10th–14th day. Human chorionic gonadotropin (hCG) increases to peak at 60th–70th day, then drops progressively.
Hydatidiform mole, choriocarcinoma. Test negative one or more times in >60% and negative at all times in >20% of these patients, for whom more sensitive methods should be used. Quantitative titers should be performed for diagnosis and for following the clinical course of patients with these conditions. Serum is preferred test.

False Positive Due To

Drugs
- Chlorpromazine (frog, rabbit, immunologic)
- Phenothiazines (frog, rabbit, immunologic)
- Promethazine (Gravindex)
- Methadone

Bacterial contamination
Protein or blood in urine

False Negative Due To

Drugs
- Promethazine (DAP test)

Dilute urine
Missed abortion
Dead fetus syndrome
Ectopic pregnancy
With the latex agglutination type of text, only urine should be used if patient has RA.

Normal In

Nonpregnant state
Fetal death

Hematuria

Use

Screening and diagnosis of disorders of genitourinary tract (Fig. 4-2).
Screening for excess anticoagulation medication.

Interpretation

<3% of normal persons have ≥ 3 RBCs/HPF or >1000 RBCs/mL (no easy conversion formula between these two methods). Abnormal range is >3 RBCs/HPF. Hematuria found in 18% of persons after very strenuous exercise. Centrifuged fresh urine sediment should be examined under high dry magnification. Urine does not show any red color at <5,000,000 RBCs/mL.
Dipsticks (orthotolidine or peroxidase) detect heme peroxidase activity in RBCs, Hb, or myoglobin with reported sensitivity of 91–100% and specificity of 65–99%; may miss 10% of patients with microscopic hematuria. Orthotolidine test strips are sensitive to 3–10 RBCs/HPF. Are more reliable in hypotonic urine (lyses RBCs) than hypertonic

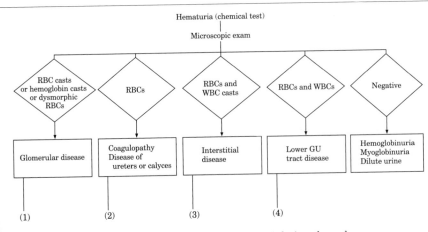

(1) Hypertension, diabetes mellitus, GN, immune-complex or postinfectious glomerular
    disease, drug reaction, endocarditis, embolic diseases. Tests: ASOT, ANA, C3, HB₅Ab, renal biopsy.
(2) Calculi, papillary necrosis, polycystic disease, sickle cell disease; GU tract trauma, neoplasm, or
    parasites. Tests: Cytology, CAT scan, ultrasonography, IVP.
(3) Pyelonephritis, tuberculosis, sarcoidosis, drug reaction. Tests: Urine cultures, lymph node biopsy.
(4) GU tract infection (e.g., prostatitis, urethritis, vaginitis), reflux, GU tract carcinoma. Tests: Urine
    cultures, cytology, cystoscopy, ultrasonography.

Fig. 4-2. Algorithm for diagnosis of microhematuria. (ANA = antinuclear antibodies; ASOT = antistreptolysin-O titer.)

URINE

urine. For detection of hematuria, specificity = 65–99% compared to microscopy; positive predictive value for significant disease = 0–2% and for possibly significant disease = 6–58%. Dipsticks exposed to air (uncapped bottles) for a week or more may give false-negative results for blood.

In microscopic hematuria, number of RBCs is not related to the significance of the causative lesion.

Presence of blood clots virtually rules out glomerular origin of blood. Large thick clots suggest bladder origin; small stringy clots suggest upper tract.

Wright's stain or phase microscopy in urine sediment is said to show distortion with crenation and uneven Hb distribution of RBCs (dysmorphic) of glomerular origin; if >80% are similar to RBCs in peripheral blood (eumorphic), the source is likely to be distal to glomeruli. Dysmorphic changes are much more apt to be found with urine osmolality >700 mOsm/kg (equivalent to specific gravity 1.017) or pH <7. With an automated RBC counter that produces size distribution curves, urine RBC size distribution has been reported less than that of venous RBCs in GN and either greater than that of venous RBCs (nonglomerular) or both (mixed) types in lower GU tract lesions.

Immunocytochemical staining (against human Tamm-Horsfall protein) is positive in >80% of RBCs of renal origin and <13.1% of RBCs of nonrenal origin.

RBC casts or Hb casts indicates blood is of glomerular origin, but their absence does not rule out glomerular disease.

Gross hematuria that is initial suggests origin in urethra distal to urogenital diaphragm; terminal suggests origin in bladder neck or prostatic urethra; total suggests origin in bladder proper or upper urinary tract.

Proteinuria may occur with gross hematuria. In nonglomerular hematuria, sufficient proteinuria to produce 2+ dipstick requires equivalent of 25 mL of blood/L urine (if Hct is normal), which would cause gross hematuria; in glomerular hematuria, proteins filter through glomerulus out of proportion to RBCs. Therefore microscopic hematuria with 2+ protein on dipstick favors glomerular origin; one exception is in papillary necrosis, which may show 2+ proteinuria with nonglomerular type of RBCs.

Pyuria or WBC casts suggest inflammation or infection of GU tract.

Persistent or intermittent hematuria should always be evaluated; one episode of micro-scopic hematuria usually does not require full evaluation (may be due to viral infec-tion, mild trauma, exercise, etc.).

Routine screening of all adults is not recommended.

Interferences

False positive
- Vaginal bleeding
- Factitious
- Bacteriuria (due to catalase production by gram-negative bacteria and *Staphylo-coccus* sp. whose action on dipsticks is similar to that of Hb peroxidase)
- Red diaper syndrome
- Drugs (e.g., rifampin, phenolphthalein, iodides, bromides, copper, oxidizing agents, permanganate)
- Foods (e.g., beets, blackberries, rhubarb)
- Pigmenturia (porphyria, hemoglobinuria, myoglobinuria)
- Oxidizing contaminants (e.g., bacterial peroxidases, povidone, hypochlorite)

False negative
- Reducing agents (e.g., high doses of ascorbic acid [vitamin C])
- pH <5.1

Nonglomerular Hematuria Due To

Trauma

Hemoglobinopathies (especially sickle cell trait and Hb sickle cell disease)

Hypercalciuria

Polycystic disease

GU tract tumors, infections

Some Causes of Hematuria in Adults[4]

	Gross (%)	Microscopic (%)
GU tract cancer	22.5	5.1
Kidney	3.6	0.5
Prostate	2.4	0.5
Ureter	0.8	0.2
Bladder	15	4
Other lesions		
GU tract infection	33	4.3
Calculi	11	5
Benign prostatic hypertrophy	13	13
Renal		2.2
Systemic (e.g., hemophilia, thrombocytopenia, dicumarol overdose)	1	
No source found	8.4	43

Hematuria in Children

Due To

Glomerular

Acute postinfectious GN

Membranoproliferative GN

IgG-IgA nephropathy (Berger's disease)

Hereditary nephritis

SLE

Henoch-Schönlein purpura

Benign familial hematuria

Benign recurrent hematuria

[4]Sutton JM. Evaluation of hematuria in adults. *JAMA* 1990;263:2475.

Nonglomerular
Polycystic kidneys
Renal tumors
Renal TB
Vascular abnormalities (e.g., renal hemangioma, essential hematuria)
Hematologic conditions (e.g., sickle cell trait, coagulation disorders)
Hydronephrosis
GU tract infection, foreign body, calculi, etc. (usually symptomatic)

Hematuria, Benign Familial or Recurrent

Asymptomatic hematuria without proteinuria
Other laboratory and clinical findings are normal.
Renal biopsy is normal on light microscopy, electron microscopy, and immunofluorescence.
Other family members may also have asymptomatic hematuria.
Should gradually clear spontaneously; annual screening for other abnormalities should be performed until condition clears.

Hemoglobinuria

Renal threshold is 100–140 mg/dL plasma.

Use

Confirms hemolyzed blood in urine from either GU tract or intravascular cause.

Due To

Hematuria (due to any cause) with hemolysis in urine
Infarction of kidney
Intravascular hemolysis due to
- Parasites (e.g., malaria, Oroya fever due to *Bartonella bacilliformis*)
- Infection (e.g., *Clostridia*, *Escherichia coli* bacteremia due to transfused blood)
- Antibodies (e.g., transfusion reactions, acquired hemolytic anemia, paroxysmal cold hemoglobinuria, paroxysmal nocturnal hemoglobinuria)
- DIC
- Inherited hemolytic disorders (e.g., sickle cell disease, thalassemias, G-6-PD deficiency, pyruvate kinase deficiency, hereditary spherocytosis)
- Fava bean sensitivity
- Mechanical causes (e.g., prosthetic heart valve)
- Hypotonicity (e.g., transurethral prostatectomy with irrigation of bladder with water, hemodialysis accidents)
- Chemicals (e.g., naphthalene, sulfonamides)
- Thermal burns injuring RBCs
- Strenuous exercise and march hemoglobinuria

Interferences

False-positive (Occultest) results may occur in the presence of pus, iodides, bromides.
Serum is pink due to free Hb but clear due to myoglobin.

Hemosiderinuria

Centrifuged specimen of random urine incubated for 10 mins with Prussian blue stain shows blue granules. Granules are located in cells, but if these have disintegrated, free granules may be predominant.
Normal—absent

Use

Present in intravascular hemolysis even when hemoglobinuria is absent (e.g., paroxysmal nocturnal hemoglobinuria).

URINE

Ketonuria

(Ketone bodies [acetone, beta-hydroxybutyric acid, acetoacetic acid] appear in urine.)

Use

Screen for ketoacidosis, especially in diabetes mellitus when blood is not immediately available
Confirm fasting in testing for insulinoma

Interferences (reagent strips)

False positive
  Drugs (e.g., levodopa)
False negative
  Volatilization of acetone
  Breakdown of acetoacetic acid

Occurs In

Metabolic conditions
  Diabetes mellitus
  Renal glycosuria
  Glycogen storage disease
Dietary conditions
  Starvation
  High-fat diets
Increased metabolic requirements
  Hyperthyroidism
Fever
  Pregnancy and lactation
  Other

Lipuria

Lipids in the urine include all fractions. Double refractile (cholesterol) bodies can be seen. Protein content is high.

Use

Rarely used.

May Occur In

Hyperlipidemia due to
  • Nephrotic syndrome
  • Severe diabetes mellitus
  • Severe eclampsia
Extensive trauma with bone fractures
Phosphorus poisoning
Carbon monoxide poisoning

Melanogenuria

Use

In some patients with malignant melanoma, when the urine is exposed to air for several hours, colorless melanogens are oxidized to melanin, and urine becomes deep brown and later black. Melanogenuria occurs in 25% of patients with malignant melanoma; it is said to be more frequent with extensive liver metastasis. It is not useful for judging completeness of removal or early recurrence.
Is also said to occur in some patients with Addison's disease or hemochromatosis and in intestinal obstruction in black persons.
Confirmatory tests
  • Ferric chloride test

- Thormählen's test
- Ehrlich's test

None of these is consistently more reliable or sensitive than observation of urine for darkening.

Interferences

Beware of false-positive red-brown or purple suspension due to salicylates.

Myoglobinuria

Renal threshold is 20 mg/dL plasma.

Use

Indicates recent necrosis of skeletal or cardiac muscle.

Interpretation

Diagnosis based on
- ♦ • Positive benzidine or *o*-toluidine test of urine, which contains few or no RBCs when urine is red or brown. This is the simplest and most practical initial test. Tests may be positive even when urine is normal in color.
  - Serum is clear (not pink) unless renal failure is present, in contrast to hemoglobinemia.
  - Serum haptoglobin is normal (in contrast to hemoglobinemia).
  - Serum enzymes of muscle origin (e.g., CK) are increased.
- ♦ • Identification of myoglobin in urine by various means.
  - Immunodiffusion is most sensitive and specific.
  - Ultracentrifugation and electrophoresis lack specificity.
  - Spectrophotometry shows similar peaks for myoglobin and hemoglobin.
  - Precipitation by ammonium sulfate may give false-negative results.

Hereditary
- Phosphorylase deficiency (McArdle's syndrome)
- Metabolic defects (e.g., associated with muscular dystrophy)

Sporadic
- Ischemic (e.g., arterial occlusion) (in AMI, levels >5 mg/mL occur within 1–2 hrs and precede ECG and serum CK and CK-MB changes). Has 100% sensitivity but is less specific than CK-MB elevation.
- Crush syndrome.
- Exertional (e.g., exercise, some cases of march hemoglobinuria, electric shock, convulsions, and seizures).
- Metabolic myoglobinuria (e.g., Haff disease, alcoholism, sea snake bite, carbon monoxide poisoning, diabetic acidosis, hypokalemia, malignant hyperpyrexia, systemic infection, barbiturate poisoning).
- ≤50% of patients with progressive muscle disease (e.g., dermatomyositis, polymyositis, SLE, others) in active stage.
- Various drugs and chemicals, especially illicit (e.g., cocaine, heroin, methadone, amphetamines, diazepam, etc.).

Odors (of Urine and Other Body Fluids)

Use

Clue to various metabolic disorders.

Condition	Odor
Maple syrup urine disease	Maple syrup, burned sugar
Oasthouse disease, methionine malabsorption	Brewery, oasthouse
Methylmalonic, propionic, isovaleric, and butyric/hexanoic acidemia	Sweaty feet
Tyrosinemia	Cabbage, fish
Trimethylaminuria	Stale fish
Hypermethioninemia	Rancid butter, rotten cabbage
Phenylketonuria	Musty, mousy

URINE

Ketosis	Sweet
Cystinuria, homocystinuria	Sulfurous

Porphyrinuria

(Due mainly to coproporphyrin)

Use

Porphyrias (see Chapter 12, p. 547)
Lead poisoning
Cirrhosis
Infectious hepatitis
Passive in newborn of mother with porphyria; lasts for several days.

Proteinuria

See Table 14-2 and Fig. 4-3.
See Microalbuminuria, p. 727.

Use

Detection of various renal disorders and Bence Jones proteinuria.

Interpretation

Found in 1–9% of cases on routine screening.
Refers to protein excretion >150 mg/day in adults and >100 mg/day in children <10 yrs or >140 mg/m^2/day. Significant proteinuria is >300 mg/day in adults. >1000 mg/day makes a diagnosis of renal parenchymal disease very likely. >2000 mg/day in adults or >40 mg/m^2 in children usually indicates glomerular etiology. >3500 mg/day or protein/creatinine ratio >3.5 points to a nephrotic syndrome.
When a 24-hr urine specimen cannot be reliably collected, a spot urine for urine protein/creatinine ratio (especially after first morning specimen and before bedtime and if renal function is not severely impaired) often correlate well. Normal value is <0.2 for adults, 0.5 for age 6–24 months, 0.2–0.25 for child >24 months. Low-grade proteinuria = 0.2–1.0. Moderate proteinuria = 1.0–5.0. Value >5 is typical of nephrosis.
Dipstick is sensitive to ~30 mg/dL of protein; 1+ = 100 mg/dL; 2+ = 300 mg/dL; 4+ = 1000 mg/dL; may be falsely negative with predominantly low-molecular-weight or nonalbumin proteins. Positive dipstick should always be followed by sulfosalicylic acid test, which is sensitive to 5–10 mg/dL of protein; may be falsely negative with very alkaline or dilute urine; may be falsely positive due to certain drugs (e.g., radiographic contrast media, high doses of penicillin, chlorpromazine, tolbutamide, sulfa drugs). *When sulfosalicylic acid test shows a significantly higher concentration than the dipstick in an adult, Bence Jones proteinuria should be ruled out. Association with hematuria indicates high likelihood of disease. For detection of proteinuria, sensitivity and specificity = 95–99%; positive predictive value for renal disease = 0–1.4% (in young populations).*
Urine electrophoresis
  Glomerular
    Selective: primarily albumin (>80%) and transferrin (mild renal injury due to dibetes mellitus, immune complex disease, minimal change disease)
    Nonselective: pattern resembles serum. Primary and secondary glomerulonephropathies (diabetes mellitus, amyloidosis, collagen diseases, dysglobulinemia, HUS).
  Tubular: principally alpha$_1$, alpha$_2$, beta, and gamma globulins; albumin is not marked. Most often seen in chronic pyelonephritis, interstitial tubular nephritis, congenital tubular nephropathies, polycystic kidneys, hypercalciuria, acute tubular necrosis due to ischemia or drugs.
  Mixed glomerular-tubular: advanced renal disease involving entire nephron (e.g., chronic renal failure, chronic pyelonephritis)
Dysglobulinemias (see Chapter 11; e.g., multiple myeloma, macroglobulinemia, heavy chain diseases)

Due To

Orthostatic (postural)
  ◆ • First morning urine before arising shows high specific gravity but no protein (protein/creatinine ratio <0.1). Protein appears only after person is upright; usually <1.5 gm/day (protein/creatinine ratio usually 0.1–1.3).

- Urine microscopy is normal.
- Is usually considered benign and slowly disappears with time but is still present in 50% of persons 10 yrs later.
- Progressive renal insufficiency does not occur.
- Occurs in 15% of apparently healthy young men and 3% of otherwise healthy persons and some patients with resolving acute pyelonephritis or GN.
- Renal biopsy, electron microscopy, and immunofluorescent stains show pathologic changes in some patients.

Transient
- Commonly found in routine urinalysis of asymptomatic healthy children and young adults initially but not subsequently.
- Progressive renal disease is not present.
- Functional occurs in 10% of hospital medical patients; associated with high fever, congestive heart failure, hypertension, stress, exposure to cold, strenuous exercise, seizures. Usually <2 gm/day; disappears with recovery from precipitating cause. Progressive renal disease is not present.

Persistent
- Glomerular (composed of large proteins, e.g., albumin, alpha$_1$-antitrypsin, transferrin)

  Idiopathic (e.g., membranoproliferative GN, membranous glomerulopathy, minimal change disease, focal segmental glomerulosclerosis, amyloidosis)

  Secondary

  Infection (e.g., poststreptococcal, hepatitis B, bacterial endocarditis, malaria, infectious mononucleosis, pyelonephritis, etc.)

  Vascular (e.g., thrombosis of inferior vena cava or renal vein, renal artery stenosis)

  Drugs (e.g., nonsteroidal antiinflammatory drugs, heroin, gold, captopril, penicillamine)

  Autoimmune (e.g., SLE, RA, dermatomyositis, polyarteritis, Goodpasture's syndrome, Henoch-Schönlein purpura, ulcerative colitis)

  Neoplasia

  Hereditary and metabolic (e.g., polycystic kidney disease, diabetes mellitus, Fabry's disease, Alport's syndrome of progressive interstitial nephritis and nerve deafness)

- Decreased tubular reabsorption (composed of low-molecular-weight proteins [e.g., alpha and beta microglobulins, free Ig light chains, retinol-binding protein, lysozyme; usually <1.5 gm/day])

  Acquired

  Drugs (e.g., phenacetin, aminoglycoside, cephalosporins, cyclosporine, high-dose analgesics, lithium, methicillin, etc.)

  Heavy metals (e.g., lead, mercury, cadmium)

  Sarcoidosis

  Acute tubular necrosis

  Interstitial nephritis

  Renal tubular acidosis

  Acute and chronic pyelonephritis

  Renal graft rejection

  Balkan nephropathy

  Congenital (e.g., Fanconi's syndrome, oculo-cerebral-renal syndrome)

  Hereditary (e.g., Wilson's disease, sickle cell disease, medullary cystic disease, oxalosis, cystinosis)

- Increased plasma levels of normal or abnormal proteins (e.g., Bence Jones proteins, myoglobin, lysozyme in monocytic or myelocytic leukemias)

Common causes of low-grade proteinuria (<1 gm/24 hrs)

- Kimmelstiel-Wilson syndrome (see p. 727)
- Idiopathic low-grade proteinuria—normal history and physical examination, renal function, and urine sediment with no hematuria.
- Nephrosclerosis
- Polycystic kidney disease
- Medullary cystic disease
- Chronic obstruction of urinary tract
- Chronic interstitial nephritis (e.g., analgesic abuse, uric acid, oxalate, hypercalcemia, hypokalemia, lead, cadmium)

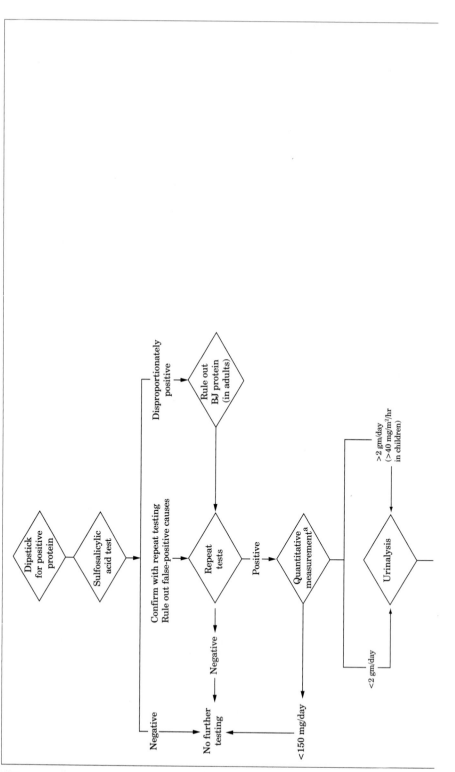

Dipstick
for positive
protein

Sulfosalicylic
acid test

Confirm with repeat testing
Rule out false-positive causes

Disproportionately
positive

Rule out
BJ protein
(in adults)

Negative

Repeat
tests

Positive

Quantitative
measurement[a]

Negative

No further
testing

<150 mg/day

>2 gm/day
(>40 mg/m²/hr
in children)

Urinalysis

<2 gm/day

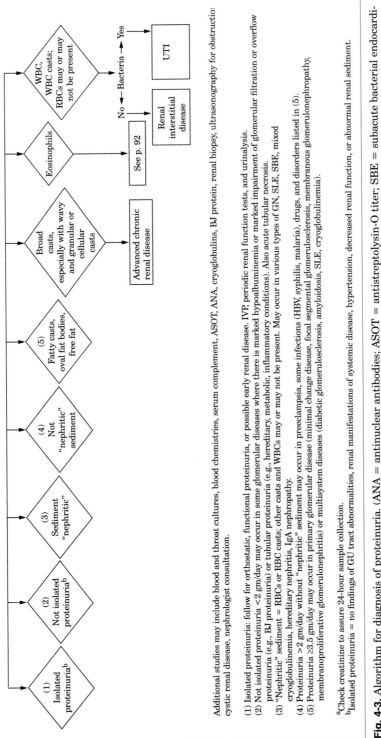

See p. 92

Additional studies may include blood and throat cultures, blood chemistries, serum complement, ASOT, ANA, cryoglobulins, BJ protein, renal biopsy, ultrasonography for obstruction, cystic renal disease, nephrologist consultation.

(1) Isolated proteinuria: follow for orthostatic, functional proteinuria, or possible early renal disease. IVP, periodic renal function tests, and urinalysis.

(2) Not isolated proteinuria <2 gm/day may occur in some glomerular diseases where there is marked hypoalbuminemia or marked impairment of glomerular filtration or overflow proteinuria (e.g., BJ proteinuria) or tubular proteinuria (e.g., hereditary, metabolic, inflammatory conditions). Also acute tubular necrosis.

(3) "Nephritic" sediment = RBCs or RBC casts; other casts and WBCs may or may not be present. May occur in various types of GN, SLE, SBE, mixed cryoglobulinemia, hereditary nephritis, IgA nephropathy.

(4) Proteinuria >2 gm/day without "nephritic" sediment may occur in preeclampsia, some infections (HBV, syphilis, malaria), drugs, and disorders listed in (5).

(5) Proteinuria ≥3.5 gm/day may occur in primary glomerular disease (minimal change disease, focal segmental glomerulosclerosis, membranous glomerulonephropathy, membranoproliferative glomerulonephritis) or multisystem diseases (diabetic glomerulosclerosis, amyloidosis, SLE, cryoglobulinemia).

[a]Check creatinine to assure 24-hour sample collection.
[b]Isolated proteinuria = no findings of GU tract abnormalities, renal manifestations of systemic disease, hypertension, decreased renal function, or abnormal renal sediment.

Fig. 4-3. Algorithm for diagnosis of proteinuria. (ANA = antinuclear antibodies; ASOT = antistreptolysin-O titer; SBE = subacute bacterial endocarditis; HBV = hepatitis B virus; UTI = urinary tract infection.)

URINE

Interferences

False Positive

	Dipstick	Sulfosalicylic Acid
Gross hematuria*	+	+
Highly concentrated urine	+	+
Highly alkaline urine (pH >8) (e.g., GU tract infection with urea-splitting bacteria)	+	−
Antiseptic contamination (e.g., benzalkonium, chlorhexidine)	+	−
Phenazopyridine	+	−
Radiopaque contrast media	−	+
Tolbutamide metabolites	−	+
High levels of cephalosporin or penicillin analogs	−	+
Sulfonamide metabolites	−	+

*Protein excretion >500 mg/m^2/day is significant. With microscopic hematuria, any amount more than an occasional trace of protein is abnormal.

False Negative
Very dilute urine

Bence Jones Proteinuria

Use
Detection of various gammopathies
80% of tests are true positive due to
  • Myeloma (70% of all positive tests)
  • Cryoglobulinemia
  • Waldenström's macroglobulinemia
  • Primary amyloidosis
  • Adult Fanconi's syndrome
  • Hyperparathyroidism
  • Benign monoclonal gammopathy
Approximately 20% of tests are false positive (i.e., urine electrophoresis does not show a spike, and immunoelectrophoresis does not show a monoclonal light chain) due to
  • Connective tissue disease (e.g., RA, SLE, scleroderma, polymyositis, Wegener's granulomatosis)
  • Chronic renal insufficiency
  • Lymphoma and leukemia
  • Metastatic carcinoma of lung, GI, or GU tracts
  • High doses of penicillin and aminosalicylic acid
  • Presence of radiographic contrast media
Positive test for Bence Jones proteinuria by heat test should always be confirmed by electrophoresis and immunoelectrophoresis/immunofiltration of concentrated urine. Heat test is not reliable and should not be used for diagnosis. Dipstick test for albumin does not detect Bence Jones protein.

Beta$_2$-Microglobulin

Normal <1 mg/day by enzyme-linked immunosorbent assay (ELISA) or RIA.

Use

Detection of various renal disorders

Increased In

Tubular disease (>50 mg/day)
  • Heavy metal poisoning (e.g., mercury, cadmium, cisplatin)
  • Drug toxicity (e.g., aminoglycosides, cyclosporine)
  • Hereditary (e.g., Fanconi's syndrome, Wilson's disease, cystinosis)
  • Pyelonephritis

- Renal allograft rejection
- Others (e.g., nephrocalcinosis)

Also increased due to increased production in hepatitis, sarcoidosis, Crohn's disease, vasculitis, and certain malignancies, which prevents diagnostic utility.

Interferences

Need 24-hr timed collection
Unstable at room temperature, with acid urine, and in presence of pyuria

Differentiation

Precipitated by 5% Sulfosalicylic Acid

On boiling, precipitate remains	*On boiling, precipitate disappears*
Albumin	Bence Jones protein
Globulin	A "proteose"
Pseudo–Bence Jones protein	

Precipitated at 40–60°C

Resuspend precipitate in normal urine and equal volume 5% sulfosalicylic acid and boil:

- Precipitate dissolves: Bence Jones protein
- Precipitate does not dissolve: Pseudo–Bence Jones protein

Now replaced by electrophoretic and immunologic procedures.

Globulin (Predominantly) Rather than Albumin

Multiple myeloma
Macroglobulinemia
Primary amyloidosis
Adult Fanconi's syndrome (some patients)

Postrenal Proteinuria

Primarily associated with epithelial tumors of bladder or renal pelvis
Degree of proteinuria related to size and invasiveness; generally <1 gm/day (similar to pyelonephritis) and includes IgM

Renal Diseases in Which Proteinuria May Be Absent

Congenital abnormalities
Renal artery stenosis
Obstruction of GU tract
Pyelonephritis
Stone
Tumor
Polycystic kidneys
Hypokalemic nephropathy
Hypercalcemic nephropathy
Prerenal azotemia

Retinol-Binding Protein

Use

Detection of various renal disorders

Increased In

Proximal tubular dysfunction. Correlates with beta$_2$-microglobulin excretion but not affected by acid urine. More sensitive than N-acetyl-beta-D-glucosaminidase excretion. May show false negative due to low serum level in vitamin A deficiency.

Reducing Substances

Use

Screening for diabetes mellitus (not recommended as primary screening modality due to poor sensitivity)

Interferences (Reagent Strips)

False positive
- Strips exposed to air (uncapped bottles) for a week or more
- Peroxidase contamination
- Oxidizing agents

False negative (found in >1% of routine urine analyses in hospital)
- Ascorbic acid >25 mg/dL
- Drugs (e.g., aspirin)
- Specific gravity >1.020
- High pH

Due To

Glycosuria
- Hyperglycemia
    Endocrine (e.g., diabetes mellitus, pituitary, adrenal, thyroid disease)
    Nonendocrine (e.g., liver, CNS diseases)
    Administration of hormones (e.g., ACTH, corticosteroids, thyroid, epinephrine)
      or drugs (e.g., morphine, anesthetic drugs, tranquilizers)
- Renal
    Tubular origin (serum glucose <180 mg/dL; oral and IV glucose tolerance test
      [GTT] are normal; ketosis is absent)
    Fanconi's syndrome
    Toxic renal tubular disease (e.g., due to lead, mercury, degraded tetracycline)
    Inflammatory renal disease (e.g., acute GN, nephrosis)
    Glomerular due to increased GFR without tubular damage
- Idiopathic

Melituria (5% of cases of melituria in the general population are due to renal glycosuria
  [incidence = 1:100,000], pentosuria [incidence = 1:50,000], essential fructosuria
  [incidence = 1:120,000])
- Hereditary (e.g., galactose, fructose, pentose, lactose)
    Galactose (classic and variant forms of galactosemia). *Galactosuria (in galactosemia) shows a positive urine reaction with Clinitest but negative with Clinistix and Tes-Tape.*
    Fructose (fructosemia, essential fructosuria, hereditary fructose intolerance)
    Lactose (lactase deficiency, lactose intolerance)
    Phenolic compounds (phenylketonuria, tyrosinosis)
    Xylulose (pentosuria)
- Neonatal (e.g., physiologic lactosuria, sepsis, gastroenteritis, hepatitis)
- Lactosuria during lactation
- Xylose (excessive ingestion of fruit)

Non–sugar-reducing substances (e.g., ascorbic acid, glucuronic acid, homogentisic acid,
  salicylates)

Renal Antigens Excretion

(Derived from proximal tubule brush borders)
Low levels in healthy persons

May Be Useful To

Distinguish cases of prerenal azotemia and glomerular disease (with low levels) from
  increased levels in acute renal failure due to proximal tubular disease
Follow course of renal transplant patients
Distinguish pyelonephritis from cystitis

Renal Enzyme Excretion

Lactate Dehydrogenase (LD)

Increased In

Carcinoma of kidney, bladder, and prostate in a high proportion of cases; may be useful for detection of asymptomatic lesions or screening of susceptible population
  groups and differential diagnosis of renal cysts

Other renal diseases
- Active GN, SLE with nephritis, nephrotic syndrome, acute tubular necrosis, diabetic nephrosclerosis, malignant nephrosclerosis, renal infarction
- Active pyelonephritis (25% of patients), cystitis, and other inflammations

Instrumentation of the GU tract (especially cystoscopy with retrograde pyelography); transient increase is <1 wk

AMI and other conditions with considerably increased serum levels

Normal In

Benign nephrosclerosis
Pyelonephritis (most patients)
Obstructive uropathy
Renal stones
Polycystic kidneys
Renal cysts

The test is not useful in routine screening for malignancy of kidney, renal pelvis, and bladder because increased levels suggest GU tract disease but do not indicate its nature. Increased values usually precede clinical symptoms.

Precautions

8-hr overnight urine collection, clean voided to prevent bacterial and menstrual contamination. Refrigerate until analysis is begun. Specimen must be dialyzed to remove inhibitors in urine. Urinalysis should be performed first, because false-positive LD may occur if there are >10 bacteria/HPF or if RBCs or hemolyzed blood is present.

L-Alanine Aminopeptidase

(Derived from proximal tubule brush borders)

Normal is 1500–3700 mU/24 hrs in women and 2000–6000 mU/24 hrs in men. Affected by diuresis and circadian rhythm but not by proteinuria or bacteriuria.

Increased by all types of proximal tubular injury and other renal diseases (e.g., glomerular disease, tumors); consequently, test too sensitive and nonspecific.

N-Acetyl-Beta-D-glucosaminidase

(Derived from proximal tubule lysozymes)

Increased in many types of renal disease causing low specificity; therefore not clinically useful.

Correlates with degree of albuminuria.

Lysozyme

Increased in acute monocytic and myelomonocytic leukemias.

Specific Gravity

Increased In

Proteinuria
Glucosuria
Sucrosuria (see p. 544)
Radiographic contrast medium (frequently 1.040–1.050)
Mannitol
Dextran
Diuretics
Antibiotics
Detergent
Temperature

Urinometer readings should be corrected by adding or subtracting 0.001 to specific gravity reading for each 3°C above or below calibration temperature, respectively. Subtract 0.003 for each 1 gm/dL of protein and 0.004 for each 1 gm/dL of glucose from temperature-compensated specific gravity. For reagent strips, add 0.005 if pH >6.5.

Specific gravity compares mass of a solution to that of an equal volume of water (i.e., it is related to but not an exact measure of number of solute particles); osmolality measures the exact number of solute particles and is a constant weight/weight relationship. Osmolarity is 1 Osm of nonelectrolyte in 1 L of water and varies with the volume-expanding effect of the dissolved substance and the proportional effect of temperature on the fluid volume. Osmolality is the preferred unit of measure.

Decreased volume of concentrated urine (specific gravity >1.030 and osmolality >500 mOsm/kg) is diagnostic of prerenal azotemia.

Urine/plasma osmolality ratio is more accurate than urine osmolality or specific gravity to distinguish prerenal azotemia (with increased ratio) from acute tubular necrosis (with decreased ratio that is rarely >1.5).

See also Urine Concentration and Dilution Tests, p. 706.

Uric Acid/Creatinine Ratio

Ratio >1.0 in most patients with acute renal failure due to hyperuricemia but lower in other causes of acute renal failure.

Urobilinogenuria

Use

Rarely useful instead of blood direct and indirect bilirubin.
Quantitative determination is not as useful as simple qualitative test.

Interferences

False-positive dipstick
    Increased pH
    Some drugs (e.g., procaine, 5-HIAA, sulfonamides)

Increased In

Increased hemolysis (e.g., hemolytic anemias)
Hemorrhage into tissues (e.g., pulmonary infarction, severe bruises)
Hepatic parenchymal cell damage (e.g., cirrhosis, acute hepatitis in early and recovery stages)
Cholangitis

Absent In

Complete biliary obstruction

Volume

Anuria
(Excretion <100 mL/24 hrs)

Due To
Bilateral complete urinary tract obstruction
Acute cortical necrosis
Necrotizing GN
Certain causes of acute tubular necrosis

Acute Oliguria

(Excretion usually <400 mL/24 hrs or ~20 mL/hr; <15–20 mL/kg/24 hrs in children)

Due To
See Acute Renal Failure, p. 739.
Prerenal causes
Postrenal causes
Renal causes
    Glomerular: urine protein >2+ (>1.5 gm/24 hrs), RBCs, RBC casts
    Tubulointerstitial: urine protein ≤ 2+ (≤ 1.5 gm/24 hrs), WBCs, WBC casts

Polyuria
(Normal or increased urine excretion in presence of increasing serum creatinine and BUN)

Due To
Diabetic ketoacidosis
Partial obstruction of urinary tract with impaired urinary concentration function
Some types of acute tubular necrosis (e.g., due to aminoglycosides)

Other Procedures

Urine findings in various diseases: see Table 14-2, p. 712.
See also specific tests on urine in various chapters (e.g., Chapter 7, Gastrointestinal Diseases; Chapter 11, Hematologic Diseases; Chapter 12, Metabolic and Hereditary Diseases; Chapter 13, Endocrine Diseases).

URINE

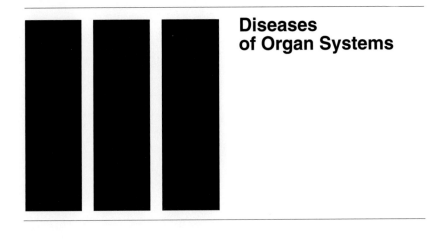

Diseases
of Organ Systems

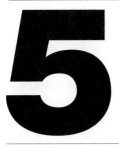

Cardiovascular Diseases

Arrhythmias

Metabolic abnormalities should always be ruled out before performing Holter monitor studies or committing to long-term antiarrhythmic therapy (e.g., hypokalemia, hypomagnesemia, anemia, hypoxemia, hypo- or hyperthyroidism).

Arteriovenous Fistulas, Angiomatous, Congenital

Platelet count may be decreased.

Behçet's Syndrome

(Systemic vasculitis involving arteries and veins characterized by triad of recurrent aphthous ulcers of mouth and genitalia, and relapsing panuveitis.)
No definitive laboratory tests
Laboratory findings due to involvement of various organ systems, e.g.,
   Large vessel occlusion (e.g., aneurysms, arthritis, meningitis) (see p. 268)
   Skin lesions

Churg-Strauss Syndrome (Allergic Granulomatosis and Angiitis)

♦ Biopsy showing granulocytes around an arteriole and venule establishes the diagnosis.[1]
ESR is high.
WBC count is increased.
Eosinophilia is usual and seems to correlate with disease activity.
Serum IgE is often increased.
p-ANCA is found in ≤ 60% of patients. c-ANCA is rare.

Cor Pulmonale

Secondary polycythemia
Increased blood CO_2 when cor pulmonale is secondary to chest deformities or pulmonary emphysema
Laboratory findings of the primary lung disease (e.g., chronic bronchitis and emphysema, multiple small pulmonary emboli, pulmonary schistosomiasis)

Coronary Heart Disease (CHD)

Increased risk factors
- Increased serum total and LDL cholesterol, decreased HDL cholesterol and various ratios (see Chapter 12, pp. 516–525).
- Recent reports suggest that apo A-I and apo B may be better discriminators of CHD than cholesterol, and low ratio of apo A-I to apo B may be best predictor. (Variation in methodology and lack of interlaboratory standardization makes this difficult to evaluate at present.)

---

[1]Included in American College of Rheumatology 1990 criteria for classification of vasculitis. *Arthritis Rheum* 1990;33:1068.

- Atherogenic index (combination of ratio of LDL to HDL × apo B with ratio of apo B to apo A-I) =

$$\frac{(\text{total cholesterol} - \text{HDL}) \times \text{apo B}}{\text{apo A-I} \times \text{HDL}}$$

- Increased serum homocysteine >15.9 μmol/L (normal = 5–15 μmol/L) triples risk of AMI. Each increase of 5 μmol/L increases risk equivalent to increased cholesterol of 20 mg/dL. Increase may be due to vitamin B deficiency or genetic deficiency of methylene-tetrahydrofolate reductase enzyme. Increased in end-stage renal disease dialysis patients and in hypothyroidism, certain drug therapies (e.g., methotrexate [transient], phenytoin and carbamazepine [mild], theophylline, nitrous oxide), cigarette smoking.
- Low plasma vitamin B_{12} and folate levels are each independent risk factors for coronary artery disease.
- Increased serum triglyceride level is a risk factor but may not be independent of other factors.
- Clinical evidence of CHD or atherosclerosis in patient <age 40, family history of premature CHD, hypertension, male gender, smoking.
- Syndrome X: insulin resistance, low HDL level, high level of very low density lipoproteins (VLDLs) and triglycerides.
- Various abnormalities of blood clotting mechanisms (e.g., fibrinogen, factor VII, antithrombin III, phospholipid antibodies, protein C, protein S).

Lipoprotein electrophoresis (see Table 13-6) shows a specific abnormal pattern in <2% of Americans (usually types II, IV). Chief purpose of test is to identify rare familial disorders (I, III, V) to anticipate problems in children.

Lipoprotein electrophoresis may be indicated if serum triglyceride level is >300 mg/dL, fasting serum is lipemic, or hyperglycemia, significant glycosuria, impaired glucose tolerance, or increased serum uric acid (>8.5 mg/dL) is present.

Perform laboratory tests to rule out diabetes mellitus, liver disease, nephrotic syndrome, dysproteinemias, hypothyroidism.

Endocarditis, Bacterial

♦ Blood culture is positive in 80–90% of patients. *Streptococcus viridans* causes 40–50% of cases; *Staphylococcus aureus,* 15–20%; *Streptococcus pneumoniae,* 5%; and *Enterococcus,* 5–10%. Other causes may be gram-negative bacteria (~10% of cases; e.g., *Escherichia coli, Pseudomonas aeruginosa, Klebsiella, Proteus*) and fungi (e.g., *Candida, Histoplasma, Cryptococcus*). *Bartonella* has been reported to cause 3% of cases, which may be culture negative.

♦ In drug addicts, *S. aureus* causes 50–60% of cases and ~80% of tricuspid infections; gram-negative bacteria cause 10–15% of cases; cases due to polymicrobial and unusual organisms appear to be increasing. ≤ 75% of patients may be HIV positive.

♦ *Proper blood cultures require adequate volume of blood, at least five cultures taken during a period of several days with temperature of 101°F or more (preferably when highest), anaerobic as well as aerobic growth, variety of enriched media, prompt incubation, prolonged observation (growth is usual in 1–4 days but may require 2–3 wks).* Beware of negative culture due to recent antibiotic therapy. Beware of transient bacteremia after dental procedures, tonsillectomy, etc., which does not represent bacterial endocarditis (in these cases, streptococci usually grow only in fluid media; in bacterial endocarditis, many colonies also occur on solid media). Blood culture is also negative in bacterial endocarditis due to *Rickettsia burnetii,* but phase 1 complement fixation test is positive.

♦ Positive blood cultures may be more difficult to obtain in prosthetic valve endocarditis (due to unusual and fastidious organisms), right-sided endocarditis, uremia, and long-standing endocarditis. A single positive culture must be interpreted with extreme caution. Aside from the exceptions noted in this paragraph, the diagnosis should be based on two or more cultures positive for the same organism.

Serum bactericidal test measures ability of serial dilutions of patient's serum to sterilize a standardized inoculum of patient's infecting organisms; it is sometimes useful to demonstrate inadequate antibiotic levels or to avoid unnecessary drug toxicity.

Progressive normochromic normocytic anemia is a characteristic feature; in 10% of patients, Hb level is <7 gm/dL. Rarely there is a hemolytic anemia with a positive Coombs' test. Serum iron is decreased. Bone marrow contains abundant hemosiderin.

WBC is normal in ~50% of patients and elevated ≤ 15,000/cu mm in the rest, with 65–86% neutrophils. Higher WBC indicates presence of a complication (e.g., cerebral, pulmonary). Occasionally leukopenia is present. Monocytosis may be pronounced. Large macrophages may occur in peripheral blood.

Platelet count is usually normal, but occasionally it is decreased; rarely purpura occurs.

Serum proteins are altered, with an increase in gamma globulin; therefore positive ESR and tests for cryoglobulins, RF, etc., are found. Often a direct correlation is seen between ESR and course and severity of disease.

Hematuria (usually microscopic) occurs at some stage in many patients due to glomerulitis, renal infarct, or focal embolic GN.

Albuminuria is almost invariably present, even without these complications. Renal insufficiency with azotemia and fixed specific gravity is infrequent now.

Nephrotic syndrome is rare.

CSF findings in various complications, meningitis, brain abscess

Laboratory findings due to underlying or predisposing diseases or complications
- Rheumatic heart disease.
- Congenital heart disease.
- Infection of genitourinary system.
- Congestive heart failure.
- Bacterial endocarditis occurs in ≤ 4% of patients with prosthetic valves.
- Other.

Giant Cell Arteritis (GCA)

(Systemic panarteritis of medium-sized elastic arteries)

♦ Biopsy of involved segment of temporal artery is diagnostic,[1] but negative biopsy does not exclude GCA because of skip lesions. Therefore, surgeon should remove at least 20 mm of artery, paraffin sections of which must be examined at multiple levels. Biopsy findings remain positive for at least 7–14 days after onset of therapy.

○Classic triad of increased ESR (≥ 50 mm/hr),[1] anemia, increased serum ALP is strongly suggestive of GCA.

Mild to moderate normocytic normochromic anemia is present in 20–50% of cases and is rough indicator of degree of inflammation.

ESR is markedly increased in virtually all patients (97%); average Westergren = 107. A normal ESR excludes the diagnosis when little clinical evidence exists for temporal arteritis. CRP test has equal sensitivity.

Serum ALP is slightly increased in ~25% of patients.

WBC is usually normal or slightly increased with shift to the left.

Platelet count may be nonspecifically increased.

Serum protein electrophoresis may show increased gamma globulins. Rouleaux may occur.

Serum CK is normal.

Laboratory findings reflect specific organ involvement.
- Kidney (e.g., GN).
- CNS (e.g., intracerebral artery involvement, which may cause increased CSF protein; stroke; mononeuritis of brachial plexus).
- Heart and great vessels (e.g., myocardial infarction, aortic dissection, Raynaud's disease).
- Mild liver function abnormalities in 20–35% of patients.
- SIADH.
- Microangiopathic hemolytic anemia.
- Polymyalgia rheumatica is presenting symptom in one-third of patients and ultimately develops in 50–90% of cases.

Heart Failure

Renal changes:
- Slight albuminuria (<1 gm/day) is common.

[1]Included in American College of Rheumatology 1990 criteria for classification of vasculitis. *Arthritis Rheum* 1990;33:1068.

- Isolated RBCs and WBCs, hyaline, and (sometimes) granular casts.
- Urine is concentrated, with specific gravity >1.020.
- Phenolsulfonphthalein (PSP) excretion and urea clearance are usually depressed.
- Moderate azotemia (BUN usually <60 mg/dL) is evident with severe oliguria; may increase with vigorous diuresis. *(Primary renal disease is indicated by proportionate increase in serum creatinine and low specific gravity of urine despite oliguria.)*
- Oliguria is a characteristic feature of right-sided failure.

ESR may be decreased because of decreased serum fibrinogen.

Plasma volume is increased. Serum albumin and total protein are decreased, with increased gamma globulin. Hct is slightly decreased, but RBC mass may be increased.

Plasma sodium and chloride tend to fall but may be normal before treatment. Urine sodium is decreased. Total body sodium is markedly increased and potassium is decreased. Plasma potassium is usually normal or slightly increased (because of shift from intracellular location); it may be somewhat reduced with hypochloremic alkalosis due to some diuretics.

Liver function changes (see pp. 217–218).

Laboratory findings due to underlying disease (e.g., rheumatic fever, viral myocarditis, bacterial endocarditis, chronic severe anemia, hypertension, hyperthyroidism, Hurler's syndrome).

- Acidosis (reduced blood pH) occurs when renal insufficiency is associated or CO_2 retention exists due to pulmonary insufficiency, low plasma sodium, or ammonium chloride toxicity.
- Alkalosis (increased blood pH) occurs in uncomplicated heart failure itself, in hyperventilation, in alveolar-capillary block due to associated pulmonary fibrosis, after mercurial diuresis that causes hypochloremic alkalosis, or because of potassium depletion.
- Alkalosis (with normal or increased blood pH) showing increased plasma bicarbonate and moderately increased pCO_2 after acute correction of respiratory acidosis is due to CO_2 retention when there is chloride deficit and usually decreased potassium.

Hypertension

(Present in 18% of adults in the United States)

Systolic hypertension
- Hyperthyroidism
- Chronic anemia with hemoglobin <7 gm/dL
- Arteriovenous fistulas—advanced Paget's disease of bone; pulmonary arteriovenous varix
- Beriberi

Diastolic hypertension
- Hypothyroidism

Systolic and diastolic hypertension
- Essential (primary) hypertension (causes >90% of cases of hypertension).
- Secondary hypertension (causes <10% of cases of hypertension). Laboratory findings due to the primary disease. These conditions are often unsuspected and should always be ruled out, because many of them represent curable causes of hypertension.

Due To

- Endocrine diseases
  - Adrenal
    - Pheochromocytoma (<0.64% of cases of hypertension) (see p. 658)
    - Aldosteronism (<1% of cases of hypertension) (see p. 643)
    - Cushing's syndrome (see p. 649)
    - Congenital adrenal hyperplasia (CAH; see p. 635)
  - Pituitary disease
    - Signs of hyperadrenal function
    - Acromegaly
  - Hyperthyroidism
  - Hyperparathyroidism
- Renal diseases

Vascular (4% of cases of hypertension)
  Renal artery stenosis (usually due to atheromatous plaque in elderly patients
      and to fibromuscular hyperplasia in younger patients) (0.18% of cases of
      hypertension)
  Nephrosclerosis
  Embolism
  Arteriovenous fistula
  Aneurysm
  Aortitis or coarctation of aorta with renal ischemia
Parenchymal
  Glomerulonephritis
  Pyelonephritis
  Polycystic kidneys
  Kimmelstiel-Wilson syndrome
  Amyloidosis
  Collagen diseases
  Renin-producing renal tumor (Wilms' tumor; renal hemangiopericytoma)
  Miscellaneous
  Urinary tract obstructions
• Central nervous system diseases
  Cerebrovascular accident
  Brain tumors
  Poliomyelitis
• Other
  Toxemia of pregnancy
  Polycythemia
  Acute porphyria
• Drugs, toxins
  Oral contraceptives, tricyclic antidepressants
  Lead, alcohol
  Licorice ingestion

In children <18 yrs of age	
Renal disease	61–78%
Cardiovascular disease (e.g., coarctation of aorta)	13–15%
Endocrine (e.g., mineralocorticoid excess, pheochro-mocytoma, hyperthyroidism, hypercalcemia)	6–9%
Miscellaneous (e.g., induced by traction, after GU tract surgery, associated with sleep apnea)	2–7%
Essential	1–16%

In neonates and young infants
  Most common
    Renal artery thrombosis after umbilical artery catheterization
    Coarctation of aorta
    Congenital renal disease
    Renal artery stenosis
  Less common
    Bronchopulmonary dysplasia
    Patent ductus arteriosus
    Intraventricular hemorrhage

Laboratory findings indicating the functional renal status (e.g., urinalysis, BUN, creatinine, uric acid, serum electrolytes, PSP, creatinine clearance, radioisotope scan of
kidneys, renal biopsy). The higher the uric acid in uncomplicated essential hypertension, the less the renal blood flow and the higher the renal vascular resistance.
Laboratory findings due to complications of hypertension (e.g., congestive heart failure, uremia, cerebral hemorrhage, myocardial infarction)
Laboratory findings due to administration of some antihypertensive drugs
  • Oral diuretics (e.g., benzothiadiazines)
      Increased incidence of hyperuricemia (to 65–75% of hypertensive patients from
          incidence of 25–35% in untreated hypertensive patients)
      Hypokalemia
      Hyperglycemia or aggravation of preexisting diabetes mellitus

Less commonly, bone marrow depression, aggravation of renal or hepatic insufficiency by electrolyte imbalance, cholestatic hepatitis, toxic pancreatitis
- Hydralazine
  Long-term dosage of >200 mg/day may produce syndrome not distinguishable from SLE. Usually regresses after drug is discontinued. Antinuclear antibody may be found in ≤ 50% of asymptomatic patients.
- Methyldopa
  ≤ 20% of patients may have positive results on direct Coombs' test, but relatively few have hemolytic anemia. When drug is discontinued, Coombs' test may remain positive for months but anemia usually reverses promptly. Abnormal liver function tests indicate hepatocellular damage without jaundice associated with febrile influenza-like syndrome. RA and SLE tests may occasionally be positive (see Chapter 17). Rarely, granulocytopenia or thrombocytopenia may occur.
- Monoamine oxidase inhibitors (e.g., pargyline hydrochloride)
  Wide range of toxic reactions, most serious of which are
    Blood dyscrasias
    Hepatocellular necrosis
- Diazoxide
    Sodium and fluid retention
    Hyperglycemia (usually mild and manageable by insulin or oral hypoglycemic agents)

When hypertension is associated with decreased serum potassium, rule out
- Primary aldosteronism
- Pseudoaldosteronism (due to excessive ingestion of licorice)
- Secondary aldosteronism (e.g., malignant hypertension)
- Hypokalemia due to diuretic administration
- Potassium loss due to renal disease
- Cushing's syndrome

Kawasaki Syndrome (Mucocutaneous Lymph Node Syndrome)

(Variant of childhood polyarteritis of unknown etiology, with high incidence of cardiac complications; diagnosis is based on clinical criteria)
♦ Diagnosis is confirmed by histologic examination of coronary artery (same as in polyarteritis nodosa).
♦ Laboratory changes due to acute myocardial infarction
Acute phase reactants are increased (e.g., ESR, CRP, alpha-1-antitrypsin); usually return to normal after 6–8 wks.
Leukocytosis (20,000–30,000/cu mm) with shift to left during first week; lymphocytosis thereafter; peaks at end of second week; this is a hallmark of the illness.
Anemia occurs in ~50% of patients; reaches nadir about end of second week; improves during recovery.
CSF shows increased mononuclear cells with normal protein and sugar.
Increased mononuclear cells in urine; dipstick negative.
Increased WBC (predominantly PMNs) in joint fluid in patients with arthritis.

Löffler's Parietal Fibroplastic Endocarditis

○Eosinophilia ≤ 70%; may be absent at first but appears sooner or later.
WBC frequently increased.
Laboratory findings due to frequent
- Mural thrombi in heart and embolization of spleen and lung
- Mitral and tricuspid regurgitation

Myocardial Contusion

(90% due to motor vehicle accident)
♦ Increased serum CK-MB (>3%) alone in 15% of cases; combined with ECG changes in 20% of cases; ECG changes alone in 65% of cases
♦ Increased serum cardiac troponin I (cTnI) implies some myocardial necrosis and differentiates increased CK-MB due to skeletal muscle damage. Specificity = 90% but

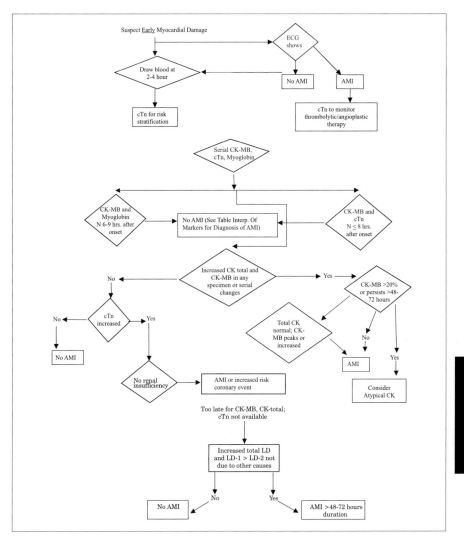

Fig. 5-1. Algorithm for diagnosis of acute myocardial infarction.

sensitivity = only 30% and positive predictive value = only 16%. Cardiac troponin T (cTnT) may be increased due to muscle necrosis.

Myocardial Infarction, Acute (AMI)

See Figs. 5-1 and 5-2 and Tables 5-1, 5-2, and 5-3.

Includes the whole spectrum of acute coronary syndromes, from silent ischemia, unstable angina, and "non–Q wave" infarction, to typical AMI.

◆ Diagnostic Criteria for AMI

Two of the following three findings:
- History of ischemic chest discomfort for ≥ 30 mins
- Characteristic evolution of ECG changes

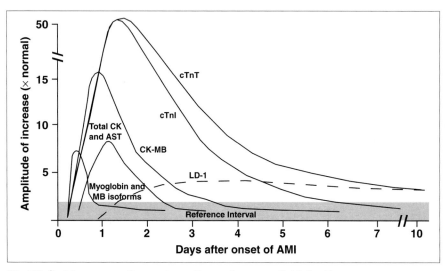

Fig. 5-2. Serial serum cardiac markers after acute myocardial infarction.

- Typical rise and fall of cardiac enzymes. Blood should be drawn promptly after onset of symptoms. Repeat determinations should be made at appropriate intervals (e.g., 4, 8, and 12 hrs) and also if symptoms recur or new signs or symptoms develop. Changes may indicate extension or additional myocardial infarction (MI) or other complications (e.g., pulmonary infarction).

Use of Laboratory Determinations
- For diagnosis when ECG changes are nondiagnostic (occurs in ~50% of AMI patients) on admission to emergency room (e.g., masked by bundle branch block or Wolff-Parkinson-White syndrome) or may not reveal intramural or posterior or lateral infarcts. False-positive ECG occurs in >10–20% of cases.
- For differential diagnosis of chest pain.
- To follow the course of the patient with AMI.
- To estimate prognosis (e.g., marked elevation of serum enzyme [4–5× normal] correlates with increased incidence of ventricular arrhythmia, shock, and heart failure, and with higher mortality).
- For noninvasive assessment of coronary reperfusion after thrombolytic therapy.
- *Utility of each enzyme depends on time of specimen's collection after onset of AMI.*
- Combination of markers (e.g., serum myoglobin, CK-MB, cTn) and (ratios of) serial changes are most effective because of uncertainty as to actual duration of myocardial damage.

Serum Total Creatine Kinase (CK)
Use
- Replaced by serum cTn, CK-MB, myoglobin in various combinations.
- May allow early diagnosis because increased levels appear 3–6 hrs after onset and persist ≤ 48 hrs.
- Sensitive indicator because of large amplitude of change (6–12× normal).
Interpretation
- Serial total CK has sensitivity of 98% early in course of MI but false-positive rate of 15% due to many causes of increased CK.
- Returns to normal by third day; a poorer prognosis is suggested if the increase lasts more than 3–4 days. Reinfarction is indicated by an elevated level after the fifth day after previous return to normal.

Table 5-1. Summary of Increased Serum Marker Levels After Acute
Myocardial Infarction (AMI)

Serum Marker	Earliest Increase (hrs)[a]	Peak (hrs)[a]	Duration of Increase (hrs)[a]	Amplitude of Increase (× normal)	Specificity (%)[b]	Sensitivity at Peak (%)[b]
Troponin T	3–4	10–24	10–14 days		80%	>98%
Troponin I	4–6	10–24	4–7 days		95%	>98%
CK total	4–8	24–36	36–48	6–12	57–88%	93–100%
CK-MB	3–4	15–24	24–36	16	93–100%	94–100%
CK-MB-2/ MB-1	2–4	4–6	16–24		94%	95%
Myoglobin	1–3	6–9	12–24	10	70%	75–95%
CK-MM-3/ MM-1	6	10	~2			
Myosin light chain	3–8	24–35	10–15			
ECG					100%	63–84%
LD[c]	10–12	48–72	11	3	88%	87%
LD-1[c]	8–12	72–144	8–14		85%	40–90%
LD-1/LD-2[c]	>6		>3		94–99%	61–90%
AST[d]	6–8	24–48	4–6	5	48–88%	89–97%
ALT[d]	Usually normal unless liver damage is present (e.g., congestive heart failure)					

High degree of myocardial perfusion in cardiac surgery or contusion patients may lead to earlier and higher peaks and faster washout, causing shorter duration of increased values.
[a]Time periods represent average reported values.
[b]Depends on time after onset of AMI. Sensitivity is lower at earlier or later times after myocardial damage.
[c]Replaced by cardiac troponin for diagnosis of AMI.
[d]Not used for diagnosis of AMI.
Note: Range of reported values because different studies used different time periods after onset of symptoms, size of infarct, benchmarks for establishing the diagnosis, patient populations, instrumentation, etc.

CARDIOVASC

- Useful in differential diagnosis of chest pain due to diseases often associated with MI or difficult to distinguish from MI.

Serial Serum CK-MB Concentrations
Use
- Present gold standard for diagnosis within 24 hrs of onset of symptoms.
- Detect *re*infarction or extension of MI after 72 hrs.
- Document reperfusion after thrombolytic therapy.
Interpretation
◆ • In AMI, CK-MB usually is evident at 4–8 hrs, peaks at 15–24 hrs (mean peak = 16× normal), with sensitivity and specificity each >97% within the first 48 hrs. By 72 hrs, two-thirds of patients still show some increase in CK-MB. More frequent sampling (every 6 hrs) is more likely to identify a peak value. False-negative results may be due to sampling timing (e.g., only once in 24 hrs or sampling <4 hrs or >72 hrs after AMI).

◆ • Diagnosis of AMI is usually confirmed by 8–12 hrs, and sampling beyond 24 hrs is usually not needed except to detect early reinfarction (especially in patients receiving thrombolytic therapy).

◆ • Diagnosis of AMI should not be based on only a single enzyme value. One criterion for AMI is serial CK-MB measurements 4 hrs apart that show ≥ 50% increase with at least one sample greater than upper reference value.

Table 5-2. Interpretation of Markers for Diagnosis of Acute Myocardial Infarction (AMI)

ECG	cTn	CK total	CK-MB	Myoglobin	Interpretation
+	+	+	+	+	AMI.
+	±	±	±	±	AMI. Confirm with cTn for risk stratification and to monitor angioplastic/thrombolytic therapy.
–	+	–	–	–	AMI or unstable angina with increased risk of subsequent coronary event.
–	–	–	+	–	AMI or unstable angina. Confirm with serial CK-MB, ECG, and cTn.
–	+	±	±	±	AMI or unstable angina.
–	–	–	–	+	Follow up cTn or CK-MB to rule out early AMI. See p. 124 for other causes of increased myoglobin.
–	–	+	–	–	Not AMI. See pp. 52–53 for other causes of increased total CK.

+ indicates increased; – indicates not increased.

Table 5-3. Characteristics of Serum Markers for Myocardial Damage

Early appearance: Myoglobin, CK isoforms, glycogen phosphorylase isoenzyme BB, heart fatty acid–binding protein
High specificity: cTnI, cTnT, CK-MB, CK isoforms
Wide diagnostic window: cTnT, cTnI, LD, myosin light and heavy chains
Risk stratification: cTnT, cTnI, CK-MB
Predicts reperfusion: Myoglobin, cTnI, cTnT, CK isoforms
Indicates reinfarction after 2–4 days: CK-MB

◆ • In ~5% of AMI patients (especially in older age groups) a peak CK-MB may be the only abnormality, with total CK and CK-MB still within reference ranges. This is because normal serum total CK values decline with decreased muscle mass (e.g., with age and sedentary or bedridden status).
 • Rapid return to normal makes CK-MB a poor marker >72 hrs after symptoms.
 • Increased CK-MB with normal total CK may indicate non–Q wave AMI.
 • MB index (CK-MB/total CK) should be calculated; normal <2.5. For example, with extreme skeletal muscle injury (e.g., trauma, perioperative condition), total CK may be >4000 U/L and CK-MB may be ≤ 40 U/L.
 • CK-MB should be reported in units as well as percentage, because if injury of both cardiac and skeletal muscle (e.g., perioperative AMI) is present, CK-MB percentage may not appear increased.
 • CK-MB mass immunoassays (preferred method) at 0, 3, and 6 hrs can measure small but significant serial changes that may still be within the normal range. CK-MB mass ≥ 10 μg/L indicates AMI. Serum CK-MB can now be measured directly in the emergency room with or without total CK, cTn, and myoglobin.
 • Thrombolytic therapy should be given within 4–6 hrs of the acute event, at which time CK-MB may not yet be increased. CK-MB, cTn, and myoglobin measured initially and at 60 and/or 90 mins after thrombolytic therapy can document *failed reperfusion*.[2]

[2]Stewart JT, et al. Early noninvasive identification of failed reperfusion after intravenous thrombolytic therapy in acute myocardial infarction. *J Am Coll Cardiol* 1998;31:1499.

		60 min			90 min	
		Sensitivity	**Specificity**		**Sensitivity**	**Specificity**
CK-MB	(1.5)	33%	85%	(5)	82%	66%
	(5)	93%	60%	(10)	91%	49%
cTnT	(1.5)	70%	65%	(5)	82%	67%
	(5)	97%	43%	(10)	95%	58%
Myoglobin	(1.5)	42%	89%	(5)	84%	73%
	(5)	92%	59%	(10)	88%	65%

Numbers in parentheses are ratios of marker values after thrombolytic therapy to pretreatment values.

CK and CK-MB May Also Be Increased In

- Diagnostic value of CK-MB and total CK are diminished after cardiac surgery. A diagnosis of AMI cannot be made until >12–24 hrs after cardiac surgery; typically AMI patients have higher peak values of CK, CK-MB, and myoglobin; patients without AMI have earlier peaks that return to base values more rapidly.
- Increases common after angioplasty of coronary arteries; may indicate reperfusion.
- Cardiac trauma and contusions, electrical injury, and inflammatory myocarditis may produce enzyme changes that cannot be distinguished from those due to AMI. CK-MB and total CK can be increased with long-term exercise and in chronic disease.
- No significant increase after pacemaker implantation or electrical cardioversion.
- If CK-MB is >20% or persists >48–72 hrs, consider atypical CK-MB.
- Other causes of CK and CK-MB changes are noted on pp. 52–54.
- In one protocol the criteria for AMI are an increasing (above reference range) and then decreasing CK total and CK-MB in serial specimens drawn on admission and at 8- or 12-hr intervals; this is considered almost pathognomonic in patients in whom AMI is strongly suspected; no blood need be collected after 48 hrs in patients with uneventful course.
- CK-MB in pericardial fluid may be helpful for postmortem diagnosis of AMI.

Increased Serum Cardiac Troponins T and I

Use
- Increased cTn implies some myocardial necrosis (e.g., anoxia, contusion, inflammation) even without ECG changes.
- Replace LD testing for late diagnosis of AMI. May replace CK-MB as gold standard.
- Risk stratification in patients with chest pain. Sensitive marker for minor myocardial injury in unstable angina without AMI. Patients with chest pain, normal CK-MB, nondiagnostic ECG, and detectable cTn have greater risk of later coronary events.
- Diagnosis of perioperative AMI when CK-MB may be increased by skeletal muscle injury.
- Serial measurements to assess reperfusion after thrombolytic therapy. Peak cTn after reperfusion is related to infarct size.
- Serial values may be indicator of cardiac allograft rejection.

Interpretation
- ◆ • cTn is about as sensitive as CK-MB during first 48 hrs after AMI; sensitivity = 33% from 0 to 2 hrs, 50% from 2 to 4 hrs, 75% from 4 to 8 hrs, and approaches 100% from 8 hrs after onset of chest pain. >85% concordance with CK-MB. Specificity approaches 100%. High sensitivity for 6 days; may remain increased for ~7–10 days.
- With rapid ELISA for cTnT, AMI was present in
    1% of cases with cTnT <0.1 μg/L
    28% of cases with cTnT 0.1–0.19 μg/L
    88% of cases with cTnT 0.2–0.29 μg/L
    100% of cases with cTnT >4.0 μg/L[3]

---

[3]Gerhardt W, et al. An improved rapid troponin T test with a decreased detection limit: a multicentre study of the analytical and clinical performance in suspected myocardial damage. *Scand J Clin Lab Invest* 1997;57:549.

- cTnT may be increased in some patients with skeletal muscle injury, myotonic dystrophy, and chronic renal failure. cTnI is not increased by skeletal muscle injury, which makes it more highly specific for myocardial injury; may be detected in some patients with renal failure.
- Normal values exclude myocardial necrosis in patients with increased CK of skeletal muscle origin (e.g., after arduous physical exercise).
- Not increased by uncomplicated coronary angioplasty or electrical cardioversion.
- Not increased by pulmonary or orthopedic surgery.
- Long duration of increase provides a longer diagnostic window than with CK-MB but may make it difficult to recognize reinfarction.
- cTnI increases ~4–6 hrs after AMI and remains increased for ≤ 7 days. Rapid (20 mins) test kit using whole blood is now available.

Time after symptom onset in AMI	Comparative Sensitivity[4]		
	Rapid cTnI	CK-MB mass	CK-MB activity
3.5±2.7 hrs	60%	48%	36%
4 hrs later	98%	91%	61%
Unstable angina	38%	4%	2%

Serum Myoglobin

Use
- Earliest marker for AMI

♦ Interpretation
Increased within 1–3 hrs in >85% of AMI patients, peaks in ~8–12 hrs (may peak within 1 hr) to ~10× upper reference limit, and becomes normal in ~24–36 hrs or less; reperfusion causes peak 4–6 hrs earlier.
- May precede release of CK-MB by 2–5 hrs.
- Sensitivity >95% within 6 hrs of onset of symptoms.
- Myoglobinuria often occurs (see p. 99).

Disadvantages
- Two or three blood samples should be drawn at ~1-hr intervals (myoglobin may be released in multiple short bursts).
- Wide normal range (6–90 ng/mL).
- Low specificity for AMI (may also be increased in renal failure, shock, open heart surgery, and skeletal muscle damage or exhaustive exercise, or in patients and carriers of progressive muscular dystrophy, but not by cardioversion, cardiac catheterization, or congestive heart failure). Values are usually much higher in patients with uremia and muscle trauma than in those with AMI.

CK Isoforms

CK-MB and CK-MM are sequentially converted in the serum by a carboxypeptidase (CK-MM→MM-3→MM-2→MM-1; CK-MB→MB-2→MB-1).

Interpretation
♦ • CK-MM and CK-MB isoforms parallel CK-MB but rise and peak earlier. MB-2/MB-1 and MM-3/MM-1 isoform ratios appear to be the most useful, but methodology for rapid turnaround time is not widely available. Because serum MM-3 is normally so low, its release from damaged cardiac muscle is readily evident.
- Diagnostic MM isoform changes are independent of amount of tissue damage, whereas total CK activity depends on infarct size.
- MM-3/MM-1 isoform ratio shows a large change because MM-1 is continually cleared from the blood. Ratio is ~1.3 in controls but >14 in AMI patients (1.0 is a useful cutoff value).
- MB-2 >1.0 U/L and MB-2/MB-1 ratio >1.5 (normal ratio = 1) is specific for AMI within 4–8 hrs of infarct. Ratio is >1.5 within 2–4 hrs in >50% of cases, within 4–6 hrs in 92%, and by 8 hrs in 100%. MB-2/MB-1 ratio ≤ 1.0 by 4–6 hrs or normal CK-MB by 10 hrs rules out AMI in 95% of cases.
- MM-3 and MM-3/MM-1 ratio also increase 2 hrs after intense brief exercise and in marathon runners.

---

[4]Heeschen C, et al. Analytical performance and clinical application of new rapid bedside assay for the detection of serum cardiac troponin I. *Clin Chem* 1998;44:1925.

- CK-MB subforms may also be increased in severe skeletal muscle damage (e.g., rhabdomyolysis) and muscular dystrophy.
- Isoform ratios return to normal by 24 hrs in most patients.

Glycogen Phosphorylase BB

Use
- More sensitive early marker for AMI and unstable angina within 4 hrs after onset of pain than is CK-MB, cTnT, or myoglobin
- Sensitive marker of perioperative myocardial injury in coronary artery bypass surgery

Interpretation
- Returns to normal within 24–36 hrs.
- Not widely available. Additional studies are needed.

Also being investigated are serum cardiac myosin heavy and light chains, fatty acid–binding protein, alpha-actin, calcitonin gene-related peptide.

Serum Lactate Dehydrogenase (LD)

Use
- Replaced by cTn.
- Prolonged elevation lasting 10–14 days was formerly used for late diagnosis.

Interpretation
- Increases in 10–12 hrs, peaks in 48–72 hrs (~3× normal).
- Increased CK-MB and LD-1/LD-2 ratio >1 ("flipped" LD) both within 48 hrs (not necessarily at the same time) is virtually diagnostic of AMI.
- Increased total LD with flipped LD may also occur in acute renal infarction, hemolysis (e.g., hemolytic anemia, pernicious anemia, prosthetic heart valves), some muscle disorders (e.g., polymyositis, muscular dystrophies, rhabdomyolysis), pregnancy, some neoplasms (e.g., small cell of lung, prostate, testicular germ cell); LD >2000 U suggests a poorer prognosis.

Serum Aspartate Aminotransferase (AST)

Use
- Replaced by other enzymes in diagnosis of AMI.

Interpretation
- AST is increased in >95% of the patients when blood is drawn at the appropriate time.
- Increase appears within 6–8 hrs, peaks in 24 hrs; level usually returns to normal in 4–6 days.
- Peak level is usually ~200 U (5× normal). Value >300 U and a more prolonged increase suggest a poorer prognosis.
- Reinfarction is indicated by a rise that follows a return to normal.

Serum ALT is usually not increased unless there is liver damage due to congestive heart failure, drug therapy, etc.

Serum ALP (from vascular endothelium) is increased during reparative phase (4–10 days after onset). Serum GGT is also increased.

Leukocytosis is almost invariable; commonly detected by second day but may occur as early as 2 hrs. WBC is usually 12,000–15,000; ≤ 20,000 is not rare; sometimes it is very high. Usually 75–90% PMNs with only a slight shift to the left. Leukocytosis is likely to develop before fever.

ESR is increased, usually by second or third day (may begin within a few hrs); peak rate is in 4–5 days, persists for 2–6 mos. ESR is sometimes more sensitive than WBC, as increase may occur before fever and persists after temperature and WBC have returned to normal. Degree of ESR increase does not correlate with severity or prognosis.

CRP is usually normal in unstable angina patients who have a normal cTnT (<0.1 μg/L). Peak CRP correlates with peak CK-MB.

Blood lactate is increased; sensitivity = 55%, specificity = 96% in patients presenting with acute chest pain.

Glycosuria and hyperglycemia occur in ≤ 50% of patients.

Glucose tolerance is decreased.

Laboratory findings due to underlying coronary heart disease.

Laboratory findings due to sequelae (e.g., congestive heart failure).

CARDIOVASC

Myocarditis, Viral

(Routine autopsy incidence of 1.2–3.5%)

Due To

Coxsackievirus B (causes most cases in United States) and coxsackievirus A, echovirus, poliomyelitis, influenza A and B, cytomegalovirus (CMV), EBV, adenovirus, rubeola, mumps, rubella, variola, vaccinia, varicella-zoster virus (VZV), rabies, lymphocytic choriomeningitis, chikungunya, dengue, yellow fever
♦ Serologic tests for viral antigen, IgM antibody, or changed titer using acute and convalescent paired sera
♦ Endomyocardial biopsy of right ventricular muscle showing >5 lymphocytes/HPF and degeneration of muscle fibers has become major diagnostic tool to establish diagnosis of myocarditis and rules out other lesions (e.g., sarcoidosis).
Increased serum markers of myocardial damage is common only in early stages
  • cTn sensitivity = 53%, specificity = 93%
  • CK-MB and CK total <10% sensitivity
Increased acute phase reactants (e.g., ESR, CRP, mild to moderate leukocytosis)

Myxoma of Left Atrium

○Anemia that is hemolytic in type and mechanical in origin (due to local turbulence of blood) should be sought and may be severe. Bizarre poikilocytes may be seen in blood smear. Reticulocyte count may be increased. Other findings may reflect effects of hemolysis or compensatory erythroid hyperplasia. The anemia is recognized in ~50% of patients with this tumor. Increased serum LD reflects hemolysis.
Serum gamma globulin is increased in ~50% of patients. IgG may be increased.
Increased ESR is a reflection of abnormal serum proteins.
Platelet count may be decreased (possibly the cause here also is mechanical) with resultant findings due to thrombocytopenia.
Negative blood cultures differentiate this tumor from bacterial endocarditis.
Occasionally WBC is increased, and CRP may be positive.
Laboratory findings due to complications
  • Emboli to various organs (increased AST may reflect many small emboli to striated muscle)
  • Congestive heart failure
These findings are reported much less frequently in myxoma of the right atrium, which is more likely to be accompanied by secondary polycythemia than by anemia.

Pericardial Effusion, Chronic

See Table 6-2 on body fluids.
Laboratory findings due to underlying disease (e.g., TB, myxedema, metastatic tumor, uremia, SLE). Rarely due to severe anemia, scleroderma, polyarteritis nodosa, Wegener's granulomatosis, RA, irradiation therapy, mycotic or viral infections, primary tumor of heart, African endomyocardial fibrosis, idiopathic causes.

Pericarditis, Acute

Laboratory Findings Due to Primary Disease

Active rheumatic fever (40% of patients)
Bacterial infection (20% of patients)
Other infections (e.g., viral [especially coxsackievirus B], rickettsial, parasitic, mycobacterial, fungal)
  Viruses are most common infectious causes.
Uremia (11% of patients)
Benign nonspecific pericarditis (10% of patients)
Neoplasms (3.5% of patients)
Collagen disease (e.g., SLE, polyarteritis nodosa) (2% of patients)
Acute myocardial infarction, postcardiac injury syndrome

Trauma
Myxedema
Others (e.g., hypersensitivity, unknown origin or in association with various syndromes)
WBC is usually increased in proportion to fever; normal or low in viral disease and
tuberculous pericarditis; markedly increased in suppurative bacterial pericarditis
Examination of aspirated pericardial fluid (see Table 6-1)

Phlebothrombosis

Tests indicate recent extensive clotting of any origin (e.g., postoperative status).
- D-dimer test (see Pulmonary Embolism and Infarction, pp. 154–155).
- Staphylococcal clumping test measures breakdown products of fibrin in serum;
  these indicate the presence of a clot that has begun to dissolve. Sensitivity = 88%,
  specificity = 66% using venography as gold standard.
- Serial dilution protamine sulfate test measures the presence of a fibrin monomer
  that is one of the polymerization products of fibrinogen. It is less sensitive than
  the staphylococcal clumping test but indicates clotting earlier.
Laboratory findings of pulmonary infarction (see pp. 154–155) should be sought as evidence of embolization.

Polyarteritis Nodosa

♦ Tissue biopsy is basis for diagnosis
- Findings on biopsy of small or medium-sized artery.
- Findings in random skin and muscle biopsy are confirmatory in 25% of patients;
  most useful when taken from area of tenderness; if no symptoms are present, pec-
  toralis major is the most useful site.
- Testicular biopsy is useful when local symptoms are present.
- Lymph node and liver biopsies are usually not helpful.
- Renal biopsy is not specific; often shows glomerular disease.
Increased BUN or creatinine; uremia occurs in 15% of patients.
Hepatitis B surface antigen (HBsAg) is present in 20–40% of adult patients.
p-ANCA is positive in 70% of patients; rarely reflects disease activity.
Increased WBC (≤ 40,000/cu mm) and PMNs. A rise in eosinophils takes place in 25%
of patients and is sometimes very marked; it usually occurs in patients with pul-
monary manifestations.
ESR and CRP are increased.
Mild anemia is frequent; it may be hemolytic anemia with positive Coombs' test.
Urine is frequently abnormal.
- Albuminuria (60% of patients)
- Hematuria (40% of patients)
- "Telescoping" of sediment (variety of cellular and noncellular casts)
Serum globulins are increased.
Abnormal serum proteins occasionally occur. Biological false-positive test for syphilis,
circulating anticoagulants, cryoglobulins, macroglobulins, etc., occurs.
Laboratory findings due to organ involvement by arteritis may be present (e.g., GU,
pulmonary, GI, neurologic in >75% of patients).

Prosthetic Heart Valves

Complications
- Hemolysis—increased serum LD, decreased haptoglobin, reticulocytosis are usual.
  Severe hemolytic anemia is uncommon and suggests leakage due to partial dehis-
  cence of valve or infection.
- Prosthetic valve infection
  Early (<60 days after valve replacement)—usually due to *Staphylococcus epi-
  dermidis*, *S. aureus*, gram-negative bacteria, diphtheroids, fungi; occasion-
  ally due to *Mycobacteria* and *Legionella*. 30–80% mortality.
  Late (>60 days postoperatively)—usually due to streptococci. *S. epidermidis* is
  common up to 12 mos after surgery. 20–40% mortality.
♦ • Blood culture positive in >90% of patients unless received antibiotic therapy, infection involves fastidious organism (e.g., HACEK [*Haemophilus-Actinobacillus-Car-*

diobacterium-Eikenella-Kingella]), or identification requires special technique (e.g., *Rickettsia*, fungi, mycobacteria, *Legionella*).

Surgery is indicated if blood culture is positive after 5 days of appropriate antimicrobial therapy or infection is recurrent. Infection with organisms other than *Streptococcus* usually require valve replacement.

- Complications of anticoagulant therapy

Rheumatic Fever, Acute[5]

♦ Increased serum cTn implies some myocardial necrosis due to myocarditis.

♦ Laboratory confirmation of preceding group A streptococcal infection
- Increased titer of antistreptococcal antibodies
- Positive throat culture for group A *Streptococcus* and recent scarlet fever
- Serologic tests—see below

♦ Serologic titers: one of the following is elevated in 95% of patients with acute rheumatic fever; if all are normal, a diagnosis of rheumatic fever is less likely. (See p. 38.)

ASOT increase indicates recent group A *Streptococcus* pharyngitis within the last 2 mos. Increased titer develops only after the second week and reaches a peak in 4–6 wks. Increasing titer is more significant than a single determination. Titer is usually >250 U; more significant if >400–500 U. A normal titer helps to rule out clinically doubtful rheumatic fever. Sometimes ASOT is not increased even when other titers are increased. Height of titer is not related to severity; rate of fall is not related to course of disease.

Anti–DNase B assay should also be performed because >15% of patients with acute rheumatic fever do not have an increased ASOT. This assay is superior to ASOT in detecting antibodies after group A streptococcal skin infections and is less prone to false-positive reactions; longer period of reactivity is helpful in patients with isolated chorea or carditis, who may have a long latent period before manifesting rheumatic fever during which ASOT may have returned to normal.

Antihyaluronidase titer of 1000–1500 U follows recent group A streptococcal disease and ≤ 4000 U with rheumatic fever. Average titer is higher in early rheumatic fever than in subsiding or inactive rheumatic fever or nonrheumatic streptococcal disease or nonstreptococcal infections. Antihyaluronidase titer is increased as often as ASOT and antifibrinolysin titer.

Antifibrinolysin (antistreptokinase) titer is increased in rheumatic fever and in recent hemolytic streptococcus infections.

♦ Acute phase reactants (ESR, CRP, increased WBC) are minor manifestations.
- ESR increase is a sensitive test of rheumatic activity; ESR returns to normal after adequate treatment with ACTH or salicylates. It may remain increased after WBC becomes normal. It is said to become normal with onset of congestive heart failure even in the presence of rheumatic activity. It is normal in uncomplicated chorea alone.
- CRP parallels ESR.
- WBC may be normal but usually is increased (10,000–16,000/cu mm) with shift to the left; increase may persist for weeks after fever subsides. Count may decrease with salicylate and ACTH therapy.

Serum proteins are altered, with decreased serum albumin and increased $alpha_2$ and gamma globulins. (*Streptococcus group A infections do not increase $alpha_2$ globulin.*) Fibrinogen is increased.

Anemia (Hb usually 8–12 gm/dL) is common; gradually improves as activity subsides; microcytic type. Anemia may be related to increased plasma volume that occurs in early phase of acute rheumatic fever.

Urine: A slight febrile albuminuria is present. Often mild abnormality of protein, casts, RBCs, WBCs indicates mild focal nephritis. Concomitant GN appears in ≤ 2.5% of cases.

[5]Special Writing Group, Committee on Rheumatic Fever, Endocarditis, and Kawasaki Disease, Council on Cardiovascular Disease in the Young, American Heart Association. Guidelines for the diagnosis of rheumatic fever: Jones Criteria, 1992 update. *JAMA* 1992;268:2069.

Blood cultures are usually negative. Occasional positive culture is found in 5% of patients (bacteria usually grow only in fluid media, not on solid media), in contrast to bacterial endocarditis.

Throat culture is often negative for group A streptococci.

Serum AST may be increased, but ALT is normal unless the patient has cardiac failure with liver damage.

Determine clinical activity—follow ESR, CRP, and WBC. Return to normal should be seen in 6–12 wks in 80–90% of patients; it may take ≤ 6 mos. Normal findings do not prove inactivity if patient is receiving hormone therapy. When therapy is stopped after findings have been suppressed for 6–8 wks, a mild rebound may be seen for 2–3 days followed by a return to normal. Relapse after cessation of therapy occurs within 1–8 wks.

Shock

Leukocytosis is common, especially with hemorrhage. Leukopenia may be present when shock is severe, as in gram-negative bacteremia. Circulating eosinophils are decreased.

Hemoconcentration (e.g., dehydration, burns) or hemodilution (e.g., hemorrhage, crush injuries, and skeletal trauma) takes place.

Acidosis appears when shock is well developed, with increased blood lactate, low serum sodium, low CO_2-combining power with decreased alkaline reserve.

Blood pH is usually relatively normal but may be decreased. BUN and creatinine may be increased.

Serum potassium may be increased.

Hyperglycemia occurs early.

Urine examination
- Volume: Normovolemic patients have output ≥ 50 mL/hr; cause should be investigated if <25–30 mL/hr. In hypovolemia, normal kidney may lower 24-hr urine output to 300–400 mL.
- Specific gravity: >1.020 with low urine output suggests patient is fluid depleted. <1.010 with low urine output suggests renal insufficiency. Specific gravity depends on weight rather than concentration of solutes; therefore it is more affected than osmolarity by high-molecular-weight substances such as urea, albumin, and glucose.
- Osmolarity: Hypovolemia is suggested by high urine osmolarity and urine-plasma osmolarity ratio of ≥ 1:2. Renal failure is suggested by low urine osmolarity with oliguria and urine/plasma osmolarity ratio of ≤ 1:1.

Systemic Capillary Leak Syndrome[6]

(Very rare recurring idiopathic disorder in adults with sudden transient extravasation of <70% of plasma; very high morbidity and mortality; hypotension is part of triad)

Hemoconcentration (e.g., leukocytosis; Hb may be ~25 gm/dL)

Hypoalbuminemia

Monoclonal gammopathy (especially IgG with kappa or lambda light chain) without evidence of multiple myeloma is often present. Some patients may progress to multiple myeloma.

Laboratory findings due to complications (e.g., rhabdomyolysis, acute tubular necrosis, pleural/pericardial effusion)

Takayasu's Syndrome (Arteritis)

Increased ESR in ~75% of cases during active disease but normal in only one-half during remission

WBC usually normal

Serum proteins abnormal with increased gamma globulins (mostly composed of IgM)

Female patients have a continuous high level of urinary total estrogens (rather than the usual rise during luteal phase after a low excretion during follicular phase).

Laboratory tests not useful for diagnosis or to guide management.
- ◆ Diagnosis is established by characteristic arteriographic changes or histologic examination.

[6]Tahirkheli NK, Greipp PR. Treatment of the systemic capillary leak syndrome with terbutaline and theophylline. *Ann Intern Med* 1999;130:905.

CARDIOVASC

Thromboangiitis Obliterans (Buerger's Disease)

(Vascular inflammation and occlusion of intermediate-sized arteries and veins of extremities)
Laboratory tests are usually normal.

Thrombophlebitis, Septic

Laboratory findings due to associated septicemia
* Increased WBC (often >20,000/cu mm) with marked shift to left and toxic changes in neutrophils.
* DIC may be present (see p. 464).
* Respiratory alkalosis due to ventilation-perfusion abnormalities with hypoxia. Significant acidosis indicates shock.
* Azotemia.
* Positive blood culture (*S. aureus* is most frequent organism; others are *Klebsiella, Pseudomonas aeruginosa,* enterococci, *Candida*).
Laboratory findings due to complications (e.g., septic pulmonary infarction)
Laboratory findings due to underlying disease

Transplant Rejection (Acute) of Heart

♦ Endocardial biopsy to determine acute rejection and follow effects of therapy has no substitute.
Increasing ESR and WBC
Increased isoenzyme LD-1 as amount (>100 IU) and percentage (35%) of total LD during first 4 wks after surgery
These findings are reversed with effective immunosuppressive therapy. Total LD continues to be increased even when LD-1 becomes normal.
Chronic rejection is accelerated coronary artery atherosclerosis.

Valvular Heart Disease

Laboratory findings due to associated or underlying or predisposing disease (e.g., syphilis, rheumatic fever, carcinoid syndrome, genetic disease of mucopolysaccharide metabolism, congenital defects)
Laboratory findings due to complications (e.g., heart failure, bacterial endocarditis, embolic phenomena)

Vasculitis, Classification

By Etiology

Primary
* Polyarteritis nodosa
* Wegener's granulomatosis
* Giant cell arteritis
* Hypersensitivity vasculitis
Secondary
* Infections
    Bacteria (e.g., septicemia due to *Gonococcus* or *Staphylococcus*)
    Mycobacteria
    Viruses (e.g., CMV, HBV)
    Rickettsia (e.g., Rocky Mountain spotted fever)
    Spirochetes (e.g., syphilis, Lyme disease)
* Associated with malignancy (e.g., multiple myeloma, lymphomas)
* Connective tissue diseases
    RA
    SLE
    Sjögren's syndrome
* Diseases that may simulate vasculitis (e.g., ergotamine toxicity, cholesterol embolization, atrial myxoma)

By Size of Involved Vessel (Noninfectious Vasculitis)

Large vessel
  • Takayasu's arteritis
  • Giant cell (temporal) arteritis
Medium-sized vessel
  • Polyarteritis nodosa
  • Kawasaki's disease
  • Primary granulomatous CNS vasculitis
Small vessel
  • ANCA-associated vasculitis
      Wegener's granulomatosis
      Churg-Strauss syndrome
      Drug induced
      Microscopic polyangiitis
  • Immune complex–type vasculitis
      Henoch-Schönlein purpura
      Cryoglobulinemia
      Rheumatoid vasculitis
      SLE
      Sjögren's syndrome
      Goodpasture's syndrome
      Behçet's disease
      Drug induced
      Serum sickness
  • Paraneoplastic vasculitis (lymphoproliferative, myeloproliferative, carcinoma)
  • Inflammatory bowel disease

Wegener's Granulomatosis[7]

(Necrotizing granulomatous vasculitis affecting respiratory tract; disseminated form shows renal involvement)
♦ Diagnosis is established by biopsy of affected tissue with cultures and special stains that exclude mycobacterial and fungal infection.

Antineutrophil Cytoplasmic Antibodies (ANCA)

Use
Aid in diagnosis and classification of various vasculitis-associated and autoimmune disorders.

Interpretation
♦ **c-ANCA** (anti-proteinase 3; coarse diffuse cytoplasmic pattern) is highly specific (>90%) for active Wegener's granulomatosis. Sensitivity >90% in systemic vasculitic phase, ~65% in predominantly granulomatous disease of respiratory tract, ~30% during complete remission. Height of ELISA titer does not correlate with disease activity; high titer may persist during remission for years. Also occasionally found in other vasculitides (polyarteritis nodosa, microscopic polyangiitis [e.g., lung, idiopathic crescentic and pauci-immune GN], Churg-Strauss vasculitis).

p-ANCA (against various proteins [e.g., myeloperoxidase, elastase, lysozyme], perinuclear pattern) occurs only with fixation in alcohol, not formalin. Positive result should be confirmed by ELISA. Has poor specificity and 20–60% sensitivity in a variety of autoimmune diseases (microscopic polyangiitis, Churg-Strauss vasculitis, SLE, inflammatory bowel disease, Goodpasture's syndrome, Sjögren's syndrome, idiopathic GN, chronic infection). However, pulmonary small vessel vasculitis is strongly linked with myeloperoxidase antibodies.

Both p-ANCA and c-ANCA may be found in non–immune mediated polyarteritis and other vasculitides.

Atypical pattern (neither c-ANCA or p-ANCA; unknown target antigens) has poor specificity and unknown sensitivity in various conditions (e.g., HIV infection, endocarditis, cystic fibrosis, Felty's syndrome, Kawasaki syndrome, ulcerative colitis, Crohn's disease).

[7]Included in American College of Rheumatology 1990 criteria for classification of vasculitis. *Arthritis Rheum* 1990;33:1068.

CARDIOVASC

Laboratory findings reflecting specific organ involvement
- Kidneys—renal disease in ~80% of cases. Hematuria (>5 RBCs/HPF), proteinuria, azotemia. Nephrosis or chronic nephritis may occur. Most patients develop renal insufficiency. Biopsy most frequently shows focal necrotizing GN with crescent formation; coarse granular pattern with immunofluorescent staining. Biopsy is important to define extent of disease.
- CNS.
- Respiratory tract.
- Heart.

Nonspecific laboratory findings
- Normochromic anemia, thrombocytosis, and mild leukocytosis occur in 30–40% of patients; eosinophilia may occur but is not a feature. Leukopenia or thrombocytopenia occur only during cytotoxic therapy.
- ESR is increased in 90% of cases, often to very high levels; CRP level correlates with disease activity even better than ESR.
- Serum globulins (IgG and IgA) are increased in up to 50% of cases.
- Serum C3 and C4 complement levels may be increased.
- RF may be present in low titer in two-thirds of cases.
- ANA is negative.

Laboratory findings due to secondary infection (usually staphylococcal) of sinus, mucosal, pulmonary lesions.

Laboratory findings due to therapy (e.g., bladder cancer and sterility due to cyclophosphamide therapy).

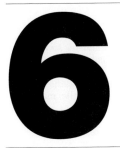

Respiratory Diseases

Laboratory Tests for Respiratory System Disease

Bronchoscopy and Bronchoalveolar Lavage (BAL)[1]
(Saline lavage of lung subsegment via fiberoptic bronchoscope)

Use

For biopsy of endobronchial tumor in which obstruction may cause secondary pneumonia with effusion but still a resectable tumor

To obtain bronchial washings for
- Diagnosis of nonresectable tumors that may be treated with radiation (e.g., oat cell carcinoma, Hodgkin's disease), metastatic tumors, peripheral lesions that cannot be reached by bronchoscope.
- Diagnosis of pulmonary infection, especially when sputum examination is not diagnostic. Quantitative bacterial culture and cytocentrifugation for staining slides provides overall diagnostic accuracy of 79% for pulmonary infection. Negative predictive value = 94%.

Giemsa stain
- Healthy persons show <3% neutrophils, 8–18% lymphocytes, 80–89% alveolar macrophages.
- >10% neutrophils: indicates acute inflammation (e.g., bacterial infection, including Legionella, acute respiratory distress syndrome [ARDS], drug reaction).
- >1% squamous epithelial cells: indicates that a positive culture may reflect saliva contamination.
- >80% macrophages: common in pulmonary hemorrhage. Aspergillosis is the only infection associated with significant alveolar hemorrhage, which may also be found in >10% of patients with hematologic malignancies.
- >30% lymphocytes: may indicate hypersensitivity pneumonitis (often up to 50–60% with more cytoplasm and large irregular nucleus).
- >10% neutrophils and >3% eosinophils: characteristic of idiopathic pulmonary fibrosis; alveolar macrophages predominate. Lymphocyte percentage may be increased.
- >10^5 colony-forming bacteria/mL indicates bacterial infection if <1% squamous epithelial cells are present on Giemsa stain.

Gram stain
- Many bacteria suggests bacterial infection if there are <1% squamous epithelial cells, especially if culture shows >10^4 bacteria/mL.
- No bacteria suggests that bacterial infection is unlikely but *Legionella* should be ruled out with direct fluorescent antibody (DFA) test if Giemsa stain shows increased neutrophils.
- Combined with methenamine silver or Pap stain, 94% sensitivity for diagnosis of *Pneumocystis* infection; increased to 100% when BAL is combined with transbronchial biopsy.

Acid-fast stain: positive result may indicate *Mycobacterium tuberculosis* or *Mycobacterium avium-intracellulare* infection.

RESPIRATORY

---

[1]Kahn FW, Jones JM. Bronchoalveolar lavage in the rapid diagnosis of lung disease. *Lab Manage* June 1986:31.

Toluidine blue stain: may show *Pneumocystis carinii* cysts in *Pneumocystis* pneumonia or *Aspergillus* hyphae in immunocompromised host with invasive aspergillosis.

Prussian blue–nuclear red stain: strongly positive result indicates severe alveolar hemorrhage; moderately positive indicates some hemorrhage; absent indicates no evidence of alveolar hemorrhage.

DFA stain for *Legionella*, herpes simplex virus (HSV) I and II (stains bronchial epithelial cells and macrophages), and CMV (stains mononuclear cells) may indicate infection with corresponding organism.

Pap stain: atypical cytology may be due to cytotoxic drugs, radiation therapy, viral infection (intranuclear inclusions of herpesvirus or CMV), tumor.

Oil red O stain: shows many large intracellular fat droplets in one-third to two-thirds of cells in some patients with fat embolism due to bone fractures but in <3% of patients without embolism.

Gases, Blood

See Chapter 12.

Decreased pO_2 (Anoxemia)

Hypoventilation (e.g., chronic airflow obstruction): due to increased alveolar CO_2, which displaces O_2

Alveolar hypoxia (e.g., high altitude, gaseous inhalation)

Pulmonary diffusion abnormalities (e.g., interstitial lung disease): supplemental O_2 usually improves pO_2

Right-to-left shunt: supplemental O_2 has no effect; requires positive end-expiratory pressure
  • Congenital anomalies of heart and great vessels
  • Acquired (e.g., ARDS)

Ventilation-perfusion mismatch: supplemental O_2 usually improves pO_2
  • Airflow obstruction (e.g., chronic obstructive pulmonary disease [COPD], asthma)
  • Interstitial inflammation (e.g., pneumonia, sarcoidosis)
  • Vascular obstruction (e.g., pulmonary embolism)

Decreased venous oxygenation (e.g., anemia)

Increased pCO_2 (Hypercapnia)

Decreased ventilation
  • Airway obstruction
  • Drug overdose
  • Metabolic disorders (e.g., myxedema, hypokalemia)
  • Neurologic disorders (e.g., Guillain-Barré syndrome, multiple sclerosis)
  • Muscle disorders (e.g., muscular dystrophy, polymyositis)
  • Chest wall abnormalities (e.g., scoliosis)

Increased dead space in lungs (perfusion decreased more than ventilation decreased)
  • Lung diseases (e.g., COPD, asthma, pulmonary fibrosis, mucoviscidosis)
  • Chest wall changes affecting lung parenchyma (e.g., scoliosis)

Increased production (e.g., sepsis, fever, seizures, excess carbohydrate loads)

Lymph Node (Scalene) Biopsy

(Biopsy of scalene fat pad even without palpable lymph nodes)

Positive in 15% of bronchogenic carcinoma cases. May also be positive in various granulomatous diseases (e.g., TB, sarcoidosis, pneumoconiosis).

Pleural Needle Biopsy (Closed Chest)

(Whenever cannot diagnose otherwise)

Positive for tumor in ~6% of malignant mesothelioma cases and ~60% of other cases of malignancy.

Positive for tubercles in two-thirds of cases on first biopsy with increased yield on second and third biopsies; therefore repeat biopsy if suspicious clinically. Can also culture biopsy material for TB. Fluid culture alone establishes diagnosis of TB in 25% of cases.

Sputum

Color in various conditions

• Rusty	Lobar pneumonia
• Anchovy paste (dark brown)	Amebic liver abscess rupture into bronchus
• Red currant jelly	*Klebsiella pneumoniae*
• Red (pigment, not blood)	*Serratia marcescens*; rifampin overdose
• Black	*Bacteroides melaninogenicus* pneumonia; anthracosilicosis
• Green (with WBCs, sweet odor)	*Pseudomonas* infection
• Milky	Bronchioalveolar carcinoma
• Yellow (without WBCs)	Jaundice

Smears and cultures for infections (e.g., pneumonias, TB, fungi) must be adequate samples of sputum showing ciliated cells, macrophages; neutrophils (usually >25/LPF in good specimen) if acute inflammation is present unless patient is neutropenic; monobacterial population if due to bacterial infection; acute inflammation without a definite bacterial pattern may be due to *Legionella* or RSV or influenza viruses. *Must be promptly refrigerated.* Saliva contamination may show squamous epithelial cells (>19/LPF = poor specimen; 11–19/LPF = fair specimen; <10/LPF = good specimen), extracellular strands of streptococci, clumps of anaerobic *Actinomyces*, candidal budding yeasts with pseudohyphae. For possible anaerobic aspiration, fine needle aspiration (FNA) or alveolar lavage is needed.

Cytology for carcinoma
- Positive in 40% on first sample
- Positive in 70% with three samples
- Positive in 85% with five samples
- False-positive in <1%

Cytology in bronchogenic carcinoma
- Positive in 67–85% of squamous cell carcinoma
- Positive in 64–70% of small-cell undifferentiated carcinoma
- Positive in 55% of adenocarcinoma

Thoracoscopy/Open Lung Biopsy

Use

Diagnosis of pleural malignancy
- Accuracy = 96%; sensitivity = 91%, specificity = 100%; negative predictive value = 93%[2]

Diagnosis of pulmonary infection or neoplasm when BAL is not diagnostic

Respiratory Diseases

Abscess, Lung

◆Sputum: marked increase; abundant, foul, purulent; may be bloody; contains elastic fibers.
- Gram stain is diagnostic—sheets of PMNs with a bewildering variety of organisms.
- Bacterial cultures (including tubercle bacilli)—anaerobic as well as aerobic; rule out amebas, parasites.
- Cytologic examination for malignant cells.

Blood culture: may be positive in acute stage.
Increased WBC in acute stages (15,000–30,000/cu mm)
Increased ESR
Normochromic normocytic anemia in chronic stage
Albuminuria is frequent.
Findings of underlying disease—especially bronchogenic carcinoma; also drug addiction, postabortion state, coccidioidomycosis, amebic abscess, TB, alcoholism

RESPIRATORY

---

[2]Menzies R, Charbonneau M. Thoracoscopy for the diagnosis of pleural disease. *Ann Intern Med* 1991;114:271.

Adult Respiratory Distress Syndrome (ARDS)

Defined As[3]

Ratio of pO_2 (partial pressure arterial O_2)/FiO_2 (fraction inspired O_2 concentration) ≤ 200 regardless of positive end-expiratory pressure. This ratio correlates with patient's outcome. In acute lung injury (change in lung function) this ratio is ≤ 300.
Bilateral pulmonary infiltrates on frontal radiography
Pulmonary wedge pressure ≤ 18 mm Hg or no evidence of increased left atrial pressure

Preceding or associated event (e.g., sepsis [most common], aspiration, infection, pneumonia, pancreatitis, shock, fat emboli, trauma, DIC, etc.; more than one cause is often present). Infection is more likely due to due to gram-negative than gram-positive organisms. Occurs in 23% of cases of gram-negative bacteremia.
Static pulmonary compliance <50 mL/cm H_2O that markedly reduces vital capacity, total lung capacity, functional residual capacity.
Initially there is respiratory alkalosis and varying degrees of hypoxemia resistant to supplementary O_2; then profound anoxemia with pO_2 <50 mm Hg on room air.
BAL shows increased PMNs ($\leq 80\%$). Eosinophilia occurs occasionally. Opportunistic organisms may be found if presents as ARDS.

Asthma, Bronchial

Earliest change is decreased pCO_2 with respiratory alkalosis with normal pO_2. Then pO_2 decreases before pCO_2 increases.
With severe episode
  - Hyperventilation causes decreased pCO_2 in early stages (may be <35 mm Hg).
  - Rapid deterioration of patient's condition may be associated with precipitous fall in pO_2 and rise in pCO_2 (>40 mm Hg).
  - pO_2 <60 mm Hg may indicate severe attack or presence of complication.
  - Normal pCO_2 suggests that the patient is tiring.
  - Acidemia and increased pCO_2 suggest impending respiratory failure.
Mixed metabolic and respiratory acidosis occurs.
When patient requires hospitalization, arterial blood gases should be measured frequently to assess status.
Eosinophilia may be present.
Sputum is white and mucoid without blood or pus (unless infection is present).
Eosinophils, crystals (Curschmann's spirals), and mucus casts of bronchioles may be found.
Laboratory findings due to underlying diseases that may be primary and that should be ruled out, especially polyarteritis nodosa, parasitic infestation, bronchial carcinoid, drug reaction (especially to aspirin), poisoning (especially by cholinergic drugs and pesticides), hypogammaglobulinemia.

Bronchiectasis

WBC usually normal unless pneumonitis is present.
Mild to moderate normocytic normochromic anemia with chronic severe infection
Sputum abundant and mucopurulent (often contains blood); sweetish smell
Sputum bacterial smears and cultures
Laboratory findings due to complications (pneumonia, pulmonary hemorrhage, brain abscess, sepsis, cor pulmonale)
Rule out cystic fibrosis of the pancreas and hypogammaglobulinemia or agammaglobulinemia.

Bronchitis, Acute

Due To

Viruses (e.g., rhinovirus, coronavirus, adenovirus, influenza) cause most cases.
Mycoplasma pneumoniae, Chlamydia pneumoniae, Bordetella pertussis, Legionella spp.

WBC and ESR may be increased.

[3]Bernard GR, Artigas A, Brigham KL, et al. The American-European Consensus Conference on ARDS: definitions, mechanisms, relevant outcomes and clinical trial coordination. *Am J Respir Crit Care Med* 1994;149:818.

Bronchitis, Chronic

WBC and ESR normal or increased
Eosinophil count increased if there is allergic basis or component
Smears and cultures of sputum and bronchoscopic secretions
Laboratory findings due to associated or coexisting diseases (e.g., emphysema, bronchiectasis)
Acute exacerbations are most commonly due to
- Viruses
- *M. pneumoniae*
- *Haemophilus influenzae*
- *S. pneumoniae*
- *Moraxella (Branhamella) catarrhalis*

Carcinoma, Bronchogenic

♦ Cytologic examination of sputum for malignant cells—positive in 40% of patients on first sample, in 70% with three samples, in 85% with five samples. False-positive tests are <1%.
♦ Sputum cytology gives highest positive yield with squamous cell carcinoma (67–85%), intermediate with small cell undifferentiated carcinoma (64–70%), lowest with adenocarcinoma (55%).
♦ Biopsy of scalene lymph nodes for metastases to indicate inoperable status—positive in 15% of patients
♦ Biopsy of bronchus, pleura, lung, metastatic sites in appropriate cases
♦ Cytology of pleural effusion (see p. 149)
♦ Needle biopsy of pleura is positive in 58% of cases with malignant effusion; indicates inoperable status.
♦ Transthoracic needle aspiration provides definitive cytologic diagnosis of cancer in 80–90% of cases; useful when other methods (e.g., sputum cytology, bronchoscopy) fail to provide a microscopic diagnosis.
♦ Cancer cells in bone marrow and rarely in peripheral blood
○ Biochemical tumor markers (see pp. 146, 148)
- Serum CEA is increased in one-third to two-thirds of patients with all four types of lung cancer. Principal uses are to monitor response to therapy and to correlate with staging. Values <5 ng/mL correlate with survival over 3 yrs compared to values >5 ng/mL. Values >10 ng/mL correlate with higher incidence of extensive disease and extrathoracic metastases. A fall to normal suggests complete tumor removal. A fall to still elevated values may indicate residual tumor. An elevated unchanged value suggests residual progressive disease. A value that falls and then rises during chemotherapy suggests that resistance to drugs has occurred.
- Serum neuron-specific enolase may be increased in 79–87% of patients with small cell cancer and in 10% of those with non–small cell cancer and nonmalignant lung diseases (see p. 908). Pretreatment level correlates with stage of small cell cancer. May be used to monitor disease progression; falls in response to therapy and becomes normal in complete remission but not useful for initial screening or detecting early recurrence.
Paraneoplastic syndromes
- Endocrine and metabolic (primarily due to small cell cancer)
    ACTH (Cushing's syndrome) is most commonly produced ectopic hormone (50% of patients with small cell cancer)
    Hypercalcemia occurs in >12% of patients (mostly in epidermoid carcinoma); correlates with large tumor mass that is often incurable and quickly fatal. (See Humoral Hypercalcemia of Malignancy, p. 598.)
    Serotonin production by carcinoid of bronchus. (See p. 688.)
    SIADH occurs in 11% of patients with small cell cancer.
    Prolactin usually due to anaplastic tumors.
    Gonadotropin production predominantly with large cell carcinoma
    Renal tubular dysfunction with glycosuria and aminoaciduria
    Hyponatremia due to massive bronchorrhea in bronchoalveolar cell carcinoma
    Others (e.g., melanocyte-stimulating hormone, vasoactive intestinal peptides)
- Coagulopathies, e.g.,
    DIC

RESPIRATORY

Migratory thrombophlebitis
Chronic hemorrhagic diathesis
- Neuromuscular syndromes (most commonly with small cell cancer), e.g.,
  Myasthenia
  Encephalomyelitis—antineuronal antibodies and small cell cancer associated
    with limbic encephalitis
- Cutaneous, e.g.,
  Dermatomyositis
  Acanthosis nigricans

Syndromes due to metastases (e.g., liver metastases with functional hepatic changes,
  Addison's disease, diabetes insipidus)
Findings of complicating conditions (e.g., pneumonitis, atelectasis, lung abscess)
Normochromic, normocytic anemia in <10% of patients

Croup (Epiglottitis, Laryngotracheitis)

Group B *H. influenzae* causes >90% of cases of epiglottitis; other bacteria include beta-
  hemolytic streptococci and pneumococci.
Cultures, smears, and tests for specific causative agents
Blood cultures should be taken at the same time as throat cultures.
Neutrophilic leukocytosis is present.
Clinical picture in infectious mononucleosis or diphtheria may resemble epiglottitis.
Laryngotracheitis is usually viral (especially parainfluenza) but rarely bacterial in origin.

Dysplasia, Bronchopulmonary

Usually seen in infants recovering from respiratory distress syndrome (RDS) in whom
  endotracheal tube and intermittent positive pressure ventilation have been used for
  >24 hrs.
Stage I (first days of life)—severe RDS is present.
Stage II (late in first week)—clinical improvement but not asymptomatic
Stage III (second week of life)—clinical deterioration, increasing hypoxemia, hypercapnia, acidosis, diffuse radiographic changes in lungs
Stage IV (after 1 mo of age)—chronic healing phase with further radiographic changes.
  25% die, usually due to pneumonia. Symptoms usually resolve by 2 yrs but abnormal pulmonary function tests and right ventricular hypertrophy may persist for several years.

Emphysema, Obstructive

Laboratory findings of underlying disease that may be primary (e.g., pneumoconiosis,
  TB, sarcoidosis, kyphoscoliosis, marked obesity, fibrocystic disease of pancreas, alpha-
  1-antitrypsin deficiency)
Laboratory findings of associated conditions, especially duodenal ulcer
Laboratory findings due to decreased lung ventilation
- pO_2 decreased and pCO_2 increased
- Ultimate development of respiratory acidosis
- Secondary polycythemia
- Cor pulmonale

Goodpasture's Syndrome

**(Alveolar hemorrhage and GN [usually rapidly progressive] associated with anti-
  body against pulmonary alveolar and glomerular basement membranes)**
Proteinuria and RBCs and RBC casts in urine
Renal function may deteriorate rapidly or renal manifestations may be mild.
- ◆ Renal biopsy may show characteristic linear immunofluorescent deposits of IgG and
  often complement and focal or diffuse proliferative GN.
- ◆ Serum may show antiglomerular basement membrane IgG antibodies by enzyme
  immunoassay (EIA). Titer may not correlate with severity of pulmonary or renal disease.
Eosinophilia absent and iron-deficiency anemia more marked than in idiopathic pul-
  monary hemosiderosis
Sputum or BAL showing hemosiderin-laden macrophages may be a clue to occult pulmonary hemorrhage.

Other causes of combined pulmonary hemorrhage and GN are
- Wegener's granulomatosis
- Hypersensitivity vasculitis
- SLE
- Polyarteritis nodosa
- Endocarditis
- Mixed cryoglobulinemia
- Allergic angiitis and granulomatosis (Churg-Strauss syndrome)
- Behçet's syndrome
- Henoch-Schönlein purpura
- Pulmonary-renal reactions due to drugs (e.g., penicillamine)

Hantavirus Pulmonary Syndrome

See p. 848.

Hernia, Diaphragmatic

Microcytic anemia (due to blood loss) may be present.
Stool may be positive for blood.

Histiocytosis X

(See also p. 696.)
♦ Diagnosis is established by open lung biopsy.
Pulmonary disorder is the major manifestation of this disease; bone involvement in
   minority of cases with lung disease. Pleural effusion is rare.
BAL shows increase in total number of cells; 2–20% Langerhans' cells, small numbers
   of eosinophils, neutrophils, and lymphocytes, and 70% macrophages.
Most adults do not have positive gallium citrate 67 (^{67}Ga) scans.
Mild decrease in pO_2, which falls with exercise

Interstitial Pneumonitis, Diffuse

Serum LD is increased.

Larynx Diseases

♦ Culture and smears for specific organisms (e.g., tubercle bacilli, fungi)
♦ Biopsy for diagnosis of visible lesions (e.g., leukoplakia, carcinoma)
May be due to any respiratory viruses.

Legionnaires' Disease

See Chapter 15, p. 805.

Nasopharyngitis, Acute

Due To

Bacteria (e.g., Group A beta-hemolytic *streptococci* [causes 10–30% of cases seen by doc-
   tors], *H. influenzae, M. pneumoniae,* etc.). *(Mere presence of staphylococci, pneumo-
   cocci, alpha- and beta-hemolytic streptococci [other than groups A, C, and G] in throat
   culture does not establish them as cause of pharyngitis and does not warrant antibi-
   otic treatment.)*
Virus (e.g., EBV, CMV, adenovirus, RSV, HSV, coxsackievirus)
M. pneumoniae
C. pneumoniae (formerly TWAR agent)
Fungus, allergy, foreign body, trauma, neoplasm
Idiopathic (no cause is identified in ~50% of cases)

Microscopic Examination of Stained Nasal Smear

○Large numbers of eosinophils suggest allergy. Does not correlate with blood eosinophilia.
   Eosinophils and neutrophils suggest chronic allergy with superimposed infection.
○Large numbers of neutrophils suggest infection.
○Gram stain and culture of pharyngeal exudate may show significant pathogen.

Neonatal Respiratory Distress Syndrome (RDS)

Hypoxemia
Hypercapnia and acidosis in severe cases
pO_2 is maintained between 50–70 mm Hg to minimize retinal damage.
Laboratory findings due to complications (e.g., hypoglycemia, hypocalcemia, acidosis, anemia)

Pleural Effusion

See Fig. 6-1 and Tables 6-1, 6-2, and 6-3.

Normal Values

Specific gravity	1.010–1.026
Total protein	
Albumin	0.3–4.1 gm/dL
Globulin	50–70%
Fibrinogen	30–45%
pH	6.8–7.6

The underlying cause of an effusion is usually determined by first classifying the fluid as an exudate or a transudate. A transudate does not usually require additional testing but *exudates always do.*

Transudate

Congestive heart failure (causes 15% of cases)—acute diuresis can result in pseudoexudate
Cirrhosis with ascites (pleural effusion in ~5% of these cases)—rare without ascites
Nephrotic syndrome
Early (acute) atelectasis
Pulmonary embolism (some cases)
Superior vena cava obstruction
Hypoalbuminemia
Peritoneal dialysis—occurs within 48 hrs of initiating dialysis
Early mediastinal malignancy
Misplaced subclavian catheter
Myxedema (rare cause)
Constrictive pericarditis—effusion is bilateral
Urinothorax—due to ipsilateral GU tract obstruction

Exudate

Pneumonia, malignancy, pulmonary embolism, and GI conditions (especially pancreatitis and abdominal surgery, which cause 90% of all exudates)
Infection (causes 25% of cases)
- Bacterial pneumonia
- Parapneumonic effusion (empyema)
- TB
- Abscess (subphrenic, liver, spleen)
- Viral, mycoplasmal, rickettsial
- Parasitic (ameba, hydatid cyst, filaria)
- Fungal effusion (*Coccidioides, Cryptococcus, Histoplasma, Blastomyces, Aspergillus*; in immunocompromised host, *Aspergillus, Candida, Mucor*)

Pulmonary embolism/infarction
Neoplasms (metastatic carcinoma, especially breast, ovary, lung; lymphoma, leukemia, mesothelioma, pleural endometriosis) (causes 42% of cases)
Trauma (penetrating or blunt)
- Hemothorax, chylothorax, empyema, associated with rupture of diaphragm

Immunologic mechanisms
- Rheumatoid pleurisy (5% of cases)
- SLE
- Other collagen vascular diseases occasionally cause effusions (e.g., Wegener's granulomatosis, Sjögren's syndrome, familial Mediterranean fever, Churg-Strauss syndrome, mixed connective tissue disease)

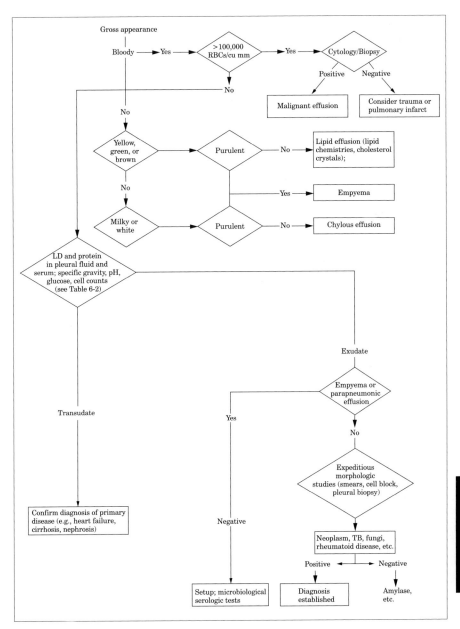

Fig. 6-1. Algorithm for pleural effusion.

- After myocardial infarction or cardiac surgery
- Vasculitis
- Hepatitis
- Sarcoidosis (rare cause; may also be transudate)
- Familial recurrent polyserositis
- Drug reaction (e.g., nitrofurantoin hypersensitivity, methysergide)

Chemical mechanisms
- Uremic

RESPIRATORY

Table 6-1. Pleural Fluid Findings in Various Clinical Conditions

Disease	Appearance	Total WBC (1000/cu mm)	Predominant Type WBC	Total RBC (1000/cu mm)	pH	Glucose mg/dL	Glucose PF:S	Protein PF:S	LD PF:S	LD IU/L	Amylase PF:S	Comments
Transudates												
Congestive heart failure	Clear, straw	<1	M	0–1	>7.4	>60	1	<0.5	<0.6	<200	≤1	If right side not involved, rule out pulmonary infarct.
Cirrhosis	Clear, straw	<0.5	M	<1	>7.4	>60	1	<0.5	<0.6	<200	≤1	Occurs in 5% of cirrhotics with clinical ascites.
Pulmonary embolus; atelectasis	Clear, straw	5–15	M	<5	>7.3	>60	1	<0.5	<0.6		≤1	
Exudates												
Pulmonary embolus; infarction	Turbid to hemorrhagic Small volume	5–15	P May show many mesothelial cells	Bloody in one-third to two-thirds of patients	>7.3	>60	1	>0.5	>0.6		≤1	Occurs in 15% of patients; often no characteristic findings.
Pneumonia[a]	Turbid	5–40	P	<5	≥7.3	>60	1	>0.5	>0.6		≤1	Occurs in 50% of bacterial pneumonias and Legionnaires' disease, 5–20% of viral and mycoplasma pneumonias.
Empyema[b]	Turbid to purulent	25–100	P	<5	5.50–7.29	<60	<0.5	>0.5	>0.6	May be >1000/L	≤1	Most commonly due to anaerobic bacteria, *Staphylococcus aureus*,

	Appearance				pH	Glucose		Protein ratio	LDH ratio		Comments
TB	Straw; serosanguineous in 15%	5–10	M	<10	<7.3 in 20%	30–60 in 20%	1	>0.5	>0.6	≤1	AFB stain positive in 15–20% and culture of fluid positive in 30% of cases. Biopsy for histologic examination and culture of pleura are diagnostic in 75–85% of cases. Often presents as effusion; pulmonary disease may be absent.
Malignancy[c]	Straw to turbid to bloody	<10	M	1 to >100	<7.3 in 30%	<60 in 30%	1	>0.5	>0.6	≤1	
RA effusion[d]	Turbid or green or yellow	1–20	P in acute M in chronic	<1	<7.3; usually ~7.0	<30 in 95%	Often >1000/L	>0.5	>0.6	≤1	Biopsy is useful, especially in men with rheumatoid nodules and high RF titer.
SLE	Straw to turbid		P in acute M in chronic		<7.3 in 30%	<60 in 30%		>0.5	>0.6	>2	PF may show LE cells, ANA titer, and low complement. Usually found only when lupus is active.
Rupture of esophagus	Purulent		P		6.0	N or D		>0.5	>0.6	Salivary type	

(continued)

Table 6-1. (continued)

Disease	Appearance	Total WBC (1000/cu mm)	Predominant Type WBC	Total RBC (1000/cu mm)	pH	Glucose mg/dL	PF:S	Protein PF:S	LD PF:S IU/L	Amy-lase PF:S	Comments
Pancreatitis	Serous to turbid to serosan-guineous	5–20	P	1–10	>7.3	>60	1	>0.5	>0.6	>2	Occurs in 15% of acute cases. Left-sided in 70% of cases.

Note: Blood specimens should always be drawn at the same time as serous fluid for determination of glucose, protein, LD, amylase, pH, etc. Pleural fluid for pH should be collected in the same way as arterial blood samples (i.e., heparinized syringe, maintained anaerobically on ice, analyzed promptly). Pleural fluid pH should normally be at least 0.15 greater than arterial blood pH. Normal pH is alkaline and may approach 7.6.

PF:S = ratio of pleural fluid to serum; PF = pleural fluid.

[a]Parapneumonic effusions (exudate type of effusion associated with lung abscess, bronchiectasis; ~5% of bacterial pneumonias).

Aerobic gram-negative organisms (Klebsiella, Escherichia coli, Pseudomonas) are associated with a high incidence of exudates (with 5000–40,000/cu mm, high protein, normal glucose, normal pH) and resolve with antibiotic therapy.

Nonpurulent fluid with positive Gram stain, positive blood culture, or low pH suggests that effusion will become or behave like empyema.

Streptococcus pneumoniae causes parapneumonic effusions in 50% of cases, especially with positive blood culture.

Staphylococcus aureus has effusion in 90% of infants, 50% of adults.

Streptococcus pyogenes in 90% of cases; massive effusion, greenish color.

Haemophilus influenzae has effusion in 50–75% of cases.

[b]pH <7.0 and glucose <40 mg/dL indicate need for closed chest tube drainage even without grossly purulent fluid.
  pH of 7.0–7.2 is a questionable indication and should be repeated in 24 hrs, but tube drainage is favored if pleural fluid LD >1000 IU/L. Tube drainage is also indicated if there is grossly purulent fluid or positive Gram stain or culture.
  In Proteus mirabilis empyema, high ammonia level may cause a pH ~8.0.

[c]Usually is large; frequently hemorrhagic (50% have RBC >10,000/cu mm).
  Cytology establishes the diagnosis in approximately 50% of patients. Cytology plus biopsy is diagnostic in about 90% of cases.
  Lung and breast cancer and lymphoma cause 75% of malignant effusions; in 6%, no primary tumor is found. Pleural or ascitic effusion occurs in 20–30% of patients with malignant lymphoma.
  In some instances of suspected lymphoma with negative conventional test results, flow cytometry of pleural fluid showing a monoclonal lymphocyte population can establish the diagnosis.
  Mucopolysaccharide level may be increased in mesothelioma.

[d]Decreased glucose is the most useful finding clinically; may be 0.
  RA cells may be found. RF may be present but may also be found in other effusions (e.g., TB, cancer, bacterial pneumonia).
  Needle biopsy usually may show characteristic rheumatoid nodule.
  Protein level is >3 gm/dL.

Table 6-2. Comparison of "Typical"[a] Findings in Transudates and Exudates[b]

Findings	Transudates	Exudates
Specific gravity[c]	<1.016	>1.016
Protein (gm/dL)[d]	<3.0	>3.0
Pleural fluid:serum ratio[e]	<0.5	>0.5
LD[f]		
IU	<200	>200
Pleural fluid:serum ratio[e]	<0.6	>0.6
Ratio pleural fluid:upper limit normal serum[e]	<2:3	>2:3
WBC count	<1000/cu mm	>1000/cu mm
	Mainly lymphocytes	May be grossly purulent
RBCs	Few	Variable; few or may be grossly bloody
Glucose	Equivalent to serum	May be decreased because of bacteria or many WBCs
Cholesterol (mg/dL)	<55	Usually >55
Pleural fluid:serum ratio	<0.32	>0.32
pH	Usually 7.4–7.5	Usually 7.35–7.45
Appearance	Clear	Usually cloudy
Color	Pale yellow	Variable

[a]"Typical" means 67–75% of patients.
[b]Isoenzymes not useful for differentiating.
[c]Long-standing transudates, however, can produce a high specific gravity.
[d]Protein level of 3.0 gm/dL misclassifies ~15% of effusions if it is the only criterion.
[e]Each of these three criteria has been used to define pleural fluid exudate and transudate. *All three* constitute the best differential of exudate and transudate. Transudate meets none of these criteria, and exudate meets at least one criterion. Unequivocal criteria of transudate precludes the need for pleural biopsy in most cases unless two mechanisms are suspected (e.g., nephrotic syndrome with miliary TB, congestive heart failure with malignancy). It would be uncommon for use of diuretics in congestive heart failure to change characteristics of transudate to that of exudate.
[f]If nonhemolyzed, nonbloody effusion.

- Pancreatic (pleural effusion occurs in ~10% of these cases)
- Esophageal rupture (high *salivary* amylase and pH <7.30 that approaches 6.00 in 48–72 hrs)
- Subphrenic abscess

Lymphatic abnormality
- Irradiation
- Milroy's disease
- Yellow nail syndrome (rare condition of generalized hypoplasia of lymphatic vessels)

Injury
- Asbestosis

Altered pleural mechanics
- Late (chronic) atelectasis
- Trapped lung

Endocrine
- Hypothyroidism

Movement of fluid from abdomen to pleural space
- Meigs' syndrome (protein and specific gravity are often at transudate-exudate border but usually not transudate)
- Urinothorax
- Cancer
- Pancreatitis, pancreatic pseudocyst

Table 6-3. Comparison of Tumor Markers in Various Pleural Effusions

	CA-125	CEA[a]
Benign effusion	−	−
Mesothelioma	−	−
Melanoma	−	−
Lymphoma	−	−
Carcinosarcoma	−	−
Breast	−	+
Lung	−	+
GI tract	−	+
Ovary (mucinous)	−	+
Ovary (serous)[b]	+	−
Fallopian tube[b]	+	−
Endometrium[b]	+	−

CA-125 = C125 tumor antigen; CEA = carcinoembryonic antigen; + indicates value increased; − indicates value not increased.
[a]CEA not increased <5 ng/mL.
[b]CA-125 >1000 units/mL has 85% sensitivity and 96% specificity.
Source: Pinto MM, et al. Immunoradiometric assay of CA-125 in effusions: comparison with carcinoembryonic antigen. *Cancer* 1987;59:218.

Unknown (~15% of all exudates)
Cirrhosis, pulmonary infarct, trauma, and connective tissue diseases comprise ~9% of all cases.

Exudates That Can Present as Transudates

Pulmonary embolism (>20% of cases)—due to atelectasis
Hypothyroidism—due to myxedema heart disease
Malignancy—due to complications (e.g., atelectasis, lymphatic obstruction)
Sarcoidosis—stage II and III
Pleural fluid analysis results in definitive diagnosis in ~25% and a probable diagnosis in another 50% of patients; may help to rule out a suspected diagnosis in 30%.

Location

Typically left-sided—ruptured esophagus, acute pancreatitis, RA. Pericardial disease is left-sided or bilateral; rarely exclusively right-sided.
Typically right-sided or bilateral—congestive heart failure (if only on left, consider that right pleural space may be obliterated or patient has another process, e.g., pulmonary infarction).
Typically right-sided—rupture of amebic liver abscess.

Gross Appearance

Clear, straw-colored fluid is typical of transudate.
Cloudy, opaque appearance indicates more cell components.
Bloody fluid suggests malignancy, pulmonary infarct, trauma, postcardiotomy syndrome; also uremia, asbestosis, pleural endometriosis. Bloody fluid from traumatic thoracentesis should clot within several minutes, but blood present more than several hours has become defibrinated and does not form a good clot. Nonuniform color during aspiration and absence of hemosiderin-laden macrophages and some crenated RBCs also suggest traumatic aspiration.
Chylous (milky) fluid is usually due to trauma (e.g., auto accident, postoperative) but may be obstruction of duct (e.g., especially lymphoma; metastatic carcinoma, granulomas). Pleural fluid triglyceride >110 mg/dL or triglyceride pleural fluid to serum

ratio >2 occurs only in chylous effusion (seen especially within a few hours after eating). After centrifugation, supernatant is white due to chylomicrons, which also stain with Sudan III. Equivocal triglyceride levels (60–110 mg/dL) may require a lipoprotein electrophoresis of fluid to demonstrate chylomicrons diagnostic of chylothorax. Triglyceride <50 mg/dL excludes chylothorax.

"Pseudochylous" in chronic inflammatory conditions (e.g., rheumatoid pleurisy, TB, chronic pneumothorax therapy for TB) due to either cholesterol crystals (rhomboid shaped) in sediment or lipid-containing inclusions in leukocytes. Distinguish from chylous effusions by microscopy. Fluid may have lustrous sheen.

White fluid suggests chylothorax, cholesterol effusion, or empyema.

Black fluid suggests *Aspergillus niger* infection.

Greenish fluid suggests biliopleural fistula.

Purulent fluid indicates infection.

Anchovy (dark red-brown) color is seen in amebiasis, old blood.

Anchovy paste in ruptured amebic liver abscess; amebas found in <10%.

Turbid and greenish yellow fluid is classical for rheumatoid effusion.

Turbidity may be due to lipids or increased WBCs; after centrifugation, a clear supernatant indicates WBCs as cause; white supernatant is due to chylomicrons.

Very viscous (clear or bloody) fluid is characteristic of mesothelioma.

Debris in fluid suggests rheumatoid pleurisy; food particles indicate esophageal rupture.

Color of enteral tube food or central venous line infusion due to tube or catheter entering pleural space.

Odor

Putrid due to anaerobic empyema
Ammonia due to urinothroax

Protein, Albumin, Lactate Dehydrogenase

See Table 6-2.

When exudate criteria are met by LD but not by protein, consider malignancy and parapneumonic effusions.

Very high pleural fluid LD (>1000 U/L) occurs in empyema, rheumatoid pleurisy, paragonimiasis; sometimes with malignancy; rarely with TB.

Glucose

Same concentration as serum in transudate

Usually normal but 30–55 mg/dL or pleural fluid to serum ratio <0.5 and pH <7.30 may be found in TB, malignancy, SLE; also esophageal rupture; lowest levels may occur in empyema and RA. Therefore, only helpful if very low level (e.g., <30). 0–10 mg/dL highly suspicious for RA (see Rheumatoid Effusion, p. 149).

pH

Low pH (<7.30) always means exudate, especially empyema, malignancy, rheumatoid pleurisy, SLE, TB, esophageal rupture. Esophageal rupture is only cause of pH close to 6.0; collagen vascular disease is only other cause of pH <7.0. pH <7.10 in parapneumonic effusion indicates need for tube drainage. In malignant effusion, pH <7.30 is associated with short survival time, poorer prognosis, and increased positive yield with cytology and pleural biopsy; tends to correlate with pleural fluid glucose <60 mg/dL.

Amylase

Increased (pleural fluid to serum ratio >1.0 and may be >5 or pleural fluid greater than upper limit of normal for serum)
- Acute pancreatitis—may be normal early with increase over time.
- Pancreatic pseudocyst—always increased, may be >100,000 U/L.
- Also perforated peptic ulcer, necrosis of small intestine (e.g., mesenteric vascular occlusion); 10% of cases of metastatic cancer and esophageal rupture.

Isoenzyme studies
- *Pancreatic* type amylase is found in acute pancreatitis and pancreatic pseudocyst.

RESPIRATORY

• *Salivary* type amylase is found in esophageal rupture and occasionally in carcinoma of ovary or lung or salivary gland tumor. Should be determined in undiagnosed left pleural effusions.

Other Chemical Determinations

♦ Cholesterol <55 mg/dL is said to be found in transudates and >55 mg/dL in exudates.
♦ CEA >10 ng/mL has specificity of >95% and sensitivity of 54–100% for lung cancer, 83% for breast cancer, 100% for GI tract cancers (see p. 906). May also be increased in empyema and parapneumonic effusions.
♦ C125 tumor antigen (CA-125; see p. 905) has sensitivity of 71% and specificity of 99% for non-mucinous epithelial ovarian carcinoma.

Combined CEA and CA-125 have sensitivity for detection of malignant effusions due to carcinomas of lung, breast, GI tract, and ovary of 75–100% and specificity of 98%. May indicate primary site when the source is unknown or cytology is negative (Table 6-3).

Other tumor markers have been suggested for diagnosis of cancer, but value not established (e.g., acid phosphatase in prostatic cancer, hyaluronic acid in mesothelioma, beta 2-microglobulin, etc.)

Acid mucopolysaccharides (especially hyaluronic acid) may be increased (>120 μg/mL) in mesotheliomas.

Immune complexes (measured by Raji cell, C1q component of C, RIA, etc.) are often found in exudates due to collagen vascular diseases (SLE, RA). RA latex agglutination tests show frequent false-positives and should not be ordered.

Occasionally latex agglutination for bacterial antigens is useful. Gas-liquid chromatography has been reported to show butyric, isobutyric, propionic, and isovaleric acids in anaerobic acute bacterial infection and increased lactic and acetic acid levels in aerobic infections.

Cell Count

Total WBC count is almost never diagnostic.
• >10,000/cu mm indicates inflammation, most commonly with pneumonia, pulmonary infarct, pancreatitis, postcardiotomy syndrome.
• >50,000/cu mm is typical only in parapneumonic effusions, usually empyema.
• Chronic exudates (e.g., malignancy and TB) are usually <5000/cu mm.
• Transudates are usually <1000/cu mm.

5000–6000 RBCs/cu mm needed to give red appearance to pleural fluid
• Can be caused by needle trauma producing 2 mL of blood in 1000 mL of pleural fluid.

>100,000 RBCs/cu mm is grossly hemorrhagic and suggests malignancy, pulmonary infarct, or trauma but occasionally seen in congestive heart failure alone.

Hemothorax (pleural fluid to venous Hct ratio >2) suggests trauma, bleeding from a vessel, bleeding disorder, or malignancy but may be seen in same conditions as above.

Smears

Wright's stain differentiates PMNs from mononuclear cells; cannot differentiate lymphocytes from monocytes.

Mononuclear cells predominate in transudates and chronic exudates (lymphoma, carcinoma, TB, rheumatoid conditions, uremia). >50% is seen in two-thirds of cases due to cancer. >85–90% suggests TB, lymphoma, sarcoidosis, rheumatoid causes.

PMNs predominate in early inflammatory effusions (e.g., pneumonia, pulmonary infarct, pancreatitis, subphrenic abscess).

After several days, mesothelial cells, macrophages, lymphocytes may predominate.

Large mesothelial cells >5% are said to rule out TB (must differentiate from macrophages).

Lymphocytes
• >85% suggests TB, lymphoma, sarcoidosis, chronic rheumatoid pleurisy, yellow nail syndrome, chylothorax.
• 50–75% in >50% of cases of carcinoma.

Eosinophils in pleural fluid (>10% of total WBCs) is not diagnostically significant.
• May mean blood or air in pleural space (e.g., pneumothorax [most common], repeated thoracenteses, traumatic hemothorax).

- It also is said to be associated with asbestosis, pulmonary infarction, polyarteritis nodosa.
- Parasitic disease (e.g., paragonimiasis, hydatid disease, amebiasis, ascariasis).
- Fungal disease (e.g., histoplasmosis, coccidioidomycosis).
- Drug-related (e.g., nitrofurantoin, bromocriptine, dantrolene).
- Idiopathic effusion (in approximately one-third of cases; may be due to occult pulmonary embolism or asbestosis).
- Uncommon with malignant effusions.
- Rare with TB.
- Not usually accompanied by striking blood eosinophilia. Many diseases associated with blood eosinophilia infrequently cause pleural effusion eosinophilia.

Basophils >10% only in leukemic involvement of pleura.

Occasionally lupus erythematosus (LE) cells make the diagnosis of SLE.

Gram stain for early diagnosis of bacterial infection.

Acid-fast smears are positive in 20% of tuberculous pleurisy.

Culture is often positive in empyema but not in parapneumonic effusions.

♦ **Bacterial antigens** may detect *H. influenzae* type b, *Streptococcus pneumoniae*, several types of *Neisseria meningitidis*. Useful when viable organisms cannot be recovered (e.g., due to prior antibiotic therapy).

♦ Cytology

Positive in 60% of malignancies on first tap, 80% by third tap. Therefore should repeat taps with cytologic examinations if cancer is suspected. Is more sensitive than needle biopsy. Combined with needle biopsy, increases sensitivity by <10%.[4] (See Carcinoma, Bronchogenic, p. 137.) High yield with adenocarcinoma, low yield with Hodgkin's disease.

Rheumatoid effusions: cytologic triad of slender elongated and round giant multinucleated macrophages and necrotic background material with characteristically low glucose is said to be pathognomonic. Mesothelial cells are nearly always absent.

Flow cytometry assay for DNA aneuploidy and staining with monoclonal antibodies (e.g., CEA, cytokeratin) to distinguish malignant mesothelioma, metastatic tumor, and reactive mesothelial cells can be performed (note: some malignant cells may be diploid).

Pleural Fluid Findings in Various Clinical Conditions

See Fig. 6-1.

Tuberculosis

High protein content—almost always >4.0 gm/dL

Increased lymphocytes

♦ Acid-fast smears are positive in <20%, and culture is positive in ~67% of cases; culture combined with histologic examination establishes the diagnosis in 95% of cases.

♦ Needle biopsy can be performed without hesitation.

Large mesothelial cells >5% are said to rule out TB (must differentiate from macrophages).

TB often presents as effusion, especially in youth; pulmonary disease may be absent; risk of active pulmonary TB within 5 yrs is 60%.

Malignancy

Can cause effusion by metastasis to pleura, causing exudate-type fluid, or by metastasis to lymph nodes, obstructing lymph drainage and giving transudate-type fluid. Low pH and glucose indicate a poor prognosis with short survival time.

Characteristic effusion is moderate to massive, frequently hemorrhagic, with moderate WBC count with predominance of mononuclear cells; however, only half of malignant effusions have RBC >10,000/cu mm.

♦ Cytology establishes the diagnosis in ~50% of patients.

♦ Combined cytology and pleural biopsy give positive results in 90%.

♦ In some instances of suspected lymphoma with negative conventional test results, flow cytometric analysis of pleural fluid showing a monoclonal lymphocyte population can establish the diagnosis.

Mucopolysaccharide level may be increased (normal <17 mg/dL) in mesothelioma.

[4]Prakesh UBS, Reiman HM. Comparison of needle biopsy with cytologic analysis for the evaluation of pleural effusion: Analysis of 414 cases. *Mayo Clin Proc* 1985;60:158.

Lung and breast cancer and lymphoma cause 75% of malignant effusions; in 6%, no primary tumor is found. Pleural or ascitic effusion occurs in 20–30% of patients with malignant lymphoma.

CEA, CA-125—see Table 6-3 and pp. 905, 906.

Pulmonary Infarct

Effusion occurs in 50% of patients with pulmonary infarct; is bloody in one-third to two-thirds of patients; often no characteristic diagnostic findings occur.

Small volume, serous or bloody, predominance of PMNs, may show many mesothelial cells; this "typical pattern" is seen in only 25% of cases.

Congestive Heart Failure

Is predominantly right-sided or bilateral. If unilateral or left-sided in patients with congestive heart failure, rule out pulmonary infarct.

Pneumonias

Parapneumonic effusions (exudate type of effusion associated with lung abscess, bronchiectasis; ~5% of bacterial pneumonias).

Aerobic gram-negative organisms (*Klebsiella, Escherichia coli, Pseudomonas*) are associated with a high incidence of exudates (with 5000–40,000/cu mm, high protein, normal glucose, normal pH) and resolve with antibiotic therapy. Nonpurulent fluid with positive Gram stain or positive blood culture or low pH suggests that effusion will become or behave like empyema.

S. pneumoniae causes parapneumonic effusions in 50% of cases, especially with positive blood culture.

Staphylococcus aureus has effusion in 90% of infants, 50% of adults; usually widespread bronchopneumonia.

Streptococcus pyogenes has effusion in 90% of cases; massive effusion, greenish color.

Haemophilus influenzae has effusion in 50–75% of cases.

Viral or *Mycoplasma* pneumonia—pleural effusions develop in 20% of cases.

Legionnaires' disease—pleural effusion occurs in up to 50% of patients; may be bilateral.

P. carinii pneumonia cases often have pleural effusion to serum LD ratio >1.0 and pleural effusion to serum protein ratio <0.5.

pH <7.0 and glucose <40 mg/dL indicate need for closed chest tube drainage even without grossly purulent fluid.

pH of 7.0–7.2 is questionable indication and should be repeated in 24 hrs, but tube drainage is favored if pleural fluid LD >1000 U/L. Tube drainage is also indicated if fluid is grossly purulent or Gram stain or culture is positive.

Normal pH is alkaline and may approach 7.6.

Empyema

Usually WBCs >50,000/cu mm, low glucose, and low pH. Suspect clinically when effusion develops during adequate antibiotic therapy.

In *Proteus mirabilis* empyema, high ammonia level may cause a pH ~8.0.

Rheumatoid Effusion

See Table 6-4.

Found in ~70% of RA patients at autopsy.

○Exudate is frequently turbid and may be milky. Classic picture is cloudy greenish fluid with 0 glucose level. Level is <50 mg/dL in 80% and <25 mg/dL in 66% of patients; is the most useful finding clinically. Failure of level to increase during IV glucose infusion distinguishes RA from other causes. *Nonpurulent, nonmalignant effusions not due to TB or RA almost always have glucose level >60 mg/dL.*

RF may be present but may also be found in other effusions (e.g., TB, cancer, bacterial pneumonia). RF titer ≥ 1:320 or equal to or greater than serum level suggests rheumatoid pleurisy.

RA cells may be found (see Cytology, p. 149).

Cytologic examination for malignant cells and smears and cultures for bacteria, tubercle bacilli, and fungi are negative.

♦ Needle biopsy usually shows nonspecific chronic inflammation but may show characteristic rheumatoid nodule microscopically. One-third of cases have parenchymal lung disease (e.g., interstitial fibrosis).

Other laboratory findings of RA are found (see p. 313).

Protein level is >3 gm/dL.

Table 6-4. Comparison of Pleural Fluid in Rheumatoid Arthritis and Systemic Lupus Erythematosus (SLE)

Test	Rheumatoid Arthritis	SLE
pH >7.2	≤ 7.2	>7.2
Glucose	<30 mg/dL	Normal
Lactate dehydrogenase	>700 IU/L	<700 IU/L
Rheumatoid factor	Strongly positive	Negative or weakly positive
Ratio pleural fluid to serum	>1.0	<1.0
Rheumatoid arthritis cells (ragocytes)	May be present	Absent
Epithelioid cells	Present	Absent
C4	Markedly decreased ($<10 \times 10^5$ gm/gm of protein)	Moderately decreased ($<30 \times 10^6$ gm/gm of protein)
Clq–binding assay	Moderately positive	Weakly positive
Ratio pleural fluid to serum	>1.0	<1.0

Increased LD (usually higher than in serum) is commonly found in other chronic pleural effusions and is not useful in differential diagnosis.

Systemic Lupus Erythematosus
◆ • LE cells are specific for SLE but test has poor sensitivity.
○ • ANA titer ≥ 160 or pleural fluid to serum ratio >1.0 is suggestive but not diagnostic.

Pneumoconiosis

◆ Biopsy of lung, scalene lymph node—histologic, chemical, spectrographic, and radiographic diffraction studies, electron microscopy (e.g., silicosis, berylliosis; also metastatic tumor, sarcoidosis, TB, fungus infection)
Bacterial smears and cultures of sputum (especially for tubercle bacilli) should be done.
Cytologic examination of sputum and bronchoscopic secretions for malignant cells, especially squamous cell carcinoma of bronchus and mesothelioma of pleura
Asbestos bodies sometimes occur in sputum after exposure to asbestos dust even without clinical disease.
Acute beryllium disease may show occasional transient hypergammaglobulinemia.
Chronic beryllium disease
• Secondary polycythemia
• Increased serum gamma globulin
• Increased urine calcium
• Increased beryllium in urine long after beryllium exposure has ended
Increased WBC if associated infection
Secondary polycythemia or anemia
Silicosis
Associated conditions
• ≤ 25% have mycobacterial infections, half of which are nontuberculous.
• Increased incidence of nocardiosis, cryptococcosis, sporotrichosis.
• 10% have connective tissue diseases (e.g., progressive systemic sclerosis, RA, SLE).
• Increased incidence of ANA, RF, hypergammaglobulinemia. ACE increased in one-third of patients.

Pneumonia

See Table 6-5.

RESPIRATORY

Table 6-5. Opportunistic Pulmonary Infections

Organism	Preferred Specimen[a]	Direct Stain	Antigen or Nucleic Acid	Culture Turnaround Time
Usual bacteria	1	Gram stain	NA	Routine 3–4 days
Legionella spp.	2	DFA	Urine antigen only for sero-type 1 PCR[b]	Special media[d] 2–7 days
Fungi	2	Wet mount	Cryptococcal and histoplasmal antigens	Mycologic media, 6–8 wks
		Calcofluor white	Commercial DNA probes for *Histoplasma capsulatum, Coccidioides immitis, Blastomyces dermatitidis*	
Mycobacteria spp.	2	Acid fast		Mycobacterial media ≥ 8 wks
Nocardia spp.	2	Modified acid fast	NA	Blood agar 4–6 wks
Pneumocystis spp.	2, 3	FAB, Giemsa, toluidine blue O	PCR	Noncultivable
Viruses	2, 4	FAB for specific viruses	FAB for CMV, HSV, VZV	Shell vial 1–2 days; ≥ 2 wks for traditional
Chlamydia spp.	2	None	PCR[c]	Cell culture[d] 3–5 days
Mycoplasma spp.	2	None	PCR[c]	Special media[d] 7–10 days

CMV = cytomegalovirus; DFA = direct fluorescent antibody stain; FAB = fluorescent antibody; HSV = herpes simplex virus; NA = not applicable; PCR = polymerase chain reaction; VZV = varicella-zoster virus.
[a]1 = sputum; 2 = bronchoalveolar lavage, brushings, bronchial biopsy, open lung biopsy, percutaneous needle biopsy; 3 = saline-induced sputum; 4 = nasopharyngeal swab or wash.
[b]Not generally available.
[c]Research laboratories only.
[d]Culture is difficult; not routinely offered by clinical laboratories.
See also Chapter 15.
Source: Shelhamer JH, et al. The laboratory evaluation of opportunistic pulmonary infections. *Ann Intern Med* 1996;124:585.

Due To

Bacteria

S. pneumoniae causes 60–70% of bacterial pneumonia in patients requiring hospitalization. May cause ~25% of hospital-acquired cases of pneumonia. Blood culture positive in 25% of untreated cases during first 3–4 days.

Staphylococcus causes <1% of all acute bacterial pneumonia with onset outside the hospital but more frequent after outbreaks of influenza; may be secondary to measles, mucoviscidosis, prolonged antibiotic therapy, debilitating diseases (e.g., leukemia, collagen diseases). Frequent cause of nosocomial pneumonia. Bacteremia in <20% of patients.

H. influenzae is important in 6- to 24-mo age group; rare in adults except for middle-aged men with chronic lung disease and/or alcoholism and patients with immuno-deficiency (HIV, multiple myeloma, chronic lymphocytic leukemia [CLL]). Can mimic pneumococcal pneumonia; may be isolated with *S. pneumoniae.*

Gram-negative bacilli (e.g., *K. pneumoniae,* enterobacteria, *E. coli, P. mirabilis, Pseudomonas aeruginosa*) are common causes of hospital-acquired pneumonia but unlikely outside the hospital. *K. pneumoniae* causes 1% of primary bacterial pneu-monias, especially in alcoholic patients and patients with upper lobe pneumonia; tenacious red-brown sputum is typical.

Tubercle bacilli

Legionella pneumophila—see p. 805

M. pneumoniae—most common in young adult male population (e.g., armed forces camps)

C. pneumoniae, Chlamydia psittaci

Others (e.g., streptococcosis, tularemia, plague)

See Table 6-5.

Viruses

Influenza, parainfluenza, adenoviruses, RSV, echovirus, coxsackievirus, reovirus, CMV, viruses of exanthems, herpes simplex, hantavirus

Rickettsiae

Q fever is most common in endemic areas; typhus.

Fungi

P. carinii, Histoplasma, and *Coccidioides* in particular; *Blastomyces, Aspergillus.*

Protozoans

Toxoplasma

Underlying Condition	Organism
Obstructive cancer	*S. pneumoniae, H. influenzae, M. catarrhalis,* anaerobes
Alcoholism	*S. pneumoniae, H. influenzae, Klebsiella* spp., *Legionella* spp., anaerobes, *M. tuberculosis*
HIV infection	*S. pneumoniae, H. influenzae, S. aureus,* gram-negative bacilli, *P. carinii, M. tuberculosis* and *MAI (mycobac-terium avium-intracellulare), Toxoplasma gondii, Cryp-tococcus, Nocardia,* CMV, histoplasmosis, *Coccidioides immitis, Legionella, M. catarrhalis, Rhodococcus equi*
Atypical pneumonia	*M. pneumoniae, C. psittaci, C. pneumoniae, Coxiella bur-netii, Francisella tularensis,* many viruses

Laboratory Findings

WBC is frequently normal or slightly increased in nonbacterial pneumonias; considerable increase in WBC is more common in bacterial pneumonia. *In severe bacterial pneumo-nia, WBC may be very high or low or normal. Because individual variation is consider-able, it has limited value in distinguishing bacterial and nonbacterial pneumonia.*

Urine protein, WBCs, hyaline and granular casts in small amounts are common. Ketones may occur with severe infection. *Check for glucose to rule out underlying diabetes mellitus.*

♦ Sputum reveals abundant WBCs in bacterial pneumonias. Gram stain shows abun-dant organisms in bacterial pneumonias (e.g., *Pneumococcus, Staphylococcus*). Cul-ture sputum for appropriate bacteria. *Sputum that contains many organisms and WBCs on smear but no pathogens on aerobic culture may indicate aspiration pneu-monia. Sputum is not appropriate for anaerobic culture.*

♦ In all cases of pneumonia, blood culture and sputum culture and smear for Gram stain should be performed before antibiotic therapy is started. Optimum specimen of sputum shows >25 PMNs and ≤ 5 squamous epithelial cells/LPF (10× magnifica-tion), but >10 PMNs and <25 epithelial cells may be considered acceptable sputum specimen. >25 epithelial cells indicate unsatisfactory specimen from oropharynx which should not be submitted for culture. If good sputum specimen is obtained, fur-ther diagnostic microbiological tests are usually not performed.

Nasopharyngeal aspirate may identify *S. pneumoniae* with few false positives but *S. aureus* and gram-negative bacilli often represent false-positive findings.

RESPIRATORY

In *H. influenzae* pneumonia, sputum culture is negative in >50% of patients with positive cultures from blood, pleural fluid, or lung tissue, and may be present in the sputum in the absence of disease.

♦ Transtracheal aspiration (puncture of cricothyroid membrane) generally yields a faster, more accurate diagnosis.

♦ Protected brush bronchoscopy and BAL have high sensitivity.

♦ Diagnostic lung puncture to determine specific causative agent as a guide to antibiotic therapy may be indicated in critically ill children.

♦ Open lung biopsy is gold standard with 97% accuracy but 10% complication rate.

For pleural effusions that are aspirated, Gram stain and culture should also be performed.

♦ Respiratory pathogens isolated from blood, pleural fluid, or transtracheal aspirate (except in patients with chronic bronchitis) or identified by bacterial polysaccharide antigen in urine may be considered the definite causal agent.

♦ Urine testing for capsular antigen from *S. pneumoniae* or type B *H. influenzae* by latex agglutination may be helpful. Positive in ~90% of bacteremic pneumococcal pneumonias and 40% of nonbacteremic pneumonias. May be particularly useful when antibiotic therapy has already begun.

Acute phase serum should be stored at onset. If causal diagnosis is not established, a convalescent phase serum should be taken. A 4× increase in antibody titer establishes the causal diagnosis (e.g., *L. pneumophila*, *Chlamydia* spp., respiratory viruses [including influenza and RSV]), *M. pneumoniae*. Serologic tests to determine whether pneumonia is due to *Histoplasma*, *Coccidioides*, etc.

Pneumonia, Lipid

○ Sputum shows fat-containing macrophages that stain with Sudan. *They may be present only intermittently; therefore, examine sputum more than once.*

Pulmonary Alveolar Proteinosis

(Rare disease characterized by amorphous, lipid-rich, proteinaceous material in alveoli)

○ PAS–positive material appears in sputum.

○ PSP dye injected intravenously is excreted in sputum for long periods of time.

BAL fluid contains increased total protein, albumin, phospholipids, and CEA.

♦ Recently antibodies to surfactant protein A (ELISA assay) in sputum and BAL have been reported to be highly specific.

○ Serum CEA is increased and correlates with BAL findings. Reflects severity of disease and decreases with response to treatment.

○ Routine laboratory test findings are nonspecific.

- Serum LD increases when protein accumulates in lungs and becomes normal when infiltrate resolves; correlates with serum CEA.
- Decreased arterial O_2.
- Secondary polycythemia may occur.

♦ Diagnosis usually requires open lung biopsy. Electron microscopy shows many lamellar bodies.

Laboratory findings due to superinfection.

Pulmonary Embolism and Infarction

No laboratory test is diagnostic.

<10% of emboli lead to infarction

Measurement of arterial blood gases (obtained when patient is breathing room air) is the most sensitive and specific laboratory test.

○ • pO_2 <80 mm Hg in 88% of cases but normal pO_2 does not rule out pulmonary embolus. In appropriate clinical setting, pO_2 <88 mm Hg (even with a normal chest radiograph) is indication for lung scans and search for deep vein thromboses. pO_2 >90 mm Hg with a normal chest radiograph suggests a different diagnosis. Normal complete lung scans exclude the diagnosis.

- Hypocapnia and slightly elevated pH.

Increased WBC in 50% of patients but is rarely >15,000/cu mm (whereas in acute bacterial pneumonia is often >20,000/cu mm).

Increased ESR

Triad of increased LD and bilirubin with normal AST is found in only 15% of cases.
Serum enzymes differ from those in acute myocardial infarction.
- Increased serum LD (due to isoenzymes LD-2 and LD-3) in 80% of patients rises on first day, peaks on second, normal by tenth day.
- Serum AST is usually normal or only slightly increased.
- cTn not increased.

Serum indirect bilirubin is increased (as early as fourth day) to ~5 mg/dL in 20% of cases.
Pleural effusion may occur (see p. 150).

◆ Plasma D-dimer (ELISA or Latex Agglutination Kits)

Use

Detects lysis of fibrin clot only, whereas fibrinogen degradation products test detects lysis of both fibrin clot and fibrinogen (see Chapter 11). At appropriate cutoff level, has >80% sensitivity but only ~30% specificity. Negative predictive value >90%; normal test useful in excluding pulmonary embolism in patients with low pretest probability. Value less than cutoff level (which varies with assay kit) obviates need for pulmonary angiography.

Increased In
- Deep venous thrombosis
- DIC with fibrinolysis
- Renal, liver, or cardiac failure
- Major injury or surgery
- Inflammation (e.g., arthritis, cellulitis), infection (e.g., pneumonia)
- Thrombolytic therapy

Measurements of serum CK, LD, and fibrin products are not indicated routinely as they do not have sufficient sensitivity or specificity to be of diagnostic value.
Increased serum ALP (heat labile derived from vascular endothelium) during reparative phase 4–10 days after onset. Serum GGT may similarly increased.
Pleural effusion occurs in one-half of patients; bloody in one-third to two-thirds of cases; typical pattern in only one-fourth of cases.
These laboratory findings depend on the size and duration of the infarction, and the tests must be performed at the appropriate time to detect abnormalities.
Laboratory findings due to predisposing conditions, e.g.,
- Malignant tumors.
- Pregnancy.
- Use of estrogens.
- Hypercoagulable conditions, e.g.,
  Polycythemia vera
  Dysfibrinogenemias
  Protein C or S deficiency
  Antithrombin III deficiency
  Splenectomy with thrombocytosis
- See discussion of fat embolism (p. 303) and phlebothrombosis of leg veins (p. 127).

Sinusitis, Acute

Due To

Often precipitated by obstruction due to viral URI, allergy, foreign body.
S. pneumoniae and *H. influenzae* cause >50% of cases; also anaerobes, *S. aureus*, *S. pyogenes* (group A).
M. catarrhalis causes ~20% of cases in children
Viruses cause ~10–20% of cases
P. aeruginosa and *H. influenzae* are predominant organisms in cystic fibrosis patients.
Mucor spp., *Aspergillus* spp. should be ruled out in patients with diabetes or acute leukemia and in renal transplant recipients.
Anaerobes (e.g., streptococci, *Bacteroides* spp.) occur in ~50% of cases of chronic sinusitis.

Needle aspiration of sinus is required for determination of organism. Culture of nose, throat, and nasopharynx specimens do not correlate well.
Mucosal biopsy may be indicated if aspirate is not diagnostic in unresponsive patient with acute infection.

RESPIRATORY

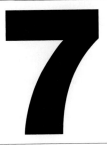

Gastrointestinal Diseases

Laboratory Tests of Gastrointestinal Function

Bentiromide

Bentiromide (Chymex), 500 mg taken orally after overnight fast, is acted on by pancreatic chymotrypsin, releasing para-aminobenzoic acid, which is measured in a 6-hr urine sample (normal value is >50%) and (in some procedures) 1- to 2-hr serum sample. Sensitivity of 6-hr test is ≤ 100% in severe chronic pancreatitis (with steatorrhea) and 40–50% in mild to moderate chronic pancreatitis (without steatorrhea).

Use

Initial test gauges pancreatic exocrine activity to rule out pancreatic disease in patients with chronic diarrhea, weight loss, or steatorrhea.
In conjunction with D-xylose tolerance test for differentiation of pancreatic exocrine insufficiency from intestinal mucosal disease.

Interference

False-negatives may occur due to drugs (e.g., thiazides, chloramphenicol, sulfonamides, acetaminophen, phenacetin, sunscreens, procaine anesthetics) and certain foods (prunes, cranberries).

Decreased In

Renal insufficiency, diabetes mellitus gastric emptying, severe liver disease, or gut mucosal disease (malabsorption such as celiac sprue)

Biopsy, Colon

Rectal biopsy is particularly useful in diagnosis of
- Cancer of colon
- Polyps of colon
- Secondary amyloidosis
- Amebic ulceration
- Schistosomiasis (even when no lesions are visible)
- Hirschsprung's disease
- Ulcerative colitis

Biopsy, Small Intestine

Use

Verifies mucosal lesions or establishes the diagnosis of various causes of malabsorption.
Confirms deficiency of various enzymes in intestinal mucosal cells (e.g., lactase deficiency).
Diagnosis of neoplasms of small intestine
Differential diagnosis of some cases of diarrhea
Differential diagnosis of some nutritional deficiencies
Monitoring of intestinal allografts

GI

Biopsy is diagnostic (diffuse lesion, diagnostic histology):
- Whipple's disease
- Agammaglobulinemia
- Abetalipoproteinemia (see p. 528: acanthotic RBCs, steatorrhea, failure of beta-lipoprotein manufacture, neurologic findings)
- Celiac sprue (becomes normal after dietary gluten withdrawal and abnormal after challenge)
- *Mycobacterium avium-intracellulare* infection

Biopsy may or may not be of specific diagnostic value (patchy lesions, diagnostic histology):
- Amyloidosis
- Intestinal lymphangiectasia
- Malignant lymphoma of small bowel
- Eosinophilic gastroenteritis
- Regional enteritis
- Systemic mastocytosis
- Hypogammaglobulinemia and dysgammaglobulinemia
- Parasitic infestations (giardiasis, coccidiosis, strongyloidiasis, capillariasis)

Biopsy may be abnormal but not diagnostic (diffuse lesions; histology not diagnostic):
- Celiac sprue
- Tropical sprue
- Severe prolonged folate and vitamin B_{12} deficiency
- Z-E syndrome
- Stasis with intraluminal bacterial overgrowth
- Drug-induced lesions (neomycin, antimetabolites)
- Malnutrition
- Bacterial overgrowth of small bowel
- Graft-versus-host reaction
- Viral enteritis

Biopsy may be abnormal but not diagnostic (patchy lesions; histology abnormal but not diagnostic):
- Acute radiation enteritis
- Dermatitis herpetiformis enteropathy

Biopsy is normal:
- Cirrhosis
- Pancreatic exocrine insufficiency
- Postgastrectomy malabsorption without intestinal mucosal disease
- Functional bowel disease (irritable colon, nonspecific diarrhea)

Biopsy taken using radiographic localization, prompt fixation of tissue, proper orientation of tissue for histologic sectioning, and serial sectioning of specimen are all necessary for proper interpretation. Multiple biopsies may be necessary for patchy lesions.

D-Xylose Tolerance Test

Normal: With 25 gm D-xylose dose, 30–52 mg/dL in blood at 2 hrs or ~25% in urine in 5 hrs. Up to age 9 yrs, use 5 gm dose and 1-hr serum sample; urine collection is not reliable. Normal 1-hr blood level ≥ 25 mg/dL, ≥ 20 mg/dL in children ≤ 9 yrs, ≥ 15 mg/dL in infants. Reference ranges may vary between laboratories.

Use

Follow response to gluten-free diet

Replaced by biopsy except in diseases with patchy distribution of lesions

Screening for intestinal malabsorption. Chief value was to distinguish proximal small intestinal malabsorption due to impaired transport across diseased mucosa, in which values are decreased, from pancreatic steatorrhea (impaired digestion in lumen), in which values are normal.

Urine test has poor sensitivity in mild mucosal disease.

False-positive and false-negative rates of 20–30%

Decreased In

Steatorrhea due to proximal small intestinal malabsorption (e.g., sprue, some cases of
Giardia lamblia infestation, bacterial overgrowth, viral gastroenteritis; may not be
useful in adult celiac disease)
Decreased glomerular filtration, e.g.,
- Elderly persons
- Myxedema
- Ascites
- Increased portal pressure
- Renal insufficiency
- Delayed gastric emptying
- Vomiting
- Dehydration
- Drugs (e.g., NSAIDs)

Normal In

Steatorrhea due to pancreatic disease
Postgastrectomy state
Malnutrition

Gastric Analysis

Use

Determine status of acid secretion in hypergastrinemia patients being treated for gastrinoma.
Determine if patients who have undergone surgery for ulcer disease and who have complications are secreting acid.

Interpretation

1-hr basal acid

<2 mEq	Normal, gastric ulcer, or carcinoma
2–5 mEq	Normal, gastric or duodenal ulcer
>5 mEq	Duodenal ulcer
>20 mEq	Z-E (Zollinger-Ellison) syndrome

1 hr after stimulation by pentagastrin

0 mEq	Achlorhydria, gastritis, gastric carcinoma
1–20 mEq	Normal, gastric ulcer, or carcinoma
20–35 mEq	Duodenal ulcer
35–60 mEq	Duodenal ulcer, high normal, Z-E syndrome
>60 mEq	Z-E syndrome

Ratio of basal acid to poststimulation outputs

20%	Normal, gastric ulcer, or carcinoma
20–40%	Gastric or duodenal ulcer
40–60%	Duodenal ulcer, Z-E syndrome
>60%	Z-E syndrome

Achlorhydria[1]

Chronic atrophic gastritis (serum gastrin is frequently increased)

PA	100% of patients
Vitiligo	20–25%
Alopecia areata	6%
RA	10–20%
Thyrotoxicosis	10%

GI

[1]Wolfe MM, Soll AH. The physiology of gastric acid secretion. *N Engl J Med* 1988;319:1707.

Gastric carcinoma (50% of patients) even after pentagastrin stimulation. Hypochlorhydria occurs in 25%, hydrochloric acid is normal in 25%, hyperchlorhydria is rare in patients with gastric carcinoma.

Gastric ulcer	Common
Adenomatous polyps of stomach	85% of patients
Ménétrier's disease	75%
Chronic renal failure	13% (usually normal; occasionally increased)
Iatrogenic	
Postvagotomy, postantrectomy	>90%
Measure acid output after IV insulin to demonstrate adequacy of vagotomy (see Insulin Test Meal, p. 161).	
Medical (e.g., potent H_2 receptor antagonists, substituted benzimidazoles)	>80%

Occurs in normal persons: 4% of children, increasing to 30% of adults older than age 60 years.

True achlorhydria excludes duodenal ulcer.

Hyperchlorhydria and Hypersecretion[2]

Duodenal ulcer	40–45%
Z-E syndrome (see p. 629)	100%

Twelve-hour night secretion shows acid of >100 mEq/L and volume >1500 mL.

Basal secretion is >60% of secretion caused by histamine or betazole stimulation.

Hyperplasia/hyperfunction of antral gastrin cells >90% (unusual condition with marked hyperchlorhydria, severe peptic ulceration, moderately increased fasting serum gastrin with exaggerated postprandial increase [>200% above fasting levels], no gastrin-secreting tumors).

Hypertrophic hypersecretory gastropathy	100%
Massive resection of small intestine (transient)	50%
Systemic mastocytosis	Rare

When basal serum gastrin level is equivocal, serum gastrin level should be measured after stimulation with infusion of secretin or calcium.

Gastrin, Serum

Normal levels: 0 to ≤ 200 pg/mL serum
Elevated levels: >500 pg/mL

Condition	Serum Gastrin	Serum Gastrin After Intragastric Administration of 0.1 N HCl
Peptic ulcer without Z-E syndrome	Normal range	—
Z-E syndrome	Very high	No change
PA	High level may approach that in Z-E syndrome	Marked decrease

Secretin infusion (IV of 2 U/kg body weight) with blood specimens drawn before and at intervals.
- Secretin test is preferred first test because of greater sensitivity and simplicity.
- Normal persons and patients with duodenal ulcer show no increase in serum gastrin.
- Patients with Z-E syndrome show increased serum gastrin that usually peaks in 45–60 mins (usually >400 pg/mL). With fasting gastrin <1000 pg/mL, sensitivity = 85% for an increased serum gastrin >200 pg/mL.
- With other causes of hypergastrinemia associated with hyperchlorhydria (e.g., retained antrum syndrome, gastric outlet obstruction, small bowel resection, renal insufficiency), serum gastrin is unchanged or decreases.

Calcium infusion (IV calcium gluconate, 5 mg/kg body weight/hr for 3 hrs) with preinfusion blood specimen compared to specimens every 30 mins for up to 4 hrs.

---

[2]Rosenfeld L. Gastric tubes, meals, acid and analysis: rise and decline. *Clin Chem* 1997;43:837.

- Recommended when secretin test is negative in patients in whom Z-E syndrome is suspected.
- Normal patients and those with ordinary duodenal ulcer show minimal serum gastrin response to calcium.
- Patients with antral G cell hyperfunction may or may not show serum gastrin increase >400 pg/mL.
- Patients with Z-E syndrome show increase in serum gastrin >400 pg/mL in 2–3 hrs (sensitivity = 43% for an increase of 395 pg/mL in serum gastrin). Positive in one-third of patients with a negative secretin test.[3]

Indications for measurement of serum gastrin and gastric analysis include
- Atypical peptic ulcer of stomach, duodenum, or proximal jejunum, especially if multiple, in unusual location, poorly responsive to therapy, or multiple, with rapid onset, or showing severe recurrence after adequate therapy
- Unexplained chronic diarrhea or steatorrhea with or without peptic ulcer
- Peptic ulcer disease with associated endocrine conditions (see Multiple Endocrine Neoplasia, p. 697)

Serum gastrin levels are indicated with any of the following:
- Basal acid secretion >10 mEq/hr in patients with intact stomachs.
- Ratio of basal to poststimulation output >40% in patients with intact stomachs.
- All patients with recurrent ulceration after surgery for duodenal ulcer.
- All patients with duodenal ulcer for whom elective gastric surgery is planned.
- Patients with peptic ulcer associated with severe esophagitis or prominent gastric or duodenal folds or hypercalcemia or extensive family history of peptic ulcer disease.
- Measurement for screening of all peptic ulcer patients would not be practical or cost effective.

Increased Serum Gastrin without Gastric Acid Hypersecretion

Atrophic gastritis, especially when associated with circulating parietal cell antibodies
PA in ~75% of patients
Some cases of carcinoma of body of stomach, a reflection of the atrophic gastritis that is present
Gastric acid inhibitor therapy
After vagotomy

Increased Serum Gastrin with Gastric Acid Hypersecretion

Z-E syndrome
Hyperplasia of antral gastrin cells
Isolated retained antrum (a condition of gastric acid hypersecretion and recurrent ulceration after antrectomy and gastrojejunostomy that occurs when the duodenal stump contains antral mucosa)

Increased Serum Gastrin with Gastric Acid Normal or Slight Hypersecretion

RA
Diabetes mellitus
Pheochromocytoma
Vitiligo
Chronic renal failure with serum creatinine >3 mg/dL; occurs in 50% of patients.
Pyloric obstruction with gastric distention
Short-bowel syndrome due to massive resection or extensive regional enteritis
Incomplete vagotomy

Insulin Test Meal

Aspirate gastric fluid and measure gastric acid every 15 mins for 2 hrs after IV administration of sufficient insulin (usually 15–20 U) to produce blood sugar <50 mg/dL.

[3]Frucht H, et al. Secretin and calcium provocative tests in the Zollinger-Ellison syndrome. *Ann Intern Med* 1989;111:713.

GI

Use

Differentiate causes of hypergastrinemia (see Table 13-14)
Supplanted by other tests; formerly used to
    Aid in distinguishing benign and malignant gastric ulcers
    Aid in diagnosis of PA
    Evaluate patients with ulcer dyspepsia but normal radiographs

Interpretation

Normal: Increased free HCl due to hypoglycemia.
Successful vagotomy produces achlorhydria.

Stool, Laboratory Examination

Normal Values

Bulk	100–200 gm
Water	Up to 75%
Total osmolality	200–250 mOsm
pH	7.0–7.5 (may be acid with high lactose intake)
Nitrogen	<2.5 gm/day
Potassium	5–20 mEq/kg
Sodium	10–20 mEq/kg
Magnesium	<200 mEq/kg
Coproporphyrin	400–1000 mg/24 hrs
Trypsin	20–950 U/gm
Urobilinogen	50–300 mg/24 hrs

Microscopic Examination

RBCs absent
Epithelial cells present (increased with GI tract irritation); absence of epithelial cells in meconium of newborn may aid in diagnosis of intestinal obstruction in the newborn.
Few WBCs present (increased with GI tract inflammation).
Crystals of calcium oxalate, fatty acid, and triple phosphate commonly present.
Hematoidin crystals sometimes found after GI tract hemorrhage.
Charcot-Leyden crystals sometimes found in parasitic infestation (especially amebiasis).
Some undigested vegetable fibers and muscle fibers sometimes found normally.
Neutral fat globules (stained with Sudan), normal 0–2+

Color Changes

Normal: brown
Clay color (gray-white): biliary obstruction
Tarry: >100 mL of blood in upper GI tract
Red: blood in large intestine or undigested beets or tomatoes
Black: blood
Silver: combination of jaundice and blood (cancer of ampulla of Vater)
Various colors: depending on diet

Due to Drugs	Resulting Color
Alkaline antacids and aluminum salts	White discoloration or speckling
Anticoagulants (excess)	Due to bleeding
Anthraquinones	Brown staining
Bismuth salts	Black
Charcoal	Black
Diathiazine	Green to blue
Indomethacin	Green (due to biliverdin)
Iron salts	Black
Mercurous chloride	Green
Phenazopyridine	Orange-red
Phenolphthalein	Red

Phenbutazone and oxyphenbutazone	Black (due to bleeding)
Pyrvinium pamoate	Red
Rhubarb	Yellow
Salicylates	Due to bleeding
Santonin	Yellow
Senna	Yellow to brown
Tetracyclines in syrup (due to glucosamine)	Red

Occult Blood

Use

Screening for asymptomatic ulcerated lesions of GI tract, especially carcinoma of the colon and large adenomas, is generally recommended now.

Interpretation

Kits (e.g., Hemoccult cards) use guaiac; detect blood losses of ~20 mL/day; "normal" amount of blood lost in stool daily is <2 mL/day or 2 mg Hb/gm of stool, but sensitivity is only 20% at this level and 90% at Hb concentration >25 mg/gram of stool. ~50% of colon cancers shed enough blood to produce a positive test. Hemoccult gives 1–3% false-positives even with strict protocol for stool collection. Sensitivity of Hemoccult and HemoQuant is only ~20–30% for colorectal cancer and ~13% for polyps; most of these lesions are missed.[4]

Benzidine reaction is too sensitive; yields too many false-positive results. Guaiac test yields too many false-negative results.

In various screening programs, 2–6% of participants have positive tests; of these, carcinoma is found in 5–10% and adenoma in 20–40%. Sensitivity = 81% for left colon cancer, 47% for colon and cecum cancer, 45% for rectal cancer. ~90% of positives are false-positives.

Adenomas <2 cm in size are less likely to bleed. Upper GI tract bleeding is less likely than lower GI tract bleeding to cause a positive test.

Long-distance running is associated with positive guaiac test in up to 23% of runners.

Recommendations for testing
- Test two areas from each of three consecutive stool samples.
- Test all samples within 7 days of collection.
- Rehydration of slide before development is controversial.
- Use of fecal sample obtained during digital rectal examination is not recommended.
- For 3 days before test, avoid large doses of aspirin (>325 mg/day) and other NSAIDs, ascorbic acid (false-negative may occur with >500 mg/day), oral iron, red meat, poultry, fish, and certain fruits and vegetables that contain catalases and peroxidases (e.g., cucumbers, horseradish, cauliflower), especially if slides are rehydrated.
- Even one positive result is considered a positive test even without dietary restriction.[5,6]

Other tests for occult blood
- Quantitative HemoQuant test kit (uses fluorescence to assay stool-derived porphyrins) doubles sensitivity of guaiac tests; may be affected by red meat and aspirin (for up to 4 days) but not by other substances mentioned above. Manual test performed in a laboratory requires 90 mins (<2 mg/gm is normal; >4 mg/gm is increased; 2–4 mg/gm is borderline).
- Immunochemical tests (e.g., HemeSelect) specifically detect human hemoglobin, do not require diet or chemical restrictions (do not react with animal heme or foods), are stable for up to 30 days, detect ~0.3 mg Hb/gm of stool whereas 5–10× this amount is required to cause a positive guaiac test.
- Samples from *upper* GI tract should not be tested for blood using urine dipsticks or stool occult blood test kits (low pH may cause false-negative and oral drug use false-positive results).[7,8]

GI

[4]Ahlquist DA. Accuracy of fecal occult blood screening for colorectal neoplasia. A perspective study using Hemoccult and HemoQuant tests. *JAMA* 1993;269:1262.

[5]Ransohoff DH, Lang CA. Suggested technique for fecal occult blood testing and interpretation in colorectal cancer screening. *Ann Intern Med* 1997;126:808.

[6]Ransohoff DH, Lang CA. Screening for colorectal cancer with the fecal occult blood test: a background paper. *Ann Intern Med* 1997;126:811.

[7]Knight KK, et al. Occult blood screening for colorectal cancer. *JAMA* 1989;261:587.

[8]Fleischer DE, et al. Detection and surveillance of colorectal cancer. *JAMA* 1989;261:580.

^{51}Cr Test for Bleeding

Tag 10 mL of the patient's blood with 200 μCi of ^{51}Cr, and administer it IV.
Collect daily stool specimens for radioactivity measurement and also measure simultaneous blood samples.

Use

Measure GI blood loss in ulcerative diseases (e.g., ulcerative colitis, regional enteritis, peptic ulcer).

Interpretation

Radioactivity in the stool establishes GI blood loss. Comparison with radioactivity measurements of 1 mL of blood indicates the amount of blood loss.

Electrolytes

	Sodium (mEq/24 hrs)	Chloride (mEq/24 hrs)	Potassium (mEq/24 hrs)
Normal*	7.8±2.0	3.2±0.7	18.2±2.5
Idiopathic proctocolitis	22.3	19.8	Normal
Ileostomy	30	19.0	4.1
Cholera	Increased	Increased	

*Average values for eight healthy individuals. Variable but considerably lower than simultaneous concentrations in serum.

Normal calcium ≈0.6 gm/24 hrs

Fat

See Malabsorption, pp. 185–189.

Osmotic Gap

(Osmotic gap = measured osmolality minus 2 × [Na + K] or 290 mOsm/kg H$_2$O minus 2 × [Na + K])

Increased In

Osmotic diarrhea (see p. 173)
See Factitious Disorders (p. 893).

Stool Findings	**Possible Diagnosis**
Osmotic gap <50 mOsm/kg H$_2$O and Na >90 mEq/L	Secretory diarrhea or osmotic diarrhea due to Na$_2$SO$_4$ or Na$_2$PO$_4$*
Osmotic gap >100 mOsm/kg H$_2$O and Na <60 mEq/L	Osmotic diarrhea; if fasting does not return stool volume to normal, consider factitious Mg ingestion†
Osmolality >375 mOsm/kg H$_2$O and Na <60 mEq/L	Possible contamination with concentrated urine
Osmolality <200–250 mOsm/kg H$_2$O	Possible contamination with dilute urine or water. Stool osmolality considerably lower than plasma osmolality; useful only if <250 mOsm/kg.

*Stool sulfate and phosphate increased; chloride <20 mEq/L.
†Mg usually >50 and often >100 mmol/L; normal during fasting is <10 mmol/L; normal on regular diet is 10–45 mmol/L.

Other Procedures

Alkalinization of stool to pH of 10 turns stool blue due to phenolphthalein in certain laxatives. Useful in cases of laxative abuse.
Examination for ova and parasites
Trypsin digestion (see Cystic Fibrosis of Pancreas, p. 254)
See Malabsorption, pp. 185–189.

Urobilinogen

(Normal = 50–300 mg/24 hrs; 100–400 Ehrlich units/100 gm)
Increased In
Hemolytic anemias
Decreased In
Complete biliary obstruction
Severe liver disease
Oral antibiotic therapy altering intestinal bacterial flora
Decreased hemoglobin turnover (e.g., aplastic anemia, cachexia)

Latex Agglutination Test Kit for Leukocytes

**(Detects fecal lactoferrin, a marker protein for fecal leukocytes; uses frozen or fresh
   stool.)**
Use
Detection of bowel inflammation not evident by endoscopy or radiographic studies
Interpretation
In one study, a stool dilution of 1:50 had a negative predictive value of 94% for the presence of invasive enteropathogens. Positive and negative predictive values of 93% and
   88% compared to stool microscopy for leukocytes are reported. At 1:200 dilution, sensitivity is <70%; therefore if test is negative when infectious diarrhea must be ruled
   out with considerable certainty (e.g., in immunocompromised patient), stool should
   be cultured.
Leukocytes labeled with [111]indium have been used as quantitative index of fecal leukocyte loss in research laboratory.

Microscopic Examination of Diarrheal Stools for Leukocytes

Primarily PMNs—any number of PMNs found in less than two-thirds of cases
  • Shigellosis: 70% have >5 PMNs/oil immersion field
  • Salmonellosis: 30% have >5 PMNs/oil immersion field
  • Campylobacter infection: 30% have >5 PMNs/oil immersion field
  • Rotavirus infection: 11% have >5 PMNs/oil immersion field
  • Invasive *Escherichia coli* colitis
  • *Yersinia* infection
  • Ulcerative colitis
  • *Clostridium difficile* infection (pseudomembranous colitis, see p. 172)
Primarily mononuclear leukocytes
  • Typhoid
Leukocytes absent
  • Cholera
  • Noninvasive *E. coli* diarrhea
  • Other bacterial toxins (e.g., *Staphylococcus*, *Clostridium perfringens*)
  • Viral diarrheas
  • Parasitic infestations (e.g., *Giardia lamblia*, *Entamoeba histolytica*, *Dientamoeba
    fragilis*)
  • Drug effects

Diseases of the Gastrointestinal Tract

Anticoagulant Therapy, Gastrointestinal Complications

Hemorrhage into gastrointestinal tract occurs in 3–4% of patients on anticoagulant
   therapy; may be spontaneous or secondary to unsuspected disease (e.g., peptic ulcer,
   carcinoma, diverticula, hemorrhoids). Occasionally hemorrhage occurs into the wall
   of the intestine with secondary ileus. PT may be in the therapeutic range or, more
   commonly, is increased. *Coumarin drug action is potentiated by administration of
   aspirin, antibiotics, phenylbutazone, and thyroxine and T-tube drainage of the common bile duct, especially if pancreatic disease is present.*

GI

Hypersensitivity to phenindione may cause hepatitis or steatorrhea.
Stool is positive for occult blood.

Appendicitis, Acute

Increased WBC (12,000–14,000/cu mm) with shift to the left in acute catarrhal stage;
   higher and more rapid rise with suppuration or perforation
ESR may be normal during first 24 hrs.
CRP <2.5 mg/dL 12 hrs after onset of symptoms has been said to exclude acute appendicitis.
Later—laboratory findings due to complications (e.g., dehydration, abscess formation,
   perforation with peritonitis)

Ascites

(See also Pleural Effusion, pp. 140–149, for differential diagnosis of effusions.)
Chronic liver disease: To differentiate ascites due to malignancy from that due to
   chronic liver disease
   • Albumin gradient (= serum albumin minus ascitic fluid albumin) reflects portal
      pressure (replaces terms *transudate* and *exudate*).
         Almost always ≥ 1.1 in cirrhosis (most common cause), alcoholic hepatitis, mas-
            sive liver metastases, fulminant hepatic failure, portal vein thrombosis, Budd-
            Chiari syndrome, cardiac ascites, acute fatty liver of pregnancy, myxedema,
            mixed (e.g., cirrhosis with peritoneal TB). May be falsely low if serum albu-
            min <1.1 gm/dL or patient in shock. May be falsely high with chylous ascites
            (lipid interferes with albumin assay).
         <1.1 gm/dL in >90% of cases of peritoneal carcinomatosis (most common cause)
            or TB, pancreatic or biliary ascites, nephrotic syndrome, bowel infarction or
            obstruction, serositis in patients without cirrhosis.
   • Ascitic fluid to serum albumin ratio <0.5 in cirrhosis (>90% accuracy).
   • Total protein >2.5 mg/dL in cancer is only 56% accurate because of high protein
      content in 12–19% of these ascites cases as well as changes due to albumin infu-
      sion and diuretic therapies.
   • Ascitic fluid to serum ratio for LD (>0.6) or protein (>0.5) is not more accurate
      (~56%) than total protein only for diagnosis of exudate.
   • Ascitic fluid cholesterol is <55 mg/dL in cirrhosis (94% accuracy).
   • Total WBC is usually <300/cu mm (one-half of cases) and PMN is usually <25%
      (two-thirds of cases).
   • Findings cannot distinguish neoplasia from TB etiology.
   • Cirrhosis findings similar with or without hepatocellular carcinoma.
Cardiac ascites is associated with a blood–ascitic fluid albumin gradient >1.1 gm/dL
   but malignant ascitic fluid shows blood–ascitic fluid albumin gradient <1.1 gm/dL
   in 93% of cases.
Infected ascitic fluid
   ♦ • WBC >250/cu mm (sensitivity = 85%, specificity = 93%) and neutrophils >50%
      and are presumptive of bacterial peritonitis.
   ♦ • pH <7.35 and arterial–ascitic fluid pH difference >0.10; both these findings are
      virtually diagnostic of bacterial peritonitis and absence of the above findings vir-
      tually excludes bacterial peritonitis.
   • Ascitic fluid lactate >25 mg/dL and arterial–ascitic fluid difference >20 mg/dL are
      often present.
   • Ascitic fluid LD is markedly increased.
   • Ascitic fluid glucose is unreliable for diagnosis.
   • Ascitic fluid phosphate, potassium, and GGT may also be increased.
   ♦ • Gram stain is positive in 25% of cases.
   ♦ • Ascitic fluid in *blood culture bottles* has 85% sensitivity.
   ♦ • Acid-fast stains and culture establish the diagnosis of TB in only 25–50% of cases
      of TB.
   • Total protein <1.0 gm/dL indicates high risk for spontaneous bacterial peritonitis.
Secondary peritonitis shows polymicrobial infection, total protein ≥ 1.0 gm/dL, ascitic
   fluid LD greater than serum upper limit of normal, and glucose <50 mg/dL compared

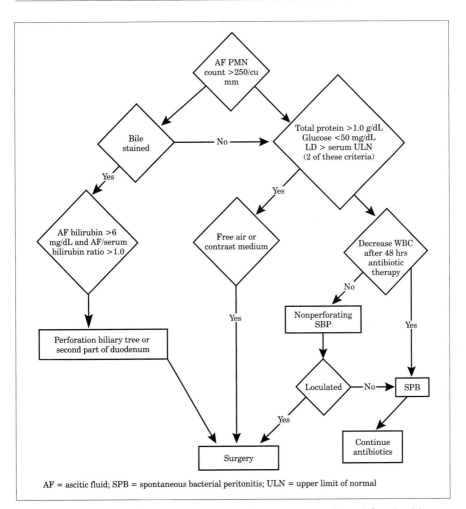

Fig. 7-1. Algorithm for differentiating secondary from spontaneous bacterial peritonitis (SBP).

to spontaneous bacterial peritonitis. Spontaneous bacterial peritonitis has prevalence of ~15%; due to *E. coli* ~50%, due to *Klebsiella* and other gram-negative or gram-positive bacteria, ~25% (especially streptococci).

In continuous ambulatory peritoneal dialysis, monitor dialysate for (see Figs. 7-1 and 7-2):

♦ • Infection: Peritonitis is defined as WBC >100/cu mm, usually with >50% PMNs (normal value is <50 WBC/cu mm, usually mononuclear cells), or positive Gram stain or culture (most prevalent: coagulase-negative staphylococci, *Staphylococcus aureus*, *Streptococcus* spp.; multiple organisms, especially mixed aerobes and anaerobes, occur with bowel perforation). Successful therapy causes fall in WBC within first 2 days and return to <100/cu mm in 4–5 days; differential returns to predominance of monocytes in 4–7 days with increased eosinophils in 10% of cases. Patients check outflow bags for turbidity. Turbid dialysate can occasionally occur without peritonitis during first few months of placing catheter (due to catheter hypersensitivity) with WBC 100–8000/cu mm and 10–95% eosinophils, sometimes increased PMNs, and negative cultures. Occasional RBCs

GI

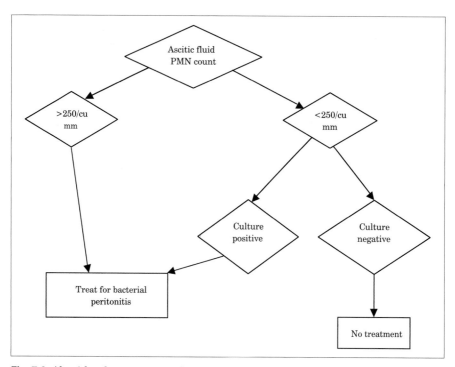

Fig. 7-2. Algorithm for spontaneous bacterial peritonitis.

may be seen during menstruation or with ovulation at midcycle. *Because of low WBC decision level, manual hemocytometer count rather than an automated instrument must be used.*
- Metabolic change: Assay dialysate for creatinine and glucose; calculate ultrafiltrate volume by weighing dialysate fluid after 4-hr dwell time and subtracting it from preinfusion weight using specific gravity of 1.0.
♦ Pancreatic disease: Ascitic fluid amylase greater than serum amylase is virtually specific for pancreatic disease, but both levels are normal in 10% of cases. Methemalbumin in serum or ascitic fluid and total protein >4.5 gm/dL indicate poor prognosis.
Chylous ascites: Triglyceride is 2–8× serum level. Protein is 2–3 gm/dL. Due to lymphatic obstruction (e.g., lymphoma or carcinoma [60% of cases]), inflammation or obstruction of small intestine, trauma to chest or abdomen, filariasis; in pediatric patients, is often due to congenital lymphatic defects.
♦ Malignant ascites: Increased fluid cholesterol (>45 mg/dL) and fibronectin (>10 mg/dL) have sensitivity of 90% and specificity of 82%. Positive cytology has sensitivity of 70% and specificity of 100%. Increased ascitic fluid CEA (>2.5 mg/dL) has sensitivity of 45% and specificity of 100%.
♦ Criteria to diagnose *penetrating* abdominal wounds by peritoneal lavage
- >10,000 RBC/cu mm (>5000 RBC/cu mm for gunshot wounds).
- >500 WBC/cu mm or
- Bacteria, fecal, or vegetable matter on Gram stain or bile (Ictotest) or
- Detection of endotoxin by limulus amoebocyte lysate assay for ileocolic perforation or
- Amylase or ALP level has been used to detect small bowel or pancreatic injury.
- Increases in WBC, amylase, and ALP are often delayed >3 hrs.
- RBC and WBC counts of lavage fluid have most clinical utility.
♦ Criteria to diagnose *blunt* abdominal trauma by peritoneal lavage with 10,000 mL of normal saline; falsely low RBC count if <600–800 mL of fluid is recovered.

- Grossly bloody fluid or
- >100,000 RBC/cu mm (newspaper print is unreadable through lavage tubing if RBC count is this high); negative test = <50,000 RBC/cu mm; equivocal results = 50,000–100,000; or
- >500 WBC/cu mm or
- Amylase >2.5× normal

♦ Criteria to diagnose *intestinal injury* in blunt abdominal trauma by peritoneal lavage with 10,000 mL of normal saline, especially 3–18 hrs after injury
  - If bloody ascites is not present, may signal solid organ injury
  - >10,000 WBC/cu mm and
  - WBC/cu mm ≥ (RBC/cu mm divided by 150)

♦ To differentiate urine from ascitic or pleural fluid (in cases of possible GU tract fistula or accidental aspiration of bladder)
  - Urine creatinine is >2× serum level.
  - Uncontaminated ascitic or pleural fluid creatinine is usually same as serum level but always <2× serum level.
  - Urea nitrogen also greater in urine.

Increased serum inorganic phosphate in 25% of cases of ischemic bowel disease; >5.5 mg/dL indicates extensive bowel injury, acute renal failure, metabolic acidosis, and poorer prognosis.

Peritoneal fluid bicarbonate value to differentiate site of penetrating wounds of GI tract:

Wound Site	Effect on Bicarbonate Value
Stomach or duodenum proximal to pancreatic duct	Decrease
Duodenum just distal to pancreatic duct	Increase
Third part of duodenum, jejunum, or ileum	Probably no effect

Fluid Source	Bicarbonate Values (mEq/L) (Reference Values)
Peritoneal	24.0–29.0
Pancreatic	66.0–127.0
Duodenal	4.0–21.0
Jejunal	2.0–32.0
Ileal	2.3
Gastric	—
Plasma/venous blood	20.0–30.0

Ascites in Fetus or Neonate

Due To

Nonimmune (occur in 1:3000 pregnancies)

	% of cases
Cardiovascular abnormalities causing congestive heart failure (e.g., structural, arrhythmias)	40
Chromosomal (e.g., Turner's and Down syndromes are most common; trisomy 13, 15, 16, 18)	10–15
Hematologic disorders (any severe anemia)	10

    Inherited, e.g.,
        Alpha-thalassemia
        Hemoglobinopathies
        G-6-PD deficiency
        Other RBC enzyme defects
    Acquired, e.g.,
        Fetal-maternal hemorrhage
        Twin-to-twin transfusion
        Congenital infection (parvovirus B19)
        Methemoglobinemia
Congenital defects of chest and abdomen
    Structural, e.g.,
        Diaphragmatic hernia
        Cystic adenomatoid malformation of lung
        Jejunal atresia
        Fetal lymphatic dysplasia

GI

Midgut volvulus
Intestinal malrotation
Peritonitis due to
 GI tract perforation
 Congenital infection (e.g., syphilis, TORCH [*t*oxoplasma, *o*ther agents, *r*ubella, *c*ytomegalovirus, *h*erpes simplex] syndrome, hepatitis)
 Meconium peritonitis due to complications of cystic fibrosis
Lymphatic duct obstruction
Biliary atresia
Bile ascites (rare) due to biliary tree perforation caused by congenital stenosis, choledochal cyst or stone.
• Intermittent acholic stools, dark urine, fluctuating hyperbilirubinemia.
• Bile-stained ascitic fluid with increased protein (2–4 gm/dL).
• IV administration of iodine 131 (^{131}I)–labeled rose bengal appearing in ascitic fluid makes the diagnosis early before bile staining occurs.
Nonstructural, e.g.,
 Congenital nephrotic syndrome
 Cirrhosis
 Cholestasis
 Hepatic necrosis
 GI tract obstruction
Lower GU tract obstruction (e.g., usually due to posterior urethral valves, urethral atresia, ureterocele) is most common cause.
Inherited skeletal dysplasias (enlarged liver causing extramedullary hematopoiesis)
Fetal tumors, most often teratomas and neuroblastomas
Vascular placental abnormalities
Genetic metabolic disorders, e.g.,
   Hurler's syndrome
   Gaucher's disease
   Niemann-Pick disease
   GM_1 gangliosidosis type I
   I-cell disease
   Beta-glucuronidase deficiency
Immune (maternal antibodies reacting to fetal antigens, e.g., Rh, C, E, Kell)

Celiac Disease (Gluten-Sensitive Enteropathy, Nontropical Sprue, Idiopathic Steatorrhea)

See Fig. 7-3.
♦ Steatorrhea demonstrated by positive Sudan stain on ≥ 2 stool samples or quantitative determination of fat in 72-hr pooled stool sample (see p. 185).
♦ Xylose tolerance test distinguishes malabsorption due to impaired transport across diseased mucosa from impaired pancreatic digestion in lumen (see p. 188).
♦ Biopsy of small intestine shows characteristic although not specific mucosal lesions. Establishing the diagnosis is essential; patients should not be committed to gluten-free diet without first assessing intestinal mucosal histology.
♦ Firm diagnosis requires definite clinical response to gluten-free diet, preferably with histologic documentation that mucosa has reverted to normal by repeat biopsy in 6–12 mos. If no response to rigid dietary control, GI lymphoma should be ruled out.
♦ Gluten challenge is performed if diagnosis is uncertain and not documented by biopsy before gluten withdrawal, to determine if symptoms recur and mucosal changes occur. (Baseline biopsy followed by one-half slice bread, doubled every 3 days up to four slices daily for 4 wks or until symptoms recur, followed by repeat biopsy.)
♦ Antigliadin antibodies (IgG is more sensitive but less specific than IgA) and antiendomysial antibodies (IgA is most specific; sensitivity = 80–100%) in serum of untreated patients. Is especially useful in patients in whom index of suspicion is very low or who have atypical features but consistent biopsy findings. Also present in patients with other small intestine mucosal diseases (e.g., Crohn's disease), 25% of patients with dermatitis herpetiformis, and rarely in those with autoimmune diseases. Decreased in celiac patients on gluten-free diet. Serial measurement to monitor compliance and therapy. Antireticulin antibodies are less sensitive (<50%) but more specific than antigliadin antibodies.

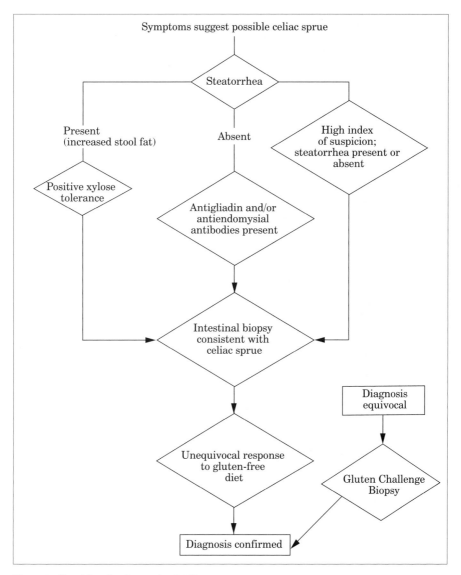

Fig. 7-3. Algorithm for diagnosis of celiac sprue.

Laboratory findings due to frequently associated diseases (e.g., especially lymphoma of
 intestine and elsewhere; also dermatitis herpetiformis, insulin-dependent diabetes,
 selective IgA deficiency, carcinoma of esophagus, small intestine, and breast; possibly IgA nephropathy, ulcerative colitis, thyroid disease, primary biliary cirrhosis, sclerosing cholangitis). In any such patients with unexplained diarrhea or malabsorption,
 celiac sprue should be ruled out.
○Should always be considered in cases of iron-deficiency anemia without demonstrable bleeding, unexplained folate deficiency, or unexplained osteopenic bone disease.

GI

Chloridorrhea, Congenital

(Rare autosomal recessive condition characterized by profound watery diarrhea beginning at birth due to ion transport defect in ileum and colon.)
♦ Hypochloremic, hypokalemic acidosis with volume depletion
♦ Copious acidic chloride-rich diarrhea
Normal intestinal mucosal histology.
Maternal hydramnios is almost always present.

Similar rarer autosomal recessive condition of congenital sodium diarrhea with sodium-rich alkaline stool and systemic acidosis.

Colitis, Collagenous

♦ Diagnosis is established by biopsy of colon in patients thought to have irritable bowel syndrome. Incidence ~3:1000 in such patients.
ESR increased in some patients.
Eosinophil count increased in some patients.

Colitis, Pseudomembranous

(Antibiotic-related diarrhea and colitis due to *C. difficile*)
♦ Tissue culture assay is gold standard (>94% sensitivity, 99% specificity). Level of toxin is not related to clinical severity.
♦ Diagnosis depends on detection of cytotoxin in stool. Demonstration of toxins (toxin A) or antigens by rapid immunoassays (EIA) show good sensitivity (64–87%) and specificity (99%). Rapid results make these tests useful for screening.
Latex agglutination has variable and poor sensitivity and is not recommended as a single test.
Glutamate dehydrogenase enzyme by latex agglutination or immunoassay lacks good specificity (enzyme found in other organisms).
Stool assay for glutamate dehydrogenase enzyme combined with toxin A assay in one test may be more useful.
For *C. difficile*–associated diarrhea both culture and cytotoxin assay should be performed.
Counterimmunoelectrophoresis (CIE), gas-liquid chromatography (GLC), and Gram stain of stool have high false-negative and false-positive results.
Stool culture is less efficient because some strains are nontoxigenic. >50% of healthy neonates, 2–5% of healthy adults, 25% of adults recently treated with antibiotics are carriers. Nontoxigenic strains may be found in 10–20% of hospitalized patients. Toxin testing alone does not detect 20–30% of *C. difficile*–associated diarrhea.
PCR of stool for toxin A and/or B may be available.
Fecal leukocytes in stool (see p. 165); large numbers in <50% of cases; bloody diarrhea in ≤ 10% of cases.
WBC >15,000/cu mm in <50% of cases.
Hypoalbuminemia in ≤ 24% of cases.
Laboratory findings due to dehydration and electrolyte imbalance in severe cases.

Colitis, Ulcerative, Chronic Nonspecific

Laboratory findings parallel severity of the disease
• Anemia due to blood loss (frequently Hb = 6 gm/dL).
• WBC usually normal unless complication occurs (e.g., abscess).
• ESR often normal or only slightly increased.
• With diarrhea and fever, Hb <7.5 gm/dL and ESR >30 mm/hr indicate severe disease.
• Hypoalbuminemia indicates severe disease of longer duration.
Stools
• Positive for blood (gross and/or occult)
• Negative for usual enteric bacterial pathogens and parasites; high total bacterial count
Changes in liver function
• Microscopic changes in needle biopsy of liver.
• Serum ALP often increased slightly.
• Other liver function tests usually normal.
Changes in serum electrolytes due to diarrhea or to therapy with adrenal steroids or ACTH

Laboratory changes due to complications or sequelae (e.g., malabsorption due to involvement of small intestine, perforation, abscess formation, hemorrhage, carcinoma, arthritis, sclerosing cholangitis)
○Rectal biopsy

Colon, Carcinoma

Blood in stool (occult or gross)
Evidence of inflammation
  • Increased WBC and ESR
Anemia—usually hypochromic
  • May be the only symptom of carcinoma of right side of colon (present in >50% of these patients)
  • Stools sometimes negative for occult blood
Laboratory evidence of liver metastases
♦Biopsy of colon lesion establishes the diagnosis
Serum CEA (see p. 906)
○ *Villous tumor of rectum may cause secretory diarrhea with potassium loss and decreased serum potassium. Carcinoid tumors may cause increased 5-HIAA in urine.*
Laboratory findings due to underlying condition (e.g., hereditary polyposis, chronic nonspecific ulcerative colitis)
Laboratory findings due to complications (e.g., hemorrhage, perforation, obstruction)

Diarrhea, Acute

Osmotic (Malabsorptive) Diarrhea

(Increased osmotically active solutes in bowel; diarrhea usually stops during fasting.)
Due To
Exogenous
  • Laxatives (e.g., magnesium sulfate, milk of magnesia, sodium sulfate [Glauber's salt], sodium phosphate, polyethylene glycol/saline)
  • Drugs (e.g., lactulose, colchicine, cholestyramine, neomycin, PAS)
  • Foods (e.g., mannitol, sorbitol [in diet candy, chewing gum, soda])
Endogenous
Congenital malabsorption
  • Specific (e.g., lactase deficiency, fructose malabsorption)
  • General (e.g., abeta- and hypobetalipoproteinemia, congenital lymphangiectasia, cystic fibrosis)
Acquired malabsorption
  • Specific (e.g., pancreatic disease, celiac sprue, parasitic infestation, rotavirus enteritis, metabolic disorders [thyrotoxicosis, adrenal insufficiency], jejunoileal bypass, bacterial overgrowth, short-bowel syndrome, inflammatory disease [mastocytosis, eosinophilic enteritis])

Secretory (Abnormal Electrolyte Transport) Diarrhea

(Increased water and chloride secretion; normal water and sodium absorption may be inhibited.)
Due To
Exogenous
Laxatives (e.g., aloe, anthraquinones, bisacodyl, castor oil, dioctyl sodium sulfosuccinate, phenolphthalein, senna)
Drugs
  Diuretics (e.g., furosemide, thiazides), asthma drugs (theophylline), thyroid drugs
  Cholinergic drugs, e.g.,
    Myasthenia gravis (cholinesterase inhibitors)
    Cardiac (quinidine) and antihypertensives (ACE inhibitors)
    Antidepressants (clozapine)
    Gout (colchicine)
Toxins (e.g., arsenic, mushrooms, organophosphates, alcohol)
Bacterial toxins (e.g., *S. aureus, E. coli, Vibrio cholerae, Bacillus cereus, Campylobacter jejuni, Yersinia enterocolitica, Clostridium botulinum* and *perfringens*)

GI

Endogenous
Hormones
- Serotonin (carcinoid)
- Calcitonin (medullary carcinoma of thyroid)
- Villous adenoma
- Vipoma

Gastric hypersecretion
- Z-E syndrome
- Systemic mastocytosis
- Basophilic leukemia
- Short-bowel syndrome

Bile salts (e.g., disease or resection of terminal ileum)
Fatty acids (e.g., disease of small intestine mucosa, pancreatic insufficiency)
Congenital (e.g., congenital chloridorrhea, congenital sodium diarrhea)

Watery stool
Volume >1 L/day
Blood and pus are absent.
Stool osmolality close to plasma osmolality with no anion gap.
Diarrhea usually continues during 24–48 hr fasting except for fatty acid malabsorption.

Exudative Diarrhea

(Active inflammation of bowel mucosa)
Due To
Inflammation
- Infectious (e.g., *Shigella, Salmonella, Campylobacter, Yersinia, C. difficile*, TB organisms, amebae)
- Idiopathic (e.g., ulcerative colitis, Crohn's disease)
- Injury (e.g., radiation)
- Ischemia (e.g., mesenteric thrombosis)
- Vasculitis
- Abscess (e.g., diverticulitis)

Stool contains blood and pus.
Some features of osmotic diarrhea may be present.
20–40% of cases of acute infectious diarrhea remain undiagnosed.

Motility Disturbances

Due To
Decreased small intestinal motility (e.g., hypothyroidism, diabetes mellitus, amyloidosis, scleroderma, postvagotomy)
Increased small intestinal motility (e.g., hyperthyroidism, carcinoid syndrome)
Increased colonic motility (e.g., irritable bowel syndrome)

Diarrhea, Chronic

Due To

Infection (e.g., giardiasis, amebiasis, infection with *Cryptosporidium, Isospora, Strongyloides, C. difficile*)
Inflammatory bowel disease (e.g., Crohn's disease, ulcerative colitis, collagenous colitis)
Carbohydrate malabsorption (e.g., lactase or sucrase deficiency)
Foods (e.g., ethanol, caffeine, sweeteners such as sorbitol, fructose)
Drugs (e.g., antibiotics, antihypertensives, antiarrhythmics, antineoplastics, colchicine, cholestyramine; see previous Diarrhea, Acute)
Laxative abuse (see p. 893); factitious
Endocrine (e.g., diabetes mellitus, adrenal insufficiency, hyper- or hypothyroidism)
Hormone-producing tumors (e.g., gastrinoma, VIPoma, villous adenoma, medullary thyroid carcinoma, pheochromocytoma, ganglioneuroma, carcinoid tumor, mastocytosis, somatostatinoma, ectopic hormone production by lung or pancreatic carcinoma)

Injury due to radiation, ischemia, etc.
Infiltrations (e.g., scleroderma, amyloidosis, lymphoma)
Colon carcinoma
Previous surgery (e.g., gastrectomy, vagotomy, intestinal resection)
Immune system disorders (e.g., systemic mastocytosis, eosinophilic gastroenteritis)
Intraluminal maldigestion
   Bile duct obstruction, cirrhosis
   Bacterial overgrowth
   Pancreatic exocrine insufficiency
Celiac sprue
Whipple's disease
Abetalipoproteinemia
Dermatitis herpetiformis
Intestinal lymphangiectasia
Allergy
Idiopathic

Diverticula of Jejunum, Multiple

Laboratory findings due to malabsorption syndrome

Diverticulitis, Acute

Increased WBC and ESR
Hypochromic microcytic anemia (some patients)
Occult blood in stool
Cytologic examination of stool—negative for malignant cells
Laboratory findings due to complications (e.g., hemorrhage, perforation, obstruction)

Dumping Syndrome

(Occurs in ≤ 70% of post–subtotal gastrectomy patients.)
During symptoms may have
- Rapid prolonged alimentary hyperglycemia
- Decreased plasma volume
- Decreased serum potassium
- Increased blood and urine serotonin
- Hypoglycemic syndrome (occurs in <5% of post–subtotal gastrectomy patients)
   Prolonged alimentary hyperglycemia followed after 2 hrs by precipitous hypo-
   glycemia
   Late hypoglycemia shown by 6-hr oral glucose tolerance test (OGTT)
- Stomal gastritis—anemia due to chronic bleeding
- Postgastrectomy malabsorption
- Postgastrectomy anemia (due to chronic blood loss, malabsorption, vitamin B_{12} deficiency, etc.)
- Afferent-loop obstruction—marked increase in serum amylase to >1000 U
Laboratory findings due to complications of gastric or duodenal ulcer e.g., hemorrhage, perforation, obstruction.
Gastric analysis
- True achlorhydria after maximum stimulation rules out duodenal ulcer.
- Normal secretion or hypersecretion does not prove the presence of an ulcer.

Duodenal Ulcer, Chronic

○*Helicobacter pylori*–associated gastritis is present in ~95% of all patients with duo-
   denal ulcer except those with Z-E syndrome.
Laboratory findings due to associated conditions
- Z-E syndrome
- MEN type I

GI

- Chronic renal failure
- Kidney stones
- Alpha₁-antitrypsin deficiency
- Systemic mastocytosis
- Chronic pancreatitis
- Mucoviscidosis
- RA
- Chronic pulmonary disease (e.g., pulmonary emphysema)
- Cirrhosis
- Certain drugs (e.g., ACTH)
- Crohn's disease
- Hyperparathyroidism
- Polycythemia vera

Duodenal ulcer is absent in patients with ulcerative colitis (unless under steroid therapy), carcinoma of stomach, PA, pregnancy.

Laboratory findings due to treatment

- Milk-alkali (Burnett's) syndrome—alkalosis, hypercalcemia, azotemia, renal calculi, or nephrocalcinosis
- Inadequate vagotomy—use insulin test meal (see p. 161).
- Gastric acidity shows late response >4.5 mEq total free acid in 30 mins or any early response. *To obtain valid collection, tube must be correctly placed fluoroscopically.*

Enteritis, Regional (Crohn's Disease)

No findings that are pathognomonic for this disease or distinguish it from ulcerative colitis.

Increased WBC, ESR, CRP, other acute-phase reactants. Mild increase of WBC indicates activity, but marked increase suggests suppuration (e.g., abscess). ESR tends to be higher in disease of colon than of ileum.

Anemia due to iron deficiency or vitamin B_{12} or folate deficiency or chronic disease

Decreased serum albumin, increased gamma globulins

Diarrhea may cause hyperchloremic metabolic acidosis, dehydration, decreased sodium, potassium, magnesium.

Mild liver function test changes due to pericholangitis (especially increased serum ALP)

Serum CEA may be increased.

○Biopsy may show granulomas in ~50% of cases.

Laboratory changes due to complications or sequelae (e.g., malabsorption, perforation and fistula formation, abscess formation, arthritis, sclerosing cholangitis)

Enterocolitis, Acute Membranous

Laboratory findings due to antecedent condition
    Disease for which antibiotics are administered
    Myocardial infarction
    Surgical procedure
    Other
Laboratory findings due to shock, dehydration
♦Culture of staphylococci from stool or rectal swab

Enterocolitis, Necrotizing, in Infancy

(Syndrome of acute intestinal necrosis of unknown etiology especially associated with prematurity and exchange transfusions)

No specific laboratory tests

Bloody stools; no characteristic organisms

Oliguria, neutropenia, anemia may be present.

Persistent metabolic acidosis, severe hyponatremia, and DIC are a common triad in infants.

In infants, significant organisms are often found by frequent repeated cultures of blood, urine, and stool.

Enteropathy, Protein-Losing

Secondary (i.e., disease states in which clinically significant protein-losing enteropathy may occur as a manifestation)
- Giant hypertrophy of gastric rugae (Ménétrier's disease)
- Eosinophilic gastroenteritis
- Gastric neoplasms
- Infections (e.g., Whipple's disease, bacterial overgrowth, enterocolitis, shigellosis, parasitic infestation, viral infection, *C. difficile* infection)
- Nontropical sprue
- Inflammatory and neoplastic diseases of small and large intestine, including ulcerative colitis, regional enteritis
- Constrictive pericarditis
- Immune diseases (e.g., SLE, milk allergy)
- Lymphatic obstruction (e.g., lymphoma, sarcoidosis, mesenteric TB)

Primary (i.e., hypoproteinemia is the major clinical feature)
- Intestinal lymphangiectasia
- Nonspecific inflammatory or granulomatous disease of small intestine

Serum total protein, albumin, and gamma globulin decreased
Serum alpha and beta globulins normal
Serum cholesterol usually normal
Mild anemia
Eosinophilia (occasionally)
Serum calcium decreased
Steatorrhea with abnormal tests of lipid absorption
Increased permeability of GI tract to large molecular substances shown by IV ^{131}I-polyvinylpyrrolidone test (see section on protein malabsorption, p. 192)
Proteinuria absent

Esophagus, Carcinoma

♦ Cytologic examination of esophageal washings is positive for malignant cells in 75% of patients. It is falsely positive in <2% of patients.
♦ Diagnosis is confirmed by biopsy of tumor.

Esophagus, Infections

Due To

Fungi
- *Candida albicans* (most common)
- Other *Candida* species
- *Torulosis glabrata*
- *Aspergillus* species
- *Histoplasma capsulatum*
- *Blastomyces dermatitidis*

Viruses
- HSV (especially in AIDS patients)
- CMV (especially in AIDS patients)
- HIV-1
- EBV
- VZV

Bacteria
- Gram-positive, usual oral flora (e.g., *Streptococcus viridans*, *Staphylococcus*)
- Gram-negative cocci, rods, enteric bacilli
- Tubercle bacilli (rare; usually no evidence of active pulmonary disease)
- *Actinomyces israelii*
- *Treponema pallidum*

Predisposing factors
- Immunosuppression (e.g., HIV infection)
- Drugs (e.g., corticosteroids, anticancer chemotherapy, radiation, broad-spectrum antibiotics)

GI

- Debilitating illnesses or conditions (e.g., diabetes mellitus, chronic renal failure, burns, old age)
- Trauma (e.g., insertion of nasogastric tubes, tracheal intubation)
♦ Diagnosis by cytologic brushings, biopsy, bacterial smears and cultures obtained via endoscope.

Esophagus, Spontaneous Perforation

♦ Gastric contents in thoracocentesis fluid

Esophagus Involvement Due to Primary Systemic Diseases

Scleroderma *(esophageal involvement in >50% of patients with scleroderma)*
Esophageal varices (cirrhosis of liver)
Malignant lymphoma
Bronchogenic carcinoma
Infections (see p. 177)
Sarcoidosis
Crohn's disease
Behçet's disease
Graft-versus-host disease
Pemphigus vulgaris
Bullous pemphigoid
Benign mucous membrane pemphigoid
Epidermolysis bullosa dystrophica

Gallstone Ileus

Laboratory findings due to preceding chronic cholecystitis and cholelithiasis
Laboratory findings due to acute obstruction of terminal ileum *(accounts for 1–2% of patients)*

Gastric Adenomatous Polyp

♦ Diagnosis is confirmed by biopsy of tumor.
Gastric analysis—achlorhydria in 85% of patients
Sometimes evidence of bleeding
Polyps occur in 5% of patients with PA and 2% of patients with achlorhydria.

Gastric Carcinoma

♦ Exfoliative cytology positive in 80% of patients; false-positive in <2%.
♦ Biopsy of lesions confirms diagnosis.
♦ Lymph node biopsy for metastases; needle biopsy of liver, bone marrow, etc.
Tumor markers are not useful for early detection.
- Increased serum CEA (>5 ng/dL) in 40–50% of patients with metastases and 10–20% of patients with surgically resectable disease. May be useful for postoperative monitoring for recurrence or to estimate metastatic tumor burden.
- Increased serum alpha-fetoprotein (AFP) and CA 19-9 in 30% of patients, usually incurable.
Gastric analysis
- Achlorhydria after histamine or betazole in 50% of patients
- Hypochlorhydria in 25% of patients
- Normal in 25% of patients
- Hyperchlorhydria rare
Anemia due to chronic blood loss
Occult blood in stool
○ *Carcinoma of the stomach should always be searched for by periodic prophylactic screening in high-risk patients, especially those with PA, gastric atrophy, gastric polyps.*

Gastric Leiomyoma, Leiomyosarcoma, Malignant Lymphoma

♦Diagnosis is confirmed by biopsy of tumor.
May show evidence of bleeding

Gastric Peptic Ulcer

Laboratory findings due to underlying conditions
- Administration of ACTH and adrenal steroids
- Various drugs (e.g., NSAIDs)
- Acute burns (Curling's ulcer)
- Cerebrovascular accidents and trauma, and inflammation (Cushing's ulcer)
- Uremia
- Cirrhosis

Laboratory findings due to complications
Gastric retention—dehydration, hypokalemic alkalosis
Perforation—increased WBC with shift to the left, dehydration, increased serum amylase, increased amylase in peritoneal fluid
Hemorrhage
See *Helicobacter pylori*, p. 804.
Curling's ulcer—hemorrhage 8–10 days and perforation 30 days after burn; causes death in 15% of fatal burn cases.
Recurrent ulcer after partial gastrectomy (≤ 3% of patients) may be due to inadequacy of operation, but acid secretory syndrome should be considered (e.g., gastrinoma, retained antrum syndrome) and serum gastrin should be assayed.

Gastritis, Benign Giant Hypertrophic (Ménétrier's Disease)

○Serum protein and albumin decreased in 80% of cases due to loss of plasma proteins through gastric mucosa; gamma globulins may be decreased. Serum calcium may be low due to decreased serum albumin. Protein loss is nonselective in contrast to loss through glomerular membrane, in which loss of low-molecular-weight proteins is greater than loss of high-molecular-weight proteins.
Hypochlorhydria by gastric analysis in 75% of cases. Gastric fluid taken during endoscopy shows increased protein concentration (normal level is 0.8–2.5 g/L) and protein electrophoresis resembles pattern of serum electrophoresis. Increased pH of gastric fluid (normal value is <2).
Protein loss can also be determined by injecting ^{51}Cr-labeled albumin and measuring radioactivity in stool. Alpha$_1$-antitrypsin clearance (calculated by measuring trypsin in blood and stool) can also be used to measure protein loss because alpha$_1$-antitrypsin resists digestion by trypsin; this method can only be used if acid hyposecretion is present because the protein is destroyed by pH <3.
♦Diagnosis is confirmed by full-thickness gastric biopsy showing thickening of gastric mucosa due to hyperplasia of mucus-secreting glands (parietal and chief cells are usually diminished or absent); superficial biopsy may appear normal.
Laboratory findings due to complications (e.g., iron-deficiency anemia due to chronic GI hemorrhage, edema due to hypoalbuminemia)
Liver function tests are normal.
Proteinuria is absent.

Gastritis, Chronic

Type A gastritis (autoimmune type; gastric antrum spared)
Parietal cell antibodies and intrinsic factor antibodies help define those patients prone to PA.
Achlorhydria
Vitamin B$_{12}$ deficient megaloblastosis
Hypergastrinemia (due to hyperplasia of gastrin-producing cells)
Gastric carcinoids
Low serum pepsinogen I concentrations

GI

Laboratory findings due to other autoimmune diseases (e.g., Hashimoto's thyroiditis, Addison's disease, Graves' disease, myasthenia gravis, hypoparathyroidism, insulin-dependent diabetes mellitus)

Type B gastritis (gastric antrum involved)

H. pylori infection; is detectable in ~80% of patients with peptic ulcer and chronic gastritis. Diagnosis by biopsy, culture, direct Gram stain, urease test, serologic tests (see p. 804)

Hypogastrinemia (due to destruction of gastrin-producing cells in antrum)

Chronic antral gastritis is consistently present in patients with benign gastric ulcer.

♦Diagnosis depends on biopsy of gastric mucosa.

Anemia due to iron deficiency and malabsorption may occur.

Gastric acid studies are of limited value. Severe hypochlorhydria or achlorhydria after maximal stimulation usually denotes mucosal atrophy.

Due To

H. pylori infection
Other infections (other bacteria, viruses, parasites, fungi)
Chemical effects (e.g., NSAIDs, bile reflux)
Metaplastic atrophic disease (e.g., autoimmune)
Eosinophilic gastroenteritis
Crohn's disease
Sarcoidosis
Lymphocytic gastritis
Ménétrier's disease

Gastroenteritis, Eosinophilic

♦Diagnosis requires histologic evidence of predominant eosinophilic infiltration of GI tract in absence of parasitic infection or extraintestinal disease.

Laboratory findings due to
- Diarrhea, malabsorption, protein-losing enteropathy with predominant disease of mucosal layer
- GI tract obstruction with predominant disease of muscular layer
- Eosinophilic ascites with predominant disease of serosal layer

Gastrointestinal Diseases, Genetic

Atrophic gastritis (PA)	
MEN types I and II	AD
Gastric cancer	
Colon cancer	
Cancer family syndrome (cancer of colon, breast, endometrium)	AD
Familial polyposes (see Polyposis, Hereditary, p. 194)	
Celiac disease	
Cystic fibrosis	AR
Shwachman syndrome	AR
Hereditary hemorrhagic telangiectasia (Osler-Weber-Rendu disease)	AD
Hereditary pancreatitis	AD
Ehlers-Danlos syndrome type IV (bowel rupture)	AD
Tylosis (esophageal cancer; hyperkeratosis of palms and soles)	AD
Hereditary hollow visceral myopathy (intestinal pseudoobstruction)	AD
Familial Mediterranean fever (recurrent polyserositis)	AR
Hermansky-Pudlak syndrome (inflammatory bowel disease, platelet dysfunction, oculocutaneous albinism, pulmonary fibrosis)	AR
Lactase deficiency	AR
Sucrase-isomaltase deficiency	AR
Hartnup's disease	AR
Cystinuria	AR
Pancreatic lipase deficiency	AR
Congenital PA	AR
Imerslund-Graesback syndrome	AR

Congenital chloride diarrhea	AR
Hirschsprung's megacolon	
Acrodermatitis enteropathica	AR

AD = autosomal dominant; AR = autosomal recessive.

Gastrointestinal Tract: Conditions with No Useful Laboratory Findings

Chronic esophagitis
Diverticula of esophagus and stomach
Esophageal spasm
Prolapse of gastric mucosa
Foreign bodies in stomach

Hemorrhage, Gastrointestinal

Due To

Duodenal ulcer (25% of patients)
Esophageal varices (18% of patients)
Gastric ulcer (12% of patients)
Gastritis (12% of patients)
Esophagitis (6% of patients)
Mallory-Weiss syndrome (5% of patients)
Other (22% of patients)
In addition to the main cause of bleeding, 50% of patients have an additional lesion that
   could cause hemorrhage (especially duodenal ulcer, esophageal varices, hiatus hernia).
   40% of patients with previously known GI tract lesions bled from a different lesion.

Hernia, Diaphragmatic

Microcytic anemia (due to blood loss) may be present.
Stool may be positive for blood.

Hirschsprung's Disease (Aganglionic Megacolon)

Rectal biopsy to include muscle layers shows absence of myenteric plexus ganglia in
   muscle layers. Only diagnostic if ganglia are present to rule out this diagnosis.
Up to 15% of all infants with delayed passage of meconium have Hirschsprung's disease.

Infections of Gastrointestinal Tract

(See also Chapter 15, Infectious Diseases.)

AIDS Gastrointestinal Involvement

Mouth—*Candida*
Esophagus—CMV, *Candida*, HSV
Small intestine—CMV, *Cryptosporidia, Giardia, Isospora belli, Microsporidia, M.
   avium-intracellulare*
Colon—*Candida*, amebae, *Campylobacter, Chlamydia trachomatis, C. difficile,* CMV,
   Histoplasma, M. avium-intracellulare, Salmonella, Shigella
Rectum—HSV, *C. trachomatis*
Liver and biliary tract—CMV hepatitis, ampullary stenosis, cryptosporidiosis, *M.
   avium-intracellulare* infection

Agents of Infectious Gastroenteritis

See Fig. 7-4.

Agent	Frequency (%) in Traveler's Diarrhea
Enterotoxigenic *E. coli*	40–60
Shigella species	5–10

GI

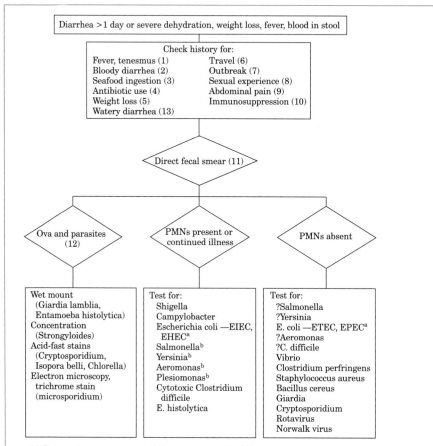

(1) Fever or tenesmus suggests inflammatory proctocolitis.

(2) Diarrhea with blood, especially without fecal WBCs, suggests EHEC *E. coli* 0157 or amebiasis in which WBCs are destroyed by parasite.

(3) Eating inadequately cooked seafood suggests *Vibrio* or Norwalk-like viruses.

(4) Stop antibiotics if possible; consider cytotoxigenic *C. difficile*; may also predispose to other infections (e.g., salmonellosis).

(5) Diarrhea > 10 days with weight loss suggests giardiasis or cryptosporidiosis.

(6) Travel to tropical regions: consider ETEC *E. coli*, viral (Norwalk-like or rotaviral), parasitic (*Giardia, Entamoeba, Strongyloides, Cryptosporidium*), or invasive bacterial infections.

(7) Outbreaks suggest anisakiasis, infection with *S. aureus*, *B. cereus* (incubation period < 6 hours), *C. perfringens*, ETEC *E. coli, Vibrio, Salmonella, Campylobacter, Shigella*, EIEC *E. coli*.

(8) Sigmoidoscopy in symptomatic gay men should distinguish proctitis in distal 15 cm (due to HVS, gonococcal, *Chlamydia*, syphilitic infections) from colitis (*Campylobacter, Shigella, C. difficile, Chlamydia* infections) or noninflammatory diarrhea (giardiasis).

(9) Appendicitis-like syndrome or persistent abdominal pain and fever suggest culture for *Yersinia enterocolitica* with cold enrichment.

(10) In immunocompromised hosts, consider many viral (CMV, HVS, Coxsackievirus, rotavirus), bacterial (*Salmonella, Mycobacterium avium-intracellulare*), or parasitic (*Cryptosporidium isopora, Strongyloides, Entamoeba, Giardia*) causes.

(11) Some inflammatory pathogens (e.g., cytotoxigenic *C. difficile, E. histolytica*) may destroy fecal WBC morphology.

(12) Especially if diarrhea > 10 days or recurrent.

(13) Consider viruses (e.g., rotavirus, Norwalk and Norwalk-like, adenovirus), protozoa (e.g., *Giardia lamblia, Cryptosporidium*), bacteria (e.g., *Vibrio cholerae*, those listed in [2]).

[a]Special tests (*E. coli* samples for serotyping and testing for heat-labile and heat-stable toxin, invasiveness, adherence). Stools and paired serum samples for Norwalk-like virus or toxin testing.

[b]Rare.

Salmonella species	<5
Campylobacter species	<5
Unknown agents	30–40
G. lamblia	Rare
E. histolytica	Rare
Enteropathogenic *E. coli*	NA
Enteroinvasive *E. coli*	NA
Enterohemorrhagic *E. coli*	NA
Rotavirus, groups A, B, C	NA
Norwalk viruses	NA
Enteric adenovirus	
Astrovirus	
Calicivirus	
Cryptosporidium species	NA
Balantidium coli	
I. belli	

Other bacteria to consider
  Y. enterocolitica
  V. cholerae, Vibrio parahaemolyticus
  Aeromonas hydrophila
  C. difficile, C. perfringens type A
  S. aureus
  B. cereus
Helminths (see Chapter 15)
NA = data on frequency not available.

Parasites, Gastrointestinal

See Chapter 15.

Inflammatory Disorders of the Intestine

Idiopathic, e.g., ulcerative colitis, regional enteritis, colitis of indeterminate type (e.g., collagenous colitis)
Infectious
  • Bacteria (e.g., *C. jejuni, C. difficile, Salmonella, Shigella sonnei,* enteropathic *E. coli, Yersinia, Aeromonas*)
  • Tubercle bacilli
  • *Chlamydiae*
  • Viruses (e.g., rotavirus, CMV, HSV)
  • Parasites (*E. histolyticum, G. lamblia*)
  • Fungi (e.g., *Cryptosporidium*)
Motility disorders (e.g., diverticulitis, solitary rectal ulcer syndrome)
Circulatory disorders (e.g., ischemic colitis, associated with obstruction of colon)
Iatrogenic
  • Use of enemas, laxatives, drugs
  • Radiation exposure
  • After small intestine bypass and diversion of fecal stream
  • Graft-versus-host disease
Specific disease association
  • Chronic granulomatous disease of childhood
  • Immunodeficiency syndromes
  • Hemolytic uremic syndrome

GI

◄ **Fig. 7-4.** Algorithm for etiology of infectious diarrhea. Bacteria cause the severest forms of infectious diarrhea; viruses (e.g., rotaviruses, Norwalk viruses) are most common causes. (PMNs = polymorphonuclear neutrophil leukocytes; EIEC = enteroinvasive; EHEC = enterohemorrhagic; ETEC = enterotoxigenic; EPEC = enteropathogenic; HVS = herpes simplex virus; CMV = cytomegalovirus.) (Adapted from Guerrant RL, Bobak DA. Bacterial and protozoal gastroenteritis. *N Engl J Med* 1991;325:327.)

- Behçet's disease

Miscellaneous
- Collagenous colitis
- Eosinophilic colitis and allergic proctitis
- Necrotizing enterocolitis
- Idiopathic ulcer of colon

Intestinal Obstruction

WBC is normal early. Later it tends to rise, with increase in PMNs; 15,000–25,000/cu mm suggests strangulation; >30,000/cu mm suggests mesenteric thrombosis.

Hb and Hct concentrations are normal early but later increase, with dehydration.

Urine specific gravity increases, with deficit of water and electrolytes unless pre-existing renal disease is present. Urinalysis helps rule out renal colic, diabetic acidosis, etc.

Gastric contents
- Positive guaiac test suggests strangulation; gross blood may be present if strangulated segment is high in jejunum.

Rectal contents—gross rectal blood suggests carcinoma of colon or intussusception.

Decreased serum sodium, potassium, chloride, and pH and increased CO_2 are helpful indications to follow the course of the patient and to guide therapy.

Increased BUN suggests blood in intestine or renal damage.

Serum amylase may be moderately increased in absence of pancreatitis.

Increased serum LD, AST, CK, and phosphorus may indicate infarction of small intestine.

In Neonate

Due To
Congenital mechanical
- Intrinsic (e.g., pyloric stenosis, meconium ileus, atresia, imperforate anus)
- Extrinsic (e.g., volvulus, malrotation, congenital bands, hernia)

Acquired mechanical (e.g., intussusception, necrotizing enterocolitis, meconium plugs, adhesions, mesenteric thrombosis)

Functional
- Hirschsprung's disease
- Paralytic ileus (e.g., sepsis, *Pseudomonas* enteritis, maternal drugs such as heroin, hypermagnesemia)
- Endocrine (e.g., hypothyroidism, adrenal insufficiency)
- Other (e.g., sepsis, CNS disease, meconium plug syndrome)

Laboratory Findings in Neonate
Gastric aspirate >15 mL or is bile stained.

Vomitus is colorless when obstruction proximal to ampulla of Vater (e.g., pyloric atresia) but bile stained and alkaline with obstruction distal to ampulla. *Bile-stained vomitus in a neonate is always abnormal and is to be considered a surgical problem until proved otherwise.*

Findings due to complications (e.g., perforation, infarction, enterocolitis, peritonitis, changes in fluid and electrolytes)

Laboratory findings due to associated conditions
- Duodenal atresia is associated with
  Down syndrome (30% of cases)
  Intestinal malrotation (20% of cases)
  Congenital heart disease (17% of cases)
  Annular pancreas (20% of cases)
  Renal anomalies (5% of cases)
  Tracheoesophageal anomalies (7% of cases)
- Polyhydramnios in 50% of cases of duodenal obstruction; 40% show hyperbilirubinemia
- Cystic fibrosis is associated with
  Meconium ileus
  Increased incidence of intestinal atresia

Lymphangiectasia, Intestinal

♦ Biopsy of small bowel or lymphangiography confirms the diagnosis.
Decreased serum protein.
IV infusion of ^{51}Cr-labeled albumin demonstrates excessive protein loss in stools.
May manifest abnormal lymph nodes (inguinal, pelvic, retroperitoneal) and lymphedema between early infancy and childhood.

Malabsorption

See Fig. 7-5.

Due To

Inadequate mixing of food with bile salts and lipase (e.g., pyloroplasty, subtotal or total gastrectomy, gastrojejunostomy)
Inadequate lipolysis due to lack of lipase (e.g., cystic fibrosis of the pancreas, chronic pancreatitis, cancer of the pancreas or ampulla of Vater, pancreatic fistula, vagotomy)
Inadequate emulsification of fat due to lack of bile salts (e.g., obstructive jaundice, severe liver disease, bacterial overgrowth of small intestine, disorders of terminal ileum)
Primary absorptive defect in small bowel
Inadequate absorptive surface due to extensive mucosal disease (e.g., regional enteritis, tumors, amyloid disease, scleroderma, irradiation)
Biochemical dysfunction of mucosal cells (e.g., celiac sprue syndrome, severe starvation, intestinal infections or infestations, or administration of drugs such as neomycin sulfate, colchicine, or PAS)
Obstruction of mesenteric lymphatics (e.g., by lymphoma, carcinoma, Whipple's disease, intestinal TB)
Inadequate length of normal absorptive surface (e.g., surgical resection, fistula, shunt)
Miscellaneous (e.g., "blind loops" of intestine, diverticula, Z-E syndrome, agammaglobulinemia, endocrine and metabolic disorders)
Chronic infection (e.g., in common variable hypogammaglobulinemia, 50–55% of patients have chronic diarrhea and malabsorption due to specific pathogen such as *G. lamblia* or overgrowth of bacteria in small bowel)
Factitious (see p. 893)

♦ *Fat absorption indices* (steatorrhea)
Direct qualitative stool examination
≥ 2 random stool samples are collected on diet of >80 gm of fat daily.
Interpretation
• Gross—oil droplets, egg particles, buttery materials
• Microscopic examination after staining for fat (e.g., oil red O, Sudan)
Sensitivity >94% in moderate/severe fat malabsorption (>10% of ingested fat excreted); ~75% in mild/moderate fat malabsorption (6–10% of ingested fat excreted); positive in ~14% of normal persons.
4+ fat in stool means excessive fat loss.
Interference
Neutral fat
Mineral and castor oil ingestion
Dietetic low-calorie mayonnaise ingestion
Rectal suppository use
Quantitative determination of fecal fat is gold standard test to establish the diagnosis of fat malabsorption.
Interpretation
Normal is <7 gm/24 hrs when a 3-day pooled stool sample is collected on diet of 80–100 gm of fat/day. <5 gm/24 hrs (or <4% of measured fat intake) on diet of <50 gm of fat/day for a 3-day period.
Determination parallels but is more sensitive than triolein ^{131}I test in chronic pancreatic disease.
Increased In
Chronic pancreatic disease (>9.5 gm/24 hrs)

GI

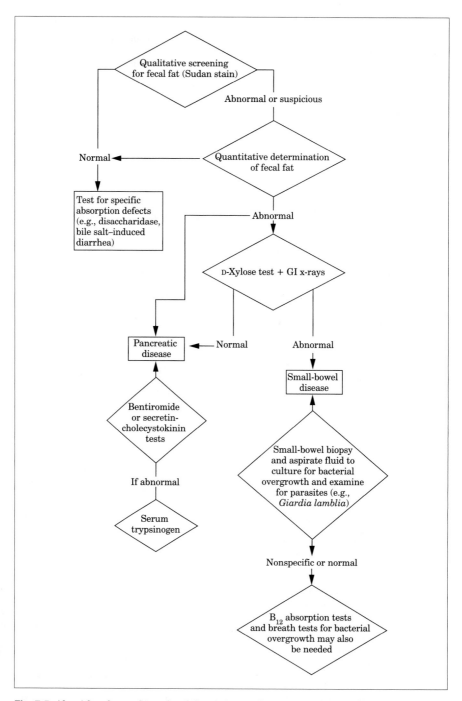

Fig. 7-5. Algorithm for workup of malabsorption. (Adapted from Roberts IM. Workup of the patient with malabsorption. *Postgrad Med* 1987;8:32.)

May also be increased in
- High fiber diet (>100 gm/day).
- When dietary fat is ingested in solid form (e.g., whole peanuts).
- Neonatal period.
- Weight—much heavier (>300 gm/24 hrs) than normal (normal weight is <200 gm/24 hrs or normal fecal solids of 25–30 gm/24 hrs).

Serum trypsinogen <10 ng/mL in 75–85% of patients with severe chronic pancreatitis (those with steatorrhea) and 15–20% of those with mild to moderate disease; occasionally low in patients with cancer of pancreas; normal (10–75 ng/mL) with non-pancreatic causes of malabsorption.

Bentiromide used to differentiate pancreatic exocrine insufficiency (abnormal result) from intestinal mucosal disease (normal result) (see p. 157).

♦ Secretin-cholecystokinin is the most sensitive and reliable test of chronic pancreatic disease.

Indirect indices of fat absorption; these lack sensitivity and specificity for routine screening.
- Serum cholesterol may be decreased.
- PT may be prolonged due to malabsorption of vitamin K.
- Serum carotene is always abnormal in steatorrhea unless therapy is successful. Not recommended for screening; poor precision at lower end of reference range. May also be low in liver disease, high fever, hyperthyroidism, chronic illness, and decreased dietary intake (blood level falls within 1 wk but vitamin A level is unaffected by dietary change for 6 mos because of much larger body stores). May be increased in hyperlipidemia and hypothyroidism. Normal level is 70–290 μg/dL; 30–70 μg/dL indicates mild depletion; <30 indicates severe depletion.
- Carotene tolerance test: Measure serum carotene after daily oral loading of carotene for 3–7 days. Low values for serum carotene levels are usually associated with steatorrhea. Increase of serum carotene by >35 μg/dL indicates previously low dietary intake of carotene and/or fat.

Decreased In

Steatorrhea. Serum carotene increases >30 μg/dL. Patients with sprue in remission with normal fecal fat excretion may still show low carotene absorption.

Mineral oil interferes with carotene absorption. On a fat-free diet only 10% is absorbed.
- Vitamin A tolerance test (for screening steatorrhea)
  Measure plasma vitamin A level 5 hrs after ingestion.
  Normal rise is 9× fasting level.
  Flat curve in liver disease
  Not useful after gastrectomy
  With vitamin A as ester of long-chain fatty acid, flat curve occurs in both pancreatic disease and intestinal mucosal abnormalities; when water-soluble forms of vitamin A are used, the curve becomes normal in patients with pancreatic disease but remains flat in those with intestinal mucosal abnormalities.
- Triolein ^{131}I and oleic acid ^{131}I absorption with measurement of blood, breath, or fecal radioactivity; sensitive and specific for screening but may not be routinely available.

Triolein ^{131}I absorption test used to screen patients with steatorrhea.
- Normal: ≥ 10% of administered radioactivity appears in the blood within 6 hrs; <5% appears in the feces; indicates that digestion of fat in the small bowel and absorption of fat in the small bowel are normal.
- Abnormal: perform an oleic acid ^{131}I absorption test.

Triolein ^{14}C breath test
^{14}C-labeled triolein is administered and ^{14}CO$_2$ is measured in collected breath. Said to have >85% sensitivity and specificity for fat malabsorption.

Interferences

False-positives
- Poor gastric emptying (e.g., gastric surgery, diabetes mellitus)
- CO_2 retention (e.g., chronic lung disease)
- Impaired metabolism (e.g., severe liver disease)
- Dilution of ^{14}CO$_2$ (e.g., hyperlipidemia, ascites, obesity)
- Apparently healthy persons

False-negatives
- Increased CO_2 production (e.g., hyperthyroidism, fever)

GI

• Mild degree of fat malabsorption

Oleic acid ^{131}I absorption test: normal values same as for the triolein absorption test.

Interpretation

An abnormal result indicates a defect in small bowel mucosal absorption function (e.g., sprue, Whipple's disease, regional enteritis, tuberculous enteritis, collagen diseases involving the small bowel, extensive resection). Abnormal pancreatic function does not affect the test.

Most common laboratory abnormalities are decreased serum carotene, albumin, and iron, increased ESR, increased stool weight (>300 gm/24 hrs) and stool fat (>7 gm/24 hrs), anemia.

♦ Normal D-xylose test, low serum trypsinogen, pancreatic calcification on radiograph of abdomen establish diagnosis of chronic pancreatitis. If calcification is absent (as occurs in 70–80% of cases), abnormal contents of pancreatic secretion after secretin-cholecystokinin stimulation or abnormal bentiromide tests establishes diagnosis of chronic pancreatitis.

Anemia is due to deficiency of iron, folic acid, vitamin B_{12}, or various combinations, depending on their decreased absorption.

Carbohydrate absorption indices

• Oral GTT—limited value

Flat curve or delayed peak occurs in celiac disease and nontropical sprue.
Curve is normal in pancreatic insufficiency.

• D-Xylose tolerance test of carbohydrate absorption

Measure total 5-hr urine excretion; may also measure serum levels at 2 hrs.

Accuracy is 90% in distinguishing normal levels in pancreatic disease from decreased levels in intestinal mucosal disease and intestinal bacterial overgrowth, but opinions vary on usefulness. Also decreased in renal disease, myxedema, and the elderly although absorption is normal.

• Disaccharide malabsorption

Due To

Primary malabsorption (congenital or acquired) due to absence of specific disaccharidase in brush border of small intestine mucosa

• Isolated lactase deficiency (also called milk allergy, milk intolerance, congenital familial lactose intolerance, lactase deficiency) is most common of these defects; occurs in ~10% of whites and 60% of blacks; infantile type shows diarrhea, vomiting, failure to thrive, malabsorption, etc.; often appears first in adults; become asymptomatic when lactase is removed from diet.

• Sucrose-isomaltose malabsorption (inherited recessive defect)

Oral sucrose tolerance curve is flat, but glucose plus fructose tolerance test is normal. Occasionally an associated malabsorption is noted with increased stool fat and abnormal D-xylose tolerance test although intestinal biopsy is normal.

Hydrogen breath test after sucrose challenge.

Intestinal biopsy with measurement of disaccharidase activities.

Sucrose-free diet causes cessation of diarrhea.

• Glucose-galactose malabsorption (inherited autosomal recessive defect that affects kidney and intestine)

Oral glucose or galactose tolerance curve is flat, but intravenous tolerance curves are normal. Glucosuria is common. Fructose tolerance test is normal.

Secondary malabsorption

• Resection of >50% of disaccharidase activity

Lactose is most marked, but there may also be sucrose. Oral disaccharide tolerance (especially lactose) is abnormal, but intestinal histology and enzyme activity are normal.

• Diffuse intestinal disease—especially celiac disease in which activity of all disaccharidases may be decreased, with later increase as intestine becomes normal on gluten-free diet; also cystic fibrosis of pancreas, severe malnutrition, ulcerative colitis, severe *Giardia* infestation, blind-loop syndrome, beta-lipoprotein deficiency, effect of drugs (e.g., colchicine, neomycin, birth control pills).

Oral tolerance tests (especially lactose) are frequently abnormal, with later return to normal with gluten-free diet. Tolerance tests with monosaccharides may also be abnormal because of defect in absorption as well as digestion.

• Bacterial overgrowth—see Table 7-1

Culture of duodenal aspirate showing $>10^5$ colony-forming units of anaerobic organisms is considered diagnostic.

[^{14}C]D-xylose breath test has good specificity.

Hydrogen breath tests (glucose-H$_2$, lactulose-H$_2$)—not recommended due to limited sensitivity and specificity.

Laboratory tests for lactase deficiency

(Similar tests for other disaccharide deficiencies can be performed.)

- Oral lactose tolerance curve is flat (blood glucose rises <20–25 mg/dL in blood drawn 15, 30, 60, and 90 mins after 50–100 gm dose of lactose) but tolerance test is normal using constituent monosaccharides (25 gm each of glucose and galactose) indicating isolated lactase deficiency rather than general mucosal absorptive defect.

  Normal: Blood glucose increases >24 mg/dL above fasting level; may increase >20–25 mg/dL in diabetics despite impaired lactose absorption.

  Abnormal: glucose increases <20 mg/dL above fasting level. False abnormal test may be due to delayed gastric emptying or small bowel transit or delayed blood collection. Poor sensitivity—largely replaced by breath hydrogen lactose test.

- Stool examination

  After ingestion of 50–100 gm of lactose, frothy diarrheal stools typically show low pH (4.5–6.0; normal is >7.0), high osmolality, positive test for reducing substances (e.g., Clinitest tablets; >0.5% is abnormal; 0.25–0.5% is suspicious; 0.25% is normal); found in children but rarely in adults.

  Chromatography detects specific carbohydrates.

  Fecal studies are of limited value.

Table 7-1. Infectious Foodborne Diseases

Organism	Identification	Cases of Foodborne Gastroenteritis (%)
Bacterial[a]		88.6
Bacillus cereus gastroenteritis	Isolation of $\geq 10^5$ *B. cereus*/gm of suspected food Isolation of same-serotype *B. cereus* from other ill patients but not from control persons Detection of enterotoxin by special tests (e.g., immunogel diffusion)	0.03
Botulism	Isolation of *Clostridium botulism* from stool of patients Detection of toxin in stool, serum, or food by mouse test	0.4
Brucellosis	Isolation of *Brucella* organism from blood	0.1
Campylobacteriosis	Increase in blood agglutination titer of fourfold or greater at onset and 3–6 wks later Isolation of same strain of organism from patients' stool Isolation of organism from suspected food Increase in blood agglutination titer of fourfold or greater at onset and 2–4 wks later	
Cholera	Isolation of organism from vomitus or stool Isolation of organism from suspected food Demonstration that organism is enterotoxigenic by special biological tests	
Clostridium perfringens enteritis	Isolation of same serotype of *C. perfringens* from food and from patients but not from control persons	18.5

(*continued*)

GI

Table 7-1. (continued)

Organism	Identification	Cases of Foodborne Gastroenteritis (%)
	Isolation of ≥10^5 organisms from suspected food	
	Fecal spore count >10^6/gm in most patients within a few days of onset	
	Demonstration of toxin in feces (fluorescent antibody test)	
Escherichia coli	Isolation of same serotype *E. coli* from suspected food and from patients but not from control persons	
	Demonstration that organism strain is enteropathogenic	
Listeriosis	Isolation of organism from tissue of fatal case	
	Isolation of same phage type and serogroup from patient and food	
	Demonstration of virulence by biological tests	
Salmonellosis	Isolation of organism from stool or rectal swab, urine, or blood	31.9
	Isolation of same organism serovar from suspected food	
Shigellosis	Isolation of organism from stool or rectal swab	18.0
	Isolation of same organism serovar from suspected food	
Staphylococcal poisoning or intoxication	Detection of enterotoxin in suspected food (serological assay)	16.5
	Isolation of same phage type of organism from patient and suspected food	
	Isolation of ≥10^5 organisms/gm of suspected food	
Streptococcus, Group A	See Chapter 15	3.2
Vibrio parahaemolyticus	See Chapter 15	0.03
Yersiniosis	Isolation of *Yersinia enterocolitica* or *Yersinia pseudotuberculosis* from stool or blood or from suspected food	5.5
Viral[b]		
Hepatitis A and E	See Tables 8.5, 8.6	
Norwalk and parvo-like	Fourfold or greater increase of blood antibody titer from acute to convalescent phase	
	Immunoelectron microscopy	
Rotavirus	See footnote	
Chemical (scroboid)		5.1
Amebae (e.g., *Entamoeba histolytica, Blastocystis hominis*)	Identification of cysts or trophozoites in feces, biopsy, aspirate; serology	
Parasitic		0.8
Cryptosporidiosis	Demonstration of organisms in stool or suspected food	
	Detection of antigen in stool	
Giardiasis	Recognition of organism in stool, duodenal contents, or small bowel	
	Detection of antigen in stool	

(continued)

Table 7-1. (continued)

Organism	Identification	Cases of Foodborne Gastroenteritis (%)
Balantidium coli infestation	Recognition of organism in stool, tissue biopsy Rarely recovered in USA	
Helminthic		
Cestodiasis (e.g., due to *Diphyllobothrium latum, Taenia saginata, Taenia solium*)	Eggs and proglottids in stool	
Trichinosis	Recognition of cysts in muscle biopsy Demonstration of larvae in suspected food Demonstration of adults and larvae in stool only during first 1–2 wks Detection of antigen in stool Serological tests for antibody	
Trematodiasis (e.g., due to *Clonorchis sinensis, Fasciola hepatica, Paragonimus westermani*)	Eggs in stool	
Fungal		
Mushroom poisoning	Demonstration of toxin in urine and suspected gathered mushrooms	

[a]Confirm by culture of food, patient's stool, or food handler's stool.

[b]Suspected by exclusion by negative tests for other causes of the symptoms (e.g., failure to find *Entamoeba histolytica, Shigella, Salmonella*). Fecal white blood cells in 20% of rotavirus cases; absent in Norwalk, Norwalk–like, and adenovirus cases.

Antigen detection: Commercial monoclonal-based antibody kits for rotavirus (enzyme immunoassay [EIA], latex agglutination, enzyme-linked immunosorbent assay) are inexpensive, permit rapid diagnosis, require only small amounts of stool, which may be frozen until testing. Detection of viral antigen in stool may be negative due to brief period of excretion. Sensitivities of 70–100% and specificities of 50–100% are reported. False-positive rates are high in newborn and breast-feeding children. Less useful in adults and outside of rotavirus season, when confirmatory testing should be performed. Kits also available for adenovirus. Rapid assays for other viruses are under development.

Antibody detection (e.g., to Norwalk virus, especially due to ingestion of raw oysters) can be diagnosed by presence of serum immunoglobulin M or by 4× rise in specific IgG antibody titers (EIA) drawn at the first week (acute phase serum) and after the second week (convalescent serum). Patient will have long since recovered from self-limited illness. Chief use is to identify cause of an outbreak. Stool antigen and serum antibody assay for Norwalk virus only available in research laboratories at present. Monoclonal antibodies for adenovirus 40 and 41.

Direct electron microscopy of stool can detect (≤ 90% sensitivity) and identify all the morphologic types of enteric viruses (e.g., rotaviruses, adenoviruses, astroviruses, caliciviruses, Norwalk virus) by characteristic morphology. Detection requires ≥ 1 million viruses/mL of stool; usually present only during first 48 hrs of viral diarrhea. Required for conclusive diagnosis of Norwalk virus. Immune electron microscopy improves sensitivity by 10–100 times but technology limits this to few laboratories.

Culture: Rotavirus, adenovirus, astrovirus culture available in research centers; not useful for routine diagnosis. Other viruses cannot be cultured.

Electropherotyping: Detection of rotavirus RNA in stool by gel electrophoresis pattern is 100% specific and >90% sensitive in first days of illness; chiefly research tool in United States.

Dot-hybridization probes for rotavirus are more sensitive and specific than antigen detection but only available in research centers.

Polymerase chain reaction techniques are being developed.

See appropriate sections in Chapter 15.

Source: Steele JCH Jr, ed. Food-borne diseases. *Clin Lab Med* 1999;19:469–703.

GI

- Hydrogen breath test measures (by gas chromatography) amount of H_2 exhaled at 2 hrs after ingestion of 50 gm of lactose in fasting state. Normal is 0 to 0.11 mL/min; in lactase deficiency, 0.31 to 2.50 mL/min. Peak or cumulative 4-hr values also differentiates these patients. Based on production of H_2 by bacteria in colon from unabsorbed lactose. False-negative test due to absence of H_2-producing bacteria in colon or prior antibiotic therapy in ~20% of patients. Similar test can be used to detect disaccharidase deficiency and small intestine bacterial overgrowth.
- Endoscopic intestinal biopsy for histologic examination and enzyme activity assay is now considered obsolete.

Protein absorption indices
- Normal fecal nitrogen is <2 gm/day. Marked increase is seen in sprue and severe pancreatic deficiency.
- Measure plasma glycine or urinary excretion of hydroxyproline after gelatin meal. Plasma glycine increases 5× in 2 hrs in normal persons. In those with cystic fibrosis of the pancreas, the increase is <2.5×.
- Serum albumin may be decreased.

[131]I-Polyvinylpyrrolidone test
Give 15–25 μCi of ^{131}I-polyvinylpyrrolidone IV and collect all stools for 4–5 days.
Interpretation
Normal: <2% is excreted in feces when the mucosa of the GI tract is intact. In protein-losing enteropathy, >2% of administered radioactivity appears in stool.

Electrolyte absorption indices
- Serum calcium, magnesium, potassium, and vitamin D may be decreased.

[51]Cr albumin test (IV dose of 30–50 μCi) shows increased excretion in 4-day stool collection due to protein-losing enteropathy.

Biopsy of small intestine mucosa is excellent for verification of sprue, celiac disease, and Whipple's disease.

Culture for bacterial overgrowth should be considered in malabsorption associated with abnormal intestinal motility (e.g., scleroderma) or anatomic abnormalities (e.g., diverticula). Positive if >10^5–10^6 organisms/mL from upper intestinal contents but may vary from one location to another; should be collected for anaerobic and aerobic culture. Perform with peroral intestinal biopsy. If breath tests using ^{14}C–bile acid or ^{14}C–D-xylose or hydrogen are available, they are more sensitive and specific for bacterial overgrowth.

Breath test for bile acid malabsorption: Oral radiolabeled ^{14}C-glycocholate undergoes bacterial deconjugation in colon. [14]CO_2 derived from glycine is absorbed in bowel, excreted by lungs, and measured in breath. This simulates secretion of bile acids into duodenum and 95% resorption in terminal ileum. Identifies bacterial overgrowth or impaired ileal absorption of bile acids.
Interpretation
Normal: ~5% enters the colon.
Increased:
- Bacterial overgrowth in small intestine allows earlier bacterial deconjugation and therefore more [14]CO_2 appears in breath.
- Disease or resection of terminal ileum allows more bile acids into colon, where they undergo bacterial conjugation.

Schilling test: Performed before and after administration of antibiotics; is a useful adjunct to intestinal culture to detect bacterial overgrowth. (See Table 7-2.)

Mallory-Weiss Syndrome

(Spontaneous cardioesophageal laceration after retching)
Laboratory findings due to hemorrhage from cardioesophageal laceration

Meckel's Diverticulum

Laboratory findings due only to complications
- Gastrointestinal hemorrhage
- Intestinal obstruction
- Perforation or intussusception (~20% of patients; the other 80% of patients are asymptomatic)

○Should be suspected when GI tract bleeding and symptoms of appendicitis occur together.

Table 7-2. Interpretation of Schilling Test

Disorder	Vitamin B$_{12}$ Absorption Normal	
	Without Intrinsic Factor	With Intrinsic Factor
Pernicious anemia	No	Yes
Congenital deficiency of intrinsic factor	No	Yes
Gastrectomy	No	Yes
Intestinal malabsorption (e.g., ileal diseases, bacterial overgrowth, pancreatic disease, fish tapeworm)	No	No
Renal failure	No	No
Incomplete urine collection	No	No
Folate deficiency	Yes	Yes

Megacolon, Toxic

(Atonic dilatation of colon due to transmural inflammation)

Due To

Severe ulcerative colitis (most common cause)
Crohn's disease
Pseudomembranous colitis
Ischemic colitis
Bacterial colitis
Amebiasis

Laboratory findings due to sepsis (e.g., increased WBC and PMNs)
Bloody diarrhea

Peritonitis, Acute

See Figs. 7-1 and 7-2.

Primary

Laboratory findings due to nephrotic syndrome and postnecrotic cirrhosis and occasionally bacteremia in children and cirrhosis with ascites in adults.
♦ Gram stain of direct smear and culture of peritoneal fluid usually shows streptococci in children. In adults is due to *E. coli* (40–60%) or *Streptococcus pneumoniae* (15%), other gram-negative bacilli, and enterococci; usually one organism. May be due to *Mycobacterium tuberculosis*.
♦ Diagnostic peritoneal lavage fluid shows WBC count >200/cu mm in 99% of cases.
Marked increase in WBC (≤ 50,000/cu mm) and PMN (80–90%).

Secondary

Laboratory findings due to perforation of hollow viscus (e.g., appendicitis, perforated ulcer, volvulus). Usually more than one organism is found.
♦ Occurs and recurs very frequently in continuous ambulatory peritoneal dialysis. Suggested by turbid dialysate (indicates >300 WBC/cu mm); Gram stain and culture may be negative and leukocytosis may be absent. Due to gram-positive bacteria in ~70%, enteric gram-negative bacilli and *Pseudomonas aeruginosa* in 20–30%, others in 10–20%, sterile in 10–20%. *If more than one pathogen, rule out perforated viscus.*

Plummer-Vinson Syndrome

Hypochromic anemia associated with dysphagia and cardiospasm in women

GI

Table 7-3. Comparison of Some Inherited Gastrointestinal Polyps

Syndrome	Type	Location	Cancer Predisposition and Mode of Inheritance	Associated Abnormalities
Familial polyposis	Adenoma	Colon; also stomach, small bowel	Yes (~100%) AD	Osteomas of mandible
Gardner's syndrome	Adenoma	Colon; also stomach, small bowel; may develop before puberty; 100% become malignant	Yes (~100%) AD	Multiple osteomas of jaw and skull, fibrous and fatty tumors of skin and mesentery, epidermoid inclusion cysts of skin
Turcot's syndrome	Adenoma	Colon	Yes AR	Brain tumors usually within first two decades of life
Peutz-Jeghers syndrome	Hamartoma	Small bowel; also stomach, colon	Yes (risk <3–6%, especially stomach, duodenum) AD	Pigmented foci on buccal and perianal mucosa, hands, feet are characteristic; bladder and nasal polyps
Juvenile polyps	Hamartoma Adenoma	Colon; also stomach, small bowel	Rare AD	
Neurofibromatosis	Neurofibroma	Stomach, small bowel	No	Skin
Cronkhite-Canada syndrome	Inflammatory	Small bowel; also stomach, colon	~15% risk Sporadic	Alopecia, dystrophic nails, hyperpigmentation, enteropathy

AD = autosomal dominant; AR = autosomal recessive.
Source: Eastwood GL, Avunduk C. *Manual of gastroenterology*, 2nd ed. Boston: Little, Brown, 1994.

Polyposis (Gastrointestinal), Hereditary

See Table 7-3.
Laboratory findings due to intestinal polyps and due to associated lesions
- Familial polyposis of colon
- Occasional discrete polyps of colon and rectum
- Peutz-Jeghers syndrome
- Gardner's syndrome (see next section)
- Turcot's syndrome (CNS tumors)
- Oldfield's syndrome (extensive sebaceous cysts)

- Z-E syndrome
- Generalized juvenile polyposis

Laboratory findings due to complications (e.g., bleeding, intussusception, obstruction, malignancy)

Proctitis, Acute

♦ Rectal Gram stain preparation shows >1 PMN/HPF (1000×).

In homosexual men, specific cause can be found in 80% of cases completely studied. The most common causes are *C. trachomatis* (non–lymphogranuloma venereum strains) in >75% of cases, *N. gonorrhoeae*, lymphogranuloma venereum, HSV type II, *T. pallidum*.

Histopathology of rectal biopsy in acute proctocolitis due to C. trachomatis *is indistinguishable from Crohn's disease; culture and serologic tests for* C. trachomatis *and serologic tests for lymphogranuloma venereum strains should be performed in such cases. Primary or secondary syphilitic proctitis may be very severe and of variable appearance; serologic test for syphilis should be performed.*

Sprue, Tropical

(Probably an infectious disease due to persistent toxicogenic coliform bacteria in small intestine, e.g., *Klebsiella pneumoniae*, *Enterobacter cloacae*, *E. coli*; responds to antibiotic therapy.)

Initial bout of acute watery diarrhea followed by persistent, progressive course if untreated.

Malabsorption, e.g.,
- Steatorrhea in 50–90% of cases
- Deficiency of folate and vitamin B_{12} (not corrected by adding intrinsic factor)
- Abnormal xylose tolerance in most cases
- Oral GTT abnormal in ~50% of cases

Histologic changes seen in jejunal biopsy.

Systemic Diseases, Gastrointestinal Manifestations

AIDS
Allergy
Amyloidosis
Bacterial infection (lymphogranuloma venereum)
Cirrhosis (esophageal varices, hemorrhoids, peptic ulcer)
Collagen diseases (e.g., scleroderma, polyarteritis nodosa, SLE)
Cystic fibrosis of pancreas
Embolic accidents in rheumatic heart disease, bacterial endocarditis
Hemolytic crises (e.g., sickle cell disease)
Henoch's purpura
Hirschsprung's disease
Ischemic vascular disease
Lead poisoning
Lymphoma and leukemia
Metastatic carcinoma
Osler-Weber-Rendu disease
Parasitic infestation (schistosomiasis)
Peptic ulcer associated with other diseases (in 8–22% of patients with hyperparathyroidism, 10% of patients with pituitary tumor, etc.)
Porphyria
Uremia
Z-E syndrome (peptic ulcer)

Systemic Diseases, Oral Manifestations

Hematologic diseases
- Acute leukemia—edema and hemorrhage
- Granulocytopenia—ulceration and inflammation
- Iron-deficiency anemia—atrophy

GI

Table 7-4. Comparison of Two Major Types of Lymphoma

	Western Type	Alpha Chain Disease
Population	Western world	Middle East
Sex distribution	Equal	Preponderance in males
Age	<10 or >50 yrs	10–30 yrs
Location	Ileum	Duodenum, jejunum
Therapy	Excision, radiation, chemotherapy	Antibiotics, chemotherapy
Laboratory findings	Anemia, obstruction, intussusception, perforation	Paraproteinemia, anemia, steatorrhea

- PA—glossitis
- Polycythemia—erosions

Infections
- Bacterial (e.g., diphtheria, scarlet fever, syphilis, Vincent's angina)
- Fungal (e.g., actinomycosis, histoplasmosis, mucormycosis, moniliasis)
- Viral (e.g., HSV infection, herpangina, measles, infectious mononucleosis)

Systemic diseases (e.g., SLE, primary amyloidosis, Osler-Weber-Rendu disease)
Vitamin deficiencies (e.g., pellagra, riboflavin deficiency, scurvy, folate deficiency)

Systemic Manifestations in Some Gastrointestinal Diseases

Anemia (e.g., due to bleeding occult neoplasm)
Arthritis, uveitis, etc., in ulcerative colitis
Carcinoid syndrome
Endocrine manifestations due to replacement by metastatic tumors of GI tract
Vitamin deficiency (e.g., sprue, malabsorption)

Tumors of Small Intestine

See Table 7-4.
♦ Biopsy of lesions confirms the diagnosis.
Laboratory findings due to complications, e.g., hemorrhage, obstruction, intussusception, malabsorption
Laboratory findings due to underlying condition, e.g., Peutz-Jeghers syndrome, carcinoid syndrome
Laboratory findings due to conditions with increased risk of small bowel tumor

GI Tract Condition	Tumor
Celiac sprue	Non-Hodgkin's lymphoma, adenocarcinoma
Crohn's disease	Adenocarcinoma
Familial adenomatous polyposis	Adenocarcinoma, adenoma
Postcolectomy ileostomy	Adenocarcinoma
Neurofibromatosis	Adenocarcinoma, leiomyoma
AIDS	Non-Hodgkin's lymphoma
Nodular lymphoid hyperplasia	Non-Hodgkin's lymphoma
Immunoproliferative small bowel disease	Non-Hodgkin's lymphoma

Vascular Occlusion, Mesenteric

Chronic (mesenteric arterial insufficiency)
- Laboratory findings due to malabsorption and starvation

Acute
- Marked increase in WBC (≥ 15,000–25,000/cu mm) with shift to the left.
- Infarction of intestine may cause increased serum LD, AST, CK, BUN, and phosphorus.

- Increased plasma lactate with metabolic acidosis has been suggested as indicator for surgery in patients with acute abdomen.
- Laboratory findings due to intestinal hemorrhage, obstruction, shock.

Villous Adenoma of Rectum

Stool contains large amount of mucus tinged with blood; frequent watery diarrhea.
Serum potassium may be decreased due to secretory diarrhea.
♦ Biopsy of lesion establishes the diagnosis.

Whipple's Disease (Intestinal Lipodystrophy)

(Multiorgan disease due to *Tropheryma whippleii*)

♦ Characteristic biopsy of proximal intestine (especially duodenum) and mesenteric lymph nodes establishes the diagnosis by light (using special stains) and characteristic electron microscopy showing bacilli. Has also been observed in other tissues (e.g., liver, lymph nodes, heart, CNS, eye, kidney, synovium, lung). Organism has not been cultured.
♦ PCR to amplify bacterial 16S ribosomal RNA in infected tissues, mononuclear cells of peripheral blood, cells of pleural effusion.
Anemia of chronic disease in 90% of cases; occasionally due to iron deficiency; rarely due to folate or B_{12} deficiency.
Hypogammaglobulinemia is usual.
Many patients are anergic with impaired immune function.
Laboratory findings due to involvement of various organs, e.g., malabsorption syndrome with steatorrhea in most patients, wasting syndrome, seronegative arthritis, sarcoid-like illness.

GI

8

Hepatobiliary Diseases and Diseases of the Pancreas

Liver Function Tests

Common Test Patterns

See Table 8-1.

See Figs. 8-1 through 8-3.

Patterns of abnormalities rather than changes in single test results are particularly useful despite sensitivities of only 65% in some cases.

Test results may be abnormal in many conditions that are not primarily hepatic (e.g., heart failure, sepsis, infections such as brucellosis, SBE), and individual test results may be positive in conditions other than liver disease. Results on individual tests are normal in a high proportion of patients with proven specific liver diseases, and normal values may not rule out liver disease.

Serum bilirubin (direct/total ratio)

- <20% direct.

    Constitutional (e.g., Gilbert's disease, Crigler-Najjar syndrome).

    Hemolytic states.

- 20–40% direct.

    Favors hepatocellular disease rather than extrahepatic obstruction.

    Disorders of bilirubin metabolism (e.g., Dubin-Johnson, Rotor's syndromes).

- 40–60% direct: Occurs in either hepatocellular or extrahepatic type.

- >50% direct: Favors extrahepatic obstruction rather than hepatocellular disease.

Serum total bilirubin

- Not a sensitive indicator of hepatic dysfunction; may not reflect degree of liver damage.

- Must be >2.5 mg/dL to produce clinical jaundice.

- >5 mg/dL seldom occurs in uncomplicated hemolysis unless hepatobiliary disease is also present.

- Is generally less markedly increased in hepatocellular jaundice (<10 mg/dL) than in neoplastic obstructions (≤ 20 mg/dL) or intrahepatic cholestasis.

- In extrahepatic biliary obstruction, bilirubin may rise progressively to a plateau of 30–40 mg/dL (due in part to balance between renal excretion and diversion of bilirubin to other metabolites). Such a plateau tends not to occur in hepatocellular jaundice, and bilirubin may exceed 50 mg/dL (partly due to concomitant renal insufficiency and hemolysis).

- Concentrations are generally higher in obstruction due to carcinoma than that due to stones.

- In viral hepatitis, higher serum bilirubin suggests more liver damage and longer clinical course.

- In acute alcoholic hepatitis, >5 mg/dL suggests a poor prognosis.

- Increased serum bilirubin with normal ALP suggests constitutional hyperbilirubinemias or hemolytic states.

- Normal serum bilirubin, AST, and ALT with increased ALP (of liver origin) and LD suggests obstruction of one hepatic duct or metastatic or infiltrative disease of liver. Metastatic and granulomatous lesions of liver cause 1.5–3.0× increase of serum ALP and LD.

Table 8-1. Increased Serum Enzyme Levels in Liver Diseases

Serum Enzyme	Acute Viral Hepatitis		Complete Biliary Obstruction		Cirrhosis		Liver Metastases	
	Frequency[a]	Amplitude[b]	Frequency	Amplitude	Frequency	Amplitude	Frequency	Amplitude
AST	>95%	14	>95%	3	75%	2	50%	1–2
ALT	>95%	17	>95%	4	50%	1	25%	1–2
ALP	60%	1–2	>95%	4–14	55%	1–2	50%	1–10 (TB)
							40%	1–3 (sarcoidosis)
							80%	1–14 (carcinoma)
							Frequently	1–20 (amyloidosis)
Leucine aminopeptidase	80%	1–2	85%	3	30%	1	70%	2–3
Isocitrate dehydrogenase	>95%	6	10%	1	20%	1	40%	2
5'-Nucleotidase	70%	1–2	>95%	6	50%	1–2	65%	3–4

[a]Frequency = average percentage of patients with increased serum enzyme level when blood taken at optimal time.
[b]Amplitude = average number of times normal that serum level is increased.

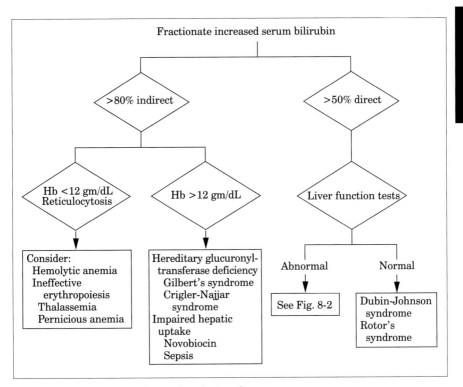

Fig. 8-1. Algorithm illustrating workup for jaundice.

- Due to renal excretion, maximum bilirubin = 10–35 mg/dL; if renal disease is present, level may reach 75 mg/dL.
- Direct bilirubin >1.0 mg/dL in an infant always indicates disease.

AST and ALT

- Most sensitive tests for acute hepatocellular injury (e.g., viral, drug related). >500 U/L suggests such a diagnosis. Seldom >500 U/L in obstructive jaundice, cirrhosis, viral hepatitis in AIDS, alcoholic liver disease.
- Most marked increase (100–2000 U/L) occurs in viral hepatitis, drug injury, carbon tetrachloride poisoning.
- >4000 indicates toxic injury, e.g., from acetaminophen.
- Patient is rarely asymptomatic with level >1000 U/L.
- AST >10× normal indicates acute hepatocellular injury but lesser increases are nonspecific and may occur with virtually any other form of liver injury.
- Usually <200 U/L in posthepatic jaundice and intrahepatic cholestasis.
- <200 U/L in 20% of patients with acute viral hepatitis.
- Usually <50 U/L in fatty liver.
- <100 U/L in alcoholic cirrhosis; ALT is normal in 50% and AST is normal in 25% of these cases.
- <150 U/L in alcoholic hepatitis (may be higher if patient has delirium tremens).
- <200 U/L in 65% of patients with cirrhosis.
- <200 U/L in 50% of patients with metastatic liver disease, lymphoma, and leukemia.
- Normal values may not rule out liver disease: ALT is normal in 50% of cases of alcoholic cirrhosis and AST is normal in 25% of cases.
- AST soaring to peak of 1000–9000 U/L and declining by 50% within 3 days and to <100 U/L within a week suggests shock liver with centrolobular necrosis (e.g., due to congestive heart failure, arrhythmia, sepsis, GI hemorrhage); serum bilirubin and ALP reflect underlying disease.

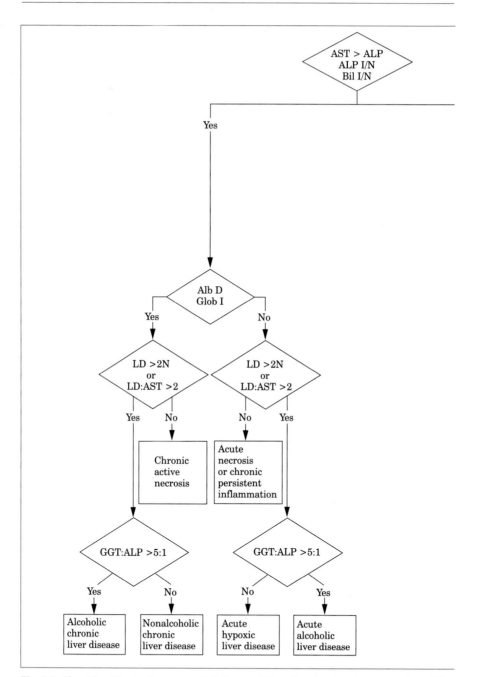

Fig. 8-2. Algorithm illustrating sequential abnormal liver function test interpretation. (Alb = albumin; Bil = bilirubin; CHF = congestive heart failure; Glob = globulin; I = increased; N = normal. Enzymes all in same U/L.) (Adapted from Henry JB. *Clinical diagnosis and management by laboratory methods,* 16th ed. Philadelphia: WB Saunders, 1979.)

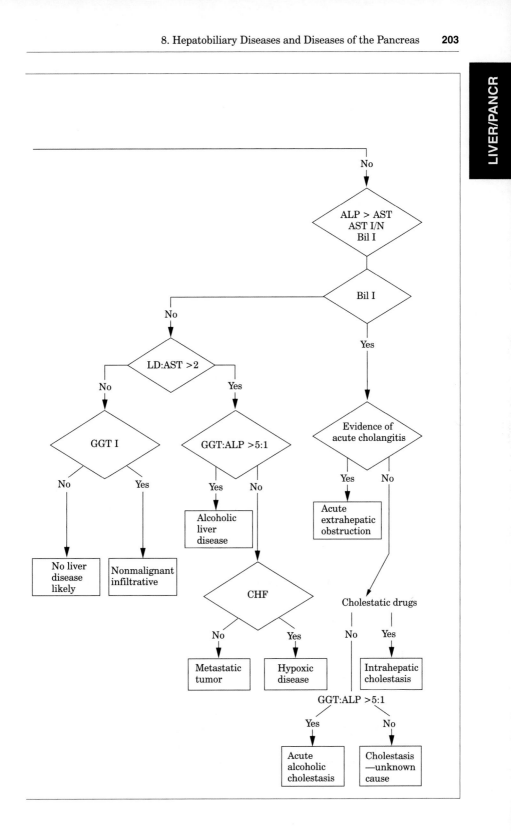

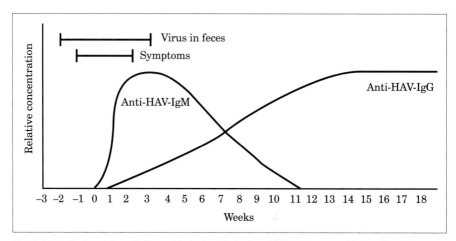

Fig. 8-3. Antibody markers in hepatitis A virus infection. (IgG = immunoglobulin G; IgM = immunoglobulin M.) (Reproduced with permission of Abbott Laboratories, Pasadena, CA.)

- Rapid rise of AST and ALT to very high levels (e.g., >600 U/L and often >2000 U/L) followed by a sharp fall in 12–72 hrs is said to be typical of acute biliary duct obstruction.
- Abrupt AST rise may also be seen in acute fulminant viral hepatitis (rarely >4000 U and declines more slowly; positive serologic tests) and acute chemical injury.
- Degree of increase has low prognostic value.
- Serial determinations reflect clinical activity of liver disease.
- Mild increase of AST and ALT (usually <500 U/L) with ALP increased >3× normal indicates cholestatic jaundice, but more marked increase of AST and ALT (especially >1000 U/L) with ALP increased <3× normal indicates hepatocellular jaundice.
- Increased concentration has poor correlation with extent of liver cell necrosis and has little prognostic value.

AST/ALT ratio >2 with ALT <300 U/L is suggestive of alcoholic hepatitis, and ratio >3 is highly suggestive, in cases of liver disease. Greater increase in AST than in ALT also occurs in cirrhosis and metastatic liver disease. In patients with cirrhosis or portal hypertension, AST/ALT ratio ≥ 3 suggests primary biliary cirrhosis. Greater increase in AST than in ALT favors viral hepatitis, posthepatic jaundice, intrahepatic cholestasis. *AST is increased in AMI and in muscle diseases, but ALT is normal. ALT is more specific for liver disease than AST.*

Serum ALP
- Is the best indicator of biliary obstruction but does not differentiate intrahepatic cholestasis from extrahepatic obstruction. Is increased out of proportion to other liver function tests.
- Increases before jaundice occurs.
- High values (>5× normal) favor obstruction and normal levels virtually exclude this diagnosis.
- Markedly increased in infants with congenital intrahepatic bile duct atresia but is much lower in extrahepatic atresia.
- Increase (3–10× normal) with only slightly increased transaminases may be seen in biliary obstruction and the converse in liver parenchymal disease (e.g., cirrhosis, hepatitis).
- Increased (2–10× normal) in early infiltrative (e.g., amyloid) and space-occupying diseases of the liver (e.g., tumor, granuloma, abscess).
- Increased >3× normal in ≤ 5% of acute hepatitis.
- <3× normal is nonspecific and may occur in all types of liver diseases (e.g., infiltrative liver diseases, cirrhosis, chronic hepatitis, viral hepatitis) and in diseases affecting the liver (e.g., congestive heart failure).

GGT/ALP ratio >5 favors alcoholic liver disease.

Isolated increase of GGT is a sensitive screening and monitoring test for alcoholism. Increased GGT due to alcohol or anticonvulsant drugs is not accompanied by increased ALP.

Serum 5'-NT and LAP levels parallel the increase in ALP in obstructive type of hepatobiliary disease, but the 5'-NT is increased only in the latter and is normal in pregnancy and bone disease, whereas the LAP is increased in pregnancy but usually normal in bone disease. GGT is normal in bone disease and pregnancy. Therefore, these enzymes are useful in determining the source of increased serum ALP. Although serum 5'-NT usually parallels ALP in liver disease, it may not increase proportionately in individual patients.

Serum Enzyme	Biliary Obstruction	Pregnancy	Childhood; Bone Disease
ALP	I	I	I
5'-NT	I	N	N
LAP	I	I	N
GGT	I	N	N

I = increased; N = normal.

Test for antimitochondrial antibodies to rule out primary biliary cirrhosis in females (present in >90% of cases; see p. 211) and radiologic studies to rule out primary sclerosing cholangitis (see pp. 207–208).

Bilirubin ("bile") in urine implies increased serum direct bilirubin and excludes hemolysis as the cause. Often precedes clinical icterus. May occur without jaundice in anicteric or early hepatitis, early obstruction, or liver metastases. (Tablets detect 0.05–0.1 mg/dL; dipsticks are less sensitive; test is negative in normal persons.)

Complete absence of urine urobilinogen strongly suggests complete bile duct obstruction; level is normal in incomplete obstruction. Decreased in some phases of hepatic jaundice. Increased in hemolytic jaundice and subsiding hepatitis. Increase may indicate hepatic damage even without clinical jaundice (e.g., some patients with cirrhosis, metastatic liver disease, congestive heart failure). Presence in viral hepatitis depends on phase of disease. (Normal is <1 mg or 1 Ehrlich unit per 2-hr specimen.)

Serum cholesterol
- May be normal or slightly decreased in hepatitis.
- Markedly decreased in severe hepatitis or cirrhosis.
- Increased in posthepatitic jaundice or intrahepatic cholestasis.
- Markedly increased in primary biliary cirrhosis.

PT
- May be prolonged due to lack of vitamin K absorption in obstruction or lack of synthesis in hepatocellular disease. Not useful when only slightly prolonged.
- Corrected within 24–48 hrs by parenteral administration of vitamin K (10 mg/day for 3 days) in obstructive but not in hepatocellular disease. Failure to correct suggests poor prognosis; extensive hepatic necrosis should be considered.
- Markedly prolonged PT is a good index of severe liver cell damage in hepatitis and cirrhosis and may herald onset of fulminant hepatic necrosis.

Serum gamma globulin
- Tends to increase with most forms of chronic liver disease.
- Increases are not specific; found in other chronic inflammatory and neoplastic diseases.
- Moderate increases (e.g., >3 gm/dL) are suggestive of chronic active hepatitis; marked increases are suggestive of autoimmune chronic hepatitis.
- Polyclonal increases in IgG and IgM are found in most cases of cirrhosis.
- Increased IgM alone may suggest primary biliary cirrhosis.
- Increased IgA may occur in alcoholic cirrhosis.
- Immunoglobulins are usually normal in obstructive jaundice.

Serum albumin is slow to reflect liver damage.
- Is usually normal in hepatitis and cholestasis.
- Increase toward normal by 2–3 gm/dL in treatment of cirrhosis implies improvement and more favorable prognosis than if no increase with therapy.

Some patients do not present the usual pattern.
- Liver function test abnormalities may occur in systemic diseases, e.g., SLE, sarcoidosis, TB, SBE, brucellosis, sickle cell disease.
- A confusing pattern may occur in mixed forms of jaundice (e.g., sickle cell disease producing hemolysis and complicated by pigment stones causing duct obstruction).

Disorders of the Liver, Gallbladder, Biliary Tree, and Pancreas

Abscess of Liver, Pyogenic

Due To

Biliary tract infection, 33%
Direct extension, 25%
Trauma, 15%
Bacteremia, 10%
Pyelophlebitis, 6%
Unknown, 10%

♦ Gram stain and culture
   • Gram-negative bacilli (e.g., *Escherichia coli, Klebsiella* spp.)
   • Anaerobes (e.g., *Bacteroides fragilis*)
   • *Staphylococcus aureus* or streptococci are found in children with bacteremia.
♦ Abnormalities of liver function tests
   • Decreased serum albumin in 50% of cases; increased serum globulin
   • Increased serum ALP in 75% of cases
   • Increased serum bilirubin in 20–25% of cases; >10 mg/dL usually indicates pyo-
     genic rather than amebic origin and suggests poorer prognosis because of more
     tissue destruction
   • See Space-Occupying Lesions, p. 248
Increase in WBC due to increase in granulocytes in 70% of cases
Anemia in 60% of cases
Ascites is unusual compared to other causes of space-occupying lesions.
Laboratory findings due to complications (e.g., right pleural effusion in 20% of cases,
   subphrenic abscess, pneumonia, empyema, bronchopleural fistula)
♦ Patients with amebic abscess of liver due to *Entamoeba histolytica* also show positive
   serologic tests for ameba (see p. 870).
         Stools may be negative for cysts and trophozoites.
         Needle aspiration of abscess may show *E. histolytica* in 50% of patients.
            *Characteristic brown or anchovy-sauce color may be absent; secondary bacte-
            rial infection may be superimposed.*
See *Echinococcus granulosus* cyst, p. 870.

Biliary Atresia, Extrahepatic, Congenital

○Direct serum bilirubin is increased in early days of life in some infants but not until
   second week in others. Level is often <12 mg/dL during first months, with subsequent rise later in life.
○Laboratory findings as in Biliary Obstruction, Complete (see next section).
♦ Liver biopsy to differentiate from neonatal hepatitis.
Laboratory findings due to sequelae (e.g., biliary cirrhosis, portal hypertension, frequent infections, rickets, hepatic failure)
[131]I-rose bengal excretion test (see Neonatal Hepatitis, p. 241)
Most important to differentiate this condition from neonatal hepatitis, for which
   surgery may be harmful.
>90% of cases of extrahepatic biliary obstruction in newborns are due to biliary atre-
   sia; occasional cases may be due to choledochal cyst (causes intermittent jaundice in
   infancy), bile plug syndrome, or bile ascites (associated with spontaneous perforation of the common bile duct).

Biliary Obstruction, Complete (Intrahepatic or Extrahepatic)

○Typical pattern of extrahepatic obstruction includes increased serum ALP (>2–3×
   normal), AST <300 U/L, increased direct serum bilirubin.
In extrahepatic type, the increased ALP is related to the completeness of obstruction.
   Normal ALP is extremely rare in extrahepatic obstruction. Very high levels may also
   occur in cases of intrahepatic cholestasis.
Serum LAP parallels ALP.

AST is increased (≤ 300 U) and ALT is increased ≤ 200 U); levels usually return to normal in 1 wk after relief of obstruction. In *acute* biliary duct obstruction (e.g., due to common bile duct stones or acute pancreatitis), AST and ALT are increased >300 U (and often >2000 U) and decline 58–76% in 72 hrs without treatment; simultaneous serum total bilirubin shows less marked elevation and decline, and ALP changes are inconsistent and unpredictable.

Direct serum bilirubin is increased; indirect serum bilirubin is normal or slightly increased.

Serum cholesterol is increased (acute, 300–400 mg/dL; chronic, ≤ 1000 mg/dL).

Serum phospholipids are increased.

PT is prolonged, with response to parenteral vitamin K more frequent than in hepatic parenchymal cell disease.

Urine bilirubin is increased; urine urobilinogen is decreased.

Stool bilirubin and urobilinogen are decreased (clay-colored stools).

Laboratory findings due to underlying causative disease are noted (e.g., stone, carcinoma of duct, metastatic carcinoma to periductal lymph nodes).

Bile Duct Obstruction (One)

○Characteristic pattern is serum bilirubin that remains normal in the presence of markedly increased serum ALP.

Breast-Milk Jaundice

(Due to the presence in mother's milk of 5-β-pregnane-3-α-20-β-diol, which inhibits glucuronyl transferase activity)

○Severe unconjugated hyperbilirubinemia. Develops in 1% of breast-fed infants by fourth to seventh day. Reaches peak of 15–25 mg/dL by second to third week, then gradually disappears in 3–10 wks in all cases. If nursing is interrupted, serum bilirubin falls rapidly by 2–6 mg/dL in 2–6 days and may rise again if breast-feeding is resumed; if interrupted for 6–9 days, serum bilirubin becomes normal.

No other abnormalities are present.

Kernicterus does not occur.

Cholangitis, Acute

Marked increase in WBC (≤ 30,000/cu mm) with increase in granulocytes

○Blood culture positive in ~30% of cases; 25% of these are polymicrobial.

○Laboratory findings of incomplete duct obstruction due to inflammation or of preceding complete duct obstruction (e.g., stone, tumor, scar). See Choledocholithiasis (p. 208).

○Laboratory findings of parenchymal cell necrosis and malfunction

Increased serum AST, ALT, etc.

Increased urine urobilinogen

Cholangitis, Primary Sclerosing

(Chronic fibrosing inflammation of intra- and extrahepatic bile ducts predominantly in men younger than age 45 years; rare in pediatric patients; ≤ 75% of cases are associated with inflammatory bowel disease, especially ulcerative colitis; slow, relentless, progressive course of chronic cholestasis to death [usually from liver failure]. 25% of patients are asymptomatic at time of diagnosis.)

♦Diagnosis should not be made if there is previous bile duct surgery, gallstones, suppurative cholangitis, bile duct tumor, or damage due to floxuridine, AIDS, congenital duct anomalies.

♦Characteristic cholangiogram is required for diagnosis; distinguishes it from primary biliary cirrhosis (see p. 211).

○Cholestatic biochemical profile for >6 mos
  • Serum ALP may fluctuate but is always increased >1.5× upper limit of normal (usually ≥ 3× upper limit of normal).
  • Serum GGT is increased.
  • Serum AST is mildly increased in >90%. ALT is greater than AST in three-fourths of cases.

- Serum bilirubin is increased in one-half of patients; occasionally is very high; may fluctuate markedly; gradually increases as disease progresses. Persistent value >1.5 mg/dL is poor prognostic sign that may indicate irreversible, medically untreatable disease.

Increased gamma globulin in 30% of cases and increased IgM in 40–50% of cases

ANCAs in ~65% of cases and ANAs in <35% are present at higher levels than in other liver diseases, but diagnostic significance is not yet known.

In contrast to primary biliary cirrhosis, antimitochondrial antibody, smooth-muscle antibody and RF are negative in >90% of patients.

HBsAg is negative.

○Liver biopsy provides only confirmatory evidence in patients with compatible history, laboratory, and radiographic findings. Liver copper is usually increased but serum ceruloplasmin is also increased.

Laboratory findings due to sequelae

- Cholangiocarcinoma in 10–15% of patients may cause increased serum CA 19-9.
- Portal hypertension, biliary cirrhosis, secondary bacterial cholangitis, steatorrhea and malabsorption, cholelithiasis, liver failure.

Laboratory findings due to underlying disease, e.g.,

- ≤ 7.5% of ulcerative colitis patients have this disease; many fewer patients with Crohn's disease. Associated with syndrome of retroperitoneal and mediastinal fibrosis.

Cholecystitis, Acute

Increased ESR, WBC (average 12,000/cu mm; if >15,000 suspect empyema or perforation), and other evidence of acute inflammatory process

Serum AST is increased in 75% of patients.

Increased serum bilirubin in 20% of patients (usually <4 mg/dL; if higher, suspect associated choledocholithiasis)

Increased serum ALP (some patients) even if serum bilirubin is normal

Increased serum amylase and lipase in some patients

Laboratory findings of associated biliary obstruction if such obstruction is present

Laboratory findings of preexisting cholelithiasis (some patients)

Laboratory findings of complications (e.g., empyema of gallbladder, perforation, cholangitis, liver abscess, pyelophlebitis, pancreatitis, gallstone ileus)

Cholecystitis, Chronic

May be mild laboratory findings of acute cholecystitis or no abnormal laboratory findings.
May be laboratory findings of associated cholelithiasis.

Choledocholithiasis

During or soon after an attack of biliary colic

- Increased WBC
- Increased serum bilirubin in approximately one-third of patients
- Increased urine bilirubin in approximately one-third of patients
- Increased serum and urine amylase
- Increased serum ALP

○Laboratory evidence of fluctuating or transient cholestasis (see p. 209). Persistent increase of WBC, AST, ALT suggests cholangitis.

Laboratory findings due to secondary cholangitis, acute pancreatitis, obstructive jaundice, stricture formation, etc.

In duodenal drainage, crystals of both calcium bilirubinate and cholesterol (some patients); 50% accurate (only useful for nonicteric patients)

Cholelithiasis

Laboratory findings of underlying conditions causing hypercholesterolemia (e.g., diabetes mellitus, malabsorption) may be present.

Laboratory findings of causative chronic hemolytic disease (e.g., hereditary spherocytosis)

Laboratory findings due to complications (e.g., cholecystitis, choledocholithiasis, gallstone ileus)

Table 8-2. Comparison of Various Types of Cholestatic Disease

Disorder	Bilirubin (mg/dL)	ALP	AST	ALT	Albumin
			Serum Values*		
CBD obstruction					
Stone	0–10	N–10	N–10	N–10	N
Cancer	5–20	2–10	N	N	N
Intrahepatic					
Drug–induced	5–10	2–10	N–5	10–50	
Acute viral hepatitis	0–20	N–3	10–50	10–50	N
Alcoholic liver disease	0–20	5	<10	<50% of AST	N/sl D

CBD = common bile duct; N = normal; sl D = slightly decreased.
*Serum value = times normal.

Cholestasis

See Table 8-2.
○Increased serum ALP
○Increased GGT, 5'-NT, and LAP parallel ALP and confirm the hepatic source of ALP.
○Increased serum cholesterol and phospholipids but not triglycerides
○Increased fasting serum bile acid (>1.5 μg/mL) with ratio of cholic acid to chenodeoxycholic acid >1 in primary biliary cirrhosis and many intrahepatic cholestatic conditions but <1 in most chronic hepatocellular conditions (e.g., Laënnec's cirrhosis, chronic active hepatitis). *(Relatively little experience exists with this test.)*
Cholestasis may occur without hyperbilirubinemia.

Due To

Canalicular
Drugs (e.g., estrogens, anabolic steroids)—most common cause (see Table 8-3)
Normal pregnancy
Alcoholic hepatitis
Infections, e.g.,
    Acute viral hepatitis
    Gram-negative sepsis
    Toxic shock syndrome
    AIDS
    Parasitic, fungal infection
Sickle cell crisis
Postoperative state after long procedure and multiple transfusions
Benign recurrent familial intrahepatic cholestasis (rare)
Non-Hodgkin's lymphoma more often than Hodgkin's disease
Amyloidosis
Sarcoidosis
Interlobular Bile Ducts
Sclerosing pericholangitis (associated with inflammatory bowel disease)
Primary biliary cirrhosis
Postnecrotic cirrhosis (20% of cases)
Congenital intrahepatic biliary atresia
Interlobular and Larger Intrahepatic Bile Ducts
Multifocal lesions (e.g., metastases, lymphomas, granulomas)
Larger Intrahepatic Bile Ducts
Sclerosing cholangitis
Intraductal stones
Intraductal papillomatosis
Cholangiocarcinoma
Caroli's disease (congenital biliary ectasia)

Table 8-3. Comparison of Three Main Types of Liver Disease Due to Drugs

	Predominantly Cholestatic	Predominantly Hepatitic	Mixed Biochemical Pattern
Laboratory findings	Obstructive type of jaundice (see p. 206) Average duration for jaundice = 2 wks; may last for years Serum bilirubin may be >30 mg/dL ALP and LAP are markedly increased; may remain increased for years after jaundice has disappeared AST, ALT, LD show mild to moderate increase	Less markedly increased More markedly increased	Some aspects of each type, but one may be more marked
Some causative drugs	Organic arsenicals Anabolic steroids* Estrogens* Sulfonylurea derivatives (including sulfonamides, phenothiazine tranquilizers, antidiabetic drugs, oral diuretics) Antithyroid drugs (e.g., methimazole) Chlorpromazine PAS (usually this type but may be mixed) Erythromycin	Cinchophen Monoamine oxidase inhibitors (particularly iproniazid) Isonicotinic acid hydrazide	Phenytoin Phenylbutazone PAS and other anti-tuberculosis agents
Pathology	Centrilobular bile stasis Low incidence High mortality (20%)	Same as acute viral hepatitis	

PAS = p-aminosalicylic acid.
*ALP, AST, and ALT are not increased as much compared with other drugs.

Extrahepatic Ducts (Surgical or Extrahepatic Jaundice)

Carcinoma (e.g., pancreas, ampulla, bile ducts, gallbladder)
Stricture, stone, cyst, etc., of ducts
Pancreatitis (acute, chronic), pseudocysts

Increased risk of cholangiocarcinoma in progressive cholestatic diseases.

Cholestasis, Benign Recurrent Intrahepatic

(Familial condition; attacks begin after age 8 yrs, last weeks to months, complete resolution between episodes, may recur after months or years; exacerbated by estrogens.)
Increased serum ALP
Transaminase usually <100 U.
Serum bilirubin may be normal or ≤ 10 mg/dL.
Liver biopsy shows centrolobular cholestasis without inflammation.

Cholestasis, Neonatal

Due To

Idiopathic neonatal hepatitis	50–60%
Extrahepatic biliary atresia	20%
Metabolic disease	
Alpha$_1$-antitrypsin deficiency	15%
Cystic fibrosis	
Tyrosinemia	
Galactosemia	
Niemann-Pick disease	
Defective bile acid synthesis	

Infection (e.g., CMV infection, syphilis, sepsis, GU tract infection)
Toxic causes (e.g., drugs, parenteral nutrition)
Other conditions
    Paucity of bile ducts (Alagille syndrome)
    Indian childhood cirrhosis
    Hypoperfusion/shock

Cirrhosis, Primary Biliary (Cholangiolitic Cirrhosis, Hanot's Hypertrophic Cirrhosis, Chronic Nonsuppurative Destructive Cholangitis, etc.)

(Multisystem autoimmune disease; chronic nonsuppurative inflammation and destruction of small intrahepatic bile ducts producing chronic cholestasis and cirrhosis)

♦ Diagnostic Criteria

Laboratory findings of
- Cholestatic pattern (increased ALP) of long duration (may last for years) not due to known cause (e.g., drugs).
- Antimitochondrial autoantibodies present.
- Confirmed patency of bile ducts (e.g., with ultrasonography or computed tomographic [CT] scan).
- Compatible liver biopsy is highly desirable.

♦Serum ALP is markedly increased; is of liver origin. Reaches a plateau early in the course and then fluctuates within 20% thereafter; changes in serum level have no prognostic value. 5'-NT and GGT parallel ALP. *This is one of the few conditions that elevates both serum ALP and GGT to striking levels.*

♦Serum mitochondrial antibody titer is strongly positive (1:40–1:80) in ~95% of patients and is hallmark of disease (98% specificity); titer >1:160 is highly predictive of primary biliary cirrhosis (PBC) even in absence of other findings. Does not correlate with severity or rate of progression. Titers differ greatly in patients. Similar titers occur in 5% of patients with chronic hepatitis; low titers occur in 10% of patients with other liver disease; rarely found in normal persons. Titer usually decreases after liver transplantation but generally remains detectable.

♦Serum bilirubin is normal in early phase but increases in 60% of patients with progression of disease and is a reliable prognostic indicator; an elevated level is a poor prognostic sign. Direct serum bilirubin is increased in 80% of patients; levels >5 mg/dL in only 20% of patients; levels >10 mg/dL in only 6% of patients. Indirect bilirubin is normal or slightly increased.

♦Laboratory findings show relatively little evidence of parenchymal damage.
  • AST and ALT may be normal or slightly increased (up to 1–5× normal), may fluctuate within a narrow range, and have no prognostic significance.
  • Serum albumin, globulin, and PT normal early; abnormal values indicate advanced disease and poor prognosis; not corrected by therapy.

♦Marked increase in total cholesterol and phospholipids with normal triglycerides; serum is not lipemic; serum triglycerides become elevated in late stages. Associated with xanthomas and xanthelasmas. In early stages, LDL and VLDL are mildly elevated and HDL is markedly elevated (thus atherosclerosis is rare). In advanced stage, LDL is markedly elevated with decreased HDL and presence of lipoprotein X (nonspecific abnormal lipoprotein seen in other cholestatic liver disease).

○Serum IgM is increased in ~75% of patients; levels may be very high (4–5× normal). Other serum immunoglobulins are also increased.

Hypocomplementemia

Polyclonal hypergammaglobulinemia

♦Biopsy of liver categorizes the four stages and helps assess prognosis, but needle biopsy is subject to sampling error because the lesions may be spotty; findings consistent with all four stages may be found in one specimen.

○Serum ceruloplasmin is characteristically elevated (in contrast to Wilson's disease).

Liver copper may be increased 10–100× normal; correlates with serum bilirubin and advancing stages of disease.

ESR is increased 1–5× normal in 80% of patients.

Urine contains urobilinogen and bilirubin.

Laboratory findings of steatorrhea, including the following:
  • Serum 25-hydroxyvitamin D and vitamin A are usually low.
  • PT is normal or restored to normal by parenteral vitamin K.

Laboratory findings due to associated diseases
  • >80% of patients have at least one other and >40% have at least two other circulating antibodies to autoimmune disease (e.g., RA, autoimmune thyroiditis [hypothyroidism in 20% of patients], Sjögren's syndrome, scleroderma) although not useful diagnostically.

Laboratory findings due to sequelae and complications
  • Portal hypertension, hypersplenism
  • Treatment-resistant osteoporosis
  • Hepatic encephalopathy, liver failure
  • Renal tubular acidosis (due to copper deposition in kidney) is frequent but usually subclinical.
  • Increased susceptibility to urinary tract infection is associated with advanced disease.

Should be ruled out in an asymptomatic female with elevated serum ALP without obesity, diabetes mellitus, alcohol abuse, use of some drugs.

Cirrhosis of Liver

♦ **Criteria for diagnosis** liver biopsy or at least three of the following:
  • Hyperglobulinemia, especially with hypoalbuminemia
  • Low-protein (<2.5 g/dL) ascites
  • Evidence of hypersplenism (usually thrombocytopenia, often with leukopenia and less often with Coombs'-negative hemolytic anemia)
  • Evidence of portal hypertension (e.g., varices)
  • Characteristic "corkscrew" hepatic arterioles on celiac arteriography
  • Shunting of blood to bone marrow on radioisotope scan
  • *Abnormality of serum bilirubin, transaminases, or ALP is often not present and therefore not required for diagnosis.*

○Serum bilirubin is often increased; may be present for years. Fluctuations may reflect liver status due to insults to the liver (e.g., alcoholic debauches). Most bilirubin is of the indirect type unless cirrhosis is of the cholangiolitic type. Higher and more stable levels occur in postnecrotic cirrhosis; lower and more fluctuating levels occur in Laënnec's cirrhosis. Terminal icterus may be constant and severe.

○Serum AST is increased (<300 U) in 65–75% of patients. Serum ALT is increased (<200 U) in 50% of patients. Transaminases vary widely and reflect activity or progression of the process (i.e., hepatic parenchymal cell necrosis).

Serum ALP is increased in 40–50% of patients.

○Serum total protein is usually normal or decreased. Serum albumin parallels functional status of parenchymal cells and may be useful for following progress of liver disease; but it may be normal in the presence of considerable liver cell damage. Decreasing serum albumin may reflect development of ascites or hemorrhage. Serum globulin level is usually increased; it reflects inflammation and parallels the severity of the inflammation. Increased serum globulin (usually gamma) may cause increased total protein, especially in chronic viral hepatitis and posthepatitic cirrhosis.

Serum total cholesterol is normal or decreased. Progressive decrease in cholesterol, HDL, LDL with increasing severity. Decrease is more marked than in chronic active hepatitis. LDL may be useful for prognosis and selection of patients for transplantation. Decreased esters reflect more severe parenchymal cell damage.

Urine bilirubin is increased; urobilinogen is normal or increased.

BUN is often decreased (<10 mg/dL); increased with GI hemorrhage.

Serum uric acid is often increased.

Electrolytes and acid-base balance are often abnormal and reflect various combinations of circumstances at the time, such as malnutrition, dehydration, hemorrhage, metabolic acidosis, respiratory alkalosis. In cirrhosis with ascites, the kidney retains increased sodium and excessive water, causing dilutional hyponatremia.

Blood ammonia is increased in liver coma and cirrhosis and with portacaval shunting of blood.

Anemia reflects increased plasma volume and some increased destruction of RBCs. If more severe, rule out hemorrhage in GI tract, folic acid deficiency, excessive hemolysis, etc.

WBC is usually normal with active cirrhosis; increased (<50,000/cu mm) with massive necrosis, hemorrhage, etc.; decreased with hypersplenism.

○Laboratory findings due to complications or sequelae, often in combination
- Portal hypertension.
   Ascites.
   Esophageal varices.
   Portal vein thrombosis.
- Liver failure.
- Hepatocarcinoma.
- Abnormalities of coagulation mechanisms (see Chapter 11), e.g.,
   Prolonged PT (does not respond to parenteral vitamin K as frequently as in patients with obstructive jaundice).
   Prolonged bleeding time in 40% of cases due to decreased platelets and/or fibrinogen (see Chapter 11).
- Hepatic encephalopathy.
   Increased arterial ammonia.
   CSF glutamine >35 mg/dL (due to conversion from ammonia); correlates with depth of coma and more sensitive than arterial ammonia.
- Spontaneous bacterial peritonitis—in ≤ 10% of alcoholic cirrhosis cases. 70% have positive blood culture; usually single organism, especially *E. coli, Pneumococcus, Klebsiella.*
- Hepatorenal syndrome (see p. 725).
- Most commonly death is due to liver failure, bleeding, infections.

Laboratory findings due to causative/
associated diseases or conditions   **Frequency in USA**
- Chronic viral hepatitis (HBV with or without   10%
   HDV, HCV)
- Alcoholism   60–70%
- Wilson's disease   Rare
- Autoimmune chronic active hepatitis
- Hemochromatosis   5%

**Laboratory findings due to causative/
associated diseases or conditions**   **Frequency in USA**
- Mucoviscidosis
- Glycogen-storage diseases
- Galactosemia
- Alpha$_1$-antitrypsin deficiency   Rare
- Porphyria
- Fructose intolerance
- Tyrosinosis
- Infections (e.g., congenital syphilis, schistosomiasis)
- Gaucher's disease
- Ulcerative colitis
- Osler-Weber-Rendu disease
- Venous outflow obstruction (e.g., Budd-Chiari syndrome, venoocclusive disease, congestive heart failure)
- Biliary disease (e.g., primary biliary cirrhosis, sclerosing   5–10%
  cholangitis
- Cryptogenic   10–15%

Crigler-Najjar Syndrome (Hereditary Glucuronyl Transferase Deficiency)

(Rare familial autosomal recessive disease due to marked congenital deficiency or absence of glucuronyl transferase, which conjugates bilirubin to bilirubin glucuronide in hepatic cells [counterpart is the homozygous Gunn rat])
See Table 8-4.

Type I

Indirect serum bilirubin is increased; it appears on first or second day of life, rises in 1 wk to peak of 12–45 mg/dL, and persists for life. No direct bilirubin in serum or urine.
Fecal urobilinogen is very low.
Liver function tests are normal; sulfobromsulfophthalein (BSP) is normal.
Liver biopsy is normal.
No evidence of hemolysis is found.
Untreated patients often die of kernicterus by age 18 mos.
Nonjaundiced parents have diminished capacity to form glucuronide conjugates with menthol, salicylates, and tetrahydrocortisone.
Type I should always be ruled out when persistent unconjugated bilirubin levels of 20 mg/dL are seen after 1 wk of age without obvious hemolysis and especially after breast-milk jaundice has been ruled out.
This syndrome has been divided into two groups:

	Type I	Type II
Transmission	Autosomal recessive	Autosomal dominant
Hyperbilirubinemia	More severe (usually >20 mg/dL)	Less severe and more variable (usually <20 mg/dL)
Kernicterus	Frequent	Absent
Bile	Essentially colorless	Normal color
Bilirubin-glucuronide	Totally absent	Present
Bilirubin concentration	Very low (<10 mg/dL) Only traces of conjugated bilirubin	Nearly normal (50–100 mg/dL)
Stool color	Pale yellow	Normal
Parents	Normal serum bilirubin in both parents Partial defect (~50%) in glucuronide conjugation in both parents	One parent usually shows minimal to severe icterus Defect in glucuronide conjugation may be present in only one parent

Table 8-4. Differential Diagnosis of Hereditary Jaundice with Normal Liver Chemistries and No Signs or Symptoms of Liver Disease

	Conjugated Hyperbilirubinemias		Unconjugated Hyperbilirubinemias		
				Crigler-Najjar Syndrome	
	Dubin-Johnson Syndrome	Rotor's Syndrome	Gilbert's Disease	Type I	Type II
Incidence	Uncommon	Rare	≤ 7% of population	Very rare	Uncommon
Inheritance mode	AR	AR	AD	AR	AD
Serum bilirubin usual total (mg/dL)	2–7; ≤ 25 Direct ~60%	2–7; ≤ 20 Direct ~60%	<3; ≤ 6 Mostly indirect; increases with fasting	>20 All indirect	<20 All indirect
Defect in bilirubin metabolism	Impaired biliary excretion of conjugated organic anions and bilirubin		Hepatic UDP–glucuronyl transferase activity Decreased	Absent	Marked decrease
Impaired excretion of dyes requiring conjugation (e.g., BSP)	Yes; initial rapid fall, then rise in 45–90 mins	Yes; slow clearance; no later increase	May be slightly impaired in ≤ 40% of patients		
Effect of phenobarbital			Decrease to normal	None	Marked decrease
Urine coproporphyrin Total I/III*	Normal >80%	Increased <80%			
Age at onset of jaundice	Childhood, adolescence	Adolescence, early adulthood	Adolescence	Infancy	Childhood, adolescence
Usual clinical features	Asymptomatic jaundice in young adults	Asymptomatic jaundice	Appear in early adulthood; often first recognized with fasting; very mild hemolysis in ≤ 40% of patients	Jaundice, kernicterus in infants, young adults	Asymptomatic jaundice; kernicterus rare
Oral cholecystogram	GB usually not visualized	Normal	Normal	Normal	Normal
Liver biopsy	Characteristic pigment	No pigment	Normal	Normal	Normal
Treatment	Not needed	None	Not needed	Liver transplant; no response to phenobarbital	Phenobarbital
Animal model	Corriedale sheep			Gunn rat	

AD = autosomal dominant; AR = autosomal recessive; BSP = sulfobromsulfophthalein; GB = gallbladder; UDP-glucuronyl transferase = uridine-diphosphate glucuronosyl-transferase.
*Normally coproporphyrin III = 75% of total.

Type II

Patients have partial deficiency of glucuronyl transferase (autosomal dominant with incomplete penetrance). Not related to type I syndrome; may be homozygous form of Gilbert's disease. Patient may not become jaundiced until adolescence. Neurologic complications are rare.

Serum indirect bilirubin = 6–25 mg/dL. Increases with fasting or removal of lipid from diet. May decrease to <5 mg/dL with phenobarbital treatment.

Dubin-Johnson Syndrome (Sprinz-Nelson Syndrome)

(Autosomal recessive disease due to inability to transport bilirubin-glucuronide through hepatocytes into canaliculi, but conjugation of bilirubin-glucuronide is normal. Characterized by mild chronic, recurrent jaundice; hepatomegaly and right upper quadrant abdominal pain may be present. Usually is compensated except in periods of stress. Jaundice [innocuous and reversible] may be produced by estrogens, birth control pills, or last trimester of pregnancy. May resemble mild viral hepatitis.)

See Table 8-4.

○Serum bilirubin is increased (3–10 mg/dL; rarely ≤ 30 mg/dL); significant amount is direct.

Urine contains bile and urobilinogen.

♦BSP excretion is impaired with late (1.5- to 2-hr) increase; virtually pathognomonic.

○Other liver function tests are normal.

♦Urine total coproporphyrin is usually normal but ~80% is coproporphyrin I (normally 75% is coproporphyrin III); diagnostic of Dubin-Johnson syndrome. Not useful to detect individual heterozygotes.

○Liver biopsy shows large amounts of yellow-brown or slate-black pigment in centrolobular hepatic cells (lysosomes) and small amounts in Kupffer's cells.

Fatty Liver

Laboratory findings are due to underlying conditions (most commonly alcoholism; nonalcoholic fatty liver is commonly associated with non–insulin dependent diabetes mellitus [≤ 75%], obesity [69–100%], hyperlipidemia [20–81%]; malnutrition, toxic chemical exposure)

♦Biopsy of liver establishes the diagnosis.

Nonalcoholic fatty liver is distinguished by negligible history of alcohol consumption and negative random blood alcohol assays.

Liver function tests
  Most commonly, serum AST and ALT are increased 2–3×; usually ALT >AST.
  Serum ALP is normal or slightly increased in <50% of patients.
  Increased serum ferritin (≤ 5×) and transferrin saturation in ~60% of cases.
  Other liver function tests are usually normal.
  Serologic tests for viral hepatitis are negative.

Cirrhosis occurs in ≤ 50% of alcoholic and ≤ 17% of nonalcoholic cases.

Biochemically different form occurs in acute fatty liver of pregnancy, Reye's syndrome, tetracycline administration.

Fatty liver may be the only postmortem finding in cases of sudden, unexpected death.[1]

Fatty Liver of Pregnancy, Acute

(Incidence of 1 per 13,328 deliveries; usually occurs after 35th week of pregnancy. Medical emergency because of high maternal and fetal mortality, which is markedly improved by termination of pregnancy.)

Often associated with toxemia (see p. 763)

Increased AST and ALT to ~300 U (rarely >500 U) are used for early screening in suspicious cases; ratio is not helpful in differential diagnosis.

Increased WBC in >80% of cases (often >15,000/cu mm)

Evidence of DIC in >75% of patients (see p. 464)

[1]Sheth SG, Gordon FD, Chopra S. Nonalcoholic Steatohepatitis. *Ann Intern Med* 1997;126:137.

Serum uric acid is increased disproportionately to BUN and creatinine, which may also be increased.

Serum bilirubin may be normal early but will rise unless pregnancy terminates.

Blood ammonia is usually increased.

Blood glucose is often decreased, sometimes markedly.

Neonatal liver function tests are usually normal, but hypoglycemia may occur.

♦Biopsy of liver confirms the diagnosis.

Gallbladder and Bile Duct Cancer

Laboratory findings reflect varying location and extent of tumor infiltration that may cause partial intrahepatic duct obstruction or obstruction of hepatic or common bile duct (see pp. 206–207), metastases in liver (see p. 248), or associated cholangitis (see pp. 207–208); 50% of patients have jaundice at the time of hospitalization.

Laboratory findings of duct obstruction are of progressively increasing severity in contrast to the intermittent or fluctuating changes due to duct obstruction caused by stones. A papillary intraluminal duct carcinoma may undergo periods of sloughing, producing the findings of intermittent duct obstruction.

Anemia is present.

♦Cytologic examination of aspirated duodenal fluid may demonstrate malignant cells.

○Silver-colored stool due to jaundice combined with GI bleeding may be seen in carcinoma of duct or ampulla of Vater.

Laboratory findings of the preceding cholelithiasis are present (gallbladder cancer occurs in ~3% of patients with gallstones).

Gilbert's Disease

(Chronic, benign, intermittent, familial [autosomal dominant with incomplete penetrance], nonhemolytic unconjugated hyperbilirubinemia with evanescent increases of indirect serum bilirubin, which is usually discovered on routine laboratory examinations; due to defective transport and conjugation of unconjugated bilirubin. Jaundice is usually accentuated by pregnancy, fever, exercise, and various drugs, including alcohol and birth control pills. Rarely identified before puberty. May be mildly symptomatic. 3–7% prevalence in total population.)

See Table 8-4.

♦Presumptive diagnostic criteria

Exclusion of other diseases.

Unconjugated hyperbilirubinemia on several occasions.

Liver chemistries and hematologic parameters are normal.

♦Indirect serum bilirubin is increased transiently and has been previously normal at least once in ≤ 33% of patients. It may rise to 18 mg/dL but usually is <4 mg/dL. Considerable daily and seasonal fluctuation. Fasting (<400 calories/day) for 72 hrs causes elevated indirect bilirubin to increase >100% in Gilbert's disease but not in healthy persons (increase <0.5 mg/dL) or those with liver disease or hemolytic anemia. Fasting bilirubin returns to baseline 12–24 hrs after resumption of normal diet. Combination of basal total bilirubin >1.2 mg/dL and fasting increase of unconjugated bilirubin >1 mg/dL has sensitivity of 84%, specificity of 78%, positive predictive value of 85%, negative predictive value of 76%. Provocative tests are rarely needed. Direct serum bilirubin is normal but may give elevated results by liquid diazo methods but not by dry methods or chromatography. Enzyme inducers (e.g., phenobarbital) normalize unconjugated bilirubin in 1–2 wks. Prednisone administration reduces bilirubin concentration.

Liver function tests are usually normal.

Fecal urobilinogen usually normal but may be decreased.

Urine shows no increased bilirubin.

Liver biopsy is normal.

Heart Failure (Congestive), Liver Function Abnormalities

Pattern of abnormal liver function tests is variable depending on severity of heart failure; the mildest cases show only slightly increased ALP and slightly decreased serum albumin; moderately severe cases also show slightly increased serum bilirubin and GGT; one-fourth to three-fourths of the most severe cases also show increased AST and ALT (≤ 200 U/L) and LD (≤ 400 U/L). All return to normal when heart failure responds to treatment. Serum ALP is usually the last to become normal, and this may occur weeks to months later.

Serum bilirubin is frequently increased (indirect more than direct); usually 1–5 mg/dL. It usually represents combined right- and left-sided failure with hepatic engorgement and pulmonary infarcts. Serum bilirubin may suddenly rise rapidly if superimposed myocardial infarction occurs.

AST and ALT are disproportionately increased compared with other liver function tests in left-sided heart failure.

PT may be slightly increased, with increased sensitivity to anticoagulant drugs.

Serum cholesterol and esters may be decreased.

Urine urobilinogen is increased. Urine bilirubin is increased in the presence of jaundice.

These findings may occur with marked liver congestion due to other conditions (e.g., Chiari's syndrome [occlusion of hepatic veins] and constrictive pericarditis).

Hemochromatosis[2-4]

See Fig. 8-4.

Due To

Hereditary hemochromatosis is an autosomal recessive defect in the ability of the duodenum to regulate iron absorption; abnormal gene present in 10% of white Americans; frequency of homozygosity >3 in 1000. 1–3% of heterozygotes develop iron overload; may be due to coincidental condition with altered iron absorption or metabolism.

Other primary causes of iron overload (may have one hemochromatosis allele)
- Neonatal hemochromatosis
- Juvenile hemochromatosis
- African iron overload
- Aceruloplasminemia

Secondary
- Increased intake (e.g., excessive medicinal iron ingestion, long-term frequent transfusions, Bantu siderosis)
- Anemias with increased erythropoiesis (especially thalassemia major; also thalassemia minor, some other hemoglobinopathies, paroxysmal nocturnal hemoglobinuria, sideroblastic anemias, refractory anemias with hypercellular bone marrow, pyruvate kinase deficiency, pyridoxine-responsive anemia, X-linked iron-loading anemia, etc.)
- Chronic hemodialysis
- Porphyria cutanea tarda (minor)
- Alcoholic liver disease (minor; deposited in Kupffer's cells, not hepatocytes)
- After portal-systemic shunt
- Congenital atransferrinemia

♦ Increased transferrin saturation (= serum iron ÷ total iron-binding capacity × 100); usually >70% and frequently approaches 100%; repeat fasting transferrin saturation >60% in men and >50% in women without other known causes probably represents hemochromatosis; 50–62% usually indicates heterozygous state but occasionally found in homozygous persons. Most heterozygotes have no detectable changes unless a secondary cause (e.g., thalassemia) is present. If value is increased, patient should be retested (fasting) twice at weekly intervals. Screening discovers hemochromatosis in 2–3 of 1000 persons; should be sought especially in patients with diabetes mellitus, congestive heart failure, idiopathic cardiomyopathy, arthritis, alcoholic cirrhosis, bronze skin, hypogonadism.

♦ Increased serum ferritin (usually >1000 μg/L); increased in approximately two-thirds of patients with hemochromatosis. Is good index of total body iron but has limited

[2]Mendlein J, et al. Iron overload, public health and genetics. *Ann Intern Med* 1998;129:921.
[3]Edwards CQ, Kushner JP. Screen for hemochromatosis. *N Engl J Med* 1993;328:1616.
[4]Press RD, et al. Hepatic iron overload. *Am J Clin Pathol* 1998;109:577.

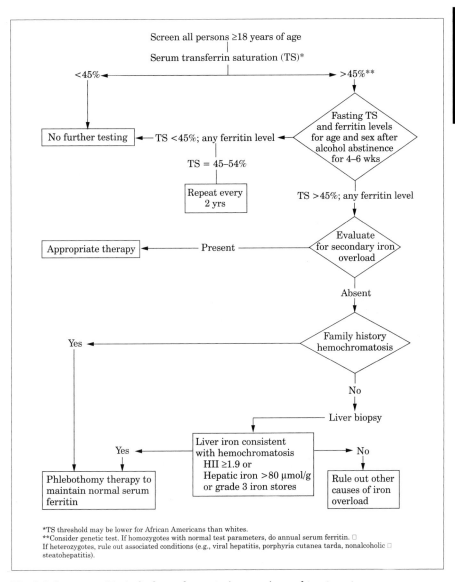

Fig. 8-4. Sequence of tests for hemochromatosis screening and treatment.

value for screening because may be increased in acute inflammatory conditions and less sensitive than transferrin saturation in early cases. May not be increased in patients who have not yet accumulated excess amounts of iron (e.g., children, young adults, premenopausal women). >5000 μg/L indicates tissue damage (e.g., liver degeneration) with release of ferritin into circulation. >350 μg/L in fasting men and >250 μg/L in women is recommended for screening. Critical threshold associated with cirrhosis is unknown. Liver biopsy is probably not indicated if serum ferritin is normal.
♦ Serum iron is increased (usually >200 μg/dL in women and >300 μg/dL in men and typically >1000 μg/dL) but should not be only screening test because of many other conditions in which it occurs. Confirm by measuring repeat fasting sample at least two more times. *Serum iron levels may show marked diurnal variation, with lowest values in evening and highest between 7 a.m. and noon.*

- ◆TIBC is decreased (~200 μg/dL; often approaches zero; generally higher in secondary than primary type).
- ◆Liver biopsy is needed to confirm or refute diagnosis, grade amount of iron, and assess tissue damage (presence of fibrosis/cirrhosis, other liver diseases). Is indicated when repeat fasting serum ferritin (>750 mg/L) and transferrin saturation are increased after 4–6 wks of abstinence from alcohol. Histologic examination confirms increased stainable iron (special stain) in perilobular hepatocytes and biliary epithelium in hereditary hemochromatosis with little in Kupffer's cells (in contrast to secondary iron overload) or bone marrow, with or without inactive cirrhosis. In later stages, liver biopsy alone does not distinguish hereditary hemochromatosis from secondary hemochromatosis. Liver iron is increased (normal 200–2000 μg/gm in men and 200–1600 μg/gm in women). >1000 μg/100 mg of dry liver is consistent with homozygous state but level may reach 5000. Some heterozygotes may reach 1000 μg/100 mg but do not progress beyond this level. Fibrosis or cirrhosis usually does not occur at levels <2000 μg/100 mg dry liver unless alcoholism is also present. For chemical analysis of iron, use acid-washed needle and place specimen in iron-free container. Liver iron and serum ferritin may also be increased in alcoholic cirrhosis but levels are not as abnormal (<2× normal) as in hemochromatosis. Liver iron must be related to patient age: hepatic iron index (micrograms/gram divided by 55.8 × age) in homozygotes is ≥ 1.9; in heterozygotes usually ≤ 1.5. False negative may be due to phlebotomy treatment; false positive may be due to secondary hemosiderosis. Another calculation is liver iron (micromoles/gram dry weight) divided by patient age; value >2 in homozygotes; <2 in heterozygotes, healthy persons, patients with alcoholic liver disease.

Other tests to assess iron stores (when liver biopsy is not possible)
- Chelating agent (0.5 gm IM deferoxamine mesylate) causes urinary excretion >5 mg/24 hrs in hereditary hemochromatosis but <2 mg/24 hrs in normal persons. Measures only chelatable iron rather than total iron stores so may underdiagnose hereditary hemochromatosis; not a useful diagnostic test.
- Weekly phlebotomy for 5–10 wks causes iron deficiency in alcoholic liver disease but >50 weekly phlebotomies are required in hereditary hemochromatosis.

○Presence of excess iron in other tissue biopsy sites (e.g., synovia, GI tract) should arouse suspicion of hereditary hemochromatosis; iron stains should be done.

Bone marrow biopsy stained for iron is not useful for diagnosis of hereditary hemochromatosis.

Liver function tests depend on presence and degree of liver damage (e.g., cirrhosis).

On average, women have serum ferritin concentrations 1000 μg/L less than men; men have twice the incidence of cirrhosis (25%) and diabetes (15%) compared with women.

Laboratory findings due to involvement of various organs
- Insulin-dependent diabetes mellitus in 40–75% of cases; glucose intolerance
- Osteoarthritis and chondrocalcinosis (pseudogout) in 50% of cases
- Cardiomyopathy in 33% of cases (congestive heart failure)
- Hypogonadism/pituitary dysfunction in ~50% of cases
- Skin pigmentation
- Underlying diseases (see previous diseases)

○Laboratory findings due to complications and sequelae
- Increased susceptibility to severe bacterial infection, especially *Yersinia* sepsis (also occurs in other iron overload conditions).
- Cirrhosis in 69% of cases. Does not resolve with phlebotomy. Increased risk of hepatocellular carcinoma. Associated alcoholism.
- Hepatocellular carcinoma develops in ≤ 30% of cases and has become the chief cause of death in hereditary hemochromatosis (see p. 242).
- Portal hypertension.

○When diagnosis of hereditary hemochromatosis is established, other family members should be screened; one-fourth of siblings have the disease; 5% of patients' children are homozygous for hemochromatosis gene. Relatives with negative results should be rescreened every 5 yrs.

○Genotyping is not used for screening to discover sporadic cases but useful to identify patient's siblings at risk because HLA-identical sibs almost always are also homozygous for hemochromatosis gene and at high risk for developing clinical disease. May be useful to distinguish patients with primary hereditary hemochromatosis from cirrhotic patients with secondary iron overload and siderosis.

DNA test for hereditary hemochromatosis gene is available, but diagnostic role is being evaluated. C282Y or H63D present in 69–97% of affected patients; would not identify ≤ 31% of clinically affected patients. May ultimately replace HLA typing.

Adequate treatment with phlebotomy (1–3 U/wk) sufficient to maintain a mild anemia is determined by Hct (37–39%) before each phlebotomy. If >40%, an additional treatment may be scheduled. Serum iron and ferritin are used only when anemia become refractory to establish whether iron stores are exhausted. Maintenance phlebotomy (4–6 U/yr) can be monitored with serum ferritin to indicate normal amount of storage iron. Insulin requirement decreases in more than one-third of diabetics; liver function tests often improve; arthritis, impotence, and sterility usually do not improve. Removal of 450–500 mL of blood causes loss of 200–250 mg of iron.

Hemochromatosis, Neonatal

(Severe iron overload disorder with onset in utero. Death usually occurs soon after birth.)

Oligohydramnios or less commonly polyhydramnios may indicate intrauterine growth retardation or fetal hydrops.

○Fulminant liver failure including hyperbilirubinemia, decreased transaminases, glucose, and albumin. Increased AFP. Variable fibrinogen consumption, thrombocytopenia, anemia, acanthocytosis.

♦Marked hepatic and extrahepatic (e.g., heart, pancreas, adrenal; not spleen) siderosis with relative lack in RE cells.

Liver iron analysis not useful because high in healthy newborn.

Hepatic Encephalopathy

(Neurologic and mental abnormalities in some patients with liver failure)

○Blood ammonia is increased in 90% of patients but does not reflect the degree of coma. Normal level in comatose patient suggests another cause of coma. Not reliable for diagnosis but may be useful to follow individual patients. May be increased by tight tourniquet or vigorously clenched fist; thus arterial specimen may be preferable.

Respiratory alkalosis due to hyperventilation is frequent.

Hyponatremia and iatrogenic hypernatremia are frequent complications and are associated with a higher mortality rate.

Hypokalemic metabolic alkalosis may occur due to diuretic excess.

Serum amino acid profile is abnormal. All serum amino acids are markedly increased in coma due to acute liver failure.

CSF is normal except for increased glutamine level.

♦Diagnosis is clinical; characteristic laboratory findings are supportive but not specific.

Hepatic Failure, Acute

Due To

Infection
- Viral hepatitis (e.g., hepatitis A, B, C, D, E; HSV 1, 2, 6; EBV, CMV).
   Acute liver failure related to HSV is usually associated with immunosuppressive therapy.
   Develops in ~1–3% of adults with acute icteric type B hepatitis with resultant death.
- Other causes rare (e.g., amebic abscesses, disseminated TB).

Drugs (e.g., acetaminophen, methyltestosterone, isoniazid, halothane, idiosyncratic reaction)

Toxins (e.g., phosphorus, death-cap mushroom [*Amanita phalloides*])

Acute fatty liver
- Pregnancy (see p. 216)
- Reye's syndrome (see p. 290)
- Drugs (e.g., tetracycline)

Ischemic liver necrosis
- Shock
- Budd-Chiari syndrome (acute)
- Wilson's disease with intravascular hemolysis (see p. 250)

- Congestive heart failure
- Extracorporeal circulation during open heart surgery

Marked infiltration by tumor
  - Acute leukemia
  - Lymphoma
      Hodgkin's disease
      Non-Hodgkin's lymphoma
      Burkitt's lymphoma
      Malignant histiocytosis

○Serum bilirubin progressively increases; may become very high.

Increased serum AST, ALT, may fall abruptly terminally; serum ALP and GGT may be increased.

Serum cholesterol and esters are markedly decreased.

Decreased albumin and total protein

Electrolyte abnormalities, e.g.,
  - Hypokalemia (early)
  - Metabolic alkalosis due to hypokalemia
  - Respiratory alkalosis
  - Lactic acidosis
  - Hyponatremia, hypophosphatemia

Hypoglycemia in ~5% of patients

○Laboratory findings associated with
  - Hepatic encephalopathy (see p. 221)
  - Hepato-renal syndrome (see p. 725)
  - Coagulopathy
      Decreased factors II, V, VII, IX, X cause prolonged PT and aPTT (PT is never normal in acute hepatic failure). (See p. 221.)
      Decreased antithrombin III.
      Platelet count <100,000 in two-thirds of patients.
  - Hemorrhage, especially in GI tract
  - Bacterial and fungal infections, especially streptococci and *S. aureus*
  - Ascites

As patient deteriorates, titers of HBsAg, and HBeAg may often fall and disappear.

Hepatitis, Acute Viral

See Table 8-5 and Fig. 8-5.

Different types of viral hepatitis cannot be distinguished by clinical features or routine chemistries; serologic tests are needed.

Prodromal Period

♦Serologic markers appear in serum (Table 8-6).

Bilirubinuria occurs before serum bilirubin increases.

Increase in urinary urobilinogen and total serum bilirubin just before clinical jaundice occurs.

○Serum AST and ALT both rise during the preicteric phase and show very high peaks (>500 U) by the time jaundice appears.

ESR is normal.

Leukopenia (lymphopenia and neutropenia) is noted with onset of fever, followed by relative lymphocytosis and monocytosis; may find plasma cells and <10% atypical lymphocytes (in infectious mononucleosis level is >10%).

Asymptomatic Hepatitis

Biochemical evidence of acute hepatitis is scant and often absent.

Acute Icteric Period

(Tests show parenchymal cell damage.)

Serum bilirubin is 50–75% direct in the early stage; later, indirect bilirubin is proportionately more.

Serum AST and ALT fall rapidly in the several days after jaundice appears and become normal 2–5 wks later.
- *In hepatitis associated with infectious mononucleosis*, peak levels are usually <200 U and peak occurs 2–3 wks after onset, becoming normal by the fifth week.
- *In toxic hepatitis*, levels depend on severity; slight elevations may be associated with therapy with anticoagulants, anovulatory drugs, etc.; poisoning (e.g., carbon tetrachloride) may cause levels ≤ 300 U.
- *In severe toxic hepatitis (especially carbon tetrachloride poisoning)*, serum enzymes may be 10–20× higher than in acute hepatitis and show a different pattern, i.e., increase in LD > AST > ALT.
- *In acute hepatitis*, ALT > AST > LD.

Other liver function tests are often abnormal, depending on severity of the disease—bilirubinuria, abnormal serum protein electrophoresis, ALP, etc.

Serum cholesterol/ester ratio is usually depressed early; total serum cholesterol is decreased only in severe disease.

Serum phospholipids are increased in mild but decreased in severe hepatitis. Plasma vitamin A is decreased in severe hepatitis.

Urine urobilinogen is increased in the early icteric period; at peak of the disease it disappears for days or weeks; urobilinogen simultaneously disappears from stool.

ESR is increased; falls during convalescence.

Serum iron is often increased.

Urine: Cylindruria is common; albuminuria occurs occasionally; concentrating ability is sometimes decreased.

Defervescent Period

Diuresis occurs at onset of convalescence.
Bilirubinuria disappears, whereas serum bilirubin is still increased.
Urine urobilinogen increases.
Serum bilirubin becomes normal after 3–6 wks.
ESR falls.

Anicteric Hepatitis

Laboratory findings are the same as in the icteric type, but abnormalities are usually less marked and serum bilirubin shows slight or no increase.

Acute Fulminant Hepatitis with Hepatic Failure

See p. 221.

Cholangiolitic Hepatitis

Same as acute hepatitis, but evidence of obstruction is more prominent (e.g., increased serum ALP and direct serum bilirubin), and tests of parenchymal damage are less marked (e.g., AST increase may be 3–6× normal).

Chronic Hepatitis

See Table 8-7.
Occurs in 5–10% of adults with acute HBV.
HBV hepatitis is generally divided into three stages:
- Stage of acute hepatitis: Usually lasts 1–6 mos with mild or no symptoms.
  AST and ALT are increased >10×.
  Serum bilirubin is usually normal or only slightly increased.
  HBsAg gradually rises to high titers and persists; HBeAg also appears.
  Gradually merges with next stage.
- Stage of chronic hepatitis: Transaminases increased >50% for >6 mos duration; may last only 1 yr or for several decades with mild or severe symptoms; most cases resolve, but some develop cirrhosis and liver failure.
  AST and ALT fall to 2–10× normal range.
  HBsAg usually remains high, and HBeAg remains present.
- Chronic carrier stage: Patients are usually, but not always, healthy and asymptomatic.
  AST and ALT fall to normal or <2× normal.

Table 8-5. Comparison of Different Types of Viral Hepatitis

	A	B	C	D	E
Genome	ssRNA	dsDNA	ssRNA	ssRNA	ssRNA
Classification	Picornaviridae	Hepadnaviridae	Flaviviridae	Unclassified	Caliciviridae ?
Cause of hepatitis (% in U.S.)	~30	~40	~20	Always associated with HBV; 4% of acute HBV cases have HDV coinfection	Rare; occurs in travelers to endemic areas
Incubation period (days)	15–60	45–160	14–180	42–180	15–64
Transmission					
Enteric	Yes	No	No	No	Yes
Sexual	No	Yes	Possible	Possible	No
Perinatal	No	Yes	Possible	Possible	No
Parenteral	Rare	Yes	Yes	Yes	No
Postransfusion incidence (%)	None	0.002	1–4		None
Viremia	Transient	Prolonged	Prolonged	Prolonged	Transient?
Fecal excretion of virus	+	–	–	–	+
Onset	Abrupt	Insidious	Insidious	Abrupt	Abrupt
Course	Mild, often subclinical	Insidious ———	—— See text	Abrupt ———	Mild, self-limited[a]
Asymptomatic	Most children	Most children; 50% adults[b]	~75%	Rare	Often
Jaundice	Child: 10% Adult: 70–80%	15–40%[c]	10–25%	Varies	25–50%
Fulminant	1% Causes 5% of fulminant cases	0.2–2.0%	~0.5%	High	May cause one-third of fulminant cases with 90% mortality

Carrier state	No	Adult: 6-10% Child: 25-50% Infant: 70-90% ≤1% of U.S. donors	50-70% ≤1% of U.S. donors addicts and hemophiliacs	10-15% 1-10% of drug	No Unknown
Chronic hepatitis	No	5-10% of acute infections	>50%	<5% coinfection; 80% superinfection	No
Hepatocellular	No	Yes	Yes	Yes	Unknown; not likely
Mortality	1-2%	1-2%	1-2%	≤30% in chronic cases	1-2%; 20% in pregnancy

[a] Resembles hepatitis A. Case fatality = 1-2% except ≤ 20% in pregnancy. Usually milder infection and biochemical abnormalities than HBV or HAV infection.

[b] ≤ 20% have serum sickness–like prodroma.

[c] Nonicteric patient is more likely to progress to chronic hepatitis. 1% of icteric cases become fulminant (<8 weeks) and 90% die within 2-4 weeks; associated with encephalopathy; renal, electrolyte, acid–base imbalances; hypoglycemia; coagulation derangements.

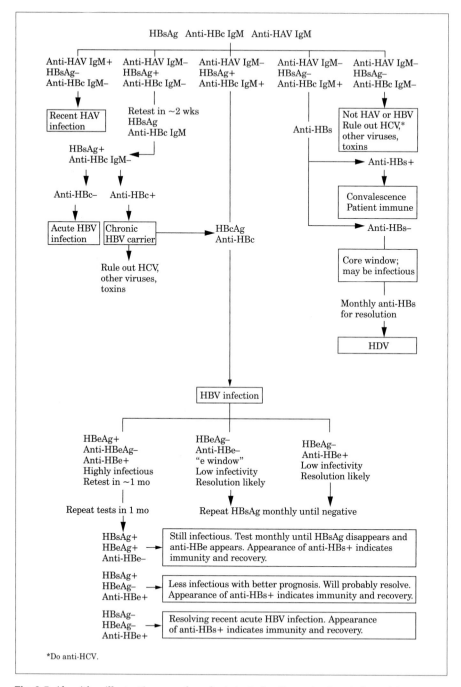

Fig. 8-5. Algorithm illustrating use of serologic tests for diagnosis of acute hepatitis.

Table 8-6. Serologic Markers of Viral Hepatitis

Stage of Infection	HAV	HBV	HCV	HDV	HEV
Acute disease	Anti-HAV-IgM	HBcAb-IgM	Anti-HCV	HDAg	Anti-HEV[a]
Chronic disease	NA	HBsAg	Anti-HCV	Anti-HDV	NA
Infectivity	HAV-RNA[b]	HBeAg, HBsAg, HBV-DNA[c]	Anti-HCV, HCV-RNA	Anti-HDV, HDV-RNA[b]	HEV-RNA[b]
Recovery	None	HBeAb, HBsAb	None	None	None
Carrier state	NA	HBsAg	None	Anti-HDV, HDAg	NA
Immunity screen	Anti-HAV-total (includes anti-HAV-IgG)	HBsAb, HBcAb-total	None	None	Anti-HEV[a]

[a]Not available in United States.
[b]Only available in research laboratories.
[c]Only for investigational use.

Table 8-7. Comparison of Types of Hepatitis D Virus (HDV) Infections

	Coinfection	Superinfection	Chronic HDV
HBV infection	Acute	Chronic	Chronic
HDV infection	Acute	Acute to chronic	Chronic
Chronicity rate	<5%	>75%	Cirrhosis in >70%
Serology			
HBsAg	+	Usually persistent	Persistent
HBcAb-IgM	+	Negative	Negative
Anti-HDV-total	Negative or low titer	+	+
Anti-HDV-IgM*	Transient +	Transient	High titer
HDV-RNA (HDAg)	Transient +	Usually persistent	Persistent
Liver HDAg	Transient +	Usually persistent	Persistent

+ = positive.
*Decrease in anti-HDV-IgM usually predicts resolution of acute HDV. Persistent anti-HDV-IgM typically predicts progression to chronic HDV infection. High titer correlates with active liver inflammation.

HBeAg disappears, and anti-HBe appears.
HBsAg titer falls although may still be detectable; anti-HBs subsequently develops, marking the end of carrier stage.
Anti-HBc is usually present in high titer (>1:512).
Laboratory findings due to sequelae, e.g.,
- GN or nephrotic syndrome due to deposition of HBeAg or HBcAg in glomeruli, which often progresses to chronic renal failure.

Hepatitis, Alcoholic[5]

♦ Diagnosis is established by liver biopsy and history of alcohol intake. Liver biopsy should be performed for any alcoholic patient with enlarged liver as the only way to make definite diagnosis of alcoholic hepatitis. Many alcoholics have normal liver biopsies.
○ Increased serum GGT and MCV >100 together or separately are useful clues for occult alcoholism.
Ratio of desialylated transferrin to total transferrin >0.013 has been reported to have 81% sensitivity and 98% specificity for ongoing alcohol consumption.
Serum AST is increased (rarely >300 U/L), but ALT is normal or only slightly elevated.
AST and ALT are more specific but less sensitive than GGT. Levels of AST and ALT do not correlate with severity of liver disease. AST/ALT ratio >1 associated with AST <300 U/L will identify 90% of patients with alcoholic liver disease; is particularly useful for differentiation from viral hepatitis, in which increase of AST and ALT are about the same.
Cholestasis in ≤ 35% of patients.
In acute alcoholic hepatitis, GGT level is usually higher than AST level. GGT is often abnormal in alcoholics even with normal liver histology. Is more useful as index of occult alcoholism or to indicate that elevated serum ALP is of bone or liver origin than to follow course of patient, for which AST and ALT are most useful.
Serum ALP may be normal or moderately increased in 50% of patients and is not useful as a diagnostic test.
Serum bilirubin may be mildly increased except with cholestasis; is not useful as a diagnostic test. However, if bilirubin continues to increase during a week of therapy in the hospital, a poor prognosis is indicated.
Decreased serum albumin and increased polyclonal globulin with disproportionately increased IgA are frequent. Decreased albumin means long-standing or relatively severe disease.
Increased PT that is not corrected by parenteral administration of 10 mg/day of vitamin K for 3 days is best indicator of poor prognosis.
Discriminant function to assess severity of alcoholic hepatitis = 4.6 × (PT [secs] – control PT) + serum bilirubin. Discriminant function >32 is equated with severe disease.

[5]Sheth SG, Gordon FD, Chopra S. Nonalcoholic steatohepatitis. *Ann Intern Med* 1997;126:137.

Increased WBC (>15,000) in up to one-third of patients with shift to left (WBC is decreased in viral hepatitis); normal WBC may indicate folic acid depletion.

Anemia in >50% of patients may be macrocytic (folic acid or vitamin B_{12} deficiency), microcytic (iron or pyridoxine deficiency), mixed, or hemolytic.

Metabolic alkalosis may occur due to K^+ loss with pH normal or increased, but pH <7.2 often indicates that disease is becoming terminal.

In terminal stage of chronic alcoholic liver disease (last week before death), there is often decrease of serum sodium and albumin and increase of PT and serum bilirubin; AST and LD decrease from previously elevated levels.

Indocyanine green (50 mg/kg) is abnormal in 90% of patients.

Compared to nonalcoholic patients, alcoholic patients as a group show an increase in a number of blood components (e.g., AST, phosphorus, ALP, GGT, MCV, MCH, Hb, WBC) and a decrease in others (e.g., total protein, BUN); however, these variations usually remain within the reference range. These changes may last for >6 wks after abstaining from alcohol.

Laboratory findings due to sequelae or complications
    Fatty liver
    Cirrhosis
    Portal hypertension
    Infections (e.g., GU tract, pneumonia, peritonitis)
    DIC
    Hepatorenal syndrome
    Encephalopathy

Hepatitis, Autoimmune Chronic Active

♦ **Criteria for diagnosis** (all must be present for definite diagnosis)[6]

	Probable	Definite
Increased serum AST or ALT concentrations	X	X
Increased serum ALP <3× normal concentration		X
Increased serum total or gamma globulin or IgG		
>1.5× upper limit of normal		X
1.0–1.5× upper limit of normal	X	
Antibody titers to nucleus, smooth muscle or liver/kidney		X
microsome type 1 >1:80 (adults) or >1:20 (children)		
Lower titers or presence of other antibodies	X	
Absence of markers for viral hepatitis (HAV, HBV, HCV,	X	X
CMV, EBV)		
Absence of excess alcohol consumption		
<25 gm/day (women) or <35 gm/day (men)		X
<40 gm/day (women) or <50 gm/day (men)	X	
Exposure to blood products		
No		X
Yes, but unrelated to disease	X	
Exposure to hepatotoxic drugs		
No		X
Yes, but unrelated to disease	X	
Compatible histologic findings and absence of biliary	X	X
lesions, copper deposits or other changes suggestive		
of other causes of lobular hepatitis		

Hepatitis, Chronic Active

(Inflammatory liver disease present >6 mos.)

Due To

Viruses
- HBV (with or without HDV)
- HCV (with or without hepatitis G virus [HGV])

[6]Czaja AJ. The variant forms of autoimmune hepatitis. *Ann Intern Med* 1996;125:588.

Metabolic disorders
- Wilson's disease
- Alpha$_1$-antitrypsin deficiency
- Hemochromatosis
- Primary biliary cirrhosis
- Sclerosing cholangitis

Drugs, e.g.,
- Methyldopa
- Nitrofurantoin
- Isoniazid
- Oxyphenacetin

Nonalcoholic fatty liver
Alcoholic hepatitis
Autoimmune causes
- Type I (lupoid) (anti–smooth muscle; antiactin)
- Type II (anti–kidney-liver-microsomal)
- Type III (anti–soluble liver antigen)

Hepatitis A

Serum bilirubin usually 5–10× normal. Jaundice lasts a few days to 12 wks. Usually not infectious after onset of jaundice.
Serum AST and ALT increased to hundreds for 1–3 wks.
Relative lymphocytosis is frequent.

Serologic Tests for Viral Hepatitis A (HAV)[7]

See Tables 8-5 and 8-6, and Figs. 8-3, 8-5, and 8-6.
♦ Anti-HAV IgM appears at the same time as symptoms in >99% of cases, peaks within first month, becomes nondetectable in 12 mos (usually 6 mos). Presence confirms diagnosis of recent acute infection.
♦ Anti-HAV–total is predominantly IgG except immediately after acute HAV infection, when it is mostly IgM and IgA. Almost always positive at onset of acute hepatitis and is usually detectable for life; found in 45% of adult population; indicates previous exposure to HAV, recovery, and immunity to type A hepatitis. Negative anti-HAV–total effectively excludes acute HAV. Positive anti-HAV–total does not distinguish recent from past infection, for which anti-HAV IgM test is needed. Test for anti-HAV–total is relatively insensitive (minimum detection amount = 100 mU/mL) and may not detect protective antibody response after one dose of inactivated HAV vaccine (minimum protective antibody is <10 mU/mL).
Serial testing is usually not indicated.
Tests for anti-HAV–total and anti-HAV IgM are not influenced by normal doses of immune globulin.
HAV antigen and HAV RNA are available only as research tools.

Hepatitis B

See Tables 8-5 and 8-6, and Figs. 8-5, 8-6.

Serologic Tests for Viral Hepatitis B (HBV)

See Table 8-6 and Tables 8-8 through 8-12.

Use

Differential diagnosis of hepatitis
Screening of blood and organ donors
Determination of immune status for possible vaccination

[7]Lemon SM. Type A viral hepatitis: epidemiology, diagnosis, and prevention. *Clin Chem* 1997; 43:1494.

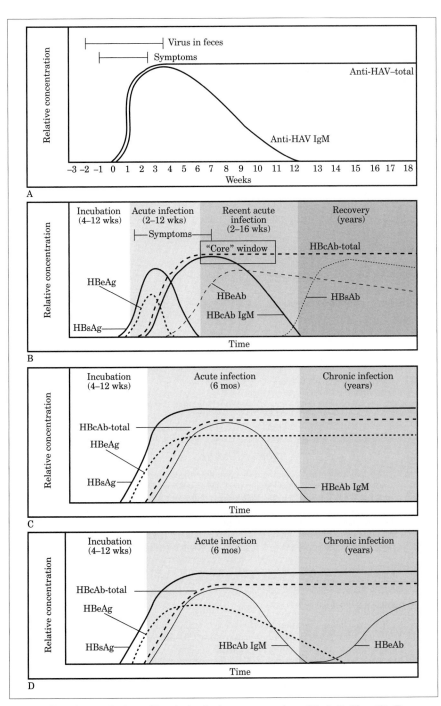

Fig. 8-6. Hepatitis serologic profiles. **A:** Antibody response to hepatitis A. **B:** Hepatitis B core window identification. **C, D:** Hepatitis B chronic carrier profiles: no seroconversion (**C**); late seroconversion (**D**). (Reproduced with permission of Hepatitis Information Center, Abbott Laboratories, Abbott Park, IL.)

Table 8-8. Serologic Tests for Hepatitis B Virus Infections

Test						Interpretation
HBsAg	HBsAb	HBeAg	HBeAb	HBcAb-Total	HBcAb-IgM	
+	–	–	–	–	–	Late incubation or early acute HBV
+	–	+	–	–	–	Early acute HBV; highly infectious
+	–	+	–	+	+	Acute HBV
+	–	–	+	+	+	"Serologic window/ gap" or acute HBV
–	–	–	–	+	+	Serologic gap
–	–	–	+	+	+	Convalescence
–	+	–	+	+	+	Early recovery
–	+	–	+	+	–	Recovery[a]
+	–	±	±	+	–	Chronic infection (chronic carrier)[a]
–	+	–	–	–	–	Old previous HBV with recovery and immunity or HBV vaccination or passive transfer antibody[b]
–	–	–	–	–	–	Not HBV infection

+ = positive; – = negative.
[a]Chronic carriers of HBV may have clinical hepatitis due to non-A, non-B hepatitis rather than HBV.
[b]Various serologic patterns may occur after blood transfusion or injection of immune (gamma) globulin by passive transfer. Anti-HBs can be found for up to 6–8 months after injection of high-titer HB immunoglobulin because of 25-day half-life.

Hepatitis B Surface Antigen (HBsAg)

♦ Earliest indicator of HBV infection. Usually appears in 27–41 days (as early as 14 days). Appears 7–26 days before biochemical abnormalities. Peaks as ALT rises. Persists during the acute illness. Usually disappears 12–20 wks after onset of symptoms or laboratory abnormalities in 90% of cases. Is the most reliable serologic marker of HBV infection. Persistence >6 mos defines carrier state. May also be found in chronic infection. Hepatitis B vaccination does not cause a positive HBsAg. Titers are not of clinical value. Present sensitive assays detect <1.0 ng/mL of circulating antigen, which is the level needed to find 10–15% of reactive blood donors who carry antigen but express only low levels. Is never detected in some patients, and diagnosis is based on presence of HBc IgM.

HBsAg and Blood Transfusions

Transfusion of blood containing HBsAg causes hepatitis or appearance of HBsAg in blood in >70% of recipients; needle stick with such blood causes hepatitis in 45% of cases. Transfusion of blood not containing HBsAg causes anicteric hepatitis in 16% of recipients and icteric hepatitis in 2%.
Screening out of blood donors with HBsAg reduces posttransfusion hepatitis by 25–40%.
When HBsAg carriers are discovered (e.g., in screening program), 60–80% show some evidence of hepatic damage.
Persons with a positive test for HBsAg should never be permitted to donate blood or plasma.
HBsAg is found in

Chronic persistent hepatitis	50%
Chronic active hepatitis	25%
Cirrhosis	3%

Table 8-9. Serologic Tests for Hepatitis B Virus Infection Follow-Up

Test				Interpretation	Follow-Up
HBsAg	HBsAb	HBeAg	HBeAb		
+	–	–	–	Acute HBV infection	Repeat serology for resolution or chronicity. Serum ALT to monitor disease activity.
+	–	+	–	Early acute HBV infection; highly infectious	Repeat serology for resolution or chronicity. Serum ALT to monitor disease activity.
+	–	+	+	Decreasing infectivity	Repeat serology for resolution. Serum ALT to monitor disease activity.
+	–	–	+	Early seroconversion; HBsAb not yet detected	Repeat for HBsAb and disappearance of HBsAg.
–	+	–	+	Recovery; immune	None needed for HBV.
–	–	–	–	No evidence of prior HBV infection	Test for other cause of hepatitis.

+ = positive; – = negative.

Patients undergoing multiple transfusions	3.8%
Drug addicts	4.2%
Blood donor population	<0.1%
Prevalence in United States	0.25%

Antibody to HBsAg (Anti-HBsAg)

♦ Presence of antibody (titer ≥ 10 mU/mL); (without detectable HBsAg) indicates recovery from HBV infection, absence of infectivity, and immunity from future HBV infection; patient does not need gamma globulin administration if exposed to infection; this blood can be transfused.

Table 8-10. Serologic Tests for Prenatal Screening for Hepatitis B Virus

Test			Interpretation	Follow-Up
HBsAg	HBeAg	HBsAb		
–	–	+	Mother is HBV immune.	Not needed.
–	–	–	No evidence of HBV infection.	Not needed unless other evidence of hepatitis.
+	+	–	Mother is HBV carrier. Infant at high risk of acquiring HBV infection during delivery and developing chronic hepatitis.	Infant must be vaccinated within 12 hrs of birth.
+	–	–	Mother is HBV carrier. Infant at high risk of acquiring HBV infection during delivery and developing chronic hepatitis.	Infant must be vaccinated within 12 hrs of birth.

Table 8-11. Serologic Tests for Candidate for Hepatitis B Virus Vaccination

	Test			
HBsAg	HBsAb	HBcAb	Interpretation	Follow-Up
+	−	−	Acute HBV infection	See Table 8-9
−	−	+	Acute HBV or carrier	Previous HBV infection; vaccinate
−	+	+	Immune; previous HBV infection or vaccination	None
+	−	+	Previous HBV infection; may not be immune	Vaccinate
−	−	−	Not immune	Vaccinate

+ = positive; − = negative.

- May also occur after transfusion by passive transfer.
- Found in 80% of patients after clinical cure. Appearance may take several weeks or months after HBsAg has disappeared and after ALT has returned to normal, causing a "serologic gap" during which time (usually 2- to 6-wk "window") only IgM–anti-HBsAg can identify patients who are recovering but may still be infectious.
- Presence can be used to show efficiency of immunization program. Appears in ~90% of healthy adults after three-dose deltoid muscle immunization; 30–50% of these lose antibodies in 7 yrs and require boosters. Revaccination of nonresponders produces adequate antibody in <50% after three additional doses.
- A few persons acquire HBV infection after developing high titers of anti-HBsAg due to a mutant HBV virus.

In fulminant hepatitis—antibody is produced early and may coexist with low antigen titer. In chronic carriers—no IgM antibody is present but antigen titers are very high.

Hepatitis Be Antigen (HBeAg)

♦ Indicates highly infectious state. Appears within 1 wk after HBsAg; in acute cases disappears before disappearance of HBsAg; is found only when HBsAg is found. Occurs early in disease before biochemical changes and disappears after serum ALT peak. Usually lasts 3–6 wks. Is a marker of active HBV replication in liver; with few exceptions, is present only in persons with circulating HBV DNA and is used as alternative to HBV DNA assay.

Is useful to determine resolution of infection. Persistence >20 wks suggests progression to chronic carrier state and possible chronic hepatitis. Presence in HBsAg-positive mothers indicates 90% chance that infant will acquire HBV infection.

Absence of HBeAg is not indicator of benign nonprogressive disease.

May be HBeAg negative and HBV DNA positive in patients infected with an HBV mutant who do not synthesize HBeAg.

Antibody to HBe (Anti-HBe)

♦ Appears after HBeAg disappears and remains detectable for years. Indicates decreasing infectivity, suggests good prognosis for resolution of acute infection. Association with anti-HBc in absence of HBsAg and anti-HBs confirms recent acute infection (2–16 wks).

Table 8-12. Serologic Tests for Hepatitis B Virus Vaccination Follow–Up

HBsAb	Interpretation	Follow-Up
+	Effective immunization	Repeat in future years to ensure immunity
−	No evidence of immunity	Await appearance of HBsAb or repeat vaccination

+ = positive; − = negative.

Antibody to Hepatitis B Core Antigen–Total (Anti-HBc–Total)

♦Occurs early in acute infection, 4–10 wks after appearance of HBsAg, at same time as clinical illness; persists for years or for lifetime. Anti-HBc–total and HBsAg are always present and anti-HBsAg is absent in chronic HBV infection.

♦**Anti-HBc IgM** is the earliest specific antibody; usually occurs 2 wks after HBsAg. Is found in high titer for a short time during the acute disease stage that covers the serologic window and then declines to low levels during recovery (see Fig. 8-6); may be detectable ≤ 6 mos. May be the only serologic marker present after HBsAg and HBeAg have subsided but before these antibodies have appeared (serologic gap or window). Because this is the only test unique to recent infection, it can differentiate acute from chronic HBV. It is the only serologic test that can differentiate recent and remote infection with one specimen. However, because some patients with chronic hepatitis B infection become positive for anti-HBc IgM during flares, it is not an absolutely reliable marker of acute illness. Before anti-HBc IgM disappears, anti-HBc IgG appears and lasts indefinitely.

Anti-HBc detects virtually all persons who have been previously infected with HBV and can therefore serve as surrogate test for other infectious agents (e.g., HCV). Exclusion of anti-HBc–positive donors reduces the incidence of posttransfusion hepatitis and possibly of other virus infections (e.g., AIDS) due to the frequency of dual infection. Present without other serologic markers and with normal AST in ~2% of routine blood donors; 70% of cases are due to recovery from subclinical HBV (and individual may be infectious) and the rest are considered false-positives. False-positive anti-HBc can be confirmed by immune response pattern to hepatitis B vaccination. Anti-HBc is not protective (unlike anti-HBsAg) and therefore cannot be used to distinguish acute from chronic infection.

♦**HBV DNA** (by PCR) is the most sensitive and specific assay for early evaluation of HBV and may be detected when all other markers are negative (e.g., in immunocompromised patients). May become negative before HBeAg becomes negative. Measures HBV replication even when HBeAg is not detectable. Marked decrease in patients who respond to therapy; those with concentrations <200 ng/L are more likely to respond to therapy.

Other Laboratory Findings

○Very high serum ALT and bilirubin are not reliable indicators of patient's clinical course, but prolonged PT, especially >20 secs, indicates the likely development of acute hepatic insufficiency; therefore the PT should be performed when patient is first seen.
- Acute fulminant hepatitis may be indicated by triad of prolonged PT, increased PMNs, and nonpalpable liver with likely development of coma.
- Acute viral hepatitis B completely resolves in 90% of patients within 12 wks with disappearance of HBsAg and development of anti-HBs.
- Relapse, usually within 1 yr, has been recognized in 20% of patients by some elevation of ALT and changes in liver biopsy.
- Chronic hepatitis (disease for >6 mos and ALT >50% above normal): 70% of these patients have benign chronic persistent hepatitis and 30% have chronic active hepatitis that can progress to cirrhosis and liver failure.
- Effective treatment of chronic HBV hepatitis causes ALT, HBeAg, and HBV DNA to become normal.
- Chronic carriers have also been defined as those who are either HBsAg positive on two occasions >6 mos apart or have one specimen that is HBsAg positive and anti-HBc IgM negative but anti–HBc-positive.
- 10% of adults and 90% of children ≤ 4 yrs old become chronic carriers; 25% of these develop cirrhosis and high risk of hepatoma. HBV carriers should be screened periodically with serum AFP and ultrasonography or CT scan of liver for hepatoma.

Laboratory indicators for favorable response to interferon:
- Pretreatment serum ALT >100 U/L (high ALT may indicate better host immune response to HBV)
- HBV DNA <200 ng/L (pg/mL)
- Absence of HIV
- Also duration <4 yrs and acquisition of infection after 6 yrs of age

Laboratory effects of interferon treatment:
- Serum ALT may increase to >1000 U/L.

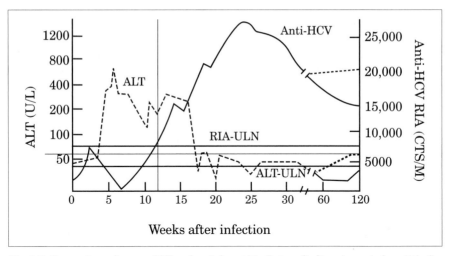

Fig. 8-7. Comparison of serum ALT and anti–hepatitis C virus findings in acute hepatitis C. Chronic infection is indicated by broken lines. (CTS/M = counts/minute; RIA = radioimmunoassay; ULN = upper limit of normal.)

- 10% of patients show sustained disappearance of HBV DNA and clearance of HBeAg.
- If serum ALT is persistently increased despite lack of HBeAg, presence of an HBeAg-negative mutant that may have emerged during treatment is suggested.
- 5–10% of patients with seroconversion due to therapy will have reactivation in next 10 yrs; this is usually transitory.

Laboratory contraindications to interferon therapy for chronic hepatitis B:
- Liver decompensation
  Serum albumin <3.0 gm/L
  Serum bilirubin >3.0 mg/dL
  PT increased >3×
- Portal hypertension (e.g., ascites, bleeding esophageal varices, encephalopathy)
- Hypersplenism
  WBC <2000/cu mm
  Platelet count <70,000
- Autoimmune disease (e.g., RA, polyarteritis nodosa)
- Major system impairment
- Other (e.g., pregnancy, current IV drug abuse, psychiatric)

Hepatitis C (Formerly Non-A, Non-B Hepatitis)[8,9]

See Fig. 8-7 and Tables 8-5 and 8-6.
Can remain infectious for years.
~85% of acute cases become chronic with viremia.
    Of chronic carriers with or without abnormal ALT values,
- 15% experience resolution.
- 70% develop chronic hepatitis (average time = 10 yrs).
- 10–20% develop cirrhosis despite normal liver function tests (average time = 20 yrs).
- ~50% die of consequences of HCV infection.

[8]*MMWR Recommendations for prevention and control of hepatitis C virus infection and HCV-related chronic disease.* US Department of Health and Human Services, Centers for Disease Control and Prevention; 1998 Oct 16; 47/no RR-19.
[9]Fairfax MR, Merline JR, Podzorski RP. *Am Soc Clin Pathol.* Check Sample Microbiology No. 97-1.

- Fulminant hepatitis is rare.
- Hepatocellular carcinoma may occur in ~20% of cirrhosis patients (average time = 30 yrs) and 1–5% of those with HCV infections.
- 50–75% of all liver cancers are HCV associated.
- ~40% of liver transplantations in United States are performed to treat chronic hepatitis C with cirrhosis.

Routine screening for HCV should be performed and HCV should be ruled out in hepatitis in persons who

- Ever injected illegal drugs.
- Received clotting factor concentrates produced before 1987 (70–90% of severe hemophiliacs are infected with HCV).
- Ever were on long-term hemodialysis.
- Ever received blood from donor who later tested positive for HCV (2–7% of blood donors in United States are asymptomatic carriers).
- Ever received blood or components or organ transplant before July 1992.
- Have persistently abnormal serum ALT.

Causes ≤ 25% of sporadic cases of acute viral hepatitis in adults, 90% of cases of post-transfusion hepatitis.

Source of infection: injected drug use = 42%; occupational exposure = ~5%; transfusion = <1%; dialysis = 0.6%; household contact = 3%; heterosexual transmission = 6% (cumulative risk may be 18%); unidentified = 42%.

Perinatal infection at time of birth in 5% of infants of HCV-infected mothers.

Biochemical and histologic evidence of abnormality occurs in 7% of sporadic cases, ≤ 60% of posttransfusion cases, and ≤ 80% of immunosuppressed patients.

Occult HBV infection is present in approximately one-third of patients with chronic HCV liver disease by HBV DNA analysis of liver biopsy.[10]

○May be associated with mixed cryoglobulinemia with vasculitis (see Chapter 11), thyroiditis, Sjögren's syndrome, membranoproliferative GN, and porphyria cutanea tarda, which should be ruled out in cases of hepatitis C, and HCV infection should be ruled out in patients with those disorders. Patients with alcoholic liver disease have more rapidly progressive disease with higher ALT values and more severe histologic changes.

Increased Serum Transaminases

○Levels characteristically show unpredictable waxing and waning pattern, returning to almost normal levels (formerly called acute "relapsing" hepatitis); pattern is highly suggestive but only occurs in 25% of cases.

May be extreme (>10× normal).

Patients with monophasic ALT response usually recover completely with no biopsy evidence of residual disease.

ALT is usually <800 U. ALT cannot be relied on to determine whether to perform liver biopsy in chronic hepatitis C; biopsy is needed to define severity.

ALT is primary marker to monitor therapy. In chronic HCV, AST/ALT ratio >1 has specificity and positive predictive value of 100% for cirrhosis although sensitivity is 52%. Ratio does not correlate with serum ALP, bilirubin, albumin, or PT.

Anicteric patients with ALT >300 U/L are at high risk for progressing to chronic hepatitis.

Liver Biopsy

Use

Diagnose chronic active hepatitis

Assess disease progression and indication for antiviral therapy

No consistent correlation between serum ALT and severity of liver pathology; significant liver damage can occur with normal ALT.

Exclude coexisting or alternative (e.g., alcohol-related) diseases

---

[10]Cacciola I, et al. Occult hepatitis B virus infections in patients with chronic hepatitis C liver disease. *N Engl J Med* 1999;341:22.

♦ Antibody to Hepatitis C Virus (anti-HCV) (by EIA)

Use
Screening of populations with low and high prevalence, including blood donors

Initial evaluation of patients with liver disease, including those with increased serum ALT

Positive results should be verified by a supplemental assay (i.e., recombinant immunoblot assay [RIBA]) showing reactivity with ≥ 2 viral antigens; indeterminate in ≤ 10% of cases.

Interpretation
Indicates past or present infection but does not differentiate between acute, chronic, and resolved infection.

Sensitivity ≥ 97%; only ~80% in chronic carriers. Low positive predictive value in low-prevalence population.

Seroconversion: average time after exposure = 2–3 wks with EIA-3. Detected in 80% of patients within 15 wks, in >90% within 5 mos, in >97% by 6 mos after exposure or 2–3 mos after increase in ALT. Therefore serial assay of anti-HCV and ALT for up to 1 yr after suspected acute hepatitis may be needed for diagnosis. Negative EIA rules out HCV infection in low-risk group.

Present in 70–85% of cases of chronic posttransfusion NANB hepatitis but is relatively infrequent in acute cases. Present in 70% of IV drug abusers, 20% of hemodialysis patients, and only 8% of homosexual men positive for HIV.

Prevalence in normal blood donors is 0.5–2.0%. In routine blood donor screening, estimates are that 40–70% of initial reactors prove not to be true positives. Surrogate markers fail to detect one-third to one-half of blood units positive for anti-HCV. Found in 7–10% of transfusion recipients. Only one-third of anti-HCV donors had increased ALT and 54% were positive for anti-HBc.

In one study, anti-HCV was positive in 75% of patients with hepatocellular carcinoma, 56% of patients with cirrhosis, and 7% of controls.

Present in various quality assurance and calibration sera; overall rate = 43% with much higher rates in some proficiency samples.

Because resolves slowly, is considered chronic only with evidence of activity >12 mos.

Interferences
False-positive
- Autoimmune diseases (≤ 80% of cases of autoimmune chronic active hepatitis).
- EIA and RIBA are also found in polyarteritis nodosa (~10%) and SLE (~2%).
- RF.
- Hypergammaglobulinemia.
- Paraproteinemia.
- Passive antibody transfer.
- Anti-idiotypes.
- Anti–superoxide dismutase (a human enzyme used in the cloning process).
- Repeated freezing and thawing or prolonged storage of blood specimens.

False-negative
- Early acute infection
- Immunosuppression
- Immunoincompetence
- Repeated freezing and thawing or prolonged storage of blood specimens

RIBA

Positive EIA should be evaluated with RIBA-2; negative RIBA indicates false-positive EIA.

Positive RIBA indicates past or previous exposure.

Confirms positive EIA in >50% of cases; in high-risk population RIBA confirms diagnosis in >88% of cases.

Increasingly replaced by HCV RNA.

HCV RNA Assay

(By reverse transcriptase PCR [RT-PCR])

Qualitative tests

Use

Diagnose acute HCV infection before seroconversion; can detect virus as early as 1–2 wks after exposure.

Detection may be intermittent; one negative RT-PCR is not conclusive.

Monitor patients on antiviral therapy

Evaluate indeterminate RIBA results

False-positive and false-negative results may occur.

Quantitative Tests

(RT-PCR and branched DNA; not presently approved by U.S. Food and Drug Administration.)

Quantitative tests from different manufacturers do not yield identical results.

Determines concentration of HCV RNA.

Large spontaneous fluctuations in RNA level; therefore should measure two times or more to evaluate changes due to therapy.

RT-PCR yields positive results for 75–85% of persons positive for anti-HCV and >95% of persons with acute or chronic HCV hepatitis.

Use

May be used to assess likelihood of response to antiviral therapy. Patients with pre-treatment level <2 million copies/mL (by PCR or quantitative branched DNA) are most likely to respond to interferon therapy. Positive test after 12 wks of interferon therapy predicts failed response; negative test has ~30% predictive value for sustained response.

Less sensitive than qualitative test RT-PCR.

Earliest marker for diagnosis of fulminant hepatitis C. Negative test in patient with fulminant hepatitis rules out HCV infection.

Confirm persistent HCV infection after liver transplantation when anti-HCV is positive and serum ALT is normal.

Diagnose chronic hepatitis patients with
  Negative anti-HCV
  False-positive serologic tests due to autoantibodies

Not used to exclude diagnosis of HCV infection.

Not used to determine treatment end point.

HCV Genotyping

Presently a research tool with no clinical utility. At least six genotypes and >90 subtypes. A correlation may exist between genotype and disease. Mixed infections often occur.

HCV Genotype	Occurrence (%)	
1a	37	Higher rate of chronic hepatitis; poorer response to interferon therapy and higher likelihood of relapse
1b	30	More severe liver disease; higher risk of hepatocellular carcinoma

Other genotypes have various geographic distributions.

Antiviral therapy is recommended for patients with greatest risk of progression to cirrhosis
  • Positive anti-HCV with
  • Persistently increased ALT
  • Detectable HCV RNA
  • Liver biopsy showing at least moderate inflammation and necrosis or fibrosis
Indicators of response to antiviral therapy
  • ~50% show normal serum ALT.
  • 33% lose detectable HCV RNA in serum; loss associated with remission. Presence after sustained response to interferon indicates late relapse.
  • 50% relapse after therapy ends.
Decreased interferon response occurs in <15% of patients; indicated by
  • Higher serum HCV RNA titers
  • HCV genotype 1

Laboratory contraindications to interferon therapy
- Persistently increased serum ALT
- Cytopenias
- Hyperthyroidism
- Renal transplantation
- Evidence of autoimmune disease

No tests are routinely available for other HCV viruses.

Hepatitis D (Delta)

See Tables 8-5, 8-6, and 8-7.

Hepatitis D is due to a transmissible virus that depends on HBV for expression and replication. It may be found for 7–14 days in the serum during acute infection. Delta agent can be an important cause of acute or chronic hepatitis. The course depends on the presence of HBV infection. HDV hepatitis is often severe with relatively high mortality in acute disease and frequent development of cirrhosis in chronic disease. Chronic HDV infection is more severe and has higher mortality than other types of viral hepatitis. Prevalence in United States is 1–10% of HBsAg carriers, principally in high-risk groups of IV drug abusers and multiply transfused patients but uncommon in other groups at risk for HBV infection (e.g., health care workers, male homosexuals).

Serologic Tests for HDV

See Tables 8-5, 8-6, 8-7, and 8-13.

Serum HDAg and HDV-RNA appear during incubation period after HBsAg and before rise in AST, which often shows a biphasic elevation. HBsAg and HDAg are transient; HDAg resolves with clearance of HBsAg. Anti-HDV appears soon after clinical symptoms but titer is often low and short-lived. Anti-HDV–total test is commercially available; HDAg and anti-HDV-IgM testing is available only in research laboratories.

Coinfection means simultaneous acute HBV and acute HDV infection; usually causes acute limited illness with additive liver damage due to each virus, followed by recovery. Usually is self-limited; <5% of cases become chronic. ~3% have fulminant course.

Superinfection means acute HDV infection in a chronic HBV carrier. Mortality = 2–20%; >80% develop chronic hepatitis. Serum anti-HDV appears and rises to high sustained titers indicating continuing replication of HDV; intrahepatic HDAg is present. HDV-RNA persists in low titers.

♦ Diagnosis of HDV hepatitis is made by presence of anti-HDV in patient with HBsAg-positive hepatitis. Anti-HDV assay should not be performed unless diagnosis of HBV is confirmed.

♦ Acute coinfection is distinguished from superinfection by presence of serum HBsAg and anti-HBc-IgM, which indicate acute HBV.

♦ Chronic HDV infection occurs in ≤ 80% of acute cases; shows presence of HBsAg and high titer of anti-HDV (RIA titer >1:100 suggests chronic HDV hepatitis) and absence of anti-HBc-IgM in serum. Confirm by liver biopsy showing HDAg by immunofluorescence or immunoperoxidase.

♦ Serum anti-HDV-IgM documents acute HDV infection; low levels remain in persistent infection.

Western blot can demonstrate serum HDV-Ag when RIA is negative. Persistence correlates with development of chronic HDV hepatitis and viral antigen in liver biopsy.

DNA probe for HDV-RNA in serum to monitor HDV replication.

Serum anti-HDV may be sought in patients with HBsAg-positive chronic or acute hepatitis in high-risk group or with severe disease or with biphasic acute hepatitis or acute onset in chronic hepatitis.

Hepatitis E

See Tables 8-5 and 8-6.

Recent travel to certain areas (e.g., Mexico, India, Africa, Burma, Russia)

♦ Serologic markers for hepatitis A, B, and C and other causes of acute hepatitis (e.g., EMB, CMV) are absent.

♦ Antibody to hepatitis E can be detected by fluorescent antibody blocking assay and by Western blot; not commercially available.

Table 8-13. Serologic Diagnosis of Hepatitis B Virus (HBV) and Hepatitis D Virus (HDV)

	Test			
HBsAg	HBcAb-IgM	Anti-HDV-IgM	Anti-HDV-IgG	Interpretation
Transient +	+ High titer	Transient +	Transient low titer	Acute HBV and acute HDV[a]
Transient decrease due to inhibitory effect of HDV on HBV synthesis	Negative or low titers	High titer first, low titer later	Increasing titers	Acute HDV and chronic HBV[b]
May remain + in chronic HBV	Replaced by anti-HBc-IgG in chronic HBV	+ correlates with HDAg in hepato-cytes	High titers corre-late with active infection; may remain + for years after infection resolves	Chronic HDV and chronic HBV[c]

+ = positive.
[a]Clinically resembles acute viral hepatitis; fulminant hepatitis is rare, and progression to chronic hepatitis is unlikely. If HBV does not resolve, HDV can continue to replicate indefinitely.
[b]Clinically resembles exacerbation of chronic liver disease or of fulminant hepatitis with liver failure.
[c]Clinically resembles chronic liver disease progressing to cirrhosis.

Hepatitis G[11–13]

(Due to single-stranded RNA virus of Flaviviridae family. HGV RNA found in ~1–2% of American blood donors; higher in multiply transfused persons, those with hepatitis B or C, drug addicts. Benign course; more studies needed to determine if causes acute or chronic hepatitis.)
Infection tends to persist for many years.
Serum ALT is persistently normal; increase is due to concomitant HCV infection.
Serologic assays under development.
Detected by RT-PCR.
Of hemodialysis patients
  • ≤ 5% are HGV positive.
  • ~25% have anti-HCV and ~15% are PCR positive for HCV.
  • ~5% are HBsAg positive.
  • >50% had anti-HBs or anti-HBc (representing resolved HBV infection).

Hepatitis, Neonatal

Infectious Causes

Adenovirus	Rubella
Coxsackievirus B	Syphilis
CMV	Toxoplasmosis
HAV and HBV	Varicella
HSV	Unknown agent
Listeria	

[11]Masuko K, et al. Infection with hepatitis GB virus C in patients on maintenance hemodialysis. *N Engl J Med* 1996;334:1485.
[12]Alter HJ. The cloning and clinical implications of HGV and HGBV-C. *N Engl J Med* 1996;334:1536.
[13]De Lamballerie X, Charrel RN, Dussol B. Hepatitis GB virus C in patients on hemodialysis. *N Engl J Med* 1996;334:1549.

Metabolic Causes

Alpha$_1$-antitrypsin deficiency—causes 20–35% of cases of neonatal liver disease.
Cystic fibrosis rarely presents as prolonged neonatal jaundice.
Dubin-Johnson syndrome
Fructosemia
Galactosemia
Gaucher's disease
Glycogen storage disease type IV
Histiocytosis X
Hypothyroidism
Hypopituitarism
Leprechaunism
Niemann-Pick disease
Tyrosinemia
Zellweger syndrome
Jaundice in infants receiving parenteral alimentation—many are premature and have various complications (e.g., RDS, septicemia, acidosis, congenital heart disease).
  • Increased AST, ALT, ALP
  • Serum proteins normal
  • Increased serum bile acids
  • Increased serum ammonia
  • Abnormal plasma amino acid patterns (increased threonine, serine, methionine)

Associated with Hemolytic Disease of Newborn

Occurred in 10% of cases ("inspissated bile" syndrome) before modern prevention of Rh disease.
  • Cord blood direct bilirubin ≥ 2 mg/dL indicates that syndrome will develop.
  • Jaundice may persist for 3–4 wks.
  • Most cases have required exchange transfusion.

Clinical and Laboratory Findings

Jaundice at birth, or days or weeks later. Both direct and indirect bilirubin levels are increased in variable proportions.
Mild hemolytic anemia is usual.
Increased AST, ALT, etc.; may be marked and usually greater than in biliary atresia, but increases are not useful for differentiating the two conditions.
Laboratory findings as in acute viral hepatitis (p. 222).
Liver biopsy to differentiate from biliary atresia and to avoid unnecessary surgery is useful in ~65% of patients but it may be misleading.
^{131}I-rose bengal excretion test indicates complete biliary obstruction if <10% of the radioactivity is excreted in stools during 48–72 hrs and incomplete obstruction if >10%. Complete obstruction is found in all infants with biliary atresia and in ~20% with neonatal hepatitis and severe cholestasis. Administration of phenobarbital and cholestyramine increases the ^{131}I-rose bengal excretion in neonatal hepatitis but not in extrahepatic atresia. Some authors have suggested a repeat test in 3–4 wks before exploratory surgery if rose bengal test indicates complete obstruction.
Laboratory tests for various causal agents.
Laboratory findings of chronic liver disease, which develops in 30–50% of these infants.
Whenever mother has hepatitis during pregnancy or is HBsAg positive, test cord blood and baby's blood every 6 mos. If baby develops HBsAg or anti-HBs, measure liver chemistries at periodic intervals. Infants who acquire hepatitis in utero or at time of birth may develop clinical acute hepatitis with abnormal liver chemistries, benign course, or development of HBsAb. Infants who are asymptomatic but develop HBsAg often become chronic carriers with biochemical and liver biopsy evidence of chronic hepatitis and increased likelihood of hepatoma. (See Serologic Tests for HBV, p. 230.)

Hepatocellular Carcinoma (Hepatoma)

  ♦ Serum AFP present in 50% of white and 75–90% of nonwhite patients; may be present for up to 18 mos before symptoms; is sensitive indicator of recurrence in treated patients but a normal postoperative level does not ensure absence of metastases. Levels >500 ng/dL in adults strongly suggest primary carcinoma of liver.

♦Serum GGT hepatoma-specific band (HSBs I', II, II') by electrophoresis activity >5.5 U/L has sensitivity of 85%, specificity of 97%, accuracy of 92%. Does not correlate with AFP or tumor size.[14]

Laboratory findings associated with underlying disease (>60% occur with preexisting cirrhosis).

* Hemochromatosis (≤ 20% of patients die of hepatoma).
* HBV, HCV.
* More frequent in postnecrotic than in alcoholic cirrhosis.
* Cirrhosis associated with alpha$_1$-antitrypsin deficiency and other inborn errors of metabolism, e.g., tyrosinemia.
* *Clonorchis sinensis* infection is associated with cholangiosarcoma.
* Relative absence of hepatoma associated with cirrhosis of Wilson's disease.

Sudden progressive worsening of laboratory findings of underlying disease (e.g., increased serum ALP, LD, AST, bilirubin).

♦Hemoperitoneum—ascites in ~50% of patients but tumor cells found irregularly.

Laboratory findings due to obstruction of hepatic veins (Budd-Chiari syndrome), portal veins, or inferior vena cava may occur.

Occasional marked hypoglycemia unresponsive to epinephrine injection; occasional hypercalcemia.

ESR and WBC sometimes increased.

Anemia is common; polycythemia occurs occasionally.

Serologic markers of HBV frequently present.

CEA in bile is increased in patients with cholangiocarcinoma and intrahepatic stones but not in patients with benign stricture, choledochal cysts, sclerosing cholangitis. Increases with progression of disease and declines with tumor resection. Does not correlate with serum bilirubin or ALP.

Serum CEA is usually normal.

Hyperbilirubinemia, Neonatal

Due To

Unconjugated

Increased destruction of RBCs

* Isoimmunization (e.g., incompatibility of Rh, ABO, other blood groups)
* Biochemical defects of RBCs (e.g., G-6-PD deficiency, pyruvate deficiency, hexokinase deficiency, congenital erythropoietic porphyria, alpha and gamma thalassemias)
* Structural defects of RBCs (e.g., hereditary spherocytosis, hereditary elliptocytosis, infantile pyknocytosis)
* Infection
  Viral (e.g., rubella)
  Bacterial (e.g., syphilis)
  Protozoal (e.g., toxoplasmosis)
* Extravascular blood (e.g., subdural hematoma, ecchymoses, hemangiomas)
* Erythrocytosis (e.g., maternal-to-fetal or twin-to-twin transfusion, delayed clamping of umbilical cord)

Increased enterohepatic circulation

* Any cause of delayed bowel motility
  Pyloric stenosis—unconjugated hyperbilirubinemia >12 mg/dL develops in 10–25% of infants, usually during second or third week, at which time vomiting begins; jaundice is due to decreased hepatic glucuronyl transferase activity of unknown mechanism.
  Duodenal and jejunal obstruction may also be associated with exaggerated unconjugated hyperbilirubinemia; level becomes normal 2–3 days after surgical relief.
  In Hirschsprung's disease, unconjugated hyperbilirubinemia is usually more mild.
  Meconium ileus, meconium plug syndrome.
  Hypoperistalsis (e.g., induced by drugs, fasting)

---

[14]Yao DF, et al. Diagnosis of hepatocellular carcinoma by quantitative detection of hepatoma-specific bands of serum γ-glutamyltransferase. *Am J Clin Pathol* 1998;110:743.

Endocrine and metabolic
- Neonatal hypothyroidism—associated with prolonged and exaggerated unconjugated hyperbilirubinemia in 10% of cases and is promptly alleviated by thyroid hormone therapy.

Always rule out congenital hypothyroidism in cases of unexplained persistent or excessive unconjugated hyperbilirubinemia; may be the only manifestation of hypothyroidism.

- Infants of diabetic mothers—associated with higher incidence of prolonged and exaggerated unconjugated hyperbilirubinemia of unknown mechanism; not related to severity or duration of diabetes.
- Drugs and hormones (e.g., breast-milk jaundice, Lucey-Driscoll syndrome, novobiocin).
- Galactosemia.
- Tyrosinosis.
- Hypermethionemia.
- Heart failure.
- Hereditary glucuronyl-transferase deficiency.
- Gilbert's syndrome.

Interference of albumin binding of bilirubin
- Drugs (e.g., aspirin, sulfonamides)
- Severe acidosis
- Hematin
- Free fatty acids (e.g., periods of stress, inadequate caloric intake)
- Prematurity (serum albumin may be 1–2 gm/dL less than in full-term infants)

Neonatal physiologic hyperbilirubinemia

Conjugated

Premature infants with these conditions have more severe hyperbilirubinemia than full-term infants.

Biliary obstruction—usually due to extrahepatic biliary atresia but may be due to choledochal cyst, obstructive inspissated bile plugs, or bile ascites

Neonatal hepatitis (see pp. 241–242)

Sepsis, especially *E. coli* pyelonephritis (moderate azotemia, acidosis, increased serum bilirubin, slight hemolysis, normal or slightly increased AST)

Hereditary diseases (e.g., galactosemia, alpha$_1$-antitrypsin deficiency, cystic fibrosis, hereditary fructose intolerance, tyrosinemia, infantile Gaucher's disease, familial intrahepatic cholestasis [Byler's disease])

In the course of hemolytic disease of the newborn—due to liver damage of unknown cause.

Differential Diagnosis

Unconjugated hyperbilirubinemia is serum level >1.5 mg/dL. Conjugated hyperbilirubinemia is direct-reacting serum level >1.5 mg/dL when this fraction is >10% of total serum bilirubin (because in newborn with marked elevation of unconjugated bilirubin level, ≤ 10% of the unconjugated bilirubin will act as direct reacting in the van den Bergh reaction).

Mixed hyperbilirubinemia shows conjugated bilirubin as 20–70% of total and usually represents disorder of hepatic cell excretion or bile transport.

Visible icterus before 36 hrs of age indicates hemolytic disorder.

Diagnostic studies should be performed whenever serum bilirubin is >12 mg/dL.

After hemolytic disease and hepatitis, the most frequent cause of hyperbilirubinemia is enterohepatic circulation of bilirubin.

Visible icterus persisting after seventh day is usually due to impaired hepatic excretion, most commonly due to breast-milk feeding or congenital hypothyroidism.

Increase in direct bilirubin usually indicates infection or inflammation of liver, but can also be seen in galactosemia and tyrosinosis.

Hyperbilirubinemia, Neonatal Nonphysiologic

See Fig. 8-8.

Cause should be sought for underlying pathologic jaundice if:
- Total serum bilirubin is >7 mg/dL during first 24 hrs or increases by >5 mg/dL/day or visible jaundice.
- Peak total serum bilirubin is >12.5 mg/dL in white or black full-term infants or >15 mg/dL in Hispanic or premature infants.

- Direct serum bilirubin is >1.5 mg/dL.
- Clinical jaundice lasts longer than 7 days in full-term or 14 days in premature infants or occurs before age 36 hrs or with dark urine (containing bile).

Initial tests in unconjugated hyperbilirubinemia:
- Serial determinations of total and direct bilirubin
- CBC including RBC morphology, platelet count, normoblast and reticulocyte counts
- Blood type, mother and infant
- Direct Coombs' test
- Maternal blood for antibodies and hemolysins
- Blood cultures
- Urine microscopy and culture
- Serologic tests for infection
- Serum thyroxine (T_4) and thyroid-stimulating hormone (TSH)
- Urine for non–glucose reducing substances

Hyperbilirubinemia, Neonatal Physiologic

(Transient unconjugated hyperbilirubinemia ["physiologic jaundice"] that occurs in almost all newborns)

In normal full-term neonate, average maximum serum bilirubin is 6 mg/dL (up to 12 mg/dL is in physiologic range), which occurs during the second to fourth days and then rapidly falls to ~2.0 mg/dL by fifth day (phase I physiologic jaundice). Declines slowly to <1.0 mg/dL during fifth to tenth days, but may take 1 mo to fall to <2 mg/dL (phase II physiologic jaundice). Phase I due to deficiency of hepatic bilirubin glucuronyl transferase activity and sixfold increase in bilirubin load presented to liver. In Asian and American Indian newborns, the average maximum serum levels are approximately double (10–14 mg/dL) the levels in non-Asians, and kernicterus is more frequent. Serum bilirubin >5 mg/dL during first 24 hrs of life is indication for further workup because of risk of kernicterus.

In older children (and adults) icterus is apparent clinically when serum bilirubin is >2 mg/dL, but in newborns clinical icterus is not apparent until serum bilirubin is >5–7 mg/dL; therefore only half of full-term newborns show clinical jaundice during first 3 days of life.

In premature infants—average maximum serum bilirubin is 10–12 mg/dL and occurs during the fifth to seventh days. Serum bilirubin may not fall to normal until 30th day. Further workup is indicated in all premature infants with clinical jaundice because of risk of kernicterus in some low-birth-weight infants with serum levels of 10–12 mg/dL.

In postmature infants and half of small-for-date infants—serum bilirubin is <2.5 mg/dL and physiologic jaundice is not seen. When mothers have received phenobarbital or used heroin, physiologic jaundice is also less severe.

When a pregnant woman has unconjugated hyperbilirubinemia, similar levels occur in cord blood, but when the mother has conjugated hyperbilirubinemia (e.g., hepatitis), similar levels are not present in cord blood.

Hyperbilirubinemia; Neonatal, Transient Familial (Lucey-Driscoll Syndrome)

Syndrome is due to progestational steroid in mother's serum only during last trimester of pregnancy, which inhibits glucuronyl transferase activity; disappears ~2 wks postpartum.

Newborn infants have severe nonhemolytic unconjugated hyperbilirubinemia, usually up to 20 mg/dL during first 48 hrs, and a high risk of kernicterus.

Hyperbilirubinemia in Older Children
Due To

All cases of conjugated hyperbilirubinemia also show some increase of unconjugated serum bilirubin.

Unconjugated
Gilbert's disease
Administration of drugs (e.g., novobiocin)
Occasionally other conditions (e.g., thyrotoxicosis, after portacaval shunt in cirrhosis)

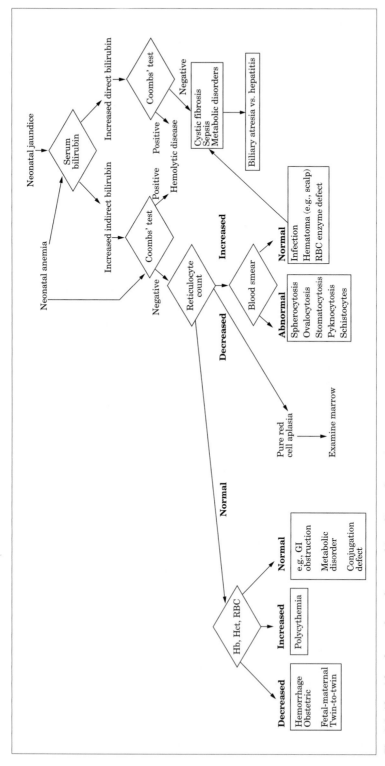

Fig. 8-8. Algorithm for workup of neonatal jaundice and anemia.

Conjugated

Dubin-Johnson syndrome
Rotor's syndrome
Acute viral hepatitis causes most cases in children.
Cholestasis due to chemicals and drugs or associated with other diseases (e.g., Hodgkin's disease, sickle cell disease)

Jaundice (Cholestatic and Hepatocellular), Comparison

	Hepatocellular	Cholestasis	Infiltration
Disease example	Acute viral hepatitis	Common duct stone	Metastatic tumor
Serum bilirubin (mg/dL)	4–8	6–20*	Usually <4, often normal
AST, ALT (U/mL)	Markedly increased, often 500–1000	May be slightly increased, <200	May be slightly increased, <100
Serum ALP	1–2× normal	3–5× normal[†]	2–4× normal
PT	Increased in severe disease	Increased in chronic cases	Normal
Response to parenteral vitamin K	No	Yes	

*Serum bilirubin >10 mg/dL is rarely seen with common duct stone and usually indicates carcinoma.
[†]Increased serum ALP <3× normal in 15% of patients with extrahepatic biliary obstruction, especially if obstruction is incomplete or due to benign conditions.

Occasionally AST and LD are markedly increased in biliary obstruction or liver cancer.

Metabolism, Inborn Errors, Causing Liver Disorder

Inborn Errors of Carbohydrate Metabolism

Glycogen storage diseases
Galactosemia
Fructose intolerance

Inborn Errors of Protein Metabolism

Tyrosinemia
Urea cycle enzyme defects

Inborn Errors of Lipid Metabolism

Gaucher's disease
Gangliosidosis
Cholesterol ester storage disease
Niemann-Pick disease
Lipodystrophy
Wolman's disease

Others

Mucopolysaccharidoses
Wilson's disease
Hepatic porphyria
Alpha$_1$-antitrypsin deficiency
Byler's disease
Cystic fibrosis

Pylephlebitis, Septic

Increased WBCs and PMNs in >90% of patients; usually >20,000/cu mm
Anemia of varying severity
Moderate increase in serum bilirubin in ~33% of patients

Other liver function tests positive in ~25% of patients
Needle biopsy of liver not helpful; contraindicated
Blood culture sometimes positive
Laboratory findings due to preceding disease (e.g., acute appendicitis, diverticulitis, ulcerative colitis)
Laboratory findings due to complications (e.g., portal vein occlusion)

Rotor's Syndrome

(Autosomal recessive, familial, asymptomatic, benign defective uptake and storage of conjugated bilirubin and possibly in transfer of bilirubin from liver to bile or in intra-hepatic binding; usually detected in adolescents or adults. Jaundice may be produced or accentuated by pregnancy, birth control pills, alcohol, infection, surgery.)
See Table 8-4.
○Mild chronic fluctuating nonhemolytic conjugated hyperbilirubinemia (usually <10 mg/dL).
BSP excretion is impaired.
Other liver function test are normal.
Liver biopsy is normal; no pigment is present.
○Urine coproporphyrins are markedly increased especially coproporphyrin I (increased more than III).

Space-Occupying Lesions

Due To

Neoplasms (e.g., primary hepatocellular carcinoma, metastasis)
Cysts
- *Echinococcus*
- ≤ 40% of patients with autosomal dominant polycystic renal disease
Abscesses (amebic, pyogenic)
Granulomas
- Sarcoidosis
- Infections (e.g., TB, cat-scratch bacillus, Q fever, Lyme disease, secondary syphilis)
- Drugs (e.g., gold, quinidine, diltiazem, hydralazine, methimazole, tocainide)
○Increased serum ALP is the most useful index of partial obstruction of the biliary tree in which serum bilirubin is usually normal and urine bilirubin is increased.
- Increased in 80% of patients with metastatic carcinoma.
- Increased in 50% of patients with TB.
- Increased in 40% of patients with sarcoidosis.
- Increased frequently in patients with amyloidosis.

Increase in serum LAP parallels that in ALP but is not affected by bone disease.
Whenever the ALP is increased, a simultaneous increase of 5'-NT establishes biliary disease as the cause of the elevated ALP.
AST is increased in 50% of patients (≤ 300 U).
ALT is increased less frequently (≤ 150 U).
○Detection of metastases by panel of blood tests (ALP, LD, transaminase, bilirubin) has sensitivity of 85%. ALP or GGT alone has sensitivity of 25–33% and specificity of ≤ 75%. Serum LD is often increased in cancer even without liver metastases.
Radioactive scanning of the liver has 65% sensitivity.
♦Blind needle biopsy of the liver is positive in 65–75% of patients.
○Laboratory findings due to primary disease (e.g., increased serum CEA in colon carcinoma, carcinoid syndrome, pyogenic liver abscess)

Transplantation of Liver

Indications

Liver Failure Due To
Arterial thrombosis
Autoimmune liver disease
Biliary atresia (infants)
Budd-Chiari syndrome
Cirrhosis

- Alcoholic
- Postnecrotic
- Primary biliary
- Secondary biliary

Hepatitis

Inborn errors of metabolism
- Alpha$_1$-antitrypsin deficiency
- Protein C deficiency
- Crigler-Najjar syndrome type I
- Cystic fibrosis
- Erythropoietic protoporphyria
- Glycogen storage diseases type I and IV
- Hemophilias A and B
- Homozygous type II hyperlipoproteinemia
- Hyperoxaluria type I
- Niemann-Pick disease
- Tyrosinemia
- Urea cycle enzyme deficiencies
- Wilson's disease

Laboratory indications, e.g.,
- Portal hypertension with intractable ascites
- Hypersplenism and/or bleeding esophageal varices
- Poor synthesis function (e.g., decreased albumin, fibrinogen, prolonged PT)
- Progressive hyperbilirubinemia

Liver trauma

Polycystic liver disease

Rejection of liver transplant (causes 20% of retransplants)

Reye's syndrome

Sclerosing cholangitis

Unresectable liver neoplasms confined to liver

Venoocclusive disease

Contraindications

Extrahepatic neoplasms

Positive serology for HBsAg, HBcAb, HIV

Sepsis other than of hepatobiliary system

Stage 4 hepatic coma

Unrelated failure of other organ systems

Postoperative Complications

Early	**Reported Incidence**
Primary nonfunction due to graft ischemia	5–10%
Portal vein thrombosis	
Hepatic artery thrombosis	5–10%
Hyperacute rejection	
Early acute rejection	
Immunosuppressant therapy toxicity	
Hepatorenal syndrome	$\leq 9.8\%$
Hepatopulmonary syndrome	$\leq 13.2\%$
Infection/sepsis	

Later

Acute and chronic rejection

Side effects of immunosuppressant therapy

Biliary stenosis

Recurrence of disease (especially hepatitis B, hepatitis C, EBV-associated lymphopro-liferative disorders)

Vanishing bile duct syndrome

Rejection

Most episodes occur within first 3 mos; patients are usually asymptomatic.

Electrolytes must be monitored rapidly to treat cardiac arrest due to sudden release of large amounts of potassium from perfused liver and to monitor IV fluid replacement. Ionized calcium is lost due to chelation by citrate in transfused blood; left ventricular dysfunction may occur when serum level is <1.2 mEq/L. Serum sodium is monitored to avoid postoperative neurologic complications due to rapid increase during transplant and postoperative periods (e.g., central pontine myelinolysis). Normalization of serum HCO_3^- and anion gap signifies early function of liver transplant and of kidneys.

○Serum GGT is the most sensitive marker for rejection; rises early during rejection before serum ALP and bilirubin. Is more specific than other markers because other complications (e.g., CMV infection) cause relatively low levels compared with AST and ALT.

○Serum ALP lags behind serum GGT and bilirubin indicators of rejection. In uncomplicated cases, serum ALP and GGT remain within reference range.

○AST and ALT rise after reperfusion of the allograft; increase to >4–5× upper limit of reference range even in uncomplicated cases. Persistent or late increases may be due to rejection or to other causes such as viral infections (e.g., CMV, HSV, adenovirus), occlusion of hepatic artery, liver abscess.

○Serum total and direct bilirubin are monitored with enzymes and are useful to help differentiate between biliary obstruction (suggesting rejection) and hepato-cellular disease. Increase may be early sign of rejection but less useful than enzymes.

Monitoring of serum cyclosporine is important because it is metabolized in the liver and proportion of cyclosporine and its metabolites may be altered when postoperative liver function is not maintained.

PT and aPTT monitor synthesis of coagulation factors; specific factor measurements are not needed.

Cultures from appropriate sites are performed for evidence of infection.

♦Liver biopsy is gold standard for diagnosis.
  • Distinguish causes of rejection that have no specific biochemical pattern (e.g., acute rejection, chronic rejection, opportunistic viral infection, recurrence of HBV infection, CMV, changes in hepatic blood perfusion, unrecognized disease in donor liver).
  • Differentiate from cholangitis, hepatitis, ischemic injury, which may mimic rejection.
  • Substantial number of false-positives occur.

Laboratory findings due to immunosuppression therapy
  • Nephrotoxicity
  • Liver toxicity (e.g., serum cyclosporine concentration >1200 ng/dL)
  • Infection (e.g., bacterial, fungal, HBV, CMV, HSV, EBV)
  • Cancer (e.g., non-Hodgkin's lymphoma, Kaposi's sarcoma, carcinomas of cervix, perineum, lip)
  • Complications of hypertension

In rare cases, genetic defects (e.g., factor XI deficiency) can be transmitted to the recipient and cause postoperative complications.

Trauma

Serum LD is frequently increased (>1400 U) 8–12 hrs after major injury. Shock due to any injury may also increase LD.

Other serum enzymes and liver function tests are not generally helpful.

Findings of abdominal paracentesis
  • Bloody fluid (in ~75% of patients) confirming traumatic hemoperitoneum and indicating exploratory laparotomy.
  • Nonbloody fluid (especially if injury occurred >24 hrs earlier).
      Microscopic—some red and white blood cells.
      Determine amylase, protein, pH, presence of bile.

Wilson's Disease[15]

(Autosomal recessive defect impairs copper excretion by liver, causing copper accumulation in liver.)

Heterozygous gene for Wilson's disease occurs in 1 of 200 in the general population; 10% of these have decreased serum ceruloplasmin; liver copper is not increased (<250

---

[15]Stremmel W, et al. Wilson disease: clinical presentation, treatment, and survival. *Ann Intern Med* 1991;115:720.

μg/gm of dry liver). Serum copper and ceruloplasmin and urine copper levels are inadequate to detect heterozygous state.

Homozygous gene (clinical Wilson's disease) occurs in 1 of 200,000 in the general population. Screening with DNA probes may become useful to detect homozygous infants.

Serum Ceruloplasmin

Decreased (<20 mg/dL) In
Wilson's disease. (*It is normal in 2–5% of patients with overt Wilson's disease.*) May not be decreased in Wilson's disease with acute or fulminant liver involvement (ceruloplasmin is an acute-phase reactant).

Healthy infants (therefore cannot use test for Wilson's disease in first year of life)

10–20% of persons heterozygous for Wilson's disease

Renal protein loss (e.g., nephrosis)

Malabsorption (e.g., sprue)

Malnutrition

Inherited ceruloplasmin deficiency (rare)

♦ *Serum ceruloplasmin (<20 mg/dL) with increased hepatic copper (>250 μg/gm) occurs only in Wilson's disease or normal infants aged <6 mos.*

Increased In
Pregnancy

Use of estrogen or birth control pills

Thyrotoxicosis

Cirrhosis

Cancer

Acute inflammatory reactions (e.g., infection, RA)

(May cause green color of plasma.)

Total serum copper is decreased and generally parallels serum ceruloplasmin. Not a good indicator because changes during course of disease.

♦ *Free (nonceruloplasmin)* copper in serum is increased and causes excess copper deposition in tissues and excretion in urine. Calculated from difference between total serum copper and ceruloplasmin-bound copper. Free copper (μg/dL) = total serum copper (μg/dL) – ceruloplasmin (mg/dL) × 3. Is virtually 100% sensitive and specific.

Urinary copper is increased (>100 μg/24 hrs; normal <50 μg/24 hrs); may be normal in presymptomatic patients and increased in other types of cirrhosis.

♦ Liver biopsy shows high copper concentration (>250 μg/gm of dry liver; normal = 20–45) and should be used to confirm the diagnosis. (Special copper-free needle should be used.) Copper concentrations may vary between nodules; thus extensive sampling may be necessary to confirm diagnosis. May also be elevated in cholestatic syndromes (e.g., primary biliary cirrhosis, primary sclerosing cholangitis, extrahepatic biliary cirrhosis, Indian childhood cirrhosis), which are easily differentiated from Wilson's disease by increased serum ceruloplasmin.

○ Histochemical staining of paraffin-embedded liver specimens for copper and copper-associated protein is diagnostic in appropriate clinical context but may be negative in Wilson's disease and present in other hepatic disorders.

Liver biopsy may show no abnormalities, moderate to marked fatty changes with or without fibrosis, or active or inactive cirrhosis.

○ Findings of liver function tests may not be abnormal, depending on the type and severity of disease. *In patients presenting with acute fulminant hepatitis, Wilson's disease is suggested if a disproportionately low serum ALP and relatively mild increase in AST and ALT are seen. Should also be ruled out in any patient <30 yrs with hepatitis (with negative serology for viral hepatitis), Coombs'-negative hemolysis, or neurologic symptoms to allow early diagnosis and treatment of Wilson's disease.*

♦ Radiocopper loading test: ^{64}Cu is administered IV or by mouth and serum concentration is plotted against time. Serum ^{64}Cu disappears within 4–6 hrs and then reappears in persons without Wilson's disease; secondary reappearance is absent in Wilson's disease because incorporation of ^{64}Cu into ceruloplasmin is decreased. Useful test in patients with normal ceruloplasmin levels or increased hepatic copper due to other forms of liver disease, or heterozygous carriers of Wilson's disease gene, or when liver biopsy is contraindicated.

Aminoaciduria (especially cystine and threonine), glucosuria, hyperphosphaturia, hypercalciuria, uricosuria, and decreased serum uric acid and phosphorus may occur due to renal proximal tubular dysfunction; distal renal tubular acidosis is less common.

Coombs'-negative nonspherocytic hemolytic anemia may occur.

Other tests that have been used in diagnosis of heterozygotes may not be available locally:
- D-penicillamine administration induces increased urinary copper excretion.
- Excretion of radioactive copper.
- Conversion of ionic radioactive copper to radioactive ceruloplasmin.
- Copper content of cultured fibroblasts.
- DNA markers have been used for detection of homozygous and heterozygous patients.

Laboratory findings due to complications
- Cirrhosis and sequelae (e.g., ascites, esophageal varices, liver failure).
- Hypersplenism (e.g., anemia, leukopenia, thrombocytopenia).
- Acute liver failure characterized by very high serum bilirubin (often >30 mg/dL) and decreased ALP; ALP/bilirubin ratio <2.0 is said to distinguish this from other causes of liver failure.

Laboratory findings due to effects of therapeutic agents
- Long-term treatment with copper-depleting agents may sometimes cause a mild sideroblastic anemia and leukopenia due to copper deficiency.
- Penicillamine toxicity (e.g., nephrotic syndrome, thrombocytopenia, etc.).

All transplant recipients have complete reversal of underlying defects in copper metabolism.

Tests for Pancreatic Disease

Amylase, Serum

See Fig. 8-9.

(Composed of pancreatic and salivary types of isoamylases; distinguished by various methodologies; nonpancreatic etiologies are almost always salivary; both types may be increased in renal insufficiency.)

Increased In

Acute pancreatitis. Urine levels reflect serum changes by a time lag of 6–10 hrs.

Acute exacerbation of chronic pancreatitis

Drug-induced acute pancreatitis (e.g., aminosalicylic acid, azathioprine, corticosteroids, dexamethasone, ethacrynic acid, ethanol, furosemide, thiazides, mercaptopurine, phenformin, triamcinolone)

Obstruction of pancreatic duct by
- Stone or carcinoma
- Drug-induced spasm of Oddi's sphincter (e.g., opiates, codeine, methyl choline, cholinergics, chlorothiazide) to levels 2–15× normal
- Partial obstruction plus drug stimulation (see discussion of cholecystokinin-secretin test, p. 260)

Biliary tract disease
- Common bile duct obstruction
- Acute cholecystitis

Complications of pancreatitis (pseudocyst, ascites, abscess)

Pancreatic trauma (abdominal injury; after ERCP)

Altered GI tract permeability
- Ischemic bowel disease or frank perforation
- Esophageal rupture
- Perforated or penetrating peptic ulcer
- Postoperative upper abdominal surgery, especially partial gastrectomy (up to 2× normal in one-third of patients)

Acute alcohol ingestion or poisoning

Salivary gland disease (mumps, suppurative inflammation, duct obstruction due to calculus, radiation)

Malignant tumors (especially pancreas, lung, ovary, esophagus; also breast, colon); usually >25× ULN, which is rarely seen in pancreatitis

Advanced renal insufficiency. Often increased even without pancreatitis.

Macroamylasemia

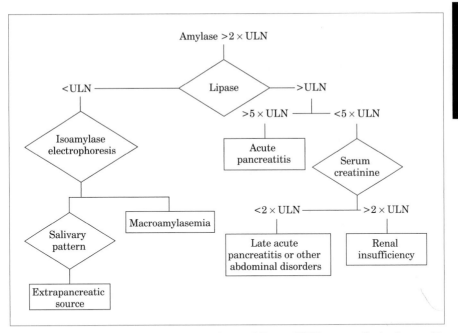

Fig. 8-9. Algorithm for increased serum amylase and lipase. (ULN = upper limit of normal.)

- Others, e.g., chronic liver disease (e.g., cirrhosis; ≤ 2× normal), burns, pregnancy (including ruptured tubal pregnancy), ovarian cyst, diabetic ketoacidosis, recent thoracic surgery, myoglobinuria, presence of myeloma proteins, some cases of intracranial bleeding (unknown mechanism), splenic rupture, dissecting aneurysm
- It has been suggested that a level >1000 U/L is usually due to surgically correctable lesions (most frequently stones in biliary tree), the pancreas being negative or showing only edema; but 200–500 U is usually associated with pancreatic lesions that are not surgically correctable (e.g., hemorrhagic pancreatitis, necrosis or pancreas).
- *Increased serum amylase with low urine amylase* may be seen in renal insufficiency and macroamylasemia. Serum amylase ≤ 4× normal in renal disease only when creatinine clearance is <50 mL/min due to pancreatic or salivary isoamylase but rarely >4× normal in absence of acute pancreatitis.

Decreased In

Extensive marked destruction of pancreas (e.g., acute fulminant pancreatitis, advanced chronic pancreatitis, advanced cystic fibrosis). Decreased levels are clinically significant only in occasional cases of fulminant pancreatitis.

Severe liver damage (e.g., hepatitis, poisoning, toxemia of pregnancy, severe thyrotoxicosis, severe burns)

Methodologic interference by drugs (e.g., citrate and oxalate decrease activity by binding calcium ions)

Amylase–creatinine clearance ratio = (urine amylase concentration ÷ serum amylase concentration) × (serum creatinine concentration ÷ urine creatinine concentration) × 100

Normal: 1–5%
Macroamylasemia: <1%; very useful for this diagnosis.
Acute pancreatitis: >5%; use is presently discouraged for this diagnosis.

May Be Normal In

Patients with relapsing chronic pancreatitis
Patients with hypertriglyceridemia (technical interference with test)

Frequently normal in patients with acute alcoholic pancreatitis.

Lipase, Serum[16]

(Method should always include colipase in reagent.)
See Fig. 8-9.

Increased In

Acute pancreatitis
Perforated or penetrating peptic ulcer, especially with involvement of pancreas
Obstruction of pancreatic duct by
• Stone
• Drug-induced spasm of Oddi's sphincter (e.g., codeine, morphine, meperidine, methacholine, cholinergics), to levels 2–15× normal
• Partial obstruction plus drug stimulation
Chronic pancreatitis
Acute cholecystitis
Small bowel obstruction
Intestinal infarction
Acute and chronic renal failure (increased 2–3× in 80% of patients and 5× in 5% of patients)
Organ transplant (kidney, liver, heart), especially with complications (e.g., organ rejection, CMV infection, cyclosporin toxicity)
Alcoholism
Diabetic ketoacidosis
After ERCP
Some cases of intracranial bleeding (unknown mechanism)
Macro forms in lymphoma, cirrhosis
Drugs
• Induced acute pancreatitis (see preceding section on serum amylase)
• Cholestatic effect (e.g., indomethacin)
• Methodologic interference (e.g., pancreozymin [contains lipase], deoxycholate, glycocholate, taurocholate [prevent inactivation of enzyme], bilirubin [turbidimetric methods])
Chronic liver disease (e.g., cirrhosis) (usually ≤ 2× normal)

Decreased In

Methodologic interference (e.g., presence of hemoglobin, calcium ions)

Usually Normal In

Mumps
Values are lower in neonates.
Macroamylasemia

Diseases of the Pancreas

Cystic Fibrosis of Pancreas[17]

(Autosomal recessive disorder with abnormal ion transport due to failure of chloride regulation; incidence of 1 in 1500 to 1 in 2000 in whites with a carrier frequency of 1 in 20; 1 in 17,000 in American blacks; marked heterogeneity among patients.)

Quantitative Pilocarpine Iontophoresis Sweat Test (Properly Performed)

♦Striking increase in sweat sodium (>60 mEq/L) and chloride (>60 mEq/L) and, to a lesser extent, potassium is present in virtually all homozygous patients; value is 3–5×

[16]Tietz NW, Shuey DF. Lipase in serum—the elusive enzyme: an overview. *Clin Chem* 1993;39:746.
[17]Stern RC. The diagnosis of cystic fibrosis. *N Engl J Med* 1997;336:487.

higher than in healthy persons or in those with other diseases. Is consistently present throughout life from time of birth, and degree of abnormality is not related to severity of disease or organ involvement. Sensitivity = 98%, specificity = 83%, positive predictive value = 93%. *Sweat chloride is somewhat more reliable than sodium for diagnostic purposes.*
- In children, chloride >60mEq/L is considered positive for cystic fibrosis.
- 40–60 mEq/L is considered borderline and requires further investigation.
- <40 mEq/L is considered normal.
- ≤ 80 mEq/L may be normal for adults.
- On occasion 1–2% of cystic fibrosis patients have normal, borderline, or variable values.
- Rare patients with borderline values have only mild disease.
- Sweat potassium is not diagnostically valuable because of overlap with normal controls.
- Increased sweat sodium and chloride are not useful for detection of heterozygotes (who have normal values) or for genetic counseling.

♦ Sweat chloride ≥ 80 mEq/L on repeated occasions with characteristic clinical manifestations or family history confirm diagnosis of cystic fibrosis.

A broad range of sweat values is seen in patients with this disease and in normal persons but overlap is minimal.

Sweat values (mEq/L)

	Chloride		Sodium		Potassium	
	Mean	**Range**	**Mean**	**Range**	**Mean**	**Range**
Cystic fibrosis	115	79–148	111	75–145	23	14–30
Normal	28	8–43	28	16–46	10	6–17

Note that one instrument (Wescor; Logan, Utah) measures sweat conductivity, not sweat chloride, which is not equivalent. Sweat conductivity measurement is considered a screening test; patients with values ≥ 50 mEq/L should have quantitative sweat chloride test.

Interferences

Sweat testing is fraught with problems and technical and laboratory errors are very frequent; should be performed in duplicate and repeated at least once on separate days on samples >100 mg of sweat.

Values may be increased to cystic fibrosis range in healthy persons when sweat rate is rapid (e.g., exercise, high temperature), but pilocarpine test does not increase sweating rate.

Mineralocorticoids decrease sodium concentration in sweat by ~50% in normal subjects and 10–20% in cystic fibrosis patients, whose final sodium concentration remains abnormally high.

Increased In

Endocrine disorders
- Untreated adrenal insufficiency (Addison's disease)
- Hypothyroidism
- Vasopressin-resistant diabetes insipidus
- Familial hypoparathyroidism
- Pseudohypoaldosteronism

Metabolic disorders
- Malnutrition
- Glycogen storage disease type I (von Gierke's disease)
- Mucopolysaccharidosis IH and IS
- Fucosidosis

Genitourinary disorders
- Klinefelter's syndrome
- Nephrosis

Allergic/immunologic disorders
- Hypogammaglobulinemia
- Prolonged infusion with prostaglandin E_1
- Atopic dermatitis

Neuropsychologic disorders
- Anorexia nervosa
- Autonomic dysfunction

Others
- Ectodermal dysplasia
- G-6-PD deficiency

Serum chloride, sodium, potassium, calcium, and phosphorus are normal unless complications occur (e.g., chronic pulmonary disease with accumulation of CO_2; massive salt loss due to sweating causing hyponatremia). Urine electrolytes are normal. Submaxillary saliva has slightly increased chloride and sodium but not potassium; considerable overlap with results for normal persons prevents diagnostic use.

Submaxillary saliva is more turbid, with increased calcium, total protein, and amylase. These changes are not generally found in parotid saliva.

Serum protein electrophoresis shows increasing IgG and IgA with progressive pulmonary disease; IgM and IgD are not appreciably increased.

Serum albumin is often decreased (because of hemodilution due to cor pulmonale; may be found before cardiac involvement is clinically apparent).

○Laboratory changes secondary to complications that *should also suggest diagnosis of cystic fibrosis*

Salt-loss syndromes
- Hypochloremic metabolic alkalosis and hypokalemia due to excessive loss of electrolytes in sweat and stool
- Acute salt depletion

Respiratory abnormalities
- Chronic lung disease (especially upper lobes) with laboratory changes of decreased pO_2, accumulation of CO_2, metabolic alkalosis, severe recurrent infection, secondary cor pulmonale, etc. Nasal polyps, pansinusitis; normal sinus radiographs are strong evidence against cystic fibrosis.
- BAL usually shows increased PMNs (>50% in cystic fibrosis; ~3% in normal persons) with high absolute neutrophil count; is strong evidence of cystic fibrosis even in absence of pathogens.
- Bacteriology: Special culture techniques should be used in these patients. Before 1 yr of age, *S. aureus* is found in 25% and *Pseudomonas* in 20% of respiratory tract cultures; in adults *Pseudomonas* grows in 80% and *S. aureus* in 20%. *Haemophilus influenzae* is found in 3.4% of cultures. *Pseudomonas aeruginosa* is found increasingly often after treatment of staphylococcal infection, and special identification and susceptibility tests should be performed on *P. aeruginosa*. *Pseudomonas cepacia* is becoming more important in older children. Increasing serum antibodies against *P. aeruginosa* can document probable infection when cultures are negative.

Gastrointestinal abnormalities
- Chronic/recurrent pancreatitis.
- Pancreatic enzyme activity is lost in 80% of patients, decreased in 10%, and normal in 10% of patients. Protein-calorie malnutrition, hypoproteinemia, fat-soluble vitamin deficiency (see Malabsorption, pp. 185–188). Stool and duodenal fluid show lack of trypsin digestion of radiographic film gelatin; useful screening test up to age 4; decreased chymotrypsin production (see bentiromide test, p. 157). Impaired glucose intolerance in ~40% of patients, with glycosuria and hyperglycemia in 8%, precedes diabetes mellitus.
- Cirrhosis (in >25% of patients at autopsy), especially before age 30 years; hypersplenism; cholelithiasis.
- Meconium ileus during early infancy; causes 20–30% of cases of neonatal intestinal obstruction; present at birth in 8% of these children. Almost all of them will develop the clinical picture of cystic fibrosis.

GU tract abnormalities
- Aspermia in 98% due to obstructive changes in vas deferens and epididymis, confirmed by testicular biopsy.

♦ Neonatal screening using dried filter paper blood test that measures immunoreactive trypsin has been used. Normal in ≤ 10% of cystic fibrosis infants. Increased false-negative rate in meconium ileus.

♦ DNA genotyping (using blood; can use buccal scrapings) to confirm diagnosis based on two mutations is highly specific but not very sensitive. Supports diagnosis of cys-

tic fibrosis, but failure to detect gene mutations does not exclude cystic fibrosis because of large number of alleles. Substantial number of cystic fibrosis patients have unidentified gene mutation. Helpful when sweat test is borderline or negative. Can also be used for prenatal diagnosis and carrier screening. Identical genotypes can be associated with different degrees of disease severity.
♦ Nasal electrical potential-difference measurements may be more reliable than sweat tests but are much more complex to perform.

Macroamylasemia

♦ Serum amylase *persistently* increased (often 1–4× normal) without apparent cause. Serum lipase is normal. Normal pancreatic to salivary amylase ratio.
Urine amylase normal or low.
○ Amylase–creatinine clearance ratio <1% with normal renal function is very useful for this diagnosis; should make the clinician suspect this diagnosis.
♦ Macroamylase is identified in serum by special gel filtration or ultracentrifugation technique.
May be found in ~1% of randomly selected patients and 2.5% of persons with increased serum amylase. Same findings may also occur in patients with normal-molecular-weight hyperamylasemia in which excess amylase is principally salivary gland isoamylase types 2 and 3.
When associated with pancreatic disease, serum lipase may be elevated.

Pancreatic Carcinoma[18]

Body or Tail

Laboratory tests are often normal.
○ Serum markers for tumor CA 19-9, CEA, etc. (see Chapter 16)
  • In carcinoma of pancreas, CA 19-9 has sensitivity of 70%, specificity of 87%, positive predictive value of 59%, negative predictive value of 92%. No difference in sensitivity between local disease and metastatic disease. Often normal in early stages, therefore not useful for screening. Increased value may help differentiate benign disease from cancer. Declines to normal in 3–6 mos if cancer is completely removed, so may be useful for prognosis and follow-up. Detects tumor recurrence 2–20 wks before clinical evidence appears. Not specific for pancreas because high levels may also occur in other GI cancers, especially those affecting colon and bile duct.
  • Testosterone/dihydrotestosterone ratio is <5 (normal = ~10) in >70% of men with pancreatic cancer (due to increased conversion by tumor). Less sensitive but more specific than CA 19-9; present in higher proportion of stage I tumors.
♦ The most useful diagnostic test is ultrasonography or CAT scanning followed by ERCP (at which time fluid is also obtained for cytologic and pancreatic function studies). This combination correctly diagnoses or rules out cancer of pancreas in ≥ 90% of cases. ERCP with brush cytology has sensitivity ≤ 25% and specificity ≤ 100%.
CEA level in bile (obtained by percutaneous transhepatic drainage) was reported increased in 76% of a small group of cases.
Serum amylase and lipase may be slightly increased in early stages (<10% of cases); with later destruction of pancreas, they are normal or decreased. They may increase after secretin-pancreozymin stimulation before destruction is extensive; therefore, the increase is less marked with a diabetic glucose tolerance curve. Serum amylase response is less reliable.
○ Glucose tolerance curve is of the diabetic type with overt diabetes in 20% of patients with pancreatic cancer. Flat blood sugar curve with IV tolbutamide tolerance test indicates destruction of islet cell tissue. *Unstable, insulin-sensitive diabetes that develops in an older man should arouse suspicion of carcinoma of the pancreas.*
♦ Secretin-cholecystokinin stimulation (see p. 260) evidences duct obstruction when duodenal intubation shows decreased volume of duodenal contents (<10 mL/10-min collection period) with usually normal bicarbonate and enzyme levels in duodenal contents. Acinar destruction (as in pancreatitis) shows normal volume (20–30 mL/10-min collection period), but bicarbonate and enzyme levels may be decreased. Abnor-

[18]Warshaw AL, Fernandez-del Castillo C. Pancreatic cancer. *N Engl J Med* 1992;326:455.

mal volume, bicarbonate, or both is found in 60–80% of patients with pancreatitis or cancer. In carcinoma, the test result depends on the relative extent and combination of acinar destruction and of duct obstruction. Cytologic examination of duodenal contents shows malignant cells in 40% of patients. Malignant cells may be found in up to 80% of patients with periampullary cancer.

Serum LAP is increased (>300 U) in 60% of patients with carcinoma of pancreas due to liver metastases or biliary tract obstruction. *It may also be increased in chronic liver disease.*

♦ Triolein ^{131}I test demonstrates pancreatic duct obstruction with absence of lipase in the intestine causing flat blood curves and increased stool excretion.

Radioisotope scanning of pancreas may be done (selenium 75) for lesions >2 cm.

♦ Needle biopsy has reported sensitivity of 57–96%; false-positives are rare.

Head

The abnormal pancreatic function tests and increased tumor markers that occur with carcinoma of the body of the pancreas may be evident.

♦ Laboratory findings due to complete obstruction of common bile duct
  • Serum bilirubin increased (12–25 mg/dL), mostly direct (increase persistent and nonfluctuating).
  • Serum ALP increased.
  • Urine and stool urobilinogen absent.
  • Increased PT; normal after IV vitamin K administration.
  • Increased serum cholesterol (usually >300 mg/dL) with esters not decreased.

Other liver function tests are usually normal.

Pancreatitis, Acute[19]

♦ Serum lipase increases within 3–6 hrs with peak at 24 hrs and usually returns to normal over a period of 8–14 days. Is superior to amylase; increases to a greater extent and may remain elevated for up to 14 days after amylase returns to normal. In patients with signs of acute pancreatitis, pancreatitis is highly likely (clinical specificity = 85%) when lipase ≥ 5× ULN, if values change significantly with time, and if amylase and lipase changes are concordant. (*Lipase should always be determined whenever amylase is determined.*) New methodology improves clinical utility. Urinary lipase is not clinically useful. It has been suggested that a lipase/amylase ratio >3 (and especially >5) indicates alcoholic rather than nonalcoholic pancreatitis. Acute pancreatitis or organ rejection is highly likely if lipase is ≥ 5× ULN, but unlikely if <3× ULN. (See Fig. 8-9 and p. 254.)

♦ Serum amylase increase begins in 3–6 hrs, rises rapidly within 8 hrs in 75% of patients, reaches maximum in 20–30 hrs, and may persist for 48–72 hrs. >95% sensitivity during first 12–24 hrs. The increase may be ≤ 40× normal, but the height of the increase and rate of fall do not correlate with the severity of the disease, prognosis, or rate of resolution; however, an increase of >7–10 days suggests an associated cancer of pancreas or pseudocyst, pancreatic ascites, or nonpancreatic cause. *Similar high values may occur in obstruction of pancreatic duct; they tend to fall after several days. >10% of patients with acute pancreatitis (especially when seen more than 2 days after onset of symptoms) may have normal values, even when dying of acute pancreatitis.* May also be normal in patients with relapsing chronic pancreatitis and patients with hypertriglyceridemia (technical interference with test). Frequently normal in acute alcoholic pancreatitis. Acute abdomen due to GI infarction or perforation rather than acute pancreatitis is suggested by only moderate increase in serum amylase and lipase (<3× ULN), evidence of bacteremia. 10–40% of patients with acute alcoholic intoxication have elevated serum amylase (about half of amylases are salivary type); patients often present with abdominal pain, but increased serum amylase is usually <3× ULN. Levels >25× ULN indicate metastatic tumor rather than pancreatitis. (See p. 252.)

♦ Serum pancreatic isoamylase can distinguish elevations due to salivary amylase, which may account for 25% of all elevated values. (In healthy persons, 40% of total serum amylase is pancreatic type and 60% is salivary type.)

---

[19]Ranson JHC. Etiological and prognostic factors in human acute pancreatitis: a review. *Am J Gastroenterol* 1982;77:633.

Only slight increase in serum amylase and lipase values suggests a different diagnosis than acute pancreatitis. *Many drugs increase both amylase and lipase in serum.*

Serum calcium is decreased in severe cases 1–9 days after onset (due to binding to soaps in fat necrosis). The decrease usually occurs after amylase and lipase levels have become normal. Tetany may occur. (*Rule out hyperparathyroidism if serum calcium is high or fails to fall in hyperamylasemia of acute pancreatitis.*)

Increased urinary amylase tends to reflect serum changes by a time lag of 6–10 hrs, but sometimes increased urine levels are higher and of longer duration than serum levels. The 24-hr level may be normal even when some of the 1-hr specimens show increased values. Measurement of amylase levels in hourly samples of urine may be useful. Ratio of amylase clearance to creatinine clearance is increased (>5%) and its use avoids the problem of timed urine specimens; also increased in any condition that decreases tubular reabsorption of amylase (e.g., severe burns, diabetic ketoacidosis, chronic renal insufficiency, multiple myeloma, acute duodenal perforation). Considered not specific; its use now discouraged by some but still recommended by others.

Serum bilirubin may be increased when pancreatitis is of biliary tract origin but is usually normal in alcoholic pancreatitis. Serum ALP, ALT, and AST may increase and parallel serum bilirubin rather than amylase, lipase, or calcium levels. Marked amylase increase (e.g., >2000 U/L) also favors biliary tract origin. Fluctuation >50% in 24 hrs of serum bilirubin, ALP, ALT, and AST suggests intermittent biliary obstruction.

○Serum trypsin (by RIA) is increased. High sensitivity makes a normal value useful for excluding acute pancreatitis. But low specificity (increased in large proportion of patients with hepatobiliary, bowel, and other diseases and renal insufficiency; increased in 13% of patients with chronic pancreatitis and 50% with pancreatic carcinoma) and RIA technology limit utility.

WBC is slightly to moderately increased (10,000–20,000/cu mm).

Hemoconcentration occurs (increased Hct). Hct may be decreased in severe hemorrhagic pancreatitis.

Glycosuria appears in 25% of patients.

Methemalbumin may be increased in serum and ascitic fluid in hemorrhagic (severe) but not edematous (mild) pancreatitis; may distinguish these two conditions but not useful in diagnosis of acute pancreatitis.

Hypokalemia, metabolic alkalosis, or lactic acidosis may occur.

Laboratory findings due to predisposing conditions (may be multiple)
- Alcohol abuse accounts for ~36% of cases.
- Biliary tract disease accounts for 17% of cases.
- Idiopathic origin accounts for >36% of cases.
- Infections (especially viral such as mumps, coxsackievirus and CMV infections, AIDS).
- Trauma and postoperative condition account for >8% of cases.
- Drug effects (e.g., steroids, thiazides, azathioprine, estrogens, sulfonamides; valproic acid in children) account for >5% of cases.
- Hypertriglyceridemia (hyperlipidemia types V, I, IV) accounts for 7% of cases.
- Hypercalcemia from any cause.
- Tumors (pancreas, ampulla).
- Anatomic abnormalities of ampullary region causing obstruction (e.g., annular pancreas, Crohn's disease, duodenal diverticulum).
- Hereditary.
- Renal failure; renal transplantation.
- Miscellaneous (e.g., collagen vascular disease, pregnancy, ischemia, scorpion bites, parasites obstructing pancreatic duct [*Ascaris*, fluke], Reye's syndrome, fulminant hepatitis, severe hypotension, cholesterol embolization).

Laboratory findings due to complications
- Pseudocysts of pancreas.
- Pancreatic abscess.
- Polyserositis (peritoneal, pleural, pericardial, synovial surfaces). Ascites may develop, cloudy or bloody or "prune juice" fluid, 0.5–2.0 L in volume, containing increased amylase with a level higher than that of serum amylase. No bile is evident (unlike in perforated ulcer). Gram stain shows no bacteria (unlike in infarct of intestine). Protein >3 gm/dL and marked increase in amylase.
- ARDS (with pleural effusion, alveolar exudate, or both) may occur in ~40% of patients; arterial hypoxemia is present.

- DIC.
- Hypovolemic shock.
- Others.

Prognostic laboratory findings
- On admission
    - WBC >16,000/cu mm
    - Blood glucose >200 mg/dL
    - Serum LD >350 U/L
    - Serum AST >250 U/L
    - Age >55 yrs
- Within 48 hrs
    - Serum calcium <8.0 mg/dL
    - Decrease in Hct >10 points
    - Increase in BUN >5 mg/dL
    - Arterial pO$_2$ <60 mm Hg
    - Metabolic acidosis with base deficit >4 mEq/L
- Mortality
    - 1% if three signs are positive
    - 15% if three or four signs are positive
    - 40% if five or six signs are positive
    - 100% if seven or more signs are positive
- Degree of amylase elevation has no prognostic significance.

Pancreatitis, Chronic

See also Malabsorption, pp. 185–188.

♦ Cholecystokinin-secretin test measures the effect of IV administration of cholecystokinin and secretin on volume, bicarbonate concentration, and amylase output of duodenal contents and increase in serum lipase and amylase. This is the most sensitive and reliable test (gold standard) for chronic pancreatitis, especially in the early stages. Is technically difficult and is often not performed accurately; gastric contamination must be avoided. Some abnormality occurs in >85% of patients with chronic pancreatitis. Amylase output is the most frequent abnormality. When all three are abnormal, there is a greater frequency of abnormality in the tests listed below.

Normal duodenal contents
- Volume: 95–235 mL/hr
- Bicarbonate concentration: 74–121 mEq/L
- Amylase output: 87,000–267,000 mg

Serum amylase and lipase increase after administration of cholecystokinin and secretin in ~20% of patients with chronic pancreatitis. They are more often abnormal when duodenal contents are normal. Normally serum lipase and amylase do not rise above normal limits.

Fasting serum amylase and lipase are increased in 10% of patients with chronic pancreatitis.

Serum pancreolauryl test

Fluorescein dilaurate taken with breakfast is acted on by a pancreas-specific cholesterol ester hydrolase, releasing fluorescein, which is absorbed from gut and measured in serum; preceded by administration of secretin and followed by administration of metoclopramide. Reported sensitivity = 82%, specificity 91%.[20]

Diabetic OGTT results in 65% of patients with chronic pancreatitis and frank diabetes in >10% of patients with chronic relapsing pancreatitis. When GTT is normal in the presence of steatorrhea, the cause should be sought elsewhere than in the pancreas.

♦ Laboratory findings due to malabsorption (occurs when >90% of exocrine function is lost) and steatorrhea.
- Bentiromide test is usually abnormal with moderate to severe pancreatic insufficiency.
- Schilling test may show mild malabsorption of Vitamin B$_{12}$.
- Xylose tolerance test and small bowel biopsy are not usually done but are normal.

---

[20]Dominguez-Munoz JE, Malfertheiner P. Optimized serum pancreolauryl test for differentiating patients with and without chronic pancreatitis. *Clin Chem* 1998;44:869.

Chemical analysis of fecal fat demonstrates steatorrhea. It is more sensitive than tests using triolein [131]I.

Triolein ^{131}I testing is abnormal in one-third of patients with chronic pancreatitis.

Starch tolerance test is abnormal in 25% of patients with chronic pancreatitis.

Laboratory findings due to causes of chronic pancreatitis and pancreatic exocrine insufficiency
  • Alcoholism in 60–70%
  • Idiopathic in 30–40%
  • Obstruction of pancreatic duct (e.g., trauma, pseudocyst, pancreas divisum, cancer or obstruction of duct or ampulla)
  • Other causes occasionally (e.g., cystic fibrosis, primary hyperparathyroidism, heredity, protein caloric malnutrition, miscellaneous [Z-E syndrome, Shwachman syndrome, alpha$_1$-antitrypsin deficiency, trypsinogen deficiency, enterokinase deficiency, hemochromatosis, parenteral hyperalimentation])

♦ Radioactive selenium scanning of pancreas yields variable findings in different clinics.

CT, ultrasonography, ERCP are most accurate for diagnosing and staging chronic pancreatitis.

Pseudocyst of Pancreas

Serum direct bilirubin is increased (>2 mg/dL) in 10% of patients.

Serum ALP is increased in 10% of patients.

Fasting blood sugar is increased in <10% of patients.

Duodenal contents after secretin-pancreozymin stimulation usually show decreased bicarbonate content (<70 mEq/L) but normal volume and normal content of amylase, lipase, and trypsin.

♦ Findings of pancreatic cyst aspiration[21]
  • Best when panel of tests is used.
  • High fluid viscosity and CEA indicate mucinous differentiation and exclude pseudocyst, serous cystadenoma, other nonmucinous cysts or cystic tumors.
  • Increased CA 72-4, CA 15-3, and tissue polypeptide antigen are markers of malignancy; if all are low, pseudocyst or serous cystadenoma is most likely.
  • CA 125 is increased in serous cystadenoma.
  • Pancreatic enzymes, leukocyte esterase, and NB/70K are increased in pseudocysts.
  • Cytologic examination.

Laboratory findings of preceding acute pancreatitis (this is mild and unrecognized in one-third of patients). Persistent increase of serum amylase and lipase after an episode of acute pancreatitis may indicate formation of a pseudocyst.

Laboratory findings due to conditions preceding acute pancreatitis (e.g., alcoholism, trauma, duodenal ulcer, cholelithiasis).

Laboratory findings due to complications
  • Infection
  • Perforation
  • Hemorrhage by erosion of blood vessel or into a viscus

[21]Centeno BA. Fine needle aspiration biopsy of the pancreas. *Clin Lab Med* 1998;18:401.

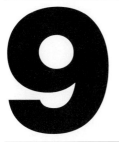

Central and Peripheral Nervous System Disorders

Laboratory Tests for Disorders of the Nervous System

Cerebrospinal Fluid (CSF), Abnormal

See Table 9-1.

Gross Appearance

Viscous CSF may occur with metastatic mucinous adenocarcinoma (e.g., colon), large numbers of cryptococci, severe meningeal infection, or, rarely, injury to annulus fibrosus with release of nucleus pulposus fluid.

Turbidity may be due to increased WBCs (>200/cu mm) or RBCs (>400/cu mm), or presence of bacteria (>10^5/mL) or other microorganisms (fungi, amebae), contrast media, or epidural fat aspirated during lumbar puncture.

Clots or pellicles indicate protein >150 mg/dL.

CSF with RBC >6000/cu mm appears grossly bloody; with RBC = 500–6000/cu mm appears cloudy, xanthochromic, or pink-tinged (in bright light in clear glass tubes containing >1 mL of CSF).

Xanthochromia caused by bilirubin, may be due to

Bleeding within 2–36 hrs. Minimum period for bilirubin detection is 12 hrs.
  * Traumatic lumbar puncture >2 hrs earlier.
  * Hemorrhage into CSF (e.g., subarachnoid or intracerebral hemorrhage). Is present in all patients for ≤ 2 wks and 70% of patients at 3 wks.

Serum bilirubin >6 mg/dL.

Protein >100 mg/dL usually causes CSF to look faintly yellow.

WBCs

CSF WBCs may be corrected for presence of blood (e.g., traumatic tap, subarachnoid hemorrhage) by subtracting 1 WBC for each 700 RBCs/cu mm counted in CSF if the CBC is normal.

If significant anemia or leukocytosis is present:

$$\text{Corrected WBC} = \text{WBC in bloody CSF} - \frac{[\text{WBC (blood)} \times \text{RBC (CSF)}]}{[\text{RBC (blood)}]}$$

(RBC and WBC are cells/cu mm)

In normal CSF, minimal blood contamination may cause ≤ 2 PMN/25 RBCs, or ≤ 10 PMN/25–100 RBCs.

CSF WBC count (>3000/cu mm) with predominantly PMNs strongly suggests bacterial cause and is >2000/cu mm in 38% of cases. When WBC <1000/cu mm in bacterial meningitis, one-third of cases have >50% lymphocytes or mononuclear cells. *However, WBCs are usually PMNs in early stages of all types of meningitis; mononuclear cells only appear in a second specimen 18–24 hrs later.* Low WBC counts do not rule out acute bacterial meningitis.

Neutrophilic leukocytes are found in:
  * Bacterial infections (e.g., *Nocardia, Actinomyces, Arachnia, Brucella*)

Table 9-1. Cerebrospinal Fluid (CSF) Findings in Various Conditions

	Appearance	Protein (mg/dL)	Glucose (mg/dL)	WBC/cu mm	Microbiology/Serology/Other
Normal					
Ventricular	C, colorless no clot	5–15	45–80	0–10	
Cisternal		10–25			
Lumbar		10–45			
TB meningitis	O, sl yellow, delicate clot	45–500	10–45	10–1000, chiefly L	Acid-fast stain 25% sensitive Culture 60–80% sensitive PCR 100% specific
Tuberculoma		I		Small number of cells	
Acute pyogenic meningitis	O to Pu, sl yellow, delicate clot	50–1500	0–45	25–10,000, chiefly P	Gram stain 60–90% sensitive Culture 80% sensitive, 100% specific Direct antigen/PCR 50–90% sensitive, 100% specific
Aseptic meningitis[a]	C, T, or X	20 to >200	N	≤500, occ 2000; first PMNs, later mononuclear cells	All cultures negative
Viral meningitis		I	N	10–1000, mostly L	Seroconversion Specific IgM Antigens PCR Culture 40–70% sensitive
AIDS		50–100	N	≤300	Culture 40–70% sensitive HIV antibodies, antigens
Acute anterior polio	C or sl O, may be sl yellow, may be delicate clot	20–350	N	10 to >500, L > P	Serologic tests Stool culture AST in CSF is always I
Mumps	N or O	20–125	N	0 to >2000	IgM and IgG in blood and CSF Culture of CSF
Measles	N or O	sl I	N	≤500	Blood serology
Herpes zoster	N	20–110	N	≤300 in 40% of patients	PCR

Disease	Pressure	Protein	Glucose	Cells	Tests
Equine, St. Louis encephalitis, choriomeningitis	N or sl T	20 to >200	N	10–200; occ to 3000	Blood serologic tests
Herpes simplex		I	N	10–1000, chiefly L	CSF culture in congenital infection CSF serologic tests; brain biopsy
Rabies		N or sl I	N	N or ≤ 100 mononuclear cells	Serologic tests Cultures of brain or saliva Animal brain Tissue examination
Postinfectious	N	15–75	N	5–200, rarely ≤ 1000	Serologic tests for specific viruses
Fungal Coccidioidomycosis	I	I	N early, then D	≤ 200 early; may be higher later	Antigen assay Culture 50% sensitive CF in CSF 75–90% sensitive Wet preparation in 20% KOH
Cryptococcal meningitis	N	≤ 500 in 90%	Moderate D in 55%	≤ 800 (L >P)	India ink ~50% sensitive Cryptococcal antigen assay ~90% sensitive Culture ~90% sensitive
Toxoplasmosis	X	≤ 2000	N	50–500; chiefly monocytes	Serologic tests in serum PCR Organism identified in sediment smear See p. 866, Chapter 15.
Histoplasmosis					
Syphilis					Positive serologic test in blood and positive CSF VDRL PCR can detect treponemal DNA in CSF
Tabes dorsalis	N	25–100; I gamma globulin less marked than in general paresis	N	10–80	Early: VDRL titer may be low Late: ~25% of patients may have normal CSF and negative VDRL in blood and CSF

(continued)

CNS

265

Table 9-1. (continued)

	Appearance	Protein (mg/dL)	Glucose (mg/dL)	WBC/cu mm	Microbiology/Serology/Other
General paresis[b]	N	≤ 100; marked I in gamma globulin	N	≤ 175, mononuclear	VDRL titer usually high
Meningo-vascular syphilis	N	≤ 260 in 66%; I gamma globulin in 75% of cases	N	10–100, N in 60%	
Syphilitic meningitis				≤ 2000 L	
Asymptomatic CNS lues		I protein and cell count are index of activity			Serologic test may be negative in blood but positive in CSF
Leptospirosis		I ≤ 80	N	≤ 500 M	
Lyme disease		I IgG and oligoclonal bands		≤ 450 L	*Borrelia burgdorferi* antibodies higher in CSF than in serum
Primary amebic (*Naegleria*) meningitis	Sanguino-purulent, may be T or Pu	I	Usually D	400–21,000, mostly P; also RBC	Amebas seen on Wright's stain of CSF
Chronic meningitis[c] Symptoms for 1–4 wks		Moderate to marked I	D	100–400, mostly L	
Cavernous sinus thrombophlebitis	Usually N; may be B		Usually N		
Brain abscess[d]		May be ≤ 75–300	N	25–300; PMN, L, RBCs	CSF cultures sterile Positive blood cultures in 10% Can be caused by almost any

Extradural abscess		100–400	N	Relatively few PMNs and L	organism including fungi, *Nocardia*
Subdural empyema		I	N	Few hundred or less, mostly PMNs	Negative smears and cultures Peripheral WBC I (≤ 25,000/cu mm)
Cord tumor	C, occ X	≤ 3500 in 85%; N in 15%	N	≤ 100, chiefly L; N in 60%	
Brain tumor[e]	C, occ X; B if hemorrhage into tumor	≤ 500	May be D if cells are present	≤ 150; N in 75%	Tumor cells in 20–40% of solid tumors; absence does not exclude meningeal tumor
Leukemia		I	D to 50% of blood		Tumor cells identified by special methods
Pseudotumor cerebri	N	N	N		
Cerebral thrombosis	N	≤ 100, N in 60%	N	≤ 50, N in 75%, rarely ≤ 2000	
Cerebral embolism[f] Bland	Sl X in one-third of cases in a few days; may be B			May be 10,000 RBC	
Septic	Sl X	I	N	≤ 200 with varying L and PMNs; ≤ 1000 RBCs	
Cerebral hemorrhage	N in 15%, X in 10%, B in 75%	Usually ≤ 2000	N	Same as in blood; N in 10%	
Subarachnoid hemorrhage	B; X in 24 hrs; no clot	Usually ≤ 1000	N	Same as in blood	
Hypertensive encephalopathy		≤ 100			
Postoperative neurosurgery (especially posterior fossa)		I	<40	1000–2000, mostly PMNs	CSF sterile unless postoperative infection

(continued)

Table 9-1. (continued)

	Appearance	Protein (mg/dL)	Glucose (mg/dL)	WBC/cu mm	Microbiology/Serology/Other
Traumatic tap	B	I by blood	N	Same as in blood	
Head trauma	N, B, or X	I if bloody	N	Same as in blood	
Acute epidural hemorrhage	C unless associated injuries				
Subdural hematoma	C, B, or X, depending on associated injuries	N or sl I			Infants are often anemic
Chronic subdural hematoma	Usually X	300–2000			
Multiple sclerosis	N				
Polyneuritis; Polyarteritis; porphyria; beriberi; alcohol effect; arsenic poisoning	N, X if protein very I	Usually N	N	N but albumino-cytologic dissociation in Guillain-Barré syndrome that may occur in heavy metal poisoning, infection, etc.	
Diabetes mellitus	Same as polyarteritis, etc.	Often ≤ 300	N	Same as polyarteritis, etc.	
Acute infection	Same as polyarteritis, etc.	≤ 1500	N	Same as polyarteritis, etc.	
Lead encephalopathy	N or sl yellow	≤ 100	N	0–100	
Sarcoidosis (findings in ≤ 50%)		sl I; oligoclonal bands may be present	D in 10%	I in 40% Typically 10–100 but ≤ 6000	I ACE in serum or CSF in 50–70%

Condition					
Behçet's disease (25% have meningoencephalitis)	I			N	I
Alcoholism	N		N	N	Usually N
Diabetic coma	N		N	N	Usually N
Uremia	N		N	N or I	Usually N
Epilepsy	N		N	N	N
Eclampsia	May be B	Usually ≤ 200	N	N	May be RBCs	Uric acid I ≤ 3× N reflecting marked I in serum
Guillain-Barré syndrome		50–100 average; albuminocytologic dissociation	N	N	

ACE = angiotensin-converting enzyme; AIDS = acquired immunodeficiency syndrome; B = bloody; C = clear; CF = complement fixation; D = decreased; I = increased; L = lymphocytes; N = normal; O = opalescent; occ = occasionally; P = polymorphonuclear leukocyte; PCR = polymerase chain reaction; Pu = purulent; sl = slightly; T = turbid; X = xanthochromic.

aPossible underlying disorders:
- Infections (e.g., viral, bacterial [such as incompletely treated or very early bacterial meningitis], spirochetal [leptospirosis, syphilis, Lyme disease], tuberculosis, fungal, amebic, mycoplasma, rickettsial, helminthic)
  - Chemical meningitis
  - Drug-induced meningitis
- Systemic disorders
  Vasculitis
  Collagen vascular disease
  Sarcoidosis
- Neoplasm (e.g., leukemia, metastatic carcinoma)
- SLE

bCSF always abnormal in untreated general paresis.
cPossible underlying disorders:
- Various infections: tuberculosis (most common cause), bacteria, spirochetes, fungi, protozoa, amebae, *Mycoplasma*, *Rickettsia*, helminths
- Systemic disorders (e.g., vasculitis, collagen vascular disease, sarcoid, neoplasm)

dFindings depend on stage and duration of abscess.
eProtein is particularly increased with meningioma of the olfactory groove and with acoustic neuroma. Usually normal in brainstem gliomas and diencephalic syndrome of infants due to glioma of hypothalamus.
fUsually same as in cerebral thrombosis.

- Fungal infections (*Blastomyces, Coccidioides, Candida, Aspergillus, Zygomycetes, Cladosporium, Allescheria*)
- Chemical meningitis (see p. 284)
- Other conditions (e.g., SLE)

Lymphocytic cells are found in:

- Bacterial infections (e.g., *Treponema pallidum, Leptospira, Actinomyces israelii, Arachnia propionica*, 90% of *Brucella* cases, *Borrelia burgdorferi* [Lyme disease], *Mycobacterium tuberculosis*)
- Fungal infections (e.g., *Cryptococcus neoformans, Candida* spp., *Coccidioides immitis, Histoplasma capsulatum, Blastomyces dermatitides, Sporotrichum schenckii, Allescheria boydii, Cladosporium trichoides*)
- Parasitic diseases (e.g., toxoplasmosis, cysticercosis)
- Viral infections (e.g., mumps, lymphocytic choriomeningitis, infection with human T-cell leukemia virus [HTLV] type III or echovirus)
- Parameningeal disorders (e.g., brain abscess)
- Noninfectious disorders (e.g., neoplasms, sarcoidosis, multiple sclerosis, granulomatous arteritis)

Eosinophils may be found in:

- Lymphoma
- Helminth infection (e.g., angiostrongyliasis, cysticercosis)
- Rarely other infections (e.g., TB, syphilis, Rocky Mountain spotted fever, coccidioidomycosis)

Microbiology/Serology

Smears for Gram and acid-fast stains must be routinely *centrifuged* on all CSF specimens because other findings may be normal in meningitis. Occasionally animal inoculations may be required. Gram stain of CSF sediment is negative in 20% of cases of bacterial meningitis because at least 10^5 bacteria/mL of CSF must be present to demonstrate 1–2 bacteria/100× microscopic field. Gram stain is positive in 90% of cases due to pneumococci, 85% of cases due to *Haemophilus influenzae*, 75% of cases due to meningococci, and 50% of cases due to *Listeria monocytogenes*, but only 30–50% of cases due to gram-negative enteric bacilli. If antibiotics have been given before CSF obtained, Gram stain may be negative. Stains are positive in <60% of cases of treated bacterial meningitis, <5% of cases of TB meningitis, 20–70% of cases of fungal meningitis and <2% of cases of brain abscess. Sensitivity of Gram stain is increased by using fluorescent techniques with acridine orange.

Positive CSF culture has sensitivity of 92%, specificity of 95%, false-negative rate of 8%, and false-positive rate of 5%.

Limulus amebocyte lysate is a rapid specific indicator of endotoxin produced by gram-negative bacteria (*Neisseria meningitidis, H. influenzae* type b, *Escherichia coli, Pseudomonas*). Is not affected by prior antibiotic therapy; is more rapid and sensitive than CIE. Often is not routinely available.

Serologic methods are often preferred (e.g., positive in 85% of coccidioidal cases compared with culture, which is positive in 37% of cases) especially in syphilis, brucellosis, Lyme disease.

Blood and CSF serology are positive in CNS syphilis (see pp. 266, 816–822); positive in 7–10% of active cases of infectious mononucleosis.

PCR to detect HSV and human enteroviruses in meningitis and encephalitis.

Antigen detection (latex agglutination) for *H. influenzae* type b, *C. neoformans, N. meningitidis, Streptococcus pneumoniae, Streptococcus agalactiae* has replaced CIE.

Use

- Abnormal CSF chemistries or cell count with negative Gram stain and culture (e.g., prior antibiotic therapy).
- Not indicated for screening or if chemistry is normal and CSF cell count is <50/cu mm unless patient is immunocompromised. Not indicated if Gram stain is positive.

Interpretation

- Negative results are not conclusive; positive results should be confirmed by culture, especially to determine antibiotic susceptibility. Test for *H. influenzae* type b antigen in CSF has reported sensitivity of 74%, specificity of 100%, positive predictive value of 100%, negative predictive value of 99%.

- Antigen detection is less sensitive in urine and serum than in CSF specimens.
- Specific antigens have also been detected in urine and other body fluids in non-meningeal infections (e.g., pneumococcal pneumonia, *H. influenzae* epiglottitis, legionnaire's disease).

Interferences

- False-positive results for group B streptococci may occur due to colonization of perineum.
- Misleading positive results with *H. influenzae* type b may occur in both urine and CSF due to recent immunization with *H. influenzae* type b vaccine.

CSF Chemistries

CSF glucose

- Decreased by utilization by bacteria (pyogens or tubercle bacilli), WBCs, or occasionally cancer cells in CSF.
- Lags behind blood glucose by ~1 hr.
- May rapidly become normal after onset of antibiotic therapy.
- Is decreased in only ~50% of cases of bacterial meningitis.
- <45 mg/dL is almost always abnormal; <40 mg/dL is always abnormal.
- Normally is ~50–65% of blood glucose, which should *always* be drawn simultaneously. In acute bacterial meningitis, CSF/serum ratio of glucose is usually <0.5; a ratio <0.4 has 80% sensitivity and 96% specificity for distinguishing acute bacterial meningitis from acute viral meningitis; a ratio <0.25 is found in <1% of acute viral meningitis cases and in 44% of acute bacterial meningitis cases, even when CSF glucose is normal. A ratio of <8.0 is significant in infants.
- May also be decreased in acute infection due to syphilis, Lyme disease, 10–20% of cases of lymphocytic choriomeningitis, and encephalitis due to mumps or HSV but generally rare in viral infections or parameningeal processes. May also be decreased in rheumatoid meningitis, lupus myelopathy, and other causes of chronic meningitis such as bacterial infection (e.g., *Brucella*, *M. tuberculosis*), syphilis, fungal infection (*Cryptococcus*, *Coccidioides*), parasitic infection (e.g., cysticercosis), granulomatous meningitis (e.g., sarcoid), chemical meningitis, carcinomatous meningitis, hypoglycemia, and subarachnoid hemorrhage.

CSF protein, glucose, and WBC levels may not return to normal in ~50% of patients with clinically cured bacterial meningitis and therefore are not recommended as a test of cure.

CSF protein

- Total protein may be corrected for presence of blood (e.g., due to traumatic tap or intracerebral hemorrhage) by subtracting 1 mg/dL of protein for each 1000 RBCs/cu mm if serum protein and CBC are normal and CSF protein and cell count are determined on same tube of CSF. *Serum protein levels must be normal to interpret any CSF protein values and should therefore always be measured concurrently.*
- May not be increased in early stages of many types of meningitis.
- Normal in 10% of patients with bacterial meningitis (20% of cases of meningococcal meningitis).
- Usually >150 mg/dL in bacterial meningitis. Increase occurs especially with *S. pneumoniae*.
- >100 mg/dL distinguishes bacterial from aseptic meningitis (82% sensitivity and 98% specificity).
- >172 mg/dL occurs in 1% of acute viral meningitis cases and 50% of acute bacterial meningitis cases but may be normal in 10% of acute bacterial meningitis cases).
- >200 mg/dL distinguishes bacterial from aseptic meningitis (86% sensitivity and 100% specificity).
- >500 mg/dL is infrequent and occurs chiefly in bacterial meningitis, bloody CSF, or cord tumor with spinal block and occasionally in polyneuritis and brain tumor.
- >1000 mg/dL suggests subarachnoid block; with complete spinal block, the lower the level of the cord tumor, the higher the protein concentration.
- Rarely >200 mg/dL in viral meningitis.
- When antibiotic treatment of bacterial meningitis is started before CSF is obtained, protein may be only slightly elevated.
- May show mild to moderate elevation in myxedema (25% of cases), uremia, connective tissue disorders, or Cushing's syndrome.

CNS

- Decreased CSF protein (3–20 mg/dL) may occur in hyperthyroidism, one-third of patients with benign intracranial hypertension, after removal of large volumes of CSF (e.g., during pneumoencephalography), in children 6–24 mos of age.

CSF and serum ACE are increased in 50–70% of cases of neurosarcoidosis.

CSF lactate has been reported useful to differentiate bacterial from viral meningitis; is independent of serum concentrations. Due to sequelae of increased WBC.
- If <3 mmol/L (normal range), viral meningitis is most likely.
- If >4.2 mmol/L, bacterial (including TB) or fungal meningitis is most likely.
- If 3–6 mmol/L with negative Gram stain and prior antibiotic therapy, partially treated bacterial meningitis is most likely. In bacterial meningitis, level is still high after 1–2 days of antibiotic therapy.
- In cases with mild symptoms and negative Gram stain with few PMNs, CSF lactate may differentiate mild bacterial from very early viral meningitis.
- May also be increased in non-Hodgkin's lymphoma with meningeal involvement, severe cerebral malaria, head injury, and anoxia.

CSF chloride reflects only blood chloride level, but in tuberculous meningitis a decrease of 25% may exceed the serum chloride decrease because of dehydration and electrolyte loss. It is not useful in diagnosis of tuberculous meningitis.

CSF glutamine >35 mg/dL is associated with hepatic encephalopathy (due to conversion from ammonia).

CSF Enzymes

Normal CSF is not permeable to serum enzymes. Changes in AST are irregular and generally of limited diagnostic value. If determinations of AST, LD, and CK in CSF are all performed, at least one shows marked increase in 80% of patients with cortical stroke (usually due to emboli), but this is not noted in patients with lacunar stroke (usually due to small-vessel hypertensive disease). Generally are not useful in diagnosis of CNS diseases.

Transaminase (AST)
Increased In
Large infarcts of brain during first 10 days. In severe cases, serum AST may also be increased; occurs in ~40% of patients.

~40% of CNS tumors (various benign, malignant, and metastatic), depending on location, growth rate, etc.; chiefly useful as indicator of organic neurologic disease.

Some other conditions (e.g., head injury, subarachnoid hemorrhage)

Lactate Dehydrogenase
Increased In
Cerebrovascular accidents—increase occurs frequently, reaches maximum level in 1–3 days, and is apparently not related to xanthochromia, RBC, WBC, protein, sugar, or chloride levels. Subarachnoid and subdural hemorrhage cause increase of all LD isoenzymes especially LD-3, LD-4, and LD-5 (not due only to hemolysis).

CNS tumors—LD-5 >9% and decreased LD-1/LD-5 ratio <2.5 in absence of infection or hemorrhage suggests tumor in meninges. LD-5 >10% suggests higher grade malignancy. Increase in LD-3, LD-4, and occasionally LD-5 may occur in leukemic and lymphomatous infiltration.

Meningitis—is sensitive indicator of meningitis (in specimen with no blood); normal or mild increase in viral meningitis; more marked increase in bacterial meningitis. Bacterial meningitis shows increase of LD-4 and LD-5; viral meningitis shows increase of LD-1 and LD-2; TB meningitis shows increase of LD-1, LD-2, LD-3 (especially LD-3); HIV alone does not alter LD isoenzyme pattern; isoenzyme changes may appear only in later stage and are of low sensitivity.

Creatine Kinase (CK Total)
Not Useful Because
Does not consistently increase in various CNS diseases.

No relationship to CSF protein, WBC, or RBC values

No pattern of relationship to LD and AST in CSF

No correlation of serum CK and CSF CK

In global anoxic or ischemic brain insults due to respiratory or cardiac arrest, CK-BB level 24–72 hrs after injury can be used to estimate overall extent of brain damage; good correlation with neurologic prognosis after resuscitation. Less correlation with outcome in head trauma and stroke. Not recommended for estimating stroke size.

CSF CK-BB levels association with neurologic injury
- Higher levels indicate poorer prognosis.
- <5 U/L: Only mild injury; most patients awaken, some minimal deficit.
- >10 U/L: Substantial brain injury; guarded prognosis.
- 5–20 U/L: Mild to moderate; often moderate to severe impairment; guarded prognosis.
- 21–50 U/L: Severe impairment; poor prognosis; few patients awaken; most die in hospital.
- >50 U/L: Patients rarely regain minimal reflexes or responsiveness; poor prognosis; usually die in hospital.

CSF CK-MM is normally absent and, if present, indicates blood contamination due to traumatic tap or subarachnoid hemorrhage.

Mitochondrial CK is found with high CK-BB levels; not used to estimate prognosis or brain damage.

Tumor Markers

- Increased CSF CEA has been reported to be helpful in diagnosis of suspected metastatic carcinoma (from breast, lung, bowel) with negative cytology.
- Beta-glucuronidase has been reported to be increased in 75% of patients with metastatic leptomeningeal adenocarcinoma and 60% of patients with acute myeloblastic leukemia involving CNS. Normal = <49 mU/L, indeterminate = 49–70 mU/L, suspicious = >70 mU/L.
- Lysozyme (muramidase) is increased in various CNS tumors, especially myeloid and monocytic leukemias, but is also increased when neutrophils are increased (e.g., bacterial meningitis).

Gamma-aminobutyric acid is decreased in CSF in Huntington's disease.

Colloidal gold test is no longer used; replaced by electrophoresis/immunofixation of CSF. IgG in CSF is increased 14–35% in two-thirds of patients with neurosyphilis. IgG oligoclonal bands are seen in neurosyphilis and multiple sclerosis.

In eclampsia, CSF shows gross or microscopic blood and increased protein (up to 200 mg/dL) in most cases. Glucose is normal. Uric acid is increased (to 3× normal level) in all cases, reflecting the marked increase in serum level. (In normal pregnancy, CSF values have same reference range as in nonpregnant women.)

CSF, Normal

Found In

Korsakoff's syndrome
Wernicke's encephalopathy
Alzheimer's disease
Jakob-Creutzfeldt disease
Tuberous sclerosis (protein rarely increased)
Idiopathic epilepsy (If protein is increased, rule out neoplasms; if cell count is increased, rule out neoplasm or inflammation.)
Narcolepsy, cataplexy, etc.
Parkinson's disease
Hereditary cerebellar degenerations
Huntington's disease
Migraine
Ménière's syndrome
Psychiatric conditions (e.g., neurocirculatory asthenia, hysteria, depression, anxiety, schizophrenia) *(Rule out psychiatric condition as a manifestation of primary disease, e.g., drugs, porphyria, primary endocrine diseases.)*
Transient cerebral ischemia
Amyotrophic lateral sclerosis
Muscular dystrophy
Progressive muscular atrophy
Syringomyelia
Vitamin B_{12} deficiency with subacute combined degeneration of spinal cord
Pellagra
Beriberi

CNS

Subacute myelo-opticoneuropathy
Minimal brain dysfunction of childhood
Cerebral palsies
Febrile convulsions of childhood
See Chapter 12 for metabolic and hereditary diseases that affect the nervous system
  (e.g., gangliosidosis, mucopolysaccharidoses, glycogen storage disease).

CSF, Normal Values

Measurement of these components should always be performed **on simultaneously
  drawn blood samples.**

Appearance	**Clear, colorless: no clot**
Total cell count	
Adults, children	0–6/cu mm (all mononuclear cells)
Infants	<19/cu mm
Neonates	<30/cu mm
Glucose	45–80 mg/dL (20 mg/dL less than blood level)
	Ventricular fluid 5–10 mg/dL higher than lumbar fluid
Total protein	Cisternal: 15–25 mg/dL
	Ventricular: 5–15 mg/dL
	Lumbar: 15–45 mg/dL 3 mos–60 yrs
	15–100 mg/dL neonates
	15–60 mg/dL >60 yrs
Albumin	10–35 mg/dL
Protein electrophoresis	
Transthyretin (prealbumin)	2–7%
Albumin	56–76%
Alpha$_1$ globulin	2–7%
Alpha$_2$ globulin	4–12%
Beta globulin	8–18%
Gamma globulin	3–12%
IgG	<4.0 mg/dL
	<10% of total CSF protein
Albumin index (ratio)	<9.0
IgG synthesis rate	0.0–8.0 mg/day
IgG index (ratio)	0.28–0.66
CSF IgG/albumin ratio	0.09–0.25
Oligoclonal bands	Negative
Myelin basic protein	0.0–4.0 ng/mL
Chloride	120–130 mEq/L
	(20 mEq/L above serum values)
Sodium	142–150 mEq/L
Potassium	2.2–3.3 mEq/L
Carbon dioxide	25 mEq/L
pH	7.35–7.40
Transaminase (AST)	7–49 U
LD	~10% of serum level
LD-1	38–58% (LD-1 > LD-2)
LD-2	26–36%
LD-3	12–24%
LD-4	1–7%
LD-5	0–5%
CK	0–5 U/L
Bilirubin	0
Urea nitrogen	5–25 mg/dL
Amino acids	30% of blood level
Xanthochromia	0
Total volume (adults)	~140 mL
Generation rate	0.35 mL/min = 500 mL/day

Dexamethasone Suppression Test (DST)

Blood is drawn at 11 p.m., 8 a.m., 12 noon, 4 p.m., and 11 p.m. for plasma cortisol. 1 mg of dexamethasone is given immediately after the first sample is taken. An abnormal test result is failure of suppression of plasma cortisol to $\leq 5~\mu g/dL$ in any sample after the first. Plasma dexamethasone should also be measured to avoid false values due to aberrant clearance of dexamethasone.

Use

A positive DST result "rules in" the diagnosis of melancholia (endogenous depression), but a negative DST result does not rule it out, because results may be positive in only 40–50% of such patients.

In the presence of a positive DST result, appropriate drug treatment (e.g., tricyclic antidepressants) that results in normalization of DST with clinical recovery is a good prognostic sign, whereas failure of DST to normalize suggests a poor prognosis and the need for continued antidepressant therapy. Despite clinical improvement, treatment should be continued until DST results become negative (usually within 10 days). With relapse, DST may become abnormal when symptoms are still mild, before fully developed syndrome is present. The need to continue treatment is indicated if a positive DST result that became negative with therapy reverts to positive after drug treatment is discontinued or the drug dosage is lowered.

Interference

Certain drugs or substances that cause nonsuppression, especially phenytoin, barbiturates, meprobamate, carbamazepine, and alcohol (chronic high doses or withdrawal within 3 wks) can interfere with DST.

Enhanced suppression may be caused by benzodiazepines (high doses), corticosteroids (spironolactone, cortisone, artificial glucocorticoids such as prednisone [topical and nasal forms]), and dextroamphetamine.

Other drugs that are said to interfere include estrogens (not birth control pills), reserpine, narcotics, and indomethacin.

Medical conditions including weight loss to 20% below ideal body weight, pregnancy or abortion within 1 mo, endocrine diseases, systemic infections, serious liver disease, cancer, and other severe physical illnesses may also cause false-positive test results.

Lithium maintenance therapy does not interfere with DST.

With a 50% prevalence of melancholia in the population studied and fulfillment of certain medical criteria, DST was found to have a sensitivity of 67%, a specificity of 96%, and a confidence level of 94% in determining diagnosis. When only the 4 p.m. blood sample was used, the sensitivity was ~50%. However, there are still no clear indications for routine use of DST in clinical psychiatry, and many of the routine methods are not accurate at the decision level.

Response of TSH to administration of thyrotropin-releasing hormone (TRH) has also been suggested as useful in the diagnosis of unipolar depression and prediction of relapse. These patients have a maximum rise in serum TSH level of $<7~\mu U/mL$ (normal $= 17\pm9~\mu U/mL$). Use of this test with DST is said to add confidence to diagnosis of major unipolar depression; abnormal response to either test before treatment suggests that patient is particularly liable to have early relapse, unless there is laboratory proof as well as clinical evidence of recovery after treatment.

Diseases of the Nervous System

See Table 9-1.

Abscess, Brain

○CSF shows WBC ~25–300/cu mm and increased neutrophils, lymphocytes, and RBCs.
  • Protein may be increased (75–300 mg/dL).
  • Glucose is normal.
  • Bacterial cultures are negative.

- Findings depend on stage and duration of abscess.
♦ • With rupture, acute purulent meningitis with many organisms
○Positive blood cultures in ~10% of patients.
○Laboratory findings due to associated primary disease
- 10% of cases are due to penetrating skull trauma.
- 50% of cases are due to contiguous spread from sinuses, mastoids, middle ear.
- 20% of cases are cryptogenic.
- 20% of cases are due to hematogenous spread.
  Dental infections
  Primary septic lung disease (e.g., lung abscess, bronchiectasis, empyema)
  Cyanotic congenital heart disease (e.g., septal defects)
  Other causes

Due To

Usually mixed anaerobic (e.g., streptococci or *Bacteroides*) and aerobic (e.g., strepto-
cocci, staphylococci, or *S. pneumoniae*) organisms and gram-negative species (e.g.,
Proteus, Klebsiella, Pseudomonas)
Staphylococcus predominates when due to penetrating trauma.
Toxoplasma and *Nocardia* infections may be due to underlying AIDS.
20% of cultures are sterile.
May be caused by almost any organism, including fungi and *Nocardia*.

Abscess, Epidural of Spinal Cord/Extradural, Intracranial

CSF protein is increased (usually 100–400 mg/dL), and relatively few WBCs are present (lymphocytes and neutrophils).
Most common organism is *S. aureus*, followed by *Streptococcus* and gram-negative
bacilli.
Laboratory findings due to preceding condition (e.g., adjacent osteomyelitis; bacteremia
due to dental, respiratory, or skin infections)

Acquired Immunodeficiency Syndrome (AIDS), Neurologic Manifestations

See Acquired Immunodeficiency Syndrome, Chapter 15.
Dementia (also called subacute encephalitis) is most common neurologic syndrome in
AIDS; occurs in >50% of cases; may be initial or later manifestation.
- CSF abnormalities in 85%
  Increased protein (50–100 mg/dL) in 60% of patients
  Mild mononuclear pleocytosis (5–50 cells/cu mm) in 20% of patients
♦ HIV antibodies
Aseptic meningitis—may occur early or late, or be chronic recurrent.
- CSF may show
  20–300 cells/cu mm
  Increased protein (may be 50–100 mg/dL)
  ♦ HIV culture is usually positive.
  ♦ Increased CSF/serum antibody ratio, indicating local antibody production
Myelopathy—gradual onset; usually associated with dementia.
- Polymyositis is most common type
Peripheral neuropathies, some of which may resemble Guillain-Barré syndrome
- CSF may show
  Increased protein (50–100 mg/dL)
  Pleocytosis of 10–50 cells/cu mm
Opportunistic infections of CNS
- Viral (e.g., CMV, HSV-I and HSV-II, papovavirus)
- Nonviral (e.g., *Cryptococcus, Toxoplasma, Aspergillus fumigatus, Candida albi-
  cans, Coccidioides immitis, Mycobacterium avium-intracellulare,* and *M. tubercu-
  losis, Nocardia asteroides, Listeria*)
Neoplasms (e.g., Kaposi's sarcoma, non-Hodgkin's lymphoma)
Vascular (e.g., infarction, hemorrhage, vasculitis)
Associated diseases (e.g., neurosyphilis)

Arachnoiditis, Chronic Adhesive

(Due to spinal anesthesia, syphilis, etc.)
CSF protein may be normal or increased.

Arteritis, Cranial

♦ ESR is markedly increased.

Bassen-Kornzweig Syndrome

○Abnormal RBCs (acanthocytes) are present in the peripheral blood smear.
○There may be
  • Marked deficiency of serum beta-lipoprotein and cholesterol
  • Marked impairment of GI fat absorption
  • Low serum carotene levels (see p. 507)
  • Abnormal pattern of RBC phospholipids

Cerebellar Ataxia, Progressive, with Skin Telangiectasias (Louis-Bar's Syndrome)

(Autosomal recessive multisystem disease with cerebellar ataxia and oculocutaneous telangiectasia)
See also Table 11-22, p. 421.
Some patients have
  • Glucose intolerance.
  • Abnormal liver function tests.
  • Decreased or absent serum IgA and IgE causing recurrent pulmonary infections; IgM is present.
  • Increased serum AFP. See also Table 11-7, p. 355.

Cerebrovascular Accident (Nontraumatic)

Due To

Hemorrhage
  • Ruptured berry aneurysm (45% of patients)
  • Hypertension (15% of patients)
  • Angiomatous malformations (8% of patients)
  • Miscellaneous causes (e.g., brain tumor, blood dyscrasia)—infrequent
  • Undetermined cause (remainder of patients)
Occlusion (e.g., thrombosis, embolism, etc.) in 80% of patients
Especially if blood pressure is normal, always rule out ruptured berry aneurysm, hemorrhage into tumor, and angioma.

Berry Aneurysm

  • In early subarachnoid hemorrhage (<8 hrs after onset of symptoms), the test for occult blood may be positive before xanthochromia develops. After bloody spinal fluid occurs, WBC/RBC ratio may be higher in CSF than in peripheral blood.
  • Bloody CSF clears by tenth day in 40% of patients. CSF is persistently abnormal after 21 days in 15% of patients. ~5% of cerebrovascular episodes due to hemorrhage are wholly within the parenchyma and CSF findings are normal.

Embolism, Cerebral

Laboratory findings due to underlying causative disease
  • Bacterial endocarditis
  • Nonbacterial thrombotic vegetations on heart valves
  • Chronic rheumatic mitral stenosis with atrial thrombi
  • Mural thrombus due to underlying myocardial infarction
  • Myxoma of left atrium
  • Fat embolism in fracture of long bones
  • Air embolism in neck, chest, or cardiac surgery

Table 9-2. Differentiation between Bloody Cerebrospinal Fluid (CSF) Due to Subarachnoid Hemorrhage and Traumatic Lumbar Puncture

CSF Finding	Subarachnoid Hemorrhage	Traumatic Lumbar Puncture
CSF pressure	Often increased	Low
Blood in tubes for collecting CSF	Mixture with blood is uniform in all tubes	Earlier tubes more bloody than later tubes; RBC count decreases in later tubes
CSF clotting	No clots	Often clots
Xanthochromia	Present if >8–12 hrs since subarachnoid hemorrhage	Absent unless patient is icteric; may appear if CSF examination delayed ≥ 2 hrs
Immediate repeat of lumbar puncture at higher level	CSF same as initial puncture	CSF clear

CSF
- Usually findings are the same as in cerebral thrombosis.
- Hemorrhagic infarction develops in one-third of patients, usually producing slight xanthochromia several days later; some of these patients may have grossly bloody CSF (10,000 RBCs/cu mm).
- Septic embolism (e.g., bacterial endocarditis) may cause increased WBC (≤ 200/cu mm with variable lymphocytes and PMNs), increased RBC (≤ 1000/cu mm), slight xanthochromia, increased protein, normal glucose, and negative culture.

Hemorrhage, Cerebral

Increased WBC (15,000–20,000/cu mm); higher than in cerebral infarct (e.g., embolism, thrombosis)
Increased ESR
Urine
- Transient glycosuria
- Laboratory findings of concomitant renal disease
Laboratory findings due to other causes of intracerebral hemorrhage (e.g., leukemia, aplastic anemia, purpuras, hemophilias, anticoagulant therapy, SLE, polyarteritis nodosa)
CSF
- See Tables 9-1 and 9-2.
Laboratory findings due to other diseases that occur with increased frequency in association with berry aneurysm (e.g., coarctation of the aorta, polycystic kidneys, hypertension)

Thrombosis, Cerebral

Laboratory findings due to some diseases that may be causative
- Hematologic disorders (e.g., polycythemia, sickle cell disease, thrombotic thrombopenia, macroglobulinemia)
- Arterial disorders (e.g., polyarteritis nodosa, Takayasu's syndrome, dissecting aneurysm of aorta, syphilis, meningitis)
- Hypotension (e.g., myocardial infarction, shock)
CSF
- Protein may be normal or increased to ≤ 100 mg/dL.
- Cell count may be normal or ≥ 10 WBC/cu mm during first 48 hrs and rarely ≥ 2000 WBC/cu mm transiently on third day.

Cobalamin Deficiency Causing Neuropsychiatric Disorders

See pernicious anemia, p. 366.
More than 25% of patients may present with neuropsychiatric findings (e.g., paresthesias, sensory loss, ataxia and abnormal gait, mental or psychiatric disturbances) with some normal hematologic findings (e.g., Hct, MCV, WBC, platelet count, serum biliru-

bin, serum LD) and some abnormal findings (e.g., hypersegmentation of PMNs, macroovalocytes, mild megaloblastic bone marrow).
♦ Serum cobalamin and Schilling test results may occasionally be only borderline decreased or even normal.
♦ Increased serum methylmalonic acid and total homocysteine, which return to normal after cyanocobalamin therapy, confirm diagnosis.

Coma and Stupor

Due To

Poisons, drugs, or toxins
  • Sedatives (especially alcohol, barbiturates)
  • Enzyme inhibitors (especially salicylates, heavy metals, organic phosphates, cyanide)
  • Other (e.g., paraldehyde, methyl alcohol, ethylene glycol)
Cerebral disorders
  • Brain contusion, hemorrhage, infarction, seizure, or aneurysm
  • Brain mass (e.g., tumor, hematoma, abscess)
  • Subdural or epidural hematoma
  • Venous sinus occlusion
  • Hydrocephalus
  • Hypoxia
      Decreased blood O_2 content and tension (e.g., lung disease, high altitude)
      Decreased blood O_2 content with normal tension (e.g., anemia, carbon monoxide poisoning, methemoglobinemia)
  • Infection (e.g., meningitis, encephalitis)
Vascular abnormalities (e.g., subarachnoid hemorrhage, hypertensive encephalopathy, shock, AMI, aortic stenosis, Adams-Stokes syndrome, tachycardias)
Metabolic abnormalities
  • Acid-base imbalance (acidosis, alkalosis)
  • Electrolyte imbalance (increased or decreased sodium, potassium, calcium, magnesium)
  • Porphyrias
  • Aminoacidurias
  • Uremia
  • Hepatic encephalopathy
  • Other disorders (e.g., leukodystrophies, lipid storage diseases, Bassen-Kornzweig syndrome)
Nutritional deficiencies (e.g., vitamin B_{12}, thiamine, niacin, pyridoxine)
Endocrine
  • Pancreas (diabetic coma, hypoglycemia)
  • Thyroid (myxedema, thyrotoxicosis)
  • Adrenal gland (Addison's disease, Cushing's syndrome, pheochromocytoma)
  • Pituitary gland (panhypopituitarism)
  • Parathyroid (hypofunction or hyperfunction)
Psychogenic conditions that may mimic coma
  • Depression, catatonia
  • Malingering
  • Hysteria, conversion disorder

Dementia, Senile (Alzheimer-Pick Disease; Cerebral Atrophy)[1]

No abnormal laboratory findings are characteristic, but laboratory tests are useful to rule out other diseases that may resemble these syndromes but are amenable to therapy.
Recommended tests in all patients with new onset of dementia should include: CBC, urinalysis, electrolyte and blood chemistry panel, screening metabolic panel, serum vitamin B_{12} and folate measurements, thyroid function tests (chemistry panel screens for some other endocrine disorders), serologic test for syphilis.

---

[1]Larson EB, et al. Diagnostic tests in the evaluation of dementia. A prospective study of 200 elderly outpatients. *Arch Intern Med* 1986;146:1917.

In 200 patients >60 yrs with dementia, the causes were:

Alzheimer's type	74.5%
Due to drugs	9.5%
Alcohol related	4.0%
Hypothyroidism	3.0%
Multiple infarcts	1.5%
Hyperparathyroidism	1.0%
Hyponatremia	1.0%
Hypoglycemia	0.5%
Unknown cause	3.5%
Referred for dementia but diagnosis not confirmed	7.5%

Other newly recognized conditions were low serum iron, folate, or cobalamin (8%), urinary tract infection (2.5%). BUN was also useful for diagnosis.

Empyema, Subdural, Acute

CSF
- Cell count is increased to a few hundred, with predominance of PMNs.
- Protein is increased.
- Glucose is normal.
- Bacterial smears and cultures are negative.

WBC is usually increased ($\leq$ 25,000/cu mm).

Laboratory findings due to preceding diseases
- Ear, nose, and throat infections, especially acute sinusitis or otitis media
- Intracranial surgery

Streptococci are the most common organisms when preceding condition is sinusitis. S. aureus or gram-negative organisms are the most common organisms after trauma or surgery.

Encephalopathy, Hypertensive

Laboratory findings due to changes in other organ systems and to other conditions
- Cardiac
- Renal
- Endocrine
- Toxemia of pregnancy

Laboratory findings due to progressive changes that may occur (e.g., focal intracerebral hemorrhage)

CSF frequently shows increased pressure and protein $\leq$ 100 mg/dL.

Glomus Jugulare Tumor

CSF protein may be increased.

Guillain-Barré Syndrome

♦ CSF shows albumino-cytologic dissociation with normal cell count and increased protein (average 50–100 mg/dL). Protein increase parallels increasing clinical severity; increase may be prolonged. CSF may be normal at first.

Laboratory findings due to preceding disease may be present (e.g., acute infections of respiratory or GI tract [e.g., EBV, *Campylobacter*, VZV, *M. pneumoniae*, CMV, hepatitis, other viral, and rickettsial infections], Refsum's disease, immune disorders, endocrine disturbances, exposure to toxins, neoplasms).

Leukemic Involvement of CNS

Intracranial hemorrhage is principal cause of death in leukemia (may be intracerebral, subarachnoid, subdural)

More frequent when WBC is >100,000/cu mm and with rapid increase in WBC, especially in blastic crises

Platelet count frequently decreased.

Evidence of bleeding elsewhere
CSF findings of intracranial hemorrhage (see p. 278)
♦ Meningeal infiltration of leukemic cells
  • CNS is involved in 5% of patients with ALL at diagnosis and is the major site of relapse.
  • Meninges are involved in <30% of patients with malignant lymphoma; most prevalent in diffuse large cell ("histiocytic"), lymphoblastic, and immunoblastic leukemia; occurs in one-third to one-half of patients with Burkitt's lymphoma and 15–20% of patients with non-Hodgkin's lymphoma.
  • Hodgkin's disease seldom involves CNS.
  • Involvement by CLL, well-differentiated lymphocytic lymphoma, and plasmacytoid lymphomas is very rare.
CSF may show
  • Increased pressure and protein.
  • Glucose decreased to <50% of blood level.
♦ • Increased cells that are often not recognized as blast cells because of poor preservation and that may be identified by cytochemical, immunoenzymatic, immunofluorescent, and flow cytometry techniques.
♦ • Malignant cells are found in 60–80% of patients with meningeal involvement.
Complicating meningeal infection (e.g., various bacteria, opportunistic fungi)

Leukodystrophy, Metachromatic

(Rare lipidosis due to deficiency of arylsulfatase A; infantile and adult forms)
○Urine sediment may contain metachromatic lipids (from breakdown of myelin products).
CSF protein may be normal or increased ≤ 200 mg/dL.
♦ Biopsy of dental or sural nerve stained with cresyl violet showing accumulation of metachromatic sulfatide is diagnostic. Also increased in brain, kidney, liver.
♦ Conjunctival biopsy shows metachromatic inclusions within Schwann cells.
See Metabolic and Hereditary Diseases, Chapter 12, for other conditions that affect the CNS.

Lindau-von Hippel Disease (Hemangioblastomas of Retina and Cerebellum)

Laboratory findings due to associated conditions (e.g., polycythemia, pheochromocytomas, renal cell carcinoma, cysts of kidney and epididymis, benign cysts and nonfunctional neuroendocrine tumors of pancreas).

Meningitis, Aseptic

CSF
  • Protein is normal or slightly increased.
  • Increased cell count shows predominantly PMNs at first, mononuclear cells seen later.
  • Glucose is normal.
  • Bacterial cultures are negative.
If glucose levels are decreased, rule out TB, cryptococcosis, leukemia, lymphoma, metastatic carcinoma, sarcoidosis, drug induction.

Due To

Infections
  • Viral (especially poliomyelitis; infection with coxsackievirus, echovirus, HIV, EBV; lymphocytic choriomeningitis; and many others). Culture positive in ~40% of cases, especially with enteroviruses.
  • Bacterial (e.g., incompletely treated or very early bacterial meningitis, bacterial endocarditis, parameningeal infections such as brain abscess, epidural abscess, paranasal sinusitis).
  • Spirochetal (e.g., leptospirosis, syphilis, Lyme disease).
  • Tuberculous (CSF glucose levels may not be decreased until later stages).
  • Fungal (e.g., *Candida*, *Coccidioides*, *Cryptococcus*).

CNS

- Protozoan (e.g., *Toxoplasma gondii*).
- Amebic (e.g., *Naegleria*).
- Mycoplasmal.
- Rickettsial (e.g., Rocky Mountain spotted fever).
- Helminthic.

Chemical meningitis

Drug-induced meningitis (e.g., ibuprofen, trimethoprim, immune globulin, sulfadiazine, azathioprine, antineoplastic drugs)—onset usually within 24 hrs of drug ingestion

Systemic disorders
- Vasculitis, collagen vascular disease
- Sarcoid
- Behçet's syndrome
- Vogt-Koyanagi syndrome
- Harada syndrome
- Mollaret's meningitis (see p. 285)
- Neoplasm (e.g., leukemia, metastatic carcinoma)
- SLE

Meningitis, Bacterial

See Table 9-3.

♦ Bacteria can be identified in CSF in only 90% of patients.
- Culture is more reliable than Gram stain, although results of the stain offer a more immediate guide to therapy.
- Gram stain is positive in ~70% of patients; sensitivity is increased by cytocentrifugation of specimen. When Gram stain is positive, CSF is more likely to show decreased glucose, increased protein, and increased RBCs. 75% of cases are due to *N. meningitidis, S. pneumoniae, H. influenzae*.
- In *Listeria* meningitis, the Gram stain is usually negative and the cellular response is usually monocytic, which may cause this meningitis to be mistakenly diagnosed as due to virus, syphilis, TB, Lyme disease, etc.
- Gram stain of scrapings from petechial skin lesions demonstrate pathogen in ~70% of patients with meningococcemia; Gram stain of buffy coat of peripheral blood and, less often, peripheral blood smear may reveal this organism.

♦ Detection of bacterial antigen (rapid latex agglutination assay has largely replaced CIE) in CSF for *S. pneumoniae*, group B *Streptococcus* (*S. agalactiae*), *H. influenzae*, some strains of *N. meningitidis*.
- Not affected by previous antimicrobial therapy that might inhibit growth in culture.
- *H. influenzae* infection is now rare due to routine immunization of children.
- Not likely to be useful if CSF chemistry and cell count are normal unless patient is immunocompromised.
- False-positive for *H. influenza* may occur due to recent immunization; should not be performed if patient recently vaccinated.
- False-positive for group B *Streptococcus* antigen in urine is common due to its colonization of perineum.

♦ Blood culture is usually positive if patient has not received antibiotics.

Laboratory findings due to presence of infection (e.g., increased number of band forms, toxic granulations, Döhle's bodies, vacuolization of PMNs).

Laboratory findings due to preceding diseases
- Pneumonia, otitis media, sinusitis, skull fracture before pneumococcal meningitis
- *Neisseria* epidemics before this meningitis
- Bacterial endocarditis, septicemia, etc.
- *S. pneumoniae* in alcoholism, myeloma, sickle cell anemia, splenectomy, immunocompromised state
- *Cryptococcus* and *M. tuberculosis* in steroid therapy and immunocompromised state
- Gram-negative bacilli in immunocompromised state
- *H. influenzae* in splenectomy
- Lyme disease

Table 9-3. Etiology of Bacterial Meningitis by Age

	Newborns	Younger Than 1 Yr	1–5 Yrs	5–14 Yrs	Older Than 15 Yrs	Elderly
Most frequent	*Escherichia coli*	*Haemophilus influenzae*		*Neisseria meningitidis*	*Streptococcus pneumoniae*	*Streptococcus pneumoniae* *Neisseria meningitidis*
Common	*Klebsiella-Aerobacter* Beta-hemolytic streptococcus *Listeria monocytogenes* *Staphylococcus aureus*	*Neisseria meningitidis* *Streptococcus pneumoniae*		*Haemophilus influenzae* *Streptococcus pneumoniae*	*Neisseria meningitidis* *Staphylococcus aureus*	Gram-negative bacilli *Listeria monocytogenes*
Uncommon	Paracolon bacilli *Pseudomonas* species *Haemophilus influenzae*	*Pseudomonas* species *Staphylococcus aureus* Beta-hemolytic streptococcus *Escherichia coli*		Beta-hemolytic streptococcus	*Escherichia coli* *Pseudomonas* species	
Rare	*Neisseria meningitidis*	*Klebsiella-Aerobacter*; paracolons, various other gram-negative organisms			*Haemophilus influenzae*	

The frequency of different organisms may vary from year to year; in presence of epidemics, or by geographic location.
Occasionally more than one organism is recovered.
Haemophilus influenzae (almost always type b) causes most cases between 6 mos and 3 yrs of age but is unusual before 2 mos. Enteric bacteria are so rarely found in older children that, in their presence, immunologic defect or congenital dermal sinus should be ruled out. If surgery has not been performed and *Staphylococcus aureus* is present, congenital dermal sinus should be ruled out.
Gram stain of CSF should always be done in addition to culture because it provides a more immediate clue to the causative agent and the proper therapy and because the culture may be negative if the patient received antibiotics soon before the lumbar puncture. Cultures should also be obtained from blood and from petechial skin lesions if present. Gram stain of buffy coat of blood is often useful.
CSF glucose is very useful in differentiating bacterial from viral meningitis and is a good index to the severity of the infection, with a lower level in more severe infections.
Newborns with overwhelming pneumococcal infections may have no decrease in glucose or increase of cells.
CSF should be reexamined in 24 hrs as a guide to therapeutic response; a good response shows negative Gram–stained smear and culture, increased glucose, and a changing cell count from predominance of PMNs to predominance of mononuclear cells; total cell count and protein may show an initial rise. CSF should be reexamined when therapy is to be stopped; treatment should not be stopped unless CSF is normal except for slight increase of cells (≤ approximately 20 lymphocytes).

CNS

Laboratory findings due to complications (e.g., Waterhouse-Friderichsen syndrome, subdural effusion)

♦ Most frequent and important differential diagnosis is between acute bacterial meningitis and acute viral meningitis. The most useful test results that favor the diagnosis of acute bacterial meningitis rather than acute viral meningitis are[2,3]:
  • CSF positive by bacterial stain, culture, or antigen detection.
  • Decreased CSF glucose.
  • Decreased CSF/serum ratio of glucose (<0.25 in <1% of acute viral meningitis cases and 44% of acute bacterial meningitis cases), even if CSF glucose is normal.
  • Increased CSF protein >1.72 gm/L (1% of acute viral meningitis and 50% of acute bacterial meningitis cases).
  • CSF WBC >2000/cu mm in 38% of acute bacterial meningitis cases and PMN >1180/cu mm, but low counts do not rule out acute bacterial meningitis.
  • Peripheral WBC is useful only if WBC (>27,200/cu mm) and total PMN (>21,000/cu mm) counts are very high, which occurs in relatively few patients; leukopenia is common in infants and elderly patients.
  • Combination of findings can exclude acute viral meningitis and rule in acute bacterial meningitis, but none of them can establish the diagnosis of acute viral meningitis, and absence of these findings cannot exclude acute bacterial meningitis.

Meningitis, Chemical

(Due to injection of anesthetic, antibiotic, radiopaque dye, etc., or to rupture into CSF of contents of epidermoid tumor or craniopharyngioma)
CSF
  • Pleocytosis is mild to moderate, largely lymphocytic.
  • Protein shows variable increase.
  • Glucose is usually normal.

Meningitis, Chronic

(Symptoms for >4 wks)
CSF
  • WBC of 100–400 WBC/cu mm, preponderance of lymphocytes.
  • Glucose often decreased.
  • Protein is usually moderately or markedly increased.

Due To

Various infections
  • TB is most common cause.
  • Bacteria (e.g., Brucella).
  • Spirochetes (e.g., leptospirosis, syphilis, Lyme disease).
  • Fungus (e.g., *Candida*, *Coccidioides*, *Cryptococcus*).
  • Protozoa (e.g., *T. gondii*).
  • Ameba (e.g., *Naegleria*).
  • *Mycoplasma.*
  • *Rickettsia.*
  • Helminths.
Systemic disorders
  • Vasculitis, collagen vascular disease
  • Sarcoid
  • Neoplasm (e.g., leukemia, lymphoma, metastatic carcinoma)
  • Mollaret's meningitis (see p. 285)

[2]Spands A, Harrell FE, Durack DT. Differential diagnosis of acute meningitis. an analysis of the predictive value of initial observations. *JAMA* 1989;262:2700.
[3]Bailey EM, Domenico P, Cunha, BA. Bacterial or viral meningitis. *Postgrad Med* 1990;88:217.

Meningitis, Mollaret's

♦ Numerous recurrent episodes (2–7 days each) of aseptic meningitis occur over several years with symptom-free intervals in which mild leukopenia and eosinophilia are seen. Other organ systems are not involved. The patient frequently has a history of previous severe trauma with fractures and concussions.

CSF

♦ • During first 12–24 hrs may contain up to several thousand cells/cu mm, predominantly PMNs and 66% of a large type of mononuclear cell. The mononuclear cells (sometimes called "endothelial" cells) are of unknown origin and significance and are characterized by vague nuclear and cytoplasmic outline with rapid lysis, even while being counted in the hemocytometer chamber; they may be seen only as "ghosts" and are usually not detectable after the first day of illness. After the first 24 hrs, the PMNs disappear and are replaced by lymphocytes, which, in turn, rapidly disappear when the attack subsides.
• Protein may be increased ≤ 100 mg/dL.
• Glucose is normal or may be slightly decreased.

Meningitis, Tuberculous

See Chapter 15.

Meningitis/Encephalomyelitis, Acute Viral

For infectious, postvaccinal, postexanthematous, and postinfectious, encephalomyelitis/ meningitis see Chapter 15.

In the United States, HSV and rabies are most common endemic causes of encephalitis; outside of North America, Japanese B encephalitis is most common epidemic infection.

Postinfectious encephalomyelitis patients have an invariable, irreversible demyelinating syndrome; it is most commonly associated with varicella and URI (especially influenza) in the United States but measles is the most common cause worldwide.

Vaccination has reduced the incidence of acute and postinfectious encephalitis due to measles, mumps, rubella, and yellow fever.

Vaccination has greatly decreased incidence of poliomyelitis, but a few cases of vaccine-associated infections occur.

Coxsackievirus and echovirus usually cause benign aseptic meningitis.

CSF shows increased protein and lymphocytes.

Laboratory findings due to preceding condition (e.g., measles) are noted.

♦ PCR of CSF or fresh brain tissue for panel detection of HSV, VZV, enteroviruses, eastern equine encephalitis virus, St. Louis encephalitis virus, CMV, EBV, California serogroup viruses, and rabies (in saliva) makes 72-hr diagnosis possible on one sample and should replace culture, mouse inoculation, immunoassay, serology, and brain biopsy.

♦ Paired serum samples during acute and convalescent periods may show seroconversion or fourfold increase in specific antibody titers.

♦ ELISA to detect IgM in CSF is sensitive and specific for Japanese B encephalitis; IgM is usually present at hospitalization and almost always present by third day of illness.

♦ HSV can be cultured from CSF in 50–75% of patients with meningitis and <5% with encephalitis.

♦ Detection of HSV antigen in CSF is reported to be 80% sensitive and 90% specific if performed within 3 days of onset of illness. Brain biopsy is most sensitive and specific for HSV and its mimics.

♦ Brain biopsy is currently reserved for patients who do not respond to acyclovir therapy and have unknown abnormality on CT scan or magnetic resonance image (MRI).

♦ Brain biopsy is also required for diagnosis of progressive multifocal leukoencephalopathy.

Meningoencephalitis, Primary Amebic

(Due to free-living amebas—*Naegleria*)
Increased WBC, predominantly neutrophils
CSF findings

- Fluid may be cloudy, purulent, or sanguinopurulent.
- Protein is increased.
- Glucose is usually decreased; may be normal.
- Increased WBCs are chiefly PMNs. RBCs are frequently present also. Motile amebas are seen in hemocytometer chamber or on wet mount using phase or diminished light.
- ◆ • Amebas are seen on Wright's, Giemsa, hematoxylin-eosin stains. Gram stain and cultures are negative for bacteria and fungi.
- ◆ • Culture of tissue or CSF on agar or cell culture demonstrates organisms.
- ◆ • Electron microscopy allows precise classification of amebas.
- ◆ • Indirect immunofluorescent antibody (IFA) and immunoperoxidase assays are reliable methods to identify amebas in tissue sections.

Multiple Sclerosis (MS)

◆ Diagnosis should not be made on the basis of CSF findings unless there are multiple clinical lesions over time and in anatomic location.

No changes of diagnostic value yielded by peripheral blood studies or routine CSF tests.
- CSF WBC is slightly elevated in ~25% of patients but usually <20 mononuclear cells/cu mm; >25 cells/cu mm in <1% of cases. >50 cells/cu mm should cast doubt on diagnosis.
- Albumin, glucose, and pressure are normal.

CSF changes are found in >90% of MS patients.

CSF total protein
- May be mildly increased in ~25% of patients; not very useful test by itself.
- Decreased values and values >100 mg/dL should cast doubt on diagnosis.
- CSF gamma globulin is increased in 60–75% of patients regardless of whether the total CSF protein is increased. Gamma globulin ≥ 12% of CSF total protein is abnormal if no corresponding increase in serum gamma globulin is seen; but may also be increased in other CNS disorders (e.g., syphilis, subacute panencephalitis, meningeal carcinomatosis) and may also be increased when serum electrophoresis is abnormal due to non-CNS diseases (e.g., RA, sarcoidosis, cirrhosis, myxedema, multiple myeloma).

CSF IgG concentration
- ◆ • Increased (reference range <4.0 mg/dL) in ~70% of cases, often when total protein is normal.
- ◆ • Increase in *production* of IgG is expressed as ratio of CSF to serum albumin to rule out increased IgG due to disruption of blood–brain barrier (see Table 9-4).
- CSF IgG does not correlate with duration, activity, or course of MS.
- May also be increased in patients with other inflammatory demyelinating diseases (e.g., neurosyphilis, acute Guillain-Barré syndrome), in 5–15% of patients with miscellaneous neurologic diseases, and in a few normal persons; recent myelography is said to invalidate the test.

◆ *CSF IgG/albumin ratio* indicates in situ production of IgG. Abnormal in 90% of MS patients and 18% of non–MS neurologic patients.

◆ *CSF IgG synthesis rate* is increased in 90% of MS patients and 4% of non–MS patients.

◆ *IgG index* indicates IgG synthesis in CNS. Occurs in 90% of MS patients; may also occur in other neurologic diseases (e.g., meningitis). CSF IgM and IgA may also be increased but are not useful for diagnosis.

Albumin index

Increase

Indicates CSF contaminated with blood (e.g., traumatic tap) or increased permeability of blood–brain barrier (e.g., aged persons, obstruction of CSF circulation, diabetes mellitus, SLE of CNS, Guillain-Barré syndrome, polyneuropathy, cervical spondylosis).

Use

To prevent misinterpretation of falsely increased CSF IgG concentrations
◆ *Oligoclonal proteins* (due to abnormal gamma globulins) by high-voltage electrophoresis or isoelectric focusing of concentrated CSF shows discrete bands.

Table 9-4. Formulas for Central Nervous System Immunoglobulin G (IgG) Synthesis

$$\text{Albumin index} = \frac{\text{CSF albumin}}{\text{Serum albumin}} \times 1000 \text{ (reference range} = 0.09\text{--}0.25)$$

$$\text{IgG/albumin ratio} = \frac{\text{CSF IgG}}{\text{CSF albumin}} \text{ (reference range} < 9)$$

$$\text{IgG synthesis rate} = \left(\text{CSF IgG} - \frac{\text{Serum IgG}}{369}\right) - \left(\text{CSF albumin} - \frac{\text{Serum albumin}}{230}\right) \times$$

$$\left(\frac{0.43 \text{ Serum IgG}}{\text{Serum albumin}}\right) \text{ (reference range} = 0\text{--}8.0 \text{ mg/day)}$$

$$\text{IgG index} = \frac{\text{CSF IgG} \div \text{Serum IgG}}{\text{CSF albumin} \div \text{Serum albumin}} \text{ (reference range} = 0.28\text{--}0.66)$$

Note: All serum and CSF analytes drawn simultaneously, reported in mg/dL.

CNS

- Should always be performed on paired CSF and serum samples.
- Found in 85–95% of patients with definite MS and 30–40% with possible MS (specificity = 79%); it is the most sensitive marker of MS.
- Positive results also occur in ≤ 10% of patients with noninflammatory neurologic disease (e.g., meningeal carcinomatosis, cerebral infarction) and ≤ 40% of patients with inflammatory CNS disorders (e.g., neurosyphilis, viral encephalitis, progressive rubella encephalitis, subacute sclerosing panencephalitis, bacterial meningitis, toxoplasmosis, cryptococcal meningitis, inflammatory neuropathies, trypanosomiasis).
- Oligoclonal bands in serum may occur in leukemias, lymphomas, some infections and inflammatory diseases, immune disorders.
- Not known to correlate with severity, duration, or course of MS.
- Persists during remission.
- During steroid treatment, prevalence of oligoclonal bands and other gamma globulin abnormalities may be reduced by 30–50%.
- 90% of MS patients have oligoclonal bands in CSF, at least two of which are not present in simultaneously examined serum.
- A few patients with definite multiple sclerosis may have normal CSF immunoglobulins and lack oligoclonal bands.

♦ *Myelin basic protein*
- Indicates recent myelin destruction; it is increased in 70–90% of MS patients during an acute exacerbation and usually returns to normal within 2 wks.
- Useful for following course of MS but not for screening.
- May be helpful very early in course of MS before oligoclonal bands have appeared or in ~10% of patients who do not develop these bands.
- It is frequently increased in other causes of demyelination and tissue destruction (e.g., meningoencephalitis, leukodystrophies, metabolic encephalopathies, SLE of CNS, brain tumor, head trauma, amyotrophic lateral sclerosis, cranial irradiation and intrathecal chemotherapy, 45% of patients with recent stroke) and other disorders (e.g., diabetes mellitus, chronic renal failure, vasculitis, carcinoma of vasculitis, immune complex diseases, pancreas).
- Falsely increased by contamination with blood.
- Increased association with certain histocompatibility antigens (e.g., whites with B7 and Dw2 antigen).

Myelitis

CSF may be normal or may show increased protein and cells (20–1000/cu mm—lymphocytes and mononuclear cells).

Laboratory findings due to causative condition (e.g., poliomyelitis, herpes zoster, TB, syphilis, parasitosis, abscess, multiple sclerosis, postvaccinal myelitis)

Neuritis/Neuropathy, Multiple

Laboratory findings due to causative disease
Infections, e.g.,
- EBV (mononucleosis associated: CSF shows increased protein and up to several hundred mononuclear cells).
- Diphtheria: CSF protein is 50–200 mg/dL.
- Lyme disease.
- HIV-1.
- Hepatitis.
- Leprosy.

Postvaccinal effect
Metabolic conditions (e.g., pellagra, beriberi, combined systemic disease, pregnancy, porphyria)—CSF usually normal. In ~70% of patients with diabetic neuropathy, CSF protein is increased to >200 mg/dL.
Uremia—CSF protein is 50–200 mg/dL; occurs in a few cases of chronic uremia.
Collagen disease
- Polyarteritis nodosa—CSF usually normal; nerve involvement in 10% of patients
- SLE

Neoplasm (leukemia, multiple myeloma, carcinoma)—CSF protein often increased; may be associated with an occult primary neoplastic lesion outside CNS.
Amyloidosis
Sarcoidosis
Toxic conditions due to drugs and chemicals (especially lead, arsenic, etc.)
Alcoholism—CSF usually normal
Bassen-Kornzweig syndrome
Refsum's disease
Chédiak-Higashi syndrome
Guillain-Barré syndrome

Cranial Nerve, Multiple

Laboratory findings due to causative conditions
- Trauma
- Aneurysms
- Tumors (e.g., meningioma, neurofibroma, carcinoma, cholesteatoma, chordoma)
- Infections (e.g., herpes zoster)
- Benign polyneuritis associated with cervical lymph node tuberculosis or sarcoidosis

Neuritis of One Nerve or Plexus

Laboratory findings due to causative disease
- Infections (e.g., diphtheria, herpes zoster, leprosy)
- Sarcoidosis
- Tumor (leukemia, lymphoma, carcinomas)—may find tumor cells in CSF.
- Serum sickness
- Bell's palsy
- Idiopathic

Facial Palsy, Peripheral Acute

Laboratory findings due to causative disease
- Idiopathic (Bell's palsy)—occasional slight increase in cells in CSF
- Infection
  Viral (e.g., VZV, HSV, HIV, EBV infection, poliomyelitis, mumps, rubella)
  Bacterial (e.g., Lyme disease, syphilis, leprosy, diphtheria, cat-scratch disease, *M. pneumoniae* infection)
  Parasitic (e.g., malaria)
  Meningitis
  Encephalitis
  Local inflammation (otitis media, mastoiditis, osteomyelitis, petrositis)
- Trauma
- Tumor (acoustic neuromas, tumors invading the temporal bone)
- Granulomatous (e.g., sarcoidosis) and connective tissue diseases

- Diabetes mellitus
- Hypothyroidism
- Uremia
- Drug reaction
- Postvaccinal effect
- Paget's disease of bone
- Melkersson-Rosenthal syndrome

Lyme disease and Guillain-Barré syndrome may produce bilateral palsy.

Hemianopsia, Bitemporal

Laboratory findings due to causative disease
- Usually pituitary adenoma
- Also metastatic tumor, sarcoidosis, Hand-Schuller-Christian disease, meningioma of sella, and aneurysm of circle of Willis

Ophthalmoplegia

Laboratory findings due to causative disease
- Diabetes mellitus
- Myasthenia gravis
- Hyperthyroid exophthalmos

Trigeminal Neuralgia (Tic Douloureux)

Laboratory findings due to causative disease
- Usually idiopathic.
- May also stem from multiple sclerosis or herpes zoster.

Retrobulbar Neuropathy

CSF is normal or may show increased protein and ≤ 200/cu mm lymphocytes.
◯*Multiple sclerosis ultimately develops in 75% of these patients.*

Prion Diseases

(Due to proteinaceous infectious particles that do not use nucleic acids to mediate transmission)

Causes

Creutzfeldt-Jakob disease, variant Creutzfeldt-Jakob disease, kuru, Gerstmann-Sträussler-Scheinker disease, fatal familial insomnia
Scrapie (sheep)
Mad cow disease (bovine spongiform degeneration)
♦ Diagnosis based on biopsy showing pathologic changes and demonstration of prions or a known prion gene mutation.

Pseudotumor Cerebri

(Benign intracranial hypertension with neurologic complex of headache and papilledema without mass lesion or ventricular obstruction)
CSF normal except for increased pressure
Laboratory findings due to associated conditions (only obesity has been reported consistently) (e.g., Addison's disease, infection, metabolic conditions [acute hypocalcemia and other electrolyte disturbances, empty sella syndrome, pregnancy], drugs [psychotherapeutic drugs, sex hormones and oral contraceptives, corticosteroid administration, usually after reduction of dosage or change to different preparation], immune diseases [SLE, polyarteritis nodosa, serum sickness], other conditions [sarcoidosis, Guillain-Barré syndrome, head trauma, various anemias])

Refsum's Disease

(Rare hereditary recessive lipidosis of the nervous system with retinitis pigmentosa, peripheral neuropathy, cerebellar ataxia, nerve deafness, and ichthyosis)

CSF shows albuminocytologic dissociation (normal cell count with protein usually increased to 100–700 mg/dL).

Retardation, Mental

Laboratory findings due to underlying causative condition (see appropriate separate sections)

Prenatal

Infections (e.g., syphilis, rubella, toxoplasmosis, CMV infection)
Metabolic abnormalities (e.g., diabetes mellitus, eclampsia, placental dysfunction)
Chromosomal disorders (e.g., Down syndrome, trisomy 18, cri du chat syndrome, Klinefelter's syndrome)
Metabolic abnormalities
* Amino acid metabolism (e.g., phenylketonuria, maple syrup urine disease, hemocystinuria, cystathioninuria, hyperglycemia, argininosuccinicaciduria, citrullinemia, histidinemia, hyperprolinemia, oasthouse urine disease, Hartnup's disease, Joseph's syndrome, familial iminoglycinuria)
* Lipid metabolism (e.g., Batten disease, Tay-Sachs disease, Niemann-Pick disease, abetalipoproteinemia, Refsum's disease, metachromatic leukodystrophy)
* Carbohydrate metabolism (e.g., galactosemia, mucopolysaccharidoses)
* Purine metabolism (e.g., Lesch-Nyhan syndrome, hereditary orotic aciduria)
* Mineral metabolism (e.g., idiopathic hypercalcemia, pseudohypoparathyroidism and pseudopseudohypoparathyroidism)
* Other syndromes (e.g., tuberous sclerosis, Louis-Bar's syndrome)

Perinatal

Kernicterus
Prematurity
Anoxia
Trauma

Postnatal

Poisoning (e.g., lead, arsenic, carbon monoxide)
Infections (e.g., meningitis, encephalitis)
Metabolic abnormalities (e.g., hypoglycemia)
Postvaccinal encephalitis
Cerebrovascular accidents
Trauma

Reye's Syndrome

(Acute noninflammatory encephalopathy with fatty changes in liver and kidney and rarely in heart and pancreas. Occurs typically in child recovering from influenza, varicella, or nonspecific viral illness and is associated with use of aspirin.)

◆*Diagnostic Criteria*

CSF shows <8 WBC/cu mm.
Serum AST, ALT, or ammonia ≥ 3× ULN
Fatty liver seen histologically.
See Hepatic Failure, Acute (p. 221).

Seizures That May Be Accompanied by Laboratory Abnormalities

Associated Conditions

Neoplasms
Circulatory disorders (e.g., thrombosis, hemorrhage, embolism, hypertensive encephalopathy, vascular malformations)

Hematologic disorders (e.g., sickle cell anemia, leukemia)
Metabolic abnormalities
  • Carbohydrate metabolism (e.g., hypoglycemia, glycogen storage disease)
  • Amino acid metabolism (e.g., phenylketonuria, maple syrup urine disease)
  • Lipid metabolism (e.g., leukodystrophies, lipidoses)
  • Electrolyte balance (e.g., decreased sodium, calcium, and magnesium, increased sodium)
  • Other disorders (e.g., porphyria)
Allergic disorders (e.g., drug reaction, postvaccinal)
Infections
  • Meningitis, encephalitis
  • Postinfectious encephalitis (e.g., measles, mumps)
  • Fetal exposure (e.g., rubella, measles, mumps)
Degenerative brain diseases

Spinal Cord, Infarction

CSF changes same as in cerebral hemorrhage or infarction.
Laboratory findings due to causative condition
  • Polyarteritis nodosa
  • Dissecting aneurysm of aorta
  • Arteriosclerosis of aorta with thrombus formation
  • Iatrogenic causes (e.g., aortic arteriography, clamping of aorta during cardiac surgery)

Spinal Cord Tumor

♦ CSF protein is increased. It may be very high and associated with xanthochromia when a block of the subarachnoid space is present.
With complete block, for cord tumors located at lower levels, protein concentration is higher.
See Table 9-2.

Spondylosis, Cervical

CSF shows increased protein in some cases.

Thrombophlebitis, Cavernous Sinus

CSF is usually normal unless associated subdural empyema or meningitis is present, or it may show increased protein and WBC with normal glucose, or it may be hemorrhagic. Mucormycosis may cause this clinical appearance in diabetic patients.
Laboratory findings due to preceding infections, complications (e.g., meningitis, brain abscess), or other causes of venous thromboses (e.g., sickle cell disease, polycythemia, dehydration).

Trauma, Head

Laboratory findings due to single or various combinations of brain injuries
  • Contusion, laceration, subdural hemorrhage, extradural hemorrhage, subarachnoid hemorrhage
Laboratory findings due to complications (e.g., pneumonia, meningitis)
In possible skull fractures,
  ♦ • CSF transferrin shows a double band but only a single transferrin band is seen in other fluids (serum, nasal secretions, saliva, tears, lymph).
  ♦ • If enough (100 µL) fluid can be obtained to perform immunofixation, IgM is 5× higher, prealbumin is 12× higher, and transferrin is 2× higher in CSF than in serum.
  • The suggestion has been made that nasal secretions may be differentiated from CSF by absence of glucose (measured using test tapes or tablets) in nasal secretions, but this is not reliable because nasal secretions may normally contain glucose.

Hemorrhage, Acute Epidural

CSF is usually under increased pressure; it is clear unless associated cerebral contusion, laceration, or subarachnoid hemorrhage is present.

Hematoma, Subdural

CSF findings are variable—clear, bloody, or xanthochromic, depending on recent or old associated injuries (e.g., contusion, laceration).

Chronic subdural hematoma fluid is usually xanthochromic; protein content is 300–2000 mg/dL.

Anemia is often present in infants.

Tuberculoma of Brain

CSF shows increased protein with small number of cells. The tuberculoma may be transformed into TB meningitis with increased protein and cells (50–300/cu mm), and decreased glucose.

Laboratory findings due to TB elsewhere.

Tumor of Brain

CSF

- CSF is clear but is occasionally xanthochromic or bloody if there is hemorrhage into the tumor.
- WBC may be increased ≤ 150 cells/cu mm in 75% of patients; normal in others.
- Protein is usually increased. *Protein is particularly increased with meningioma of the olfactory groove and with acoustic neuroma.*
- ♦ • Tumor cells may be demonstrable in 20–40% of patients with all types of solid tumors, but failure to find malignant cells does not exclude meningeal neoplasm.
- Glucose may be decreased if cells are present.
- Brain stem gliomas, which are characteristically found in childhood, are usually associated with normal CSF.
- Usually normal in diencephalic syndrome of infants due to glioma of hypothalamus.

Laboratory findings due to underlying causative disease (e.g., primary brain tumors, metastatic tumors, leukemias and lymphomas, infections [tuberculoma, schistosomiasis, cryptococcosis, hydatid cyst], pituitary adenomas [CSF protein and pressure usually normal])

Laboratory findings due to associated genetic conditions (e.g., tuberous sclerosis, neurofibromatosis, Turcot's syndrome)

Von Recklinghausen's Disease (Multiple Neurofibromas)

CSF findings of brain tumor if acoustic neuroma occurs.

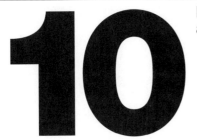

Musculoskeletal and Joint Diseases

Laboratory Tests for Skeletal Muscle Diseases

Creatine and Creatinine

Increased blood creatinine, decreased creatinine excretion, increased creatine excretion

Occurs In

Progressive muscular dystrophy
Decreased muscle mass in
- Neurogenic atrophy
- Polymyositis
- Addison's disease
- Hyperthyroidism
- Male eunuchoidism

Creatine Tolerance Test

(Ingestion of 1–3 gm creatine)
Normal: Creatine is not increased in blood or urine.
Decreased muscle mass: Blood and urine creatine increases in
- Neurogenic atrophy
- Addison's disease
- Male eunuchoidism
- Polymyositis
- Hyperthyroidism
- Other disorders

Enzymes (Serum) in Diseases of Muscle[1]

See Table 10-1.
Creatine kinase (CK) is the test of choice. It is more specific and sensitive than AST and LD and more discriminating than aldolase, but AST is more significantly associated with inflammatory myopathy and more useful in these cases. (See Chapter 3.)

Increased In

Polymyositis (see p. 301)
Muscular dystrophy (see pp. 295, 298)
Myotonic dystrophy (see p. 298)
Some metabolic disorders (see p. 300)
Malignant hyperthermia (see p. 299)
Prolonged exercise; peak 24 hrs after extreme exercise (e.g., marathon); smaller increases in well-conditioned atheletes

[1]Rosalki SB. Serum enzymes in diseases of skeletal muscle. *Clin Lab Med* 1989;9:767.

Table 10-1. Increased Serum Enzyme Levels in Muscle Diseases

	Muscular Dystrophy							Myotonic Dystrophy	Polymyositis
	Duchenne's		Limb–Girdle		Facioscapulohumeral				
Enzyme	Frequency (%)	Amplitude	Frequency (%)	Amplitude	Frequency (%)	Amplitude		Frequency (%)	Frequency (%)
CK	>95	65	75	25	80	5		50	70
ALD	90	9	25	3	30	2		20	75
AST	90	4	25	2	25	1.5		15	25
LD	90	4	15	1.5	10	1		10	25

Frequency = average percentage of patients with increased serum enzyme level when blood is taken at optimal time. Amplitude = average number of times normal level that serum level is increased.

Normal In

Scleroderma
Acrosclerosis
Discoid LE
Muscle atrophy of neurologic origin (e.g., old poliomyelitis, polyneuritis)
Hyperthyroid myopathy

Decreased In

RA (approximately two-thirds of patients)

Skeletal Muscle Disorders That May Cause Increased Serum CK-MB

Drugs (e.g., alcohol, cocaine, halothane [malignant hyperthermia], ipecac)
Dermatomyositis/polymyositis
Muscular dystrophy (Duchenne's, Becker's)
Exercise myopathy; slight-to-significant increases in 14–100% of persons after extreme
    exercise (e.g., marathons); smaller increases in well-conditioned athletes
Familial hypokalemic periodic paralysis
Endocrine (e.g., hypothyroid, hypoparathyroid, acromegaly; hypothyroidism rarely increases CK-MB
    ≤ 6% of total)
Rhabdomyolysis
Infections
  • Viral (e.g., HIV, EBV, influenza virus, picornaviruses, coxsackievirus, echovirus,
    adenoviruses)
  • Bacterial (e.g., *Staphylococcus*, *Streptococcus*, *Clostridium*, *Borrelia*)
  • Fungal
  • Parasitic (e.g., trichinosis, toxoplasmosis, schistosomiasis, cysticercosis)
Skeletal muscle trauma (severe)

Myoglobinemia and Myoglobinuria

See pp. 99, 124.

Diseases of Skeletal Muscles

Adynamia Episodica Hereditaria (Gamstorp's Disease)

♦ Transient increase in serum potassium occurs during the attack; attack is induced
    by administration of potassium.
Urine potassium excretion is unchanged before or during the attack.

Dystrophy, Muscular

(Genetic primary myopathies)
See Table 10-2 and Fig. 10-1.
♦ Serum enzymes (CK is most useful) are increased, especially in
  • Young patients. Highest levels (≤ 50× normal) are found at onset of disease in
    infancy or childhood, with gradual return to normal.
  • The more rapidly progressive dystrophies (such as the Duchenne type). They may be
    slightly or inconsistently increased in the limb-girdle and facioscapulohumeral types.
  • The active early phase. Increased levels are not constant and are affected by patient's
    age and duration of disease. Enzymes may be increased before disease is clinically
    evident. Elevated serum enzyme levels are not affected by steroid therapy.
Preclinical diagnosis of Duchenne's and Becker's dystrophies in families with history
    of disease or for screening.
  Serum CK is always increased in affected children (5–100× ULN of adults) to peak by
    2 yrs of age; then begins to fall as disease becomes manifest. Persistent normal CK
    virtually rules out this diagnosis. Begin testing at 2–3 mos of age. (Note: Normal
    children have very high CK levels during first few days, which fall to 3× ULN by
    fourth day and fall to 2–3× adult level during first month of life; levels remain
    higher than adult levels during first 2 yrs.) Neonatal screening that is positive with

Table 10-2. Laboratory Findings in the Differential Diagnosis of Some Muscle Diseases

Disease	Complete Blood Cell Count	ESR	Thyroid Function Tests	Percentage of Patients with Increase in Various Serum Enzyme Levels	Muscle Biopsy	Comment
Myasthenia gravis	N	N	N	N	Lymphorrhages	Cancer of lung should always be ruled out; high frequency of associated diabetes mellitus, especially in older patients Serum electrolytes N
Polymyositis	Total eosinophil count frequently I	Moderately to markedly I; occasionally N	N	CK in 65%; levels may vary greatly and become N with steroid therapy; marked increase may occur in children LD in 25%, AST in 25%	Necrosis of muscle with phagocytosis of muscle fibers; infiltration of inflammatory cells	Associated cancer in ≤17% of cases (especially lung; also breast) Serum alpha$_2$ and gamma globulins may be I
Muscular dystrophy	N	N	N	In active phase, CK in 50%, LD in 10%, AST in 15%	Various degenerative changes in muscle; late muscle atrophy; no cellular infiltration	

N = normal; I = increased.

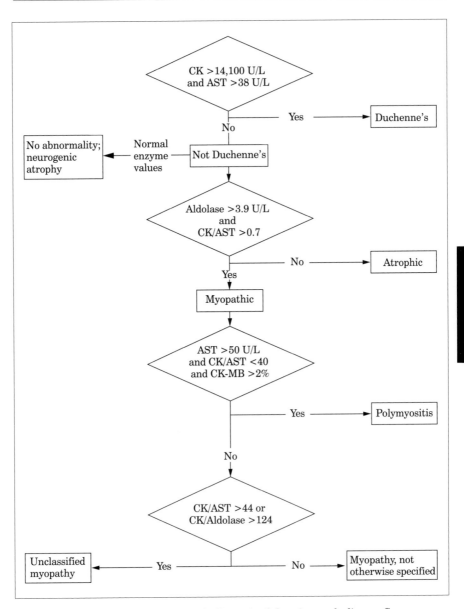

Fig. 10-1. Algorithm for serum enzymatic diagnosis of chronic muscle disease. Serum enzymes are not useful diagnostically in patients receiving immunosuppressive therapy in which the cause of muscle weakness is uncertain and muscle biopsy is required. (From Hood D, Van Lente F, Estes M. Serum enzyme alterations in chronic muscle disease: a biopsy-based diagnostic assessment. *Am J Clin Pathol* 1991;95:402.)

whole blood should be confirmed with serum. CK is >3× ULN for age in all boys with Duchenne's dystrophy and >2× ULN in those with Becker's dystrophy. Sex-linked dystrophy is virtually the only cause of high values in normal neonates. High values persist in patients with dystrophy but not in those with false-positive results. Neonatal screening of girls has been discontinued. Prenatal screening at 18–20 wks

MUSCULOSKEL

of gestation by placental aspiration of fetal blood has been abandoned due to false-negative and false-positive results.

Clinical diagnosis.

CK is increased in almost all patients with Duchenne's dystrophy (average 30× ULN) and Becker's dystrophy (average 10× ULN). Diagnosis is in doubt if CK is normal. Highest levels occur in young patients and decrease with age so that level is ~50% less at 7 yrs of age; levels usually consistently exceed 5× ULN but in terminal cases may decline further. Except for polymyositis, CK is normal or <5× ULN in other myopathies and neurogenic atrophy. CK-MB of up to 10% of total is sometimes seen in Becker's and limb-girdle dystrophies. In Duchenne's dystrophy CK-MB is increased (10–15% of total) in 60–90% of patients; CK-BB may be slightly increased; CK-MM is chief fraction. CK-MB may be slightly increased (usually <4%) in carriers with increased total CK.

Serum aldolase is increased in ~20% of patients.

Serum LD is increased in ~10% of patients. AST is increased in ~15% of patients.

Identify female carriers.

CK is increased in carriers with two affected sons or one affected son and one affected male relative in ~70% of cases of Duchenne's dystrophy and 50% of cases of Becker's dystrophy. Highest levels and greatest frequency occur in younger carriers; may only be present during childhood and not in later life. Levels may be up to 10× ULN but usually <3× ULN; average = 1.5× ULN. Values overlap with those of normal females; therefore, special precautions are needed: draw blood after normal activity in afternoon or evening but not after vigorous or prolonged exercise or IM injections or during pregnancy; recheck three times at weekly intervals; values are higher in blacks than in whites.

◆ Dystrophin protein determined by Western blot on punch biopsy of muscle is absent in Duchenne's dystrophy and decreased or abnormally formed in Becker's dystrophy.

◆ Immunofluorescence performed on open biopsy specimen of muscle is used to confirm Western blot results in males or to diagnose females with suspected dystrophinopathy.

◆ Recombinant DNA technology (Southern blot and PCR) allows
  • Prenatal diagnosis by chorionic villous sampling at 12th week of gestation
  • Diagnosis of carriers
  • Diagnosis and differential diagnosis (e.g., differentiation from limb-girdle dystrophy)

Muscle biopsy specimen shows muscle atrophy but no cellular infiltration.

Urine creatine is increased; urine creatinine is decreased. These changes are less marked in limb-girdle and facioscapulohumeral dystrophies than in Duchenne's dystrophy.

ESR is usually normal.

Thyroid function tests are normal.

Laboratory findings due to myocardial damage in most female carriers older than age 16 yrs.

Limb-Girdle Dystrophy

(Heterogeneous group of disorders in both sexes; autosomal recessive disorder that begins in second decade and progresses to disability by 30 yrs of age and death by 50 yrs of age)

Serum CK is increased in 70% of patients to average of 10× ULN. Not useful to detect carriers. Not useful to distinguish it from other autosomal recessive forms of dystrophy, myopathy, or neurologic disorders (e.g., hereditary proximal spinal muscular atrophy).

Facioscapulohumeral Dystrophy

(Begins in late adolescence; normal life span)

Serum CK is increased in 75% of patients to average 3× ULN. Frequently normal by 50 yrs of age.

Dystrophy, Myotonic

(Autosomal dominant disorder that presents in adolescence)

Serum CK is increased in 50% of patients to average of 3× ULN.

Increased creatine in urine may occur irregularly.

Findings due to atrophy of testicle and androgenic deficiency are noted.

Urine 17-KS are decreased.

Thyroid function may be decreased.

Eosinophilia-Myalgia Syndrome

(Associated with ingestion of L-tryptophan; patient may also have arthralgias, fatigue, fever, edema, and skin, lung, and neurologic changes.)

♦ *Diagnostic Criteria*

- Eosinophil count >1000/cu mm.
- Muscle biopsy specimen shows inflammation.
- No evidence of trichinosis on biopsy or serologic tests.
- Absence of infection, neoplasm, or primary connective tissue disease that could cause myalgia.
- Generalized myalgia sufficiently severe to impair daily activity.

Moderate increase of serum aldolase and LD but serum CK shows minimal or no increase.
Mild to moderate increase of AST, ALT, GGT.
ESR is normal or increased.
CRP, serum globulin, serum protein electrophoresis, IgE are normal.

Hyperthermia, Malignant[2]

(Rare autosomal dominant syndrome triggered by various inhalational and local anesthetic agents, muscle relaxants [e.g., succinylcholine, tubocurarine], and various types of stress causing hyperthermia, muscle rigidity, and 70% fatality)

Due To

Excess heat production
- Exertional
- Heat stroke
- Malignant hyperthermia of anesthesia
- Neuroleptic malignant syndrome (in ~0.2% of patients who receive various phenothiazines, butyrophenones, or thioxanthenes; most often haloperidol)
- Lethal catatonia
- Thyrotoxicosis
- Pheochromocytoma
- Drugs (e.g., salicylate intoxication, cocaine, amphetamines)
- Delirium tremens
- Status epilepticus
- Generalized tetanus

Decreased heat dissipation
- Heat stroke
- Dehydration
- Anticholinergic agents
- Autonomic dysfunction
- Extensive occlusive dressings
- Neuroleptic malignant syndrome

Disorders of hypothalamic function
- Encephalitis
- Cerebrovascular accidents
- Trauma
- Neuroleptic malignant syndrome
- Granulomatous lesions (e.g., sarcoidosis, infections)

♦ Combined metabolic and respiratory acidosis is the most consistent abnormality and is diagnostic in the presence of muscle rigidity or rising temperature. pH is often <7.2, base excess is > –10, hypoxia is present, and arterial pCO_2 is 70–120 mm Hg. *Immediate* arterial blood gas analysis should be performed.

♦ Increased serum potassium (>7 mEq/L) and calcium initially with below-normal values later.

♦ Serum CK, LD, and AST are markedly increased with peak in 24–48 hrs after surgery; CK is often 20,000–100,000 U/L.

[2]Simon HB. Hyperthermia. *N Engl J Med* 1993;329:483.

♦ Myoglobinemia and myoglobinuria due to rhabdomyolysis may be present early. Oliguria with acute renal shutdown may occur later.

Coagulopathy, including DIC, may occur later but is infrequent.

Resting serum CK may be elevated in relatives. However, the sensitivity and specificity of serum CK are too low to warrant its use for diagnosis or screening and should not be used to diagnose susceptibility to malignant hyperthermia.

♦ Diagnosis confirmed by in vitro exposure of biopsied skeletal muscle to incremental doses of caffeine and halothane. Test is done at very few laboratories.

Muscle, Metabolic Diseases

Endocrine
- Hypothyroidism (rarely associated with myotonia)
    Increased serum CK in 60–80% of patients to average 4–8× ULN; becomes normal 4–6 wks after treatment. CK-MB is rarely increased ≤ 6% of total.
    Decreased urine creatine
    Increased creatine tolerance
    Other serum enzyme levels are normal.
- Hyperthyroidism
    Normal serum enzyme levels
    Increased urine creatine
    Decreased creatine tolerance
    Normal muscle biopsy findings
    Causes some cases of hypokalemic periodic paralysis.
- Acromegaly
    Serum CK may be increased to average of 2× ULN.
- Cushing's syndrome and adrenal corticosteroid therapy
    Increased serum enzymes—uncommon and may be due to the primary disease.
    Muscle biopsy—degenerative and regenerative changes in scattered muscle fibers; no inflammatory cell infiltration
    Increased urine creatine
- Other endocrinopathies (e.g., hypoadrenalism, hyperparathyroidism)

Inherited metabolic myopathies (see Chapter 12)
- Glycogen storage diseases (types II, III, V, VII)
- Disordered lipid metabolism (muscle carnitine deficiency)

Myasthenia Gravis (MG)

See Table 10-2.
♦ Acetylcholine receptor (AChR)–binding antibodies
- Present in >85% of patients with generalized MG
- Present in >70% of patients with ocular MG
- Present in >80% of patients in remission
♦ AChR-blocking antibodies
- Present in >50% of patients with generalized MG
- Present in 30% of patients with ocular MG
- Present in 19% of patients in remission
- Present in only 1% of MG patients without AChR-binding antibodies
- Not detected by AChR-modulating antibody assay
- More often associated with more severe forms of disease
♦ AChR-modulating antibodies
- Highest activity (>90%) in MG patients with thymoma
- Present in >70% of patients with ocular MG
- Does not distinguish between AChR-binding and AChR-blocking antibodies
- Useful when AChR-binding antibodies are not detected (e.g., in patients with recent, mild, or ocular MG)
♦ Striational antibodies to skeletal muscle cross striations are found in
- 30% of adult MG patients.
- ~90% of myasthenia gravis patients with thymoma; absence argues against thymoma.
- ≤ 25% of patients with thymoma without MG. May be useful to predict risk of MG in patients with thymoma and to predict recurrence of thymoma.
- ~5% of patients with Lambert-Eaton myasthenic syndrome.
- Less frequent within 1 yr of onset of MG.
- Less frequent in patients receiving immunosuppressive drug therapy.

- Rare in MG patients <20 yrs old; increased frequency with each decade of disease after onset.
- Absent in congenital MG.
- 25% of patients treated with D-penicillamine.
- Graft-versus-host disease in marrow transplant recipients. Can be used for monitoring autoimmune complications of marrow transplantation.
- Autoimmune liver diseases: >90% of seropositive patients, have more than one type of autoantibody.

Other immunologic abnormalities are frequent.

- Anti-DNA antibodies in 40% of cases.
- ANA, anti–parietal cell, anti–smooth muscle, antimitochondrial, antithyroid antibodies, RF, etc., may be found.

Thymic tumor develops in up to 15–20% of generalized MG patients; 70% of patients have thymic hyperplasia with germinal centers in medulla. (See p. 445.)

CBC, ESR, thyroid function tests, serum enzymes, and electrolyte levels are normal.

May be associated with thyrotoxicosis, RA, PA, SLE.

High frequency of associated diabetes mellitus is seen, especially in older patients; therefore GTT should be performed with or without cortisone.

Always rule out cancer of lung.

Myopathy Associated with Alcoholism

Acute

- Increased serum CK, AST, and other enzymes. Serum CK increased in 80% of patients; rises in 1–2 days; reaches peak in 4–5 days; lasts ~2 wks. CK in CSF is normal, even when serum level is elevated.
- Gross myoglobinuria.
- Acute renal failure (some patients).

Chronic—may show some or all of the following changes.

- Increased serum CK in 60% of patients to average of 2× ULN
- Increased AST and other enzymes due to liver as well as muscle changes
- Increased urine creatine
- Diminished ability to increase blood lactic acid with ischemic exercise
- Abnormalities on muscle biopsy (support the diagnosis)
- Myoglobinuria

Myopathy: Myotubular, Mitochondrial, and Nemaline (Rod)

Routine laboratory studies including serum enzymes are normal.

♦ Muscle biopsy with histochemical staining establishes the diagnosis.

Paralysis, Familial Periodic

See Table 10-3.

♦ Serum potassium is decreased during the attack.

Urine potassium excretion decreases at the same time.

Serum enzymes are normal.

Polymyositis

(Nongenetic primary inflammatory myopathy; may be idiopathic or due to infection or may be associated with skin disease [dermatomyositis] or collagen or malignant disease; 10–20% of patients older than 50 yrs of age have a neoplasm.)

○Serum enzymes

- Serum CK is the most useful. Increased in 70% of patients. Levels may vary greatly (≤ 50× normal). Degree of increase is highest in children and usually reflects the activity of the disease but can be normal in active disease; decrease usually occurs 3–4 wks before improvement in muscle strength and increase occurs 5–6 wks before clinical relapse; the level frequently becomes normal with steroid therapy (in ~3 mos) or in chronic myositis.
- Serum aldolase is increased in 75% of patients.
- Serum LD is increased in 25% of patients.
- Serum AST is increased in ~25% of the patients.
- Serum alpha-hydroxybutyric dehydrogenase may be increased, paralleling the increased LD.

Table 10-3. Types of Periodic Paralysis

	Hypokalemic (Familial, Sporadic, Associated with Hyperthyroidism)	Hyperkalemic (Adynamia Episodica Hereditaria)	Normokalemic
Induced by	Glucose and insulin, ACTH, DOCA, epinephrine	KCl	KCl
Serum potassium during attack	Decreased	Transiently increased	Normal or slightly decreased
Urine potassium excretion	Decreased	Normal	Decreased

ACTH = corticotropin; DOCA = deoxycorticosterone acetate; KCl = potassium chloride.

♦ Muscle biopsy findings are definitive; also for dermatomyositis and inclusion-body myositis. They also help to exclude other types of myositis.

Total eosinophil count is frequently increased. WBC may be increased in fulminant disease. Mild anemia may occur.

ESR is moderately to markedly increased; may be normal; not clinically useful.

Thyroid function tests are normal.

Urine shows a moderate increase in creatine and a decrease in creatinine. Myoglobinuria occurs occasionally in severe cases.

Increased ANA titers are found in 20% of patients. RF tests may be positive in 50% of patients.

Serum gamma globulins may be increased.

Associated carcinoma is present in ≤ 20% of patients and in ≤ 5% of patients older than 40 yrs (especially those with cancer of lung or breast). The polymyositis may antedate the neoplasm by up to 2 yrs.

Other types of inflammatory myositis

♦ • Inclusion-body myositis shows characteristic biopsy finding of basophilic rimmed vacuoles with intranuclear filaments on electron microscopy. Serum CK is normal or only slightly increased.

Laboratory Tests for Bone Diseases

Alkaline Phosphatase (ALP), Bone-Specific, Serum

Use

Marker for bone formation

Increased In

Paget's disease; may be more sensitive than total ALP, especially when activity is low.
Primary hyperparathyroidism
Osteomalacia
Osteoporosis
Pregnancy

Calcium, Serum

See Chapter 3, pp. 45–47, and Chapter 13.

Hydroxyproline, Urine

Use

Marker of collagen (including bone) turnover
Limited diagnostic value; largely replaced by following tests.

Increased In

Increased collagen catabolism (e.g., especially Paget's disease; hyperparathyroidism, acromegaly, psoriasis, burns)

Certain inborn errors of metabolism (e.g., hydroxyprolinemia, familial aminoglycinuria)

Osteocalcin

Use

Marker of bone turnover rather than just of resorption or formation
Assess patients at risk for osteoporosis
Classify patients with established osteoporosis
Determine efficacy of therapy in osteoporosis or bone metastases

Increased In

Increased bone formation (e.g., Paget's disease, primary hyperparathyroidism, healing fractures, osteogenic sarcoma, hyperthyroidism, effective therapy for osteoporosis)

Decreased In

Hypoparathyroidism
Cushing's syndrome

Pyridinium Cross-Links and Deoxypyridinoline, Urine

(Stabilizing factors to type I bone collagen within organic matrix of mineralized bone; released into circulation; now measured by immunoassay.)

Use

Increase is marker of increased osteoclastic activity and bone demineralization.

Telopeptide, N-Terminal and C-Terminal Telopeptide, Urine

(Antibodies to intermolecular cross-links of type I bone collagen are recently developed markers of bone resorption.)

Use

Serial changes decide course of therapy and monitor response to therapy. Failure to change >30% after 4–8 wks of therapy may suggest need to change therapy.
More specific to bone than pyridinoline, hydroxyproline, or calcium
Not for diagnosis of osteoporosis

Increased In (Indicates Bone Resorption)

Paget's disease
Osteoporosis
Primary hyperparathyroidism
Metastatic bone cancer

Diseases of Skeletal System

Embolism, Fat

(Occurs after trauma [e.g., fractures, insertion of femoral head prosthesis])
Unexplained decrease in Hb in 30–60% of patients
Decreased platelet count in 80% of patients with rebound in 5–7 days
○Free fat in urine in 50% of patients and in stained blood smear
○Fat globules in sputum (some patients) and BAL washings
○Fat globulinemia in 42–67% of patients and in 17–33% of controls
Decreased arterial pO_2 with normal or decreased pCO_2

Arterial blood gas values are always abnormal in clinically significant fat embolism syndrome; are the most useful and important laboratory data. Patients show decreased lung compliance, abnormal ventilation-perfusion ratios, and increased shunt effect.
Increased serum lipase in 30–50% of patients; 3–4 days after injury; increased free fatty acids; not of diagnostic value
Increased serum triglycerides
Normal CSF
Hypocalcemia is a common nonspecific finding (due to binding to free fatty acids).
♦ *Laboratory findings alone are inadequate for diagnosis, prognosis, or management.*

Hypophosphatemia, Primary (Familial Vitamin D–Resistant Rickets)

(Hereditary metabolic defect in phosphate transport in renal tubules and possibly intestine)
○Serum phosphorus is markedly decreased.
Serum calcium is relatively normal.
Serum ALP is moderately increased.
Stool calcium is increased, and urine calcium is decreased.
♦ Administration of vitamin D does not cause serum phosphorus to increase (in contrast to ordinary rickets), but urine and serum calcium may be increased with sufficiently large dose.
Serum phosphorus usually remains low; increase of >4 mg/dL may indicate renal injury due to vitamin D toxicity.
Treatment is monitored by choosing dose of vitamin D that does not increase serum calcium by >11 mg/dL or urine calcium by >200 mg/day.
Renal aminoaciduria is absent, in contrast to ordinary rickets.

Osteoectasia, Familial

(Uncommon inherited disorder of membranous bone characterized by painful swelling of the periosteal soft tissue and spontaneous fractures)
Serum ALP is increased.
Serum acid phosphatase and aminopeptidase are also increased.

Osteomyelitis

♦ Organism is identified by culture of bone biopsy material in 50–70% of patients; blood culture is positive in ~50% of patients; results of sinus drainage cultures in chronic osteomyelitis do not correlate with causative organism unless *Staphylococcus aureus* is cultured from sinus.
○Microbiology
  • *S. aureus* causes almost all infections of hip and two-thirds of infections of skull, vertebrae, and long bones. Other bacteria may be present simultaneously and contribute to infection.
  • *S. aureus* causes 90% of cases of hematogenous osteomyelitis, which occurs principally in children, but only 50% of blood cultures are positive.
  • Group B streptococci, *S. aureus,* and *Escherichia coli* are chief organisms in neonates. *Haemophilus influenzae* type b, *S. aureus*, group A *Streptococcus,* and *Salmonella* are chief organisms in older children. *S. aureus*, coagulase-negative staphylococci, gram-negative bacilli (especially *Pseudomonas aeruginosa, Serratia marcescens, E. coli*) are most frequent organisms.
  • *Staphylococcus epidermidis* is the most common organism involved in total hip arthroplasty infection.
  • Gram-negative bacteria cause most infections of mandible, pelvis, and small bones.
  • *Salmonella* is more commonly found in patients with sickle cell and some other hemoglobinopathies.
  • Diabetic patients with foot ulcers and surgical infections that extend to bone usually have polymicrobial infection, often including anaerobic infection.
  • Most infections due to *Candida, Aspergillus*, and other fungi occur in diabetic and immunocompromised patients. *Candida* infection also occurs in patients with central and hyperalimentation lines. Patients are often on steroid and antibiotic therapy.
  • Mucor occurs in patients with poorly controlled diabetes.

- IV drug abusers frequently have osteomyelitis of sternoclavicular joints due most commonly to *P. aeruginosa* and *S. aureus*.
- Puncture wounds of calcaneus usually involve pseudomonal organisms.
- Cranial involvement in neonates after scalp fetal monitoring during labor is mainly associated with group B *Streptococci*, *E. coli*, and staphylococci.
- Histoplasmosis is described in AIDS patients. HSV infection and vaccinia have been described in immunocompromised patients.
- *Coccidioides immitis* infection may occur in endemic areas.

WBC may be increased, especially in acute cases.

ESR is increased in <50% of patients but may be an important clue in occult cases (e.g., intervertebral disk space infection).

Laboratory findings due to underlying conditions (e.g., postoperative status, radiotherapy, foreign body, tissue gangrene, contiguous infection)

○Vertebral osteomyelitis
- May be due to unusual organisms (e.g., *Mycobacterium tuberculosis*, fungi, *Brucella*).
- Increased WBC in <50% of patients.
- Increased ESR in >80% of patients.
- Blood culture may be positive.
- Aspiration of involved site with stains, cultures, and histologic examination. Gram-positive cocci, especially *S. aureus,* are most common.
  Gram-negative enteric bacilli, especially *E. coli* and *Salmonella*, cause ~30% of cases, especially in sickle cell disease.
  P. aeruginosa infection is associated with IV drug abuse.
  Brucella infection occurs in certain parts of the world.

Laboratory findings due to predisposing factors (e.g., diabetes, IV drug abuse, GU tract infection) or complications (e.g., epidural or subdural abscess, aortic involvement)

Osteopenia

(Generic term for decreased mineralized bone on radiographic study, but radiographic study cannot distinguish osteomalacia from osteoporosis in most patients unless pseudofractures are seen.)

All serum chemistry values may be normal in any form of osteopenia.

All chemistry values are commonly normal in osteomalacia, especially that coexisting with osteoporosis, which occurs in 20% of patients.

Serum vitamin D level that is below normal (e.g., 15 ng/mL of 25-hydroxy–vitamin D) suggests osteomalacia

♦Diagnosis is established by bone biopsy, which may be combined with tetracycline labeling.

During therapeutic trial of calcium and vitamin D, serum and urine calcium should be monitored monthly to avoid toxicity.

Urine calcium is maintained at <300 mg/gm of creatinine and serum calcium at <10.2 mg/dL by reducing dose of vitamin D.

Osteopetrosis (Albers-Schönberg Disease; Marble Bone Disease)

Normal serum calcium, phosphorus, and ALP
Serum acid phosphatase increased (some patients)
Myelophthisic anemia (some patients)
Laboratory findings due to complications (e.g., osteomyelitis)

Paget's Disease of Bone (Osteitis Deformans)

♦Marked increase in serum ALP (in 90% of cases) is directly related to severity and extent of disease; sudden additional increase with development of osteogenic sarcoma occurs in ~1% of patients. May be normal in patients with monostotic disease (~15% of symptomatic patients). Bone-specific serum ALP is more sensitive marker of bone formation.

Serum calcium increased during immobilization (e.g., due to intercurrent illness or fracture).

Normal or slightly increased serum phosphorus

Frequently increased urine calcium; renal calculi common.

Increase in urinary pyridinium cross-link pyridinoline is better indicator of bone resorption than the increase in urinary hydroxyproline, which may be marked.

Osteocalcin is often normal.

Biochemical response to calcitonin therapy
- Initial decrease of serum ALP and urinary hydroxyproline followed by return to former values despite continued therapy—occurs in ~20% of cases.
- Serum ALP and urinary hydroxyproline decrease 30–50% in 3–6 mos and maintain those values for duration of therapy—occurs in >50% of cases.
- Serum ALP and urinary hydroxyproline become normal only in previously untreated patients with only small increase in bone turnover—occurrence is unusual.

♦ Radionuclide scan shows areas of heavy uptake in affected bones.

Rickets

Due To

Low serum calcium-phosphorus product
- Vitamin D deficiency
- Hypophosphatemia
    Vitamin D–resistant rickets
    Fanconi's syndrome
    Excess intake of phosphate-binding antacids
    Hypophosphatemic nonrachitic bone disease
    Tumor-induced osteomalacia
- Renal tubular acidosis

Normal or high serum calcium-phosphorus product
- Renal osteomalacia
- Hypophosphatasia

○Serum ALP is increased. This is the earliest and most reliable biochemical abnormality; it parallels the severity of the rickets. It may remain elevated until bone healing is complete.

Serum calcium is usually normal or slightly decreased.

Serum phosphorus is usually decreased. In some persons, serum calcium and phosphorus may be normal.

Generalized renal aminoaciduria is present; it disappears when adequate vitamin D is given.

Serum calcium and phosphorus rapidly become normal after institution of vitamin D therapy.

♦ Serum 25-hydroxy–vitamin D is low (usually <5 ng/mL; normal = 10–20 ng/mL).

Vitamin D–deficient state is suggested by
- Low serum phosphorus
- Severe liver disease
- Malabsorption
- Anticonvulsant therapy

Rickets, Vitamin D Dependent

♦ Blood level of 1,25-dihydroxyvitamin D is very low in type I (autosomal recessive deficiency of 1-α-hydroxylase enzyme in kidney) and increased in type II (group of genetic disorders causing increased end-organ resistance to 1,25-dihydroxyvitamin D).

Serum calcium is frequently decreased, sometimes causing tetany.

Serum phosphorus is decreased but not as markedly or as consistently as in hypophosphatemic rickets.

Increased serum ALP, parathormone, and urinary cyclic adenosine monophosphate.

Urine calcium is decreased.

Generalized renal aminoaciduria is present.

♦ Findings return to normal after adequate vitamin D is given (may require very large doses).

Sarcoma, Osteogenic

Marked increase in serum ALP (≤ 40× normal); reflects new bone formation and parallels clinical course (e.g., metastasis, response to therapy); is said to occur in only 50% of patients.

Laboratory findings due to metastases—80% of patients have lung metastases at time of diagnosis.

Laboratory findings due to preexisting diseases (e.g., Paget's disease).

♦ Histologic examination of lesion establishes diagnosis.

Tumor of Bone, Metastatic

♦ Biopsy confirms the diagnosis

Osteolytic metastases (especially from primary tumor of bronchus, breast, kidney, or thyroid)

- Urine calcium is often increased; marked increase may reflect increased rate of tumor growth.
- Serum calcium and phosphorus may be normal or increased.
- Serum ALP is usually normal or slightly to moderately increased.
- Serum acid phosphatase is often slightly increased, especially in prostatic metastases.

Osteoblastic metastases (especially from primary tumor in prostate)

- Serum calcium is normal; it is rarely increased.
- Urine calcium is low.
- Serum ALP is usually increased.
- Serum acid phosphatase is increased in prostatic carcinoma.
- Serum phosphorus is variable.

○ Increased concentration of markers of bone turnover (pyridinoline and deoxypyridinoline, and associated N-telopeptides, serum bone ALP), which may predict metastases in breast, prostate, lung cancers.

Tumor of Bone, Osteolytic

(E.g., Ewing's sarcoma)

Usually normal serum calcium, phosphorus, and ALP.

♦ Biopsy establishes the diagnosis.

Normal Values—Synovial Fluid

Volume	1.0–3.5 mL
pH	Parallels serum
Appearance	Clear, pale yellow, or straw-colored; viscous, does not clot
Fibrin clot	0
Mucin clot	Good
WBC (per cu mm)	<200 (even in presence of leukocytosis in blood)
Neutrophils	<25%
Crystals	
Free	0
Intracellular	0
Fasting uric acid, bilirubin	Approximately the same as in serum
Total protein	~25–30% of serum protein
	Mean = 1.8 gm/dL
	Abnormal if >2.5 gm/dL; inflammation is moderately severe if >4.5 gm/dL
Glucose	<10 mg/dL lower than serum level of simultaneously drawn blood
Culture	No growth

Laboratory Tests for Joint Diseases

Acute-phase reactants, e.g., ESR (see pp. 55–57), CRP (see pp. 50–52)

Anti–*Borrelia burgdorferi* antibodies (see p. 808)

Anticardiolipin antigens

Anticytoplasmic antigens (see p. 63)

MUSCULOSKEL

ANA (see Table 17-1)
Complement (C3, C4, CH50)
Cryoglobulins
Immune complexes (C1q binding, Raji cell assay)
RF (see p. 128)
Synovial fluid examination (see Tables 10-4, 10-5)

Diseases of Joints

Arthritis, Associated with Hemochromatosis

♦ Laboratory findings of hemochromatosis
Negative RF
No subcutaneous nodules
♦ Biopsy of synovia: iron deposits in synovial lining but not in cartilage; little iron in
  deep macrophages.
   • Hemarthrosis—iron diffusely distributed in macrophages (e.g., in hemophilia,
     trauma, and pigmented villonodular synovitis).
   • Osteoarthritis—small amount of iron that is limited to deep macrophages.
   • RA—iron in both deep macrophages and lining cells.
Frequently associated with chondrocalcinosis.

Arthritis, Associated with Ulcerative Colitis/Regional Enteritis

RA, ankylosing spondylitis (in ≤ 20% of patients with Crohn's disease), or acute synovitis (monoarticular or polyarticular—absent RF) may be present.
Joint fluid is sterile on the basis of both bacteriologic and microscopical findings. It is
  similar to fluid of RA and Whipple's disease (in cell count, differential count, specific
  gravity, viscosity, protein, glucose, poor mucin clot formation). Joint fluid examination is principally useful in evaluating monarticular involvement to rule out suppurative arthritis.
Synovial biopsy findings are similar to RA biopsy findings.
Abnormal laboratory results (e.g., increased ESR, WBC, platelets) are related to activity of bowel disease.
Absent RF and ANAs.

Arthritis, Associated with Whipple's Disease

Findings of a nonspecific synovitis

Arthritis, Infective

♦ Joint fluid (see Table 10-4)
   • Bacterial
      In purulent arthritis, organism is recovered from joint in 90% of patients and
        from blood in 50% of patients. Most often due to S. aureus (60%) and Strep-
        tococcus species.
         Gram stain is positive in ~50% of patients; it is particularly useful for estab-
           lishing diagnosis promptly and in cases in which cultures are negative.
         Culture may be negative because of prior administration of antibiotics.
      In tuberculous arthritis
         Gram stain and bacterial cultures are negative, but acid-fast stain, culture
           for tubercle bacilli, guinea pig inoculation, and biopsy of synovia confirm
           the diagnosis.
      In children, most common organisms are H. influenzae type b, S. aureus, vari-
        ous streptococci, and gram-negative bacilli.
      In young adults, >50% of cases are due to Neisseria gonorrhoeae; rest are due
        to S. aureus, streptococci, or gram-negative bacilli.
   • Viral (e.g., mumps, rubella, HBV infection, parvovirus B19 infection)

Table 10-4. Synovial Fluid Findings in Various Diseases of Joints

Property	Normal	Noninflammatory[a]	Hemorrhagic[b]	Acute Inflammatory[c] — Acute Gouty Arthritis	RF	RA	Septic — TB Arthritis	Gonorrheal Arthritis	Septic Arthritis[e,f]
Volume	3.5 mL	I	I	I			I		
Appearance	Clear, colorless	Clear, straw	Bloody or xanthochromic	Turbid yellow			Turbid yellow		
Viscosity	High	High	V	D			D		
Fibrin clot	0	Usually 0	Usually 0	+			+		
Mucin clot[d]	Good	Good	V	Fair to poor			Poor		
WBC (no./cu mm)[g]	<200	<5000	<10,000	Range 750–45,000; Average 13,500	Range 300–98,000; Average 17,800	Range 300–75,000; Average 15,500	Range 2500–105,000; Average 23,500	Range 1500–108,000; Average 14,000	Range 15,600–213,000; Average 65,400
Neutrophils (%)	<25	<25	<50	Range 48–94; Average 83	Range 8–98; Average 46	Range 5–96; Average 65	Range 29–96; Average 67	Range 2–96; Average 64	Range 75–100; Average 95
Blood-synovia[h] glucose difference (mg/dL)[i]	<10	<10	<25	Range 0–41; Average 12	6	Range 0–88; Average 31	Range 0–108; Average 57	Range 0–97; Average 26	Range 40–122; Average 71

(continued)

Table 10-4. (continued)

Property[j]	Normal	Noninflammatory[a]	Hemorrhagic[b]	Acute Gouty Arthritis	RF	RA	TB Arthritis	Gonorrheal Arthritis	Septic Arthritis[e,f]
Culture[j]	Neg	Neg	Neg	Neg	Neg	Neg	See Infective Arthritis.		

I = increased; D = decreased; Neg = negative; V = variable; WBC = white blood count; + = positive.

[a]For example, degenerative joint disease, traumatic arthritis, some cases of pigmented villonodular synovitis.

[b]For example, tumor, hemophilia, neuroarthropathy, trauma, some cases of pigmented villonodular synovitis.

[c]For example, RA, Reiter's syndrome, acute gouty arthritis, acute pseudogout, SLE.

[d]Mucin clot test adds little additional information to WBC count.

[e]For example, pneumococcal.

[f]In purulent arthropathy of undetermined cause, very high synovial fluid lactate (>2000 mg/dL) indicates a nongonococcal septic arthritis (gram-negative bacilli, gram-positive cocci, fungi). Lactate is <100 mg/dL in gonococcal infection, gout, RA, osteoarthritis, trauma.

[g]Use saline instead of acetic acid, which clumps the joint fluid.

[h]Glucose concentration may give spurious results unless obtained after prolonged fasting, and differences between joint and blood samples may not be significant unless >50 mg/dL. Joint tap should be performed, preferably after the patient has been fasting for >4 hrs, and a blood glucose determination should be performed simultaneously.

[j]Material should be cultured aerobically and anaerobically. Culture for tubercle bacilli should be performed.

Synovial fluid analysis is primarily useful to diagnose or to rule out infectious arthritis, gout, or pseudogout.

To distinguish inflammatory from noninflammatory conditions, synovial fluid WBC >2000/cu mm and >75% PMNs have sensitivities of 84% and 75% and specificities of 84% and 92%, respectively.

Table 10-5. Synovial Fluid Findings in Acute Inflammatory Arthritis of Various Etiologies[a]

Disease	WBC	Complement Activity	Rheumatoid Factor	Crystals[b]	Other Findings
Acute gouty arthritis	I	I	0	Monosodium urate; within PMNs during acute stage	
Acute chondrocalcinosis	I	I	0	Calcium pyrophosphate	
Reiter's syndrome	Markedly I	Markedly I	0		Macrophages with ingested leukocytes
Rheumatoid arthritis	I	Low	Usually +		
Juvenile rheumatoid arthritis	I	Low	0		Abundant lymphocytes (sometimes > 50%); immature lymphocytes and monocytes present
Systemic lupus erythematosus	Usually very low	Low or 0	V	0	LE cells may be present
Arthritis associated with psoriasis, ulcerative colitis, ankylosing spondylitis	I	I			

0 = absent; + = positive; I = increased; LE = lupus erythematosus; V = variable.
[a]Measurement of rheumatoid factor and complement in synovial fluid is rarely helpful; antinuclear antibody determination is not useful.
[b]Crystals of gout and pseudogout should be identified *within* polymorphonuclear neutrophils using polarized light microscopy. Finding of characteristic crystals is diagnostic of gout and of chondrocalcinosis. Must be differentiated from crystals of corticosteroid esters and cholesterol or talc (after recent joint infections). Crystals are engulfed by WBCs during acute attack but between acute episodes may lie free in fluid.

Table 10-6. Comparison of Rheumatoid Arthritis and Osteoarthritis

Rheumatoid Arthritis	Osteoarthritis
Synovial fluid has high WBC and low viscosity	Effusions infrequent
	Synovial fluid has low WBC and high viscosity
ESR more markedly increased	ESR may be mildly to moderately increased
RF usually present	RF usually absent
Positive biopsy of subcutaneous rheumatoid nodule and synovia	Rheumatoid changes in tissue absent

ESR = erythrocyte sedimentation rate; RF = rheumatoid factor; WBC = white blood cell count.

- Fungal (e.g., *Sporothrix schenckii, C. immitis*, candida, *Blastomyces dermatitidis*)
♦ - If five biopsies are cultured, bacterial growth in two or less or only in broth media indicates contamination, but growth in all five in solid and broth media suggests infection.

Laboratory findings due to preexisting infections (e.g., SBE, meningococcic meningitis, pneumococcal pneumonia, typhoid, gonorrhea, Lyme disease, TB, rat-bite fever, syphilis)

Infection of prosthetic joints
- Early onset (within first 3 mos)
- Delayed onset (within first 2 yrs—two-thirds of patients)
   Due to organisms introduced during surgery or to those of nosocomial infection, which multiply slowly (50% of cases occur >1 yr later). Most common are skin flora (e.g., *S. epidermidis*, other coagulase-negative staphylococci, *Corynebacterium* sp.)

Table 10-7. Serologic Tests in Various Rheumatoid Diseases

Disease[a]	ANA[b]	RF[c]	Serum Complement	LE Clot[d]
SLE	100 (H)	30–40	D	70–80
Rheumatoid arthritis				
Adult	50 (L–M)	80–90	N or I	5–15
Juvenile	<5 (L–M)	15	N	<5
Mixed connective tissue disease	100 (M–H)	50	N or I	20
Dermatomyositis	25	10–15	N	<5
Scleroderma	25–40	33	N	<5
Polyarteritis nodosa	<5 (L)	5–10	N or D	<5
Sjögren's syndrome	95 (M–H)	75	N or D	20
Ankylosing spondylitis	5–10	<5	N	<5

Numbers = percentage of cases positive for each test. D = decreased; I = increased; N = normal.
[a]Normal ESR in patients with nonspecific rheumatic symptoms suggests fibromyositis rather than any of the above disorders.
[b]ANA = fluorescent antinuclear antibody; H = titer >1:200; M–H = titer 1:100–1:200; L–M = titer 1:20–1:100; ANA titer ≥ 1:160 with suggestive pattern and clinical setting is very helpful diagnostically, but when titer is negative, other laboratory tests are not productive. Anti–DNA antibodies correlate best with a diagnosis of SLE; they are positive in <5% of patients with other immunologic diseases. Diagnosis of SLE is barely credible without a positive ANA test.
[c]Positive rheumatoid factor (RF) test shows a significantly higher titer in RA than in other collagen diseases, but diagnosis is primarily clinical rather than serologic. Serial titers are not helpful to follow response to treatment since antiglobulins remain at constant levels despite clinical status. Frequently positive at low to moderate titers in polyclonal hypergammaglobulinemia (e.g., SLE, sarcoidosis, cirrhosis, active viral hepatitis, some acute viral infections).
Measurement of RF and complement in synovial fluid is rarely helpful; ANA determination is not useful. Crystals of gout and pseudogout should be identified *within* PMNs.
[d]Lupus erythematosus (LE) cells in peripheral blood clot preparation. Now rarely used.

Table 10-8. Erythrocyte Sedimentation Rate (ESR) in Differential Diagnosis of Juvenile Rheumatoid Arthritis

Disease	ESR Falls to Normal
Untreated acute rheumatic fever	9–12 wks
Salicylate-treated acute rheumatic fever	5 wks
Steroid-treated acute rheumatic fever	2 wks
Chronic rheumatic fever	Occasionally shows persistent elevation
Juvenile rheumatoid arthritis	May remain elevated for months or years despite therapy

- Late onset (after 2 yrs—one-third of cases)
   Due to hematogenous seeding from infected focus (e.g., GU tract, dental)
- Increased WBC and ESR support diagnosis of infection rather than aseptic loosening of prosthesis.

Arthritis, Juvenile Rheumatoid

See Table 10-8.
Latex fixation and other serologic tests for RF are negative, but RF and circulating immune complexes can be demonstrated by various special techniques.
Reported incidence of ANAs is 4–88% depending on clinical type and laboratory technique.

Arthritis, Rheumatoid (RA)

See Tables 10-6 and 10-7.
- ◆ American Rheumatism Association has 11 criteria for diagnosis of RA; seven are required for diagnosis of classic RA, five for definite RA, and three for probable RA. Four laboratory findings included in these criteria are positive serum test for RF (by any method; positive in <5% of normal control subjects), poor mucin clotting of synovial fluid, characteristic histologic changes in synovium, and characteristic histologic changes in rheumatoid nodules.
- ◆ Serologic tests for RF (autoantibodies to immunoglobulins) using nephelometry, latex, bentonite, or sheep or human RBCs
  - Use slide test only for screening; confirm positive result with tube dilution (nephelometry). Significant titer is ≥ 1:80. In RA, titers are often 1:640 to 1:5120 and sometimes ≤ 1:320,000. Titers in conditions other than RA are usually <1:80.
  - Gives useful objective evidence of RA, but a negative result does not rule out RA. Negative in one-third of patients with definite RA. Positive result in <50% during first 6 mos of disease. Various methods show sensitivity of 50–75% and specificity of 75–90%. Positive in 80% of "typical" cases; high titers in patients with splenomegaly, vasculitis, subcutaneous nodules, or neuropathy. Titer may decrease during remission but rarely becomes negative. Progressive increases in titer during the first 2 yrs indicate a more severe course.
  - Positive in 5–10% of healthy population; progressive increase with age in ≤ 25–30% of persons older than 70 yrs.
  - Positive in 5% of rheumatoid variants (arthritis associated with ulcerative colitis, regional enteritis, Reiter's syndrome, juvenile RA, rheumatoid spondylitis, tophaceous gout, pseudogout).
  - Positive in 5% of cases of scleroderma, mixed connective tissue disease, polymyositis, polymyalgia rheumatica.
  - Positive in 10–15% of patients with SLE.
  - Positive in 90% of patients with primary Sjögren's syndrome or cryoglobulinemic purpura.
  - Positive in 10–40% of patients with Waldenström's macroglobulinemia, chronic infections (e.g., syphilis, leprosy, brucellosis, TB, SBE), viral infections (e.g., hepati-

MUSCULOSKEL

tis, EBV infection, influenza, vaccinations [positive in ≤ 10% of cases of parvovirus B19–associated arthritis]), parasitic diseases (e.g., malaria, schistosomiasis, trypanosomiasis, filariasis), chronic liver disease, infectious hepatitis, chronic pulmonary interstitial fibrosis, etc.

- Positive in ≤ 20% of cases of psoriatic arthritis.
- Positive in 25% of cases of sarcoid arthritis.
- Negative in osteoarthritis, ankylosing spondylitis, rheumatic fever, suppurative arthritis.

ANA present in up to 28% of patients (see Table 10-7).

Serum complement is usually normal except in patients with vasculitis; depressed level is usually associated with very high levels of RF and immune complexes (see p. 49, and Table 16-1).

Immune complexes—monoclonal RF and C1q-binding assays are positive more frequently than other assays in RA but correlate poorly with disease activity. Positive test for mixed cryoglobulins indicates presence of immune complexes and is associated with increased incidence of extra-articular manifestations, especially vasculitis. Not clinically useful.

Increased ESR, CRP, and other acute-phase reactants. ESR is often used as guide to activity and to therapy but is normal in 5% of patients. Very high ESR (>100 mm/hr) is distinctly unusual in early cases.

WBC is usually normal; a slight increase may be seen early in active disease.

Mild thrombocytosis occurs frequently as an acute-phase reactant.

Serum protein electrophoresis shows increase in globulins, especially in gamma and alpha$_2$-globulins, and decreased albumin.

Moderate normocytic hypochromic anemia of chronic disease (see p. 370) with decreased serum iron, normal TIBC, and normal iron stores (serum ferritin and bone marrow iron); not responsive to iron, folic acid, vitamin B$_{12}$ administration or splenectomy. If Hct is <26%, search for other cause of anemia (e.g., GI tract bleeding). Anemia diminishes as patient goes into remission or responds to therapy.

Serum CK is decreased below normal in >60% of patients; not associated with decreased serum aldolase and myosin, which indicates that decrease is not due to general impairment of muscle function.

Serum calcium, phosphorus, ALP, uric acid, and ASOT are normal.

Synovial biopsy is especially useful in monoarticular form to rule out TB, gout, etc.

Synovial fluid glucose may be greatly decreased (<10 mg/dL); mucin clotting is fair to poor. (See Table 10-4.)

Laboratory findings due to extra-articular involvement (usually occurs late in severe disease) (e.g., pleural or pericardial effusion, interstitial pulmonary fibrosis)

Laboratory findings due to therapeutic drugs (e.g., salicylates, NSAIDs, gold, penicillamine). See Amyloidosis, p. 890.

Chondrocalcinosis ("Pseudogout")

♦Joint fluid contains crystals identified as calcium pyrophosphate dihydrate, *inside* and outside of WBCs and macrophages; differentiated from urate crystals under polarized light, which distinguishes from gout. See Tables 10-4, 10-5, and 10-9. Crystals may also be identified by other means (e.g., chemical, x-ray diffraction).

Blood and urine findings are normal.

Laboratory findings due to associated conditions (e.g., hyperparathyroidism, hypothyroidism, acromegaly, hemochromatosis, gout, hypomagnesemia, degenerative arthritis)

Felty's Syndrome

(Occurs in 5–10% of patients with far-advanced RA associated with splenomegaly and leukopenia and rheumatoid nodules)

♦Serologic tests for RF are positive in high titers.

ANAs are usually present. Titers of immune complexes are high and complement levels are lower than those in patients with RA.

Leukopenia (<2500/cu mm) and granulocytopenia are present.

Anemia and thrombocytopenia due to hypersplenism may occur and respond to splenectomy.

Table 10-9. Birefringent Materials in Synovial Fluid

Material	Usual Shape, Size	Birefringence	Cause	Location within or out of PMNs, Macrophages
Crystals				
Monosodium urate	Needle, rod, parallel edges 8–10 μm long	Strong; –	Gout	Within or out
Calcium pyrophosphate dihydrate	Rhomboid; may be rod, diamond, square, needle; <10 μm long	Weak; +	Pseudogout	Only within
Calcium oxalate	Bipyramidal	Strong; 0	Long-term renal dialysis	Within or out
Hydroxyapatite, other basic calcium phosphates	Aggregates only; small (<1 μm)	Weak; 0	Degenerating, calcifying joint	
Cholesterol	Flat, plate, corner notch; may be needle; often >100 μm			
Cartilage, collagen	Irregular, rodlike	Strong; +		
Steroids			Injection into joint	
Betamethasone acetate	Rods; blunt ends 10–20 μm	Strong; –		
Cortisone acetate	Large rods	Strong; +		
Methyl prednisone acetate	Small, pleomorphic, tend to clump	Strong; 0		
Prednisone tebutate	Small, pleomorphic, branched, irregular	Strong; +		
Triamcinolone acetonide	Small, pleomorphic fragments; tend to clump	Strong; 0		
Triamcinolone hexacetonide	Large rods, blunt ends 15–60 μm	Strong; 0		
Anticoagulants			Injection into joint	
EDTA (dry)	Small, amorphous	Weak		
Lithium heparin (not sodium)	May resemble pseudogout	Weak; +		
Other materials				
Debris	Small, irregular, nonparallel edges	Variable		
Fat (cholesterol esters)	Globules	Strong; Maltese cross		
Starch granules	Round; size varies	Strong; Maltese cross		

+ = positive birefringence; – = negative birefringence; 0 = no axis. EDTA = ethylenediaminetetraacetic acid.
Crystals are best seen in fresh, wet-mount preparations examined with polarizing light.
Hydroxyapatite complexes (diagnostic of apatite disease) and basic calcium phosphate complexes can be identified only by electron microscopy and mass spectroscopy; most cases are suspected clinically but never confirmed.
Source: Judkins SW, Cornbleet PJ. Synovial fluid crystal analysis. *Lab Med* 1997;28:774.

Gout

Due To

Primary (i.e., inborn) (30% of patients)
  Idiopathic
  Increased purine biosynthesis
    Lesch-Nyhan syndrome
Secondary (70% of patients)
  Overproduction (10% of secondary cases)
  • Neoplastic and hemolytic conditions (e.g., leukemia, polycythemia vera, secondary polycythemia, malignant lymphomas). Blood dyscrasias are found in ~10% of patients with clinical gout.
  • Psoriasis.
  Increased breakdown of adenosine triphosphate
  • Glycogen storage diseases (types I, III, V, VII)
  • Alcohol ingestion
  • Myocardial infarction
Decreased renal function (90% of secondary cases)
  • Decreased renal clearance.
      Chronic renal disease
      Chronic lead intoxication
      Increased organic acids (e.g., lactate, beta-hydroxybutyrate in diabetic ketoacidosis, acute ethanol intoxication, toxemia of pregnancy, starvation)
  • Drugs (e.g., diuretics, aspirin, cyclosporin) (≤ 20% of cases). May cause ≤ 50% of all new cases of gouty arthritis; this occurs later in life and in women is more common than primary gout.
Also associated with hypertension (in one-third of patients with gout), familial hypercholesterolemia, obesity, acute intermittent porphyria, sarcoidosis, parathyroid dysfunction, myxedema. (See Table 10-9.)

♦ Presence of crystals of monosodium urate from tophi or joint fluid viewed microscopically under polarized light—strongly negative birefringent needle-shaped crystals both *inside* and outside PMNs or macrophages establishes the diagnosis and differentiates it from pseudogout. Found in 90% of patients during an acute attack. Found in synovial fluid in 75% of patients between attacks.

○ Increased serum uric acid
  • Does *not* establish the diagnosis of gout.
  • Is normal in 30% of acute attacks. Several determinations may be required to establish increased values; beware of serum levels reduced to normal range as a result of recent aspirin use. Changes in therapy may cause wide fluctuations in serum uric acid levels. The incidence of gout occurring at various uric acid levels in men was found to be as follows: 1.1% at <6 mg/dL, 7.3% at 6–6.9 mg/dL, 14.2% at 7–7.9 mg/dL, 18.7% at 8–8.9 mg/dL, 83% at ≥ 9 mg/dL. Many gout patients have levels <8 mg/dL and more than one-third never have an elevated level. Because the mean interval between first and second gout attacks is 11.4 yrs and only 25% have a second attack within 12 yrs, therapy for this group may not be cost effective.
  • Serum uric acid is increased in ~25% of asymptomatic relatives.
  • Approximately 10% of adult males have increased serum uric acid.
  • Only 1–3% of patients with hyperuricemia have gout.
  • Secondary hyperuricemia usually produces much higher serum uric acid than primary type. If serum uric acid is >10 mg/dL, underlying malignancy should be considered after renal failure has been ruled out.

○ Uric acid stones occur 3–10 times more frequently in gouty patients than in the general population even though 75% of gouty patients have normal 24-hr excretion of uric acid. When serum uric acid is <9 mg/dL or urine level is <700 mg/24 hrs, risk of renal calculi is <21%; when serum uric acid is >13 mg/dL or urine level is >1100 mg/24 hrs, risk is >50%. With primary gout, 10–25% of patients develop uric acid stones; in 40% of them, the stones appear >5 yrs before an episode of gout.

24-hr urine uric acid excretion
  • If >600 mg/24 hrs, measurement should be repeated after 5-day purine-free diet.
  • If <600 mg/24 hrs or urine uric acid/creatinine ratio is <0.6 and patient has no history of kidney or GU tract disease, treatment of hyperuricemia is with probenecid.

- If >600 mg/24 hrs or urine uric acid/creatinine ratio is >0.8 or the patient has a history of GU tract or kidney disease, allopurinol is drug of choice.
- Uric acid/creatinine ratios of 0.6–0.8 are indeterminate; ratios of 0.2–0.6 are considered normal or indicate underexcretion.
- 700–1000 mg/24 hrs is considered borderline.
- >1000 mg/24 hrs is abnormal and is indication for treatment in patients with asymptomatic hyperuricemia.

Uric acid crystals and amorphous urates are *normal* findings in urinary sediment.
Low-grade proteinuria occurs in 20–80% of persons with gout for many years before further evidence of renal disease appears.
♦ Histologic examination of gouty nodule is characteristic.
Moderate leukocytosis and increased ESR occur during acute attacks; normal at other times.
RF is detectable in low titers in 10% of patients with gout or pseudogout; but RA rarely coexists with these conditions.
Serum triglycerides are frequently increased, resulting in a high frequency of type IIb and type IV lipoprotein patterns; HDL-cholesterol level is frequently decreased.
See Tables 10-4, 10-5, 10-7.
See sections on renal diseases (p. 725) and serum uric acid (p. 84).

Monoarthritis, Acute

Due To

Infection
- Bacteria (*N. gonorrhoeae*)
- Spirochetes (e.g., Lyme disease, syphilis)
- Mycobacteria (TB, atypical mycobacteria)
- Viruses (e.g., HIV, HBV, HSV)
- Fungi (e.g., blastomycosis, *Candida* spp.)

Crystals (e.g., monosodium urates, calcium pyrophosphate dihydrate, apatite, calcium oxalate, liquid lipid microspherules)
Prosthetic joint (infection, aseptic loosening)
Trauma
Hemarthrosis (e.g., coagulopathy, trauma)
Neoplasm (e.g., osteoid osteoma, pigmented villonodular synovitis, metastasis)
Systemic diseases (e.g., RA, Reiter's syndrome, psoriasis, inflammatory bowel disease, sarcoidosis, serum sickness, hyperlipidemias, bacterial endocarditis, AIDS)

Ochronosis

(Lumbosacral spondylitis associated with scleral pigmentation and darkening of urine on alkalinization)
See Alkaptonuria, p. 542.

Osteoarthritis

See Table 10-6.
Laboratory tests are normal and not helpful.
ESR may be slightly increased (possibly because of soft-tissue changes secondary to mechanical alterations in joints).

Polyarthritis and Fever

Type	Useful Laboratory Tests
Infectious	
Bacterial	
Septic arthritis	Blood and synovial fluid culture
Bacterial endocarditis	Blood culture

Lyme disease	Serology
Fungal and mycobacterial	Culture; biopsy
Viral	Serology
Postinfectious/reactive	
Rheumatic fever	See pp. 128–129
Reiter's syndrome	See p. 318
Inflammatory bowel disease	See p. 308
RA; Still's disease	See pp. 313–314
Systemic rheumatic disorders	
SLE	See p. 895
Systemic vasculitis	See pp. 130–131
Crystal induced	
Gout	See p. 316
Pseudogout	See p. 314
Others	
Sarcoidosis	See p. 898
Neoplasms	See p. 910
Familial Mediterranean fever	See p. 567
Mucocutaneous disorders, e.g.,	
Henoch-Schönlein purpura	See p. 478
Kawasaki's syndrome	See p. 118
Erythema nodosum	
Erythema multiforme	

Polymyalgia Rheumatica

○ESR is markedly increased; this is a criterion for diagnosis.

Mild hypochromic or normochromic anemia is commonly found.

WBC may be increased in some patients.

Abnormalities of serum proteins are frequent, although no consistent or diagnostic pattern is found. Most frequently the albumin is decreased with an increase in alpha$_1$ and alpha$_2$ globulins and fibrinogen.

Cryoglobulins are sometimes present.

RF is present in serum in 7.5% of patients.

Serum enzymes (e.g., AST, ALP) may be increased in one-third of patients.

○Muscle biopsy specimen is usually normal or may show mild nonspecific changes.

○Temporal artery biopsy findings are often positive because one-third of patients with giant cell arteritis present with polymyalgia rheumatica, which ultimately develops in 50–90% of these patients (see discussion of temporal arteritis, p. 115).

Arthritis Associated with Psoriasis

Arthritis occurs in ~2% of patients with psoriasis. No correlation is seen between skin activity and joint manifestations; either one may precede the other.

Increased serum uric acid is due to increased turnover of skin cells in psoriasis.

If serologic tests for RF are negative, should not be classified as RA.

♦No characteristic laboratory findings.

Reiter's Syndrome

(Triad of arthritis, urethritis, and conjunctivitis has additional features: dermatitis, buccal ulcerations, circinate balanitis, and keratosis blennorrhagica. Triad is initially present in only one-third of patients.)

Increased acute-phase reactants
• Increased ESR parallels the clinical course.
• Increased CRP.
• WBC is increased (10,000–20,000/cu mm), as is the granulocyte count.

Serum globulins are increased in long-standing disease.

Nonbacterial cystitis, prostatitis, or seminal vesiculitis and subclinical infection of ileum and colon may be found.

Significance of culturing various organisms or of serologic evidence of preceding infections is not determined.

HLA-B27 is found in up to 90% of white patients; not diagnostically useful.

Sjögren's Syndrome[3,4]

(Primary systemic autoimmune disease associated with decreased salivary and lacrimal gland secretion or may be secondary to RA, SLE, scleroderma, or vasculitis in one-half to two-thirds of patients. 90% of patients are female.)

♦ Diagnostic Criteria

A. Primary Sjögren's syndrome
  1. Symptoms and objective signs of dry eyes *and*
  2. Symptoms and objective signs of dry mouth, including biopsy of minor salivary gland *and*
  3. Laboratory evidence of systemic autoimmune disease
     a. Increased RF titer ≥ 1:320 (RF is present in ≤ 90% of primary and secondary Sjögren's syndrome)
     b. Increased ANA titer ≥ 1:320 *or*
     c. Presence of anti-SS-A (Ro) or anti-SS-B (La) antibodies
B. Secondary Sjögren's syndrome: above criteria plus sufficient features for diagnosis of
   • SLE—found in 4–5% of patients with Sjögren's syndrome; Sjögren's syndrome is found in 50–98% of patients with SLE.
   • RF—found in 30–55% of patients with Sjögren's syndrome; Sjögren's syndrome is found in 20–100% of patients with RA.
   • Primary biliary cirrhosis—found in 3% of patients with Sjögren's syndrome; Sjögren's syndrome is found in 50–100% of patients with primary biliary cirrhosis.
   • Polymyositis, generalized scleroderma.
C. Not due to sarcoidosis; HIV, HTLV, HBV, HCV infection; or preexisting lymphoma; fibromyalgia; or other causes of keratitis sicca or enlarged salivary glands.

♦ ANAs in speckled or homogeneous pattern are present in 65% of patients, more frequently in those with primary type. Anti-SS-A (Ro) is present in ≤ 88% of patients with primary type and <10% of those with secondary Sjögren's syndrome. Anti-SS-B (La) is present in ≤ 73% of patients with primary Sjögren's syndrome and <5% of those with secondary Sjögren's syndrome. Anti–salivary duct antibody is rare (<30%) in primary Sjögren's syndrome and frequent (76–83%) in secondary Sjögren's syndrome. Patients with primary Sjögren's syndrome also have higher levels of tissue antibodies (e.g., thyroglobulin [in 35%], gastric parietal, smooth muscle). Anti-dsDNA is not found. (See pp. 888, 890.)

Mild normochromic, normocytic anemia occurs in 50% of patients.

Leukopenia occurs in up to one-third of patients.

ESR is usually increased.

Serum protein electrophoresis shows increased gamma globulins (usually polyclonal), largely due to IgG.

Laboratory findings due to concomitant diseases

Immune complex GN may occur, but chronic tubulointerstitial nephritis is more characteristic.

Spondylitis, Ankylosing Rheumatoid (Marie-Strümpell Disease)

♦ No diagnostic laboratory test exists for this disorder.

ESR is increased in ≤ 80% of patients.

Mild to moderate hypochromic anemia develops in ≤ 30% of patients.

[3]Collins RD Jr, Ball GV. Sjögren's syndrome: distinguishing primary from secondary. *J Musculoskeletal Med* 1984;1(5):42.
[4]Fox RI. Sjögren's syndrome. Controversies and progress. *Clin Lab Med* 1997;17:431.

MUSCULOSKEL

Serologic tests for RF are positive in <15% of patients with arthritis of only the vertebral region.

CSF protein is moderately increased in ≤ 50% of patients.

Secondary amyloidosis develops in 6% of patients.

Laboratory findings due to carditis and aortitis with aortic insufficiency, which occur in 1–4% of patients.

Laboratory findings of frequently associated diseases (e.g., chronic ulcerative colitis, regional ileitis, psoriasis) are noted.

Histocompatibility antigen HLA-B27 is found in 95% of these white patients and in lesser numbers with variants of this condition. ~20% of carriers of HLA-B27 have ankylosing spondylitis, but it is not helpful in establishing the diagnosis.

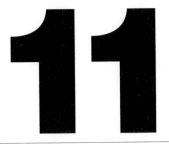

Hematologic Diseases

Hematologic Laboratory Tests

Blood Smear—Red Blood Cells (RBCs)

See Fig. 11-1.
The smear may also confirm the RBC indices or indicate leukemia or other conditions.

RBC Inclusions

Basophilic or polychromatophilic macrocytes	≤ 15 in healthy persons. Increased erythropoiesis in hemorrhage or hemolysis. Called reticulocytes if supravital stain. Due to polyribosomes producing Hb. Increased MCV.
Microcytes with stippling	Thalassemia. Lead or heavy metal poisoning
Cabot's rings	Occasional in severe hemolytic anemias and PA
Howell-Jolly bodies (dark purple spherical bodies)	Megaloblastic anemia; thalassemia; hyposplenism; postsplenectomy state
Pappenheimer bodies (siderotic granules) (purple coccoid granules at periphery)	Anemias with defect of incorporating iron into Hb (e.g., sideroblastic anemia, thalassemia, lead poisoning, pyridoxine-unresponsive and pyridoxine-responsive anemias) Iron overload
Heinz bodies* (precipitates of denatured Hb)	Congenital G-6-PD deficiency Drug-induced hemolytic anemias (e.g., dapsone, phenacetin) Unstable Hb disorders after splenectomy
Plasmodium trophozoites	Malaria
Reticulocytes*	See p. 343

Abnormally Shaped RBCs

Round	
Macrocytes	Increased erythropoiesis (reticulocytosis)
Round macrocytes	Liver disease; alcoholism; postsplenectomy; hypothyroidism; increased MCV
Oval (macro-ovalocytes)	Megaloblastic anemia; cancer chemotherapy; myelodysplastic syndromes; increased MCV
Microcytes	Hypochromic anemias; decreased MCV
Spherocytes	Hereditary spherocytosis; immunohemolytic anemia; recent blood transfusion; usually decreased MCV, increased MCHC

*Not seen with Wright's stain; requires supravital stain, e.g., cresyl violet.

HEMATOL

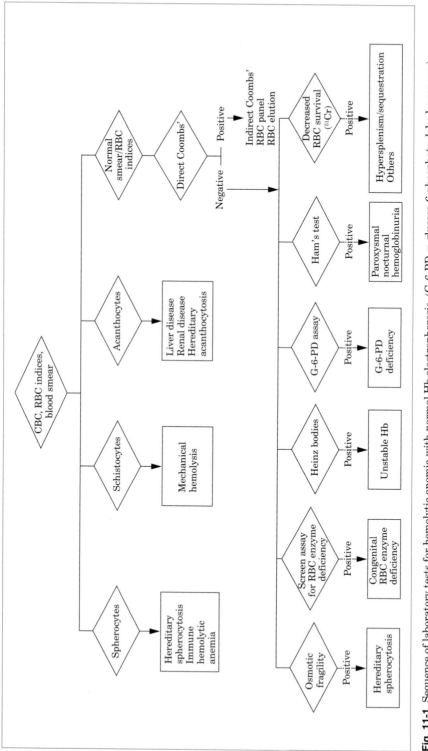

Fig. 11-1. Sequence of laboratory tests for hemolytic anemia with normal Hb electrophoresis. (G-6-PD = glucose-6-phosphate dehydrogenase.)

Stomatocytes	Hereditary stomatocytosis (see p. 439) Rh null disease (see p. 433) Acute alcoholism (transient) Certain drugs (e.g., phenothiazines) Neoplastic, cardiovascular, hepatobiliary diseases Artifactual
Target cells	HbC disease or trait; HbD; HbE; HbS; thalassemia; iron-deficiency anemia; liver disease; postsplenectomy state; artifactual; decreased osmotic fragility
Elongated	
Elliptocytes	Hereditary (>25% in smear) (see p. 374) Microcytic anemia (<25% in smear)
Ovalocytes	Megaloblastic anemia
Teardrop (dacryocyte)	Spent polycythemia Myelofibrosis Thalassemia (especially homozygous beta type)
Sickle cells	Sickle cell disorders (not in S trait)
HbC crystalloids	HbC trait or disease
Spiculated	
Acanthocytes	Abetalipoproteinemia (many are present) (p. 528) Postsplenectomy state (few are present) Fulminating liver disease (variable number)
Burr cells (echinocytes; crenated RBCs)	Usually artifactual; stomach cancer; GI bleeding; uremia; pyruvate kinase deficiency; hypophosphatemia; hypomagnesemia
Schistocytes (helmet, triangle)	Microangiopathic hemolytic anemia (e.g., DIC, thrombotic thrombocytopenic purpura [TTP]); prosthetic heart valves or severe valvular heart disease; severe burns; snakebite
"Bite" cells	Hemolysis, e.g., due to certain drugs with or without G-6-PD deficiency, unstable Hb
RBC fragmentation (seen on peripheral blood smear >10/1000 RBCs] and on histogram of RBC size with automated cell counters)	Cytotoxic chemotherapy for neoplasia; autoimmune hemolytic anemia; severe iron deficiency; megaloblastic anemia; acute leukemia; myelodysplasia; inherited structural abnormality of RBC membrane protein spectrin

HEMATOL

Blood Volume

Blood volume determination is usually done using albumin tagged with iodine 125 (^{125}I) or ^{131}I; red cell mass may be measured by labeling RBCs with ^{51}Cr.

Interferences

In the presence of active hemorrhage, the isotope is lost via the bleeding site and a false value is produced.

Use

Differential diagnosis of polycythemia
Radioisotopes should not be administered to children or pregnant women.

Bone Marrow Aspiration

Use When the Following Diagnoses Are Suspected

Aplastic anemia, agranulocytosis
Leukemia lymphomas

Megaloblastic anemias
Lipid storage diseases
Metastatic cancer
Multiple myeloma
Waldenström's macroglobulinemia
Idiopathic thrombocytopenic purpura (ITP)
Hypersplenism
Iron-deficiency anemia
Indicated for diagnosis and for posttreatment follow-up of acute leukemia and cytopenia.

Bone Marrow Biopsy

Use When the Following Diagnoses Are Suspected

Disorders in which bone marrow aspiration is indicated (see previous section)
Granulomatous diseases
Amyloidosis
TTP
Myelofibrosis—occurs in
- Agnogenic myeloid metaplasia
- Other myelodysplasias
- Hairy cell leukemia
- Metastatic carcinoma
- Miliary TB
- Granulomatous diseases
- Paget's disease
- Parathyroid disease
- After radiation therapy (e.g., for lymphoma)
- Benzene exposure

Biopsy and aspirate are both required for staging carcinoma or lymphoma.

Coombs' (Antiglobulin) Test

Positive Direct Coombs '(Antiglobulin) Test

Fig. 11-2.
Use
Detects immunoglobulin antibodies and/or complement on patient's RBC membrane (e.g., autoimmune hemolysis, hemolytic disease of newborn, drug-induced hemolysis, transfusion reactions)
Interferences
False-positive may occur in multiple myeloma and Waldenström's macroglobulinemia.
Positive In
Erythroblastosis fetalis
Most cases of autoimmune hemolytic anemia, including ≤ 15% of certain systemic diseases, especially acute and chronic leukemias, malignant lymphomas, collagen diseases. Strength of reaction may be of prognostic value in patients with lymphoproliferative disorders.
Delayed hemolytic transfusion reaction
Drug induced, e.g.,
- Alpha methyldopa (occurs in ≤ 30% of patients on continued therapy but <1% show hemolysis); rarely in first 6 mos of treatment. If not found within 12 mos, is unlikely to occur. Is dose related, with lowest incidence in patients receiving ≤ 1 gm daily. Reversal may take weeks to months after the drug is discontinued.
- L-dopa
- Others, e.g., acetophenetidin, ethosuximide, cephalosporins (most common with cephalothin; less frequent with cefazolin and cephapirin; reported in 3–50% of patients), mefenamic acid, penicillin (with daily IV dose of 20 million U/day for several weeks), procainamide, quinidine, quinine.

Healthy blood donors (1 in 4000 to 1 in 8000 persons)

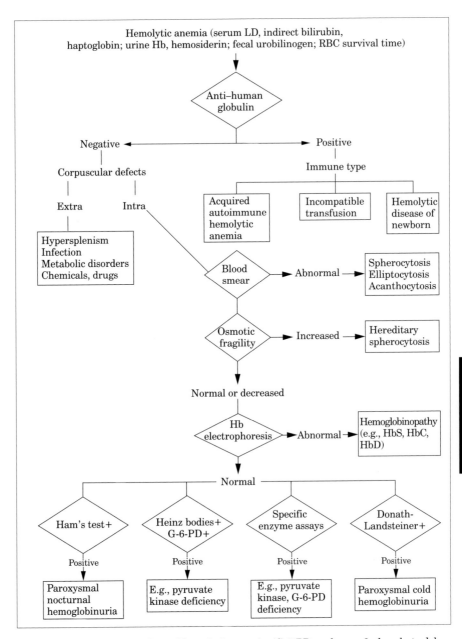

Fig. 11-2. Algorithm for workup of hemolytic anemia. (G-6-PD = glucose-6-phosphate dehydrogenase.)

May be *weakly* positive in renal disease, epithelial malignancies, RA, inflammatory bowel diseases. Weakly positive reactions are not usually clinically significant.

Negative In

Hemolytic anemias due to intrinsic defect in RBC (e.g., G-6-PD deficiency, hemoglobinopathies)

2–9% of patients with hemolytic anemia (due to smaller amount of IgG bound to RBC but similar response to splenectomy or steroid therapy or to IgM, IgA, or IgD rather than IgG). This is a diagnosis of exclusion.

Positive Indirect Coombs' Test

(Using patient's serum, which contains antibody)
Use
Cross matching for blood transfusion
Detect and identify antibodies
- Specific antibody—usually isoimmunization from previous transfusion
- "Nonspecific" autoantibody in acquired hemolytic anemia
RBC phenotyping
- In genetic and forensic medicine
- To identify syngeneic twins for bone marrow transplantation
Interferences
Beware of false-positive and false-negative results due to poor-quality test serum, failure to use fresh blood (must have complement), etc.

Erythropoietin, Plasma

(Normal = 3.7–16.0 U/L by RIA)

Use

Differential diagnosis of polycythemia vera
Indicator of need for erythropoietin therapy in patients with renal failure

Interferences

Decreased by high plasma viscosity, use of estrogens, beta-adrenergic blockers, agents that increase renal blood flow (e.g., enalapril, an inhibitor of angiotensin-converting enzyme)
Circadian rhythm in hospitalized adults, with lowest values at 0800–1200 and 40% higher values in late evening.

Increased Appropriately* In

Extremely high: usually transfusion-dependent anemia with Hct = 10–25% and Hb = 3–7 gm/dL; e.g., aplastic anemia, severe hemolytic anemia, hematologic cancers
Very high: patients have mild to moderate anemia with Hct = 25–40% or Hb = 7–12 gm/dL
High: patients are more anemic, e.g., hemolytic anemia, myelodysplasia, exposure to chemotherapeutic or immunosuppressive drugs, AIDS

Increased Inappropriately* In

Some renal disorders
- Renal cysts
- Postrenal transplant
Malignant neoplasms
- Renal adenocarcinoma (1–5% of cases)
- Juxtaglomerular cell tumor
- Nephroblastoma (Wilms' tumor)
- Hepatocellular carcinoma, or hemangiosarcoma
- Testicular carcinoma
- Malignant pheochromocytoma
- Breast carcinoma
Nonmalignant neoplasms
- Meningioma
- Hemangioblastoma of brain (20% of cases), liver, or adrenal gland
- Leiomyoma of uterus

Decreased Inappropriately* In

Renal failure
Autonomic neuropathy
AIDS before zidovudine therapy

Weeks 3 and 4 after bone marrow transplant
Polycythemia vera

Decreased Appropriately* In

Renal failure, RA, multiple myeloma, cancer

Ferritin, Serum

See Tables 11-1, 11-9, and 11-10.

Use

Diagnosis of iron deficiency or excess; correlates with total body iron stores.
Chief iron-storage protein in the body.
  • Predict and monitor iron deficiency
  • Determine response to iron therapy or compliance with treatment
  • Differentiate iron deficiency from chronic disease as cause of anemia
  • Monitor iron status in patients with chronic renal disease with or without dialysis
  • Detect iron overload states and monitor rate of iron accumulation and response
    to iron-depletion therapy
  • Population studies of iron levels and response to iron supplement

Decreased In

Iron deficiency. Is most sensitive and specific test for iron deficiency if MCV is not
    increased (e.g., pregnancy, infancy, polycythemia) or no vitamin C deficiency is present.
    *Decreases before anemia and other changes occur. No other condition causes a low level.
    Returns to normal range within few days after onset of oral iron therapy; failure to pro-
    duce serum ferritin level >50 ng/mL suggests noncompliance or continued iron loss.*
  • <18 ng/mL is associated with absent stainable iron in marrow.
  • <12 ng/mL always indicates iron deficiency and no longer corresponds to severity
    of deficiency because iron stores are essentially exhausted.
  • >80 ng/mL essentially excludes iron deficiency.

Increased In

Ferritin is an acute-phase reactant and thus is increased in many patients with vari-
    ous acute and chronic liver diseases, alcoholism (declines during abstinence), malig-
    nancies (e.g., leukemia, Hodgkin's disease), infection and inflammation (e.g.,
    arthritis), hyperthyroidism, Gaucher's disease, AMI, etc. *Serum ferritin may not be
    decreased when iron deficiency coexists with these conditions; in such cases, bone mar-
    row stain for iron may be the only way to detect the iron deficiency.*
Iron overload (e.g., hemosiderosis, idiopathic hemochromatosis). Can be used to monitor
    therapeutic removal of excess storage iron. Transferrin saturation is more sensitive to
    detect early iron overload in hemochromatosis; serum ferritin is used to confirm diag-
    nosis and as indication to proceed with liver biopsy. Ratio of serum ferritin (in ng/mL)
    to ALT (in U/L) >10 in iron-overloaded thalassemic patients but averages ≤ 2 in
    patients with viral hepatitis; ratio decreases with successful iron chelation therapy.
Anemias other than iron deficiency (e.g., megaloblastic, hemolytic, sideroblastic, thal-
    assemia major and minor, spherocytosis, porphyria cutanea tarda)
Renal cell carcinoma due to hemorrhage within tumor
End-stage renal disease; values ≥ 1000 µg/L are not uncommon. Values <200 µg/L are
    specific for iron deficiency in these patients.
Increases with age; is higher in men than in women, in women who use oral contra-
    ceptives, in persons who eat red meat compared with vegetarians.

Flow Cytometry

Use

Diagnosis of leukemias, myelodysplasia, and lymphomas by immunophenotyping
Diagnosis of DNA content and DNA synthetic activity of tumors

*Erythropoietin is normally inversely related to RBC volume, Hb, or Hct.

HEMATOL

Table 11-1. Comparison of Iron-Deficiency Anemia Alone and Combined with Thalassemia Minor or Anemia of Chronic Disease

	Iron-Deficiency Anemia Alone	Anemia of Chronic Disease Alone	Combined Anemias of Iron Deficiency and Chronic Disease	Thalassemia Minor Alone	Combined Anemias of Iron Deficiency and Thalassemia Minor
MCV	D	N or D	D	**Very D**	Very D
RDW	I	I or N	I	I or N	I
RBC count	**D**	D	D	**N or I**	N or D
Serum iron	**D**	**D**	D	N	D
Serum ferritin	D	**I or N**	N or I	N	D
Marrow iron stain	D to 0	N or I	D to 0	N	D to 0
TIBC	**I**	**D**	I or N	N	I
Hb electrophoresis	N	N	N	**Ab***	**Ab***
sTfR	I	N	I	I	I

0 = absent; Ab = abnormal; D = decreased; I = increased; N = normal; sTfR = serum transferrin receptor.
Bold type indicates most useful differences.
*Hemoglobin electrophoresis abnormal in beta-thalassemia but not alpha-thalassemia.

Enumeration of lymphocyte subsets (e.g., CD4+ T cells as surrogate marker for disease progression in AIDS)

Stem cell (counting) transplantation

Measurement of cell-bound antibody and sorting of subpopulations that differ in amount of bound antibody

Use of anti-HbF monoclonal antibodies to detect HbF (can detect <0.05% fetal RBCs)
- More accurate than Kleihauer-Betke stain for quantitation of fetal-maternal hemorrhage
- Detect increased number of RBCs containing decreased HbF ("F" cells) in patients with hemoglobinopathies, some patients with myelodysplasia

Reticulocyte counting

HLA-B27 determination

Mitogen stimulation evaluation

Neutrophil function studies (e.g., phagocytosis, oxidative burst)

Gene Rearrangement (*bcr*) Assay

♦ PCR has replaced Southern blot hybridization as preferred (more sensitive and specific) method to demonstrate reciprocal translocation of DNA from chromosome 9 (including the *abl* locus) to 22 (breakpoint cluster [*bcr*]), giving rise to shorter chromosome 22 (Ph[1]). *bcr* gene rearrangement is molecular equivalent of Ph[1] translocation. Can be done on peripheral blood as well as marrow and is more sensitive than routine cytogenetic analysis.

Use

To diagnose Ph[1]-negative cases (5% of CML patients) or to confirm Ph[1]-positive CML

To diagnose CML patients who present in blast crisis or are in blast transformation

To rule out CML in myeloproliferative disorders with similar morphologic features

To monitor CML patients treated with marrow transplant, chemotherapy, or interferon

To detect minimal-residual disease

To confirm complete remission

To provide early detection of relapse

To purge *bcr*-positive cells from autologous bone marrow before infusion

Positive *bcr* gene rearrangement in acute leukemia indicates poor prognosis, especially in ALLs.

Finding of same gene rearrangement in lymphocytes in a distant site biopsy is proof of metastasis.

To diagnose many genetic disorders (e.g., HbS, HbC, beta thalassemias).

Interferences

False-negative PCR in Ph[1]-positive patients may occur due to therapy with interferon alpha or, less commonly, with hydroxyurea.

Contamination of PCR material.

Interpretation

Found in 95% of patients with CML, 5–10% of patients with ALL, and 1–2% of patients with acute myelogenous leukemia (AML). This rearrangement of *bcr* is typical of Ph[1]-positive chronic myelogenous leukemia patients and is found in ~30% of Ph[1]-positive AML patients.

Gene Rearrangement Assay for Immunoglobulin Heavy (IgH) and Light (IgL-kappa) Chains and Gene Rearrangement Assay for Beta and Gamma T-cell Receptor

Use

Allows classification of almost all cases of ALL as T, B, or pre-B types. Used to confirm pathologic-immunologic diagnoses of T-cell and B-cell lymphomas that are difficult to classify.

HEMATOL

Interpretation

Virtually all cases of non-T, non-B leukemias are recognized as pre-B types.

≤ 90% of cases of non-Hodgkin's lymphoma are derived from B cells. Their immunophenotypic abnormalities can be used to distinguish them from benign reactions in lymph nodes.

Genetic Hematologic Diseases, Molecular Diagnosis

RBC disorders
- Hereditary spherocytosis
- Hereditary pyropoikilocytosis
- Hereditary nonspherocytic hemolytic anemia—pyruvate kinase deficiency
- Hemolytic anemia—G-6-PD deficiency
- Porphyrias

Hemoglobinopathies
- Sickle cell anemia
- HbC, HbSC, HbE, HbD diseases
- Beta- and alpha-thalassemias
- Hereditary persistence of HbF
- Hemoglobinopathies with unstable hemoglobins

Neutrophil disorders
- Chronic granulomatous disease
- Myeloperoxidase deficiency
- Glutathione reductase and synthetase deficiencies

Coagulation disorders
- Hemophilia A and B
- von Willebrand's disease
- Inherited resistance to activated protein C

Haptoglobins, Serum

Use

Indicator of chronic hemolysis (e.g., hereditary spherocytosis, pyruvate kinase deficiency). Such patients should not have splenectomy when serum haptoglobin is >40 mg/dL if infection and inflammation have been ruled out. After splenectomy, increased haptoglobin level indicates success of surgery for these conditions, e.g., haptoglobin reappears at 24 hrs and becomes normal in 4–6 days in hereditary spherocytosis patients treated with splenectomy.

Diagnosis of transfusion reaction by comparison of concentrations in pretransfusion and posttransfusion samples. Posttransfusion reaction serum haptoglobin level decreases in 6–8 hrs; at 24 hrs it is <40 mg/dL or <40% of pretransfusion level.

In paternity studies, may aid by determination of haptoglobin phenotypes.

Increased In

Conditions associated with increased ESR and alpha$_2$ globulin (haptoglobin is also an acute-phase reactant) (e.g., infection, inflammation, trauma, necrosis of tissue, scurvy, amyloidosis, nephrotic syndrome, disseminated neoplasms such as Hodgkin's disease, lymphosarcoma, collagen diseases such as rheumatic fever, RA, and dermatomyositis). *Thus these conditions may mask presence of concomitant hemolysis.*

One-third of patients with obstructive biliary disease

Therapy with steroids or androgens

Aplastic anemia (normal to very high)

Diabetes mellitus

Decreased or Absent In

Hemoglobinemia (related to the duration and severity of hemolysis) due to
  Intravascular hemolysis (e.g., hereditary spherocytosis with marked hemolysis, pyruvate kinase deficiency, autoimmune hemolytic anemia, some transfusion reactions)

Extravascular hemolysis (e.g., large retroperitoneal hemorrhage)
Intramedullary hemolysis (e.g., thalassemia, megaloblastic anemias, sideroblastic anemias)
Genetically absent in 1% of general population
Parenchymatous liver disease (especially cirrhosis)
Protein loss via kidney, GI tract, skin
Infancy

Hemoglobin, Fetal (HbF)

(Alkali denaturation method; confirmed by examination of Hb bands on electrophoresis)

Normal

>50% at birth; gradual decrease to ~5% by age 5 mos
<2% older than age 2 years

Use

Diagnosis of various hemoglobinopathies

Increased In

Various hemoglobinopathies (see Tables 11-26 and 11-27). ~50% of patients with beta-thalassemia minor have high levels of HbF; even higher levels are found in virtually all patients with beta-thalassemia major. In sickle cell disease, HbF >30% protects the cell from sickling; therefore, even infants with homozygous HbS have few problems before age 3 mos.
Hereditary persistence of HbF
Nonhereditary refractory normoblastic anemia (one-third of patients)
PA (50% of untreated patients); increases after treatment and then gradually decreases during next 6 mos; some patients still have slight elevation thereafter. Minimal elevation occurs in ~5% of patients with other types of megaloblastic anemia.
Some patients with leukemia, especially juvenile myeloid leukemia with HbF of 30–60%, absence of Ph^1, rapid fatal course, more pronounced thrombocytopenia, and lower total WBC count
Multiple myeloma
Molar pregnancy
Patients with an extra D chromosome (trisomy 13-15, D1 trisomy) or an extra G chromosome (trisomy 21, Down syndrome, mongolism)
Acquired aplastic anemia (due to drugs, toxic chemicals, or infections, or idiopathic); returns to normal only after complete remission and therefore is reliable indicator of complete recovery. Better prognosis in patients with higher initial level.
Some chronic viral infections (e.g., CMV, EBV)

Decreased In

A rare case of multiple chromosome abnormalities (probably C/D translocation)

Hemoglobin, Serum

(Normal level = <10 mg/dL; visible level = ~20 mg/dL; <30 mg/dL is not accurate technically; >150 mg/dL causes hemoglobinuria; >200 mg/dL gives clear cherry red color to serum)

Use

Increase indicates intravascular hemolysis.

Slight Increase In

Sickle cell thalassemia
HbC disease

HEMATOL

Moderate Increase In

Sickle cell–HbC disease
Sickle cell anemia
Thalassemia major
Acquired (autoimmune) hemolytic anemia

Marked Increase In

Any rapid intravascular hemolysis

Iron, Radioactive (^{59}Fe), RBC Uptake

^{59}Fe is injected IV, and blood samples are drawn in 3, 7, and 14 days for measurement of radioactivity.

Use

Study of kinetics of iron metabolism

Decreased In

Pure red cell aplasia (see p. 378)—the rate of uptake of ^{59}Fe is markedly decreased.

Iron, Serum

Use

Differential diagnosis of anemias
Diagnosis of hemochromatosis and hemosiderosis
Should always be measured with TIBC for evaluation of iron deficiency.
Diagnosis of acute iron toxicity

Interferences

Falsely increased by hemolysis, iron contamination of glassware
Falsely decreased in lipemic specimens
Iron dextran administration causes increase for several weeks (may be >1000 μg/dL)

Increased In

Idiopathic hemochromatosis
Hemosiderosis of excessive iron intake (e.g., repeated blood transfusions, iron therapy, use of iron-containing vitamins) (may be >300 μg/dL)
Decreased formation of RBCs (e.g., thalassemia, pyridoxine-deficiency anemia, PA in relapse)
Increased destruction of RBCs (e.g., hemolytic anemias)
Acute liver damage (degree of increase parallels the amount of hepatic necrosis) (may be >1000 μg/dL); some cases of chronic liver disease
Use of progesterone birth control pills (may be >200 μg/dL) and pregnancy
Premenstrual elevation 10–30%
Acute iron toxicity; ratio of serum iron/TIBC not useful for this diagnosis.

Decreased In

Iron-deficiency anemia
Normochromic (normocytic or microcytic) anemias of infection and chronic diseases (e.g., neoplasms, active collagen diseases)
Nephrosis (due to loss of iron-binding protein in urine)
PA at onset of remission
Menstruation (decreased 10–30%)
Diurnal variation—normal values in midmorning, low values in midafternoon, very low values (~10 μg/dL) near midnight. Diurnal variation disappears at levels <45 μg/dL.

Iron (Hemosiderin), Stainable, in Bone Marrow

(Present in RE cells and developing normoblasts [sideroblasts])

Use

Is the gold standard for diagnosis of iron deficiency; its presence almost invariably rules out iron-deficiency anemia. Marrow iron disappears before the peripheral blood changes. Only individuals with decreased marrow iron are likely to benefit from iron therapy.
Diagnosis of iron overload.

Interferences

May be normal or increased by injections of iron dextran (which is used very slowly) despite other evidence of iron-deficiency anemia.

Increased In

Idiopathic hemochromatosis
Hemochromatosis secondary to
- Increased intake (e.g., Bantu siderosis, excessive medicine ingestion).
- Anemias with increased erythropoiesis (especially thalassemia major; also thalassemia minor, some other hemoglobinopathies, paroxysmal nocturnal hemoglobinuria, "sideroachrestic" anemias, refractory anemias with hypercellular bone marrow, etc.). In hemolytic anemias, decrease or absence may signify acute hemolytic crisis.
- Liver injury (e.g., after portal shunt surgery).
- Atransferrinemia.

Megaloblastic anemias in relapse
Uremia (some patients)
Chronic infection (some patients)
Chronic pancreatic insufficiency

Decreased In

Iron deficiency (e.g., inadequate dietary intake, chronic bleeding, malignancy, acute blood loss). *Rapidly disappears after hemorrhage.*
Polycythemia vera (usually absent in polycythemia vera but usually normal or increased in secondary polycythemia)
PA in early phase of therapy
Collagen diseases (especially RA, SLE)
Infiltration of marrow (e.g., malignant lymphomas, metastatic carcinoma, myelofibrosis, miliary granulomas)
Uremia
Chronic infection (e.g., pulmonary TB, bronchiectasis, chronic pyelonephritis)
Miscellaneous conditions (e.g., old age, diabetes mellitus)
Myeloproliferative diseases—iron stores may be absent without other evidence of iron deficiency.
Serum iron and TIBC may be normal in iron-deficiency anemia, especially if Hb is <9 gm/dL.

Iron-Binding Capacity, Total (TIBC), Serum

(TIBC [μmol/L] = transferrin [mg/L] $\times$ 0.025)
Unsaturated iron-binding capacity = TIBC – serum iron (μg/dL).

Use

Differential diagnosis of anemias
Should always be performed whenever serum iron is measured to calculate percent saturation (see pp. 338–339) for diagnosis of iron deficiency.

Increased In

Iron deficiency
Acute and chronic blood loss
Acute liver damage

Late pregnancy
Use of progesterone birth control pills

Decreased In

Hemochromatosis
Cirrhosis of the liver
Thalassemia
Anemias of infection and chronic diseases (e.g., uremia, RA, some neoplasms)
Nephrosis
Hyperthyroidism

Kleihauer-Betke Test

(Acid-eluted stained smear of maternal blood shows pale maternal RBCs but pink fetal RBCs. Detects HbF. Quantitates amount [in mL] of fetal blood in maternal circulation. Normal <1%. Now measured more accurately by flow cytometry with anti-HbF antibodies.)

Use

In Rh-negative women with Rh-positive fetuses to determine need for and dose of RhIg, especially in presence of blunt abdominal trauma, invasive procedures (e.g., chorionic villus biopsy), placenta previa, abruptio placenta. (See Hemolytic Disease of the Newborn, p. 389.)

Interferences

False-positive in hemoglobinopathies (SS, SA, hereditary persistence of HbF)
HbF increases in pregnancy in ≤ 25% of women.

Leukocyte Alkaline Phosphatase (LAP) Staining Reaction
(In untreated diseases)

Use

Differentiation of chronic myelogenous leukemia from leukemoid reaction

Usually Increased In

Leukemoid reaction
Polycythemia vera
Essential thrombocythemia (may be normal)
Lymphoma (including Hodgkin's lymphoma, reticulum cell sarcoma)
Acute and chronic lymphatic leukemia
Multiple myeloma
Myeloid metaplasia
Aplastic anemia
Agranulocytosis
Bacterial infections
Cirrhosis
Obstructive jaundice
Pregnancy and immediate postpartum period
Administration of Enovid (mestranol and norethynodrel)
Trisomy 21
Klinefelter's syndrome (XXY)

Usually Decreased In

Chronic myelogenous leukemia
Paroxysmal nocturnal hemoglobinuria
Hereditary hypophosphatasia
Nephrotic syndrome
Progressive muscular dystrophy

11. Hematologic Diseases   **335**

Refractory anemia (siderotic)
Sickle cell anemia

Usually Normal In

Secondary polycythemia
Hemolytic anemia
Infectious mononucleosis
Viral hepatitis
Lymphosarcoma

Variable In

PA
ITP
Iron-deficiency anemia
AML and idiopathic myelofibrosis
Acute undifferentiated leukemia

Mean Corpuscular Hemoglobin (MCH)

(Hb divided by RBC count)

Use

Limited value in differential diagnosis of anemias
Instrument calibration

Interferences (Increased In)

Marked leukocytosis (>50,000/cu mm)
Cold agglutinins
In vivo hemolysis
Monoclonal proteins in blood
High heparin concentration
Lipemia

Decreased In

Microcytic and normocytic anemias

Increased In

Macrocytic anemias
Infants and newborns

Mean Corpuscular Hemoglobin Concentration (MCHC)

(Hb divided by Hct)

Use

For laboratory quality control, chiefly because changes occur very late in the course of iron deficiency when anemia is severe.
Instrument calibration

Interferences

(With automated cell counters)
Decreased
   Marked leukocytosis (>50,000/cu mm)
Increased
   Hemolysis (e.g., sickle cell anemia, hereditary spherocytosis, some cases of autoimmune hemolytic anemia) with shrinkage of RBCs, making them hyperdense
   Conditions with cold agglutinins or severe lipemia of serum
   Rouleaux or RBC agglutinates
   High heparin concentration

HEMATOL

Decreased In

(<30.1 gm/dL)
Hypochromic anemias. *Normal value does not rule out any of these anemias. Low MCHC may not occur in iron-deficiency anemia when measured with automated instruments.*

Increased In

Only in hereditary spherocytosis; should be suspected whenever MCHC is >36 gm/dL.
Infants and newborns
Not increased in PA.

Mean Corpuscular Volume (MCV)

(Hct divided by RBC count with manual methods; measured directly by automated instruments)
See Fig. 11-3 and Tables 11-2 and 11-3.

Use

Classification and differential diagnosis of anemias
Useful screening test for occult alcoholism

Interferences

Marked leukocytosis (>50,000/cu mm) (increased values)
In vitro hemolysis or fragmentation of RBCs (decreased values)
Warm autoantibodies
Cold agglutinins (increased values)
Methanol poisoning (increased values)
Marked hyperglycemia (>600 mg/dL) (increased values)
Marked reticulocytosis (>50%) due to any cause (increased values)
Presence of microcytic and macrocytic cells in same sample may result in a normal MCV.

Increased In

Macrocytic anemias (MCV >95 fL and often >110 fL; MCHC >30 gm/dL)
- Megaloblastic anemia
    PA (vitamin B_{12} or folate deficiency)
    Sprue (e.g., steatorrhea, celiac disease, intestinal resection or fistula)
    Macrocytic anemia of pregnancy
    Megaloblastic anemia of infancy
    Fish tapeworm infestation
    Carcinoma of stomach, after total gastrectomy
    Drugs, e.g.,
        Oral contraceptives
        Anticonvulsants (e.g., phenytoin, primidone, phenobarbital)
        Antitumor agents (e.g., methotrexate, hydroxyurea, cyclophosphamide)
        Antimicrobials (e.g., sulfamethoxazole, sulfasalazine, trimethoprim, zidovudine, pyrimethamine)
    Orotic aciduria
    Di Guglielmo's disease
    Nonmegaloblastic macrocytic anemias; are usually normocytic (MCV usually <110 fL).
    Alcoholism
    Liver disease
    Anemia of hypothyroidism
    Accelerated erythropoiesis (some hemolytic anemias, posthemorrhage)
    Myelodysplastic syndromes (aplastic anemia, acquired sideroblastic anemia)
    Myelophthisic anemia
    Postsplenectomy
Infants and newborns

Normal In

Normocytic anemias (MCV = 80–94 fL; MCHC >30 gm/dL)
- After acute hemorrhage

- Some hemolytic anemias
- Some hemoglobinopathies
- Anemias due to inadequate blood formation
    Myelophthisic
    Hypoplastic
    Aplastic
- Endocrinopathies (hypopituitarism, hypothyroidism, hypoadrenalism, hypogonadism)
- Anemia of chronic disease (chronic infections, neoplasms, uremia)

Decreased In

Microcytic anemias (MCV <80 fL; MCHC <30 gm/dL)
- Usually hypochromic
    Iron-deficiency anemia, e.g.,
        Inadequate intake
        Poor absorption
        Excessive iron requirements
        Chronic blood loss
    Pyridoxine-responsive anemia
    Thalassemia (major or combined with hemoglobinopathy)
    Sideroblastic anemia (hereditary)
    Lead poisoning
    Anemia of chronic diseases (less than one-third of patients)
- Usually normocytic
    Anemia of chronic diseases
    Hemoglobinopathies
Low MCV due to (in decreasing order of frequency) iron deficiency, alpha-thalassemia, heterozygous beta-thalassemias, chronic disease, abnormal HbC and HbE.

Neutrophil Function Tests

Morphology
- Light, phase, and electron microscopy (e.g., Chédiak-Higashi syndrome)
Adherence
- To glass or spreading
- Aggregometer
- Flow cytometry—anti-CD18 and anti-sialyl-Lewis X positive
Locomotion
- Random
- Chemotaxis
    Serum deficiencies (e.g., complement, immunoglobulins)
    Cell defects (e.g., hyperimmunoglobulinemia E, Chédiak-Higashi syndrome, Kartagener's syndrome, drugs, diabetes mellitus, uremia, etc.)
Phagocytosis
- Uptake of latex beads, microorganisms
- Assay hexose monophosphate shunt
Secretion
- Assay lysosome enzymes, lactoferrin B_{12}-binding protein
Bactericidal activity
- Nitroblue tetrazolium test (see following section)
- Killing of bacteria (e.g., *Staphylococcus aureus*)
- Oxygen radical production (e.g., chronic granulomatous disease, G-6-PD deficiency)

Nitroblue Tetrazolium Reduction in Neutrophils

(Usual normal values reported are <10%, but considerable variation exists, and each laboratory should establish its own normal range.)

Use

Diagnosis of poor neutrophilic function (failure of nitroblue tetrazolium reduction), particularly in chronic granulomatous disease. Prenatal diagnosis is possible with fetal blood from placental vessels.
Differentiating untreated bacterial infection from other conditions; rarely used.

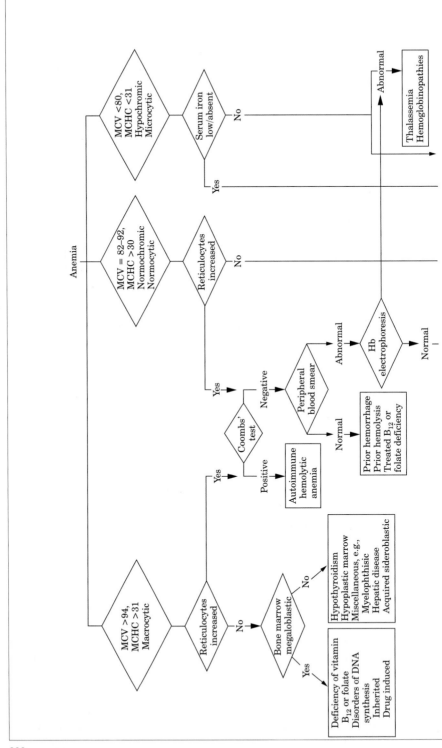

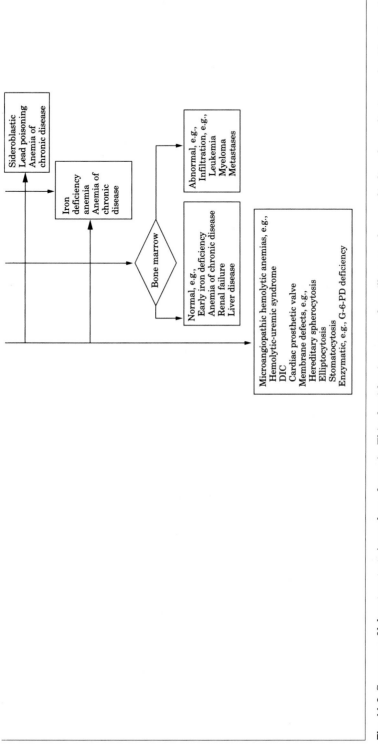

Fig. 11-3. Sequence of laboratory tests in workup of anemia. This algorithm is meant only to illustrate the use of indices for preliminary classification of anemias; many of the subsequent steps in the diagnostic workup are not included. Note also that some conditions may appear in more than one category. (DIC = disseminated intravascular coagulation; G-6-PD = glucose-6-phosphate dehydrogenase.) (Adapted from Wintrobe M, et al. *Clinical hematology*. Philadelphia: Lea & Febiger, 1974.)

HEMATOL

Increased In

Bacterial infections, including miliary TB and tuberculous meningitis
Nocardia and other systemic fungal infections
Various parasitic infections (e.g., malaria)
Chédiak-Higashi syndrome
Idiopathic myelofibrosis
Normal infants up to age 2 mos
Pregnant women
Patients taking birth control pills
Some patients with lymphoma suppressed by chemotherapy

Decreased or Normal

(In absence of bacterial infection)
Healthy persons
Postpartum state
Postoperative state (after 7–10 days)
Cancer
Tissue transplantation
Other conditions with fever or leukocytosis not due to bacterial infection (e.g., RA)

Decreased or Normal

(In presence of bacterial infection)
Antibiotic therapy—effectiveness of treatment indicated by reduction of previous elevation, sometimes in <6 hrs
Localized infection
Administration of corticosteroids and immunosuppressive drugs (contrary findings with corticosteroids have also been reported)
Miscellaneous conditions, probably involving metabolic defects of neutrophil function
  • Chronic granulomatous disease
  • Neutrophilic deficiency of G-6-PD or myeloperoxidase
  • SLE
  • Sickle cell disease
  • Chronic myelogenous leukemia
  • Lipochrome histiocytosis
  • Congenital and acquired agammaglobulinemia
  • Other

Increased

(From previously determined normal level)
Has been used to monitor development of infection in chronically ill patients; may increase before other clinical parameters change.
  • Development of wound sepsis in burn patients
  • Development of infection in uremic patients on chronic hemodialysis

Osmotic Fragility

Use

Diagnosis of hereditary spherocytic anemia

Increased In

Hereditary spherocytic anemia (can be ruled out if a normal fragility is seen after 24-hr sterile incubation)
Hereditary nonspherocytic hemolytic anemia
Acquired hemolytic anemia (usually normal in paroxysmal nocturnal hemoglobinuria)
Hemolytic disease of newborn due to ABO incompatibility
Some cases of secondary hemolytic anemia (usually normal)
After thermal injury
Symptomatic hemolytic anemia in some cases of

Table 11-2. Red Blood Cell Indices[a]

Type of Anemia	MCV[b] (fL)	MCH[c] (pg)	MCHC[d] (gm/dL)
Normal	82–92	27–31	32–36
Normocytic	82–92	25–30	32–36
Macrocytic	95–150	30–50	32–36
Microcytic (usually hypochromic)	50–80	12–25	25–30

[a]Use: Classification and differential diagnosis of anemias.
[b]MCV (fL) = Hct/RBC.
[c]MCH (pg) = Hb/RBC; represents weight of Hb in average RBC. Not as useful as MCHC.
[d]MCHC (gm/dL) = Hb/Hct; represents concentration of Hb in average RBC.
Formula for estimating Hct from Hb:
Hct = Hb (gm/dL) × 2.8 + 0.8 or Hct = 3 × Hb

- Malignant lymphoma
- Leukemia
- Carcinoma
- Pregnancy
- Cirrhosis
- Infection (e.g., TB, malaria, syphilis)

Decreased In

Early infancy
Iron-deficiency anemia
Thalassemia
Sickle cell anemia
Homozygous HbC disease
Nutritional megaloblastic anemia
Postsplenectomy
Liver disease
Jaundice

Protoporphyrin, Free Erythrocyte (FEP)

(Normal <100 µg/dL packed RBCs)

Use

Screening for lead poisoning and for iron deficiency

Increased In

Iron deficiency (even before anemia; thus is an early sensitive sign, useful for screening). Range 100–1000 µg/dL; average ~200 µg/dL.
Chronic lead poisoning
Most sideroblastic anemias (e.g., acquired idiopathic)
Anemia of chronic diseases

Normal or Decreased In

Primary disorders of globin synthesis, e.g.,
- Thalassemia minor (therefore useful to differentiate from iron deficiency)
Pyridoxine-responsive anemia
One form of sideroblastic anemia due to block proximal to protoporphyrin synthesis

RBC Indices

See Table 11-2 and Fig. 11-3.

HEMATOL

Use

Classification and differential diagnosis of anemias

RBC Survival (^{51}Cr)

Use

Confirm decreased RBC survival in various disorders affecting RBCs

Increased In

Thalassemia minor
In pure red cell anemia, one-half of the plasma radioactivity may not disappear for 7–8 hrs.
   In the healthy person, one-half of the radioactivity of plasma disappears in 1–2 hrs.

Decreased In

Idiopathic acquired hemolytic anemia
Paroxysmal nocturnal hemoglobinuria
Association with chronic lymphatic leukemia
Association with uremia
Congenital nonspherocytic hemolytic anemia
Hereditary spherocytosis
Elliptocytosis with hemolysis
HbC disease
Sickle cell–HbC disease
Sickle cell anemia
PA
Megaloblastic anemia of pregnancy

Normal In

Sickle cell trait
HbC trait
Elliptocytosis without hemolysis or anemia

Red Cell Distribution Width (RDW)

(Normal = 11.5–14.5. No subnormal values have been reported.)
Is coefficient of variation of the RBC size as determined by some newer automated blood
   cell counting instruments. Is quantitative measure of anisocytosis.

$$CV = \frac{\text{(standard deviation of RBC size)}}{\text{(MCV)}}$$

Use

Classification of anemias based on MCV and RDW is most useful to distinguish iron-
   deficiency anemia from that of chronic disease or heterozygous thalassemia and to
   improve detection of early iron or folate deficiency.
RDW is more sensitive in microcytic than in macrocytic RBC conditions. Not helpful
   for patients without anemia.
Hb distribution width and cell Hb distribution width are two other indices of RBC heterogeneity that can be obtained from newer hematology analyzers; may be useful for
   further segregation of thalassemic traits.

Classification of RBC Disorders by MCV and RDW

See Table 11-3.

Table 11-3. Classification of Red Blood Cell (RBC) Disorders by Mean Corpuscular Volume (MCV) and Red Cell Distribution Width (RDW)

		MCV		
		Low	Normal	High
RDW	Low	Thalassemia minor Thalassemia minor	Normal	Aplastic anemia
	Normal	Anemia of chronic disease	Anemia of chronic disease Hereditary sphero- cytosis (may also have high RDW) Some hemoglobin- opathy traits (e.g., AS)	Myelodysplastic syndrome
	High	Iron deficiency HbH disease S beta-thalassemia Fragmentation of RBCs Hemoglobin- opathy traits (AC) Some patients with anemia of chronic disease G-6-PD deficiency	Early deficiency of iron, or vitamin B_{12} or folate Sickle cell anemia HbSC disease	Deficiency of vita- min B_{12} or folate Immune hemolytic anemia Cold agglutinins Alcoholism

G-6-PD = glucose-6-phosphate dehydrogenase; HbH = hemoglobin H; HbSC = hemoglobin SC.

Reticulocyte Count

Use

Diagnosis of ineffective erythropoiesis or decreased RBC formation.
Increase indicates effective RBC production.
- Index of therapeutic response to iron, folate, or vitamin B_{12} therapy and to blood loss.
- Monitor treatment response after bone marrow suppression and transplantation.
- Monitor response to erythropoietin therapy.

Increased In

After blood loss or increased RBC destruction: normal increase is 3–6×.
After iron therapy for iron-deficiency anemia.
After specific therapy for megaloblastic anemias.
Possibly other hematologic conditions (e.g., polycythemia, metastatic carcinoma in bone marrow, Di Guglielmo's disease).

Decreased In

Ineffective erythropoiesis or decreased RBC formation
- Severe autoimmune type of hemolytic disease
- Aregenerative crises
- Megaloblastic disorders
Alcoholism

Myxedema

Reticulocyte index corrects count for degree of anemia:

Reticulocyte index = reticulocyte count × (patient's Hct)/45 × 1/1.85

(45 is assumed normal Hct; 1.85 is number of days required for reticulocyte to mature into an RBC)

Reticulocyte index <2% indicates hypoproliferative component to anemia.

Reticulocyte index >2–3% indicates increased RBC production.

Reticulocyte Hemoglobin[1]

(Absolute reticulocyte count multiplied by reticulocyte Hb content; in gm/L)

RBC Hb = total Hb minus reticulocyte Hb

Use

Ratio of RBC Hb to reticulocyte Hb is a rough estimate of RBC survival and severity of hemolysis.

Interpretation

Normal = 55–98

SS disease = 5.7–13.9

SS disease (with three normal genes) = 6.1–26.3

SS disease (with two normal genes) = 9.7–19.7

SC disease (no alpha genes) = 19–54

Reticulocyte Hemoglobin Content[2]

(Performed using automated hematology analyzer)

Use

These are preliminary reports that require further study

May be useful for diagnosis of iron deficiency and iron-deficiency anemia

Early indicator (within 2 wks) of response to iron therapy in cases of iron-deficiency anemia

Decreased In

Iron deficiency

Alpha- and beta-thalassemia

Interpretation

Normal = 55–98

Transferrin, Serum

See Table 11-10.

Use

Differential diagnosis of anemias

Increased In

Iron-deficiency anemia

Pregnancy, estrogen therapy, hyperestrogenism

---

[1]Brugnara C, et al. Reticulocyte hemoglobin. An integrated parameter for evaluation of erythrocyte activity. *Am J Clin Pathol* 1997;108:133.
[2]Brugnara C, et al. Reticulocyte hemoglobin content to diagnose iron deficiency in children. *JAMA* 1999;281:2225.

Decreased In

Hypochromic microcytic anemia of chronic disease
Acute inflammation
Protein deficiency or loss, e.g.,
- Thermal burns
- Chronic infections
- Chronic diseases (e.g., various liver and kidney diseases, neoplasms)
- Nephrosis
- Malnutrition

Genetic deficiency

Transferrin Receptor, Serum

(Transmembrane proteins present on surface of most cells; reference range = 0.57–2.8 µg/L; varies with assay system; higher in blacks.)

Use

Differential diagnosis of microcytic anemias; increased in iron-deficiency anemias but not increased in anemia of chronic disease
Diagnosis of iron deficiency in patients with chronic disease (Table 11-10)
Distinguish iron-deficiency erythropoiesis (iron-deficiency anemia) from physiologic depletion of iron stores (e.g., in pregnancy, childhood, adolescence)
>20% increase over baseline within 2 wks of starting or increasing erythropoietin therapy predicts response to that dosage and indicates that Hb response is likely to follow.
Evaluation of anemias when ferritin values may be increased to normal range due to acute-phase reaction if other causes of increased erythropoiesis are ruled out

Increased In

Disorders with hyperplastic erythropoiesis (e.g., iron-deficiency anemias, hemolytic anemias)
Disorders with ineffective erythropoiesis (e.g., myelodysplastic syndromes, megaloblastic anemias)
Persons living at high altitude
Erythropoietin therapy

Decreased In

Disorders with reduced erythropoiesis (e.g., aplastic anemia, after bone marrow ablation for stem cell transplantation)
Iron overload disorders

Transferrin Saturation, Serum

(Serum iron divided by TIBC; normal ≥ 16%)

Use

Differential diagnosis of anemias
Screening for hereditary hemochromatosis

Increased In

Hemochromatosis
Hemosiderosis
Thalassemia
Use of progesterone birth control pills (≤ 75%)
Ingestion of iron (≤ 100%)
Iron dextran administration causes increase for several weeks (may be >100%).

Decreased In

Iron-deficiency anemia (usually <10% in established deficiency)
Anemias of infection and chronic diseases (e.g., uremia, RA, some neoplasms)

$$\text{Transferrin saturation } (\%) = \frac{\{[\text{serum iron } (\mu g/dL)]\}}{[\text{TIBC } (\mu g/dL)]} \times 100$$

Vitamin B$_{12}$-Binding Capacity, Unsaturated
(Normal range = 870–1800 ng/L)

Use

Minor criterion in diagnosis of polycythemia vera

Increased In

Myeloproliferative diseases (especially polycythemia vera and CML)
Pregnancy
Use of oral contraceptive drugs

Decreased In

Hepatitis and cirrhosis

White Blood Cell (WBC) Differential Count

Use

Diagnosis of myeloproliferative disorders, myelodysplasias, various other hematologic
  disorders
Support diagnosis of various infections and inflammation
Is often ordered inappropriately and has almost no value as a *screening* test. The neutrophil and band counts may be useful in acute appendicitis and neonatal sepsis with
  moderate sensitivity and specificity.

Interferences

Associated with automated WBC counters (artifact is corrected when manual WBC
  counts are performed)
• Leukocyte fragility due to immunosuppressive and antineoplastic drugs
• Lymphocyte fragility in lymphocytic leukemia
• Excessive clumping of leukocytes in monoclonal gammopathies (e.g., multiple
  myeloma), cryofibrinogenemia (e.g., SLE), in presence of cold agglutinins

Causes of Neutropenia/Leukopenia

See Fig. 11-4.
**(Absolute neutrophil count [total WBC × % segmented neutrophils and bands]
<1800/cu mm; <1000 in blacks.)**
Decreased/ineffective production
• Infections, especially
    Bacterial (e.g., overwhelming bacterial infection, septicemia, miliary TB,
      typhoid, paratyphoid, brucellosis, tularemia)
    Viral (e.g., infectious mononucleosis, hepatitis, influenza, measles, rubella, psit-
      tacosis)
    Rickettsial (e.g., scrub typhus, sandfly fever)
    Other (e.g., malaria, kala-azar)
• Drugs and chemicals, especially
    Sulfonamides
    Antibiotics
    Analgesics
    Marrow depressants
    Arsenicals
    Antithyroid drugs
    Many others
• Ionizing radiation
• Hematopoietic diseases

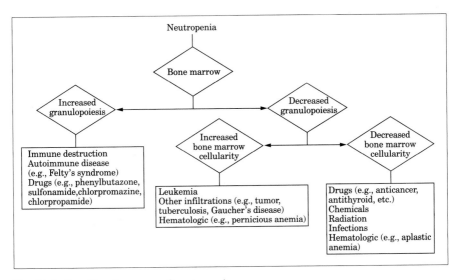

Fig. 11-4. Algorithm for causes of neutropenia.

Folic acid and vitamin B$_{12}$ deficiency
Aleukemic leukemia
Aplastic anemia
Myelophthisis
Decreased survival
- Felty's syndrome
- SLE
- Autoimmune and isoimmune neutropenias
- Splenic sequestration
- Drugs
Abnormal distribution
- Hypersplenism
Miscellaneous
- Severe renal injury

Neonatal and Infantile Causes
(Neutrophil count <5000/cu mm during first few days or <1000/cu mm by end of first week of life)

Maternal causes
- Associated with maternal neutropenia (e.g., SLE)
- Maternal drug ingestion and often associated with thrombocytopenia (e.g., sulfa drugs, thiazides, propylthiouracil, phenothiazines, trimethadione, amidopyrine)
- Associated with maternal isoimmunization to fetal leukocytes

Inborn errors of metabolism (e.g., chronic tyrosinosis, maple syrup urine disease, ketotic hyperglycinemia, methylmalonic acidemia, isovaleric acidemia, propionic acidemia)

Immune defects (e.g., X-linked agammaglobulinemia, dysgammaglobulinemia)
- Associated with phenotypic abnormalities (e.g., cartilage hair dysplasia, dyskeratosis congenita, Shwachman-Diamond syndrome [chronic hypoplastic neutropenia associated with pancreatic insufficiency])
- Infantile genetic agranulocytosis
- Disorders of uncommitted stem cell proliferation
- Cyclic neutropenia
- Reticular dysgenesis (granulocytes and lymphocytes do not develop normally, absent thymus, low immunoglobulin concentrations, platelets and RBCs are unaffected)

Table 11-4. Some Common Causes of Leukemoid Reaction

Cause	Myelocytic	Lymphocytic	Monocytic
Infections	Endocarditis Pneumonia Septicemia Leptospirosis Other	Infectious mononucleosis Infectious lymphocytosis Pertussis Varicella TB	TB
Toxic conditions	Burns Eclampsia Poisoning (e.g., mercury)		
Neoplasms	Carcinoma of colon Embryonal carci- noma of kidney	Carcinoma of stomach Carcinoma of breast	
Miscellaneous	Treatment of megalo- blastic anemia (of pregnancy, perni- cious anemia) Acute hemorrhage Acute hemolysis Recovery from agranulocytosis	Dermatitis herpetiformis	
Myeloproliferative diseases			

Disorders of myeloid stem cell proliferation
- Kostmann's agranulocytosis (moderate to severe neutropenia that may be associ-
  ated with dysgammaglobulinemia, frequent chromosomal abnormalities, normal
  granulocytic maturation up to promyelocyte or myelocyte stage)
- Benign chronic granulocytopenia of childhood
- In children
    Adult type PA (see p. 371)
    Defective secretion or type of gastric intrinsic factor (normal gastric mucosa and
      acid secretion, no antibodies to intrinsic factor or parietal cells, no associated
      endocrine deficiency)
    Imerslund-Graesbeck syndrome (see p. 371)
- Pregnancy—progressive decrease in granulocyte count during pregnancy. *Serum
  B$_{12}$ is normal in megaloblastic anemia of pregnancy.*

Causes of Neutrophilia

(Absolute neutrophil count >8000/cu mm)
See Tables 11-4 and 11-5.
Acute infections
- Localized (e.g., pneumonia, meningitis, tonsillitis, abscess)
- Generalized (e.g., acute rheumatic fever, septicemia, cholera)
Inflammation (e.g., vasculitis)
Intoxications
- Metabolic (uremia, acidosis, eclampsia, acute gout)
- Poisoning by chemicals, drugs, venoms, etc. (e.g., mercury, epinephrine, black
  widow spider)
- Parenteral (foreign protein and vaccines)
Acute hemorrhage
Acute hemolysis of red blood cells
Myeloproliferative diseases

Table 11-5. Comparison of Leukemia and Leukemoid Reaction

	Leukemia	Leukemoid Reaction
White blood cell count	May be >100,000	Usually <50,000
Neutrophils	May have myeloid cells earlier than bands	Mature; <10% bands
Leukocyte alkaline phosphatase	Decreased in CML; variable in others	Increased
Basophilia, eosinophilia, monocytosis	Frequently present	Absent
Platelets	Frequently abnormal morphology Frequently >1 million Thrombocytopenia may occur	Usually small Normal aggregation Rarely >600,000 No thrombocytopenia
Peripheral smear RBC	Nucleated RBCs, abnormal forms (teardrop, polychromatophilia) may occur	RBCs appear normal No nucleated RBCs
Bone marrow	Abnormal	Hyperplastic
Karyotype	May be abnormal Ph[1] may be present in CML	Normal Ph[1] absent
Clone demonstrated	By X-linked inactivation	No clone demonstrated
bcr-abl demonstrated	By Southern blot or PCR	Not demonstrated

Tissue necrosis, e.g.,
- AMI
- Necrosis of tumors
- Burns
- Gangrene
- Bacterial necrosis

Physiologic conditions (e.g., exercise, emotional stress, menstruation, obstetric labor)

Steroid administration (e.g., prednisone 40 mg orally) causes increased neutrophil leukocytes of 1700–7500 (peak in 4–6 hrs and return to normal in 24 hrs); no definite shift to left. Lymphocytes decrease 70% and monocytes decrease 90%.

May be accompanied by shift to left of granulocytes, toxic granulation, Döhle's bodies, and cytoplasmic vacuolization.

Causes of Lymphocytosis

(>4000/cu mm in adults, >7200/cu mm in adolescents, >9000/cu mm in young children and infants)

See Fig. 11-5.

Infections
- Pertussis
- Infectious lymphocytosis
- Infectious mononucleosis
- Infectious hepatitis
- CMV infection
- Mumps
- Rubella
- Varicella
- Toxoplasmosis
- Chronic TB
- Undulant fever
- Convalescence from acute infection

Thyrotoxicosis (relative)

Addison's disease

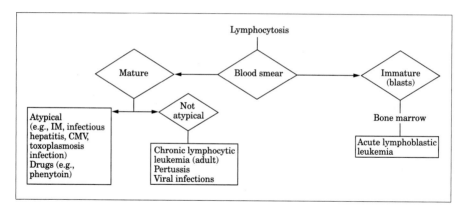

Fig. 11-5. Algorithm for causes of lymphocytosis.

Neutropenia with relative lymphocytosis
Lymphatic leukemia
Crohn's disease
Ulcerative colitis
Serum sickness
Drug hypersensitivity
Vasculitis

Causes of Lymphocytopenia

(<1500 in adults, <3000 in children)
Increased destruction
- Chemotherapy or radiation treatment
- Corticosteroids (Cushing's syndrome, stress)

Increased loss via GI tract
- Intestinal lymphectasia
- Thoracic duct drainage
- Obstruction to intestinal lymphatic drainage (e.g., tumor, Whipple's disease, intestinal lymphangiectasia)
- Congestive heart failure

Decreased production
- Aplastic anemia
- Malignancy, especially Hodgkin's disease
- Inherited immunoglobulin disorders (e.g., Wiskott-Aldrich syndrome, combined immunodeficiency, ataxia-telangiectasia)
- Infection (e.g., AIDS)

Others (e.g., SLE, renal failure, miliary TB, myasthenia gravis, aplastic anemia)

CD4 Lymphocytes

(By flow cytometry; calculated as total WBC × % lymphocytes × % lymphocytes stained with CD4)
Use
Diagnosis of immune dysfunction, especially AIDS, in which severely depressed count is the single best predictor of imminent opportunistic infection and an increase is associated with therapeutic effect of drugs. May also be expressed as CD4/CD8 lymphocyte ratio but CD8 count is more labile and may diminish the value of the CD4 counts.

Decreased In
Acute minor viral infections. Should recheck in 3 mos.
Also diurnal variation; peak evening values may be 2× morning values. Imprecision in total WBC and differential may cause 25% variability in CD4 values.

Causes of Atypical Lymphocytes

Lymphatic leukemia
Viral infections
- Infectious lymphocytosis
- Infectious mononucleosis
- Infectious hepatitis
- Viral pneumonia and other exanthems of childhood
- Mumps
- Varicella
- CMV infection

Pertussis
Brucellosis
Syphilis (in some phases)
Toxoplasmosis
Drug reactions and serum sickness
Healthy persons may show up to 12% atypical lymphocytes.
"Heterophile negative" infectious mononucleosis syndrome is most often seen in
- Early stage of infectious mononucleosis
- Toxoplasmosis
- CMV infection
- Infectious hepatitis

Basophilic Leukocytes

Use
May be first sign of blast crisis or accelerated phase of CML
Persistent basophilia may indicate unsuspected myeloproliferative disease.
Diagnosis of basophilic leukemia

Increased In (>50/cu mm or >1%)
Chronic myelogenous leukemia
Basophilic leukemia
Polycythemia
Myeloid metaplasia
Hodgkin's disease
Postsplenectomy
Chronic hemolytic anemia (some patients)
Chronic sinusitis
Varicella
Variola
Myxedema
Nephrosis (some patients)
Foreign protein injection
Ionizing radiation

Decreased In
Hyperthyroidism
Pregnancy
Period after irradiation, chemotherapy, and glucocorticoid administration
Acute phase of infection

Causes of Monocytosis

(>10% of differential count; absolute count >500/cu mm)
Monocytic leukemia, other leukemias
Other myeloproliferative disorders (myeloid metaplasia, polycythemia vera)
Hodgkin's disease and other malignant lymphomas
Lipid storage diseases (e.g., Gaucher's disease)
Postsplenectomy
Tetrachloroethane poisoning
Recovery from agranulocytosis and subsidence of acute infection
Many protozoan infections (e.g., malaria, kala-azar, trypanosomiasis)
Some rickettsial infections (e.g., Rocky Mountain spotted fever, typhus)
Certain bacterial infections (e.g., SBE, TB, brucellosis)
Chronic ulcerative colitis, regional enteritis, and sprue

HEMATOL

Sarcoidosis
Collagen diseases (e.g., RA, SLE)
Most common causes are indolent infections (e.g., mycobacteria, SBE) and recovery
 phase of neutropenia.
*Monocyte phagocytosis of RBCs in peripheral smears from earlobe is said to occur often
 in SBE.*

Plasma Cells

Increased In
Plasma cell leukemia
Multiple myeloma
Hodgkin's disease
CLL
Other neoplasias (cancer of liver, kidney, breast, prostate)
Cirrhosis
RA
SLE
Serum reaction
Bacterial infections (e.g., syphilis, TB)
Parasitic infections (e.g., malaria, trichinosis)
Viral infections (e.g., infectious mononucleosis, rubella, measles, varicella, benign lym-
 phocytic meningitis)
Decreased In
Not clinically significant

Causes of Eosinophilia

(>250/cu mm; diurnal variation with highest levels in morning)
Allergic diseases (e.g., bronchial asthma, hay fever, urticaria, drug therapy, allergic
 rhinitis, eczema)
Parasitic infestation, especially with tissue invasion (e.g., trichinosis, *Echinococcus* dis-
 ease, schistosomiasis, filariasis, fascioliasis)
Mycoses (e.g., coccidioidomycosis)
Some infectious diseases (e.g., scarlet fever, erythema multiforme, *Chlamydia* infection)
Collagen-vascular diseases (e.g., periarteritis nodosa, SLE, RA, scleroderma, dermato-
 myositis, Churg-Strauss syndrome)
Some diffuse skin diseases (e.g., pemphigus, dermatitis herpetiformis)
Some hematopoietic diseases (e.g., PA, chronic myelogenous leukemia, AML, polycythemia,
 Hodgkin's disease, T-cell lymphomas, eosinophilic leukemia); postsplenectomy
Some immunodeficiency disorders (e.g., Wiskott-Aldrich syndrome, graft-versus-host
 disease, cyclic neutropenia, IgA deficiency)
Some gastrointestinal diseases (e.g., eosinophilic gastroenteritis, ulcerative colitis,
 regional enteritis, colon carcinoma)
Some endocrine diseases (e.g., hypopituitarism, Addison's disease)
Postirradiation
Miscellaneous conditions
 • Certain tumors (ovary, involvement of bone or serosal surfaces)
 • Sarcoidosis
 • Löffler's parietal fibroplastic endocarditis
 • Familial conditions
 • Poisoning (e.g., phosphorus, black widow spider bite)
Drugs (e.g., aspirin sensitivity)
Hypereosinophilic syndrome (see p. 396)
Highest levels occur in trichinosis, *Clonorchis sinensis* infection, and dermatitis her-
 petiformis.

Hematologic Diseases

Acquired Immune Deficiency Syndrome (AIDS)
See Chapter 15, p. 828.

Table 11-6. Comparison of Some Primary Immunodeficiency Diseases

	Name	T cell	B cell	Ig
Combined lympho- cyte defects	DiGeorge syndrome	N/D	N/D	N/D
	X-linked SCID	D	N/I	D
	X-linked hyper-IgM syndrome	N	N	N/I IgM D IgA, IgG
Antibody deficiency	X-linked agamma- globulinemia	N	D/0	D/0
	Common variable immunodeficiency	N	N	D ≥ 1 sub- types
	Ig deficiency (e.g., IgA, IgG)	N	N	D ≥ 1 sub- types
	Mu heavy-chain deficiency	N	0	0
Phagocyte disorders	Chronic granulomatous disease	N	N	N
	Chédiak-Higashi syndrome	N	N	N
	Leukocyte adhesion deficiency	N	N	N
Complement deficiencies (see p. 49)	Individual complement deficiency	N	N	N
Other syndromes	Wiskott-Aldrich syndrome	N	N/D	N (some D IgM)
	Ataxia-telangiectasia	N	N	N
	Hyper-IgE syndrome	N	N	I IgE
	Bloom syndrome	N	N	N
	X-linked lymphopro- liferative syndrome	N	N	N
	Autoimmune lympho- proliferative syndrome	N/I I CD4/CD8	I	I

0 = absent; D = decreased; hyper-IgE = hyperimmunoglobulinemia E; hyper-IgM = hyperimmunoglobulinemia M; I = increased; Ig = immunoglobulin; N = normal; SCID = severe combined immunodeficiency disease.

Agammaglobulinemia, X-Linked (Bruton's Disease)

(X-linked recessive trait)
See Tables 11-6 and 11-7.

Male patients experience severe recurrent pyogenic infections (commonly due to *Streptococcus pneumoniae, Haemophilus influenzae*; also *Streptococcus pyogenes* and *S. aureus*) after age 4–6 mos. Often have persistent viral infections (e.g., chronic, progressive, fatal CNS infection with echoviruses) or parasitic infections. *Giardia lamblia* leads to chronic diarrhea. Large joint arthritis probably due to *Ureaplasma urealyticum*. Not unusually susceptible to viral infections except fulminant hepatitis.

♦ Inability to make functional antibody is the distinguishing feature; antibody responses to immunization are usually absent. Live virus vaccination may cause severe disease (e.g., paralytic polio).

♦ Serum levels of all immunoglobulins are very low (IgG <100 mg/dL; IgA, IgM undetectable).

♦ B cells in peripheral blood are absent or found in very low numbers.

♦ T cell numbers and function are intact.

Plasma cells in lymph nodes and GI tract are absent or found in very low numbers.

No markers exist for detection of heterozygotes.

Hypoplasia of tonsils, adenoids, lymph nodes. Thymus appears normal with Hassall's corpuscles and abundant lymphoid cells.

Table 11-7. Classification of Primary Immunologic Defects

Syndrome	Number of Circulating Lymphocytes	Number of Plasma Cells	Ig Changes	Thymus	Lymph Node — Germinal Center	Lymph Node — Paracortical Zone	Other Laboratory Findings
X-linked agammaglobulinemia (Bruton's disease)	N	O	Markedly D in all	N	O	N	X; increased frequency of malignant lymphoma
Selective inability to produce IgA	N	IgA-producing plasma cells, especially in lamina propria	IgA is O; others are usually N	N	N	N	May have malabsorption syndrome, steatorrhea, bronchitis.
Transient hypogammaglobulinemia of infancy	N	D	IgG is D		O or rare		X
Non–sex-linked primary immunoglobulin deficiencies (e.g., dysgammaglobulinemias—acquired, congenital)	N	V (usually D)	Present, but type and amount are V	N	Usually O Often D Reticulum hyperplasia		X, Z; increased frequency of malignant lymphoma and autoimmune diseases
Agammaglobulinemia with thymoma (Good's syndrome)	Progressively D, often to very low levels	D or O	Markedly D in all	Enlarged (stromal epithelial spindle-cell type)	D or O	May be D	X, Z; thymoma; pure red cell aplasia may occur; eosinophils O or markedly D
Wiskott-Aldrich syndrome (X-linked, recessive immune deficiency with thrombopenia and eczema)	Usually progressively D	N	Usually present, but type and amount are V (frequently IgM is D and IgA is I; IgG usually N	N	May be D	Progressively D in lymphocytes	X, Z; eczema and thrombocytopenia; increased frequency of malignant lymphoma; serum lacks isohemagglutinins; platelets one-half normal size

Syndrome							Comments
Ataxia-telangiectasia (Louis-Bar's syndrome), autosomal recessive	V (usually slightly D)	V (usually present)	Usually present, but type and amount are V (frequently IgA and IgE are D or O, and D IgG)	Embryonic type (no Hassall's corpuscles or cortical medullary organization)	May be D	Lymphocytes D	Progressive cerebellar ataxia; telangiectasia in tissues; ovarian dysgenesis; increased frequency of malignant lymphoma; frequent pulmonary infections when IgA is D
Primary lymphopenic immunologic deficiency (Gitlin's syndrome)	V–D	V	Always present, but type and amount are V	Hypoplastic (Hassall's corpuscles and lymphoid cells D)			Z
Autosomal recessive alymphocytotic agammaglobulinemia (Swiss type agammaglobulinemia; Glanzmann's and Riniker's lymphocytophthisis)	Markedly D	O	Markedly D in all	Hypoplastic (Hassall's corpuscles and lymphoid cells O)	Lymphocytes O or markedly D	Marked D in tissue lymphocytes; foci of lymphocytes may be present in spleen and lymph nodes	X, Z; increased frequency of malignant lymphoma
Autosomal recessive lymphopenia with normal immunoglobulins (Nezelof's syndrome)	D	Present	N	Hypoplastic (Hassall's corpuscles and lymphoid cells O)	May be present	Lymphocytes markedly D	Z
DiGeorge syndrome (thymic aplasia)	V (usually N)	Present	N	Absent	Present	Rare paracortical lymphocytes present	Z; absent parathyroids (tetany of the newborn); frequent cardiovascular malformations

N = normal; O = absent; D = decreased; Ig = immunoglobulin; V = variable; X = recurrent infections with pyogenic organisms; Z = frequent virus, fungus, or *Pneumocystis* infection.

Adapted from Seligmann M, Fudenberg HH, Good RA. A proposed classification of primary immunologic deficiencies. *Am J Med* 1968;45:818.

Increased frequency of lymphoreticular malignancy ($\leq 6\%$).

Prone to develop connective tissue diseases (e.g., dermatomyositis, RA-like disorder) and allergic disorders (e.g., rhinitis, asthma, eczema, drug rash)

Female carriers can be identified by examination of B cells.

Agranulocytosis

♦ In acute fulminant form, WBC is decreased to ≤ 2000/cu mm, sometimes as low as 50/cu mm. Granulocytes are 0–2%. Granulocytes may show pyknosis or vacuolization.

♦ In chronic or recurrent form, WBC is decreased to 2000/cu mm with less marked granulocytopenia.

Relative lymphocytosis and sometimes monocytosis are seen.

♦ Bone marrow shows absence of cells in granulocytic series but normal erythroid and megakaryocytic series.

ESR is increased.

Hb, RBC count and morphology, platelet count, and coagulation tests are normal.

Laboratory findings due to infection.

Due To

Peripheral destruction of PMNs (often drug related)

Overwhelming sepsis

More generalized bone marrow failure (see Anemia, Aplastic, p. 354)

Alder-Reilly Anomaly

♦ Heavy azurophilic granulation of granulocytes and some lymphocytes and monocytes associated with mucopolysaccharidoses (Table 13-12) are seen. Present in $\leq 90\%$ of neutrophils in Hurler's syndrome. Inconstant in blood but always present in marrow mononuclear phagocytes.

Alpha Heavy-Chain Disease

(Mediterranean-type abdominal lymphoma; most common heavy-chain disease)

♦ Diagnostic Criteria

Serum protein shows distinctive increase in monoclonal IgA heavy chain (alpha chain) not associated with a light chain; causes an elevated broad peak in half the cases and is normal in the other cases. Same alpha chain in jejunal fluid, lymphocytes, or plasma cells. Low concentration of alpha chains in urine.

Laboratory findings of severe malabsorption with chronic diarrhea and steatorrhea due to diffuse lymphoma-like proliferation in small intestine and mesentery. Rarely, respiratory tract involvement.

Biopsy of small intestine shows marked infiltration with abnormal plasma cells.

Bence Jones proteinuria is absent.

Bone marrow is normal.

Alpha$_1$-Antitrypsin Deficiency

(Autosomal recessive deficiency associated with familial pulmonary emphysema and liver disease. The heterozygous state occurs in 10–15% of the general population, who have serum levels of alpha$_1$-antitrypsin ~60% of normal; homozygous state occurs in 1 in 2000 persons, who have serum levels ~10% of normal; there are many alleles of alpha$_1$-antitrypsin gene.)

See Table 11-8.

♦ Absent alpha$_1$ peak on serum protein electrophoresis. Should be confirmed by assay of serum alpha$_1$-antitrypsin (electroimmunoassay) and Pi phenotyping (isoelectric focusing on polyacrylamide; DNA analysis also permits prenatal diagnosis), and functional analysis of total trypsin inhibitory capacity (90% is due to alpha$_1$-antitrypsin activity).

Table 11-8. Alleles of the AAT Gene

	Serum AAT	AAT Function	Phenotype
Normal	Normal (150–350 mg/dL)	Normal	Pi MM
Deficient severe	<50 mg/dL	Normal	Pi ZZ (>95% of cases)
			Pi SZ (rare)
			Pi SS
			Pi MZ
Null	Undetectable		Pi null–null
			Pi Z–null
Dysfunctional	Normal	Abnormal	

Z alleles are rare in Asians and blacks.
Threshold protection level for emphysema = 80 mg/dL.

Alpha$_1$-Antitrypsin May Be Decreased In

(Typically <50 mg/dL)
Prematurity
Severe liver disease
Malnutrition
Renal losses (e.g., nephrosis)
GI losses (e.g., pancreatitis, protein-losing diseases)
Exudative dermopathies
Alpha$_1$-antitrypsin deficiency should be ruled out in children with neonatal hepatitis, giant cell hepatitis, chronically abnormal liver chemistries, or juvenile cirrhosis and in adults with chronic hepatitis without serologic markers, cryptogenic cirrhosis, hepatoma.

Alpha$_1$-Antitrypsin Increased In

(Is an acute-phase reactant)
Acute or chronic infections
Neoplasia (especially cervical cancer and lymphomas)
Pregnancy
Use of birth control pills

○Liver biopsy supports the diagnosis and helps stage extent of liver damage. Shows characteristic intracytoplasmic inclusions (in both heterozygotes and homozygotes) that may be found in patients with emphysema without liver disease and in asymptomatic heterozygous relatives, but must be searched for and stained specifically, because the rest of the pathology in the liver is not specific. ~9% of adults with non-alcoholic cirrhosis are MZ phenotype. Hepatoma may occur in cirrhotic livers.

Liver disease occurs in 10–20% of children with this deficiency. Clinical picture may be neonatal hepatitis (in 15% of those with ZZ phenotype), prolonged obstructive jaundice during infancy, or cirrhosis, or patient may be asymptomatic. 5–10% of infants with undefined cholestasis have alpha$_1$-antitrypsin deficiency. In ~25% of these patients, clinical and biochemical abnormalities become normal by age 3–10 yrs; ~25% have abnormal liver function tests with or without clinical cirrhosis; ~25% survive first decade with confirmed cirrhosis; 25% die of cirrhosis between 6 mos and 17 yrs of age.

○Pulmonary emphysema occurs in heterozygotes and homozygotes; occurs in family of 25% of patients. Causes 2% of cases of emphysema. Secondary bronchitis and bronchiectasis may occur. Associated with phenotypes Pi ZZ and probably Pi SZ but not Pi MZ.

Purified alpha$_1$-antitrypsin is now available for augmentation therapy.
• Indicated when alpha$_1$-antitrypsin is severely deficient, abnormal lung function tests shows deterioration.

HEMATOL

- Not indicated when lung function is normal even if there is alpha$_1$-antitrypsin deficiency with liver disease, or when pulmonary emphysema is associated with normal or heterozygous phenotypes.

Anemia, Acute Blood Loss

RBC, Hb, and Hct level are not reliable initially because of compensatory vasoconstriction and hemodilution. They decrease for several days after hemorrhage ceases. RBC returns to normal in 4–6 wks. Hb returns to normal in 6–8 wks.

Anemia is normochromic, normocytic. (*If hypochromic or microcytic, rule out iron deficiency due to prior hemorrhages.*)

Reticulocyte count is increased after 1–2 days, reaches peak in 4–7 days (≤ 15%). Persistent increase suggests continuing hemorrhage.

Blood smear shows no poikilocytes. Polychromasia and increased number of nucleated RBCs (up to 5:100 WBCs) may be found.

Increased WBC (usually ≤ 20,000/cu mm) reaches peak in 2–5 hrs, becomes normal in 3–4 days. Persistent increase suggests continuing hemorrhage, bleeding into a body cavity, or infection. Differential count shows shift to the left.

Platelets are increased (≤ 1 million/cu mm) within a few hours; coagulation time is decreased.

BUN is increased if hemorrhage into lumen of GI tract occurs.

Serum indirect bilirubin is increased if hemorrhage into a body cavity or cystic structure occurs.

Laboratory findings due to causative disease (e.g., peptic ulcer, esophageal varices, leukemia).

Anemia, Aplastic[3]

♦ Peripheral blood pancytopenia with variable bone marrow hypocellularity in the absence of underlying myeloproliferative or malignant disease.
- Neutropenia (absolute neutrophil count <1500/cu mm) is always present; often monocytopenia is present.
- Lymphocyte count is normal; reduced helper/inducer to cytotoxic/suppressor ratio.
- Platelet count <150,000/cu mm; severity varies.
- Anemia is usually normochromic, normocytic but may be slightly macrocytic. RDW is normal. Poikilocytes are not seen on peripheral blood smear.
- Bone marrow is hypocellular; aspiration and biopsy should both be performed to rule out leukemia, myelodysplastic syndrome, granulomas, tumor.

Reticulocyte count corrected for Hct is decreased.

Serum iron is increased.

Flow cytometry phenotyping shows virtual absence of CD34 stem cells in blood and marrow.

Laboratory findings represent the whole spectrum, from the most severe condition of the classic type with marked leukopenia, thrombocytopenia, anemia, and acellular bone marrow, to cases with involvement only of erythroid elements. In some cases, the marrow may be cellular or hyperplastic.

♦ Criteria for *severe* aplastic anemia (International Aplastic Anemia Study Group)
  ≥ 2 peripheral blood criteria plus either marrow criteria
- Peripheral blood criteria
    Neutrophils <500/cu mm
    Platelets <20,000/cu mm
    Reticulocyte count <1% (corrected for Hct)
- Marrow criteria
    Severe hypocellularity
    Moderate hypocellularity with <30% of residual cells being hematopoietic

Due To

Idiopathic in 50% of cases
Chemicals (e.g., benzene family, insecticides)
Cytotoxic and antimetabolite drugs

[3]Young NS. Acquired aplastic anemia. *N Engl J Med* 1999;282:271.

Other drugs
- Antimicrobials (especially chloramphenicol, quinacrine), anticonvulsants (especially hydantoin), analgesics (especially phenylbutazone), antihistamines, antidiabetic drugs, sedatives, others (especially gold; NSAIDs, sulfonamides, antithyroid drugs)

Immunologic disorders (e.g., graft-versus-host disease, thymoma and thymic carcinoma)

Ionizing irradiation (x-rays, radioisotopes)

Malnutrition (e.g., kwashiorkor)

Viral infections in 10% of cases (especially seronegative hepatitis; EBV, CMV, HIV, parvovirus)

Constitutional, inherited (e.g., Fanconi's anemia)

Leukemia is the underlying disease in 1–5% of patients who present with aplastic anemia. 15% of aplastic anemia patients develop myelodysplasia and leukemia.

Paroxysmal nocturnal hemoglobinuria develops in 5–10% of patients with aplastic anemia, and aplastic anemia develops in 25% of patients with paroxysmal nocturnal hemoglobinuria.

Anemia, Fanconi's

(Simple autosomal recessive syndrome of pancytopenia and characteristic congenital anomalies of rudimentary thumbs, hypoplastic radii, short stature, renal anomalies, skin hyperpigmentation, chromosomal breaks)

Pancytopenia usually noted at 4–10 yrs of age but may be from infancy to 20s. Anemia, leukopenia, and thrombocytopenia may not all be present at onset.
- Profound anemia may be macrocytic and hyperchromic or normochromic.
- Increased HbF (>28%).
- Decreased granulocytes.
- Atrophic bone marrow.

Causes >20% of childhood cases of aplastic anemia.

Increased incidence of leukemia in patients and relatives.

Cytogenetic studies show normal chromosome numbers but structural instability causing breaks, gaps, constrictions, rearrangements.

Laboratory findings due to anemia, hemorrhage, infection, renal abnormalities.

Anemia, Hemolytic, Acquired

Laboratory findings due to increased destruction of RBCs
- RBC survival time differentiates intrinsic defect from factor outside RBC.
- Blood smear often shows marked spherocytosis. Anisocytosis, poikilocytosis, and polychromasia are seen.
- Slight abnormality of osmotic fragility occurs.
- Increased indirect serum bilirubin (<6 mg/dL) because of compensatory excretory capacity of liver).
- Urine urobilinogen is increased (may vary with liver function; may be obscured by antibiotic therapy altering intestinal flora). Bile is absent.
- Hemoglobinemia and hemoglobinuria are present when hemolysis is very rapid.
- Haptoglobins are decreased or absent in chronic hemolytic diseases (removed after combination with free Hb in serum).
- WBC is usually elevated.

Laboratory findings due to compensatory increased production of RBCs
- Normochromic, normocytic anemia. MCV reflects immaturity of circulating RBCs. Polychromatophilia is present.
- Reticulocyte count is increased.
- Erythroid hyperplasia of bone marrow is evident.

Laboratory findings due to mechanism of RBC destruction, e.g.,
- Positive direct Coombs' test.
- Warm antibodies.
- Cold agglutinins.
- Biological false-positive test for syphilis may occur.

Laboratory findings due to underlying conditions
- Malignant lymphoma
- Collagen diseases (e.g., SLE)
- DIC (see p. 464)

- Idiopathic pulmonary hemosiderosis
- Infections, especially *Mycoplasma* infection; infectious mononucleosis, malaria, cholera
- Paroxysmal nocturnal hemoglobinuria
- Physical/chemical (e.g., burns, drugs, toxins [phenylhydrazine, benzene])

Antibody-induced
- Drug induced (e.g., quinidine, quinine, penicillins, cephalothin, alpha methyldopa)
- Autoantibody (warm, cold)
- Alloantibody (erythroblastosis fetalis, incompatible transfusion)
- Paroxysmal cold hemoglobinuria

Anemia, Hemolytic, Microangiopathic

(Traumatic intravascular hemolysis due to fibrin strands in vessel lumens)
See Tables 11-1, 11-9, and 11-10; Fig. 11-6.
♦ Peripheral blood smear establishes the diagnosis by characteristic burr cells, schistocytes, helmet cells, microspherocytes.
Nonimmune hemolytic anemia varies in severity depending on underlying condition (see Anemia, Hemolytic, Acquired, p. 359).
Laboratory findings of hemolysis, e.g., increased serum LD, decreased haptoglobin, hemosiderinuria; hemoglobinemia and hemoglobinuria are less common.
Iron deficiency due to urinary loss of iron.
Direct Coombs' test is usually negative.
Laboratory findings due to causative disease

Due To

Renal disease (e.g., malignant hypertension, renal graft rejection)
Cardiac valvular disease (e.g., intracardiac valve prostheses, bacterial endocarditis, severe valvular heart disease)
Severe liver disease (e.g., cirrhosis, eclampsia)
DIC (see p. 464)
Autoimmune disorders (e.g., periarteritis nodosa, SLE)
TTP
Snakebite (see p. 936)
Some disseminated neoplasms

Anemia, Hemolytic, Hereditary Nonspherocytic

(This heterogeneous group may be due to pyruvate kinase deficiency, variants of G-6-PD deficiency, Hb Zurich, other rare congenital enzyme defects [e.g., glutathione])
♦ Characterized by persistent hemolysis without demonstrable autoantibodies, abnormal hemoglobins, altered RBC morphology, or other obvious findings indicating etiology. Hemolytic anemia may be severe; may begin in newborn; may be precipitated by certain drugs.
RBCs show Howell-Jolly bodies, Pappenheimer bodies, Heinz bodies, basophilic stippling; slight macrocytosis may be present.
Increase in reticulocyte count is marked, even with mild anemia.
Bone marrow shows marked erythroid hyperplasia; normal hemosiderin is present.
WBC, platelet count, Hb electrophoresis, osmotic fragility, and mechanical fragility are normal.
Autohemolysis is present in some cases but not in others; reduction by glucose is less than in normal blood.

Anemia, Iron-Deficiency

See Tables 11-1, 11-9, and 11-10 and Figs. 11-3 and 11-6.

Due To

(Usually a combination of these factors)
Chronic blood loss (e.g., menometrorrhagia; bleeding from GI tract, especially from carcinoma of colon; hiatus hernia; peptic ulcer; intestinal parasites; marathon runners)

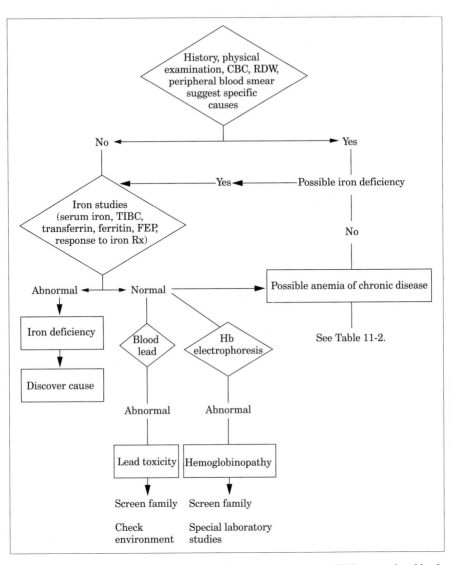

Fig. 11-6. Algorithm for workup of microcytic hypochromic anemia. (CBC = complete blood cell count; FEP = free erythrocyte protoporphyrin; Rx = therapy.)

Decreased dietary intake (e.g., poverty, emotional factors)
Decreased absorption (e.g., steatorrhea, gastrectomy, achlorhydria)
Increased requirements (e.g., pregnancy, lactation)
The cause of iron deficiency should always be ascertained to avoid overlooking occult carcinoma. In adults, iron deficiency usually means blood loss. If no GI or gynecologic cause is apparent, endoscopy must be performed.

Laboratory Findings

♦ Decreased serum ferritin is the most sensitive and specific test and is first test to reflect iron deficiency; *decreased before anemia* but may be increased when there is

Table 11-9. Laboratory Tests in Differential Diagnosis of Microcytic (MCV <80 fL) and Hypochromic (MCHC <30 gm/dL) Anemias

Type of Anemia	Serum Iron	TIBC	Transferrin Saturation	Serum Ferritin	FEP*	Marrow Hemosiderin	Sidero-blasts	Type of Hb	Anemia	RBC Count	RDW
Normal values	80–160 µg/dL in men 50–150 µg/dL in women	250–410 µg/dL	20–55%	20–150 ng/dL			30–50%	AA			11.5–14.5
Iron deficiency	D	I	D	D	I	0	D	AA	Hypochromic, normocytic, or microcytic	D	I
Normochromic, normocytic, or microcytic, of chronic disease	D	D or N	D or N	N or slightly I	I	N or I	D	AA	Normochromic, normocytic, or microcytic	D	N
Thalassemia											
Major	I	D	I	I	N	I	I	20–90% F	Hypochromic	I	N
Minor	N or I	N	N or I	I	N	N or I	I	2–8% F; A₂ is I	Microcytic	I	N
Sideroblastic	N or I	D or N	I	I	D	I	I	AA	Hypochromic and/ or microcytic with normocytic or macrocytic changes, dimorphic RBC population	D	I

0 = absent; F = decreased; FEP = free erythrocyte protoporphyrin; I = increased; N = normal.
Notes: (1) Determine serum iron and TIBC (and also perhaps do iron stain on bone marrow smear—the most reliable index of iron deficiency). (2) If serum iron and TIBC are both normal, Hb electrophoresis will establish the diagnosis of thalassemia. If serum iron is abnormal, the cause may be iron deficiency (e.g., blood loss, dietary deficiency) or normochromic microcytic anemia of chronic disease.
*FEP is useful to distinguish between iron deficiency and beta thalassemia.
Iron depletion: Early—serum iron is normal; TIBC may be increased. Later—serum iron decreases; anemia is often normocytic when mild or of rapid onset; anemia first becomes microcytic, then hypochromic.
Iron deficiency may occur without anemia (transferrin saturation <15%, decreased marrow iron and sideroblasts).

Table 11-10. Comparison of Sample Values in Iron-Deficiency States

	Normal	Early Deficiency	Early Anemia	Moderate Anemia	Moderate to Severe Anemia	Severe Anemia
MCV (fL)	82–92	N	N	D	D	D
			——————————Gradually decreases (95→80 fL)——————————			
MCH (pg)	27–31	N	N	D	D	D
Hb (gm/dL)	12–14 M 14–16 F	N	Gradually decreases to ~10		——Usually 7–10——	
RDW	11.5–14.5	N	N	——————————Gradually increases——————————		
Blood smear	N	N	Only mild microcytosis	Moderate microcytosis; ovalocytes, target cells, leptocytes	Poikilocytes, severe microcytosis, ovalocytes, elliptocytes	Schistocytes
% Cells hypochromic	N	N	N	——————————Gradually increases——————————		
Serum iron (µg/dL)	65–165	N (115)	D (<60)	D (<40)	D (<40)	D (<40)
TIBC (µg/dL)	250–450		——————————Increases to ~480——————————			
Transferrin saturation	20–50%	N (30%)	D (<15%)	D (<10%)	D (<10%)	D (<10%)
Serum ferritin (µg/L)	40–160	40–160; decreases to 20	D	<10	<10	<10
RE marrow iron	2–3+	0–1+	0–1+	0	0	0
sTfR	*	N/I	I	I	I	I
Free RBC	<100 (µg/dL)	N	I	I	I	I
Protoporphyrin	Packed RBCs	N	100 µg/dL	——————————Gradually increasing to ~200 µg/dL——————————		
RBC life span	N	N	N	——————————Gradually decreases——————————		

D = decreased; F = females; I = increased; M = males; N = normal; RDW = red cell distribution width; RE = reticuloendothelial; sTfR = serum transferrin receptor.
*Depends on method.
Source: Some data from Crosby WH. Iron deficiency anemia: signpost to blood loss. *Emerg Med* Sep 30, 1991:73–83.

HEMATOL

coexisting liver disease, inflammation, or other conditions that increase ferritin (see p. 327). Thus iron deficiency is suggested by serum ferritin <25 ng/mL in a patient with inflammation, <50 ng/mL in a hemodialysis patient, and <100 ng/mL in liver disease; <12 ng/mL always indicates iron deficiency. Serum ferritin >200 ng/mL generally indicates adequate iron stores regardless of underlying conditions. Ferritin usually distinguishes iron deficiency from thalassemia in uncomplicated cases.

♦ Hb is decreased (usually 6–10 gm/dL) out of proportion to decrease in RBC (3.5–5.0 million/cu mm); thus decreased MCV (<80 fL) is a sensitive indicator; MCH is decreased (<30 pg); decreased MCHC (25–30 gm/dL) is poor indicator as it is usually normal until anemia is severe.

♦ Increased RDW is found more often in iron deficiency than in thalassemia; increased RDW may be the first indication of iron deficiency; sensitivity = 89%; negative predictive value of normal RDW = 93%; positive predictive value = 45%; specificity = only 45%.

♦ Hypochromia and microcytosis parallel severity of anemia. Polychromatophilia and nucleated RBCs are less common than in PA or thalassemia. Diagnosis from peripheral blood smear is difficult and unreliable. Target cells may be present but are more common in thalassemias; basophilic stippling and polychromasia also favor thalassemia although absent in 50% of cases. Anisocytosis is less marked in thalassemia.

♦ Ratio of microcytic to hypochromic RBCs (measured with automated hematology analyzer) is <0.9 in iron deficiency but >0.9 in beta-thalassemia.

♦ Serum iron is decreased (usually 40 μg/dL), TIBC is increased (usually 350–460 μg/dL), and transferrin saturation is decreased (<15%). TIBC may be normal or moderately increased in many patients with uncomplicated iron deficiency. Serum transferrin may be normal or increased (calculated transferrin = TIBC × 0.7). These have limited value in differential diagnosis because they are often normal in iron deficiency and abnormal in anemia of chronic disease and may be affected by recent iron therapy.

♦ As iron deficiency progresses, decreased serum ferritin is followed in order by anisocytosis, microcytosis, elliptocytosis, hypochromia, decreases in Hb, decreases in serum iron, and decreases in transferrin saturation.

○ Serum transferrin receptor assay increases only after iron stores are depleted (i.e., decline in serum ferritin below reference range and compensatory erythropoiesis begins) but before changes are seen in other markers of tissue iron deficiency (e.g., transferrin saturation, MCV, erythrocyte protoporphyrin). Particularly useful in differentiating iron-deficiency anemia from anemia of chronic disease and in diagnosing iron-deficiency anemia in patients with chronic disease. Increased sensitivity and specificity when combined with ferritin.

♦ Bone marrow shows normoblastic hyperplasia with decreased hemosiderin, later absent, and decreased percentage of sideroblasts. Decreased to absent iron is the gold-standard test for diagnosis of iron deficiency.

Reticulocytes are normal or decreased, unless there is recent hemorrhage or administration of iron.

○ Free erythrocyte protoporphyrin is increased and is useful screening test because it can be done on fingerstick sample. Is *increased before anemia*. Also increased in lead poisoning, anemia of chronic disease, and most sideroblastic anemias but is normal in thalassemias.

WBC is normal or may be slightly decreased in 10% of cases; may be increased with fresh hemorrhage.

Serum bilirubin and LD are not increased.

Platelet count is usually normal but may be slightly increased or decreased; often increased in children.

Coagulation studies are normal.

RBC fragility is normal or (often) increased to 0.21%.

RBC life span is normal.

Laboratory finding may disclose causative factors (e.g., GI bleeding).

♦ Response to oral iron therapy is the final proof of diagnosis of iron deficiency *but primary cause must be determined.*

• Increased reticulocytes within 3–7 days with peak of 8–10% on fifth to tenth day; proportional to degree of anemia.

• Followed by increasing Hb (average 0.25–0.4 gm/dL/day) and Hct (average = 1%/day) during first 7–10 days; thereafter Hb increases 0.1 gm/dL/day to level ≥ 11 gm/dL in 3–4 wks. Should be about half corrected in 3 wks and fully corrected by

Table 11-11. Laboratory Tests in Differential Diagnosis of Vitamin B_{12} and Folic Acid Deficiencies

	Vitamin B_{12} Deficiency	Folate Deficiency	Vitamin B_{12} and Folate Deficiency
Serum folate	N or I	D	D
Serum vitamin B_{12}	D	N or D	D
RBC folate	N or D	D	D
Methylmalonic acid	I	N	I
Homocysteine	I	I	I

D = decreased; I = increased; N = normal.

8 wks. In older patients, increase of 1 gm/dL may take 1 mo, whereas in younger patients Hb increases 3 gm/dL and Hct increases 10%.
- Failure to respond suggests incorrect diagnosis, coexistent deficiencies (folic acid, vitamin B_{12}, thyroid), associated conditions (e.g., lead poisoning, bleeding, malabsorption, liver or kidney disease).

Clinical utility is not yet established for RBC ferritin (also decreased in anemia of chronic disease) and serum transferrin receptor tests.
Most difficult differential diagnosis is thalassemias and anemia of chronic disease. See Tables 11-1, 11-9, and 11-10.
In the United States, median Hb is ~ 1 gm/dL lower in blacks without iron deficiency than in whites.

Anemia, Macrocytic, of Liver Disease

♦ Increased MCV (100–125 fL) in one-third to two-thirds of patients. Indices resemble those in other megaloblastic anemias. Low MCHC may indicate associated iron deficiency.
♦ *Uniform round macrocytosis* is the cardinal finding.
Target cells and stomatocytes may be present.
Hemolytic anemia or true folate deficiency is frequent in alcoholic liver disease.
WBC and platelet count may be decreased or normal.

Anemia, Macrocytic, of Sprue, Celiac Disease, Steatorrhea

See Chapter 7.

Anemia, Megaloblastic

(Dyssynchronous nuclear and cytoplasmic maturation in all erythroid and myeloid cell lines due to aberrant DNA synthesis caused by deficiency of folate or vitamin B_{12})
See Tables 11-11 and 11-12; Fig. 11-7.
Hematologic picture is identical to that in folate or vitamin B_{12} deficiency but neurologic findings are absent in folate deficiency.
Normochromic macrocytic anemia is a relatively late event; RBC may be as low as 500,000/cu mm. Degree of anemia does not correlate with severity of neurologic signs and symptoms, which may precede hematologic abnormalities.
♦ RBC indices
- MCV is increased (95–110 fL with mild to moderate anemia, but may also be due to round macrocytes arising from nonmegaloblastic causes; 110–150 fL with more severe anemia). MCV increases many months before onset of anemia or clinical symptoms in almost all patients. MCV >95 fL should prompt further study. MCV >120 fL is most likely due to megaloblastic anemia. MCV may be normal in presence of coexisting iron deficiency, inflammatory disease, renal failure, or thalassemia trait. MCV normal in ~9% of megaloblastic patients.

Table 11-12. Pernicious Anemia (PA) (Vitamin B_{12} Deficiency) and Folate Deficiency

Most Commonly Due To	Vitamin B_{12} Deficiency	Folate Deficiency
Defective absorption	Decreased intrinsic factor (e.g., PA, congenital deficiency of intrinsic factor, 4 yrs after gastrectomy) Zollinger-Ellison syndrome Pancreatitis Ileal mucosal disease (e.g., sprue, regional enteritis, surgery) Tapeworm infestation, bacterial overgrowth in blind loop Drugs (e.g., colchicine, PAS, alcoholism)	Malabsorption due to drugs (e.g., anticonvulsants, anti-TB drugs, oral contraceptives), jejunal mucosal disease (e.g., amyloidosis, sprue, lymphoma, surgery)
Inadequate intake	Strict vegetarian diet (rare)	Malnutrition, alcoholism
Increased need	Pregnancy, lactation	Pregnancy, lactation, infancy

PAS = para-aminosalicylic acid.

- RDW is usually very increased due to marked anisocytosis/poikilocytosis but may be normal.
- MCH is increased (33–38 pg with moderate anemia; ≤ 56 pg with severe anemia).
- MCHC is normal.
♦ Large hypersegmented neutrophils (≥ 5 lobes) are the earliest morphologic sign of megaloblastic anemia (rule out congenital hypersegmentation, which occurs in 1% of white persons, and uremia); more than two 5-lobed neutrophils is strongly suggestive and any with ≥ 6 lobes is considered diagnostic. Occasionally moderate eosinophilia is present. Blood smear may show oval macrocytes, schistocytes, polychromatophilia, stippled RBCs, Howell-Jolly bodies, Cabot's rings, etc. Nucleated RBCs may be found with Hct <20%. Presence of macro-ovalocytes is a good clue, although these may also be seen in myelodysplasia in contrast to the presence of round macrocytes in nonmegaloblastic anemias.
Poikilocytosis and anisocytosis are moderate to marked; always present in relapse.
Reticulocyte count is usually decreased.
Thrombocytopenia (<150,000/cu mm) is present in 12% of cases; abnormal and giant forms may be seen.
Leukopenia is <4000/cu mm in 9% of cases.
♦ Marrow shows megaloblastic and erythroid hyperplasia and abnormalities of myeloid and megakaryocytic elements. Erythroid megaloblastosis may be masked by concomitant iron deficiency but granulocytic megaloblastic changes persist. Not indicated if diagnosis is unequivocal or treatment has been started.
♦ In PA serum vitamin B_{12} is very low, usually <100 pg/mL; 100–150 pg/mL usually signifies early vitamin B_{12} deficiency even without neuropathy or macrocytosis. May occur with neurologic symptoms but without anemia in one-third or fewer of patients with vitamin B_{12} deficiency, especially in older persons. RBC folate is low in many patients with vitamin B_{12} deficiency.

Serum Vitamin B_{12} May Also Be Decreased In

Diet deficient in folic acid (low in 10–30% of patients with simple folate deficiency; corrected by folate therapy alone). ≤ 50% of patients with pure vitamin B_{12} deficiency have falsely low RBC folate values.
Malabsorption
- Loss of gastric mucosa, e.g., partial or complete gastrectomy, atrophic gastritis, gastric irradiation. Annual assay of vitamin B_{12} should be performed because 100%

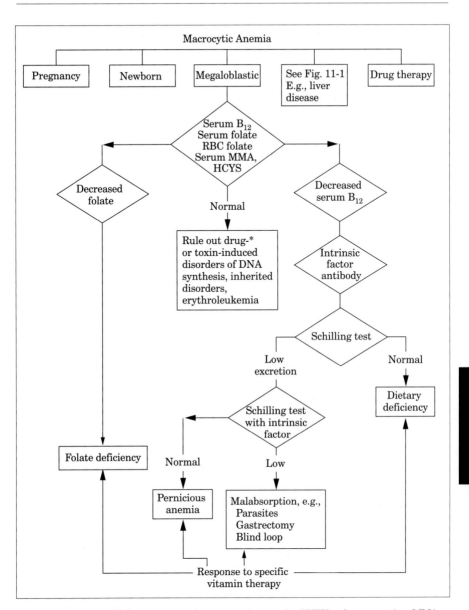

Fig. 11-7. Sequence of laboratory tests in macrocytic anemia. (HCYS = homocysteine; MMA = methylmalonic acid.)
*E.g., valproic acid, carbamazepine, phenytoin.

of patients with total resection and 10% with partial resection will be deficient within 5 yrs.
- Small bowel disease (e.g., Crohn's disease, scleroderma, lymphoma, ileal resection, tropical sprue, celiac disease, chronic pancreatic insufficiency, bacterial overgrowth).
- Primary hypothyroidism. (Almost 50% of patients have serum achlorhydria with intrinsic factor failure and low vitamin B_{12}; rarely megaloblastic anemia develops.)
- Parasites. 5% of persons infected with *Diphyllobothrium latum*.

- Blind-loop syndrome diagnosed by positive Schilling test that becomes normal after 2 wks of tetracycline therapy.

Drug effects (e.g., long-term PAS or colchicine use, use of oral contraceptives, aspirin, alcohol)

Pregnancy—progressive decrease during pregnancy *(normal serum B_{12} in megaloblastic anemia of pregnancy)*

Impaired cell utilization
- Abnormal vitamin B_{12} carrier protein (transcobalamin II deficiency, abnormal protein)
- Enzyme deficiency (e.g., congenital methylmalonicacidemias)
- Prolonged nitrous oxide exposure

One-third of patients with multiple myeloma

Other conditions
- Iron deficiency
- Vegetarian diet
- Smoking
- 15–30% of aged persons
- Cancer
- Aplastic anemia
- Folate deficiency
- Hemodialysis
- Ingestion of high doses of vitamin C

Artifactual
- Antibiotics (with microbiologic assays)
- Diagnostic radioisotopes for other tests (with RIA assays)

Serum Vitamin B_{12} May Be Increased In

Myeloproliferative diseases
- Leukemia—acute and chronic myelogenous; about one-third of the cases of chronic lymphatic; some cases of monocytic. Normal in stem cell leukemia, multiple myeloma, Hodgkin's disease.
- Polycythemia vera

Leukocytosis

Some cases of carcinoma (especially with liver metastases)

Liver disease (acute hepatitis, chronic hepatitis, cirrhosis, hepatic coma)

Ingestion of vitamin A, vitamin C, estrogens, anticonvulsants

Uremia

Serum folate is normal or increased. Decreased serum folate in folate deficiency. Decreased RBC folate in both folate and B_{12} deficiency. (See Table 11-3.)

Serum Folic Acid May Be Decreased In

Nutritional (may fall relatively quickly)
- Alcoholism is most common cause.
- Infancy, prematurity, elderly.
- Chronic disease.
- Hemodialysis.
- Anorexia nervosa.

Increased requirements due to marked cellular proliferation
- Pregnancy
- Hyperthyroidism
- Neoplasia (e.g., acute leukemia, metastatic carcinoma)
- Hemolytic anemias (e.g., sickle cell, thalassemias, hereditary spherocytosis, paroxysmal nocturnal hemoglobinuria)
- Ineffective erythropoiesis (PA, sideroblastic anemia)
- Exfoliative dermatitis, e.g., psoriasis

Malabsorption
- Small bowel disease (e.g., celiac disease, tropical sprue, Crohn's disease, lymphoma, amyloidosis, small bowel resection)

Defect in utilization due to certain enzyme deficiencies

Drug effects—folic acid antagonists (e.g., methotrexate, trimethoprim, pyrimethamine), anticonvulsants, oral contraceptives, aspirin

Decreased liver stores (e.g., cirrhosis, hepatoma)

Idiopathic
Artifactual
- Improper specimen storage (folate is labile)
- Radioactivity in blood (affects radioassays)
- Antibiotic therapy (affects microbiologic assays)

Serum folate serves to distinguish combined deficiency from vitamin B_{12} deficiency alone. Low serum folate indicates only negative folate balance, not folate deficiency. Decreased serum folate is not evidence of tissue deficiency, for which RBC folate should be assayed.

RBC Folate

Reflects folate status at time RBCs were produced; therefore more reliable indicator of tissue folate deficiency as it is not subject to daily variation due to diet, etc. Decreased in folate or vitamin B_{12} deficiency. *RBC folate does not fall below normal until all body stores are depleted. Thus, all three parameters should be measured simultaneously in suspected cases of megaloblastic anemia. RBC folate should always be measured in suspected cases of megaloblastic anemia when serum folate and vitamin B_{12} are assayed (see Table 11-11).*
Usual normal range is 5–15 ng/mL; is associated with normal hematologic findings.
3–5 ng/mL is borderline; is associated with variable hematologic findings.
<3 ng/mL is associated with positive hematologic findings.

Serum Folic Acid May Be Increased In

PA (or may be normal)
Period after folic acid administration or eating
Vegetarians
Blood transfusion
Some cases of blind-loop syndrome (due to folate synthesis by bacteria in gut)
False elevation in hemolyzed specimens (due to folate in RBCs)
Falsely increased to normal in some patients with severe iron deficiency (for unknown reason)
♦ *Iron deficiency is present in one-half of patients with folate deficiency and one-third with vitamin B_{12} deficiency. If iron deficiency is more severe than folate deficiency, results of serum and RBC folate tests are normal, and diagnosis cannot be made from these tests; hypersegmentation of PMNs in blood smear is the only clue.*
♦ Serum methylmalonic acid and homocysteine become increased very early in course of vitamin B_{12} deficiency. Patients with folate deficiency usually show only increase of homocysteine although some may have mild increase of methylmalonic acid. Are the most sensitive tests to detect early vitamin B_{12} deficiency and become positive before obvious hematologic evidence of vitamin B_{12} deficiency. Useful in patients with borderline vitamin B_{12} levels (100–300 pg/mL). Should be positive in acute neurologic disease due to vitamin B_{12} deficiency even when hematologic changes are absent. Remain positive for at least 24 hrs after onset of vitamin B_{12} therapy in cases in which therapy is begun before blood was drawn for vitamin B_{12} levels. Urine methylmalonic acid may be useful when serum methylmalonic acid is falsely high in renal insufficiency or intravascular volume depletion. Tests should be requested in cases of unexplained hematologic or neuropsychiatric abnormalities with low or borderline serum vitamin B_{12} levels. (Reference ranges: methylmalonic acid = 70–279 nmol/L, homocysteine = 5–15 μmol/L.)
♦ Serum antibodies
- **Intrinsic factor (IF) antibody**
Type I autoantibodies block binding of vitamin B_{12} to intrinsic factor; found in serum in 70% of PA patients.
Type II autoantibodies bind to site remote from vitamin B_{12} binding site; found in ~40% of PA patients; rarely occur in absence of type I antibodies. Positive test strongly supports diagnosis of PA and therefore should be performed in patients with low serum B_{12}; positive test combined with low serum B_{12} is virtually pathognomonic of PA; however, a negative test does not rule out PA because almost one-fourth of PA patients are negative for this antibody. More often found in gastric juice than in serum. False-positive results are rare (high serum B_{12} causes false-positive results).

Table 11-13. Interpretation of Schilling Test

Disorder	Without Intrinsic Factor	With Intrinsic Factor
Pernicious anemia	No	Yes
Congenital deficiency of intrinsic factor	No	Yes
Gastrectomy	No	Yes
Intestinal malabsorption (e.g., ileal diseases, bacterial overgrowth, pancreatic disease, fish tapeworm)	No	No
Renal failure	No	No
Incomplete urine collection	No	No
Folate deficiency	Yes	Yes

- **Parietal cell antibodies**
    Found in 90% of patients with PA but frequency decreases with duration of PA. Found in ~30% of their nonanemic first-degree relatives and in patients with autoimmune endocrinopathies; occur frequently in chronic gastritis. Found in 2% of normal population (third decade) increasing to >9% in eighth decade. Intrinsic antibodies are more specific but less sensitive.
- ◆ Schilling test is diagnostic of PA (shows very decreased absorption of radiolabeled B_{12}, which is corrected only by simultaneous administration of gastric intrinsic factor). Differentiates PA from other causes of vitamin B_{12} deficiency (*commonplace injection of vitamin B_{12} may make serum level temporarily normal for many weeks*) and can establish the functional absence of intrinsic factor before serum B_{12} deficiency or anemia are present or after patient has received vitamin B_{12} treatment. (See Table 11-13.)
    - Fasting patient is given oral vitamin B_{12} tagged with ^{58}Co and vitamin B_{12} tagged with ^{57}Co bound to intrinsic factor. In 1–2 hrs, a flushing dose of 1 mg of nonradioactive B_{12} is injected to saturate B_{12} binding sites, and a 24-hr urine specimen is collected.
    - In PA, the ^{58}Co in urine is low (usually <5% of the administered dose) but the ^{57}Co B_{12} bound to intrinsic factor is normally absorbed and excreted (>10% of the administered dose). A simpler method uses 1 µg of radiocobalt-labeled cobalamin followed within 1 hr by the flushing dose.
    - In intestinal malabsorption, ^{57}Co and ^{58}Co in the urine are equally low (<5%). Both become normal if underlying cause is treated (e.g., antibiotic treatment in patients with bacterial overgrowth, administration of exogenous pancreatic enzyme in patients with pancreatic insufficiency).
    - For test to be valid, patient must have normal renal function, normal intestinal mucosal absorption, complete 24-hr urine collection.
    - *Some patients (e.g., after partial gastrectomy or vagotomy) cannot absorb dietary vitamin B_{12} but can absorb crystalline vitamin B_{12} used in test, which gives false-normal result.*
    - Can probably be replaced by very high serum gastrin values[4] (see Zollinger-Ellison Syndrome, p. 629).
- ○ Increased serum gastrin with low serum vitamin B_{12} suggests PA. Vitamin B_{12} level does not predict either degree of anemia or MCV.
- ◆ Achlorhydria occurs even after administration of pentagastrin; this is virtually essential for diagnosis of PA; presence of gastric acid rules out PA. Decreased volume of gastric juice, high pH (>3.5), and decreased or absent pepsin and rennin are also found. Achlorhydria and gastric changes are rarely found in children.
- ○ Serum holotranscobalamin II (circulating protein carrier of vitamin B_{12}) falls before vitamin B_{12}.

[4]Fairbanks VF. *CAP Today* 1996;88.

♦ Recently developed deoxyuridine (dU) suppression test: patient's marrow cells are cultured with radiolabeled thymidine; in normal marrow, labeled thymidine uptake is suppressed on addition of unlabeled dU because dU can be converted to deoxythymidine, but suppression does not occur when patient is folate or B_{12} deficient due to inability to convert dU; adding either folate or B_{12} to the medium indicates specific cause. May be useful when other test results are masked by recent therapy or are equivocal. Limited availability at present but may become gold standard of megaloblastic states.

Serum iron, TIBC, ferritin, and marrow iron are almost always increased during relapse unless complicating iron deficiency is present.

Serum ALP is decreased; increases after treatment.

Serum cholesterol is moderately decreased.

Cholinesterase activity in RBC, plasma, and whole blood is decreased.

Laboratory findings due to hemolysis
- RBC survival is decreased.
- Serum LD is markedly increased (principally LD-1 and LD-2 with LD-1>LD-2).
- Serum indirect bilirubin is increased (<4 mg/dL).
- Urine urobilinogen and coproporphyrin I are increased.
- Stool urobilinogen is increased.

50% of PA patients have thyroid antibodies.

Increased frequency of gastric adenocarcinoma and gastric carcinoids.

♦ Characteristic Response of Laboratory Tests to Specific Treatment of PA or Folate Deficiency

RBC count reaches normal between 8th and 12th week regardless of severity of anemia; Hb concentration may rise at a slower rate, producing hypochromia with microcytosis. Peripheral blood is normal in 1–2 mos.

Characteristic reticulocyte response is proportional to severity of anemia. Reticulocyte count begins to rise by 4th day after treatment and reaches maximum on 8th to 9th day; returns to normal by 14th day. Daily injection of 200 μg of folinic acid or citrovorum factor causes a reticulocyte response in patients with folate deficiency but not in those with B_{12} deficiency.

Megaloblasts disappear from marrow in 24–48 hrs followed by reversal of megaloblastic changes in myeloid cells a few days later.

Serum folate decreases (in PA) at the same time reticulocytosis takes place.

Serum iron decreases to normal or less than normal at the same time reticulocytosis takes place.

Serum uric acid increases; peak precedes maximum reticulocyte count by ~24 hrs; remains increased as long as rapid RBC regeneration goes on.

Serum LD decreases but is not yet normal by eighth day.

Serum bilirubin becomes normal.

Serum ALP increases to normal.

Serum cholesterol rises to greater than normal levels; most marked at peak of reticulocyte response.

Increased urinary urobilinogen and coproporphyrin I immediately revert to normal, preceding reticulocyte response.

Achlorhydria persists.

RBC cholinesterase activity increases.

In Children

Adult type PA (very rare condition of gastric atrophy with lack of intrinsic factor production at birth; antibodies to intrinsic factor are present; parietal cell antibodies in 50% of cases; corrected by administration of intrinsic factor; frequent endocrine dysfunction such as hypoparathyroidism and hypoadrenalism)

Congenital absence of intrinsic factor (PA develops at age 12–18 mos; corrected by exogenous gastric intrinsic factor; normal gastric mucosa and acid secretion, no antibodies to intrinsic factor or parietal cells, no associated endocrine deficiency)

Imerslund-Graesbeck syndrome (rare autosomal recessive defective ileal receptor of B_{12} prevents absorption; ileum is normal histologically; normal gastric and endocrine function; proteinuria and renal tubular dysfunction are present; decreased folate and normal B_{12} concentrations; responds to parenteral B_{12} therapy)

HEMATOL

Anemia, Megaloblastic, of Pregnancy and Puerperium

Anemia may have been present during previous pregnancy with spontaneous remission after delivery.

Hematologic abnormalities are less marked than in PA.

If achlorhydria is present, it often disappears after delivery.

Therapeutic response to folic acid but usually not to vitamin B_{12}

Urinary excretion of formiminoglutamic acid is increased.

Anemia, Megaloblastic, Refractory to Folic Acid or Vitamin B_{12}

Due To

Inborn errors of metabolism
- Transcobalamin II deficiency (absence of transport protein for vitamin B_{12} with profound megaloblastic anemia in infancy; serum B_{12} is usually normal; may respond to huge doses of parenteral B_{12})
- Intrinsic factor deficiency (juvenile PA)
- Enzyme defects (e.g., congenital methylmalonicacidemia, congenital homocystinemia, 5-methyltetrahydrofolate transferase deficiency, hereditary orotic aciduria)

Drug effects
- Antifolate drugs (e.g., methotrexate, trimethoprim)
- Interference with absorption of folate (e.g., anticonvulsants, oral contraceptives, alcohol) or vitamin B_{12} (e.g., colchicine, PAS, phenformin)
- Inactivation of vitamin B_{12} by nitrous oxide
- Antimetabolites
    Mild megaloblastic anemia
        Purine inhibitors (e.g., 6-mercaptopurine, azathioprine [Imuran])
        Pyrimidine inhibitors (e.g., 5-fluorouracil)
    Severe megaloblastic anemia
        Deoxyribonucleotide inhibitors (e.g., cytosine arabinoside, hydroxyurea)
        Intercalating agents (e.g., doxorubicin)

Refractory macrocytic anemia—myelodysplastic syndromes with or without 5q(–) acquired chromosomal abnormality.

Anemia, Myelophthisic

Anemia is usually mild; not more than moderate.

Increased nucleated RBCs and normoblasts in peripheral smear, often without reticulocytosis, are out of proportion to the degree of anemia and may be found even in the absence of anemia. Polychromatophilia, basophilic stippling, and increased reticulocyte count may also occur.

WBC may be normal or decreased; occasionally it is increased up to a leukemoid picture; immature WBCs may be found in peripheral smear.

Platelets may be normal or decreased, and abnormal forms may occur. Abnormalities may occur even when WBC is normal.

♦ Bone marrow demonstrates primary disease.
- Metastatic carcinoma of bone marrow (especially breast, lung, prostate, thyroid)
- Hodgkin's disease, leukemia
- Multiple myeloma (5% of patients)
- Gaucher's disease, Niemann-Pick disease, and Hand-Schüller-Christian disease
- Osteopetrosis
- Myelofibrosis

○ *Mild anemia with normoblastemia should arouse suspicion of infiltrative disease of marrow.*

○ *Nonhemolytic normocytic anemias with no obvious cause characterized by marked RBC changes on blood smear should arouse suspicion of malignancy or marrow fibrosis.*

Anemia of Chronic Diseases

See Tables 11-1 and 11-9 and Fig. 11-6.

Due To

Subacute or chronic infections (especially TB, bronchiectasis, lung abscess, empyema, bacterial endocarditis, brucellosis, osteomyelitis)
Neoplasms
RA (anemia parallels activity of arthritis)
Rheumatic fever, SLE
Uremia (BUN >70 mg/dL)
Chronic liver diseases
Hypothyroidism
Chronic adrenal insufficiency

Laboratory Findings

♦ Anemia is usually mild (Hb >9 gm/dL) but may be as low as 5 gm/dL in uremia when other factors are present. Is insidious over 3–4 wk period, then *not progressive*. May be due to multiple mechanisms, e.g., failure of erythropoiesis, decreased RBC survival, iron deficiency, etc.
♦ Anemia is usually normocytic, normochromic. RDW and indices are usually normal. Hypochromic and/or microcytic in one-fourth to one-third of these patients, in which case it is always less marked than in iron-deficiency anemia.
Moderate anisocytosis and slight poikilocytosis are present.
Reticulocytosis, polychromatophilia, and nucleated RBCs are absent (may be present with severe anemia or uremia).
♦ Serum iron and TIBC are decreased. If TIBC is elevated, presence of iron deficiency must be ruled out, but TIBC is not sufficiently sensitive or specific to distinguish this from iron-deficiency anemia. Transferrin saturation is usually normal; >10% if decreased; <10% implies iron deficiency.
♦ Serum ferritin is increased or normal in contrast to iron deficiency. *In RA, liver disease, or neoplasms, normal serum ferritin does not exclude concomitant iron deficiency.*
Free erythrocyte protoporphyrin is increased.
Bone marrow cellular elements are generally morphologically normal. Hemosiderin is increased or normal; sideroblasts are decreased. Myeloid/erythroid ratio is usually normal.
RBC survival is slightly decreased in patient (80–90 days) but not in normal recipient.
Platelet count is normal.
Increased WBC, ESR, and other acute-phase reactants (e.g., CRP, fibrinogen, ceruloplasmin) are disproportionate to anemia and may be a useful clue to distinguish this from iron-deficiency anemia.

Hypothyroidism

♦ Occurs in one-third to two-thirds of patients with hypothyroidism; usually mild (Hct >35%). May be secondary to hypopituitarism.
Normochromic, normocytic or macrocytic (if hypochromic, rule out associated iron deficiency)
No anisocytosis or poikilocytosis
Reticulocyte count is not increased.
Serum iron is usually decreased and responds only to treatment of hypothyroidism unless concomitant iron deficiency is present.
Decreased total blood volume and plasma volume.
Normal RBC survival
Concurrent iron-deficiency anemia or PA may be present.

Hypogonadism

Normochromic, normocytic; only occurs in men.

Hypoadrenalism

Hct is pseudonormal at presentation due to plasma volume depletion; corticosteroid therapy unmasks anemia. Is corrected by 1–2 mos of therapy.

Chronic Renal Disease

Blood smear frequently shows burr cells or schistocytes.

HEMATOL

Usually normochromic, normocytic; hypochromic microcytosis may be due to chronic disease or iron deficiency. Severity of anemia roughly parallels severity of renal disease but when dialysis is required, anemia is almost always severe.

Decreased serum iron and transferrin. Serum iron, TIBC, and ferritin often are not helpful and bone marrow specimen stained for iron may be necessary for diagnosis of iron deficiency. Concurrent iron deficiency due to GI tract blood loss may be present. Anemia responds to erythropoietin therapy.

Bone marrow usually shows erythroid hypoplasia.

Decreased serum erythropoietin.

Decreased RBC survival by chromium 59 (^{59}Cr) studies.

Chronic Liver Disease

○Increased MCV (100–125 fL) in one-third to two-thirds of patients. Indices resemble those in other megaloblastic anemias. Low MCHC may indicate associated iron deficiency.

♦ *Uniform round macrocytosis* is the cardinal finding. Target cells and stomatocytes may be present. Presence of hypochromic macrocytes or microcytes may suggest misleading diagnosis of iron deficiency. Spur cell (acanthocyte) hemolysis may be due to abnormal lipid metabolism.

Hemolytic anemia or true folate deficiency is frequent in alcoholic liver disease. Reticulocyte count is usually increased.

Serum iron, TIBC, and ferritin are often not helpful, and bone marrow specimen stained for iron may be necessary for diagnosis of iron deficiency.

Decreased RBC survival by ^{59}Cr studies.

Anemia, Pathogenesis Classification

Anemias may be classified according to pathogenesis, which is convenient for understanding the mechanism or according to RBC indices and peripheral blood smear and reticulocyte count (see Fig. 11-3), which is convenient for workup of a clinical problem.

Marrow hypofunction with decreased RBC production

• Marrow replacement (myelophthisic anemias due to tumor or granulomas [e.g., TB]). *In absence of severe anemia or leukemoid reaction, nucleated RBCs in blood smear suggest miliary TB or marrow metastases.*

    Marrow injury (hypoplastic and aplastic anemias)

    Nutritional deficiency (e.g., megaloblastic anemias due to lack of vitamin B_{12} or folic acid)

    Endocrine hypofunction (e.g., pituitary, adrenal, thyroid; anemia of chronic renal failure)

• Marrow hypofunction due to decreased Hb production (hypochromic microcytic anemias)

    Deficient heme synthesis (iron-deficiency anemia, pyridoxine-responsive anemias)

    Deficient globin synthesis (thalassemias, hemoglobinopathies)

• Excessive loss of RBCs

    Hemolytic anemias due to genetically defective RBCs

        Abnormal shape (hereditary spherocytosis, hereditary elliptocytosis)

        Abnormal Hb (sickle cell anemia, thalassemias, HbC disease)

        Abnormal RBC enzymes (G-6-PD deficiency, congenital nonspherocytic hemolytic anemias)

    Hemolytic anemias with acquired defects of RBC and positive Coombs' test

        Autoantibodies, as in SLE, malignant lymphoma

        Exogenous allergens, as in penicillin allergy

• Excessive loss of normal RBCs

    Hemorrhage

    Hypersplenism

    Chemical agents (e.g., lead)

    Infectious agents (e.g., *Clostridium welchii, Bartonella*, malaria)

    Miscellaneous diseases (e.g., uremia, liver disease, cancers)

    Physical agents (e.g., burns)

    Mechanical trauma (e.g., artificial heart valves, tumor microemboli). *Blood smear shows fragmented bizarre-shaped RBCs in patients with artificial heart valves.*

Anemias are often multifactorial; the resultant characteristics depend on which factor predominates. The diagnosis must be reevaluated after the apparent causes have been treated.

Anemia, Pyridoxine-Responsive

Severe hypochromic microcytic anemia is present.

Blood smear shows anisocytosis, poikilocytosis with many bizarre forms, target cells, hypochromia. Polychromatophilia and reticulocytosis are not increased.

Serum iron is increased; TIBC is somewhat decreased; transferrin saturation is markedly increased. Marrow sideroblasts and blood siderocytes are increased. Marrow and liver biopsy show increased hemosiderin.

Bone marrow usually shows normoblastic hyperplasia; occasionally it is megaloblastic.

Response to pyridoxine is always incomplete. Even when Hb becomes normal, morphologic changes in RBCs persist.

Tryptophan tolerance test demonstrates pyridoxine deficiency. It may be positive in pyridoxine-responsive anemia, or it may be normal. A positive test produces abnormally large urinary excretion of xanthurenic acid.

Anemia, Sideroblastic

(Miscellaneous group of diseases characterized by increased sideroblasts [erythroblasts containing iron inclusions] in marrow)
See Table 11-9.

Hereditary

(X-linked transmission)

Usual onset in young adulthood but may be in childhood or infancy

Anemia is usually severe, hypochromic, microcytic; smear shows anisocytosis, poikilocytosis, elliptocytes, target cells, basophilic stippling mixed with normal-appearing RBCs (dimorphic RBC population).

WBC and platelets are usually normal.

♦ Bone marrow shows erythroid hyperplasia with normoblastic maturation; 10–40% of normoblasts are ringed sideroblasts; normal or increased iron.

• Megaloblastic changes indicate complicating folate deficiency.

Transferrin saturation is increased.

<50% of patients respond to pyridoxine therapy.

Idiopathic Refractory

Usual onset in older adulthood (rarely <50 yrs)

♦ Dimorphic anemia is usually moderate, normocytic, or macrocytic with a small population of hypochromic RBCs on blood smear, some of which show marked stippling. Reticulocytes are usually not increased.

WBCs are variable but usually normal. WBCs may show morphologic changes (hypogranular, Pelger-Huët–like neutrophils). Blasts are <1%.

Platelet counts are variable. Abnormal thrombopoiesis with abnormal morphology (e.g., hypogranular, large platelets or fragments, large nuclei).

Bone marrow shows erythroid hyperplasia; 45–95% of normoblasts are ringed sideroblasts; excessive hemosiderin. Megaloblastic changes due to complicating folate deficiency are found in 20% of patients. Dysgranulopoiesis and dysmegakaryopoiesis may be evident.

Serum ferritin and iron stores are increased due to ineffective erythropoiesis. Transferrin saturation is increased (>90% in 33% of patients). However, some patients may be iron deficient or have normal iron status. Iron overload is principal feature that determines long-term prognosis.

Acute leukemia develops in ~10% of patients.

Secondary Due To

Drugs (e.g., isoniazid, chloramphenicol, alcohol, lead, cytotoxic drugs such as nitrogen mustard and azathioprine)

Diseases

• Hematologic (e.g., leukemia, polycythemia vera, megaloblastic anemia, hemolytic anemia)

- Neoplastic (e.g., lymphoma, myeloma, carcinoma)
- Inflammatory (e.g., infection, RA, SLE, polyarteritis nodosa)
- Miscellaneous (uremia, myxedema, thyrotoxicosis, porphyria, copper deficiency)

Hereditary (pyridoxine responsive or pyridoxine refractory)
Idiopathic (pyridoxine responsive or pyridoxine refractory)

Anemia in Parasitic Infestations

Anemia due to blood loss, malnutrition, specific organ damage
Malaria: hemolytic anemia
D. latum (fish tapeworm): macrocytic anemia
Hookworm: hypochromic microcytic anemia due to chronic blood loss
Schistosoma mansoni: hypochromic microcytic anemia due to blood loss from intestine;
    macrocytic anemia due to cirrhosis of schistosomiasis
Amebiasis: due to blood loss and malnutrition

Anemia in Pregnancy

This is a normal physiologic change due to hemodilution—total blood volume and
    plasma volume increase more than red cell mass.
Onset is at eighth week; full development by 16–22 wks; rapid return to normal in puer-
    perium.
Hb averages 11 gm/dL; Hct value averages 33%.
RBC morphology is normal.
RBC indices are normal.
◯*If Hb is <10 gm/dL or hypochromic microcytic indices are abnormal, rule out iron-
    deficiency anemia, which may occur frequently during pregnancy.*
Also see p. 365

Anemias (Hemolytic), Classification[5]

See Figs. 11-1 and 11-2.
A useful approach to the diagnosis of hemolytic anemias may be based on the following:
- Site of RBC destruction (intravascular or extravascular)
- Site of etiologic defect (intracellular RBC or extracellular)
- Nature of defect (acquired or hereditary)

Hemoglobin Disorders
- Intrinsic
    Autosomal

Sickle cell (SS) disease	Common
Thalassemias	Common
HbC, HbD, HbE disease	Common
Unstable hemoglobins	Very rare

Membrane Disorders
- Intrinsic
    Congenital or familial (usually autosomal dominant)

Hereditary spherocytosis	Common (~0.02% of Northern European population)
Hereditary elliptocytosis	Rare
Hereditary stomatocytosis	Very rare
Acanthocytosis (abetalipo-proteinemia)	Very rare
Hereditary pyropoikilocytosis	Very rare
Acquired—paroxysmal nocturnal hemoglobinuria	Rare

- Extrinsic
    Acquired
        Isoimmune (blood transfusion
        reaction, hemolytic disease
        of newborn)

---

[5]Brain MC. Hemolytic anemia. *Postgrad Med* 1978;64:127.

Autoimmune hemolytic anemia   Rare
  (Coombs' test usually positive;
  spherocytes may be present)
Warm antibody 70% of auto-
  immune hemolytic anemia
Idiopathic
Secondary to disease (e.g.,
  lymphomas/leukemia, infectious
  mononucleosis, SLE)
Cold agglutinin syndrome
Idiopathic
Secondary (e.g., *Mycoplasma*
  pneumoniae infection, infectious
  mononucleosis, viral infection,
  lymphoreticular neoplasms)
Paroxysmal cold hemoglobinuria   Rare
Idiopathic
Secondary (viral illnesses, syphilis)
Atypical autoimmune hemolytic
  anemia
Coombs' test negative
Combined cold and warm auto-
  immune hemolytic anemia
Drug induced (e.g., penicillin,   Common
  methyldopa)
  ♦ Nonimmune (*usually Coombs'*
  test negative and morphologic
  changes in blood smear)
    Physical or mechanical
    Prosthetic heart valves
    Microangiopathic hemolytic disease,
      including DIC, TTP, hemolytic
      uremic syndrome, etc.
    March hemoglobinuria
    Severe burns
    Snakebite (see p. 936)
    Osmotic—distilled water used in
      prostate resection
    Infectious
    Protozoan (e.g., malaria, toxoplasmosis, leishmaniasis)
    Bacterial (e.g., sepsis, clostridial toxins, bartonellosis)
    Viral (e.g., echovirus)
Metabolic Disorders
  • Intrinsic
    G-6-PD deficiency   Common
    Pyruvate kinase deficiency   Rare
    Hexokinase deficiency
    Phosphofructokinase deficiency
    Aldolase deficiency
    Defects in nucleotide metabolism
    Erythropoietic porphyria
  • Extrinsic
    Drug effects with normal RBCs or in G-6-PD deficiency
    Marked hypophosphatemia (<1 mg/dL) may predispose to hemolysis.
    Other conditions (e.g., lead poisoning, Wilson's disease)
  ♦ 15–20% of acquired immune hemolytic anemias are related to drug therapy.
    • ~3% of patients taking penicillins and cephalosporins develop positive direct
      Coombs' test; hemolysis is infrequent and usually extravascular.
    • ~10% of patients taking methyldopa develop positive direct Coombs' test after 3–6
      mos but <1% develop hemolysis.
    • Serologic findings cannot be distinguished from those of idiopathic warm-antibody
      autoimmune hemolytic anemia.

HEMATOL

Aplasia, Congenital Pure Red Cell (Diamond-Blackfan Anemia)

(Rare familial anemia associated with congenital anomalies of kidneys, eyes, skeleton, heart; usual onset before age 12 mos; present at birth in 25% of patients. Spontaneous remissions in ~20% of patients after months or years.)

○Severe normochromic, often macrocytic, anemia that is refractory to all treatment except transfusion and sometimes prednisone.

Reticulocytes are invariably decreased or absent.

WBC and differential blood count are normal or WBC is slightly decreased.

Platelet count is normal or slightly increased.

○Bone marrow usually shows marked decrease in erythroid precursors. Myeloid cells and megakaryocytes are normal.

○Increased erythropoietin level

○Adenosine deaminase and purine nucleoside phosphorylase activity in RBCs are characteristically increased.

No evidence of hemolysis is found.

Normal serum folic acid, vitamin B_{12}, liver function tests, RBC life span; negative Coombs' test

Normal serum iron with increased saturation level

Laboratory changes due to effects of therapy, e.g.,
* Hemosiderosis
* Steroid effects (e.g., infections, diabetes mellitus, gastric ulcer)

Ataxia-Telangiectasia

(Autosomal recessive multisystem disorder of humoral and cellular defects. Cerebellar ataxia is apparent when child starts to walk. Oculocutaneous telangiectasias develop between 3 and 6 yrs of age.)

See Table 11-7.

♦Serum AFP is almost always increased.

○Selective absence of IgA in 50–80% of patients. IgE is usually low. Other immunoglobulins may be abnormal.

Decreased total T cells (CD3) and helper cells (CD4) with normal or increased suppressor cells (CD8).

○Recurrent infections in 80% of cases, usually bacterial sinopulmonary but not viral.

Delayed cutaneous anergy indicates impaired cell-mediated immunity.

Atransferrinemia

(Very rare autosomal recessive isolated absence of transferrin)

Hypochromic, microcytic, iron-deficiency anemia is unresponsive to therapy. TIBC is low (<85 μg/dL).

♦Absence of transferrin (normal = 200–400 mg/dL) is demonstrated by nephelometry or immunoelectrophoresis (see Transferrin, Serum, p. 344).

♦Serum protein electrophoresis shows marked decrease in beta globulins and absence of transferrin band.

Hemosiderosis with involvement of adrenals, heart, etc., is present.

Bisalbuminemia

♦Two albumin bands are present on serum protein electrophoresis in clinically healthy persons.
* Homozygotes or carriers

Chédiak-Higashi Syndrome

(Rare autosomal recessive lysosomal storage disease that causes hypopigmentation of skin, hair, and uvea)

See Table 11-6.

♦Neutrophils contain coarse, deeply staining, peroxidase-positive, fused large granulations in cytoplasm, which are present less frequently in other WBCs. Most prominent in marrow cells.

♦ Lysosomal inclusions also found in liver, spleen, Schwann cells.
Pancytopenia appears during the (accelerated) lymphoma-like phase.
○Laboratory findings due to frequent severe pyogenic infections and hemorrhage (which cause death by age 5 years) or to lymphoreticular malignancy in teens
Marked deficiency of natural killer cell function.
♦ Heterozygous carriers identified by a granulation anomaly in PMNs.
Treated by bone marrow transplant.

Chemicals, Hematologic Effects

(Especially benzene; also trinitrotoluene and others)
In order of decreasing frequency
- Anemia
- Macrocytosis
- Thrombocytopenia
- Leukopenia
- Other (e.g., decreased lymphocytes, increased reticulocytes, increased eosinophils)

Varying degrees of severity up to aplastic anemia
Hemolytic anemia is sometimes produced.

Cryofibrinogenemia

♦ Plasma precipitates when oxalated blood is refrigerated at 4°C overnight. Due to fibrinogen-fibrin complexes that show reversible cold precipitability in anticoagulated blood.
May cause erroneous WBC when electronic cell counter is used.
May be associated with increased alpha$_1$-antitrypsin, haptoglobin, alpha$_2$ macroglobulin (by immunodiffusion technique), and plasma fibrinogen. Not associated with cryoglobulins.
Has been reported in association with many conditions, especially
- Hematologic and solid neoplasms
- Thromboembolic conditions

Cryoglobulinemia[6]

(Presence of proteins that precipitate spontaneously and reversibly at less than body temperature within 3 days; insoluble at 4°C and may aggregate up to 30°C; can fix complement and initiate inflammatory reaction; 500–5000 mg/dL in serum; normal = <80 mg/dL)
Type I (monoclonal immunoglobulin, especially IgM kappa type)
- Causes 25% of cases.
- Most commonly associated with multiple myeloma and Waldenström's macroglobulinemia; other lymphoproliferative diseases with M components; may be idiopathic.
- Often present in large amounts (>5 mg/dL). Blood may gel when drawn.
- Severe symptoms (e.g., Raynaud's disease, gangrene without other causes).

Type II (monoclonal immunoglobulin mixed with at least one other type of polyclonal immunoglobulin, most commonly IgM and polyclonal IgG; always with RF)
- Causes up to 25% of cases.
- Associated with lymphoproliferative and autoimmune disorders, chronic HCV infection, Sjögren's syndrome, syndrome of essential mixed cryoglobulinemia, immune-complex nephritis (e.g., membranoproliferative GN, vasculitis).
- High-titer RF without definite rheumatic disease.
- C4 levels decreased.

Type III (mixed polyclonal immunoglobulin, most commonly IgM-IgG combinations, usually with RF)
- Causes ~50% of cases.
- Usually present in small amounts (<1 mg/dL serum) in normal persons.
- Most commonly associated with lymphoproliferative disorders, connective tissue diseases (e.g., SLE); vasculitis and/or nephritis in chronic inflammatory diseases of bowel or liver or rheumatic diseases or persistent infections (e.g., bacterial endocarditis, HCV, fungal, parasitic).

[6]Kallemuchikkal U, Gorevic PD. Evaluation of cryoglobulins. *Arch Pathol Lab Med* 1999;123:119.

HEMATOL

Recurrent purpura may occur.
♦Hyperviscosity syndrome is likely at IgM >4.0 gm/dL; clinically unpredictable at 2.0–4.0 gm/dL; therefore serum viscosity should be measured. Viscosity increases exponentially with IgM concentration.
○Cryoprecipitate may be seen in serum.
○May cause erroneous WBC when electronic cell counter is used.
○Rouleaux formation may occur.
ESR may be increased at 37°C but is normal at room temperature.
Laboratory findings of associated conditions
• Liver disease—e.g., serologic evidence of viral hepatitis.
• Renal disease—e.g., immune glomerular disease. Renal failure develops in ~50%, and marked proteinuria occurs in ~25%.
• Skin biopsy showing cutaneous vasculitis.

Elliptocytosis, Hereditary

(Autosomal dominant trait affecting 1 in 2500 persons in United States. >10 variants are known.)
♦Blood smear shows 25–100% elliptical RBCs. In healthy individuals, ≤ 10% of RBCs may be elliptical. Also seen frequently in thalassemias, hemoglobinopathies, iron deficiency, myelophthisic anemias, megaloblastic anemia; these must be ruled out to establish the diagnosis in a congenital hemolytic anemia with marked elliptocytosis. Only a few abnormal RBCs are present at birth with gradual increase to stable value after ~3 mos of age. Hemolysis is rare in newborns. Splenectomy does not relieve elliptocytosis despite clinical improvement.
Severity of disease varies from severe hemolytic disease to asymptomatic carrier status.
Degree of hemolysis does not correlate with proportion of abnormal RBC.
• Elliptocytes are the only hematologic abnormality seen in ~85% of patients; such patients are asymptomatic. Spherocytes are present in some forms.
• Mild normocytic normochromic anemia (Hb = 10–12 gm/dL) in 10–20% of patients.
• ~12% of patients show a chronic congenital hemolytic anemia (Hb <9 gm/dL) with decreased RBC survival time, moderate anemia, increased serum bilirubin, increased reticulocyte count, increased osmotic fragility, and autohemolysis.
• Severe in ~5% of patients (homozygous)—transfusion-dependent anemia with misshapen RBCs resembling hereditary pyropoikilocytosis.
♦Elliptocytes are found in at least one parent and may be present in siblings.
Mechanical fragility is increased.
Osmotic fragility and autohemolysis are normal in patients without hemolytic anemia.
Hb electrophoresis is normal.
Laboratory findings due to complications (e.g., gallstones, hypersplenism).

Erythrocyte Pyruvate Kinase Deficiency

(Congenital autosomal recessive nonspherocytic hemolytic anemia showing wide range of clinical and laboratory findings from severe neonatal anemia requiring transfusion to fully compensated hemolytic process in healthy adults; due to deficiency of pyruvate kinase [10–25% of normal] in RBCs)
♦Assay of RBC pyruvate kinase activity demonstrates heterozygous carrier state in persons who are hematologically normal.
○Laboratory findings due to chronic hemolysis, which may be exacerbated by pregnancy or viral infections
• Beyond early childhood Hb is usually 7–10 g/dL.
• Peripheral smear shows no characteristic changes (i.e., few or no spherocytes, occasional tailed poikilocytes, macrocytosis, reticulocytosis).
Abnormal autohemolysis test is poorly corrected by glucose.
Normal osmotic fragility.
If an infant has been transfused, the assay should be performed 3–4 mos later.
○Diagnosis is difficult to make. *May be suggested by increased Hb oxygen affinity (P_{50}) due to elevated 2,3-diphosphoglycerate.* Laboratory findings due to complications (e.g., cholelithiasis, hemosiderosis)
Other rare deficiencies of RBC enzymes also exist.

Erythrocytosis, Classification

Polycythemia vera (see p. 428)
Hereditary erythrocytosis (rare conditions)
- High oxygen-affinity hemoglobinopathies (see p. 380)
- Decreased RBC 2,3-diphosphoglycerate (due to high RBC adenosine triphosphate or autosomal recessive diphosphoglycerate mutase deficiency)
- Increased production of erythropoietin (autosomal recessive)
- Erythropoietin-receptor mutations (autosomal dominant)
- Unknown causes

Secondary polycythemia (see p. 427)
Relative polycythemia (see p. 427)
Neonatal thick blood syndrome (see p. 444)
Factitious polycythemia (due to blood doping or ingestion of steroids by athletes) (see p. 426)

Glucose 6-Phosphate Dehydrogenase (G-6-PD) Deficiency in RBC

(Inherited sex-linked disorder. Is the most frequent inherited RBC enzyme disorder.)
May be associated with several different clinical syndromes. Classes 2 and 3 represent 90% of cases. Classes 4 and 5 show no clinical findings.
- Class 1 (<5% of normal RBC enzyme activity)—rare, chronic, congenital, non-spherocytic hemolytic anemia worsened by oxidant drugs or febrile illness. Not improved by splenectomy.
- Class 2 (<10% of normal RBC enzyme activity)—episodic acute hemolytic crises induced by some oxidant drugs (e.g., primaquine, sulfonamides, acetanilid) or acidosis. Splenectomy is not helpful.
- Class 3 (RBC G-6-PD activity = 10–60% of normal)—oxidant drugs or infection (e.g., pneumonia, infectious hepatitis) induce acute self-limited (2–3 days) hemolysis in persons without previously recognized hematologic disease. Also reported in hepatic coma, hyperthyroidism, myocardial infarction (after first week), megaloblastic anemias, and chronic blood loss.
- Many other genetic and clinical variants.

♦After standard dose of primaquine in adult, intravascular hemolysis is evidenced by the following:
- Decreasing Hct usually begins in 2–4 days; reaches nadir by 8–12 days.
- Heinz bodies and increased serum bilirubin occur during first few days of hemolysis.
- Reticulocytosis begins at about fifth day; reaches maximum in 10–20 days.
- Hemolysis subsides spontaneously even if primaquine is continued.

♦*In vitro* tests of Heinz body formation when patients' RBCs are exposed to acetylphenylhydrazine.

Hb varies from 7 gm/dL to normal; is lower when due to exogenous agent; is usually normochromic, normocytic.

Peripheral smear shows varying degree of nucleated RBCs, spherocytes, poikilocytes, crenated and fragmented RBCs, and Heinz bodies but is not distinctive.

♦Diagnosis is established by RBC assay for G-6-PD (using fluorescence); heterozygotes have two RBC populations and proportions of each determine degree of deficiency detected.

○Screening test using fluorescent spot test is available.

In Newborn

5% develop neonatal jaundice after first 24 hrs (in contrast to erythroblastosis fetalis). Serum indirect bilirubin usually reaches peak at third to fifth day (often >20 mg/dL). When jaundice appears late in first week, peak serum level may occur during second week of life.
- In Asian and Mediterranean infants, neonatal jaundice and kernicterus is more common. Significant portions of the bilirubin may be conjugated.
- In American black infants at term, incidence of neonatal jaundice is not increased; occurs after exposure to certain drugs (e.g., synthetic vitamin K, naphthalene).

HEMATOL

Decreased In

American black males (13%)
American black females (3%; 20% are carriers)
Some other ethnic groups (e.g., Greeks, Sardinians, Sephardic Jews)
All persons with favism (but not all persons with decreased G-6-PD have favism)

Increased In

PA to three times normal level; remains elevated for several months, even after administration of vitamin B_{12}.
Idiopathic thrombocytopenic (ITP; Werlhof's disease); becomes normal soon after splenectomy.

Graft-Versus-Host Disease

(Due to small lymphocytes [mature marrow T cells] in transplant of donor organs or tissues to immunocompromised host [e.g., bone marrow transplant recipients, infants with congenital immunodeficiency syndromes, but not AIDS patients])

Acute

(Within days but <1–2 mos after transplantation)
♦ Laboratory findings due to selective epithelial damage involving
  • Liver: increased serum bilirubin, ALP, AST; may progress to liver failure with encephalopathy, ascites, coagulation disorders.
  • Intestine: bloody diarrhea, paralytic ileus.
  • Positive biopsy of liver, skin, colon, upper GI tract.
  • Acute condition causes persistent severe immunoincompetence with profound immunodeficiency and susceptibility to infection. Transfusion-associated graft-versus-host disease often causes bone marrow aplasia with pancytopenia; is usually severe in contrast to graft-versus-host disease after bone marrow transplant.

Chronic

♦ • >100 days but occasionally as early as 40–50 days after transplantation).
  • Liver: changes of chronic cholestasis (in 80% of cases); often resembles acute graft-versus-host disease; rarely progresses to cirrhosis.
  • Abnormalities of cellular immunity (e.g., decreased B cells, defects in number and function of $CD4^+$ T cells, increased number of nonspecific suppressor cells, impaired antibody production against specific antigens).
  • Thrombocytopenia.
  • Skin changes resemble lichen planus and, later, scleroderma.
  • Biopsy shows changes in affected organs.
In a recent report serum catalase showed sensitivity of 100%, specificity of 88% compared to 88% and 28%, respectively, for 5'-NT.[7]

Granulomatous Disease, Chronic

(Rare heterogeneous disorder characterized by chronic recurrent suppurative infections by catalase-positive organisms [e.g., S. aureus, Aspergillus spp.; also seen frequently are Serratia marcescens, Pseudomonas cepacia, Klebsiella spp., Escherichia coli, Nocardia, Chromobacterium violaceum], which usually have low virulence [e.g., Salmonella, Candida albicans]. Due to abnormality of nicotinamide-adenine dinucleotide phosphate oxidase system, PMNs and monocytes ingest normally but fail to kill certain bacteria and fungi; ~60% are X-linked membrane abnormalities, ~40% due to autosomal recessive inheritance (most are cytosol abnormalities), 5% are membrane abnormalities, <1% due to autosomal dominant inheritance.)

[7]Yasmineh WG, et al. Serum catalase as marker of graft-vs-host disease in allogeneic bone marrow transplant recipients: pilot study. *Clin Chem* 1995;41:1574.

♦ Failure of these cells to reduce nitroblue tetrazolium to purple formazan on slide test provides a simple rapid diagnosis in patients and in heterozygotes for the X-linked form (carriers). (See p. 327.) Nitroblue tetrazolium test now replaced by flow cytometry respiratory burst assay.

♦ Other confirmatory tests in reference laboratory for absent (or severely reduced) production of oxygen radicals include measurement of oxygen consumption, hydrogen peroxide or superoxide production, and chemiluminescence of phagocytes.

♦ Prenatal diagnosis has been established using nitroblue tetrazolium test on fetal blood leukocytes. Fetal DNA from chorionic villus or amniocytes can also be analyzed for specific mutation.

WBCs show morphologically normal appearance and granules on routine Wright's- and Giemsa-stained smears.

Serum complement and immunoglobulin levels are normal.

Laboratory findings due to infection (leukocytosis, anemia, increased ESR, elevated gamma globulin levels)

Laboratory findings due to abscesses of lung, liver, osteomyelitis

Laboratory findings due to granulomas causing obstruction (e.g., GI tract, GU tract)

Heavy-Chain Diseases

Gamma

(Rare disorder with excessive production of heavy-chain proteins, producing homogeneous serum and/or urine protein spike)

♦ Serum protein electrophoresis/immunofixation
- Monoclonal gamma heavy chain in serum, which may be broad or hypogammaglobulinemia.
- Localized spikes or bands may be absent.
- Normal immunoglobulins are usually decreased. Gamma globulin almost absent.

Serum tests
- Normal level of total serum protein but increased globulin (>2 gm/dL) and decreased albumin.
- Increased uric acid (>8.5 mg/dL).
- Increased BUN (30–50 mg/dL).

Urine tests
- Trace to 1+ protein (0.5–20 gm/day).
- Negative for Bence Jones protein.
- Gamma heavy chain identical to that of abnormal serum protein varies from undetectable to 20 gm/day (usually <1 gm).

Hematologic findings
- Normocytic, normochromic anemia (usually Coombs'-positive autoimmune hemolytic), leukopenia, and thrombocytopenia common (probably due to hypersplenism).
- Eosinophilia sometimes marked; relative lymphocytosis.
- Vacuolated mononuclear cells sometimes seen.
- Bone marrow and lymph nodes contain increased numbers of plasma cells, lymphocytes, and many atypical lymphoplasmacytoid cells. In terminal phase is similar to plasma cell leukemia.

○Histologic findings of associated lymphoma, e.g., extranodal non-Hodgkin's lymphoma in ~75% of cases. ~50% of cases were preceded by or associated with neoplasias (e.g., lymphoma, leukemia, carcinoma), autoimmune disorders (especially RA), or other disorders (e.g., infections, hypogammaglobulinemia, Down syndrome)

Marked susceptibility to bacterial infection.

Mu

(Usually associated with CLL or a lymphoma)
♦ Diagnostic Criteria
Serum protein electrophoresis immunofixation shows monoclonal Mu heavy chain.

Hypogammaglobulinemia with a monoclonal peak in 40% of patients.

Bence Jones proteinuria in two-thirds of patients; most excrete large amounts of kappa light chains.

Bone marrow shows vacuolated plasma cells.

Hemoglobin C (HbC) Disease
HbC Disease

♦ Hb electrophoresis demonstrates the abnormal hemoglobin.
Significant hypochromic hemolytic anemia is present.
○ Blood smear shows many target cells, variable number of microspherocytes, occasional
nucleated RBCs, a few tetragonal crystals within RBCs that increase after splenectomy.
Reticulocyte count is increased (2–10%).
Osmotic fragility is decreased.
Mechanical fragility is increased.
RBC survival time is decreased.
HbF is slightly increased.
Increase in serum bilirubin is minimal.
Normoblastic hyperplasia of bone marrow is present.

HbC Trait

(Occurs in 2% of American blacks, less frequently in other Americans.)
♦ Hb electrophoresis demonstrates the abnormal Hb.
Blood smear shows variable number of target cells.
No other abnormalities are seen.

HbC–Beta-Thalassemia

Resembles HbCC but different concentration of HbC on electrophoresis.
Usually asymptomatic but moderate hemolysis may occur if HbA is absent, in which
case family studies may be needed to differentiate from HbCC.

HbSC Disease

See p. 437.

Hemoglobin D (HbD) Disease
Homozygous HbD Disease

♦ Hb electrophoresis demonstrates the abnormal Hb at acid pH.
Mild microcytic anemia
Target cells and spherocytes
Decreased RBC survival time

Heterozygous HbD Trait

♦ Hb electrophoresis demonstrates the abnormal hemoglobin at acid pH.
No other laboratory findings are characteristic.

Hemoglobin E (HbE) Disease

**(Occurs almost exclusively in Southeast Asia; found in 3% of population in Vietnam
and up to 35% in Laos; migrates like HbA_2 on electrophoresis.)**

Homozygous HbE Disease

Mild hypochromic hemolytic anemia or no anemia
○ Marked microcytosis (MCV = 55–70 fL) and erythrocytosis (~5.5 million/cu mm)
○ Smear shows predominant target cells (25–60%), which differentiates from HbE trait
and microcytes.
♦ Electrophoresis shows 95–97% HbE and the rest is HbF. Electrophoretic mobility
same as HbA_2 but concentration is higher (15–30%).

Heterozygous HbE Trait

Asymptomatic persons found during family studies or screening programs.
Normal Hb concentration
Slight to moderate microcytosis (MCV = 65–80 fL)

Erythrocytosis (RBC = 5.0–5.34 million/cu mm)
♦ Electrophoresis shows 30–35% HbE.

HbE–Beta-Thalassemia

Is most common symptomatic thalassemia in Southeast Asia.
○ Hemolytic anemia varies in severity from moderate to marked (thalassemia major or intermedia phenotype).
○ Smear shows severe hypochromia and microcytosis, marked anisopoikilocytosis with many teardrop and target forms. Nucleated RBCs and basophilic stippling may be present.

HbE–Alpha-Thalassemia

Analogous to alpha-thalassemia 1 and 2 and HbH (see p. 444)
In American blacks, 28% have mild alpha-thalassemia without microcytosis, 3% have homozygotic alpha-thalassemia with microcytosis, 1% have microcytosis due to beta-thalassemia. Median Hb is ~ 1 gm/dL lower in blacks without iron deficiency than in whites.
Alpha- or beta-thalassemia or HbE occur in ~50% of Southeast Asians and causes microcytosis.

Hemoglobin F (HbF), Hereditary Persistence

Inherited persistence of increased HbF in adult without clinical manifestations due to many different genetic lesions (probably autosomal dominant). Incidence is <0.2%.
Decreased MCV and MCHC
♦ Hb electrophoresis shows increased HbF (20–30%) and 60–70% HbA.
♦ May be pancellular (HbF is increased in all RBCs) or heterocellular (HbF is increased only in some RBCs), as distinguished by Kleihauer-Betke stain of peripheral blood smear.
May be associated with other hemoglobinopathies but is different from the increase of HbF that is found in some hemoglobinopathies.

Hemoglobinopathies, Laboratory Screening

Normocytic normochromic RBC except in
  • Thalassemia syndromes—microcytic hypochromic
  • HbC, HbD, HbE diseases—microcytic normochromic
Osmotic fragility—normal or decreased (especially in thalassemia)
  • Symmetric shift in HbC, HbD, HbE, diseases
  • Asymmetric shift in other hemoglobin diseases
Target cells—in many of hemolytic diseases due to hemoglobinopathies; 50% of RBCs in HbC, HbD, HbE diseases
Sickle cell test (Hb solubility test may be negative with <10% HbS; or monoclonal antibody test)—recognizes HbS
Supravital stain (e.g., brilliant cresyl blue test for inclusion bodies [Heinz bodies])—these Heinz bodies may confirm suspicion of alpha-thalassemia minor in patient with microcytic anemia with normal Hb electrophoresis.
Hb electrophoresis
  • Distinguish sickle cell anemia and trait.
  • Usually cellulose acetate at alkaline pH confirmed by agar at acid pH or isoelectric focusing.
  • Electrophoresis of separated globin chains can substantiate alpha-chain abnormality.
  • Distinguish various types of Hb.
Alkali denaturation for HbF
Kleihauer-Betke stain of blood smear identifies RBCs containing HbF.
Flow cytometry (see p. 319)
Isopropanol precipitation test screen for unstable hemoglobins, which may not be detected on routine electrophoresis because they migrate with HbA.
♦ Reference laboratory tests
  • Measurement of globin-chain synthesis ratios for confirmation of alpha- and beta-thalassemias.
  • DNA analysis can detect gene deletions and point mutations, which disclose most types of alpha- and beta-thalassemia).

HEMATOL

- Prenatal diagnosis during first trimester using DNA from chorionic villi or, after 16th week, from fetal cells by amniocentesis.

Hemoglobins, Unstable

(E.g., Hb Koln, Hb Zurich)
Usually autosomal dominant inheritance
○Laboratory evidence of episodes of hemolytic anemia of varying degrees of severity precipitated by infection or drugs (e.g., antimalarials, sulfonamides, acetanilid, nitrofurantoin, nalidixic acid, toluidine blue)
Peripheral blood smear shows hypochromia, macrocytosis, anisocytosis, poikilocytosis, increased reticulocytes
Supravital stain shows preexistent Heinz bodies (precipitation of abnormal Hb); may be few or absent if spleen is present.
Excess precipitation of Hb at 37°C in 17% isopropanol compared to normal.
Hb electrophoresis is often normal.

Hemoglobins with Altered Oxygen Affinity

High-oxygen-affinity hemoglobins cause left shift in oxygen dissociation curve with less oxygen delivered to tissues; autosomal dominance.
- Erythrocytosis without splenomegaly
- Low P_{50} (see Polycythemia, p. 432)
- Due to unstable Hb (e.g., Koln, Zurich, Gun Hill) or stable Hb (e.g., Yakima, Rainer, Bethesda)
♦ May be difficult to separate from normal Hb by electrophoresis in conventional media, isoelectric focusing
○These hemoglobinopathies are discovered in patients with unexplained erythrocytosis whose Hb shows a high oxygen affinity (oxygen tension at 50% saturation). Usually <20 mm Hg (normal = 27.5 mm Hg).
Serum erythropoietin may be normal but increases after therapeutic phlebotomy.

Low-oxygen-affinity hemoglobins cause right shift in oxygen dissociation curve with more oxygen delivered to tissues; autosomal dominance; cyanosis.
- Mild hemolytic anemia in some cases.
- High P_{50}.
♦ • Identify Hb by gel electrophoresis or measure absorption spectrum at 450–750 nm.
- Due to unstable Hb (e.g., Torino, Seattle) or stable Hb Kansas.

Hemoglobinuria, Paroxysmal Cold

Due To

Original cases were due to syphilis; followed exposure to cold environment. Presently reported cases are not related to exposure to cold. May be idiopathic or associated with convalescence from an acute viral illness (e.g., mumps, measles, infectious mononucleosis).
♦ Laboratory findings of acute, transient, nonrecurring hemolytic anemia with sudden hemoglobinuria, hemoglobinemia, spherocytosis, anisocytosis, poikilocytosis, nucleated RBCs.
♦ Cold autohemolysin (IgG antibody against P blood group system) is present (Donath-Landsteiner test—only if blood is chilled and then brought to 37°C in presence of complement and type O RBCs).
Direct Coombs' test may be only weakly positive during the attack due only to complement as IgG readily elutes from RBCs.

Hemoglobinuria, Paroxysmal Nocturnal (Marchiafava-Micheli Syndrome)[8]

(Acquired clonal stem cell disorder; RBC deficiency of glycosylphosphatidylinositol-anchoring proteins causing increased sensitivity to complement-mediated lysis)

---

[8]Dunn DE, et al. Paroxysmal nocturnal hemoglobinuria cells in patients with bone marrow failure syndromes. *Ann Intern Med* 1999;131:401.

○Insidious slowly progressive hemolytic anemia (mild to moderate, often macrocytic) and cytopenia

○Evidence of hemolysis, e.g.,
- Hemoglobinuria (black urine) is evident on arising.
- Urine contains Hb, hemosiderin (in WBCs and epithelial cells of sediment), and increased urobilinogen.
- Hemoglobinemia is present; increases during sleep.
- Methemalbuminemia.
- Increased serum LD and indirect bilirubin.
- Serum haptoglobin is absent during an episode.
- Stool urobilinogen is usually increased.

Severity of hemolysis depends on number of affected RBCs, which coexist with normal cells (chimerism).
- Mild hemolysis with <20% complement-sensitive RBCs
- Sleep-related hemolysis with 20–50% affected RBCs
- Continuous hemolysis with >50% affected RBCs

◆Flow cytometry is superior to and replaces Ham's test.
- Demonstrates deficiency of glycosylphosphatidylinositol-anchored protein in RBCs and granulocytes.
- Permits concomitant diagnosis of paroxysmal nocturnal hemoglobinuria in ~20% of patients with myelodysplasia.
- CD59 analysis available commercially.

Demonstration of increased RBC sensitivity to complement
- Ham's test (RBC fragility is increased in acid medium and in hydrogen peroxide); amount of change is related to clinical severity.
- Sucrose hemolysis test is said to be more sensitive but less specific than Ham's test.

Autohemolysis is increased.

Negative direct Coombs' test.

Osmotic fragility is normal.

Serum iron may be decreased.

Platelet count usually shows mild to moderate decrease.

WBC is usually decreased.

Blood smear is not characteristic and often shows hypochromasia and polychromatophilic macrocytes (reticulocytes).

Bone marrow is not diagnostic; most often shows normoblastic hyperplasia with adequate myeloid and megakaryocytic cells, but cellularity may be decreased or aplasia may be present. Stainable iron is often absent.

Leukocyte ALP activity is decreased (as in other marrow stem cell disorders, e.g., chronic myelogenous leukemia and myelodysplastic syndromes).

RBC acetylcholinesterase activity is decreased.

Develops in 5–10% of patients with aplastic anemia, and aplastic anemia develops in 25% of patients with paroxysmal nocturnal hemoglobinuria.

Laboratory findings due to
○ • Recurrent arterial and venous thromboses, especially of GI tract, in ~30% of patients (e.g., hepatic, portal, splenic); cerebral, skin.
- Hemorrhage.
- Infection—causes death in ~10% of patients.
○ • Renal findings similar to those in sickle cell disease (e.g., papillary necrosis, multiple infarcts).
- Spontaneous clinical remission in ~15%, including negative Ham's test.

○Diagnosis should be considered in any patient with Coombs'-negative acquired chronic hemolysis, especially if hemoglobinuria, pancytopenia, or thrombosis is present.

Bone marrow transplantation is definitive therapy.

Hemolysis

Autoimmune, Extravascular, Warm

Due To
Primary (idiopathic)—55% of cases
Secondary
- Lymphoproliferative neoplasms (e.g., chronic lymphatic leukemia, Hodgkin's and non-Hodgkin's lymphoma)—20% of cases

- Drugs—20% of cases
- Viral infections
- Connective tissue diseases

Insidious onset of normochromic, normocytic anemia; nucleated RBCs, polychromasia, reticulocytosis, spherocytes; fragmented RBCs may be present.
♦ Diagnosis by positive direct antiglobulin test (negative in ≤ 4% of cases)
- RBC coating by IgG alone in 20–40% of cases (makes SLE unlikely); by complement alone in 30–50% of cases; by both in 30–50% of cases
Indirect antiglobulin test is positive in 60% of cases.
Laboratory findings due to hemolysis

Intravascular Hemolysis

♦ Anemia varies from mild (Hb = 11.5 gm/dL) to severe (Hb = 2 gm/dL). MCV is usually 80–110 fL; MCV < 70 fL in normochromic anemia suggests hemoglobinopathy or paroxysmal nocturnal hemoglobinuria; MCV > 115 fL suggests macrocytic anemia.
Peripheral smear shows macrocytes, nucleated RBCs, polychromatophilia.
Spherocytes suggest hereditary spherocytosis or autoimmune hemolytic anemia.
Microspherocytes suggest HbC disease, ABO erythroblastosis, burns.
RBC cell fragments suggest DIC, prosthetic valves, hemolytic uremic syndrome.
Target cells suggest hemoglobinopathies, postsplenectomy state.
♦ Increased reticulocyte count is a major criterion for hemolytic anemia.
♦ Plasma haptoglobin level decreases ~100 mg/dL in 6–10 hrs and lasts for 2–3 days after analysis of 20–30 mL blood. Test is relatively reliable and very sensitive.
Plasma Hb increases transiently with return to normal in 8 hrs; lacks accuracy and precision.
○ Hemoglobinuria occurs 1–2 hrs after severe hemolysis and lasts ≤ 24 hrs. It is a transient finding and is relatively insensitive. False-positive is due to myoglobinuria or to lysis of RBCs in urine.
○ Urine hemosiderin occurs 3–5 days after hemolysis with positive Prussian blue staining of renal tubular epithelial cells. It may be difficult to detect a single episode. Urine hemosiderin is commonly found in paroxysmal nocturnal hemoglobinuria.
○ Schumm's test for methemalbuminemia becomes positive 1–6 hrs after hemolysis of 100 mL blood and lasts 1–3 days. Methemalbuminemia also occurs in hemorrhagic pancreatitis.
Serum bilirubin increase depends on liver function and amount of hemolysis. With normal liver function, it is increased 1 mg/dL in 1–6 hrs to maximum in 3–12 hrs after hemolysis of 100 mL blood.
Increased serum total LD; isoenzymes may be useful to confirm RBC source. Extravascular hemolysis may cause increased serum indirect bilirubin and LD and decreased serum haptoglobin.
In compensated hemolysis, little or no increase is seen in serum LD, bilirubin, Hb, or urine hemoglobin as in acute hemolytic anemia, but urine hemosiderin may be present.
Increased urine and fecal urobilinogen are insensitive and unreliable as an index of hemolysis.
Bone marrow shows marked normoblastic erythroid hyperplasia. Iron stains show marked increase; absence of iron suggests paroxysmal nocturnal hemoglobinuria.

Combined Cold and Warm Antibody (Autoimmune Hemolytic Anemia)

In ~8% of cases of autoimmune hemolytic anemia, serologic findings satisfy criteria for both warm and cold autoimmune hemolytic anemia. SLE occurs in >25% of these cases.
Severe hemolytic anemia.

Autoimmune, Intravascular Cold

Due To

Primary (idiopathic) cold agglutinin syndrome—50% of cases
- Due to monoclonal cold antibody, usually IgM kappa anti-I (titer >1:1000), that reacts over wide temperature range and is active at skin temperature of 30–32°C.
Secondary cold agglutinin syndrome

- Usually due to polyclonal cold antibodies with low titer and narrow thermal range. Monoclonal IgM anti-I antibodies (sometimes in high titer) are associated with *Mycoplasma* pneumonia (>80% of cases), infectious mononucleosis and some viral infections. Monoclonal IgM mu, kappa antibodies (sometimes in high titer) are associated with lymphoreticular disease (e.g., non-Hodgkin's lymphoma, Waldenström's macroglobulinemia, CLL). Polyclonal anti-I antibodies in low titer (<1:64) can be found in healthy persons.

♦ Diagnosis by demonstrating cold antibody in serum.
♦ *Agglutination at room temperature that prevents performing RBC count or making blood smears should arouse suspicion of this condition.*
♦ Artifactual increased MCV and decreased RBC count due to clumps. MCH markedly increased.
○ Chronic hemolysis with exacerbations, especially when patient is chilled.
Stable mild to moderate anemia with polychromasia, rare spherocytes, occasional erythrophagocytosis.
RBC morphology is less abnormal than in warm-antibody autoimmune hemolytic anemia.
○ Direct antiglobulin test is positive due to complement.
Note difference between cold agglutinins and cryoglobulins.
- Cold agglutinins are immunoglobulins that bind RBC antigens best at 4°C; most are not cryoglobulins.
- Cryoglobulins are immunoglobulins that precipitate at low temperature; most do not bind RBC antigens. (See p. 373.)

Hemolytic Disease of the Newborn (Erythroblastosis Fetalis)

Probability of isoimmunization of Rh-negative woman by a single Rh-incompatible pregnancy is ~17%. If mother and fetus are ABO incompatible, a protective effect on Rh isoimmunization occurs (due to immediate destruction of fetal RBCs by maternal AB antibodies). An Rh-positive infant occurs in ~10% of Rh-negative white women, 5% of black women, and 1% of Asian women.
Prevalence has been markedly reduced due to prompt therapy with Rh immune globulin after abortion or delivery.

Prenatal Screening and Diagnosis

♦ Blood ABO and Rh type should be ascertained at first prenatal visit early in pregnancy. Indirect Coombs' test should always be performed regardless of Rh type because of ABO or irregular antigens.
♦ Fetal Rh D genotyping can be determined in DNA extracted from plasma buffy coat of Rh D-negative pregnant women. Occasional false-negatives occur in first trimester of pregnancy.[9]
Rh-negative women should be given anti-D immunoglobulin (RhIg) at end of second trimester and again within 72 hrs of delivery of Rh-positive baby. RhIg is also given when fetal RBCs can enter maternal circulation (see p. 386). Prevalence of hemolytic disease of the newborn has been markedly reduced due to prompt RhIg therapy.
♦ Monitor anti-D titer in maternal serum periodically to detect sensitization (titer >1:8). If increased, serial amniotic fluid indirect bilirubin is performed to determine infant's risk in severe cases, and lung maturity is determined by lecithin/sphingomyelin ratio and other studies.
♦ Amniocentesis in sensitized mothers is more reliable than anti-D titer to assess severity of disease. Indirect bilirubin reflects hemolysis. Determine prenatal umbilical vein Hct; if <18%, transfuse type O, Rh-negative RBCs in utero, which may cause infant to be typed as Rh-negative. DNA analysis of amniotic fluid by PCR can determine D-antigen status of fetus.
♦ At birth, determine cord blood Hb and bilirubin, and perform direct (Coombs') antiglobulin test on infant's RBCs. Positive direct antiglobulin test means probable

[9] Lo YMD, et al. Prenatal diagnosis of fetal RhD status by molecular analysis of maternal plasma. *N Engl J Med* 1998;339:1734.

HEMATOL

later exchange transfusions. If test results indicate fetal-maternal hemorrhage >30 mL of fetal whole blood, additional RhIg should be given.

♦ Fetal-maternal hemorrhage may be indicated by
  • Rosette test: antibody binds to fetal Rh-positive RBCs, forming rosette; detects 5 mL Rh-positive fetal RBCs (10 mL Rh-positive whole blood); negative with <2.5 mL Rh-positive fetal RBCs.
  • Kleihauer-Betke test detects HbF; is least sensitive.
  • Enzyme-linked antiglobulin test detects <12.5 mL (and as little as 3 mL) of Rh-positive whole blood.
  • Flow cytometry detects 0.1% Rh-positive RBCs equivalent to fetal-maternal hemorrhage of 15 mL whole blood.

Postnatal Diagnosis and Therapy

♦ Serum indirect bilirubin shows rapid rise to high levels. May rise 0.3–1.0 mg/hr to level of 30 mg/dL in untreated infants to maximum in 3–5 days unless they die. Increased urine and fecal urobilinogen parallels serum levels.

♦ Direct Coombs' test is strongly positive on cord blood RBCs when due to Rh, Kell, Kidd, Duffy antibodies but is usually negative or weakly positive when due to anti-A antibodies. It becomes negative within a few days of effective exchange transfusion, but may remain positive for weeks in untreated infants. Indirect Coombs' test on cord blood may be positive because of "free" immune antibody.

At birth little or no anemia is seen. Anemia may develop rapidly (RBCs may decrease by 1 million/cu mm/day) in severe cases to maximum by third or fourth day.

MCV and MCH are increased; MCHC is normal.

Nucleated RBCs in peripheral blood are markedly increased (10,000–100,000/cu mm) during first 2 days (normal = 200–2000/cu mm) and are very large. They tend to decrease and may be absent by third or fourth day. Normoblastosis is mild or absent when due to antigens other than Rh_O.

Peripheral smear shows marked polychromatophilia and anisocytosis, macrocytic RBCs, increased reticulocyte count (>6% and up to 30–40%). In ABO incompatibility, spherocytosis may be marked with associated increased osmotic fragility; *spherocytosis is slight or absent in Rh incompatibility.*

HbF is decreased and adult Hb is increased.

WBC is increased (usually 15,000–30,000/cu mm).

Platelet count is usually normal; may be decreased in severe cases but returns to normal after 1 wk. With decreased platelets, increased bleeding time, poor clot retraction, and purpura may be found. Prothrombin and fibrinogen deficiencies may occur.

Disease terminates in 3–6 wks after elimination of maternal antibodies from infant's serum.

Late anemia occurs during second to fourth week of life in 5% of those receiving exchange transfusions. Reticulocyte count is low, and marrow may not show erythroid hyperplasia.

Hypoglycemia occurs in >15% of infants with cord Hb <10 gm/dL; often asymptomatic.

Exchange Transfusion

Use mother's serum for cross match.
Use indirect Coombs' test for cross match.
Use Rh-negative donor unless both mother and baby are Rh-positive.
For subsequent transfusions, use blood compatible with that of mother and infant.
Monitor infant's glucose level during exchange with heparinized blood and after exchange with citrated blood, as high glucose content of citrated blood may cause infant hypoglycemia 1–2 hrs later.
Monitor infant's blood pH, because pH of donor is low; therefore prefer fresh heparinized blood.

In infants, Hb of 15 gm/dL corresponds to RBC volume of 30 mL/kg body weight. Transfusion of 6 mL of whole blood equals 2 mL of packed RBCs. Destruction of 1 gm of Hb produces 35 mg of bilirubin. Infant with blood volume of 300 mL can have decrease in Hb of 1 gm/dL that may be undetected but produces 105 mg of bilirubin.

Table 11-14. Criteria for Performing Exchange Transfusion

Criteria	Continue to Follow Patient	Consider Exchange	Perform Exchange
Rh antibody titer in mother	<1:64	>1:64	
Cord hemoglobin	>14 gm/dL	12–14 gm/dL	<12 gm/dL.
Cord bilirubin	<4 mg/dL	4–5 mg/dL	>5 mg/dL.
Capillary blood hemoglobin	>12 gm/dL	<12 gm/dL	<12 gm/dL and decreasing in first 24 hrs.
Serum bilirubin	<18 mg/dL	18–20 mg/dL	20 mg/dL in first 24 hrs; after 48 hrs, 22 mg/dL on two tests 6–8 hrs apart. In sick premature infants, 15 mg/dL is upper limit of normal to indicate exchange transfusion.

◆Indications for Exchange Transfusion

See Table 11-14.

Birth Weight Is (gm)	Serum Bilirubin Is (mg/dL)
<1000	10.0
1001–1250	13.0
1251–1500	15.0
1501–2000	17.0
2001–2500	18.0
>2500	20.0

Transfuse at one step earlier in presence of
- Serum protein <5 gm/dL
- Metabolic acidosis (pH <7.25)
- Respiratory distress (with O_2 <50 mm Hg)
- Certain clinical findings (e.g., hypothermia, CNS or other clinical deterioration, sepsis, hemolysis)

Other criteria for exchange transfusion are suddenness and rate of bilirubin increase and when it occurs; e.g., an increase of 3 mg/dL in 12 hrs, especially after bilirubin has already leveled off, must be followed with frequent serial determinations, especially if it occurs on the first or seventh day rather than on third day. Beware of rate of bilirubin increase >1 mg/dL during first day. Serum bilirubin of 10 mg/dL after 24 hrs or 15 mg/dL after 48 hrs in spite of phototherapy usually indicates that serum bilirubin will reach 20 mg/dL. Rate of bilirubin increase is not as great as in ABO hemolytic disease as in Rh disease; if danger level for exchange transfusion is not reached by third day, it is unlikely that it will be reached.

Laboratory Complications of Exchange Transfusion

Electrolytes—hyperkalemia, hypernatremia, hypocalcemia, acidosis
Clotting—overheparinization, thrombocytopenia
Infection—bacteremia, serum hepatitis
Other—hypoglycemia
Phototherapy of Coombs'-positive infants decreases exchange transfusions (from 25% to 10% of these infants); follow effect of therapy with serum bilirubin every 4–8 hrs. Phototherapy is not usually begun until serum bilirubin is 10 mg/dL. Skin color is disguised by phototherapy, so serum bilirubin determination is even more important.

HEMATOL

Beware of untreated anemia in these infants occurring in 1–8 wks due to short survival time of Coombs'-positive RBCs.

♦ Phototherapy is contraindicated in infants with congenital erythropoietic porphyria (see p. 547) and with significant direct-reacting bilirubinemia to avoid bronze-baby syndrome.
  • Serum, urine, and skin become bronze (bronze-black) due to some unknown pigment.
  • Onset several hours or more after phototherapy; patient usually recovers without sequelae.
  • Most patients have some preexisting liver disease.

Amniocentesis, Indications

Prior immunized pregnancy with maternal antibody titer >1:8 in albumin
History of hemolytic disease of newborn
After the first amniocentesis at 24th week, repeat every 2–3 wks to measure presence and increase in bilirubin pigments; the rise in these pigments according to age of fetus correlates with severity of disease and is indication for intrauterine transfusion, repeat examination, or immediate delivery. Lecithin/sphingomyelin ratio should also be measured to determine pulmonary maturity (see Chapter 14, p. 770).
ABO hemolytic disease alone does not cause fetal loss and therefore is not an indication for amniocentesis.

Indications for Selection of Patients for Immunosuppression of Rh Sensitization[10]

(Passive immunization using RhIg anti-D, which should be administered within hours of delivery. Less protective for ≤13 days.)
Nonimmunized mother must be Rh_O (D) negative and weak D (D+W [formerly D^u]) negative regardless of ABO blood group. 1.8% of Rh-negative women become sensitized late in pregnancy.
D+W women are classified as Rh positive and are not considered at risk for Rh immunization.
Other indications (unless the father or fetus is *known and documented* to be Rh negative) (because of prenatal typing errors ≤ 3%) include:
  • Abortion (spontaneous, therapeutic, threatened)
  • Abruptio placentae
  • Abdominal trauma during pregnancy
  • Administration of whole blood, RBCs, granulocytes, or platelet concentrates from Rh-positive donors to Rh-negative patients of childbearing age
  • Amniocentesis
  • Ectopic pregnancy
  • External cephalic version
  • Chorionic villus sampling
  • Death in utero
  • Manual removal of placenta
  • Percutaneous umbilical blood sampling
  • Placenta previa
  • Trophoblastic disease or neoplasm (not complete hydatiform mole)
  • Tubal ligation
  • Immune thrombocytopenic purpura
Whenever a positive D+W test is found in a woman known to be D+W negative before delivery, the postpartum blood should be tested to confirm fetal-maternal hemorrhage and to quantify the volume of fetal cells in maternal circulation.
Maternal serum must have no Rh antibodies. If antenatal RhIg has been administered, mother's postpartum serum will contain anti-D (usually weakly reactive [direct antiglobulin test] low titer [≤ 4]), which does not indicate existing immunization, and she should receive postpartum immunoprophylaxis.
Baby must be Rh_O (D) positive or D+W positive and have negative direct Coombs' test (cord blood).

---

[10]Hartwell EA. Use of RH immune globulin. ASCP practice parameter. *Am J Clin Pathol* 1998;1210:281.

Protocol to determine postpartum candidacy for RhIg administration:
- Test mother to determine if she is Rh negative; do not perform D+W test.
- If mother is Rh negative, test cord RBCs; if these are Rh positive or D+W positive, mother is a candidate. Even if baby (cord RBCs) is Rh_O negative, D+W typing is still necessary as D+W–positive cord RBCs can cause Rh sensitization.
- Quantitate fetal-maternal hemorrhage to determine dose of RhIg. Use microscopic D+W test for routine screening to detect Rh-positive fetal cells; detects fetal-maternal hemorrhage of ~35 mL of fetal blood in a woman of average size. This is often omitted due to difficulty in reading test and low predictive value of positive test.

RhIg half-life is 21–30 days (standard dose). Thus most women have positive antibody screen. Records must be kept of antenatal RhIg to avoid classifying this as active immunization.

Erythroblastosis, ABO

ABO incompatibility causes approximately two-thirds of cases; Rh incompatibility causes less than one-third of cases, and the latter are more severe. Minor blood factors (e.g., c, E, Kell) cause 2% of cases.
- ♦ Mother is group O with group A_1 or B infant; rarely is mother group A_2 with group A_1 or B infant.
- ♦ Infant's serum shows positive indirect Coombs' test with adult RBCs of same group varying up to moderately positive, but positive test is not dependable.

Infant's RBCs show a negative direct Coombs' test (by standard methods) due to antibody derived from mother that has crossed placenta.

Both Coombs' reactions have disappeared after the fourth day.

Marked microspherocytosis is present.

Osmotic fragility is increased.

Anti-A or anti-B titer in mother's serum is not useful because no correlation exists between the occurrence of hemolytic disease and the presence or height of the titer. If mother's serum does not hemolyze RBCs of same type as infant's, the diagnosis should be questioned.

Rapidly developing anemia is rare; serial bilirubin determinations are indicators for exchange transfusion to prevent a level of 20 mg/dL. Infants may show jaundice in first 24 hrs but rarely require exchange transfusion for anemia or hyperbilirubinemia.

For exchange transfusion, use group O, Rh-type–specific blood or group O, Rh-negative blood.

Infants born subsequently to same parents do not have more serious disease, and they may have less serious disease.

Hemorrhage, Neonatal

See Table 11-15.

Internal Hemorrhage

(E.g., intracranial, large cephalohematoma, rupture of liver or spleen, retroperitoneal hemorrhage)

Anemia without associated jaundice in first 1–3 days

Indirect hyperbilirubinemia appears after third day.

Twin-to-Twin Hemorrhage

(Occurs in ~15% of monochorial twin pregnancies.)
- ♦ Hb difference >5 gm/dL in identical twins.
- ♦ Recipient twin shows.
  - Erythrocytosis with Hb ≤ 30 gm/dL and Hct up to 82%
  - Increased indirect bilirubin
  - Laboratory findings due to congestive heart failure, venous thrombosis, respiratory distress, kernicterus
- ♦ Donor twin shows anemia with Hb as low as 4 gm/dL, increased reticulocyte count, increased number of nucleated RBCs.

HEMATOL

Table 11-15. Comparison of Neonatal Acute and Chronic Blood Loss in Fetal-Maternal Hemorrhage

	Acute	Chronic
Hemoglobin	May be normal at first, then rapid drop during first 24 hrs	Low at birth
RBC morphology	Normochromic, normocytic	Hypochromic, microcytic Anisocytosis, poikilocytosis
Serum iron	Normal at birth	Low at birth

Both types show negative direct Coombs'' test, low serum bilirubin levels, demonstrable fetal RBCs in maternal blood.

Fetal-Maternal Transfusion

Anemia varies from mild to severe.
Polychromatophilia, increased reticulocyte count, increased number of nucleated RBCs
Serum bilirubin is not increased.
Coombs' test is negative.
If chronic, then findings due to iron deficiency may occur.
♦ Diagnosis is established only by demonstrating fetal RBCs in maternal blood (e.g., Kleihauer-Betke test, flow cytometry).
This condition can be found in ~50% of mothers but in only 1% of pregnancies is infant anemic.
May not be found if there is major group incompatibility between mother and infant, in which case buffy coat smears of maternal blood may show erythrophagocytosis; or perform serial anti-A or anti-B titers in mother's blood for several weeks after birth.
Concurrent hemolytic disease of the newborn and intraplacental hemorrhage should also be ruled out.
In maternal-to-fetal transfusion, infant may show same findings as for recipient twin in twin-to-twin hemorrhage.

Histiocytosis X (Langerhans Cell Granulomatosis)

(Proliferative abnormalities of macrophages)

Eosinophilic Granuloma

♦ Biopsy of bone is diagnostic.
Blood is normal; eosinophilia is unusual.
Leukopenia and thrombocytopenia suggest poorest prognosis.

Letterer-Siwe Disease

(Rapidly progressive fatal malignant disease primarily of children)
Progressive normocytic normochromic anemia
Hemorrhagic manifestations due to thrombocytopenia
♦ Diagnostic biopsy (e.g., bone, skin, lymph nodes) shows characteristic lesions.

Hand-Schüller-Christian Disease

(Reactive proliferation of macrophages of uncertain etiology)
♦ Diagnosis by biopsy of involved tissues (especially bone)
Anemia, leukopenia, and thrombocytopenia may be present.
Diabetes insipidus may occur.

Hodgkin's Disease and Other Malignant Lymphomas

♦ Diagnosis is established by histologic findings of biopsied lymph node.
Blood findings may vary from completely normal to markedly abnormal.
Moderate normochromic normocytic anemia occurs, occasionally of the hemolytic type; may become severe.

♦ Small lymphocytic and follicular lymphomas often have malignant lymphocytes in peripheral blood; leukemic phase in 5–15% of patients. Cytopenias occur, commonly due to hypersplenism, immune effect, or lymphoma effect on marrow.

♦ Bone marrow involvement at time of diagnosis in <10% of patients with Hodgkin's disease; 50% of patients with diffuse, small cleaved lymphoma and mixed cell type; 70–80% of patients with follicular, small cleaved cell lymphoma; less frequent in those with large cell lymphomas.

Patients with large intermediate-grade lymphoma and serum LD >500 U/L are less likely to be cured.

Serum protein electrophoresis: Albumin is frequently decreased. Increased alpha$_1$ and alpha$_2$ globulins suggest disease activity. Decreased gamma globulin is less frequent in Hodgkin's disease than in lymphosarcoma. Gamma globulins may be increased, with macroglobulins present and evidence of autoimmune process (e.g., hemolytic anemia, cold agglutinins). Monoclonal gammopathy in ~20% of small lymphocytic lymphomas.

ESR and CRP are increased during active stages in ~50% of cases; may be normal during remission. ESR >30 mm/hr after radiotherapy may predict relapse.

Hodgkin's Disease

• Peripheral blood changes are common (~25% of cases at time of diagnosis) but not specific. WBC may be normal, decreased, or slightly or markedly increased (25,000/cu mm). Leukopenia, marked leukocytosis, anemia are bad prognostic signs. Eosinophilia occurs in ~20% of patients. Relative and absolute lymphopenia may occur. If lymphocytosis is present, look for another disease. Neutrophilia may be found. Monocytosis may be found. These changes may all be absent or may even be present simultaneously or in various combinations. Rarely, Reed-Sternberg cells are found in marrow or peripheral blood smears in advanced disease. Platelets may be decreased or increased.

• Patients commonly have abnormal T-cell function with deficiencies of cell-mediated immunity and increased susceptibility to bacterial, fungal, and viral infections (especially herpes zoster and varicella); these persist even after cure. Serum immunoglobulins are usually normal.

• >50% of cases show evidence of EBV in Reed-Sternberg cells.

Non-Hodgkin's Lymphoma

• Patients often have abnormalities of humoral immunity; hypogammaglobulinemia in 50% of cases and monoclonal gammopathy in ~10% of cases of small lymphocytic lymphomas.

• Autoimmune hemolytic anemia and thrombocytopenia may occur.

• Increased serum CA 125 in ~40% of cases indicates pleuropericardial or peritoneal involvement, may be useful for staging. Return of increased value to normal indicates therapeutic response with sensitivity of 100% and specificity >87%.

• Laboratory findings due to involvement of other organ systems (e.g., liver, kidney, CNS)

• Testicular non-Hodgkin's lymphoma is often aggressive and associated with CNS and bone marrow disease.

• Laboratory findings due to effects of treatment (e.g., radiation, chemotherapy, splenectomy), including acute and long-term toxicity, gonadal dysfunction, peripheral neuropathy, and second neoplasms (especially acute myelogenous leukemia).

• Occurs frequently in AIDS patients and shows rapid course, poor prognosis, frequent extranodal and CNS involvement.

Post–organ transplantation malignant lymphomas in ~2% of cases; median time ~6 mos and two-thirds within 10 mos. Occurs in 0.8% of recipients of renal allografts, 1.6% of liver allografts, 5.9% of heart allografts. Compared to spontaneous lymphomas, these tend to be more aggressive, frequently large cell type in extranodal sites, especially CNS; many are immunoglobulin negative.

♦ Gene Rearrangement

Use

In follicular lymphomas *bcl*-2 gene rearrangement is molecular counterpart of t(14;18)(q32:q21) reciprocal translocation; found in >80% by cytogenic analysis and virtually all by molecular testing and differentiates this from reactive lymph nodes.

Table 11-16. Non-Hodgkin's Lymphoma

Lymphoma	% in Adults in USA	Immunophenotype	Laboratory Findings
Small lymphocytic (SLL)	3–4	>95% B cells	In 60% blood picture resembles chronic lymphocytic leukemia; marrow involved; old age
Follicular	40	B cells	Leukemia less often than with SLL; associated with t(14;18)
Diffuse lymphomas (includes diffuse large and mixed and large immunoblastic)	40–50	~80% B cells ~20% postthymic T cells	Leukemia and involved marrow uncommon at time of diagnosis and are poor prognostic signs
Lymphoblastic	4	>95% immature intrathymic T cells	Early marrow involvement and progression to T-cell ALL; 40% of lymphomas in children
Small noncleaved (Burkitt's)	<1	B cells	Characteristic t(8;14); presents with extranodal visceral involvement; mostly children; endemic in Africa; analysis of c-*myc* oncogene by Southern blotting in lymph node, blood or bone marrow permits confirming or ruling out this diagnosis; EBV DNA is found in tumor cells in >95% of African patients but <20% of sporadic cases
Cutaneous	Uncommon	CD4⁺ T cells	See Table 11-19
Adult T-cell	Rare	CD4⁺ T cells	See Table 11-19

ALL = acute lymphoblastic leukemia; EBV = Epstein-Barr virus.

Monitor for residual lymphoma during chemotherapy, confirm remission, detect minimal residual disease, detect marrow or distant site involvement, monitor patients undergoing marrow transplantation, diagnose relapse earlier.

In B-cell diffuse lymphoma, patients positive for *bcl*-2 are less likely to have complete remission.

Detection by PCR after bone marrow has been purged before marrow transplant is indicator to predict relapse.

See Burkitt's lymphoma, Table 11-16.

Hypereosinophilic Syndrome

♦ Diagnostic Criteria

- Eosinophilia >1500/cu mm for >6 mos
- No other cause for eosinophilia
- Organ dysfunction, e.g.,

Cardiovascular in 50–75% of cases (e.g., valve insufficiency, heart failure, mural
   thrombi cause systemic embolization in 5% of cases)
Pulmonary in one-third of cases (e.g., pleural effusion, diffuse interstitial infiltrates)
Neurologic in 35–75% of patients
Cutaneous in 50% of patients
Liver function abnormalities in 15% of cases
Abnormal urine sediment in 20% of patients

Total WBC is usually <25,000 but may be >90,000/cu mm with 30–70% eosinophils.
Abnormalities in count and morphology of platelets, WBC, and RBC.
Mild anemia in ~50% of cases.
Thrombocytopenia in one-third of cases.
Hypercellular bone marrow with 25–75% eosinophils.
May be difficult to distinguish from eosinophilic leukemia.

Hyperimmunoglobulinemia E Syndrome

(Very rare autosomal dominant condition shows recurrent infections, chronic candidiasis, skeletal and dental abnormalities)
See Table 11-6.
♦ Increased eosinophils in blood (in >90% of cases), sputum, and sections of tissues. Not correlated with serum IgE.
♦ Very high serum IgE with substantial fluctuations over time.
Other immunoglobulins are usually normal.
Normal count of lymphocytes and subsets.

Hyperimmunoglobulinemia M Syndrome

(Heterogeneous group of disorders)
Male patients have history of pyogenic infections resembling those in X-linked agammaglobulinemia. Also susceptible to opportunistic infections, especially due to *Pneumocystis carinii*.
♦ Serum usually has very low concentration of IgG (<150 mg/dL) and undetectable IgA and IgE. IgM is high normal and may be ≥ 1000 mg/dL; IgD is also increased.
♦ B lymphocytes are normal in number but have only surface IgM and IgD; surface IgG and IgA are virtually absent.
Increased frequency of autoimmune disorders; neutropenia is most important and may be recurrent, severe, and prolonged; autoimmune hemolytic anemia, thrombocytopenia.
In second decade of life, IgM-producing polyclonal plasma cells may show marked proliferation with extensive invasion of GI tract, liver, and gall bladder that may be fatal.
Increased risk of abdominal cancers.

Hypoalbuminemia, Hypoanabolic

(Inherited disorder present from birth, without kidney or liver disease)
Growth and development are normal. The patient is unaffected except for periodic peripheral edema.
♦ Serum albumin is <0.3 gm/dL.
♦ Total globulins are 4.5–5.5 gm/dL.
Serum cholesterol is increased.
Albumin synthesis is decreased, with decreased catabolism of IV-injected albumin.

Hypogammaglobulinemia, Common Variable (or "Acquired")

(Heterogeneous immunodeficiency syndrome; can result from three different immunologic causes: intrinsic B-cell defects, immunoregulatory T-cell imbalances, or autoantibodies to T or B cells)
See Table 11-6.
Clinically, may resemble X-linked agammaglobulinemia but infections are less severe, sex distribution is equal. Or patients may have unusual infections (e.g., *P. carinii*, various fungi); recurrent HSV and HZV infections in ~20% of patients. Untreated

cases present with chronic lung disease and bronchiectasis and infections elsewhere due to other organisms. Many have sprue-like syndrome due to *G. lamblia*.

♦ Diagnosis by exclusion of other causes of humoral immune defects.

Serum IgG is decreased (<250 μg/μL); IgA and IgM are usually decreased.

Associated with increased incidence (~20%) of autoimmune diseases (e.g., PA occurs in ~10% of patients, SLE, RA) and malignancy (especially intestinal lymphomas and gastric adenocarcinoma)

Reactive follicular hyperplasia of lymph nodes, tonsil, spleen, and small bowel (may cause malabsorption) but lack plasma cells.

Sterile noncaseating granulomas can occur in liver, spleen, lung, skin.

T lymphocyte function may be impaired.

Number of peripheral blood B cells may be low or high but fail to differentiate into immunoglobulin antibody–secreting cells.

Immunodeficiency, Cellular, with Normal Immunoglobulins (Nezelof's Syndrome)

See Table 11-7.

♦ Lymphopenia, neutropenia, eosinophilia

♦ Marked deficiency of total T cells and T-cell subsets; normal helper/suppressor (CD4/CD8) ratio (in contrast to AIDS patients, who show marked deficiency of CD4 with reverse of ratio)

Normal or increased serum immunoglobulins; some show selective IgA deficiency, increased IgD, and marked increase in IgE.

Infants may show recurrent or chronic pulmonary infection, failure to thrive, candidiasis, gram-negative sepsis, GU tract infection, progressive varicella, etc.

Decreased lymphoid tissue with depletion of paracortical lymphocytes

Hypoplastic thymus shows abnormal architecture with no Hassall's corpuscles, few lymphocytes, poor corticomedullary distinction.

Few patients have associated enzyme deficiency causing low or absent serum uric acid.

Immunodeficiency, Classification

Primary

See Tables 11-6, 11-7, and 11-17.

Primary B-cell (antibody) deficiency disorders
- X-linked agammaglobulinemia (block in maturation of pre-B cells)
- Common variable immunodeficiency (block in differentiation of B cells to plasma cells)
- Selective IgA deficiency (block in differentiation to a specific isotype)
- Selective IgG subclass deficiency (block in differentiation to a specific isotype)
- Hyperimmunoglobulinemia M syndrome

Primary T-cell deficiency
- DiGeorge syndrome (lack of thymus development causes block in T-cell maturation)
- Chronic mucocutaneous candidiasis (probable absence of T-cell clones that respond to *Candida* infections)
- Hyperimmunoglobulinemia E syndrome

Combined T-cell/B-cell deficiency
- Severe combined immunodeficiency disease (defect in adenosine deaminase or purine nucleoside phosphorylase enzymes)
- Wiskott-Aldrich syndrome
- Ataxia-telangiectasia

Secondary, Associated With

Virus infections (e.g., HIV, CMV, EBV infection, measles)

Metabolic disorders (e.g., uremia, malnutrition, diabetes mellitus)

Protein deficiency (e.g., nephrotic syndrome)

Immunosuppression (e.g., drugs, neoplasms, splenectomy)

Respiratory tract disorders
- Anatomic (e.g., tracheoesophageal fistula, cleft palate, gastroesophageal reflux
- Other (e.g., cystic fibrosis, immotile cilia, allergy)

Prematurity

Table 11-17. Some Infectious Agents in Various Immune Deficiency Disorders

Pathogen	T-cell Defect	B-cell Defect	Granulocyte	Complement Defect
Bacteria	Sepsis	Streptococci, staphylococci, *Haemophilus*	Staphylococci, *Pseudomonas*	*Neisseria*
Viruses	CMV, EBV, severe vaccinia, chronic respiratory and intestine viruses	Enteroviral encephalitis	N/A	N/A
Fungi and parasites	*Candida, Pneumocystis carinii*	Severe giardiasis	*Candida, Nocardia, Aspergillus*	N/A
Comment	Aggressive infection with opportunistic organisms; failure to resolve infection	Recurrent sinopulmonary infections, sepsis, chronic meningitis	—	—

CMV = cytomegalovirus; EBV = Epstein-Barr virus; N/A = not applicable.

Immunodeficiency, Screening Tests

See Fig. 11-8 and Table 11-17.
Cell mediated
- HIV serology.
- Total lymphocyte count (lymphopenia usually indicates T-cell dysfunction because most circulating lymphocytes are T cells).
- T lymphocyte subsets. T cell–deficient patients tend to have chronic recurrent *Candida* infection of scalp, nails, mucous membranes.
- Anergy skin tests (purified protein derivative [tuberculin], *Candida*).
- B-cell deficiency should be suspected with recurrent, complicated, or severe pyogenic infections.
Humoral immunity
- Antibody defects
    Serum IgG, IgM, IgA, anti-A, anti-B isohemagglutinins
    Serum IgG antibody titers before and after vaccinations (e.g., diphtheria, tetanus, *Pneumococcus, H. influenzae* type b)
- Complement defects
    CH50
    C1-4 deficiencies associated with pyogenic infections and autoimmunity
    C3, C5-9 deficiencies associated with neisserial infections
- Phagocyte defects
    WBC and differential counts
    Serum IgE
    Nitroblue tetrazolium test now replaced by flow cytometry respiratory burst assay

Immunoglobulin A (IgA) Deficiency, Selective

(Immunodeficiency syndrome with lack of IgA-producing cells in intestinal lamina propria)
See Tables 11-6 and 11-7.
♦ Serum IgA is very low (<5 mg/dL).
♦ Serum IgM and IgG are usually normal.

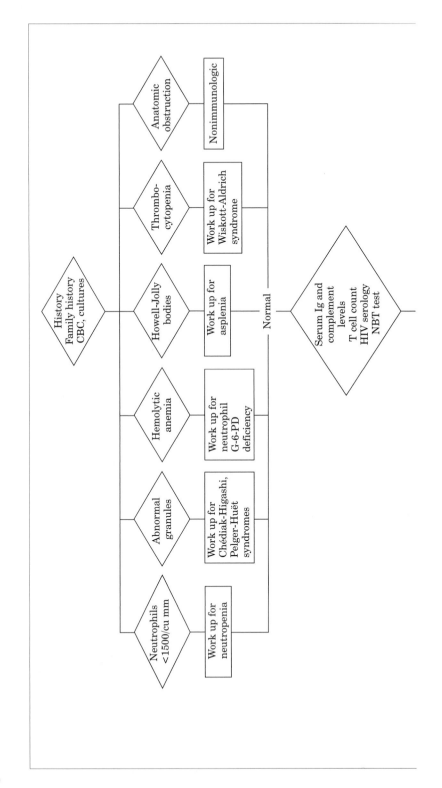

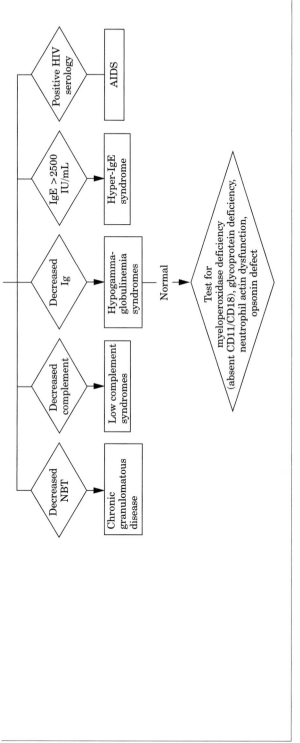

Fig. 11-8. Algorithm for workup of recurrent infections. (G-6-PD = glucose-6-phosphate dehydrogenase; hyper-IgE = hyperimmunoglobulinemia E; Ig = immunoglobulin; NBT = nitroblue tetrazolium.)

HEMATOL

Serum antibodies to IgA in >40% of patients; therefore IV or IM blood products that contain IgA (e.g., immune serum globulin) are contraindicated.

Peripheral blood lymphocytes bearing IgA, IgM, and IgG are normal.

Plasma cells producing IgA are absent in GI and respiratory epithelium.

Clinical—asymptomatic or recurrent pyogenic respiratory infections; increased incidence of allergic disease (e.g., asthma, eczema), autoimmune diseases (e.g., RA, SLE), GI complications (e.g., celiac disease, malabsorption, chronic giardiasis). Found in >1 in 400 persons in general population.

Irradiation, Hematologic Effects

(Depends on amount of irradiation received)

Severe
- Severe leukopenia with infection.
- Thrombocytopenia and increased vascular fragility, causing hemorrhage; begins in 4–7 days, peak severity in 16–22 days.
- Aplastic anemia if patient survives 3–6 wks; laboratory findings due to complications, such as hemorrhage, infection, dehydration.

Mild (<300 R)
- Increased neutrophils within a few hours with onset of irradiation sickness.
- Decreased lymphocytes after 24 hrs, causing decrease in total WBC.
- No anemia unless dose of radiation is greater; may appear in 4–8 wks. (*Early appearance of anemia with greater irradiation is due to hemorrhage and changes in fluid homeostasis rather than marrow injury.*)
- Platelets slightly decreased (some patients).

Chronic (occupational)
- Decreased granulocytes
- Increased lymphocytes, relative or absolute
- Varying degrees of leukocytosis and leukemoid reactions
- Varying degrees of anemia, normocytic or macrocytic; erythrocytosis
- Thrombocytopenia

Late
- Increased incidence of leukemia (e.g., in survivors of atomic bomb explosions)
- Increased incidence of visceral malignancy (e.g., liver cancer due to Thorotrast, bone cancer due to radium)

Jordans Anomaly

♦ Harmless rare anomaly of fatty inclusions in cytoplasm of all neutrophils, most monocytes, some basophils and eosinophils, occasional lymphocytes.

♦ 3–10 vacuoles/neutrophil stain with Sudan III. Fewer vacuoles are found in marrow myeloid cells beginning with promyelocytes.

Leukemia, Acute

In adults 20% of acute leukemias are lymphocytic (ALL) and 80% are nonlymphocytic (AML).

♦ In children, 75% of cases are ALL and 25% are AML or chronic; >80% show clonal chromosomal abnormalities. With specific genetic abnormalities, PCR can identify as few as 1 malignant cell per 10^6 normal cells and minimal residual leukemia in >90% cases of childhood ALL.

♦ Peripheral blood.
- WBC is rarely >100,000/cu mm. It may be normal and is commonly less than normal.
- Peripheral smear shows many cells that resemble lymphocytes; it may not be possible to differentiate the very young forms as lymphoblasts or myeloblasts, and special cytochemical stains may be used (blast cells are positive for peroxidase, Sudan black B, and nonspecific esterase in AML but negative in ALL; cytoplasmic acid phosphatase may be positive in T-cell ALL).
- Auer rods are diagnostic of AML; seen in 10–20% of cases.
- Special immunologic markers distinguish T-cell, B-cell, and non–T-, non–B-cell types of ALL, which is important because of different prognosis and relapse patterns in the three types.

- Prognosis is poorer in older children and adults >35 yrs and those with high initial WBC, with chromosome translocations (e.g., 9,22 in Ph[1] chromosome and 4,11-positive ALL). Favorable response to treatment is more likely if B-cell lymphoblasts are CALLA positive (common ALA antigen) but cytoplasmic mu-chain negative. Presence of leukemic lymphoblasts that express myeloid antigens is associated with an unfavorable prognosis.

Anemia is almost always present at clinical onset. Usually normocytic and sometimes macrocytic, it is progressive and may become severe. Normoblasts and polychromatophilia are common.

Platelet count is usually decreased at clinical onset and becomes progressively severe. May show poor clot retraction, increased BT, positive tourniquet test, etc.

♦ Bone marrow
- Blast cells are present even when none are found in peripheral blood. (This finding is useful to differentiate from other causes of pancytopenia.) Progressively increasing infiltration with earlier cell types (e.g., blasts, myelocytes) is seen.
- The myeloid-erythroid ratio is increased.
- Erythroid and megakaryocyte elements are replaced.
- Cultures (bacterial, fungal, viral) should be performed routinely as they may be the first clue to occult infection.

♦ Quantification of leukemic cells by molecular methods (e.g., PCR or antibody detection) in minimal residual disease ALL[11-13]
- Combinations of surface antigens semispecific for leukemic clone detect level of 10^{-4} cells.
- Various PCR techniques have limit of detection of 10^{-2} to 10^{-6} leukemic cells.
- After end of induction chemotherapy, level of minimal residual disease is useful for prognosis. >10^{-2} cells (which is below detection limit with conventional microscopic examination of bone marrow) or >10^{-3} cells at later time is associated with very high probability of relapse; <10^{-5} (<0.01% nucleated cells) is associated with very low probability of relapse.
- If <10^{-3} cells in bone marrow, sampling error may be significant because of multifocal clones; therefore use peripheral blood or multiple marrow samples.
- Considered in remission after cytotoxic therapy, <10^{10} leukemic cells and leukemic cells cannot be identified by conventional techniques.
- With 10^{11} to 10^{12} leukemic cells, clinical symptoms are present.
- With 10^{13} leukemic cells, death results.

DIC may be present at onset (especially with M3; also with M4 and M5; less commonly with other forms).

Serum uric acid is frequently increased.

Tumor lysis syndrome may cause hyperphosphatemia, hypokalemia, hypocalcemia, hypomagnesemia, etc. (See Chapter 17, p. 912.)

Increased serum creatinine and BUN reflect infiltration of kidneys, impairing renal function.

In AML serum LD is frequently but inconstantly increased; normal to slight increase in serum AST, ALT is seen. LD >400 U/L predicts shorter survival in elderly patients.

Urine lysozyme may be increased in acute nonlymphocytic leukemia (M4 and M5).

♦ Laboratory findings due to complications
- Meningeal leukemia occurs in 25–50% of children and 10–20% of adults with acute leukemia; CSF shows pleocytosis and increased pressure and LD. CSF should be examined routinely as "sanctuary" for leukemic cells during chemotherapy and to rule out occult infection. Cranial irradiation may be indicated if leukemic cells in CSF, WBC ≥ 100,000/cu mm, or Ph[1] chromosome is present.
- With large leukemic cell burden, hyperuricemia (may have urate nephropathy), hyperkalemia, hyperphosphatemia with secondary hypocalcemia are common.
- Infection causes 90% of deaths. Most important pathogens are enteric gram-negative rods (especially *Pseudomonas aeruginosa, E. coli*) and *S. aureus*. With cumu-

[11]Cave H, et al. Clinical significance of minimal residual disease in childhood acute lymphoblastic leukemia. European Organization for Research and Treatment of Cancer, Childhood Leukemia Cooperative Group. *N Engl J Med* 1998;339:591.
[12]Pui CH, et al. Acute lymphoblastic leukemia. *N Engl J Med* 1998;339:605.
[13]Morley A. Quantifying leukemia. *N Engl J Med* 1998;339:627.

HEMATOL

lative immunosuppression, fungi (especially *C. albicans*), viruses (especially VZV and other herpesviruses), and *P. carinii*.
- Hemolytic anemia.

Laboratory findings due to predisposing conditions
- Inherited syndromes
- Genetic (e.g., Down syndrome, Bloom's syndrome, Klinefelter's syndrome, Fanconi's anemia)
- Immunodeficiency (e.g., ataxia-telangiectasia, common variable immunodeficiency, severe combined immunodeficiency, Wiskott-Aldrich syndrome)
- Ionizing radiation (therapeutic or accidental)
- Chemotherapeutic drugs (e.g., alkylating agents)
- Toxins (e.g., benzene)

Complete remission is possible with drug therapy (e.g., prednisone in ALL).
- WBC falls (or rises) to normal in 1–2 wks with replacement of lymphoblasts by normal PMNs and return of RBC and platelet counts to normal; bone marrow may become normal. Maximum improvement in 6–8 wks.

Laboratory findings due to toxic effect of therapeutic agents
- Amethopterin toxicity causes a macrocytic type of anemia with megaloblasts in marrow, rather than blast cells in marrow as with leukemic normocytic anemia.
- Cyclophosphamide can cause hematuria.
- L-Asparaginase can cause coagulopathies, hyperglycemia, etc.
- Daunorubicin can cause cardiac toxicity with fibrosis.
- In childhood ALL, 7× increase in all cancers and 22× increase in CNS tumors.

Leukemia, Hairy Cell (Leukemic Reticuloendotheliosis)

(Rare condition of splenomegaly and infrequent lymphadenopathy with characteristic pathologic changes in marrow and spleen)
- ◆ Diagnosis is established by finding the characteristic mononuclear cells (that show long delicate cytoplasmic projections) in the peripheral blood (vary from 0%–90%) or bone marrow, which show a characteristic diffuse *intense* histochemical reaction of tartrate-resistant acid phosphatase (isoenzyme 5) activity (mild to moderate staining of leukocytes may be seen in Sézary syndrome, CLL, infectious mononucleosis, and in various histiocytes). Cells bear B lymphocyte markers. Isoenzyme 5 may also be increased in the serum. Hairy cells increased to frankly leukemic levels in ≤ 20% of cases.

Hypersplenism with pancytopenia in >50% of cases
- Thrombocytopenia (in 75% of cases), usually <80,000/cu mm
- Anemia (usually normochromic), usually 7–10 gm/dL
- Leukopenia (in >60% of cases), usually <4000/cu mm

Abnormal platelet function may be found.
ESR may be increased.
- ◆ Bone marrow reticulin fibrosis causes dry tap requiring core biopsy; hairy cells are readily seen.

Leukocyte ALP activity is markedly increased in some patients.
Laboratory findings due to infection (e.g., pyogenic bacteria, opportunistic organisms)

Leukemia, Lymphoblastic, Acute (ALL)

Primarily affects children; comprises >85% of childhood leukemias. Children with Down syndrome have 15× higher incidence of leukemia (especially ALL). Increased incidence also in immunodeficiency syndromes (e.g., ataxia-telangiectasia), osteogenesis imperfecta, Poland's syndrome, and sibs of ALL patients. High relapse rate.

In adults, 80% of ALL cases are B-cell and 20% are T-cell lineage.

Classified as L-1, L-2, L-3 (French-American-British [FAB] classification system) based on cell morphology; cannot be differentiated by cytochemical stains. ~25% of cells in L-1 and L-2 have T-cell antigens; rest are null cells (B-lineage ALL that lack CD10 expression). L-3 cells usually have B-cell (Burkitt's) antigens. L-1 is more common in childhood ALL and L-2 is more common in adult ALL.
- ◆ WBC increased; may be >100,000/cu mm but normal or low in some patients. Moderate to severe thrombocytopenia.

Variable degree of anemia.

Table 11-18. Comparison of Chronic Lymphocytic Leukemias

B lymphocytes

CLL	Autoimmune hemolytic anemia, hypogammaglobulinemia
Prolymphocytic leukemia (not a variant of CLL but a separate entity)	B-type lymphocytes derived from medullary cords of lymph nodes show less mature forms than in CLL extreme leukocytosis with >54% prolymphocytes with a typical phenotype, very high blast counts, prominent splenomegaly often without much lymphadenopathy
Waldenström's macro-globulinemia	Increased serum IgM
Leukemic phase of poorly differentiated lymphoma	Usually is leukemic phase of lymphoma, but ≤ 50% have marrow involvement lymphoma when first seen; occasionally may present without node involvement
Hairy cell leukemia	Pancytopenia and prominent splenomegaly; usually leukopenia with many hairy cells showing characteristic tartrate-resistant acid phosphatase

T lymphocytes

CLL	Causes <5% of cases of CLL
Adult T-cell leukemia/lymphoma	Hypercalcemia, lytic bone lesions; WBC usually >50,000/cu mm; due to HTLV-1 infection
Prolymphocytic	Morphologically identical to B-cell type, but lymph-adenopathy is more frequent in T-cell type leukemia
T-gamma–chronic lympho-proliferative disease	Severe granulocytopenia; moderate increase in WBC; recurrent infections are common; usually no lymphadenopathy or skin involvement
Cutaneous T-cell lymphoma	Sézary syndrome refers to both skin and systemic involvement; mycosis fungoides is cutaneous form, which may be present for years before clinical systemic involvement

◆ Marrow usually shows >50% lymphoblasts.
○ High incidence of meningeal involvement; CSF may show increased protein and cells (some recognized as leukemic).
○ Ph¹ chromosome is present in ~20% of adults and <5% of children. Uniformly poor prognostic sign. Most commonly in non–T-cell, non–B-cell ALL; never in T-cell ALL.
Serum LD, uric acid, ESR often increased.

Leukemia, Lymphocytic, Chronic (CLL)

(30% of all leukemias in United States; <5% are T-cell type)
See Table 11-18.

Diagnostic Criteria

◆ Lymphocyte count >15,000/cu mm in absence of other causes and marrow infiltration >30% for >6 mos. Have characteristic immunophenotype.
◆ Demonstration of monoclonality in the proper clinical context confirms the diagnosis regardless of absolute lymphocyte count. Monoclonality is determined by demonstration of light-chain restriction in B-cell lymphocytosis and rearranged T-cell receptor genes in T-cell lymphocytosis; natural killer cells do not rearrange T-cell receptor genes.
◆ Peripheral blood
  • WBC is increased (usually 50,000–250,000/cu mm) with 90% lymphocytes, which are uniformly similar, producing a monotonous blood picture of small, mature-looking lymphocytes with minimal cytoplasm indistinguishable from normal. Fre-

HEMATOL

Table 11-19. Differential Diagnosis of Chronic Myelogenous Leukemia

	Chronic Myelogenous Leukemia	Acute Myeloblastic Leukemia	Granulocytic Leukemoid Reaction	Myelo-fibrosis
WBC >100,000/cu mm	Yes	Rare	No	No
Whole spectrum of immature granulocytes	Yes	No (leukemic hiatus)	No	Yes
Myeloblasts and pro-myelocytes in blood or marrow	>30%	>30%	0	<30%
LAP scores	Usually <10	30–150	>150	Variable
Bone marrow	Granulocytic hyperplasia	>30% myelo-blasts	Granulocytic hyperplasia	Fibrosis
Philadelphia chromosome	Yes	No	No	No

quent smudge cells. Blast cells are uncommon. Granulocytopenia. Neutropenia is a late occurrence.

- Autoimmune hemolytic anemia and thrombocytopenia in 25% of patients. Hb <11 gm/dL and/or thrombocytopenia (<100000/cu mm), diffuse bone marrow infiltration, and lymphocyte doubling time <1 yr correlate with marked decrease in survival time. Progress with rising WBC but may be absent with WBC >50,000/cu mm.
- Platelet count is less likely to increase with therapy than in myelogenous leukemia.
♦ Bone marrow
- Infiltration with earlier lymphocytic cell types is progressively increased.
- There is replacement of erythroid, myeloid, and megakaryocyte series, which show normal morphology and maturation.
♦ Lymph node biopsy shows pattern of diffuse lymphoma with well-differentiated, small, noncleaved cells; aspirate or imprint shows increased number of immature leukocytes, predominantly blast cells.

Serum enzyme levels are less frequently increased and show a lesser increase than in chronic myelogenous leukemia. Even serum LD is frequently normal.

Direct Coombs' test is positive in up to one-third of patients.

Hypogammaglobulinemia occurs in two-thirds of cases depending on duration of disease; monoclonal gammapathy (most often IgM) is found in <1% of cases.

Uric acid levels are not increased but may become so during therapy.

Ph[1] chromosome is not found.

Chromosomal abnormalities in ~50% of patients, most often chromosomes 12 (especially trisomy 12) and 14 (especially 14q+).

Laboratory findings due to secondary infection (e.g., encapsulated bacteria, herpes zoster, opportunistic organisms)

Progression to more aggressive cancers in ~10% of cases, e.g., large B-cell lymphoma, prolymphocytic leukemia (>30% of cells are prolymphocytes), ALL, multiple myeloma

Leukemia, Myelogenous, Chronic

(Malignant clonal disorder of stem cells; 20% of all leukemias in United States; 90% of cases occur in adults, 10% in children)

See Table 11-19, Fig. 11-9.

Types of chronic myeloid leukemias
- Chronic myelogenous leukemia
- Chronic myelomonocytic leukemia
- Mast cell leukemia (rare)
- Chronic monocytic leukemia (rare)
- Chronic eosinophilic leukemia (rare)

Classified into chronic, accelerated, and blast crisis phases.

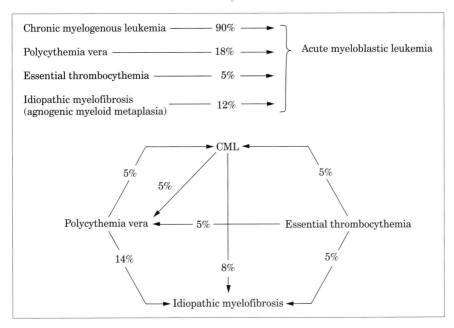

Fig. 11-9. Transformation of myeloproliferative syndromes. (CML = chronic myelogenous leukemia.)

Chronic Phase

♦WBC is usually 50,000–300,000/cu mm when disease is discovered, predominantly neutrophils and myelocytes with no leukemic hiatus. In earlier stages the more mature forms predominate, with sequentially fewer younger forms and only an occasional blast cell; later the younger cells predominate.
  • Absolute basophilia is invariably present; may precede clinical symptoms by many years.
  • Eosinophilia may be present but has less diagnostic utility than basophilia.
  • Absolute monocytosis but relative monocytopenia is typical.
  • Lymphocytes are normal in absolute number but relatively decreased.
  • Decreased leukocyte ALP score (see p. 334) in 95% of untreated cases. Leukocyte ALP score can rise to normal or high levels with infection, inflammation, or secondary malignant disease, after splenectomy, during remission due to chemotherapy, or at onset of blast crisis.
○Anemia is usually normochromic, normocytic; absent in early stage and severe in late stage. Blood smear shows few normoblasts, slight polychromatophilia, occasional stippling. Reticulocyte count is usually <3%. Anemia is due to myelophthisis; also due to bleeding (skin and GI tract), hemolysis, and insufficient compensatory hematopoiesis. Degree of anemia is a good index of extent of leukemic process and therefore of prognosis.
○Platelet count is increased in 30–50% of cases; may be normal; decreased in terminal stages with findings of thrombocytopenic purpura. Low count may increase with therapy. Bleeding manifestations are usually due to thrombocytopenia. Megakaryocytes in blood in ~25% of cases.
♦Bone marrow
  • Hyperplasia of granulocytic elements occurs, with increase in myeloid/erythroid ratio. Myeloblasts <5% of all cells initially.
  • Granulocytes are more immature than in the peripheral blood.
  • Number of eosinophils and basophils is increased.
  • Megakaryocytes may be increased.

- Hemosiderin deposits are increased.
- Focal or diffuse reticulin fibrosis in approximately one-third of cases.
- Macrophages (pseudo-Gaucher's cells) in approximately one-third of cases.
♦ Philadelphia chromosome t(9;22)(q34q11)(Ph^1) due to chimeric *bcr-abl* gene on chromosome 22 (see p. 329) is found in 95% of early chronic-phase cases; persists in chronic stable phase when marrow and blood appear normal. Presence of Ph^1 affects response to therapy and survival. Persists during blast phase when additional abnormalities may appear in ≤ 8% of cases (e.g., chronic myelomonocytic leukemias). Other cytogenic abnormalities occur in one-third of the 5% of patients who are Ph^1-negative. Ph^1 chromosome has also been found in ~20% of adults with ALL, 2% of adults with AML, 5% of children with ALL. Ph^1 chromosome in acute leukemia indicates a poor prognosis. Ph^1 is present in granulomonocytic, erythroid, and megakaryocytic lines as well as some B lymphocytes. If karyotyping is negative, Ph^1 may be revealed by Southern blot, fluorescence in situ hybridization, or RT-PCR, which are more sensitive. PCR can detect 1 Ph^1-positive cell in 10^5 to 10^6 normal cells.
Needle aspiration of spleen
- Number of immature leukocytes is increased.
- Normoblastosis is present.
- Megakaryopoiesis is increased.
Serum and urine uric acid are increased, especially with high WBC and antileukemic therapy. Urinary obstruction may develop because of intrarenal and extrarenal uric acid crystallization.
Serum LD is increased; rises several weeks before relapse and falls several weeks before remission. LD is useful for following course of therapy.
Increased serum AST and ALT show less increase than in acute leukemia; are normal in half of patients.
Serum protein electrophoresis shows decreased albumin with increased alpha and gamma globulins.
Direct Coombs' test is positive in ≤ 20% of patients at some time in course of disease; overt hemolysis in ~25% of these patients.
Laboratory findings due to leukemic infiltration of organs (e.g., kidney [hematuria common; uremia rare], heart, liver). With increasing survival in blast crisis, meningeal leukemia has become more frequent (up to 40%) with leukemic cells in CSF indicative of need for intrathecal chemotherapy.
Serum vitamin B$_{12}$ level is increased (often >1000 µg/mL); B$_{12}$-binding capacity is increased.
Peripheral blood remission due to drugs—decreased WBC to nearly normal levels (decrease in spleen size is usually parallel) with only rare immature cells, correction of anemia, control of thrombocytosis, and occasional rise of LAP score to normal; marrow continues to show granulocytic hyperplasia and Ph^1 chromosome.
Thyroid uptake of radioactive iodine is normal.

Accelerated Phase

(Experienced by ~50% of patients before a blast crisis)
♦ Combination of various criteria described in literature
- Rapidly increasing WBC (>50,000/cu mm) (doubling time <5 days) showing increasing immaturity and increased number of blasts (>5–15% in marrow, >15% in blood), basophilia (>10% in marrow, >20% in blood).
- Hb <7.0 g/dL not due to therapy.
- Platelets <100,000/cu mm not due to therapy or >1 million/cu mm despite therapy.
- Increased leukocyte ALP score.
- New karyotypic abnormalities (e.g., trisomy 8, trisomy 18, additional Ph^1 chromosomes).
- Myelofibrosis in some cases.
- Associated with clinical symptoms.
- Increasing doses of drugs are needed to lower neutrophil count.

Blast Crisis

(Occurs abruptly without an accelerated phase in 50% of cases)
♦ Diagnosed by >30% blasts in marrow or peripheral blood or extramedullary proliferation of blasts (chloroma), or large foci of blasts in bone marrow biopsy. Approxi-

mately one-third of patients with CML in blast crisis have lymphoid transformation (cells show morphologic, antigenic, enzymatic [TdT], and other lymphoid characteristics). Patients are increasingly refractory to therapy in blast phase and die of acute leukemia or complications in 3–6 mos.

Platelet count <15,000 or >1 million/cu mm, blasts in peripheral blood, absence of Ph^1, and moderate to marked myelofibrosis at time of diagnosis are poor prognostic signs. WBC <25,000/cu mm or Hb >14 gm/dL are good prognostic signs.

Juvenile Chronic Myelogenous Leukemia[14]

Differs from adult CML
- Aggressive disease.
- 95% of patients are <4 yrs old.
- Leukocytosis (usually <100,000/cu mm) with absolute monocytosis (>450/cu mm).
- Immature myeloid cells in peripheral blood in >70% of cases.
- <25% marrow blasts.
- Absent Ph^1.
- Increased HbF (typically 20–80%); is only leukemia with this increase.
- Lymphadenopathy in 20% of cases.
- Skin involvement with monocytic infiltrate is very common; may be preceded by neurofibromatosis.
- Viral studies (CMV, EBV, rubella) are usually negative.
- Leukocyte ALP is not useful; may be normal, low, or increased.

Leukemia, Plasma Cell

♦ WBC usually >15,000, with >20% plasma cells or >2000/cu mm in peripheral blood varying from typical plasmacytes to immature and atypical forms; absolute plasma cell count >2000/cu mm. Occasionally, special studies (cytochemical stains, cell surface and cytoplasmic markers, electron microscopy) are needed to confirm identity of plasma cells.

♦ Plasma cell monoclonality.

~60% of cases are primary and the rest occur in 2% of previously diagnosed cases of multiple myeloma. Primary cases have smaller M protein peak in serum, higher platelet count, younger age, and longer survival.

Other findings (see Myeloma, Multiple, p. 420)

Leukemia, Prolymphocytic

(Rare variant of CLL; may occur de novo or from CLL)

Compared to CLL, is characterized by more rapid clinical course, poorer prognosis, slightly older patient age, larger spleen, less frequent lymphadenopathy, higher prolymphocyte count (>55%), and immunologic differences (mouse erythrocytes, rosettes, surface immunoglobulin staining).

WBC >100,000/cu mm in 65% of patients.

~80% are B-cell and 20% are T-cell type, which show different chromosomal abnormalities.

Leukemia, Risk Factors

Ionizing radiation
Oncogenic viruses
Chemical agents (e.g., benzene compounds)
Genetic disorders (e.g., trisomy 21, Fanconi's syndrome, Bloom's syndrome, ataxia-telangiectasia)
Advanced maternal age

HEMATOL

[14]Hess JL, Zutter MM, Castleberry RP, Emanuel PD. Juvenile chronic myelogenous leukemia. *Am J Clin Pathol* 1996;105:238.

Leukemias, Nonlymphocytic, Acute[15,16]

♦ French-American-British (FAB) Classification

Has 85% concordance. Based on morphology and cytochemistry. Advances in
immunophenotyping and cytogenetics provide additional essential information.
M-1, M-2, M-3 leukemias are predominantly granulocytic.

M-0 Acute Myelogenous Leukemia

Incidence: ~5% of AML cases
≥ 30% blasts
Minimal differentiation.

M-1 Acute Myeloid Leukemia with Minimal Maturation

Incidence: 20% of AML cases
>90% of nonerythroid nucleated cells are blasts, predominantly type 1.
<10% of nonerythroid nucleated cells are of maturing granulocytic lineage. Occasional
Auer rods may be present

M-2 Acute Nonlymphocytic Leukemia with t(8;21)

Incidence: 30% of AML cases
Patient age: young (mean = 28 yrs)
Clinical findings: splenomegaly in 28%; chloromas, especially of face area, in 20%
Morphology: myeloblasts often with Auer rods (90%) are heterogeneous, hypogranular, and frequently show pseudo-Pelger-Huët abnormalities. Sum of type I and II
blast cells is 30–89% of nonerythroid cells (differs from M-1 in which the sum of
type I and II blast cells is >90% of nonerythroid cells and ≥ 3% of these are peroxidase or Sudan black positive); monocytic cells are <20%; granulocytes from
promyelocytes to polynuclear types are >10%. Maturation toward granulocytes is
often abnormal; eosinophil precursors are frequently increased and may contain
Auer rods.
Histochemistry: cells contain granulocyte but not monocyte enzymes; Sudan black and
myeloperoxidase is abnormal (punctate rather than diffuse).
Karyotype: t(8;21)(q22;q22); critical region 21q translocated to 8q; frequent loss of
sex chromosome. Increased predilection for this leukemia in Down syndrome (trisomy 21).
Oncogenes: c-*ets*-2 translocates from 21q to 8q but expression data for the gene are
unknown; c-*mos* remains at 8q and c-*myc* translocates to 21q but both are probably
not important.
Prognosis: 75–85% complete remission rate after chemotherapy but median survival
(9.5 mos) is of average duration.

M-3 Acute Promyelocytic Leukemia

Incidence: 10% of AML cases
Patient age: median of 31 yrs
Clinical findings: typically present with bleeding diathesis; ≤ 47% die of early fatal hemorrhage. DIC in ≤ 80% of cases.
Morphology: <30% blasts in most cases. Predominantly neoplastic promyelocytes with
coarse azurophilic granules and multiple Auer rods; a variant (**M-3V** is ~30% of M-3
cases) shows hypo/microgranular promyelocytes on electron microscopy. Leukemic
cell count in peripheral blood is usually not high (5000–15,000/cu mm).
Unusual feature: blast cells occasionally can be induced to differentiate into mature
granulocytes or macrophages by various agents.
Karyotype: t(15;17)(q22;q12) occurs frequently.
Oncogene: none known

M-4 Acute Myelomonocytic Leukemia

Incidence: 25% of AML cases
Marrow morphology: ≥ 30% of nonerythroid nucleated cells are myelomonocytic blasts;
2–80% of these are of granulocytic lineage and 20–80% are of monocytic lineage.
Peripheral blood typically shows myelomonocytic blasts and >500/cu mm monocytes;
serum lysozyme is often elevated.

[15]Koeffler HP. Syndromes of acute nonlymphocytic leukemia. *Ann Intern Med* 1987;107:748.
[16]Lauglin WR, Bick RL. Acute leukemias: FAB classification and clinical correlates. *Lab Med*
1994;25:11.

- A variant (**M-4Eo**) shows 1–30% abnormal eosinophils (precursors).

Histochemistry: very weak staining for nonspecific esterase; can be distinguished from granulocytic types by monoclonal antibodies demonstrating specific antigens.

Karyotype: almost all patients show inversion of chromosome 16 [inv(16)(p13;q22)]; <10% show balanced translocation between short arm of one chromosome 16 and long arm of other chromosome 16 [t(16;16)(p13.1;q22)].

Oncogene: unknown

Molecular oncology: disruption of metallothionein genes by the chromosomal abnormality

Prognosis: 70–90% complete remission rate, probably with prolonged median duration (>18 mos). More than one-third have relapse in CNS including myeloblastomas (compared with 5% of all patients with acute nonlymphocytic leukemia, who rarely show CNS myeloblastomas).

M-5 Acute Monocytic Leukemia with t(9;11)

Incidence: 10% of acute monoblastic leukemia patients

Patient age: often children and young adults

Clinical findings: leukemic cells may infiltrate skin or gums; serum lysozyme is often elevated.

Morphology: >30% of nonerythroid nucleated cells are blasts; >80% are of monocytic lineage. Can be distinguished from granulocytic types by monoclonal antibodies demonstrating specific antigens.

M-5a: poorly differentiated variant is 4% of AML cases; >80% of monocytic cells are blasts.

M-5b: well-differentiated variant is 6% of AML cases; <80% of monocytic cells are blasts.

Karyotype: t(9;11)(p22;q23)

Oncogene: c-*ets*-1 translocated to 9p22 in region of interferon-alpha gene; expression data not known.

M-6 Erythroleukemia

Incidence: 6% of AML cases

Marrow morphology: ≥ 50% of all nucleated cells are erythroblasts. ≥ 30% of nonerythroid nucleated cells are myeloblast cells (if <30%, the diagnosis is myelodysplastic syndrome). Erythroid hyperplasia and marked dyserythropoiesis (e.g., megaloblasts, ringed sideroblasts, Howell-Jolly bodies) are common.

Nucleated RBCs in peripheral blood smear and anemia are common.

Immunologic abnormalities are more frequent in this form, e.g., positive Coombs' test, ANA, positive RF, increased serum gamma globulins, hemolytic anemia.

M-7 Acute Megakaryocytic Leukemia

Incidence: 1% of AML cases

Marrow morphology: myelofibrosis present in almost all patients; 20–40% present with acute myelofibrosis, making blast count impossible. Blast cells are highly polymorphic and are often classified as undifferentiated. Myeloblasts and megakaryoblasts are ≥ 30% of all cells. Increased numbers of maturing megakaryocytes may be present. Megakaryocyte fragments and micromegakaryocytes and blasts are frequently present in peripheral blood.

Histochemistry: no myeloperoxidase or nonspecific esterase reaction. Unlike all other FAB subtypes, diagnosis is based on electron microscope identification of platelet peroxidase or on specific monoclonal antibodies to megakaryocyte antigens.

Karyotype: abnormalities of chromosome 21 have been reported but specificity is still uncertain.

High serum LD

Prognosis: preliminary reports of poor response to conventional anthracycline-cytarabine–based therapy

M-0 Acute Myeloid Leukemia without Differentiation

Blasts do not fulfill FAB morphologic and cytochemical classification criteria. Not included in current FAB classification.

Acute Undifferentiated Leukemia

No evidence of either myeloid or lymphoid lineage. <1% of all acute leukemia cases. Not included in current FAB classification.

Acute Mixed-Lineage Leukemia

Myeloid and lymphoid lineages in same clone. 5–10% of all acute leukemia cases. 5–10% of acute leukemias convert from one lineage to another. Not included in current FAB classification.

Therapy-Related Leukemia

Clinical findings: >70% have a preleukemic phase lasting ~11 mos; occurs several years (median = 4 yrs) after chemotherapy (most frequently with an alkylating agent, especially melphalan, chlorambucil, or cyclophosphamide) or radiation for another disease such as Hodgkin's disease (by comparison, ~20% of all acute nonlymphocytic leukemias have a preleukemic phase). Risk is 3–10% 10 yrs after therapy but may be greater after age 40. Highest risk after combined radiation and alkylating therapy; develop AML. Risk of 5–20× after exposure to nontherapeutic compounds (e.g., benzene). Unexplained pancytopenia; infection and hemorrhage.

Karyotype: >75% show deletion of chromosome 5/5q– and/or 7/7q–.

Prognosis: shorter survival compared to de novo leukemias; often refractory to therapy.

Leukemias and Lymphomas, Diagnostic Methods

♦ Based on combination of
  • Microscopic examination of blood, bone marrow and/or lymph nodes
  • Cytochemical and immunohistochemical staining
  • Immunophenotyping by flow cytometry
  • Cytogenetics
  • Molecular analysis
  • Clinical features

Chromosome Abnormalities

See Table 11-20.

At initial diagnosis, routine cytogenetic studies show chromosomal abnormality in >50% of cases.

Acute nonlymphocytic leukemia	54%
Acute lymphocytic leukemia	41%
Chronic granulocytic leukemia	94%
Myelodysplastic syndrome	39%
Lymphoma	71%

Cytogenetic studies show structural abnormalities including translocations, deletions, isochromosomes, inversions, duplications, and numeric anomalies (e.g., trisomies, monosomies). In contrast, molecular tests may detect only one or a few specific translocations.

If an abnormal chromosome clone is not observed, the analysis should be considered nondiagnostic.[17]

Risk assessment in ALL patients
  • Of children <1 yr old for whom prognosis is poor, 70–80% have MLL gene rearrangements. In adolescents and adult patients, high frequency of MLL rearrangements and bcr-abl fusion is associated with poor prognosis.
  • Favorable genetic abnormalities are hyperdiploidy (>50 chromosomes/cell), which is also associated with low WBC count, and ETV6-CBFA2 (TEL-AML1) fusion, which manifests mainly at age 1–9 yrs.
  • Markedly hypodiploid or near-haploid leukemic cells usually indicate poor prognosis regardless of age of WBC count.
  • Leukemic cells with bcr-abl fusion usually indicates high-risk.

Leukemia/Lymphoma Syndrome, Adult Human T Cell

(Recently described syndrome found chiefly in black men in United States and elsewhere with acute onset, aggressive clinical course)
♦ Increased antibody titers to HTLV-I. In Japan, ~25% of healthy persons are antibody positive.

---

[17]Dewald GW, et al. Chromosome abnormalities in malignant hematologic disorders. *Mayo Clin Proc* 1985;60:675.

Table 11-20. Chromosomal Translocations in Hematologic Malignancies

Hematologic Disorder	Chromosomal Translocation	Gene Rearrangement (Break Points)	Clinical Utility
CML	Ph[1] t(9;22) and variants	BCR/ABL (bcr break point)	D, P, M
B-cell ALL	Ph[1] t(9;22)	BCR/ABL (bcr and BCR break points)	D, P, M
	t(8;14), t(2; 8)	IgH, Ig kappa, Ig lambda, and MYC	D, M
	t(8;22)		
	t(1;19)	PBX/TCF (E2A)	D, P
	t(4;11), t(11;19) and variants	MLL/different loci	D, P
	t(5;14)	IL3/IgH	Being evaluated
T-cell ALL	t(1;14) and variants	TAL1/TCRdelta, alpha, SIL	D
B- or T-cell ALL	t(7q35), t(14q11), t(14q32)	Antigen receptor genes	D
AML-M2	t(8;21)	AML1/ETO	D, P, M
AML-M3	t(15;17)	PML/RARA	D, P, M
AML-M4 Eo	inv(16), t(16;16)	CBFB/MYHII	D, P
AML-M5	t(11q23), various partner chromosomes	MLL/different loci	D, P
AML with basophilia	t(6;9)	DEK/CAN	D, P
AML with thrombo-cytosis	t(3;3), inv (3)	EVII/?	P
Follicular, and subsets of diffuse lymphomas	t(14;18)	BCL-2/IgH	D, M
Burkitt's lymphoma	t(8;14), t(2;8), t(8;22)	IgH, Ig kappa, Ig lambda, and MYC	D, M
Mantle zone lymphoma, rare CLL cases	t(11;14)	BCL-1 (cyclin D or PRAD1)/IgH	D, M

D = diagnosis; M = monitor therapy; P = prognosis.
Source: Crisan D. Molecular diagnostics in hematology. *Advance/Laboratory* Nov 1997:45–48. Adapted from Crissan D, et al. Hematology. *Oncol Clin North Am* 1994;8(9):725–750.

♦ Leukemic phase with WBC count ≤ 190,000/cu mm, large or mixed small and large cell immunoblastic types, typical "flower" cells with indented nuclei; infrequent anemia and thrombocytopenia.
   • Bone marrow involvement in 50% of patients, correlates poorly with extent of peripheral blood involvement.
♦ Hypercalcemia in ~75% of patients is characteristic; may occur without bone involvement. May be very high.
♦ Biopsy shows lymphomatous involvement of affected sites (e.g., lymph nodes, liver, spleen, bone, skin, etc).
♦ HTLV-I can be isolated from malignant lymphoma or leukemia cells.
Laboratory findings due to involvement of various organs or systems (e.g., liver, CNS).

HEMATOL

Marked immunosuppression with opportunistic infections (e.g., cryptococcal meningitis, *P. carinii* pneumonia)

Lymphadenopathy, Angioimmunoblastic

(Rare lymphoproliferative disorder arising from mature postthymic T lymphocytes with sudden onset of constitutional symptoms and lymphadenopathy; very poor prognosis)
♦ Diagnosis requires a lymph node biopsy, which shows characteristic changes, but these alone do not permit diagnosis and the clinical findings are required.
Nonspecific polyclonal hypergammaglobulinemia in 75% of cases.
Coombs-positive hemolytic anemia in 50% of cases.
Leukocytosis with lymphopenia
Thrombocytopenia
High frequency of autoantibodies and often associated with other autoimmune syndromes, especially SLE.
Death usually due to infection associated with T-cell immune deficiency (e.g., CMV, EBV, HSV, *P. carinii*, mycobacteria, opportunistic fungi).
Lymphomas (B- or T-cell type or rarely Hodgkin's disease) develop in 5–20% of cases.
Serologic tests for HIV are negative.

Lymphocytosis (Infectious), Acute

Markedly increased WBC ($\geq$ 40,000/cu mm) is due to lymphocytosis (normal appearing, small-sized lymphocytes).
Heterophil agglutination is negative.

Lymphoma, Cutaneous T-Cell

(Derived from postthymic T helper cells)

Sézary Syndrome

♦ Syndrome of skin lesions due to infiltration of Sézary cells associated with presence of these cells in peripheral blood
♦ Increased peripheral blood lymphocyte count, >15% of which are atypical lymphocytes (Sézary cells)
Total WBC often increased.
ESR, Hb, and platelet counts usually normal.
Bone marrow, lymph nodes, and liver biopsy usually normal.

Mycosis Fungoides

♦ Biopsy of lesion (usually skin) shows microscopic findings that parallel clinical findings. Repeated periodic biopsies may be needed before diagnosis is established.
Laboratory findings are generally not helpful.
Bone marrow may show increase in RE cells, monoblasts, lymphocytes, plasma cells.
Peripheral blood may occasionally show increased eosinophils, monocytes, and lymphocytes.
♦ Mycosis fungoides cells in peripheral blood or marrow suggest extensive disease.
Laboratory findings due to involvement of virtually any other organ.

Lymphoproliferative (Autoimmune) Syndrome[18]

(Recently defined inherited disorder arising in early childhood that includes massive persistent lymphadenopathy, splenomegaly, and autoimmune features due to failure of apoptosis of lymphocytes)
♦ Absolute increase of B-cell and T-cell counts with polyclonal expansion of T cells, 25% of which are double negative.
♦ Autoimmune disease.

[18]Straus SE, et al. An inherited disorder of lymphocyte apoptosis: the autoimmune lymphoproliferative syndrome. *Ann Intern Med* 1999;130:591.

- Hemolytic anemia
- ITP
- Autoimmune neutropenia
- Polyclonal hypergammaglobulinemia
- Others (e.g., GN, primary biliary cirrhosis, Guillain-Barré syndrome)
♦ Circulating autoantibodies.
- Positive direct Coombs' test
- Anticardiolipin antibody
- Others (e.g., ANA, RF)
♦ Biopsy of lymph nodes or spleen shows characteristic benign lymphoid hyperplasia and plasmacytosis.
Marked increase in plasma interleukin-10 values
Laboratory changes due to infection after splenectomy for hypersplenism

Macroglobulinemia (Primary; Waldenström's)

(Due to monoclonal proliferation of plasmacytoid lymphocytes and lymphocytoid plasma cells of B-cell origin producing an IgM M protein)
♦ Electrophoresis/immunofixation of serum shows an intense sharp peak in globulin fraction, usually in the gamma zone, identified as IgM by immunoelectrophoresis (75% are kappa). The pattern may be indistinguishable from that in multiple myeloma. IgM protein ≥ 3.0 gm/dL. Associated decrease in normal immunoglobulins.
♦ Total serum protein and globulin are markedly increased.
○ ESR is very high.
○ Rouleaux formation is marked; positive Coombs' reaction; difficulty in cross-matching blood.
○ Severe anemia, usually normochromic normocytic; usually due to hemodilution, occasionally hemolytic. Increased plasma volume may contribute an artifactual component.
WBC is decreased, with relative lymphocytosis but no evidence of lymphocytic leukemia; monocytes or eosinophils may be increased.
♦ Bone marrow biopsy is always hypercellular and shows >30% involvement by pleomorphic infiltrate with atypical "lymphocytes" and also plasma cells. Increased number of mast cells. Similar spleen and liver involvement occurs in ~50% of patients. Marrow aspirate is often hypocellular.
♦ Lymph node may show malignant lymphoma, usually well-differentiated lymphocytic lymphoma with plasmacytoid features.
○ Flow cytometry shows that ≤ 50% of patients have circulating monoclonal B lymphocyte population.
○ 50% of patients with Waldenström's macroglobulinemia have hyperviscosity syndrome due to coagulation abnormalities caused by large IgM molecule. (Normal serum viscosity = ≤ 1.8 centipoise.) Causes persistent oronasal hemorrhage in ~75% of patients, neurologic and visual disturbances, hypervolemia, and congestive heart failure.
IgM may also cause cryoglobulinemia.
Bence Jones proteinuria is found in 10% of cases. Monoclonal light chain in 70–80% of cases.
Coagulation abnormalities: There may be decreased platelets and abnormal BT, coagulation time, PT, prothrombin consumption, etc.
Serum uric acid may be increased.
Impaired renal function is much less common than in myeloma.
Amyloidosis is rare.
♦ *Differs from multiple myeloma by absence of lytic bone lesions and of hypercalcemia. Macroglobulinemia may also be associated with neoplasms, collagen diseases, cirrhosis, chronic infections.*

Marrow Transplantation, Complications

Acute graft-versus-host disease develops in 25–30% of recipients and is fatal in 8%.
Chronic graft-versus-host disease develops in 20–30% of patients who survive >6 mos.
Most infections occur within 6 mos. Interstitial pneumonia occurs in 16% of those conditioned by cyclophosphamide and up to 50% of those conditioned with whole-body irradiation; mortality is 40–50%; one-half of cases are due to CMV and one-half are of unknown cause.

May-Hegglin Anomaly

(Rare autosomal dominant abnormality of WBCs and platelets)

♦ Large, poorly granulated platelets are associated with large abnormal Döhle's bodies in cytoplasm of most granulocytes and all neutrophils in absence of infection. (Döhle's bodies may also be found in neutrophilic response to infection.) In absence of infection, these Döhle's bodies are pathognomonic.

♦ Diagnosis is confirmed by finding Döhle's bodies in a parent or sibling.

Variable thrombocytopenia with prolonged BT and impaired clot retraction. ~50% have abnormal bleeding.

Metaplasia, Agnogenic Myeloid (Idiopathic Myelofibrosis)

(Classified as a myeloproliferative stem cell disease stimulating marrow fibroblasts)

♦ Diagnostic Criteria

Bone marrow shows fibrosis without apparent cause. Repeated bone marrow aspirations often produce no marrow elements. Surgical biopsy of bone for histologic examination shows fibrosis of marrow that is usually hypocellular.

Normocytic anemia due to hemolysis and decreased production

Leukoerythroblastic peripheral blood (see Tumor of Bone Marrow, p. 445); tailed cells (dacryocytes) present.

Splenomegaly and osteosclerosis

♦ Peripheral smear shows characteristic anisocytosis and marked poikilocytosis with teardrop RBCs (dacryocytes), polychromatophilia, and occasional nucleated RBCs. Rarely seen in other hematologic conditions.

Reticulocyte count is increased (≤ 10%).

Hypersplenism may cause thrombocytopenia and leukopenia.

WBC may be normal (50% of patients) or increased (usually ≤ 30,000/cu mm), and abnormal forms may occur. Immature cells (≤ 15%) are usual. Basophils and eosinophils may be increased.

Platelets may be normal, increased, or decreased, and abnormal and large forms may occur. Deficient platelet aggregation after collagen or epinephrine may occur.

♦ Needle puncture of spleen and a lymph node shows extramedullary hematopoiesis involving all three cell lines.

Leukocyte ALP score is usually increased (in contrast to CML); may be marked.

Serum uric acid is often increased.

Prolonged PT is found in 75% of patients.

Serum vitamin B_{12} is often increased.

Some patients have trisomies of 8, 9, and 21 (appearance during treatment is a poor prognostic sign) but Ph^1 is rare.

Laboratory findings due to complications
• Hemorrhage
• Hemolytic anemia
• Infection
• DIC (occurs in 20% of patients)

Rule out other myeloproliferative diseases, especially CML. May arise with prior polycythemia vera.

Methemoglobinemia

(>1.5 gm/dL methemoglobin)

Due To

Most common is acquired form due to drugs and chemicals, especially aniline derivatives (e.g., acetanilid, phenacetin, certain sulfonamides, various clothing dyes), nitrites, nitrates, local anesthetics (e.g., benzocaine, lidocaine), antimalarials, dapsone.

Abnormal HbM (several different types)—autosomal dominant mutation in globin chains

Autosomal recessive deficiency of methemoglobin reductase

Laboratory Findings

Normal arterial oxygen saturation in presence of apparent clinical cyanosis that does not respond to oxygen administration suggests methemoglobin level >15%. 30–40% is associated with symptoms of anoxia; >50% indicates severe toxicity; >70% is often fatal.
♦ Freshly drawn blood is chocolate-brown; does not become red after exposure to air.
♦ Reduced nicotinamide adenine dinucleotide (NADH) diaphorase activity is decreased in congenital but normal in toxic states.
♦ Starch-block electrophoresis identifies the HbM.
♦ Spectroscopic absorption analysis—band at 630 μ disappears on addition of 5% potassium cyanide.
RBC count is slightly increased; no other hematologic abnormalities are found; no jaundice is present.
G-6-PD deficiency enhances HbM production.
Oxygen dissociation curve shifted to right, causing more oxygen delivery to tissues
Patient is cyanotic clinically but in apparent good health. (Clinical cyanosis >5.0 gm/dL deoxyhemoglobin.)
♦ In newborns with cyanosis, methemoglobin level is usually >10% and may reach 60–70% in severe cases. Persistent methemoglobinemia in spite of IV methylene blue (1–2 mg/kg) suggests abnormal HbM.
  • Recurrence of methemoglobinemia without reexposure to chemicals suggests inherited enzyme deficiency.
  • Cyanosis without dyspnea in previously pink infant suggests acquired methemoglobinemia due to chemicals, but cyanosis from birth suggests inherited enzyme deficiency or abnormal HbM.
  • HbM causes cyanosis from birth only if it is alpha-chain type; cyanosis of beta-chain type appears at age 2–4 mos.

Monoclonal Gammopathies, Classification

(Clonal disorders of atypical cells of RE system. Each is a homogeneous product of a single clone of proliferating cells and is expressed as a monoclonal gammopathy.)
Monoclonal proteins consist of two heavy polypeptide chains of the same class (e.g., gamma, alpha, mu) and subclass, and two light polypeptide chains of the same type (either kappa or lambda); may be present in serum, urine, and CSF. Heavy-chain disease is production of only heavy chains without accompanying light chains; light-chain disease is the reverse. Identified by protein electrophoresis, immunoelectrophoresis, immunofixation.
Idiopathic monoclonal gammopathy of unknown significance
  • Benign (IgG, IgA, IgD, IgM; rarely free light chains).
  • Associated with neoplasms of cells now known to produce M proteins.
  • Biclonal gammopathies.
  • Only two-thirds of patients with monoclonal gammopathy are symptomatic.
Malignant
  • Multiple myeloma (IgG, IgA, IgD, and Bence Jones gammopathies are associated with classic picture)
       Symptomatic
       Smoldering (asymptomatic and indolent)
       Plasma cell leukemia
       Nonsecretory
       Osteosclerotic
  • Plasmacytoma
       Solitary of bone
       Extramedullary
  • Malignant lymphoproliferative diseases
       Waldenström's macroglobulinemia
       Malignant lymphoma
  • Heavy-chain diseases
  Gamma
  Alpha
  Mu
  Delta (very rare)

HEMATOL

Table 11-21. Comparison of Multiple Myeloma and Monoclonal Gammopathy of Unknown Significance (MGUS)

	Multiple Myeloma	MGUS
Paraprotein level	Higher	Lower (rarely <3 gm/dL)
Nonparaprotein immunoglobulins suppressed	96% of cases	12% of cases
Bence Jones proteinuria	57% of cases	17% of cases
Bone marrow plasmacytosis >20%	100% of cases	4% of cases
Plasma cell labeling index (using monoclonal antibody to 5-bromo-2-deoxyuridine)	>1%	<1%
Anemia, osteolytic bone changes	Present	Absent
Progression	Yes	No

- Amyloidosis
  - Secondary to multiple myeloma (no monoclonal protein in other secondary types)
  - Primary
- Unknown significance
  - Idiopathic
  - Others (e.g., ~10% of patients with chronic HCV liver disease)

Monoclonal Gammopathy, Idiopathic ("Benign," "Asymptomatic") (Plasma Cell Dyscrasia of Unknown Significance; Monoclonal Gammopathy of Unknown Significance)[19]

(Found in 0.5% of healthy persons >30 yrs, 3% >70 yrs, and ≤10% at 80 yrs)
See Table 11-21.

♦ The following changes are present for a period of >5 yrs.
- Monoclonal serum protein concentration usually <3 gm/dL and does not increase during follow-up; IgG type in 73% of patients, IgM in 14%, IgA in 11%, biclonal in 2%; normal immunoglobulins may be depressed. In contrast, multiple myeloma *always* shows depression of background immunoglobulins and higher monoclonal serum protein (>3 gm/dL).
- Normal serum albumin.
- Usually <10% plasma cells in bone marrow.
- Absence of Bence Jones protein (or <50 mg/day), anemia, myeloma bone lesions, lymphoproliferative disease, hypercalcemia, renal insufficiency.
- Monoclonal light-chain proteinuria may occur (up to 1 gm/24 hrs).
- May be associated with aging, cholecystitis, neoplasms, many chronic diseases (most often RA) and infections (e.g., TB).

♦ Periodic reexamination is essential because many patients develop myeloma (16%), macroglobulinemia (3%), or primary amyloidosis (3%) within 5 yrs and 25% at 10 yrs; lymphoproliferative disorders develop in 17% at 10 yrs, and 33% of patients at 20 yrs; no definite predictive factors permit recognition of this group, but more likely to become malignant if the following criteria are present and converse if these criteria are absent:
- IgG >200 mg/dL, or either IgA or IgM >100 mg/dL or IgD or IgE paraprotein is found at any concentration.
- Immunoglobulin fragments in urine (usually Bence Jones protein) or serum.
- Progressive increase in paraprotein concentration.
- Low levels of polyclonal immunoglobulin.

One study[20] in a general hospital showed the following:
- Paraproteinemia by electrophoresis was found in 730 of 102,000 samples (0.7%).

---

[19]Kyle RA. Benign monoclonal gammopathy—after 20–35 years of follow-up. *Mayo Clin Proc* 1993;68:26.

[20]Malacrida V, et al. Laboratory investigation of monoclonal gammopathy during 10 years of screening in a general hospital. *J Clin Pathol* 1987;40:793.

375 had paraprotein $\geq$ 200 mg/dL (2 g/L)
    114 of these were B lymphocytic malignancy
        96—multiple myeloma
          4—Waldenström's macroglobulinemia
          8—chronic lymphatic leukemia
          6—non-Hodgkin's lymphoma
    261 were monoclonal gammopathy of undefined significance
~50 of post–progenitor cell transplant patients for $\leq$ 2 yrs; usually low-level IgG

Myelodysplastic (Preleukemic) Syndromes

♦ Clonal proliferative disorders of bone marrow that show peripheral blood cytopenias and dysmyelopoiesis; 30–40% of cases progress to acute nonlymphocytic leukemia, 60–80% of patients die of complications (e.g., acute infection, hemorrhage) or associated diseases, 10–20% remain stable and die of unrelated causes. No detectable cause, but prior chemotherapy (especially with alkylating agents) or radiation in some. Partial or complete loss of chromosome 5 and/or 7 and trisomy 8 are very common.

French-American-British (FAB) Classification

♦ Refractory anemia
  • Persistent anemia refractory to treatment with vitamin B_{12}, folate, or pyridoxine, with decreased reticulocytes, variable dyserythropoiesis. Anemia may be macrocytic, normocytic, or dimorphic with hypochromasia with changes in size and shape of RBCs.
  • <1% blasts in peripheral blood.
  • <5% blasts in marrow.
  • <15% ringed sideroblasts in marrow (bone marrow normoblasts).
  • Hypercellular marrow with erythroid hyperplasia and/or dyserythropoiesis.
  • Normal megakaryocytes and granulocytes.
  • Dysgranulopoiesis is infrequent.
  • 5% of patients present with these findings but without anemia.
♦ Refractory anemia with ringed sideroblasts (same as acquired idiopathic sideroblastic anemia)
  • Refractory anemia (see previous section); bimorphic RBCs—oval macrocytes and hypochromic microcytes; many siderocytes
  • >15% ringed sideroblasts
  • <1% blasts in peripheral blood
  • <5% blasts in marrow
  • >10% develop acute myelocytic leukemia
♦ Refractory anemia with excess blasts (poor prognosis; usually progresses to acute leukemia within a year)
  • Cytopenia affecting $\geq$ 2 cell lines
  • <5% blasts in peripheral blood and 5–20% blasts in marrow; granulocytic maturation is present; <1% marrow sideroblasts
  • Variably cellular marrow with granulocytic or erythroid hyperplasia
  • Dysgranulopoiesis, dyserythropoiesis, and/or dysmegakaryocytopoiesis
♦ Refractory anemia with excess blasts in transformation (from myelodysplasia to overt acute nonlymphocytic leukemia)
  • >5% blasts in peripheral blood and/or 20–30% blasts in marrow (>30% blasts constitutes acute nonlymphocytic leukemia).
  • <1% marrow sideroblasts.
  • Auer rods present in myeloid precursors.
  • Does not fit into FAB M1–M7 categories (see p. 410).
  • 75% develop acute myelocytic leukemia.
♦ Chronic myelomonocytic leukemia
  • Same as refractory anemia with excess blasts but with >100 monocytes/μL in peripheral blood.
  • Neutrophilia; mature granulocytes may be increased.
  • <5% blasts in peripheral blood and usually 5–20% blasts in marrow.
  • <1% marrow sideroblasts.
  • Increased monocyte precursors in marrow (may need special stains).

HEMATOL

Abnormal and asynchronous maturation of different cell series is defined as:
♦ • Dyserythropoiesis
   Anisocytosis, poikilocytosis, oval macrocytes, nucleated RBCs, and normochromia are most common changes in RBCs on peripheral smear. RBC population may be dimorphic.
   Erythroid maturation defects with bizarre (e.g., multinucleated) forms and megaloblastic features unresponsive to folic acid, vitamin B_{12}, and iron.
♦ • Dysgranulomonopoiesis
   Increased or decreased numbers or abnormal nuclei or granulation in blood, acquired Pelger-Huët anomaly.
   Variable increase in mature granulocyte precursors (usually myelocytes) and monocytosis occur frequently in marrow.
   ♦ • Dysmegakaryocytopoiesis.
   Increased or decreased number.
   Atypical, bizarre, or giant platelets, often with giant abnormal granules, are seen in most cases. Marrow megakaryocytes are often atypical or bizarre.
   Platelet function defects with prolonged BT and aggregation abnormalities are very common.
   Other clinicopathologic forms include refractory anemias of various types, pure red cell aplasia, paroxysmal nocturnal hemoglobinuria, chronic idiopathic neutropenia, chronic idiopathic thrombocytopenia, etc.
Low granulocyte or platelet count or elevated bone marrow blast count are independent indicators of poor outcome. 5q– karyotype is often found in refractory anemia and carries a relatively good prognosis. Monosomy 7 and trisomy 8 are frequently found in other subclasses of myelodysplasia and are associated with poor prognosis.
Poor prognosis is indicated by (in decreasing order of importance) >5% blasts in marrow, circulating blasts, abnormal karyotypes, granulocytopenia (<1000/cu mL), monocytopenia, thrombocytopenia (<140,000/cu mL), ineffective erythropoiesis, presenting Hb of <9.0 gm/dL, hemolysis, <20% ringed sideroblasts in marrow, abnormal localization of blasts in center of marrow rather than in subendostial areas, circulating CD34+ cells.

Myeloma, Multiple

See Tables 11-22, 11-23, and 11-24.

♦ Diagnostic Criteria

Bone marrow shows sheets or >20% plasma cells **and**
Abnormality of immunoglobulin formation (monoclonal spike >4 gm/dL or Bence Jones proteinuria >0.5 gm/24 hrs)
   • If monoclonal spike is <4 gm/dL, then substitute criteria:
      Reciprocal depression of normal immunoglobulins or
      Panhypogammaglobulinemia and osteolytic bone lesions or
      Plasmacytosis not due to other causes (see Plasma Cells, p. 352)

Very increased serum total protein is due to increase in globulins (with decreased albumin/globulin ratio [A/G]) in one-half to two-thirds of the patients.
Serum protein immunoelectrophoresis or immunofixation characterizes protein as monoclonal (i.e., one light-chain type) and classifies disease by identifying specific heavy chain. It reveals abnormal immunoglobulins in 80% of patients. A serum or urine monoclonal paraprotein can be identified in ≤ 99% of patients with multiple myeloma.

Percent of Patients	Immunoelectrophoresis or Immunofixation Shows
≤99%	Monoclonal protein in serum or urine
90%	Serum monoclonal spike
20%	Both serum and urine monoclonal protein
20%	Monoclonal light chains in urine only
<2%	Hypogammaglobulinemia only without serum or urine paraprotein
60%	IgG myeloma protein
20%	IgA myeloma protein

Table 11-22. Comparison of Diseases with Monoclonal Immunoglobulins

	Multiple Myeloma	Macroglobulinemia	Benign Monoclonal Gammopathy	Heavy-Chain Diseases		
				Gamma	Alpha	Mu
Clinical	Bone lesions Anemia Infections	Enlarged LNN, L, S	None	Enlarged LNN, L, S	Intestinal malabsorption	Enlarged LNN, L, S
Bone marrow	Sheets of plasma cells	Lymphocytosis or lymphocytoid plasma cells	Up to 10% plasma cells	Plasma cells or lymphocytoid plasma cells	—	Lymphocytosis or lymphocytoid plasma cells with vacuoles
Monoclonal Ig in serum (electrophoresis)	80%	Present	Present	Present	Present	Present
Bence Jones protein in urine (electrophoresis)	70–80%	80–95%	Rare	Common	Rare	Common
Serum (immunoelectrophoresis)	1 type of M chain[a] 1 type of L chain[b]	Mu chain 1 type of L chain[a]	1 type of M chain[a] 1 type of L chain[b]	Gamma chain No L	Alpha chain No L	Mu chain Free kappa or lambda in two-thirds
Urine (immunoelectrophoresis)	Kappa or lambda	Kappa or lambda	Rare kappa or lambda	Gamma chain	—	Kappa or lambda in two-thirds

Ig = immunoglobulin; LNN = lymph nodes; L = liver; S = spleen.
[a]M chain is gamma, alpha, mu, delta, or epsilon.
[b]L chain is kappa or lambda.
Paraproteinemia is due to monoclonal gammopathy of unknown significance (63%), multiple myeloma (14%), primary amyloidosis (9%), indolent non-Hodgkin's lymphoma (5%), extramedullary or solitary bone plasmacytoma (4%), chronic lymphocytic leukemia (3%), Waldenström's macroglobulinemia (2%).

Table 11-23. Immunochemical Frequency of Monoclonal Gammopathies

IgG (with/without BJ)	60%
IgA (with/without BJ)	15%
IgM (with/without BJ)	10–15%
Light chain (BJ only)	15%
Rare	
IgD (with/without BJ)	1%
Heavy chain	1%
Gamma heavy-chain disease	
Alpha heavy-chain disease	
Mu heavy-chain disease	
IgE (with/without BJ)	0.1%
Biclonal (IgG + IgM)	
Triclonal	

Ig = immunoglobulin.

10%	Light chain only (Bence Jones proteinemia)
Very rare	IgE myeloma protein
<1%	IgD myeloma protein*

*IgD myeloma is difficult to recognize because serum levels are relatively low, specific antiserum is required to demonstrate IgD; on electrophoresis, IgD is often included in beta globulin peak, and clinical features are the same as in other types of myeloma. Bence Jones proteinuria is almost always present, and total protein is often normal.

♦ Bence Jones proteinuria occurs in 35–50% of patients. >50% of IgG or IgA myeloma and 100% of light-chain myelomas have Bence Jones proteinuria.
 • Dipstick tests for urine protein will miss Bence Jones protein, and heat precipitation is not a reliable test.
♦ Electrophoresis/immunofixation of both serum and urine is abnormal in almost all patients. If only serum electrophoresis is performed, kappa and some lambda light-chain myelomas will be missed. 10% of patients have hypogammaglobulinemia (<0.6 gm/dL). Free immunoglobulin light chains are rapidly filtered by glomerulus and found only in urine. Intact monoclonal Ig is identified only in serum.
♦ Bone marrow aspiration usually shows 20–50% plasma cells or myeloma cells, usually in sheets; abnormal plasma cells may be found (flaming cells, morular cells, Mott cells, thesaurocytes); multiple sites may be required.
Hematologic findings
 • Anemia (normocytic, normochromic; rarely macrocytic) in 60% of patients.
 • Usually normal WBC and platelet count; 40–55% lymphocyte frequently present on differential count, with variable number of immature lymphocytic and plasmacytic forms. Decreased WBC and platelet counts are seen in ~20% of patients, usually with extensive marrow replacement. Eosinophilia may be found.
 ○ • Rouleaux formation (due to serum protein changes) in 85% of patients, occasionally causing difficulty in cross-matching blood.
 ○ • Increased ESR in 90% of patients and other abnormalities due to serum protein changes. May be normal in light-chain myeloma. >100/hr is rare in any condition other than myeloma.
 • Cold agglutinins or cryoglobulins.
○ Hyperviscosity syndrome is characteristic of IgM and occurs in 4% of IgG and 10% of IgA myelomas and may be the presenting feature. Symptoms are usually present when relative serum viscosity = 6–7 cP (normal = <1.8 cP).
○ Clinical amyloidosis occurs in 15% of cases of multiple myeloma, but monoclonal spikes are present in urine in most, if not all, cases of primary amyloidosis. IgD myeloma and light-chain disease are associated with amyloidosis and early renal failure more frequently than in other types of myeloma. Amyloidosis is indistinguishable from primary type (see p. 890).
Serum beta$_2$-microglobulin is increased in proliferative disorders in which rapid cell multiplication or increased tumor burden is present. >6 μg/mL indicates poor prognosis (normal = <2 μg/mL); may also be increased by renal failure.

Table 11-24. Comparison of Immunoproliferative Disorders

Disease	Relative Frequency (%)	Ig Heavy Chain	Ig Light Chain	Urine BJ (%)	Complications/Associated Conditions
Myelomas					
IgG	75	Gamma	Kappa or lambda	60	Infection
IgA	15	Alpha	Kappa or lambda	70	Infection
IgD	<1	Delta	Usually lambda	100	Amyloidosis
IgE	Very rare	Epsilon	Kappa or lambda	?	Plasma cell leukemia
Light-chain myeloma	10	None	Kappa or lambda	100	Amyloid kidney, hypercalcemia
Macroglobulinemia		Mu	Kappa or lambda	30–40	Hyperviscosity
					Hemolytic anemia (cold agglutinin)
					Bleeding
Heavy-chain disease					
Gamma			None	Gamma chain	GI tract lymphoma
Alpha			None	None	Malabsorption
					Amyloidosis
Mu			None	Kappa chain	Chronic lymphocytic leukemia
				BJ	

Ig = immunoglobulin.

HEMATOL

Chromosome analysis frequently shows translocation t(11;14)(q13;q32).

Laboratory findings of repeated bacterial infections, especially those due to *Streptococcus pneumoniae*, *S. aureus*, and *E. coli*.

See bone diseases of calcium and phosphorus, Table 13-6.

- Serum calcium is markedly increased in 25–50% of cases.
- Corrected calcium (mg/dL) = serum calcium (mg/dL) – serum albumin (gm/dL) + 4.0.
- Serum phosphorus is usually normal.
- Serum ALP is usually normal or slightly increased. Increase may reflect amyloidosis of liver or bone disease.
- Hypercalciuria causing dehydration and tubular dysfunction.

See Myeloma Kidney, p. 730.

○Presymptomatic phase (may last many years) may show only
- Unexplained persistent proteinuria
- Increased ESR
- Myeloma protein in serum or urine
- Repeated bacterial infections, especially pneumonias (6× greater incidence)
- Amyloidosis (see p. 890)

♦ High tumor mass (clinical stage III) is present when any of the following are present.
- Hb <8.5 gm/dL
- Corrected calcium >12 mg/dL
- Serum IgG >7 gm/dL
- Serum IgA >5 gm/dL
- Bence Jones proteinuria >12 gm/day
- Advanced lytic bone lesions

♦ Low tumor mass (stage I) is present when all of the following are present.
- Hb >10 gm/dL.
- Normal corrected calcium.
- Serum IgG <5 gm/dL.
- Serum IgA <3 gm/dL.
- Bence Jones proteinuria <4 gm/day.
- Generalized lytic bone lesions are absent.

Stage II has intermediate values

Subclassified as A if serum creatinine <2 mg/dL or B if >2 mg/dL

Survival varies from 61 mos for stage IA patients to 15 mos for stage IIIB patients.

Serial measurement of serum globulins and/or Bence Jones proteinuria are excellent indications of efficacy of chemotherapy; decrease in Bence Jones proteinuria occurs before decrease in abnormal serum globulin peak.

Lowered AG in IgG myeloma only (due to cationic IgG paraproteins causing retention of excess chloride ion)

Increased incidence of other neoplasms (not known if related to chemotherapy)
- Acute myelomonocytic leukemia, often preceded by sideroblastic refractory anemia, is increasingly seen.
- 20% of patients develop adenocarcinoma of GI tract, biliary tree, or breast.

Myeloma, Multiple, Smoldering

(~15% of multiple myeloma patients who are asymptomatic when diagnosed)

♦ Serum M protein >3 gm/dL; uninvolved immunoglobulins are decreased.

♦ Bone marrow shows >10% atypical plasma cells.

Plasma cell labeling index is very low.

Urine frequently contains a small amount of M protein.

No anemia, renal insufficiency, or bone lesions; condition remains stable.

Myeloma, Nonsecretory

♦ 1% of multiple myeloma patients in whom no M protein in serum, urine, or monoclonal protein can be identified in plasma cells by immunofluorescence or immunoperoxidase.

Myeloma, Osteosclerotic

♦ Diagnosis based on biopsy from single or multiple osteosclerotic bone lesions

Bone marrow aspiration shows <5% plasma cells

Lambda M protein is usually present.
Absence of anemia, hypercalcemia, renal insufficiency
Erythrocytosis and thrombocytosis may occur.
CNS protein is increased.
Syndrome of POEMS (*p*olyneuropathy, *o*rganomegaly, *e*ndocrinopathy, *M* protein, *s*kin pigmentation) is rare disorder.

Neutropenia, Periodic (Cyclic)

(Rare autosomal dominant condition)
♦ Regular periodic occurrence of neutropenia every 10–35 days, lasting 3–4 days. WBC is 2000–4000/cu mm, and granulocytes are as low as 0%.
Monocytosis may occur.
Eosinophilia may occur during recovery.
Bone marrow during episode may show hypoplasia or maturation arrest at myelocyte stage.

Neutrophilia, Hereditary Giant

(Very rare innocuous autosomal dominant anomaly)
♦ 1–2% of neutrophils are ~2× normal size and contain 6–10 nuclear lobes. In females drumstick appendages are often duplicated. No associated anomalies.
Acquired form may occur in myeloproliferative disease, AML, treatment with alkylating agents.

Neutrophils, Hereditary Hypersegmentation

(Harmless autosomal dominant condition)
♦ Hypersegmentation of neutrophils resembles that seen in PA but is a permanent abnormality. Most neutrophils have ≥ 4 lobes. ≥ 5 lobes in 10% of heterozygotes and 30% of homozygotes.
A similar condition exists that affects only the eosinophilic granulocytes (hereditary constitutional hypersegmentation of the eosinophil).
An inherited giant multilobed abnormality of neutrophilic leukocytes is also seen.
Hypersegmentation is also found in almost every patient with chronic renal disease with BUN >30 mg/dL for >3 mos.

Orotic Aciduria, Hereditary

(Very rare childhood disorder of pyrimidine metabolism due to a defect in the conversion of orotic acid to uridylic acid)
♦ Severe megaloblastic anemia refractory to vitamin B_{12} and folic acid but responsive to oral prednisone and yeast extract containing uridylic and cytidylic acids.
Marked anisocytosis.
Leukopenia is present with increased susceptibility to infection.
♦ Large amounts of orotic acid in urine; crystals precipitate when urine stands at room temperature.
♦ RBC orotidylic decarboxylase activity is decreased (<5.5 U).
Iatrogenic orotic aciduria occurs during cancer chemotherapy with 6-azauridine.

Pancytopenia

♦ Anemia *plus*
♦ Leukopenia—absolute myeloid decrease may be associated with relative lymphocytosis or with lymphocytopenia *plus*
♦ Thrombocytopenia
Laboratory findings due to causative disease

Due To

Hypersplenism
• Congestive splenomegaly

- Malignant lymphomas
- Histiocytoses
- Infectious diseases (TB, kala-azar, sarcoidosis)
- Primary splenic pancytopenia

Diseases of marrow
- Metastatic carcinoma
- Multiple myeloma
- Aleukemic leukemia
- Osteopetrosis
- Myelosclerosis, myelofibrosis, etc.
- Systemic mastocytosis

Aplastic anemias
- Physical and chemical causes (e.g., ionizing irradiation, benzol compounds)
- Idiopathic causes (familial or isolated; "isolated" accounts for 50% of all cases of pancytopenia)

Megaloblastic anemias (e.g., PA)

Paroxysmal nocturnal hemoglobinuria (rare)

Pelger-Huët Anomaly

(Autosomal dominant, usually heterozygous, anomaly of WBCs)

♦ Nuclei of >80% of granulocytes lack normal segmentation but are shaped like pince-nez eyeglasses, rods, dumbbells, or peanuts; present in peripheral blood and bone marrow. Coarse chromatin is evident in nuclei of granulocytes, lymphocytes, and monocytes and in marrow metamyelocytes and bands.

Sex chromatin body is not found in affected women.

Acquired Pelger-Huët anomaly is less predominant; may occur in acute and chronic myeloproliferative disorders (may be a premonitory feature) and may be transient in various acute infections, leukemoid reactions, and reactions to certain drugs (e.g., colchicine, sulfonamides, alkylating agents). Not found in acute and rarely in chronic lymphatic leukemias.

Plasmacytoma, Solitary

♦ Diagnosis is based on histologic finding of single tumor of plasma cells, which are identical to those of multiple myeloma. No criteria of multiple myeloma are present.

♦ Bone marrow shows no evidence of multiple myeloma.

♦ Radiographs and bone scans are negative for other myeloma bone lesions.

Myeloma proteins are at low or normal concentration in serum or concentrated urine by immunofixation.

Nonmyeloma immunoglobulin concentration in serum is generally normal.

Paraprotein is detectable in 80–90% of cases of solitary plasmacytoma of bone, often at very low concentrations. IgG kappa is most common; IgA and Bence Jones protein have been described.

Solitary plasmacytoma of bone is considered to represent the earliest stage of multiple myeloma, and 50–60% of cases progress to multiple myeloma within 5 yrs. 15% remain solitary; 12% develop local recurrence; 15% develop new distant lesions.

After local radiotherapy, level of any myeloma protein is reduced and level of non-myeloma immunoglobulins may be increased above normal. ~30% remain free of disease for >10 yrs; other patients develop multiple myeloma after median of 3 yrs.

CSF total protein, albumin, and IgG may be increased if a vertebral lesion extends into the spinal canal.

Extramedullary plasmacytoma may occur, chiefly (80%) in upper respiratory tract. ~20% of patients have low level monoclonal immunoglobulin (not IgM) in urine or serum. Diagnosis is based on histologic examination of tumor and same criteria as previous section. Development of multiple myeloma is infrequent.

Polycythemia, Factitious

♦ Normal oxygen saturation.

♦ Serum erythropoietin is low in autotransfusion but increased by exogenous erythropoietin.

Due To

Use of androgens by athletes to increase muscle mass and strength

Intentional by blood doping (athlete is phlebotomized and later transfused with own stored blood before competitive event to improve performance) or administration of erythropoietin

Polycythemia, Relative (Stress Erythrocytosis)

(Recent literature questions existence of this entity[21])

Relative polycythemia is not secondary to hypoxia but results from decreased plasma volume due to unknown mechanism or to decreased fluid intake and/or excess loss of body fluids (e.g., due to diuretics, dehydration, burns) with high normal RBC mass.

Increased RBC (usually <6 million/cu mm), Hb, and Hct

Normal WBC, platelet, and reticulocyte counts

Findings of secondary polycythemia (e.g., decreased oxygen saturation) are not present (see next section).

Serum erythropoietin is normal.

Leukocyte ALP score is normal or mildly increased.

Bone marrow shows normal cellularity and megakaryocyte count; no myelofibrosis; iron may be absent.

Hypercholesterolemia is frequent.

Laboratory findings due to complications (e.g., thromboembolism)

Polycythemia, Secondary

◯Diagnosis is suggested by erythrocytosis without increased WBC, platelets, or splenomegaly; causes listed below should be sought.

Hct is slightly increased.

Leukocyte ALP score is normal or slightly increased.

Increased plasma cholesterol is frequent.

Serum erythropoietin is usually increased or normal.

Due To

Physiologically Appropriate

Hypoxia with decreased arterial oxygen saturation

- Decreased atmospheric pressure (e.g., high altitudes).
- Chronic heart disease.
    Congenital (e.g., pulmonary stenosis, septal defect, patent ductus arteriosus)
    Acquired (e.g., chronic rheumatic mitral disease)
- Arteriovenous aneurysm.
- Impaired pulmonary ventilation.
- Alveolar-capillary block (e.g., Hamman-Rich syndrome, sarcoidosis, lymphangitic cancer).
- Alveolar hypoventilation (e.g., bronchial asthma, kyphoscoliosis).
- Restriction of pulmonary vascular bed (e.g., primary pulmonary hypertension, mitral stenosis, chronic pulmonary emboli, emphysema).
- Abnormal hemoglobin pigments (methemoglobinemia or sulfhemoglobinemia due to chemicals, such as aniline and coal tar derivatives) or high-oxygen-affinity hemoglobinopathies (50% of hemoglobinopathy cases show an abnormality on standard Hb electrophoresis). (*Hb oxygen affinity [P_{50}] is the oxygen tension at which Hb becomes 50% saturated. Normal = 27.5 mm Hg. Usually <20 mm Hg in these conditions. Decreased P_{50} indicates increased oxygen affinity and increased P_{50} indicates decreased oxygen affinity. May be increased by high-affinity hemoglobinopathies, carboxyhemoglobinemia, decreased RBC 2,3-diphosphoglycerate, alkalosis. May be decreased by hemoglobinopathies, increased RBC 2,3-diphosphoglycerate, acidosis.*) Carboxyhemoglobinemia ("smoker's erythrocytosis") can be detected by oximetry but not from P_{50}.

[21]Fairbanks VF, et al. Measurement of blood volume and red cell mass: re-examination of ^{51}Cr and ^{125}I methods. *Blood Cells Mol Dis* 1996;22:169.

HEMATOL

Tables 11-25. Comparison of Polycythemia Vera, Secondary Polycythemia, and Relative Polycythemia

Test	Polycythemia Vera	Secondary Polycythemia[a]	Relative Polycythemia[b]
Hct	I	I	I
Blood volume	I	I	D or N
Red cell mass	I	I	D or N
Plasma volume	I or N	N or I	D
Platelet count	I	N	N
WBC with shift to left	I	N	N
Nucleated RBC, abnormal RBC	I	N	N
Serum uric acid	I	I	N
Serum vitamin B$_{12}$	I	N	N
Leukocyte alkaline phosphatase	I	N	N
Oxygen saturation of arterial blood	N	D	N
Bone marrow	Hyperplasia of all elements	Erythroid hyperplasia	N
Erythropoietin level	D	I	N

D = decreased; I = increased; N = normal.
[a]Diagnosis of secondary polycythemia is suggested by erythrocytosis without increased WBC, platelets, or splenomegaly; causes should be sought.
[b]Relative polycythemia is not secondary to hypoxia but results from decreased plasma volume due to unknown mechanism or to decreased fluid intake and/or excess loss of body fluids (e.g., diuretics, dehydration, burns) with high normal RBC mass.

Physiologically Inappropriate

Increased erythropoietin secretion, e.g.,
- Associated with tumors and miscellaneous conditions (may be first sign of an occult curable tumor)
- Renal disease (hypernephroma, benign tumors, hydronephrosis, cysts, renal artery stenosis, long-term hemodialysis; occurs in up to 5% of renal cell carcinomas; occurs in ≤ 17% of kidney transplant recipients)
- Hemangioblastoma of cerebellum (occurs in 15–20% of cases)
- Uterine fibromyoma
- Hepatocellular carcinoma (5–10% of cases)
- Others

Increased androgen
- Pheochromocytoma
- Cushing's syndrome (adrenocortical hyperplasia or tumor)
- Masculinizing ovarian tumor (e.g., arrhenoblastoma)
- Factitious (use of androgens by athletes)

Polycythemia Vera

See Table 11-25 and Figs. 11-9 and 11-10.

♦ Criteria for Diagnosis[22]

A1 + A2 + A3; if A3 is absent, then two of four criteria from B must be present.
A1: Increased RBC mass (≥ 36 mL/kg in men; ≥ 32 mL/kg in women)
A2: Normal arterial oxygen saturation (≥ 92%)
A3: Splenomegaly (occurs in ~75% of cases)
B1: WBC >12,000/cu mm (occurs in ~60% of cases)

[22]Polycythemia Vera Study Group. Polycythemia vera. *Semin Hematol* 1976;12:13.

B2: Platelet count >400,000/cu mm (occurs in >60% of cases)

B3: Increased leukocyte ALP score (occurs in ~70% of cases) in absence of fever or infection

B4: Increased serum vitamin B_{12} (>900 pg/mL) (occurs in ~30% of cases) or B_{12}-binding capacity (>2200 pg/mL) (occurs in ~75% of cases)

False-positive rate ~0.5% due to combination of smokers' polycythemia (causing increased RBC mass) and alcoholic hepatitis (causing splenomegaly, increased B_{12}, WBC, leukocyte ALP).

False-negative may occur in patients with (1) recent bleeding, (2) concomitant decreased arterial oxygen saturation due to concomitant chronic lung disease, (3) early or minimal polycythemia vera, (4) increased RBC mass associated with increased plasma volume resulting in normal Hb and Hct.

False-negative cases may present with portal vein thrombosis, Budd-Chiari syndrome, or unexplained thrombocytosis, leukocytosis, splenomegaly.

RBC is increased; often = 7–12 million/cu mm; may increase to >15 million/cu mm. Increased Hb = 18–24 gm/dL in males and >16 gm/dL in females residing at altitude <2000 ft, in 71% of cases.

Increased Hct >55% in 83% of cases; >60% indicates increased RBC mass but <60% may be associated with normal RBC mass.

MCV, MCH, and MCHC are normal or decreased.

Increased ^{51}Cr RBC mass is reported essential for diagnosis; blood volume is increased; plasma volume is variably normal or slightly increased. RBC mass may be difficult to perform reliably if not done frequently, and some experts omit this test when other criteria are present, especially if serum erythropoietin is decreased and marrow erythroid colony growth occurs in absence of exogenous erythropoietin.

Increased platelet count >400,000/cu mm in 62% of cases; often >1 million/cu mm.

Increased PMNs >12,000/cu mm in ~60% of cases; usually >15,000 cu mm; sometimes a leukemoid reaction is seen. Mild basophilia in ~60% of cases.

Oxygen saturation of arterial blood is normal in 84% of cases.

Increased leukocyte ALP score >100 in 79% of cases.

Increased serum vitamin B_{12} >900 pg/mL in ~30% of cases.

Increased vitamin B_{12}-binding capacity >2200 pg/mL in ~75% of cases.

♦ Erythropoietin in plasma or serum (see p. 326) is usually decreased (but occasionally normal) in polycythemia vera; usually remains normal during phlebotomy therapy. Usually increased (but may be normal) in secondary polycythemia; overlap between these. Normal level is not helpful but *increased level rules out polycythemia vera and requires search for cause of secondary erythrocytosis*. Increases may be intermittent; therefore a single normal level is unreliable. Usually normal in relative polycythemia.

ESR is decreased.

Blood viscosity is increased.

Osmotic fragility is decreased (increased resistance).

Peripheral blood smear may show macrocytes, microcytes, polychromatophilic RBCs, normoblasts, large masses of platelets, neutrophilic shift to the left.

Reticulocyte count >1.5% in 44% of cases.

○ Bone marrow shows general hyperplasia of all elements. Cellularity >75%, especially with megakaryocytic hyperplasia in presence of erythrocytosis, is strong evidence for polycythemia vera. (Mean cellularity <48% in normal persons and 48–55% in secondary cases.) Mild myelofibrosis may be present; iron may be decreased or absent.

♦ Spontaneous erythroid colony formation occurs in in vitro culture of marrow erythroid progenitors in polycythemia vera without addition of exogenous erythropoietin (seen less commonly in other myeloproliferative disorders) but not in secondary polycythemia or normal persons; test only available in special labs.

Serum uric acid increased in ~50% of cases.

Serum total bilirubin slightly increased in ~50% of cases.

Serum iron decreased in ~50% of cases.

Serum potassium may be increased (artifactual due to thrombocytosis).

BT and coagulation time are normal, but clot retraction may be poor.

Urine may contain increased urobilinogen, and occasionally albumin is present.

Laboratory findings of associated diseases (e.g., gout, duodenal ulcer, cirrhosis, hypertension).

Laboratory findings due to complications such as thromboses (e.g., cerebral, portal vein), intercurrent infection, peptic ulcer, hemorrhage, myelofibrosis, myeloid meta-

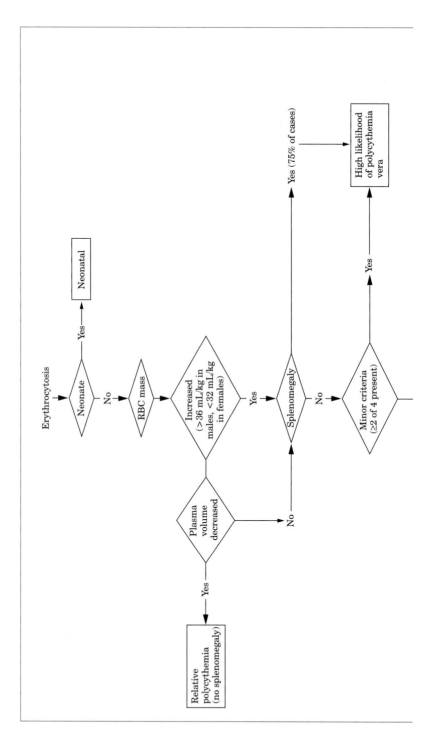

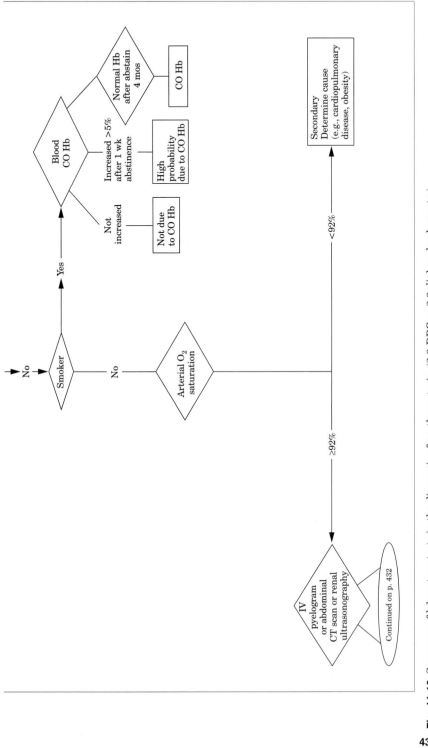

Fig. 11-10. Sequence of laboratory tests in the diagnosis of erythrocytosis. (2,3-DPG = 2,3-diphosphoglycerate.)

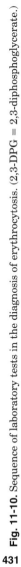

HEMATOL

Continued on p. 432

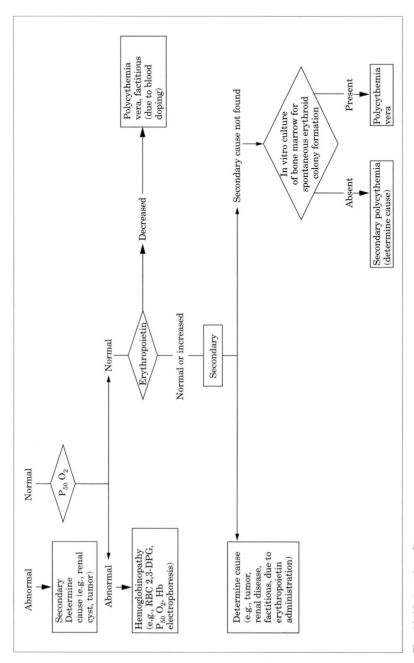

Abnormal

Secondary
Determine
cause (e.g., renal
cyst, tumor)

Normal

$P_{50} O_2$

Normal

Abnormal

Hemoglobinopathy
(e.g., RBC 2,3-DPG,
$P_{50} O_2$, Hb
electrophoresis)

Erythropoietin

Decreased

Polycythemia
vera, factitious
(due to blood
doping)

Normal or increased

Secondary

Determine cause
(e.g., tumor,
renal disease,
factitious, due to
erythropoietin
administration)

Secondary cause not found

In vitro culture
of bone marrow for
spontaneous erythroid
colony formation

Present

Polycythemia
vera

Absent

Secondary polycythemia
(determine cause)

Fig. 11-10. (continued)

plasia (develops in 3–10% of patients), chronic myelogenous leukemia (develops in 20% of patients), acute leukemia (develops in 1% of patients).

Pyropoikilocytosis, Hereditary

♦ Rare congenital severe hemolytic anemia with virtually all RBCs markedly misshapen (especially fragments, spheres, elliptocytes, pyknotic forms).
MCV is low (55–74 fL).
Increased osmotic fragility
Increased autohemolysis with or without glucose
Splenectomy greatly lessens hemolysis.

Rh$_{null}$ Disease

Mild to moderate chronic hemolytic anemia with characteristic stomatocytosis
♦ Absence of all Rh antigens on RBCs
Shortened RBC life span
Increased osmotic fragility
HbF may be increased.

Severe Combined Immunodeficiency Disorders (SCID)

(Rare disorders of many genetic causes that show congenital absence of all immune functions, with death due to infection before age 1–2 yrs. Failure to thrive. Diverse immunologic, hematologic, enzymatic, and genetic features. May be cured with bone marrow transplant.)

Autosomal Recessive SCID

♦ Marked lymphopenia (<1000 lymphocytes/cu mm) with lack of T and B cell function; very low T-cell count but CD4/CD8 ratio is rarely reversed as in AIDS. T and B cell counts very low in most autosomal recessive forms.
Eosinophilia and monocytosis are prominent features.
○ Decreased serum immunoglobulins; no antibody formation after immunization.
○ Delayed cutaneous anergy; cannot reject transplants.
○ Recurrent infections due to opportunistic organisms (persistent thrush or diaper *Monilia* rash or *P. carinii* pneumonia; viral infection from VZV, HSV, adenovirus, CMV, measles virus, progressive vaccinia) finally causes wasting and death. Graft-versus-host disease may develop.
Very small thymus (<1 gm) that fails to descend from neck shows few lymphocytes, no corticomedullary distinction, and usually no Hassall's corpuscles, but thymic epithelium appears normal.
Lymph nodes show lymphocyte depletion in both follicular and paracortical areas; tonsils, adenoids, Peyer's patches are absent or very underdeveloped.
♦ Enzyme deficiency (e.g., adenosine deaminase, purine nucleoside phosphorylase) occurs in ~40% of autosomal recessive SCID patients. Adenosine deaminase deficiency causes severe depletion of both T and B cells and lack of both cell-mediated and humoral immunity. Purine nucleoside phosphorylase deficiency preferentially affects T cells; severe defect in cell-mediated immunity but humoral immunity is intact. RBCs show adenosine deaminase deficiency and increased deoxyadenosine triphosphate and deoxyadenosine diphosphate.
SCID is most commonly X linked.

Defective Expression of Major Histocompatibility Complex Antigens

Persistent diarrhea in early infancy
Malabsorption
Susceptibility to opportunistic infection
Hypogammaglobulinemia with decreased IgM and IgA
Poor or absent antibody production
Moderate lymphopenia; decreased T-cell function; normal B cell percentage

HEMATOL

Table 11-26. Representative Laboratory Values of Some Common Hemoglobinopathies

Laboratory Test	Hemoglobinopathy				
	AS	SS	SC*	S-beta+	S-beta0
Hb (gm/dL)	N	7.5	11	11	8
Range		(6–9)	(9–14)	(8–13)	(7–10)
Hct (%)	N	22	30	32	25
Range		(18–30)	(26–40)	(25–40)	(20–36)
MCV (fL)	N	93	80	76	69
Reticulocyte count (%)	N	11	3	3	8
Range		(4–30)	(1.5–6.0)	(1.5–6.0)	(3–18)
RBC morphology	N				
Sickle cells		Many	Rare	Rare	Varies
Target cells		Many	Many		Many
Microcytosis				Mild	Marked
Hypochromia				Mild	Marked
Nucleated RBC		Many			
Hb electrophoresis (%)	N				
S	38–45	80–95	45–55	55–75	50–85
F	N	2–20	<8	1–20	2–30
A_2	1–3	<3.6	<3.6	3–6	3–6
A	55–60	0	0	15–30	0
C	0	0	45–55	0	0
Clinical severity	No symptoms	Moderate/ severe	Mild/ moderate	Mild/ moderate	Mild/ severe
Presence in U.S. blacks	10%	1:625	1:833	1:1667	1:1667

N = normal.
*Blood smear shows tetragonal crystals within RBC in 70% of patients; RBCs tend to be microcytic with low or low/normal MCV but high MCHC; typical distorted RBCs in which Hb is concentrated more in one area of cell than another.

Absent plasma cells in tissues
Severe hypoplasia of thymus and lymphoid tissues

SCID with Leukopenia

(Very rare condition in infants)
Total lack of lymphocytes
Tiny thymus (<1 gm) shows no Hassall's corpuscles or lymphocytes.

Sickle Cell Disease[23]

See Table 11-26.

Sickling of RBCs

Sickling should be confirmed with hemoglobin electrophoresis and genetic studies.
Occurs In
Sickle cell disease
Sickle cell trait
HbC-Harlem
HbC-Georgetown
HbI

[23]Steinberg MH. Management of sickle cell disease. *N Engl J Med* 1999;340:1021.

False-Positive In

First 4 mos after transfusion with RBCs having sickle cell trait
Mixture on slide with fibrinogen, thrombin, gelatin (glue)
Excessive concentration of sodium metabisulfite (e.g., $\geq 4\%$ instead of 2%)
Drying of wet coverslip preparation
Poikilocytosis

False-Negative In

First 4 mos after transfusion with normal RBCs
Heating, bacterial contamination, or prolonged washing with saline of RBCs
Newborn because HbF is high during first months of life

Sickle Solubility Test

Sodium dithionate is added to lysed RBCs to reduce the Hb.
Solution is turbid when HbS is present but remains clear with other Hb.
Does not differentiate between sickle cell anemia, sickle cell trait, and other HbS genetic
    variants.

False-Negative Results May Occur With

- Patient's Hb is <5 g/dL.
- Phenothiazine drugs.
- Unreliable for newborn screening because of high HbF.

False-Positive Results May Occur With

- Lipemic specimens
- Abnormal gamma globulins
- Polycythemia
- Increased number of Heinz bodies (e.g., postsplenectomy)
- Increased number of nucleated RBCs

Inadequate for genetic counseling because does not detect carriers of HbC and beta-
thalassemia.

Sickle Cell Trait

(Heterozygous sickle cell or HbAS disease; occurs in ~10% of American blacks)

♦ Hb electrophoresis: HbS is 20–40%, and HbA is 60–80%; normal amounts of HbA_2
    and HbF ($\leq 2\%$) may be present.
♦ Sickle cell preparation is positive.
Blood smear shows only a few target cells; sickled cells are not seen.
CBC and indices are normal; no anemia or hemolysis or jaundice is present.
Anoxia may cause systemic sickling (see following section, Sickle Cell Anemia). HbS
    concentration is too low for sickling to occur under most conditions but *beware anes-
    thesia, airplane flights, etc.*
Hematuria without any other demonstrable cause may be found.
Hyposthenuria may occur.
Sickle cells are found postmortem regardless of cause of death.

Sickle Cell Anemia

(Homozygous HbSS disease; occurs in 1 in 625 American blacks)

♦ Hb electrophoresis: HbS is 80–100%, and HbF comprises the rest (see Hemoglobin,
    Fetal, p. 331); HbA is absent.
♦ Sickle cell preparation is positive; because other Hb variants migrate with HbS on
    electrophoresis, confirming Hb as a sickle type is important. Sickle solubility test is
    positive but does not differentiate anemia from other HbS genetic variants and may
    be falsely negative if Hb <5 g/dL.
♦ Blood smear shows a variable number of RBCs with target cells (especially in HbSC
    disease), abnormal shapes, nucleated RBCs, Howell-Jolly bodies, spherical cells, poly-
    chromasia. Sickle cells in smear when RBCs contain >60% HbS (except in HbS-per-
    sistent HbF). After autosplenectomy, basophilic stippling, Pappenheimer bodies,
    nucleated RBCs also present.
Normocytic normochromic anemia (Hb = 5–10 gm/dL; normal MCV).
Reticulocyte count is increased (5–30%); may cause slight increase in MCV.
WBC is increased (10,000–30,000/cu mm) during a crisis, with normal differential or
    shift to the left. Infection may be indicated by intracellular bacteria (best seen on

HEMATOL

buffy coat preparations), Döhle's bodies, toxic granules, and vacuoles of WBCs, Westergren ESR >20 mm/hr.

Platelet count is increased (300,000–500,000/cu mm), with abnormal forms.

Bone marrow shows hyperplasia of all elements.

◯Decreased ESR becomes normal after blood is aerated. ESR in normal range may indicate intercurrent illness or crisis.

Osmotic fragility is decreased (more resistant RBCs).

Mechanical fragility of RBCs is increased.

RBC survival time is decreased (17 days in HbSS, 28 days in HbSC).

Laboratory findings of hemolysis (e.g., increased indirect serum bilirubin [≤ 6 mg/dL], increased urobilinogen in urine and stool, but urine is negative for bile).
- Hemosiderin appears in urine sediment.
- Hematuria is frequent.
- Renal concentrating ability is decreased, leading to a fixed specific gravity in virtually all patients after the first few years of life.
- Serum uric acid may be increased.
- Serum ALP is increased during crisis, representing vaso-occlusive bone injury as well as liver damage.
- Leukocyte ALP activity is decreased.

Laboratory findings due to complications
- Infections due to immunocompromised status (functional asplenia); e.g., *Salmonella* osteomyelitis (see p. 304) occurs more commonly in sickle cell syndromes; marked increase in susceptibility to pneumococcal and *H. influenzae* sepsis and meningitis, *E. coli* and meningococci infections, staphylococcal osteomyelitis, *M. pneumoniae*.
- Vaso-occlusive crisis, e.g., infarction of lungs, brain, bowel; spleen completely infarcted by middle age, causing Howell-Jolly bodies, target cells. Bone marrow necrosis causing fat emboli syndrome; bone disorders (e.g., avascular necrosis of hip; dactylitis).
- Kidney (see Nephropathy, Sickle Cell, Chapter 14, p. 732).
- Stasis and necrosis of liver—increased direct serum bilirubin ≤ 40 mg/dL, bile in urine, other findings of obstructive type of jaundice.
- Hyperhemolytic crisis—superimposed further hemolysis due to bacterial or viral infections; Hb falls from usual 6–10 g/dL to ≤ 5 g/dL in a few days with increasing reticulocyte count. When hemolysis is present, G-6-PD deficiency should be ruled out as this is also common in blacks.
- Aplastic crisis—acute, self-limited episode of erythroid aplasia lasting 5–10 days due to parvovirus B19; falling Hct and reticulocyte count may require prompt transfusion. Recovery is marked by return of reticulocytosis, usually with resolution of infection.
- Hypoplastic crisis—infection or inflammation causes brief suppression of bone marrow with accentuated brief drop in Hct and reticulocyte count.
- Splenic sequestration crisis—seen mostly in children age 5 mos to 5 yrs (before fibrosis of spleen has occurred); enormous enlargement of spleen associated with precipitous drop in Hct and hypovolemic shock. Over age 2 yrs, occurs more often with other HbS syndromes.
- Megaloblastic crisis—rare occurrence of sudden cessation of erythropoiesis due to folate depletion in persons with inadequate folate (e.g., due to pregnancy, alcoholism, poor diet).
- Bilirubin gallstones in 30% of patients by age 18 and 70% by age 30, may cause cholecystitis or biliary obstruction.

♦ • *Anemia and hemolytic jaundice are present throughout life after age 3–6 mos; hemolysis and anemia are increased only during hematologic crises.*

♦ Newborn screening by Hb electrophoresis on cord blood or filter paper spot.
- In newborns with HbSS, anemia is rarely present. May cause unexplained prolonged jaundice. May be difficult to distinguish HbSS from HbAS in neonates because of large amount of HbF, which may obscure the HbA. HbA is also not produced in HbS–beta^0-thalassemia, so an FS pattern on electrophoresis may indicate either. HbS–beta$^+$-thalassemia usually has an FSA phenotype, which requires careful differentiation from sickle cell trait (phenotype FAS). Percent of RBCs that will sickle is much lower in newborn (as low as 0.5%) than in older children. Diagnosis of HbSS is excluded by HbA on Hb electrophoresis of infant's blood or if mother has negative sickle cell preparation. *In newborn, cellulose agar elec-*

trophoresis is useless to detect HbS because of the small amount present, and acidic citrate agar gel is needed. For exchange transfusion, sickle cell test must be performed on donor blood from blacks because these RBCs may sickle in presence of hypoxia as in RDS. Hb solubility tests (e.g., Sickledex) are usually not suitable on cord blood because a positive result may be easily obscured by a large amount of HbF. Most children are anemic and symptomatic by age of 1 yr; anemia and hemolysis are present throughout life.

♦ Antenatal diagnosis is possible as early as 7–10 wks' gestation by gene analysis of fetal DNA on amniotic fluid cells or chorionic villi. Also detects HbSC disease. Diagnosis can also be made by fetal blood sampling.

HbSC Disease

(Occurs in 1 in 833 American blacks)

♦ Hb electrophoresis: HbA is absent; HbS and HbC are present in approximately equal amounts (30–60%); HbF is usually not seen (2–15%).

♦ Blood smear shows tetragonal crystals within RBC in 70% of patients; RBCs tend to be microcytic with MCV usually low or low normal but high MCHC; rare true sickle cells, occasional spherocytes, typical distorted RBCs in which Hb is concentrated more in one area of cell than another.

○ A valuable diagnostic aid is the presence of target cells with normal MCV.

♦ Other findings are the same as for sickle cell anemia, but there is less marked destruction of RBCs, anemia, etc., and the disease is less severe clinically. *Hematologic crises may cause a more marked fall in RBC than occurs in HbSS disease.*

Sickle Cell–Beta-Thalassemia Disease

(Occurs in 1 in 1667 American blacks)

♦ Hb electrophoresis: HbS is 20–90%; HbF is 2–20%.

In one syndrome, HbS may be very high and HbA synthesis is suppressed, causing a more severe disease. In the other (milder) syndrome, HbA is 25–50%; HbA_2 is increased.

Anemia is hypochromic microcytic with decreased MCV; target cells are prominent; serum iron is normal.

Other findings resemble those of sickle cell anemia.

○ Valuable diagnostic aids are: the presence of target cells with normal MCV, microcytosis or splenomegaly in patients with mild to moderate sickle cell syndrome, apparent increase in HbA_2 (HbC migrates in HbA_2 position on gel electrophoresis), microcytosis in one parent.

Sickle Cell–Persistent High Fetal Hemoglobin

(Occurs in 1 in 25,000 American blacks)

Hb electrophoresis: HbF is 20–40%; absent HbA and A_2; HbS is ~65%.

Findings are intermediate between those of sickle cell anemia and sickle cell trait, but sickle cells do not form.

Normally HbF is evenly distributed among RBCs on Kleihauer-Betke stain. In contrast, sickle cell–thalassemia patients may have high HbF values but HbF is seen in only relatively few RBCs.

Sickle Cell–HbD Disease

(Occurs in 1 in 20,000 American blacks)

Findings are intermediate between those of sickle cell anemia and sickle cell trait. Clinically mild syndrome.

♦ Hb electrophoresis demonstrates the abnormal hemoglobin at acid pH.

Spherocytosis, Hereditary

(Defective RBC membrane due to spectrin deficiency; deficiency ~30% of normal in severe cases to 80% of normal in mildest cases.)

Autosomal dominant form in ~70% of cases with moderately severe disease in which one parent and half the siblings are affected; ~20% have mild compensated hemolysis; may be sporadic and occur without a family history or may show recessive inheritance. ~10% of patients have severe debilitating disease with severe anemia that makes them transfusion dependent, with gallstones in childhood and bone changes.

♦ Abnormal peripheral blood smear is most suggestive finding. Many microspherocytes are present. Anisocytosis may be marked; poikilocytosis is slight. RBCs show Howell-Jolly bodies, Pappenheimer bodies, Heinz bodies. Polychromatophilic reticulocytes and microspherocytes are present.

♦ Hemolytic anemia is moderate (RBC = 3–4 million/cu mm), microcytic (MCV = 70–80 fL), and hyperchromic (increased MCHC = 36–40 gm/dL). *MCHC >36% means congenital spherocytic anemia if cold agglutinins and hypertriglyceridemia have been excluded.*

♦ Osmotic fragility is increased; increase generally reflects clinical severity of disease; when normal in some patients, the incubated fragility test shows increased hemolysis. Diagnosis is not established without abnormal osmotic fragility. Increased osmotic fragility does not distinguish hereditary spherocytosis from autoimmune hemolytic disease with spherocytosis but latter shows much less increased fragility with incubation.

Autohemolysis (sterile defibrinated blood incubated for 48 hrs) is increased (10–50% compared to normal of <4% of cells); very nonspecific test. May sometimes be found also in nonspherocytic hemolytic anemias.

Abnormal osmotic fragility and autohemolysis are reduced by 10% glucose; false-negative test may occur with concomitant diabetes mellitus.

♦ Direct Coombs' test must be negative (in contrast to immune hemolytic conditions in which spherocytosis is common and direct Coombs' test is positive).

Mechanical fragility is increased.

WBC and platelet counts are usually normal; may be increased during hemolysis.

♦ Evidence of hemolysis
  • Degree of reticulocytosis (usually 5–15%) is greater than in other hemolytic anemias with similar degrees of anemia.
  • Bone marrow shows marked erythroid hyperplasia except during aplastic crisis; moderate hemosiderin is present.
  • Increased serum LD and indirect bilirubin.
  • Haptoglobins are decreased or absent.
  • Hemolytic crises usually precipitated by infection (especially parvovirus) cause more profound anemia despite reticulocytosis and increased jaundice and splenomegaly.
  • Stool urobilinogen is usually increased.
  • Hemoglobinemia and hemoglobinuria only during hemolytic crises.

Laboratory findings due to complications, e.g., gallstones, aplastic crises

Diagnosis should be questioned if splenectomy does not cause a complete response.

Age at diagnosis is related to severity of hemolysis; more severe forms are diagnosed early in life.

In neonates is associated with jaundice in ~50% of cases. Serum indirect bilirubin may be >20 mg/dL. Anemia is usually mild (Hb ≥ 10 gm/dL) during first week of life. Spherocytes are present in infant and one parent and may be present in siblings. Reticulocyte count is usually 5–15%.

Spleen, Decreased Function (Hyposplenism)

Due To

Congenital absence

Splenectomy or autoinfarction (e.g., sickle cell anemia)

Infiltration (e.g., amyloidosis)

Nontropical sprue, dermatitis herpetiformis, ulcerative colitis, regional ileitis (30% of patients), but overwhelming sepsis is rare.

Irradiation

Graft-versus-host disease

♦ Howell-Jolly bodies (is the most consistent abnormality; good indicator of asplenic state), pocked cells, and target cells are seen in peripheral blood smears; also Pappenheimer bodies, a few acanthocytes, nucleated RBCs. Some Heinz bodies can be seen with special stains.

Decreased osmotic fragility may be found.

Increased risk of overwhelming infection by encapsulated bacteria (50% are due to *Streptococcus pneumonia;* another 25% are due to *H. influenzae, Neisseria meningitidis,* and group A streptococcus; *Staphylococcus, Pseudomonas,* and other gram-negative organisms are rarer). High mortality with massive bacteremia. Risk of infection is greater in infants less than 2 yrs old, within 2 yrs of splenectomy, or if underlying disorder is primary hematologic or splenic disease.

Postsplenectomy

Absence of RBC changes may suggest an accessory spleen in postsplenectomy patients.

Increased WBC (granulocytosis) for several weeks in 75% of patients and indefinitely in 25%. Lymphocytosis and monocytosis occurs in several weeks in 50% of patients; some of these may show increased eosinophils or basophils. Platelet, WBC, and reticulocyte counts may increase to peak in 5–14 days in postoperative period, then become high normal.

Spleen, Increased Function (Hypersplenism)

♦ Diagnosis is made by exclusion.
♦ Various combinations of anemia, leukopenia, thrombocytopenia are associated with bone marrow showing normal or increased cellularity of affected elements (includes primary splenic pancytopenia and primary splenic neutropenia).
  • Decreased platelet count is moderate to severe (100,000 to 30,000/cu mm).
  • Normochromic anemia (Hb = 9.0–11.0 g/dL) may occur.
  • WBCs may be decreased with a normal differential count.
  • Bone marrow is normal or shows increased cellularity of all lines with normal maturation.
Peripheral blood smear may reflect the underlying cause.
  • Spherocytes in hereditary spherocytosis
  • Target cells in liver disease
  • Atypical lymphocytes in infectious mononucleosis or chronic infection
  • Leukoerythroblastosis, nucleated RBCs, and immature granulocytes in myeloid metaplasia with extramedullary hematopoiesis
  • Teardrop and hand-mirror RBCs in myelofibrosis
Direct Coombs' test is negative.
^{51}Cr-tagged RBCs from normal person or from patient are rapidly destroyed after transfusion, and radioactivity accumulates in spleen. (Normal spleen/liver ratio = 1.0; in hypersplenism ratio is 1.5–2.0; in hemolysis ratio is >3.0.)
Laboratory findings due to underlying disease that can cause splenomegaly, e.g.,
  • Congestion (e.g., cirrhosis with portal hypertension)
  • Hematologic disorders (e.g., lymphoma/leukemia)
  • Infiltration (e.g., lipid storage disease)
  • Inflammation and infections (e.g., SBE, TB, sarcoidosis, collagen diseases, Felty's syndrome)
  • Splenic tumors and cysts

Stomatocytosis, Hereditary

♦ Rare condition of morphologic abnormality of >35% of RBCs in which one or more slit-like areas of central pallor produce a mouth-like appearance. Normally <5% of RBCs are stomacytic. ≤ 20% of RBCs are stomacytic in many acquired disorders (e.g., alcoholism, drug-induced hemolytic anemia, various neoplasms, hepatobiliary disease).
Findings resemble hereditary spherocytosis with variable degree of hemolytic anemia, but splenectomy may cause partial or no remission.

Sulfhemoglobinemia

(>0.5 gm/dL sulfhemoglobin)

Due To

Drugs, especially phenacetin (including Bromo-Seltzer) and acetanilid

HEMATOL

Table 11-27. Classification of Beta-Thalassemia Syndromes

Genotype	Anemia	Microcytosis	Hb Electrophoresis
Normal			
Beta/beta	None	None	HbA_2 <3.5%, HbF <1%
Thalassemia minima			
Beta/beta$^+$ (mild)	None	None	HbA_2 = N or slightly I HbF = I
Thalassemia minor			
Beta/beta$^+$ (severe)	Mild	Mild to moderate	HbA_2 = 3.5–7.5% HbF = N or slightly I
Beta/beta^0	Mild	Mild to moderate	HbA_2 = 3.5–7.5% HbF = N or slightly I
Beta/delta beta^0	Mild	Mild to moderate	HbA_2 = N or D HbF = 5–20%
Beta/beta Lepore	Mild	Mild to moderate	HbA_2 = N or D HbF = I Hb Lepore up to 8%
Thalassemia intermedia			
Beta$^+$ (mild)/beta$^+$ (severe)	Moderate to severe	Moderate to severe	HbA_2 = 6–8% HbF = 20–50% HbA = remainder
Delta beta^0/delta beta^0	Moderate to severe	Moderate to severe	HbF only
Thalassemia major			
Beta^0/beta^0	Severe	Severe	HbA_2 = 3–11% HbA = 0 HbF = remainder
Beta$^+$ (severe)/beta$^+$ (severe)	Severe	Severe	HbA_2 = 3–11% HbF = 10–90% HbA = remainder
Beta^0/beta$^+$ (severe)	Severe	Severe	HbA_2 = 3–11% HbF = 10–90% HbA = remainder
Beta^0/beta Lepore	Severe	Severe	HbF > 80% Hb Lepore = remainder

D = decreased; I = increased; N = normal.

Laboratory Findings

♦ Spectroscopic absorption analysis—band at 618 μ does not disappear on addition of 5% potassium cyanide.
Laboratory findings due to associated bromide intoxication.
Bromide intoxication and sulfhemoglobinemia may be due to excessive intake of Bromo-Seltzer.

Thalassemias

See Tables 11-1, 11-9, and 11-27.
Beta-chain synthesis is normally low at birth because HbA becomes predominant only after the first few months. Clinical and laboratory findings correspond to this; thus neonatal anemia occurs only with alpha- but not with beta-thalassemia.

Beta-Thalassemia Minima

Silent carrier of beta-thalassemia trait
Normal RBC morphology and Hb electrophoresis
♦ Can only be demonstrated by reduced rate of beta-globin synthesis with increased alpha/betaglobin chain ratio.

Beta-Thalassemia Trait

♦ In uncomplicated cases, Hb is normal or only slightly decreased (11–12 gm/dL), whereas RBC is increased (5–7 million/cu mm). Most nonanemic patients with microcytosis have thalassemia minor.

♦ Microcytic anemia with Hb <9.3 gm/dL is unlikely to be thalassemia minor. MCV is <75 fL whereas Hct is >30%; MCV may be as low as 55 fL. Microcytosis may be difficult to detect morphologically.

♦ Ratio of microcytic to hypochromic RBCs is >0.9 but <0.9 in iron deficiency. MCHC >31%.

Blood smear changes are less than in thalassemia major.

Anisocytosis is less marked than in iron-deficiency anemia.

Poikilocytosis is mild to moderate; more striking than iron-deficiency anemia with Hb = 10–12 gm/dL. Target cells and oval forms may be numerous.

Occasional RBCs show basophilic stippling in beta-thalassemia minor (rare in blacks but common in patients of Mediterranean descent).

Reticulocyte count is increased (2–10%).

Serum iron is normal or slightly increased; transferrin saturation may be increased. TIBC and serum ferritin are normal.

Cellular marrow contains stainable iron.

Osmotic fragility is decreased.

♦ Hb electrophoresis shows increased HbA_2 (>4%); normal value does not rule out this diagnosis.

Beta-Thalassemia Minor

(>50 forms are recognized by gene cloning)

See Table 11-28.

Slight or mild anemia. Most important differential diagnosis is iron deficiency (see p. 360).

MCV usually <75 fL and Hct >30%; RBC is often increased.

Normal iron, TIBC, serum ferritin

♦ Increased HbA_2 (3–6%) on starch or agar electrophoresis and a slight increase in HbF (2–10%). HbA_2 is often decreased in iron deficiency; thus HbA_2 level may be normal in concomitant iron deficiency and beta-thalassemia minor, and the diagnosis of beta-thalassemia trait cannot be made until iron deficiency has been treated. HbA_2 and HbF are absent in alpha-thalassemia. No specific laboratory identification of alpha-thalassemia trait (carrier). Thus, normal Hb electrophoresis and England-Fraser formula value < –6 in the absence of iron deficiency implies alpha-thalassemia minor; mild alpha-thalassemia is a clinical diagnosis.

Thalassemia Intermedia

(2–10% of thalassemia cases; may be homozygous delta-beta, beta⁰, or beta⁺, with or without an alpha gene or double heterozygous with an abnormal Hb such as S or E)

Less severe clinical and laboratory findings than in thalassemia major and occur at later age. Hb is usually >6.5 g/dL.

Combination of HbE and beta-thalassemia results in wide spectrum of clinical disorders varying from thalassemia to much milder that do not require transfusions.

Thalassemia Major (Cooley's Anemia, Mediterranean Anemia)

Several Hb electrophoretic patterns are characteristic (see Table 11-27).

♦ Classification of beta-thalassemia syndromes:
  • Homozygous beta⁰—HbA is absent; HbF and HbA_2 are present.
  • Homozygous beta⁺—HbA, HbA_2, and HbF are all detected.
  • HbF = 10–90%; HbA is decreased; HbA_2 may be normal, low, or high.

♦ Marked hypochromic microcytic regenerative hemolytic anemia is present. Often Hb = 2.0–6.5 g/dL, Hct = 10–24%, RBC = 2–3 million, indices are decreased.

♦ Blood smear shows marked anisocytosis, poikilocytosis, target cells, spherocytes, and hypochromic, fragmented, and bizarre RBCs; also many nucleated RBCs—basophilic stippling, Cabot's ring bodies, siderocytes.

Reticulocyte count is increased.

WBCs are often increased, with normal differential or marked shift to left.

Table 11-28. Differentiation of Microcytic Anemias of Iron Deficiency and Thalassemia Minor

	Iron Deficiency	No Differentiation	Thalassemia Minor	Sensitivity (%)[a]	Accuracy (%)[a]
Hb (gm/L)	<9.3 M or F	9.3–13.5 M 9.3–12.5 F	>13.5 M >12.5 F		
MCV (fL)		>68	<68	100	65
MCHC (gm/dL)	<30	>30			
RBC (per cu mm)	<4.2	4.2–5.5	>5.5		
Erythrocytosis				68	90
Mentzer formula[b] (MCV/RBC)	>13		<13	95	65
England-Fraser formula[b] (MCV – [5 × Hb + RBC + K, if K = 3.4])		Positive number	Negative number	69	77
Shine-Lal formula[b] (MCV² × MCH)			<1530	100	86
MCV of 1 parent <79				100	86
Free erythrocyte protoporphyrin = 25				60	67
HbA₂ >3.5%			>0.9	85	90
Microcytic/hypochromic ratio[c]	<0.9				

F = females; M = males.

[a] Accuracy in distinguishing anemias of thalassemia minor and iron deficiency (%).

[b] In patients with polycythemia vera who develop iron deficiency with microcytosis, a negative number results. These formulas do not account for the indeterminate zone of no differentiation.

[c] Using Technicon H-1 hematology analyzer (Technicon, Tarrytown, NY).

Source: d'Onofrio G, et al. *Arch Pathol Lab Med* 1992;116:84.

Table 11-29. Classification of Alpha-Thalassemia Syndromes

	Number of Gene Deletions	Anemia	Microcytosis	Hb Electrophoresis	
				At birth	Adulthood
Alpha-thal trait 2 (silent carrier)	1	0	0	1–2% Bart's	N
Alpha-thal trait 1 (heterozygous; or homozygous)	2	Mild	Mild	5–10% Bart's	N HbA$_2$ not I
HbH disease (alpha-thal 2 + alpha-thal 1)	3	Moderate	Marked	20–40% Bart's	HbH Small amount of HbA
Hydrops fetalis (homozygous)	4	Fatal at/before birth		>50% Bart's	Hb Bart

Alpha-thal = alpha-thalassemia; I = increased; N = normal.
Alpha-thalassemias are characterized by decreased or absent synthesis of globin chains; very common in African, Asian, and Mediterranean populations. Most prevalent genetic trait in the world.
Hb Bart disappears by age 3–6 mos. Hb Bart acts like very-high-affinity Hb with marked left-shifted oxygen dissociation curve resembling CO poisoning.
Normal Hb electrophoresis and England-Fraser of < –6 in the absence of iron deficiency implies alpha-thalassemia minor. Screening can be done for most common deletions of alpha-thalassemia using PCR amplification of specific DNA sequences.

Platelets are normal.
Bone marrow is cellular and shows erythroid hyperplasia and increased iron.
Serum iron and TIBC are increased. After age 5 yrs, iron-binding capacity is usually saturated.
Laboratory findings of hemolysis and liver dysfunction (e.g., increased serum LD, AST, ALT, and indirect bilirubin [1–3 mg/dL], urine and stool urobilinogen; serum haptoglobin and hemopexin are very decreased or absent).
  • Liver dysfunction causing disturbance of factors V, VII, IX, XI, prothrombin
RBC survival time is decreased.
Osmotic fragility is decreased.
Mechanical fragility is increased.
Laboratory findings due to complications, e.g.,
  • Secondary hypersplenism (usually occurs between age 5–10 yrs, detected when transfusion requirement is >200–250 mg/kg body weight, at which time splenectomy is indicated).
○ • Hemosiderosis (hepatic fibrosis and cirrhosis; endocrinopathies with hypofunction of pituitary, thyroid, etc.).
Proteinuria, hyposthenuria, failure to acidify urine, and increased urobilin and urobilinogen with dark color may be present.
○Beta-thalassemia trait demonstrated in both parents.
♦ Prenatal diagnosis is possible at 16 wks' gestation in 85% of cases by DNA analysis of amniotic cells; the remaining cases can be diagnosed by alpha-/beta-chain ratios in fetal blood (obtained by fetoscopy).

Alpha-Thalassemia 2

See Table 11-29.
○One alpha allele is deleted, which causes asymptomatic but transmissible trait. Occurs in ≤ 30% of black populations. Coincident with sickle cell or HbC trait, reduces the proportion of HbS or HbC below the usual 35–40% (also slightly decreasing the clinical severity); thus <35% variant Hb is good evidence for coexisting alpha-thalassemia in such patients. No clinical or hematologic findings.

HEMATOL

◆ Definitive diagnosis of older silent carrier depends on special techniques (globin synthesis rates).

Alpha-Thalassemia 1

Two copies of alpha-globin gene are deleted from same chromosome.
Minimal hypochromic, microcytic anemia, increased target cells, anisocytosis, resembling beta-thalassemia trait but without increased HbA_2

HbE–Alpha-Thalassemia

See p. 385.

HbH Disease

Inheritance of alpha-thalassemia 1 from one parent and alpha-thalassemia 2 from other causing absence of three of four alpha-globin alleles and excess of beta-globins (HbH). May also be due to deletion of two alpha-globin genes and presence of alpha-chain variant Hb Constant Spring. Acquired form may occur during course of myeloproliferative disorders due to relative suppression of alpha-chain gene.
Hypochromic, microcytic hemolytic anemia is moderate to mild (Hb = 7–11 gm/dL), accentuated by infection, drugs, pregnancy, etc.
Most RBCs are microcytic, hypochromic; many target or deformed RBCs
◆ Characteristic patterns on RBC and platelet histograms due to very small RBCs; may cause inaccurate platelet count.
○ Supravital stain shows granular inclusions (precipitated beta chains), which are very marked after splenectomy
◆ Isoelectric focusing is more sensitive than Hb gel electrophoresis for variants present in small amounts
May present with neonatal jaundice.

Hydrops Fetalis

Deletion of all four alpha-globin genes with no normal Hb causes stillbirth or prompt postnatal death due to severe hypoxemia (despite cord Hb ≤ 10 g/dL).
◆ Prenatal diagnosis by Southern blot of amniotic fluid DNA or chorionic villus sample, or by PCR techniques.

Thick Blood Syndrome, Neonatal

◆ Hct >64% in a heparinized sample or >67% in an unheparinized sample.
◆ When Hct is 60–64%, diagnosis must be made with a microviscosimeter. If <60%, hyperviscosity is not found.
Hyperbilirubinemia, hypoglycemia, platelet count <130,000/cu mm, or abnormal blood smear (burr cells, fragmented RBCs, increased erythroid elements) are found in ~50% of cases.
Therapeutic replacement of blood with plasma exchange transfusion aims to reduce Hct to 50–60% range.

Due To

Transfusion (e.g., maternal-fetal, twin to twin)
Hypoxemia (e.g., postmaturity, small-for-gestational-age neonates)
Decreased deformability of RBC membranes (e.g., sickle cell anemia, spherocytosis)

Thymic Hypoplasia (DiGeorge Syndrome)

(Hypoplasia or aplasia of thymus and parathyroid and anomalies of other structures formed at same time [e.g., cardiac defects, renal abnormalities, facial abnormalities such as cleft palate] due to chromosome band 22q11 deletions)
See Tables 11-6 and 11-7.

◆ Proposed Diagnostic Criteria

Involvement of two or more of the following organ systems:
  • Thymus

- Parathyroid
- Cardiovascular

Hypocalcemia may be transient; may cause neonatal seizures.

Serum immunoglobulins are usually near normal for age but may be decreased, especially IgA. IgE may be increased.

Decreased T cells and relative increase in B cell percentage. Normal ratio of helper and suppressor types.

With complete syndrome, susceptible to opportunistic infection (*P. carinii*, fungi, viruses) and to graft-versus-host disease from blood transfusion. In partial syndrome (with variable amount of hypoplasia), growth and response to infection may be normal.

Thymus is often absent; when found, histology appears normal.

Lymph node follicles appear normal, but paracortical areas and thymus-dependent areas of spleen show variable amount of depletion. Incidence of cancer and of autoimmune disease is not increased.

Tumor of Bone Marrow

(Due to leukemia, metastases, agnogenic myeloid metaplasia)

"Leukoerythroblastic" peripheral blood picture

- WBC may be increased, decreased, or normal.
- Peripheral blood may show left shift in myeloid series, thrombocytopenia, nucleated RBCs, schistocytes, teardrop RBCs.

◆ May show tumor cells in peripheral blood ("carcinocythemia"), especially in patients receiving high-dose chemotherapy before autologous marrow transplant and in those receiving growth factor therapy.

◆ Bone marrow examination establishes diagnosis.

Tumor of Thymus

(>40% of patients have parathymic syndromes noted in the following, which are multiple in one-third)

○Associated with

Myasthenia gravis in ~35% of cases. May appear up to 6 yrs after excision of thymoma in 5% of cases. Thymoma develops in 15% of patients with myasthenia gravis.

Acquired hypogammaglobulinemia. 7–13% of adults with this condition have an associated thymoma; does not respond to thymectomy.

Pure red cell aplasia found in approximately 5% of thymoma patients. 50% of patients with pure red cell aplasia have thymoma, of whom 25% benefit from thymectomy; onset followed thymectomy in 10% of cases. May be accompanied or followed, but not preceded, by granulocytopenia or thrombocytopenia or both in one-third of cases; thymectomy is not useful therapy. Pure red cell aplasia occurs in one-third of patients with hypogammaglobulinemia and thymoma.

Autoimmune hemolytic anemia with positive Coombs' test and increased reticulocyte count

Cushing's syndrome

MEN (usually type I)

SLE

Miscellaneous disorders (e.g., giant cell myocarditis, nephrotic syndrome)

Cutaneous disorders (e.g., mucocutaneous candidiasis, pemphigus)

Wiskott-Aldrich Syndrome

(Rare immunologic X-linked recessive condition characterized by eczema, repeated infections, and thrombocytopenia with death by age 10 due to infection, hemorrhage, or lymphoma [12% incidence]. Severe impairment of humoral and cellular immunity)

See Tables 11-6 and 11-7.

◆ Platelet count is decreased (average 15,000–30,000/cu mL) and small appearance on smear is diagnostic. Bleeding tendency (skin, GI tract) with frequent death due to intracranial hemorrhage. Decreased survival time of patients' platelets. Megakaryocytes appear normal.

Impaired maturation of hematopoietic stem cells.

Table 11-30. Comparison of Coagulation Disorders with Platelet or Vascular Disorders

	Coagulation Disorder	Platelet or Vascular Disorder
Hemarthroses and deep hematomas in muscle	Characteristic	Rare
Delayed bleeding	Characteristic	Rare
Bleeding from superficial cuts	Uncommon	Persistent; may be profuse
Petechiae	Rare	Characteristic
Ecchymoses	Common, usually single and large	Characteristic, usually multiple and large
Epistaxis, melena	Seldom predominant	Often causes significant bleeding
Hematuria	Common	Uncommon

Marked susceptibility to high-grade encapsulated organisms and to opportunistic infections (e.g., bacteria, fungi, *P. carinii*, chronic viral infections) and autoimmune disease is seen.

Highly variable immunoglobulin levels, even within the same patient; predominant pattern is decreased serum IgM, increased IgA and IgE, normal IgG.

Normal levels of circulating T and B cells; severely impaired cell-mediated and humoral immunity that decreases with age.

EBV-associated lymphoid cancers (especially B immunoblastic non-Hodgkin's lymphoma with predilection for CNS) and autoimmune disorders in older persons.

♦ Scanning electron microscopy of fetal lymphocytes from umbilical vein establishes prenatal diagnosis.

Tests of Coagulation

See Tables 11-30, 11-31, and 11-32.

Anticoagulants, Circulating

(Usually antibodies that inhibit function of specific coagulation factors, especially VIII or IX; occasionally V, XI, XIII, vWF)

May be acquired (antibodies) due to multiple transfusions for congenital deficiency of a coagulation factor, or spontaneous.

Associated with Clinical Disorders

Factor	Disorder
VIII, IX	After replacement therapy for hereditary deficiency
XI	SLE—very rare
IX	SLE—rare
VIII	SLE, RA, drug reaction, asthma, pemphigus, inflammatory bowel disease, postpartum period, advanced age
X	Amyloidosis (tissue binding rather than circulating)
V	Associated with streptomycin administration, idiopathic
X, V	SLE—common
II	Myeloma, SLE
XIII	Associated with isoniazid administration, idiopathic

Also associated with pregnancy, lymphoproliferative diseases, certain drugs (e.g., penicillin, sulfonamides, phenytoin)

Table 11-31. Screening Tests for Presumptive Diagnosis of Common Bleeding Disorders[a]

Platelet Count	BT	PT	aPTT[b]	Location of Defect	Most Frequent Causes	
					Acquired	Hereditary
N	N	I	N	Extrinsic pathway[c]	Liver disease, coumarin therapy, vitamin K deficiency, DIC (very rare)	Deficiency of factor VII (very rare)
N	N	N	I	Intrinsic pathway[d]	Heparin therapy, inhibitors	Hemophilia A or B, deficiency of factor XI, XII, prekallikrein, high-molecular-weight kininogen, Passavoy factor
N[e]	N	I	I	Common or multiple pathways	Heparin therapy, liver disease, vitamin K deficiency, DIC, fibrinogenolysis (very common)	Deficiency of factor V, X, prothrombin; dysfibrinogenemias (very rare)
D	I	N	N	Thrombocytopenia	ITP, secondary (e.g., drugs)	Wiskott-Aldrich syndrome, etc.
N or I	I	N	N	Disorder of platelet function	Thrombocythemia, drugs, uremia, dysproteinemias	Thrombasthenia, deficient release reaction
N	I	N	I	von Willebrand's disease		
N	N	N	N	Vascular abnormality	Allergic purpura, drugs, scurvy, etc.	Deficiency of factor XIII, telangiectasia

D = decreased; I = increased; N = normal; DIC = disseminated intravascular coagulation; ITP = idiopathic thrombocytopenia purpura.

[a]Screening tests may be normal in mild von Willebrand's disease that has borderline or intermittent normal bleeding time, in mild hemophilia, and in factor XIII deficiency.

[b]Concentration of factors must be decreased to ≤ 30% of normal for these tests to be abnormal.

[c]Extrinsic pathway function depends on factors VII, X, V, II (prothrombin), I (fibrinogen); is assessed by PT.

[d]Intrinsic pathway depends on factors XII, XI, IX, VIII, X, V, II, I; is assessed by aPTT.

[e]May be I in acquired disorders that produce abnormalities of platelets and multiple coagulation factors.

HEMATOL

Table 11-32. Summary of Coagulation Studies in Hemorrhagic Conditions

Condition	Screening Tests				Accessory Tests				
	Platelet Count	BT	PT	aPTT	Capillary Fragility (tourniquet test)	Coagulation Time	Clot Retraction	Prothrombin Consumption Time	Factor Assay
Thrombocytopenic purpura	D	I	N	N	+	N	Poor	I	
Nonthrombocytopenic purpura	N	N	N	N	V	N	N	N	
Glanzmann's thrombasthenia	N[a]	N or I	N	N	+ or N	N	Poor	I Corrected by platelet substitute	
von Willebrand's disease	N	I or N	N	N or I	N, + in severe	V	N	I	+
AHF (factor VIII) deficiency (hemophilia)	N	N	N	I	N	I / N in mild	N	I	+
PTC (factor IX) deficiency (hemophilia B; Christmas disease)	N	N	N	I[c]	N	I / N in mild	N	I	+
Factor X (Stuart) deficiency	N	N	I[b]	I[b]	N	N or slightly I	N	I	+
PTA (factor XI) deficiency	N	N, I in severe	N	I[c]	N	I	N	I	+
Factor XII (Hageman) deficiency	N	N	N	I[c]	N	I	N	I	+
Factor XIII deficiency	N	N	N	N	N	N	N	N	+
Fibrinogen deficiency	N	N, I in severe	I	I	N	I	N	N	+

							Lysis of clot
Hypoprothrombinemia	N	N or I	I	I	N	N	N
Excess dicumarol therapy	N	N I in severe	I	I	N	N	N
Heparin therapy	N	N to I	May be I	I	+ in severe	N in mild I	N	
Vascular purpura (e.g., Schönlein-Henoch disease, hereditary hemorrhagic telangiectasia)	N	N	N	N	N	N	N
Increased antithromboplastin	N		I		I	I	I
Increased antithrombin	N	N	I	I	N	May be I in severe	N	N^d
Increased fibrinolysin	N	N or I	N	N	N	N or I	N	N^d

+ = positive; D = decreased; I = increased; N = normal; AHF = antihemophilic factor; PTC = plasma thromboplastin components; PTA = plasma thromboplastin antecedent; V = variable.
[a]Platelets appear abnormal.
[b]Corrected by serum.
[c]Corrected by serum or plasma.
[d]Not useful; may be difficult to do.

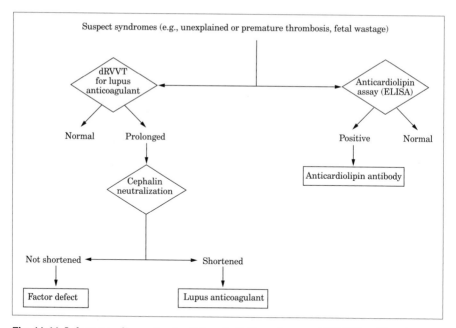

Suspect syndromes (e.g., unexplained or premature thrombosis, fetal wastage)

dRVVT for lupus anticoagulant

Anticardiolipin assay (ELISA)

Normal   Prolonged

Positive   Normal

Anticardiolipin antibody

Cephalin neutralization

Not shortened   Shortened

Factor defect   Lupus anticoagulant

Fig. 11-11. Laboratory diagnosis of antiphospholipid syndromes. (dRVRVT = dilute Russell's viper venom time; ELISA = enzyme-linked immunosorbent assay.)

♦ **Antiphospholipid-thrombosis syndrome*** defined as one or more autoantibodies (anticardiolipin antibodies, lupus anticoagulant) and/or biological false-positive for syphilis found on two occasions at least 12 wks apart associated with appropriate clinical manifestations. Most patients have positive assay for both lupus anticoagulant and anticardiolipin antibodies. May be secondary to SLE or primary (i.e., without signs of connective tissue disease). Directed against phospholipids rather than against a specific factor (Fig. 11-11).

Anticardiolipin Antibodies

Detected by ELISA against IgG, IgM, and IgA.
Common in SLE—correlates with laboratory features (e.g., thrombocytopenia, prolonged aPTT, positive direct and indirect Coombs' test); may not correlate with clinical manifestations in contrast to primary syndrome.

Lupus Anticoagulant

♦ 1. Prolonged phospholipid-dependent clotting time in a screening assay
  • Increased aPTT; 1:1 mixture with normal plasma with aPTT >4 secs longer than control aPTT establishes presence of inhibitor, but the increased aPTT is corrected if due to a clotting factor deficiency. Low factor activity increases toward normal with further dilution of test plasma.
  • Prolonged aPTT should be confirmed by a different phospholipid detection clotting system (e.g., dRVVT).
  • Abnormal dRVVT and tissue thromboplastin inhibition test. dRVVT is more specific for lupus anticoagulant than aPTT because not influenced by deficiency of

*Love PE, Santoro SA. Antiphospholipid antibodies: Anticardiolipin and the lupus anticoagulant in SLE and in non-SLE disorders. Prevalence and clinical significance. *Ann Int Med* 1990;112:682.
Bick RL. The antiphospholipid-thrombosis syndromes. *Am J Clin Path* 1993;100:470.
Riley RS, Friedline J, Rogers JS. Antiphospholipid antibodies: Standardization and testing. *Clin Lab Med* 1997;17:395.

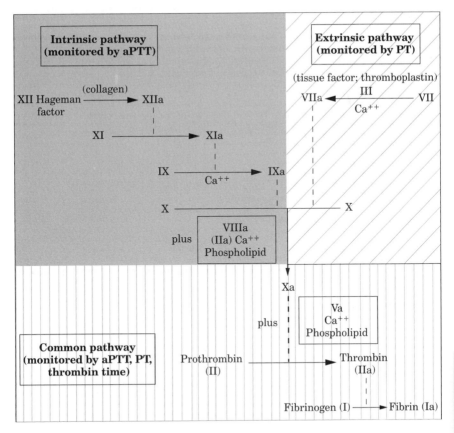

Fig. 11-12. Blood coagulation cascade.

intrinsic pathway factors or antibodies to factors VIII, IX, or XI. Heparin or warfarin can prolong dRVVT and most other tests.
- Kaolin clotting time is increased; is sensitive test for lupus anticoagulant, especially when aPTT is normal or only slightly increased.
♦ 2. Demonstration that abnormality is due to inhibitor rather than factor deficiency
- Rosner index >15 indicates an inhibitor:

$$\frac{[(\text{Clotting time of mixture of patient} + \text{normal plasma}) - (\text{normal plasma clotting time})]}{(\text{normal plasma clotting time})}$$

- Prolonged incubation with normal plasma does not increase inhibitor effect.
- Decrease in two or more factors (VIII, IX, XI, or XII) by one-stage assay but normal by two-stage assay.
♦ 3. Confirmation of inhibitor specificity for phospholipid
- Platelet neutralization procedure (addition of platelets shortens the prolonged aPTT and dRVVT due to lupus anticoagulant but not due to factor VIII inhibitors).
- Cephalin phospholipid neutralization (shortening) of prolonged test confirms lupus anticoagulant.
♦ 4. No evidence of another coagulopathy to account for abnormal coagulation reaction. PT is usually normal to slightly increased. Thrombin time is normal.

Antithrombin III

See Fig. 11-12.

Use

To detect hypercoagulable state associated with episodes of venous thrombosis; decreased in ~4.5% of patients with idiopathic venous thrombosis.

Functional tests are required because the antigen level may be normal in ~10% of cases of hereditary qualitative deficiency by immunologic method.

Decreased In

Hereditary familial deficiency (typically 40–60% of normal); autosomal dominant trait.
Chronic liver disease (>80% of cases of cirrhosis); liver cancer
Nephrotic syndrome
Protein-wasting diseases
Heparin therapy for >3 days
L-Asparaginase therapy
Active thrombotic disease (e.g., thrombophlebitis, deep venous thrombosis, pulmonary embolism) (not diagnostically useful)
AMI
DIC (not diagnostically useful)
Oral contraceptive use (slightly)
Last trimester of pregnancy (rarely <75% of normal)
Newborns (~50% of adult level, which is attained by age 6 mos)
Other conditions (e.g., acute leukemia, carcinoma, burns, postsurgical trauma, renal disease, gram-negative septicemia)

Increased In

Patients with increased ESR, hyperglobulinemia
Coumadin anticoagulation

Bleeding Time (BT)[24]

See Fig. 11-13.
Mielke modification of Ivy method; should use a standardized technique: blood pressure cuff on upper arm is inflated to 40 mm Hg; two small standardized skin incisions are made on volar surface of forearm using a specially calibrated template.
Normal = 4–7 mins. Longer in women than in men.

Use

BT is functional test of primary hemostasis.

BT is best single screening test for platelet functional or structural disorders, acquired (e.g., uremia) or congenital. Normal BT without suggestive history usually excludes platelet dysfunction. However, a normal BT does not rule out a significant defect; with clinical suspicion, platelet aggregation should be performed.

Useful as part of workup for coagulation disorders in patients who have history of excess bleeding (e.g., associated with dental extraction, childbirth, circumcision, tonsillectomy) even with a normal platelet count.

Normal in all other disorders of coagulation except vWF deficiency and some cases of very low plasma fibrinogen (because platelets contain fibrinogen).

May be useful to monitor treatment of active hemorrhage in patients with prolonged BT due to uremia, von Willebrand's disease, congenital platelet function abnormalities, or severe anemia.

No value in performing BT if platelet count is <100,000/cu mm as BT is usually prolonged. Prolonged BT with platelet count >100,000/cu mm usually indicates impaired platelet function (e.g., due to aspirin) or von Willebrand's disease.

Not recommended for prediction of bleeding in myeloproliferative diseases or neonates receiving NSAIDs.

Sensitivity, specificity, and predictive value of BT in perioperative hemorrhage are not known.

Not recommended for routine preoperative screening because
  • General surgery patients without obvious risk factors for bleeding rarely have clinically significant increase in BT.

[24]Burns ER, Lawrence C. Bleeding time. A guide to its diagnostic and clinical utility. *Arch Pathol Lab Med* 1989;113:1219.

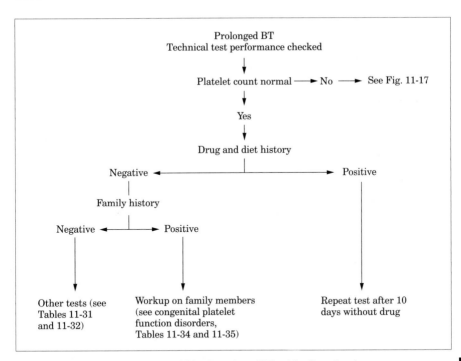

Fig. 11-13. Algorithm for prolonged bleeding time. (BT = bleeding time.)

- Even with a prolonged BT, blood loss does not exceed that of patients with normal BT.
- Prolonged BT does not necessarily cause increased bleeding.
- Therapeutic decisions are not likely to be changed by results of BT.
- Clinical history is the best preoperative screening.
- Not recommended for preoperative evaluation of patients receiving aspirin or NSAIDs, patients with liver disease, patients for coronary bypass. May be useful in preoperative screening of patients for eye, middle ear, brain, or knee surgery.

Usually Prolonged In

Thrombocytopenia
- Platelet count <100,000/cu mm and usually <80,000/cu mm before BT becomes abnormal and <40,000/cu mm before abnormality becomes pronounced. BT is almost always abnormal when platelet count is <60,000/cu mm except in conditions that have young supereffective platelets. BT may be normal in some patients with immune thrombocytopenic purpura with marked decrease in platelet count. When platelet count = 80,000/cu mm, BT should be ~10 mins; when platelet count = 40,000/cu mm, BT should be ~20 mins; when platelet count = <10,000/cu mm, BT should always be >30 mins if platelet function is normal. If results are beyond these values, patient may also have a qualitative platelet abnormality.

Platelet function disorders
- Hereditary
    Defect in plasma proteins
        von Willebrand's disease (especially 2 hrs after ingestion of 300 mg of aspirin)
        Deficient release of platelet glycoproteins
        Glanzmann's thrombasthenia
        Bernard-Soulier syndrome
    Defective release mechanisms
        Gray platelet syndrome
        Aspirin-like defect
        Storage pool deficiency

Others, e.g.,
    Wiskott-Aldrich syndrome
    Chédiak-Higashi syndrome
    Oculocutaneous albinism (Hermansky-Pudlak syndrome)
    Hereditary hemorrhagic telangiectasia
    Ehlers-Danlos syndrome
- Acquired
    Abnormal plasma factors
        Drugs
            Aspirin, NSAIDs (indomethacin, ibuprofen, phenylbutazone, etc.). Ingestion with ≤ 7 days is the most common cause of prolonged BT. Aspirin may double the baseline BT, which may still be within normal range. 325 mg of aspirin increases BT of most persons.
            Antimicrobials (especially high dose beta-lactam, e.g., carbenicillin; cephalosporins, nitrofurantoin, hydroxychloroquine)
            Anticoagulants (e.g., heparin, prostacyclin, streptokinase-streptodornase)
            Tricyclic antidepressants (e.g., imipramine, amitriptyline, nortriptyline)
            Phenothiazines (e.g., chlorpromazine, promethazine, trifluoperazine)
            Anesthetic (e.g., halothane, local)
            Methylxanthines (e.g., caffeine, theophylline, aminophylline)
        Others (e.g., dextrans, calcium channel–blocking agents, radiographic contrast agents, beta-adrenergic blockers, alcohol, aminocaproic acid, nitroglycerin)
            Uremia (may be corrected with vasopressin or cryoprecipitate)
            Fibrin degradation products (e.g., DIC, liver disease, fibrinolytic therapy)
            Macromolecules (e.g., dextran, paraproteins [myelomas, Waldenström's macroglobulinemia)
        Other immune thrombocytopenias
        Myeloproliferative diseases, including myelodysplastic syndrome, preleukemia, acute leukemia, hairy cell leukemia)
        Vasculitis
        Others (e.g., amyloidosis, viral infections, scurvy, after circulating through an oxygenator during cardiac bypass surgery)
Vascular disorders
Increased BT or BT increased out of proportion to platelet count suggests von Willebrand's disease or qualitative platelet defect.

Usually Normal In

Hemophilia
Severe hereditary hypoprothrombinemia
Severe hereditary hypofibrinogenemia

Clot Retraction

Use

Reflects platelet number and function.
Poor test of clotting function
Little value for detection of mild to moderate bleeding disorders

May Occur In

Various thrombocytopenias
Thrombasthenia

Coagulation (Clotting) Time (Lee-White Clotting Time)

Use

See Table 11-33.

Table 11-33. Effect of Anticoagulant Drugs on Coagulation Tests

Test	Heparin	Warfarin	Aspirin	Dipyridamole/ Sulfinpyrazone	Urokinase/ Streptokinase
Platelet count	N[a]	N	N	N	N
Inhibition of platelet aggregation	N or I	N	I	N	I
Bleeding time	N or I	N[b]	I	N	I
Clotting time	I	N[b]	N	N	I
Thrombin time	I	N	N	N	I
Prothrombin time	I	I	N[b]	N	I
Partial thrombo-plastin time	I	N[b]	N	N	I
Fibrinogen	N	N	N	N	D

D = decreased; I = increased; N = no change.
[a]Decreased in 25% of cases.
[b]Increased with high drug dosage.

Former routine method for control of heparin therapy but now replaced by aPTT. It is not a reliable screening test for bleeding conditions because it is not sensitive enough to detect mild conditions but only detects severe ones. Normal coagulation time does not rule out a coagulation defect. Many variables exist in the technique of performing the test. Routine preoperative bleeding and coagulation times are of little value for routine preoperative screening.

Prolonged In

Severe deficiency (<6%) of any known plasma clotting factors except factor XIII (fibrin-stabilizing factor) and factor VII
Afibrinogenemia
Presence of a circulating anticoagulant (including heparin)

Normal In

Thrombocytopenia
Deficiency of factor VII
Von Willebrand's disease
Mild coagulation defects due to any cause

Interferences

Increased In
Anticoagulants
Tetracyclines
Decreased In
Corticosteroids
Epinephrine

Fibrinogen Degradation Products

(Latex agglutination rapid test kit detects increased level [10 μg/mL] in serum and parallels results with hemagglutination inhibition [HAI] method. Detects major breakdown products of fibrin or fibrinogen. Does not distinguish between fibrinolysis and fibrinogenolysis.)

Use

Aid in diagnosis of DIC

HEMATOL

Increased in Serum

DIC

In association with fibrinolytic therapy

Thromboembolic events

- Pulmonary embolism—peak values may be transient.
- Postoperative deep venous thrombosis.
- AMI during first 24–48 hrs.
- Certain disorders of pregnancy.
- Small increases with exercise, anxiety, stress, severe liver disease.

Increased in Urine

Kidney disease

- UTI—increased in infection of upper tract but not of bladder.
- Proliferative GN—level falls during response to drug therapy.
- Rejection of renal transplant.

Conditions causing increased serum level (see previous paragraph)

Interferences

RF may cause false-positive.

Heparin, Plasma

Use

Monitor heparin therapy in selected situations.

- Combined heparin and warfarin therapy
- Combined heparin and recombinant tissue plasminogen activator therapy
- Heparin resistance in presence of a circulating anticoagulant
- Altered plasma clotting proteins (e.g., increased factor I or VIII or platelet factor 4 or decreased antithrombin III)
- When aPTT appears to be unsatisfactory for heparin therapy control (e.g., overwhelming infections, myocardial infarction, severe liver disease)
- Use of low-molecular-weight heparins

To prove unrecognized heparin administration (e.g., indwelling catheter)

Partial Thromboplastin Time, Activated (aPTT)

See Table 11-33 and Figs. 11-14, 11-15, and 11-16.

Use

Monitor heparin therapy

Screen for hemophilia A and B

Detect clotting inhibitors

aPTT is the *best single screening test* for disorders of coagulation; it is abnormal in 90% of patients with coagulation disorders when properly performed. Screens for all coagulation factors that contribute to thrombin formation except factors VII and XIII.

The test may not detect mild clotting defects (25–40% of normal levels), which seldom cause significant bleeding.

Not recommended for preoperative screening of asymptomatic adult unless patient has specific clinical indication (e.g., active bleeding, known or suspected bleeding disorders [including anticoagulant use], liver disease, malabsorption, malnutrition, other conditions associated with acquired coagulopathies, in which procedure may interfere with normal coagulation).

Prolonged By

Defect in factors (assays <30% of normal; intrinsic pathway)

- I (fibrinogen)
- II (prothrombin)

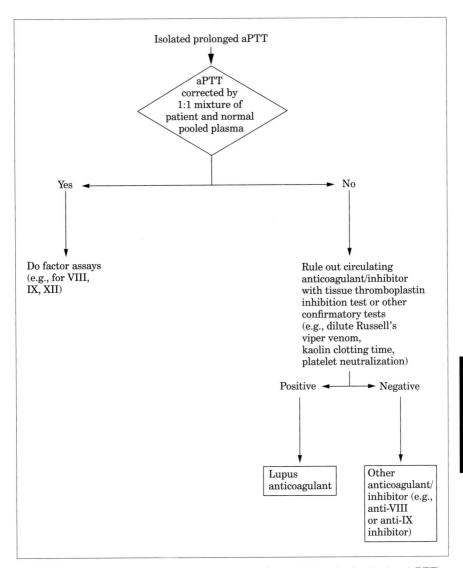

Fig. 11-14. Algorithm for isolated prolonged activated partial thromboplastin time (aPTT).

- V (labile factor)
- VIII*
- IX*
- X (Stuart-Prower factor)
- XI*
- XII (Hageman factor)

Presence of specific inhibitors of clotting factors* (most frequently antibody against factor VIII, which occurs in ~15% of multitransfused patients with severe hemophilia A and less frequently in mild/moderate hemophilia A; and against circulating lupus anticoagulant). *Mixing equal parts of patient's plasma and normal plasma corrects aPTT (or PT) if due to coagulation factor deficiency but not if due to an inhibitor.*

Heparin

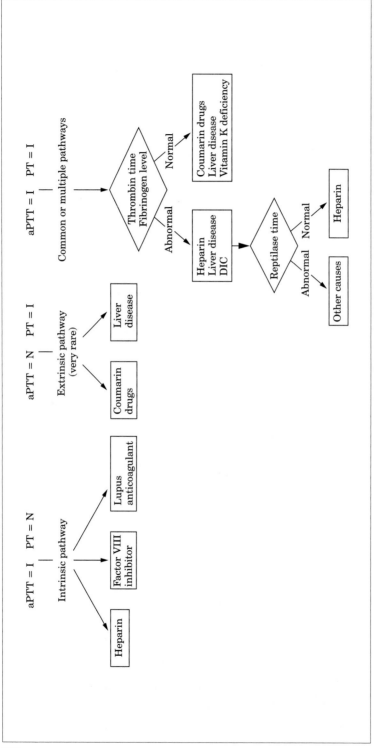

Fig. 11-15. Algorithm for acquired coagulation disorders. (I = increased; N = normal; DIC = disseminated intravascular coagulation.)

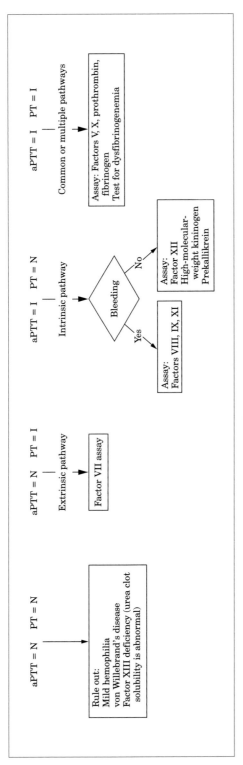

Fig. 11-16. Algorithm for hereditary coagulation disorders. (I = increased; N = normal; PT = prothrombin time; aPTT = partial thromboplastin time.)

Warfarin
Lupus anticoagulant*

*May cause isolated prolonged aPTT.

Normal In

Thrombocytopenia
Platelet dysfunction
Von Willebrand's disease (may be prolonged in some patients)
Isolated defects of factor VII

Interferences

Very increased or decreased Hct (e.g., polycythemia) that alters citrate concentration
    or inadequate citrate in collection tube
Specimen contamination with EDTA
Clots in specimen
Partially filled collection tube
Values may be falsely very high if plasma is very turbid or icteric when photoelectric
    machines are used.
Drugs other than heparin
Hirudin analogues and argatroban, warfarin
Less frequently (e.g., hematin, hydroxyethyl starch, suramin, Taularidine [an additive
    in some IV medications])
Drugs that may inhibit heparin action (e.g., antihistamines, digitalis, nicotine, peni-
    cillin (IV), protamine, tetracycline, phenothiazine)

Plasminogen

(Normal adults = 76–124% for males, 65–153% for females; infants = 27–59%)

Use

Is one indicator of fibrinolytic activity
Monitor fibrinolytic therapy with streptokinase or urokinase

May Be Decreased In

Some familial or isolated cases of idiopathic deep venous thrombosis; autosomal defi-
    ciency or dysplasminogenemia
Diabetic patients with thrombosis
DIC and systemic fibrinolysis
Behçet's disease
Cirrhosis of the liver

Platelet Aggregation Studies

**(Platelet aggregation stimulated by certain agonistic drugs is measured in vitro by
    turbidimeter, shown graphically by wave patterns.)**
See Table 11-34.

Use

Classification of congenital qualitative platelet functional abnormalities of adhesion,
    release, or aggregation (e.g., storage pool disease, Glanzmann's thrombasthenia,
    Bernard-Soulier syndrome)
Rarely useful to evaluate acquired bleeding disorders.

Interferences

Aspirin may produce characteristic abnormalities of release defects with decreased
    thromboxane A_2 synthesis.
Myeloproliferative diseases and uremia: abnormal aggregation to epinephrine, adeno-
    sine diphosphate (ADP), and collagen

Table 11-34. Congenital Functional Platelet Disorders

| | | Platelet Aggregation | | | |
| | | ADP or Epinephrine | | | |
	Platelet Retention in Glass Bead	1st Phase	2nd Phase	Ristocetin	Collagen
Bernard-Soulier syndrome	D	N	N	D	N
Glanzmann's throm-basthenia	D	D	D	N	D
Release defect	N or D	N	D	N	D
Storage pool disease	N or D	N	D	N	D
Von Willebrand's disease	D	N	N	D	N

D = depressed; N = normal; ADP = adenosine diphosphate.
Source: Bowie DJW. Recognition of easily missed bleeding mistakes. *Mayo Clin Proc* 1982;57:263.

Aggregation may also be abnormal due to dysproteinemia, lipemia, hemolysis, various drugs (e.g., NSAIDs), and cardiopulmonary bypass.

Interpretation

ADP and epinephrine produce primary and secondary waves of aggregation; collagen, arachidonic acid, and ristocetin produce only primary waves

Disorder	Decreased Aggregation
Von Willebrand's disease, Bernard-Soulier syndrome	Ristocetin
Thrombasthenia	All agents except ristocetin
Release defects	
Storage pool disease	See Table 11-34
Idiopathic	ADP, epinephrine, collagen
Abnormal thromboxane A_2 synthesis	Arachidonic acid, ADP, epinephrine, collagen
Afibrinogenemia	No primary or secondary waves to ADP

Platelet Aggregation, Ristocetin-Induced

(Not same as ristocetin cofactor assay)
Increased In
Von Willebrand's disease (type IIB)
Platelet-type von Willebrand's disease
Type I New York von Willebrand's disease

Decreased In

Von Willebrand's disease (types I, IIA, IIC, III)
ITP
Storage pool disease
Bernard-Soulier syndrome
Acute myeloblastic leukemia
Aspirin ingestion
Infectious mononucleosis
Cirrhosis

Platelet Count

See Tables 11-34, 11-35, and 11-36 and Fig. 11-17.

HEMATOL

Table 11-35. Some Congenital Hemorrhagic Diseases due to Disorders of Platelet-Vessel Wall

Platelet Defects

Bernard-Soulier syndrome	Moderate thrombocytopenia
	Bleeding time markedly increased
	Large platelets
	Decreased ristocetin-induced agglutination not corrected by vWF
Glanzmann's thrombasthenia	Normal platelet count and morphology
	Increased bleeding time
	Clot retraction absent or much decreased
	No platelet aggregation with any agonists
Pseudo-von Willebrand's disease	Variable mild thrombocytopenia
	Increased bleeding time
	Increased ristocetin-induced agglutination
	Variable plasma immunoreactive vWF
Gray-platelet syndrome	Moderate thrombocytopenia
	Large platelets
	Bleeding time slightly increased
	Platelets agranular on blood smear
	Abnormal platelet aggregation with collagen or thrombin
Dense-granule deficiency syndrome	Normal platelet count
	Normal platelet morphology on blood smear
	Bleeding time variably increased
	Abnormal aggregation with ADP and collagen
Deficiency of platelet enzyme (cyclo-oxygenase or thromboxane synthetase)	Normal platelet count and morphology
	Abnormal aggregation with ADP, collagen, and arachidonic acid
May-Hegglin anomaly	Autosomal dominant trait
	Moderate thrombocytopenia with huge platelets; normal platelet function
	Döhle's bodies in granulocytes

Plasma Defects

Von Willebrand's disease	Normal platelet count and morphology
	Increased bleeding time
	Abnormal ristocetin-induced agglutination
	Abnormal plasma vWF
Afibrinogenemia	Normal platelet morphology
	Mild thrombocytopenia occasionally
	Bleeding time variably increased
	Plasma coagulation abnormalities

Vessel Wall Defects

Genetic disorders of connective tissue	Platelets may be large
	Collagen-induced aggregation may be abnormal

ADP = adenosine diphosphate; vWF = von Willebrand's factor.

Table 11-36. Comparison of Congenital Disorders of Platelet Function

Platelet Disorder	Platelet Count	Bleeding Time	PT/aPTT	Fibrinogen	Aggregation Ristocetin	ADP
Aspirin induced	N	A	N	N	N	A
Bernard-Soulier syndrome	A	A	N	N	A	N
Congenital afibrino-genemia	N	A	A	A	N	A
Glanzmann's throm-basthenia	N	A	N	N	N	A
Storage pool deficiency	N	A	N	N	N	A
von Willebrand's disease	N	A	N/A	N	A	N

N = normal; A = abnormal; ADP = adenosine diphosphate.

Increased In

(>450,000/cu mm; <1 million/cu mm in 97% of patients)
Myeloproliferative disease (e.g., polycythemia vera, CML, agnogenic myeloid metaplasia, essential thrombocythemia)
Malignancy, especially disseminated, advanced, or inoperable, accounts for ~13% of cases in hospital patients.
Patients recently having surgery, especially splenectomy (accounts for ~19% of cases in hospital patients); or experiencing severe trauma, massive acute hemorrhage, or thrombotic episodes.
Infections account for ~31% of cases in hospital patients.
Chronic inflammation as in inflammatory bowel disease, collagen diseases, and RA
Iron-deficiency anemia
Miscellaneous disease states (e.g., cardiac disease, cirrhosis of the liver, chronic pancreatitis, ARDS in neonates, burns, hypothermia, preeclampsia, ethanol withdrawal, renal failure, splenectomy)
~50% of patients with "unexpected" increase of platelet count are found to have a malignancy.

Decreased In

(Thrombocytopenia)
Acquired
  • Decreased platelet production (e.g., aplastic anemia, myelophthisis, exposure to ionizing radiation, nutritional deficiencies [folate, vitamin B_{12}, etc.], drug effects [alcohol, chemotherapeutic agents, etc.])
  • Infections (e.g., AIDS, SBE, septicemia, typhus, rubella, infectious mononucleosis) may have several mechanisms.
  • Increased platelet destruction.
◆ *Antiplatelet antibodies* (IgG and IgM) may be found in plasma and by flow cytometry, may be detected on platelets in most patients with drug-induced thrombocytopenia (e.g., heparin, quinidine, procainamide, quinine) (sensitivity = 90%). 15–29% of patients with autoimmune thrombocytopenia have only platelet-associated IgM. Negative results in plasma and on platelets argues strongly against an immune cause of thrombocytopenia. Platelet-associated IgG may be seen in ITP (see p.473), sepsis, aplastic anemia, acute leukemia, SLE (see p. 895), immune vasculitis, drugs.
      Drug-induced immune thrombocytopenia (e.g., quinidine, quinine, gold, sulfonamides, penicillins; heparin causes thrombocytopenia in ≤ 10% of patients, usually in 5–10 days)

HEMATOL

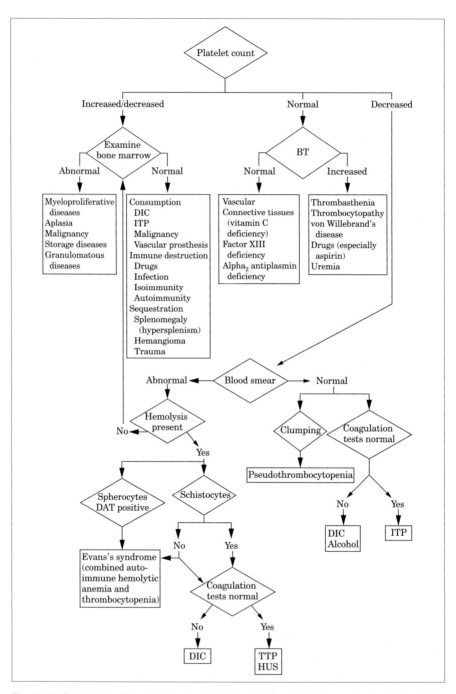

Fig. 11-17. Evaluation of hemostatic abnormalities. (Prothrombin time and activated partial thromboplastin time—see Figs. 11-15 and 11-16.) (BT = bleeding time; DAT = direct antiglobulin test [Coombs']; DIC = disseminated intravascular coagulation; HUS = hemolytic uremic syndrome; ITP = idiopathic thrombocytopenic purpura; TTP = thrombic thrombocytopenic purpura.)

Neonatal alloimmune thrombocytopenia—uncommon condition that may cause intracranial hemorrhage in utero or at birth with death or neurologic impairment. Due to maternal platelet-specific antibody against infant platelet antigen inherited from father but absent in mother. Unexplained petechiae/purpura at birth, platelet count <100,000/cu mm. Treated by transfusion of mother's platelet concentrate.

Lymphoproliferative disorders

Posttransfusion (develops in 5–10 days; complement-fixing antibody for platelet antigen P1^{A1} establishes diagnosis)

Extracorporeal circulation

- Increased platelet consumption

    TTP

    DIC

    Septicemia

    Toxemia of pregnancy (≤ 20% of cases)

    Massive blood loss

Hypersplenism

- Cirrhosis
- Dilutional (e.g., after massive transfusion)
- Renal insufficiency
- Paroxysmal nocturnal hemoglobinuria

Inherited

- Allport's syndrome
- Bernard-Soulier syndrome
- Chédiak-Higashi syndrome
- Ehlers-Danlos syndrome
- May-Hegglin anomaly
- Wiskott-Aldrich syndrome
- Glanzmann's thrombasthenia
- Hermansky-Pudlak syndrome
- TAR (*t*hrombocytopenia, *a*bsent *r*adius bones) syndrome

When associated with anemia and microangiopathy on peripheral smear, rule out DIC, TTP, hemolytic-uremic syndrome, prosthetic valve dysfunction, malignant hypertension, eclampsia, vasculitis, leaking aortic aneurysm, disseminated metastatic cancer.

Interferences

Pseudothrombocytopenia diagnosis by examination of stained blood smear

- Platelet clumping induced by EDTA blood collection tubes is the most common cause.
- Platelet satellitosis.
- Platelet cold agglutinins.
- Giant platelets.
- RBC count >6.5 million/cu mm.

Pseudothrombocytosis

- Cryoglobulinemia
- Malaria parasites
- Fragments of RBCs or WBCs
- Microspherocytes
- Howell-Jolly bodies, nucleated RBCs, Heinz bodies, clumped Pappenheimer bodies

50,000–150,000/cu mm—usually no bleeding

20,000–50,000/cu mm—minor spontaneous bleeding; postoperative bleeding

<20,000/cu mm—may have more serious bleeding.

5000/cu mm—frequently has serious bleeding.

Platelet transfusions are not used if >20,000/cu mm except preoperatively or when a specific bleeding lesion (e.g., peptic ulcer) is present.

One unit of platelet concentrate increases the platelet count by 15,000/cu mm in the average 70-kg adult; therefore minimal dose to administer is six units. No increment in 60 mins suggests that alloimmunization has occurred (should use single-donor platelets); >5000/cu mm increment suggests that alloimmunization has not occurred.

Platelet Function Defects, Acquired

Due To

Uremia

Fibrinogen degradation products (e.g., liver disease, DIC, primary fibrinolytic syndromes)

Myeloproliferative syndromes may show any combination of platelet aggregation defects that are not characteristic.

Paraprotein coating of platelet membranes (e.g., multiple myeloma, Waldenström's macroglobulinemia, essential monoclonal gammopathy)

Autoimmune diseases (e.g., collagen vascular disease, antiplatelet antibodies, immune thrombocytopenias)

Anemias (e.g., severe deficiency of iron, B_{12}, or folate)

Drug effects

- Interference with platelet membrane receptors (e.g., amitriptyline, imipramine, doxepin, chlorpromazine, cocaine, lidocaine [Xylocaine], isoproterenol, propranolol, cephalothin, ampicillin, penicillin, others)
- Inhibition of prostaglandin pathways (e.g., aspirin, indomethacin, ibuprofen, phenylbutazone, naproxen, furosemide, verapamil, others)
- Inhibition of platelet phosphodiesterase activity (e.g., caffeine, aminophylline, theophylline, papaverine, others)
- Unknown mechanisms (e.g., dicumarol, heparin, chlortetracycline, glycerol guaiacolate, others)

Platelet Volume, Mean

(Limited value when measured by routine automated hematology instruments)

Normal = 7.4–10.4 fL

Use

Indicates uniformity or heterogeneity of size of platelet population.

Study of thrombocytopenic patients

- Increased mean platelet volume with thrombocytopenia indicates that thrombopoiesis is stimulated and platelet production is increased.
- Normal mean platelet volume with thrombocytopenia indicates impaired thrombopoiesis.

Increased In

Immune thrombocytopenic purpura

Thrombocytopenia due to sepsis (recovery phase)

Myeloproliferative disorders

Massive hemorrhage

Prosthetic heart valve

Splenectomy

Vasculitis

Decreased In

Wiskott-Aldrich syndrome

Protein C, Plasma

Normal range = 70–130%

Use

Detect hypercoagulable states associated with episodes of venous thrombosis

Decreased In

Hereditary (autosomal dominant) deficiency (heterozygote levels are usually 30–65%; found in screening in 1 in 300 persons; thrombosis is not usual if level >50%). *Estab-*

lishes the diagnosis of purpura fulminans, which is seen in homozygous infants (usually <1% of normal). *Warfarin-induced skin necrosis is almost pathognomonic for protein C deficiency.*

Liver disease
DIC (not diagnostically useful)
Postoperative state
Malignancy
ARDS
Pregnancy
Oral contraceptive use
High loading dose of warfarin causes transient rapid drop in protein C levels.
L-Asparaginase therapy
Decreases with age (~4% per decade).

Protein S, Plasma

Use

Detect hypercoagulable states associated with episodes of venous thrombosis
Should be assayed whenever protein C is assayed; both are vitamin K–dependent inhibitors of coagulation. Heterozygotes with levels of 30–60% may have episodes of recurrent thrombosis. Functional rather than immunologic tests are preferred to detect qualitative as well as quantitative deficiency.

Decreased In

Pregnancy
First month of life
Oral anticoagulant or contraceptive use
Acute-phase reaction
DIC (not diagnostically useful)
Nephrotic syndrome
Liver disease
L-Asparaginase therapy
Deep venous thrombosis in some patients

Prothrombin Consumption

Impaired by

Any defect in phase I or phase II of blood coagulation
- Thrombocytopathies
- Thrombocytopenia
- Hypoprothrombinemia
- Hemophilias
- Circulating anticoagulants
- Other

Prothrombin Time (PT)

See Table 11-33 and 11-36.

Use

Primarily for three purposes:
- Control of long-term oral anticoagulant therapy with coumarins and indanedione derivatives.
- Evaluation of liver function—PT is the most useful test of impaired liver synthesis of prothrombin complex factors (factors II, VII, X, proteins C and S).
- Evaluation of coagulation disorders—screen for abnormality of factors involved in extrinsic pathway (factors V, VII, X, prothrombin, fibrinogen). Should be used with aPTT.

Prolonged by Defect In

(Assays <30% of normal; extrinsic pathway)
Factor I (fibrinogen)
Factor II (prothrombin)
Factor V (labile factor)
Factor VII (stable factor)
Factor X (Stuart-Prower factor)

Prolonged In

Inadequate vitamin K in diet
Premature infants
Newborn infants of vitamin K–deficient mothers (hemorrhagic disease of the newborn)
Poor fat absorption (e.g., obstructive jaundice, fistulas, sprue, steatorrhea, celiac disease, colitis, chronic diarrhea)
Severe liver damage (e.g., poisoning, hepatitis, cirrhosis)
Drugs (e.g., coumarin-type drugs for anticoagulant therapy, salicylates)
Factitious ingestion of warfarin
Idiopathic familial hypoprothrombinemia
Circulating anticoagulants
Hypofibrinogenemia (acquired or inherited)
Heparin
Lupus anticoagulant

Reporting

PT should be reported as ratio of patient results to control rather than as percentage.
PT may also be reported as INR (international normalized ratio) only for patients on oral anticoagulants for ≥ 2 wks who have stable PTs and responded appropriately to the drug. INR = ratio of patient PT to mean of PT reference range for that laboratory raised to the power of the international sensitivity index (index is provided by the thromboplastin manufacturer). Is intended to take into account differences due to different methods or thromboplastin-instrument combinations in interpretation of results. Suggested INR range = 2.0–3.0 for standard-dose therapy for treatment or prophylaxis of venous thrombosis or pulmonary or systemic embolus. Suggested INR range = 2.5–3.5 for high-risk patients with mechanical heart valves. *Note: INR is dependent on instrumentation. Sensitive thromboplastin (low international sensitivity index) leads to undertreatment and insensitive thromboplastin (high international sensitivity index) leads to overtreatment.*

Ristocetin Cofactor Activity

Use

Differential diagnosis of von Willebrand's disease

Decreased In

Von Willebrand's disease type I
Von Willebrand's disease type IIA
Cirrhosis

Thrombin Time

Use

Detects abnormal fibrinogen

Increased In

Fibrinogen levels that are very low (<80 mg/dL) or high (>400 mg/dL)
Interference with polymerization of fibrin
 • Fibrin degradation products, especially DIC.

- High concentrations of monoclonal immunoglobulins (e.g., myeloma, macroglobulinemia) interfere with fibrin monomer polymerization.
- Uremia.
- Dysfibrinogenemia (abnormal fibrinogen present).

Heparin contamination of specimen is common cause in hospital patients; however, a reptilase test is normal in presence of heparin but prolonged by other causes listed in previous section.

Antithrombin antibodies

Tourniquet Test

Use

Differential diagnosis of purpura

Positive In

Thrombocytopenic purpuras
Nonthrombocytopenic purpuras
Thrombocytopathies
Scurvy

Disorders of Coagulation

See Table 11-35.

Afibrinogenemia, Congenital

(Rare inherited autosomal recessive congenital condition)
See Tables 11-34 through 11-36.
♦ Plasma fibrinogen is absent.
BT is often increased (one-third of patients).
PT, aPTT, and thrombin time are abnormal.
Platelet-to-glass adhesiveness is abnormal unless fibrinogen is added.

Bernard-Soulier Syndrome

(Rare autosomal recessive absence or dysfunction of platelet membrane glycoproteins Ib receptor, V, IX [AQ37] that enable platelets to bind vWF)
See Tables 11-34, 11-35, and 11-36.
○Mild or moderate thrombocytopenia, usually 25,000–80,000/cu mm. Hemorrhage and increased BT are excessively severe for degree of thrombocytopenia.
Normal clot retraction.
Giant platelets on smear.
Abnormal vWF adhesion and ristocetin aggregation; other aggregations normal.
♦ Platelet membrane analysis using monoclonal antibodies with flow cytometry allows definite diagnosis.

Coagulation Disorders, Neonatal

Severe forms of factor VIII and IX deficiency cause most hemorrhagic congenital coagulation problems in newborns. In severe forms, bleeding occurs within the first week in 50% of cases (especially due to circumcision).
Congenital deficiency of factor XIII (see p. 475)
Hemorrhagic disease of the newborn (see p. 476) may be associated with anticonvulsant drug therapy (e.g., phenytoin, phenobarbital) in mother, severe liver disease in infant. *Water-soluble forms of vitamin K may precipitate hemolysis in newborns, especially in presence of G-6-PD.*
DIC (see p. 464)
In a child with excessive bleeding, the following six tests can usually be done on ≤ 2 mL of blood within 1 hr: platelet count, PT, PTT, fibrinogen level, BT, thrombin time.

Presence of large numbers of platelets and especially clumps of platelets on smear excludes thrombocytopenia as cause of bleeding in newborns.

Abnormal hemostasis is rare in the healthy full-term infant. Most of the bleeding disorders seen by primary care physicians are acquired rather than inherited abnormalities of coagulation and are expressions of underlying disease.

Incidence of Inherited Congenital Coagulation Factors

(Autosomal recessive except factors IX and VIII, which are X-linked recessive, and factor II)

XI	Rare
IX	1 in 100,000
VIII	1 in 25,000
VII	1 in 500,000
X	1 in 500,000
V	1 in 1,000,000
II (prothrombin)	Rare
I (fibrinogen)	Rare
XIII	Rare

In the sick neonate, thrombocytopenia is the most common cause of abnormal hemostasis; less common are DIC, vitamin K deficiency, inadequate liver function. The cause of neonatal thrombocytopenia (e.g., sepsis, DIC) is discovered in only 40% of the cases.

Coagulopathy due to Liver Disease

Screening tests may include any combination of abnormal PTT, aPTT, thrombin time, euglobulin or whole-blood clot lysis times, increased fibrin degradation products. These are corrected by mixture of equal parts of patient and normal plasma, except thrombin time if large amounts of fibrin degradation products are present due to hyperplasminemia or if fibrin polymerization is faulty. Special tests may show decreased antithrombin III, decrease in any coagulation factor (except factor VIII:c, which is normal or increased in liver disease but decreased in DIC), decreased $alpha_2$-antiplasmin.

Disseminated Intravascular Coagulation (DIC)[25,26]

(Widespread fibrin thrombi in microcirculation with rapid concurrent consumption of platelets and coagulation proteins and activation of thrombin; more than one mechanism is often present)

See Tables 11-37 through 11-40.

Due To

Incidence	(% of Cases)
• Infections	
Sepsis is most common cause (Gram positive and negative)	30–50%
Meningococcemia	
Rocky Mountain spotted fever	
Viremia (CMV and HIV infection, hepatitis, varicella)	
• Pregnancy and obstetric complications, e.g.,	50%
Retained dead fetus syndrome (in 50% of cases with fetus retained 5 wks)	
Eclampsia (fulminant in 10–15% of patients)	
Amniotic fluid embolism	
Abruptio placentae	
Saline-induced abortion	
• Trauma with extensive tissue injury (e.g., crush injuries, burns, extensive surgery, shock, fat embolism)	50–70%
• Metastatic neoplasms, especially prostate	10–15%
Necrosis due to chemotherapy or irradiation	
Acute leukemia, especially acute promyelocytic	15%

[25]Sirridge M. Laboratory evaluation of the bleeding patient. *Clin Lab Med* 1984;4:285.
[26]Levi M, ten Cate H. Disseminated intravascular coagulation. *N Engl J Med* 1999;341:586.

Table 11-37. Disseminated Intravascular Coagulation (Consumption Coagulopathy)

Determination	% of Cases Abnormal	Abnormal Level for DIC	Mean Values for DIC	Response to Heparin Therapy	Tests
Decreased platelet count (per cu mm)	93	<150,000	52,000	None or may take wks*	Platelet count, PT, fibrinogen level are performed first as screening tests; if all three are positive, diagnosis is considered established. If only two of these are positive, diagnosis should be confirmed by at least one of the tests for fibrinolysis.
Increased PT (secs)	90	>15	18.0	Becomes normal or falls >5 secs in few hrs to 1 day	
Decreased fibrinogen level (mg/dL)	71	<160	137	Rises significantly (>40 mg) in 1–3 days	
Latex test for fibrinogen degradation products (titer)	92	>1:16	1:52	Begins to fall in 1 day; if very high, may take >1 wk to become normal	Tests for fibrinolysis.
Prolonged thrombin time (secs)	59	>25	27		
Euglobulin clot lysis time (mins)	42	<120		Returns to normal	

DIC = disseminated intravascular coagulation.
*Platelet count is not a satisfactory indicator of response to heparin therapy.
Adapted from Colman RW, Robboy SJ, Mimna JD. Disseminated intravascular coagulation (DIC): an approach. *Am J Med* 1972;52:679.

Table 11-38. Comparison of Acute Disseminated Intravascular Coagulation (DIC) and Primary Fibrinogenolysis

	Acute DIC	Fibrinogenolysis
Platelet count	D	Usually N
Fibrinogen	D	D
Fibrin degradation products	O to very marked I	Very marked I
Protamine sulfate test	Positive	Negative
Euglobulin clot lysis time	N	D
Factor V	D	D
Factor VIII	D	N to moderate D

O = absent; D = decreased; I = increased; N = normal.

Table 11-39. Comparison of Acute and Chronic Disseminated Intravascular Coagulation (DIC)

	Acute DIC	Chronic DIC
Platelet count	D (moderate/marked)	D (mild/marked)
Prothrombin time	I	N or slight I
Activated partial thromboplastin time	I	N or D
Thrombin time	I	N or moderate I
Fibrinogen	D	I, N, or moderate D
Fibrin degradation products	Present	Present
Protamine sulfate test	Positive	Positive
Factors V and VIII	D	N

D = decreased; I = increased; N = normal.

- Vascular disorders
  Giant hemangioma of Kasabach-Merritt syndrome   25%
  Large aortic aneurism   <1%
  Cardiac, peripheral
- Connective tissue diseases
- Toxins (e.g., snakebites, brown recluse spider bite, drugs)
- Injury to platelets or RBCs (e.g., immunologic hemolytic anemias)
- Prosthetic devices (e.g., aortic balloon, LeVeen shunt)
- RE system injury—liver disease (e.g., acute hepatic failure, obstructive jaundice, cirrhosis, hepatitis), postsplenectomy

♦ *Criteria for specific diagnosis are not well defined. No single test is diagnostic, and diagnosis usually depends on combination of findings. Single normal level does not rule out DIC and a repeat test screen should be done a few hours later for changes in platelet count and fibrinogen.*
♦ Repeated aPTT and PT (if initially prolonged), platelet count, and fibrinogen levels are particularly useful for screening. Normal in 25% of cases of acute DIC. If any are abnormal, follow with tests for fibrinogen degradation products and D-dimer.
♦ Most sensitive and specific tests
  - Test for fibrin degradation products (FDP) in serum >20 μg/mL (may be >100 μg/mL; normal = 0–10 μg/mL); sensitivity = 85–100%, specificity = ~50%.
  - Positive D-dimer assay is specific for fibrin and is more reliable indicator of DIC (~100% specificity) than FDP assay because D-dimer is negative in cases of primary fibrinolysis. Thus combination of FDP and D-dimer tests = 100% sensitive and specific.

Table 11-40. Differential Diagnosis of Disseminated Intravascular Coagulation (DIC)

	DIC	Chronic Liver Disease	Primary Fibrinolysis	TTP	Hemolytic-Uremic Syndrome	Multiple Transfusion
Platelet count	D	D	N	N–D	D	D
PT	I	I	I	N	N	I
aPTT	I	N–I	I	N	N	I
FDP	I	N–I	I	N–I	N–I	N
D-Dimer assay	I	N	I	N	N	N
Fibrinogen	D	V	D	N	N	I
Schistocytes	+	O	+	+	+	O
BUN	I	N	N	I	I	N
Liver function tests	N	I	N	N	N	N
Protamine sulfate	I	N–I	I	N–I	N	N
Euglobulin clot lysis	N	N	D	N	N	N

I = increased; N = normal; + = present; aPTT = activated partial thromboplastin time; D = decreased; FDP = fibrin degradation products; O = absent; V = variable; TTP = thrombotic thrombocytopenic purpura.

- Declining serial fibrinogen levels to <150 μg/dL); specificity >95% but sensitivity only ~25%.
- Antithrombin III is useful for diagnosis and to monitor therapy but immunologic assay should not be used.
- Fibrinopeptide A is increased.
- Protamine sulfate or ethanol gelation (reflect fibrinogen degradation products but are less specific). A negative protamine test argues against ongoing DIC; ethanol test is less sensitive and may produce false-negative results.

Less sensitive and specific tests
- PT (should be done serially if prolonged)
- aPTT (increased in 50–60% of acute DIC cases)
- Decreased platelet count (in ~90% of cases) and abnormal platelet function tests (e.g., BT, platelet aggregation)
- Thrombin time

Least sensitive and specific tests
- Euglobulin clot lysis measures fibrinolytic activity in plasma
- Peripheral blood smear examination

In addition, the following abnormalities often occur:
- Schistocytes in the peripheral blood smear and other evidence of microangiopathic hemolytic anemia may be present (e.g., increased serum LD, decreased serum haptoglobin).
- Cryofibrinogen may be present.
- Observation of the blood clot may show the clot that forms to be small, friable, and wispy because of the hypofibrinogenemia.
- Plasma factors V, VIII, and XIII are usually significantly decreased but results are useless for diagnosis.
- Survival time of radioiodine-labeled fibrinogen and rate of incorporation of ^{14}C-labeled glycine ethyl ester into soluble "circulating fibrin" are sensitive indicators of DIC.

Clotting time determinations are used to monitor heparin therapy.

◯*Suspect clinically in patients with underlying conditions who show bleeding (frequently acute and dramatic), purpura or petechiae, acrocyanosis, arterial or venous thrombosis.*

HEMATOL

Dysfibrinogenemia, Congenital

(Rare congenital, autosomal dominant heterogeneous group of disorders due to synthesis of abnormal fibrinogen molecules; patients may have no bleeding diathesis)

Fibrin formation is abnormally slow with prolonged plasma thrombin time.

♦ Dysfibrinogenemia is present if immunologic fibrinogen is >2× functional fibrinogen. Other coagulation factors are normal.

Dysfibrinogenemia may also occur in liver disease, cancer, fibrinolysis, DIC.

Factor V Deficiency (Parahemophilia)

(Inherited autosomal recessive deficiency syndrome or acquired in association with severe liver disease or DIC)

PT and aPTT are increased but corrected by addition of absorbed plasma.

Congenital

Infrequent bleeding occurs only in the homozygote.

Variable increase in PT, prothrombin consumption, and coagulation time is not corrected by administration of vitamin K.

♦ Factor V assay

Factor VII Deficiency

(Inherited form is autosomal recessive trait and is rare; acquired type may be due to liver disease, vitamin K deficiency, or dicumarol therapy)

PT is increased but corrected by aged serum.

aPTT is normal.

♦ Factor VII assay

Factor VII Deficiency, Congenital

(With this infrequent autosomal trait, bleeding occurs when the gene is homozygous; heterozygotes have little or no manifestations.)

Increased PT is not corrected by administration of vitamin K (PT is normal when viper venom is used as thromboplastin; this does not correct PT in factor X deficiency).

BT, coagulation time, clot retraction, and prothrombin consumption are normal.

♦ Factor VII assay

Factor VIII (Antihemophilic Globulin) Deficiency (Hemophilia)

(X-linked recessive deficiency or abnormal synthesis of factor VIII)

♦ Classic hemophilia (factor VIII assay <1%) shows increased coagulation time, prothrombin consumption time, and aPTT; prolonged BT in ~20% of patients (see Table 11-32).

♦ Moderate hemophilia (factor VIII assay 1–5%) shows normal coagulation time and normal prothrombin consumption time but increased aPTT.

♦ In mild hemophilia (factor VIII assay <16%) and "subhemophilia" (factor VIII assay 20–30%), these laboratory tests may be normal; patients seldom bleed except after surgery.

Screening tests for factor VIII deficiency: normal PT and platelet count, prolonged aPTT, thrombin time, BT

Secondary tests: factor VIII:C, factor VIII:Ag, platelet aggregation, platelet agglutination, ristocetin cofactor

♦ Specific factor assay is required to differentiate from factor IX deficiency (hemophilia B).

Laboratory findings due to hemorrhage and anemia.

"Acquired" hemophilia may occur when an inhibitor (autoantibody) is present, usually occurring spontaneously but may be associated with autoimmune or lymphoproliferative disorders, pregnancy and postpartum states, or allergy to drugs, especially penicillin. aPTT mixing studies distinguish factor deficiency from antibody: pooled normal plasma supplies missing factor and corrects clotting time in case of deficiency, but antibody inhibits normal plasma causing incomplete correction of aPTT.

Antibodies develop in ~20% of patients receiving repeated transfusion of factor VIII products, prolonging aPTT and lowering factor VIII activity of normal plasma.

♦ Prenatal diagnosis during eighth to tenth week of pregnancy by DNA analysis of amniocytes or chorionic villus material or by analysis of fetal blood at 12–14 wks for VIII:C and VIII:Ag.

Carrier status determination by pedigree analysis and laboratory studies is 95% accurate in ~80% of women.

>75% of patients with severe hemophilia who received multiple doses of factor concentrate before 1985 are HIV positive; many have AIDS. High incidence of viral hepatitis seropositivity.

Factor IX (Plasma Thromboplastin Component) Deficiency (Christmas Disease; Hemophilia B)

(Inherited recessive X-linked deficiency)
In severe cases, increased coagulation time, BT, prothrombin consumption time, and aPTT are found.

Defect is corrected by administration of frozen plasma just as well as by bank blood.

♦ Factor IX assay

Factor X (Stuart-Prower) Deficiency

(Rare autosomal recessive defect resembles factor VII deficiency; heterozygotes show mild or no clinical manifestations)
Increased PT (not corrected by use of viper venom as thromboplastin) is not corrected by administration of vitamin K. Heterozygotes may have only slight increase in PT.

♦ Factor X assay

Acquired form may be associated with amyloidosis, coumarin anticoagulant therapy, vitamin K deficiency, liver trauma.

Factor XI (Plasma Thromboplastin Antecedent) Deficiency

(Inherited autosomal recessive deficiency is usually mild; acquired forms are recognized)
In mild form, coagulation may be normal, prothrombin consumption time is slightly increased.

In severe cases, increased coagulation time, increased prothrombin consumption time. *Postoperative bleeding may not begin until several days after surgery.*

♦ Factor XI assay

Factor XII (Hageman Factor) Deficiency

Coagulation time and prothrombin consumption time are increased.
Specific factor assay is needed to distinguish from factor XI deficiency.
No hemorrhagic symptoms occur.

Factor XIII (Fibrin-Stabilizing Factor) Deficiency

(Inherited autosomal recessive deficiency with severe coagulation defect)

Congenital
Results of all standard clotting tests appear normal.
Patient's fibrin clot is soluble in 5M urea.
Whole blood clot is qualitatively friable.

Acquired Type May Occur In
- AML
- Liver disease
- Association with hypofibrinogenemia in obstetric complications
- Presence of circulating inhibitors

HEMATOL

Table 11-41. Comparison of Hemorrhagic Diseases of the Newborn

Test	Hemorrhagic Disease of the Newborn due to Vitamin K Deficiency	Secondary Hemorrhagic Disease of the Newborn
Capillary fragility	Normal	Usually abnormal
Bleeding time	Normal	Often increased
Clotting time	Increased	Variable
One-stage prothrombin	Marked increase ($\leq$ 5%)	Moderate increase (usually 5–25%)
Factor V	Normal	Often decreased (<50%)
Fibrinogen	Normal	Occasionally marked decrease
Platelet count	Normal	Occasionally decreased
Response to vitamin K	Improvement in clotting factors appears in 2–4 hrs; almost complete correction in 24 hrs	Little or no response

Glanzmann's Thrombasthenia

(Rare autosomal recessive absence or dysfunction of glycoprotein receptor GPIIb/IIIa that enable platelets to bind a family of integrins [to generate large platelet aggregates], of which fibrinogen is most important; variant forms exist)
See Table 11-36.
Prolonged BT.
Impaired clot retraction. Normal in essential athrombia, in which other laboratory abnormalities are the same.
Normal platelet count and morphology but unusually well dispersed on smear with no clumping.
Normal coagulation time.
♦ Totally absent primary platelet aggregation induced by ADP, thrombin, collagen, or epinephrine. Decreased maximum response to ristocetin.
♦ Prothrombin consumption tests abnormal but corrected by adding platelet substitute.

HELLP Syndrome

(*h*emolysis, *e*levated *l*iver enzymes, *l*ow *p*latelets)

♦ Diagnostic Criteria

- Hemolysis (increased serum bilirubin >1.2 mg/dL, LD >600 U/L, abnormal peripheral blood smear)
- Abnormal liver enzymes (serum ALT >79 U/L)
- Platelet count <100,000/cu mm

Hemolysis and thrombocytopenia are typically milder than in TTP/hemolytic uremic syndrome.
Bone marrow shows excessive megakaryocytes.
Normal PT, aPTT, fibrinogen, fibrinogen degradation products
Occurs during pregnancy or within 48 hrs of delivery.

Hemorrhagic Disease of the Newborn

(Due to lack of vitamin K)
See Table 11-41.
PT is markedly increased.
PTT is increased.
Coagulation time is increased.

BT is normal; may be slightly increased.
Capillary fragility, prothrombin consumption, and platelet count are normal.
Laboratory findings due to blood loss.

Secondary

Due to a variety of transient defects in clotting; more commonly seen in low-birth-weight premature infants and anoxic or septic neonates.

Hemorrhagic Disorders, Classification

Vascular abnormalities
- Congenital (e.g., hereditary hemorrhagic telangiectasia [Osler-Weber-Rendu disease])
- Acquired (see Purpura, Nonthrombocytopenic, p. 480)
    Infection (e.g., bacterial endocarditis, rickettsial infection)
    Immunologic (e.g., Schönlein-Henoch disease, allergic purpura, drug sensitivity)
    Metabolic (e.g., scurvy, uremia, diabetes mellitus)
    Miscellaneous (e.g., neoplasms, amyloidosis, angioma serpiginosum)

Connective tissue abnormalities
- Congenital (e.g., Ehlers-Danlos syndrome)
- Acquired (e.g., Cushing's syndrome)

Platelet abnormalities (see sections on thrombocytopenic purpura, thrombocythemia, thrombocytopathies)
- Most useful tests are platelet count, peripheral smear examination, BT, platelet aggregation, platelet lumi-aggregation (release), platelet IgG and IgM antibodies, platelet membrane glycoproteins (flow cytometry), cyclo-oxygenase. Platelet factor 4, beta-thromboglobulin, thromboxanes for hyperactive/prethrombotic platelets.

Plasma coagulation defects
- Causing defective thromboplastin formation
    Factor VIII deficiency (hemophilia)
    Factor IX (plasma thromboplastin component) deficiency (Christmas disease)
    Factor XI (plasma thromboplastin antecedent) deficiency
    Von Willebrand's disease
- Causing defective rate or amount of thrombin formation
    Vitamin K deficiency (due to liver disease, prolonged bile duct obstruction, malabsorption syndrome, hemorrhagic disease of the newborn, anticoagulant therapy)
    Congenital deficiency of factor II (prothrombin), factor V (proaccelerin, labile factor), factor VII (proconvertin, stable factor), factor X (Stuart factor)
- Decreased fibrinogen due to intravascular clotting and/or fibrinolysis
    Obstetric abnormalities (e.g., amniotic fluid embolism, premature separation of placenta, retention of dead fetus)
    Congenital deficiency of factor XIII (fibrin-stabilizing factor), congenital afibrinogenemia, hypofibrinogenemia, etc.
    Neoplasms (e.g., leukemia, carcinoma of prostate)
    Transfusion reactions
    Gram-negative septicemia, meningococcemia
- Circulating anticoagulants
    Heparin therapy
    Dysproteinemias, SLE, postpartum state, some cases of hemophilia, etc.

Hypercoagulable State

Due To

	Estimated Frequency
Primary (inherited) risk factors	
♦ • Activated protein C resistance	25–50%

(Due to factor V Leiden mutation in >95% of cases; found in 5% of persons in the United States; confirmed by PCR-DNA testing.)
Activated protein C added to normal plasma prolongs aPTT but not in patients with activated protein C resistance, who have ratio <2.0. Normal ratio is >2.4; 2.0–2.3 is indeterminate.

Invalidated by use of oral anticoagulants with 7–14 days, other causes of prolonged clotting times (e.g., factor deficiencies or inhibitors), presence of platelets in test plasma.

- Abnormal/delayed fibrinolysis — 10–15%*†
- Protein C deficiency (see p. 466) — 2–5%
- Protein S deficiency (see p. 467) — 2–5%
- Antithrombin III deficiency (see p. 451) — 2–5%*
- Plasminogen deficiency (see p. 460) or dysplasminogen — 1–2%*†
- Dysfibrinogenemia (see p. 474) — 1%*†
- Homocystinemia (homocysteine deposits damage endothelium) — Unknown*†
- Sickle cell anemia — *†
- Prothrombin gene mutation — 3–6%*
- Factor XII deficiency — Rare

Secondary risk factors (acquired), e.g.,
- Antiphospholipid antibody syndrome (see p. 450) — 10%*†
- Pregnancy
- Oral contraceptive use
- Neoplasia
- Surgery, trauma, or immobilization
- Sepsis
- Protein loss (e.g., nephrotic syndrome)
- Myeloproliferative disorders (e.g., polycythemia vera, essential thrombocytosis, agnogenic myeloid metaplasia, paroxysmal nocturnal hemoglobinuria)
- Hyperviscosity syndromes due to abnormal proteins or increased RBC mass
- SLE
- DIC
- Antineoplastic drugs
- Coumadin necrosis syndrome
- Heparin-induced thrombocytopenia and thrombosis

*Associated with venous thrombosis.
†Associated with arterial thrombosis.

Indications for Screening

Recurrent or migratory venous thrombosis or thrombosis at unusual site (e.g., mesenteric, portal) or at age <45 yrs
Familial thrombosis
Arterial thrombosis at age <30 yrs
Unexplained neonatal thrombosis
Recurrent fetal loss

Hypofibrinogenemia, Congenital

(Inherited autosomal dominant condition)
Plasma fibrinogen is moderately decreased (usually <80 mg/dL).
Bleeding and coagulation times are normal.
Blood clots are soft and small.

Purpura, Allergic

(Called Henoch's purpura when abdominal symptoms are predominant and Schön-lein purpura when joint symptoms are predominant)
No pathognomonic laboratory findings
Platelet count, BT, coagulation time, clot retraction, and bone marrow are normal.
Tourniquet test may be negative or positive.
WBC and neutrophils may be increased; eosinophils may be increased.
ESR is usually normal or may be slightly increased.
Stool may show blood.

Table 11-42. Comparison of Acute and Chronic Forms of Immune Thrombocytopenia

	Acute	Chronic
Population	Children aged 2–9 yrs	Adults; mostly women aged 20–40 yrs
Onset	Usually follows recent infectious illness	Insidious
Platelet count (per cu mm)	Often <20,000	Usually 30,000–70,000
CBC	Mild anemia, eosinophilia, and lymphocytosis	Normal
Megakaryocytes	Increased number	Increased number and volume

Urine usually contains RBCs and slight to marked protein. Chronic urine findings in 25% of cases.

BUN and creatinine may be increased.

Renal biopsy shows minimal change pattern in mild cases and diffuse proliferative GN in severe cases with IgA deposition. <4% of patients progress to end-stage renal disease.

Serum complement is not decreased.

Purpura, Idiopathic Thrombocytopenic (ITP; Werlhof's Disease), Immune

See Table 11-42.

♦ Diagnosis By

- Exclusion of other causes of thrombocytopenia (e.g., SLE, leukemia, HIV infection, thyroid disorders, etc; see p. 463)
- Isolated low platelet count with quantitatively and qualitatively normal RBCs and WBCs
- Bone marrow—normal or increased number and volume of megakaryocytes but without marginal platelets

Decreased platelet count (<100,000/cu mm) due to markedly diminished half-life; no bleeding until <50,000/cu mm; postoperative and minor spontaneous bleeding may occur at 20,000–50,000/cu mm. Significant bleeding is unusual until count is below ~5000/cu mm and even then does not occur in most adults. Routine platelet counts have discovered many asymptomatic patients.

Normal blood count and blood smear except for decreased number of platelets; platelets may appear abnormal (small or large immature or deeply stained). Mean platelet volume is normal or increased.

Positive tourniquet test

Increased BT

Poor clot retraction

Normal PT, aPTT, and coagulation time

Laboratory findings due to hemorrhage
- Increased WBC with shift to left
- Anemia proportional to hemorrhage, with compensatory increase in reticulocytes, polychromatophilia, etc.

Platelet IgG and autoantibodies (in ~33% of ITP patients) to specific platelet-membrane glycoproteins are not important for diagnosis or treatment; platelet IgG found in ≤ 75% of patients with other immune-associated thrombocytopenias.

○A palpable spleen is evidence against ITP.

In children 80–90% of acute cases remit spontaneously in 6–12 mos; rest become chronic; in adults almost all are chronic. ≤ 80% of children have preceding viral infection.

HEMATOL

Two-thirds of children and 85% of adults with chronic ITP develop normal platelet count after splenectomy.

Platelet transfusions are indicated in ITP if
- Platelet count <5000/cu mm, even if asymptomatic.
- Severe mucosal bleeding at any platelet count.
- Bleeding after splenectomy.
- Impending/actual CNS hemorrhage at any platelet count.
- Before major surgery (other than splenectomy) that requires platelet count >50,000/cu mm.
- See p. 484.

Purpura, Nonthrombocytopenic

Due To

Abnormal platelets (e.g., thrombocytopathies, thrombasthenia, thrombocythemia)

Abnormal serum globulins (e.g., multiple myeloma, macroglobulinemia, cryoglobulinemia, hyperglobulinemia)

Infections (e.g., meningococcemia, SBE, typhoid, Rocky Mountain spotted fever)

Other diseases (e.g., amyloidosis, Cushing's syndrome, polycythemia vera, hemochromatosis, diabetes mellitus, uremia)

Drugs and chemicals (e.g., mercury, phenacetin, salicylic acid, chloral hydrate)

Allergic reaction (e.g., Schönlein-Henoch purpura, serum sickness)

Diseases of the skin (e.g., Osler-Weber-Rendu disease, Ehlers-Danlos syndrome)

Von Willebrand's disease

Avitaminosis (e.g., scurvy)

Miscellaneous (e.g., mechanical, orthostatic)

Blood coagulation factors (e.g., hemophilia)

Purpura, Thrombocytopenic

See Platelet Count, Decreased In (p. 463)

Purpura, Thrombotic Thrombocytopenic (TTP); Hemolytic Uremic Syndrome

♦ Classic pentad: consumptive thrombocytopenia, microangiopathic hemolytic anemia, neurologic involvement, fever, minor renal involvement. Diagnosis by excluding other known causes of these features:
- Diarrhea-associated form: related commonly to a verocytotoxin-producing strain of *E. coli* O157:H7 and to *Shigella* with gastroenteritis and bloody diarrhea.
- Non–diarrhea-associated form is associated with:
   Complications of pregnancy (e.g., eclampsia, abruptio placentae, amniotic fluid embolism)
   Drugs (e.g., oral contraceptives, phenylbutazone, cyclosporin, 5-fluorouracil, mitomycin C)
   Underlying systemic diseases (e.g., primary glomerulopathies, rejection of renal transplant, vasculitis, cryoglobulinemia, septicemia, hypertension, adenocarcinoma)
   Inherited disorder
   Nonenteric pathogens

Closely related hemolytic uremic syndrome showing acute renal failure is associated with other conditions:
- Bone marrow transplant (10% of patients)
- Normal pregnancy (usually postpartum)
- Drugs (e.g., oral contraceptives, mitomycin, immunosuppressive agents)
- Carcinoma (e.g., prostate, pancreas)
- Autoimmune disorders
- Immune deficiency disorders

BUN may rise 50 mg/dL/day; is often >100 mg/dL. Urine may show blood, protein, casts, or anuria. Progressive renal disease or recovery. Oliguria and acute renal failure are uncommon. Renal biopsy shows fibrin thrombi damaging primarily glomerular endothelium (usually in children, associated with gastroenteritis, bloody diarrhea) or primarily arterial changes (associated with scleroderma or malignant hypertension, and after mitomycin treatment).

Severe thrombocytopenic purpura with normal or increased megakaryocytes in bone marrow. Platelet count generally <50,000/cu mm; usually becomes normal in a few weeks.

Microangiopathic hemolytic anemia (normochromic, normocytic) is present at onset or within a few days.

- Hb usually <10 g/dL; is often <6 gm/dL; may fall 50% in 2 days.
- Numerous fragmented and misshapen RBCs (burr cells, schistocytes) on blood smear is virtually required for this diagnosis.
- Increased reticulocytes, nucleated RBCs, basophilic stippling, and polychromatophilia.
- Increased serum Hb, indirect bilirubin, and LD, and decreased serum haptoglobin.
- Negative Coombs' test.

Increased or normal WBCs and neutrophils

In contrast to DIC, PT and aPTT are usually normal or may be mildly increased, clotting and fibrinogen are normal or only slightly increased; fibrin split products are usually present in low levels.

Bone marrow is hypercellular with erythroid and megakaryocytic hyperplasia in response to hemolysis and consumptive thrombocytopenia.

Serum AST and ALT may be slightly increased.

High initial BUN and creatinine, decreasing Hb, and failure of platelet count to increase are poor prognostic signs.

Multiorgan microvascular platelet thrombi in various organ systems result in clinical manifestations, especially neurologic (in ~90% of cases) and hemorrhagic (in up to 70%). Presence in gingival biopsy supports the diagnosis but occurs in <50% of cases. Other sites (skin, liver, lymph nodes, bone marrow) are rarely useful.

Serum complement is normal.

Storage Pool Disease, Hereditary

(Hereditary platelet function defect disorder)

See Table 11-36.

BT is usually abnormal.

Abnormal aggregation to collagen

Absent second aggregation curve to ADP and epinephrine although primary waves are present.

Normal ristocetin aggregation

Arachidonate aggregation is usually normal.

Thrombocytosis, Primary (Essential Thrombocythemia)

(Classified as a myeloproliferative disorder involving the thrombocytes; see Fig. 11-9)

♦ Diagnostic Criteria

Platelet count >600,000/cu mm on two occasions (>1 million/cu mm in 90% of cases).

No cause for reactive thrombocytosis

- No iron deficiency (marrow contains stainable iron or <1 gm Hb increase after 1 mo of iron therapy)
- No evidence of leukemia in peripheral blood or marrow (and absent Ph^1 chromosome; abl-bcr rearrangement is not found).
- No evidence of polycythemia (normal Hb or RBC mass)
- Bone marrow
    Fibrosis must be minimal or absent to rule out agnogenic myeloid metaplasia, or in absence of both splenomegaly and leukoerythroblastosis, it must be less than one-half of area of biopsy specimen.
    Hypercellular with hyperplasia of all elements, with predominance of megakaryocytes and platelet masses, eosinophilia, basophilia; no evidence of masked polycythemia vera; no ring sideroblasts of myelodysplastic syndrome

Platelets appear normal early in disease; later abnormal in size and shape, and changes in structure occur. Aggregation may be abnormal with epinephrine, ADP, thrombin.

Mild anemia (10–13 gm/dL) in one-third of patients due to blood loss

WBC usually >12,000/cu mm without cells earlier than myelocyte forms in ≤ 40% of patients; leukocyte ALP score is usually normal or may be increased.

Increased serum LD, uric acid

Artifactual increase in serum potassium, calcium, oxygen

Thrombohemorrhagic disease (bleeding—skin, GI tract, nose, gums in 35% of patients but normal BT) and thromboses of major vessels, usually arterial, in ≤ 40% of patients

Thrombocytosis, Reactive

See Platelet Count, Increased In, p 463.

Transfusion of Blood

Adverse Effects[27–29]

Occurs from ~1 in 1000 components transfused in the United States. ~1 in 12,000 transfusions are given to the wrong person.

Immune Mediated

Acute	Frequency/unit
Fatal acute hemolysis (ABO) (mortality ~3.3%)	1:633,000
Nonfatal acute hemolysis (ABO)	1:33,000
Febrile nonhemolytic reaction (WBC or cytokine induced)	1:200
Allergic transfusion reaction	1:333
Acute anaphylaxis	1:20,000–1:50,000
Acute lung injury	>1:5000
Hemolytic transfusion reaction	1:200

Chronic

Alloimmunization	
RBC hemolysis	1:1500
Platelet refractoriness	1:3300–1:10,000
Delayed hemolysis	1:4000
Graft-versus-host disease (transfusion associated)	Unknown
Posttransfusion purpura	Rare to very uncommon

Non–Immune Mediated

Acute	
Volume overload	1:100–1:200
Nonimmune hemolysis (e.g., heat, cold, osmotic, mechanical)	Infrequent
Electrolyte imbalance (K^+, Mg^{++}, Ca^{++})	Uncommon
Chemical effects (e.g., citrate)	Uncommon
Coagulopathy (e.g., DIC; usually with massive transfusions)	Uncommon

Chronic

Alloimmunization	
RBC hemolysis	1:1500
Platelet refractoriness	1:3300–1:10,000
Delayed hemolysis	1:4000
Graft-versus-host disease (transfusion associated)	1:400,000
Posttransfusion purpura	Rare to very uncommon
Transfusional hemosiderosis	Uncommon

Infections

Viruses

HAV	Usually single case reports
HBV	1:60,000

[27]Simon TI, et al. Practice parameter for the use of red blood cell transfusions. *Arch Pathol Lab Med* 1998;122:130.

[28]College of American Pathologists. Practice parameter for the recognition, management, and prevention of adverse consequences of blood transfusion, June 1997.

[29]Goodnough LT, et al. Transfusion medicine. First of two parts—blood transfusion. *N Engl J Med* 1999;340:438.

HCV	1:100,000
HIV-I	1:450,000–1:660,000
HIV-II	Extremely rare
HTLV-I/II	1:600,000
CMV	3 per 100 to 12 per 100
Parvovirus B19	Rare
EBV	Rare (i.e., 3/100–12/100)

Bacteria

Syphilis	Not reported since 1976
Bacterial contamination—platelet units (e.g., *S. aureus, Klebsiella pneumoniae, S. marcescens, Staphylococcus epidermidis*)	1:12,000
Bacterial contamination—RBC units (e.g., *S. epidermidis, Bacillus cereus, Yersinia enterocolitica* are most common)	<1:1,000,000

Parasites

Plasmodium spp.	<5:1,000,000
Babesia microti	<1:1,000,000
Trypanosoma cruzi (see Chagas' disease)	<1:1,000,000
Leishmania spp.	<1:20,000,000
Borrelia burgdorferi (see Lyme disease)	Few or no cases
Toxoplasma gondii	Few or no cases
Wuchereria bancrofti (see Lymphatic Filariasis)	Few or no cases

Newly instituted nucleic acid tests may detect ≤ 2 HIV-infected and ≤ 100 HCV-infected units/yr that were previously undetected.

Transfusion Reactions

Hemolytic transfusion reactions occur in ~1 in 12,000 transfusions and are fatal in 1 in 600,000 transfusions; almost always due to ABO incompatibility (usually due to clerical error).

Isoimmune Major Transfusion Reactions

Immediate reaction
ABO-incompatible blood
Laboratory findings due to complications of hemolysis (e.g., DIC, acute renal failure, cardiovascular failure

Alloimmune Minor Transfusion Reactions

Due to sensitization of RBCs against foreign, minor, non-ABO antibodies
Delayed (3–10 days) reaction of extravascular hemolysis producing milder clinical and laboratory findings

Indications
Red Cell Transfusion
Hb <8 gm/dL (Hct <26%) and MCV within normal limits (81–100 fL; 70–125 fL if age 14 yrs or less)
Hb <8 gm/dL (Hct <26%) in patients with acute bleed or high risk*
Hb <11 gm/dL (Hct <36%) in clinically symptomatic patients*[†]
Hb <11 gm/dL (Hct <36%) or bleeding >1 U/24 hrs
Any Hb level in high-risk* patients with acute bleed
Any Hb level in symptomatic*[†] patients with acute bleed
Any Hb level in patients bleeding >2 U/24 hrs or >15% of blood volume in 24 hrs
Death is unlikely until Hb falls to 3 gm/dL or Hct to 10%.
After bleeding has stopped, one unit of packed RBCs typically increases recipient's Hct 3%; 2 U increase Hct ~6.4% and Hb ~2 gm/dL.

*High risk: e.g., coronary artery disease, chronic pulmonary disease, cerebrovascular disease, or known anemia.
[†]Symptomatic: e.g., patients with signs or symptoms of anemia (such as tachycardia, angina, ECG changes) or of respiratory distress; with known hemoglobinopathy, etc.

HEMATOL

Cryoprecipitate (Cryoprecipitated Antihemophilic Factor) Transfusion

Received massive transfusions >8 units/24 hrs

Received transfusion of >6 RBC units/case (e.g., open heart surgery)

Bleeding or invasive procedure in patients with hypofibrinogenemia or DIC

Deficient factor VIII or von Willebrand's disease (if desmopressin acetate or factor VIII are not effective or available), or abnormal or markedly decreased fibrinogen in bleeding patients or before surgery or invasive procedure

Typical bag of cryoprecipitate contains 100 U of factor VIII (the amount normally present in 100 mL of plasma)

Risk of viral transmission same as for 1 unit of packed RBCs

Fresh Frozen Plasma Transfusion

In actively bleeding patients or before surgery or invasive procedures documented by (1) increased PT >1.5× midnormal range (usually >18 sec) or (2) increased aPTT >1.5× upper normal range (usually >55–60 sec) (normal fibrinogen and no heparin in specimen) and (3) coagulation assay <25% activity:

* After massive blood transfusion (>1 blood volume within several hours with evidence of coagulation deficiency)
* Deficiency of various coagulation factors or von Willebrand's disease (if desmopressin acetate or factor VIII are not effective or available)
* Reverse warfarin effect for immediate hemostasis when PT >18 secs; INR >1.6)
* Deficiency of antithrombin III (when concentrate is not available), protein C, protein S, heparin cofactor II

Hypoglobulinemia (rarely)

Plasma exchange for TTP or hemolytic uremic syndrome

Contraindicated as volume expander

Each unit increases any clotting factor by 2–3% in average adult.

Platelet Transfusion

Platelet count >50,000/cu mm: unlikely to be needed; bleeding unlikely due to low count.

Platelet count <5000/cu mm

* Spontaneous bleeding is likely except in platelet destruction disorders; prophylactic use is indicated.

Platelet count <10,000/cu mm

* Prophylactic with minor hemorrhage; fever

Platelet count <20,000 in patients

* Without thrombotic or ITP or posttransfusion purpura or hemolytic uremic syndrome
* Prophylactic in leukemia in presence of coagulation disorders, during induction therapy
* Before minor surgical procedures

Platelet count <50,000 in patients with

* Minor bleeding
* Preoperative for a minor procedure
* Prematurity
* High blast count

Platelet count <90,000 in patients with

* Bleed requiring RBC transfusion
* Preoperative for a major procedure

Received massive RBC transfusion (>8 U/24 hrs)

BT >10 mins

Received transfusion of >6 RBC unit/case (e.g., open heart surgery)

(Unit of platelets = 5.5×10^{10} cu mm)

von Willebrand's Disease

(Heterogeneous group of inherited [>20 subtypes] and acquired disorders of vWF with mucocutaneous bleeding due to abnormal vWF quantity or quality. Most common inherited hemostatic abnormality.)

See Tables 11-36 and 11-43.

Table 11-43. Types of von Willebrand's Disease (vWD)

	Type of vWD				
	I (classic)	IIA	IIB	III	Platelet Type
Frequency	70–80%	10–12%	3–5%	1–3%	0–1
Platelet count	N	N	N or D	N	D or low N
BT	I or N	I	I	Marked I	I
Factor VIII:C	D or N	D or N	D or N	Marked D	D or N
vWF:Ag	D	D or N	D or N	0 or tiny amounts	D or N
vWF:RCoF	D (20–50%)	DDD	D or N	0	D or N
RIPA	D	D	N	0	N
RIPA (1/2)	0	0	I	0	I
Plasma SDS multimers	All present; HMW may be D	Large and intermediate A	Large A	May be A	Large A
Platelet SDS multimers	All present; HMW may be D	Large and intermediate A	N	A	N
Response to desmopressin	Hemostasis becomes N		Platelets D	No response	Platelets D; contraindicated
Genetics	AD	AD	AD	AR	AD

D = decreased; I = increased; 0 = absent; A = abnormal; AD = autosomal dominant; AR = autosomal recessive; DDD = much decreased; HMW = high molecular weight; N= normal; RCoF = ristocetin cofactor; RIPA = ristocetin-induced platelet aggregation; RIPA (1/2) = 1/2 normal concentration (0.6 mg/mL); SDS = sodium dodecyl sulfate for electrophoresis separation; vWF = von Willebrand's factor.
Types IIC–IIH now classified under type IIA.
Source: Triplett DA. Laboratory diagnosis of von Willebrand's disease. *Mayo Clin Proc* 1991;66:832.

Hereditary deficiency (types I and III) or qualitative defect (type II) of a high-molecular-weight plasma protein (vWF) that mediates adherence of platelets to injured endothelium. All show mild to moderate bleeding except type III, which is severe. Type I: decreased amount of vWF without qualitative abnormality. Type III: vWF completely or almost completely absent from plasma and platelets. Type II: qualitative abnormalities of vWF due to loss of various multimers. vWF circulates complexed to (carrier for) factor VIII:c, which also responds as an acute-phase protein. Pseudo–von Willebrand's disease is a rare platelet disorder in which platelet receptors have marked avidity for vWF, which causes spontaneous clumping, depletes the plasma of vWF, and may cause mild to moderate thrombocytopenia. Acquired von Willebrand's disease due to formation of autoantibodies (in association with autoimmune and lymphoproliferative disorders), decreased synthesis, or other mechanisms (e.g., in myeloproliferative, vascular, and congenital heart diseases), or idiopathic.

Difficulty in diagnosis arises from temporal variation in clinical and laboratory findings in an individual patient as well as from patient to patient; because many patients do not have the classic laboratory findings, a number of clinical variants have been described.

BT is prolonged using a calibrated template; in a few patients, may only be prolonged after administration of 300 mg of aspirin.

aPTT is prolonged.

Platelet adhesiveness to glass beads is decreased. Ristocetin-induced aggregation of platelets is abnormal if ristocetin cofactor activity is <30%; thus may be normal in mild von Willebrand's disease. May not identify some mild cases in which activity is >30% but less than normal value of 50–150%.

Platelet count is usually normal but may be mildly decreased in type IIB or platelet-type von Willebrand's disease.

PT and clot retraction are normal.

Tourniquet test may be positive.

Factor VIII coagulant activity (VIII:c) may range from normal to severely reduced (indicated by direct assay, aPTT, or TGT tests).

♦ Factor VIII–related antigen (vWF:Ag) measured by special electroimmunoassay is decreased.

May be increased in endothelial cell injury (e.g., trauma, surgery, surgical graft failure, clotting).

♦ Transfusion of normal plasma (or of hemophiliac plasma, cryoprecipitate, serum) causes a rise in factor VIII activity greater than the amount of factor VIII infused, which does not peak until 8–10 hrs and slowly declines for days; in contrast, hemophilia shows rapid peak and fall after infusion of normal plasma or cryoprecipitate. This response to transfusion is a good diagnostic test in patients in whom diagnosis is equivocal. Factor VIII levels may increase to normal during pregnancy or use of oral contraceptives with subsidence of hemorrhagic episodes, although BT is often unaffected. Therefore diagnostic evaluation should not be done in the presence of these two circumstances.

Screening of family members may be useful in difficult diagnostic cases, even if they are asymptomatic and have no history of unusual bleeding.

Laboratory findings due to complications, e.g., viral infections, development of antibodies to vWF (occurs in severe type III).

Platelet-type von Willebrand's disease is distinguished from type IIB by mixing studies with normal platelets and plasma.

Screening tests: aPTT, BT, platelet count

Confirmatory tests: tests for VIII:c, vWF:Ag, vWF:RCoF

Tests to confirm diagnosis and determine type: ristocetin-induced platelet aggregation (RIPA), plasma wWF multimer analysis

Comparison of Hemophilia A and Von Willebrand's Disease

	Hemophilia A	von Willebrand's Disease
BT	Normal	Prolonged
Factor VIII:Ag	Normal	Low
Factor VIII:C	Low	Prolonged-normal
Platelet adhesion	Normal	Retarded
Platelet aggregation (RIPA)	Normal	Decreased
Ristocetin cofactor	Normal	Deficient
aPTT	Prolonged	Prolonged-normal

HEMATOL

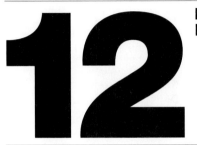

Metabolic and Hereditary Disorders

Acid-Base Disorders

In analyzing acid-base disorders, several points should be kept in mind:
- Determination of pH and blood gases should be performed on *arterial* blood. Venous blood is useless for judging oxygenation but offers an estimate of acid-base status.
- Blood specimens should be packed in ice immediately; delay of even a few minutes causes erroneous results, especially if WBC is high.
- Determination of electrolytes, pH, and blood gases ideally should be performed on blood specimens obtained simultaneously, because the acid-base situation is very labile.
- Repeated determinations may often be indicated because of the development of complications, the effect of therapy, and other factors.
- Acid-base disorders are often mixed rather than in the pure form usually described in textbooks.
- These mixed disorders may represent simultaneously occurring diseases, complications superimposed on the primary condition, or the effect of treatment.
- Changes in chronic forms may be notably different from those in the acute forms.
- For judging hypoxemia, one must also know the patient's Hb or Hct and whether the patient was breathing room air or oxygen when the specimen was drawn.
- Arterial blood gas values cannot be interpreted without clinical information about the patient.

Renal compensation for a respiratory disturbance is slower (3–7 days) but more successful than respiratory compensation for a metabolic disturbance but cannot completely compensate for pCO_2 >65 mm Hg unless another stimulus for HCO_3^- retention is present. Respiratory mechanism responds quickly but can only eliminate sufficient CO_2 to balance the most mild metabolic acidosis.

Most laboratories measure pH and pCO_2 directly and calculate HCO_3^- using the Henderson-Hasselbalch equation:

$$\text{Arterial pH} = 6.1 + \log [(HCO_3^-) \div (0.03 \times pCO_2)]$$

where 6.1 is the dissociation constant for CO_2 in aqueous solution and 0.03 is a constant for the solubility of CO_2 in plasma at 37°C.

A normal pH does not ensure the absence of an acid-base disturbance if the pCO_2 is not known.

An abnormal HCO_3^- means a metabolic rather than a respiratory problem; decreased HCO_3^- indicates metabolic acidosis, and increased HCO_3^- indicates metabolic alkalosis. Respiratory acidosis is associated with a pCO_2 of >45 mm Hg, and respiratory alkalosis is associated with a pCO_2 of <35 mm Hg. Thus mixed metabolic and respiratory acidosis is characterized by low pH, low HCO_3^-, and high pCO_2. Mixed metabolic and respiratory alkalosis is characterized by high pH, high HCO_3^-, and low pCO_2.

See Tables 12-1, 12-2, and 12-3.

In severe metabolic acidosis, respiratory compensation is limited by inability to hyperventilate pCO_2 to less than ~15 mm Hg; beyond that, small increments of H^+ ion produce disastrous changes in pH and prognosis; thus patients with lung disorders (e.g., COPD, neuromuscular weakness) are very vulnerable because they cannot compensate by hyperventilation. In metabolic alkalosis, respiratory compensation is limited

Table 12-1. Metabolic and Respiratory Acid-Base Changes in Blood

	pH	pCO_2	HCO_3^-
Acidosis			
Acute metabolic	D	N	D
Compensated metabolic	N	D	D
Acute respiratory	D	I	N
Compensated respiratory	N	I	I
Alkalosis			
Acute metabolic	I	N	I
Chronic metabolic	I	I	I
Acute respiratory	I	D	N
Compensated respiratory	N	D	D

D = decreased; I = increased; N = normal.

by CO_2 retention, which rarely causes pCO_2 levels >50–60 mm Hg (because increased CO_2 and hypoxemia stimulate respiration very strongly); thus pH is not returned to normal.

- Base excess is a value that hypothetically "corrects" pH to 7.40 by first adjusting pCO_2 to 40 mm Hg, thereby allowing comparison of resultant HCO_3^- with normal value at that pH (24 mEq/L). Base excess can be calculated from determined values for pH and HCO_3^- by the following formula:

$$\text{Base excess (mEq/L)} = HCO_3^- + 10(7.40 - pH) - 24$$

Negative base excess indicates depletion of HCO_3^-. Does not distinguish primary from compensatory derangement.

See Tables 12-1, 12-3, 12-4, and 12-5; section on metabolic and respiratory acid-base changes in blood.

Pearls

- Pulmonary embolus: Mild to moderate respiratory alkalosis is present unless sudden death occurs. The degree of hypoxia often correlates with the size and extent of the pulmonary embolus. pO_2 of >90 mm Hg when patient breathes room air virtually excludes a lung problem.

- Acute pulmonary edema: Hypoxemia is usual. CO_2 is not increased unless the situation is grave.

- Asthma: Hypoxia occurs even during a mild episode and increases as the attack becomes worse. As hyperventilation occurs, the pCO_2 falls (usually <35 mm Hg); a normal pCO_2 (>40 mm Hg) implies impending respiratory failure; increased pCO_2 in a patient with true asthma (not bronchitis or emphysema) indicates impending disaster and the need to consider intubation and ventilation assistance.

- COPD (bronchitis and emphysema): May show two patterns—"pink puffers" with mild hypoxia and normal pH and pCO_2 and "blue bloaters" with hypoxia and increased pCO_2; normal pH suggests compensation, and decreased pH suggests decompensation.

- Neurologic and neuromuscular disorders (e.g., drug overdose, Guillain-Barré syndrome, myasthenia gravis, trauma, succinylcholine administration): Acute alveolar hypoventilation causes uncompensated respiratory acidosis with high pCO_2, low pH, and normal HCO_3^-. Acidosis appears before significant hypoxemia, and rising CO_2 indicates rapid deterioration and need for mechanical assistance.

- Sepsis: Unexplained respiratory alkalosis may be the earliest sign of sepsis. It may progress to cause metabolic acidosis, and the mixed picture may produce a normal pH; low HCO_3^- is useful to recognize this situation. With deterioration and worsening of metabolic acidosis, the pH falls.

Table 12-2. Illustrative Serum Values in Acid-Base Disturbances

Condition	Sodium (mEq/L)	Chloride (mEq/L)	HCO_3^- (mEq/L)	pCO_2 (mm Hg)	pH
Normal	140	105	25	40	7.40
Metabolic acidosis	140	115	15	31	7.30
Chronic respiratory alkalosis	136	102	25	40	7.44
Mixed metabolic acidosis and chronic respiratory alkalosis (e.g., sepsis: addition of respiratory alkalosis to metabolic acidosis further decreases HCO_3^- but pH may remain normal; lactic acidosis plus respiratory alkalosis due to severe liver disease, pulmonary emboli, or sepsis)	136	108	14	24	7.39
Metabolic alkalosis	140	92	36	48	7.49
Chronic respiratory acidosis	140	100–102	28	50	7.37
Mixed metabolic alkalosis and chronic respiratory acidosis (e.g., patient with COPD receiving glucocorticoids or diuretics; pCO_2 and HCO_3^- are increased by both conditions, but pH is neutralized)	140	90	40	67	7.40

(continued)

METAB/HERED

Table 12-2. (continued)

Condition	Sodium (mEq/L)	Chloride (mEq/L)	HCO$_3^-$ (mEq/L)	pCO$_2$(mm Hg)	pH
Metabolic alkalosis	139	89	35	47	7.49
Respiratory alkalosis	136	102	20	30	7.44
Mixed alkalosis, mild	139	92	32	39	7.53
Mixed alkalosis, severe (e.g., postoperative patient with severe hemorrhage stimulating hyperventilation [respiratory alkalosis] plus massive transfusion and nasogastric drainage [metabolic alkalosis])	139	92	32	30	7.63
Mixed chronic respiratory acidosis and acute metabolic acidosis (e.g., COPD [chronic respiratory acidosis] with severe diarrhea [metabolic acidosis]. pH is too low for pCO$_2$ of 55 mm Hg in chronic respiratory acidosis, indicating low pH due to mixed acidosis, but HCO$_3^-$ effect is offset.)	136	102	22	55	7.22
Mixed metabolic acidosis and metabolic alkalosis (e.g., gastroenteritis with vomiting [metabolic alkalosis] and diarrhea [metabolic acidosis due to loss of HCO$_3^-$]; surprisingly normal findings with marked volume depletion)	140	103	25	40	7.40

Table 12-3. Illustrative Serum Electrolyte Values in Various Conditions

Condition	pH	HCO$_3^-$	Potassium	Sodium	Chloride
Normal	7.35–7.45	24–26	3.5–5.0	136–145	100–106
Metabolic acidosis					
Diabetic acidosis	7.2	10	5.6	122	80
Fasting	7.2	16	5.2	142	100
Severe diarrhea	7.2	12	3.2	128	96
Hyperchloremic acidosis	7.2	12	5.2	142	116
Addison's disease	7.2	22	6.5	111	72
Nephritis	7.2	8	4.0	129	90
Nephrosis	7.2	20	5.5	138	113
Metabolic alkalosis					
Vomiting	7.6	38	3.2	150	94
Pyloric obstruction	7.6	58	3.2	132	42
Duodenal obstruction	7.6	42	3.2	138	49
Respiratory acidosis	7.1	30	5.5	142	80
Respiratory alkalosis	7.6	14	5.5	136	112

○Salicylate poisoning: Characteristically, poor correlation is seen between serum salicylate level and presence or degree of acidemia (because as pH drops from 7.4 to 7.2, the proportion of nonionized to ionized salicylate doubles and the nonionized form leaves the serum and is sequestered in the brain and other organs, where it interferes with function at a cellular level without changing blood levels of glucose, etc.). In adults salicylate poisoning typically causes respiratory alkalosis, but in children this progresses rapidly to mixed respiratory alkalosis–metabolic acidosis and then to metabolic acidosis (in adults, metabolic acidosis is said to be a rare and a near-terminal event).

○Isopropyl (rubbing) alcohol poisoning: Produces enough circulating acetone to produce a positive nitroprusside test (it therefore may be mistaken for diabetic ketoacidosis; thus insulin should not be given until the blood glucose is known). In the absence of a history, positive serum ketone test associated with normal AG, normal serum HCO$_3^-$, and normal blood glucose suggests rubbing alcohol intoxication.

Acid-base maps (Fig. 12-1) are a graphic solution of the Henderson-Hasselbalch equation that predicts the HCO$_3^-$ value for each set of pH/pCO$_2$ coordinates. They also allow a check of the consistency of arterial blood gas and some chemical analyzer determinations, because the chemical analyzer determines the total CO$_2$ content, of which 95% is HCO$_3^-$. These maps contain bands that show the 95% probability range of values for each disorder. If the pH/pCO$_2$ coordinate is outside the 95% confidence band, then the patient has at least two acid-base disturbances. These maps are of particular use when one of the acid-base disturbances is not suspected clinically. If the coordinates lie within a band, however, there is no guarantee of a simple acid-base disturbance.

Table 12-4. Upper Limits of Arterial Blood pH and HCO_3^- Concentrations (Expected for Blood pCO_2 Values)

Arterial Blood		
pCO_2 (mm Hg)	pH	HCO_3^- (mEq/L)
20	7.66	22.8
30	7.53	25.6
40	7.57	27.3
60	7.29	27.9
80	7.18	28.9

Values shown are the upper limits of the 95% confidence bands.
Source: Coe FL. Metabolic alkalosis. *JAMA* 1977;238:2288.

Acid-Base Disturbances, Mixed

(Must always be interpreted with clinical data and other laboratory findings)
See Table 12-2.

Respiratory Acidosis with Metabolic Acidosis

Examples: Acute pulmonary edema, cardiopulmonary arrest (lactic acidosis due to tissue anoxia and CO_2 retention due to alveolar hypoventilation)
Acidemia may be extreme with
- pH <7.0 (H^+ >100 mEq/L).
○ • HCO3– <26 mEq/L. Failure of HCO3– to increase ≥ 3 mEq/L for each 10 mm Hg rise in pCO2 suggests metabolic acidosis with respiratory acidosis.
Mild metabolic acidosis superimposed on chronic hypercapnia causing partial suppression of HCO_3^- may be indistinguishable from adaptation to hypercapnia alone.

Metabolic Acidosis with Respiratory Alkalosis

Examples: Rapid correction of severe metabolic acidosis, salicylate intoxication, septicemia due to gram-negative organisms, initial respiratory alkalosis with subsequent development of metabolic acidosis.
○*Primary metabolic acidosis with primary respiratory alkalosis with an increased AG is characteristic of salicylate intoxication in absence of uremia and diabetic ketoacidosis.*

Table 12-5. Summary of Pure and Mixed Acid-Base Disorders

	Decreased pH	Normal pH	Increased pH
Increased pCO_2	Respiratory acidosis with or without incompletely compensated metabolic alkalosis or coexisting metabolic acidosis	Respiratory acidosis and compensated metabolic alkalosis	Metabolic alkalosis with incompletely compensated respiratory acidosis or coexisting respiratory acidosis
Normal pCO_2	Metabolic acidosis	Normal	Metabolic alkalosis
Decreased pCO_2	Metabolic acidosis with incompletely compensated respiratory alkalosis or coexisting respiratory alkalosis	Respiratory alkalosis and compensated metabolic acidosis	Respiratory alkalosis with or without incompletely compensated metabolic acidosis or coexisting metabolic alkalosis

Source: Adapted from Friedman HH. *Problem-oriented medical diagnosis*, 3rd ed. Boston: Little, Brown, 1983.

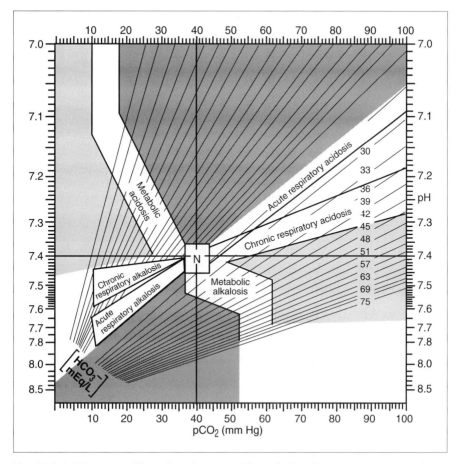

Fig. 12-1. Acid-base map. The values demarcated for each disorder represent a 95% probability range for each *pure* disorder (N = normal). Coordinates lying outside these zones suggest mixed acid-base disorders. (Adapted from Goldberg M, et al. Computer-based instruction and diagnosis of acid-base disorders. *JAMA* 1973;223:269. Copyright 1973 American Medical Association.)

pH may be normal or decreased.
Hypocapnia remains inappropriate to decreased HCO_3^- for several hours or more.

Respiratory Acidosis with Metabolic Alkalosis

Examples: Chronic pulmonary disease with CO_2 retention in which patient develops metabolic alkalosis due to administration of diuretics, severe vomiting, or sudden improvement in ventilation ("posthypercapnic" metabolic alkalosis)

○ Decreased or absent urine chloride indicates that chloride-responsive metabolic alkalosis is a part of the picture.

○ In clinical setting of respiratory acidosis but with normal blood pH and/or HCO_3^- higher than predicted, complicating metabolic alkalosis may be present.

Respiratory Alkalosis with Metabolic Alkalosis

Examples: Hepatic insufficiency with hyperventilation plus administration of diuretics or severe vomiting; metabolic alkalosis with stimulation of ventilation (e.g., sepsis, pulmonary embolism, mechanical ventilation) that causes respiratory alkalosis

♦Marked alkalemia with decreased pCO_2 and increased HCO_3^- is diagnostic.

Acute and Chronic Respiratory Acidosis

Examples: Chronic hypercapnia with acute deterioration of pulmonary function causing further rise of pCO_2
○May be suspected when HCO_3^- in intermediate range between acute and chronic respiratory acidosis (similar findings in chronic respiratory acidosis with superimposed metabolic acidosis or acute respiratory acidosis with superimposed metabolic alkalosis)

Coexistence of Metabolic Acidoses of Hyperchloremic Type and Increased AG Type

Examples: Uremia and proximal renal tubular acidosis, lactic acidosis with diarrhea, excessive administration of sodium chloride to patient with organic acidosis
○May be suspected when plasma HCO_3^- level is lower than is explained by the increase in anions (e.g., $AG = 16$ mEq/L and $HCO_3^- = 5$ mEq/L)

Coexistence of Metabolic Alkalosis and Metabolic Acidosis

Examples: Vomiting causing alkalosis plus bicarbonate-losing diarrhea causing acidosis
○May be suggested by acid-base values that are too normal for clinical picture

Acidosis, Lactic

Indicates acute hypoperfusion and tissue hypoxia.
○Should be considered in any metabolic acidosis with increased AG (>15 mEq/L).
♦Diagnosis is confirmed by exclusion of other causes of metabolic acidosis and serum lactate ≥ 5 mEq/L (upper limit of normal = 1.6 for plasma and 1.4 for whole blood). Considerable variation in literature in limits of serum lactate and pH to define lactic acidosis.
♦Exclusion of other causes by
   • Normal serum creatinine and BUN. *(Increased acetoacetic acid [but not beta-hydroxybutyric acid] causes false increase of creatinine by colorimetric assay.)*
   • Osmolar gap <10 mOsm/L.
   • Negative nitroprusside reaction. *(Nitroprusside test for ketoacidosis measures acetoacetic acid but not beta-hydroxybutyric acid; thus blood ketone test may be negative in diabetic ketoacidosis.)*
   • Urine negative for calcium oxalate crystals.
   • No known ingestion of toxic substances.
Laboratory findings due to underlying diseases (e.g., diabetes mellitus, renal insufficiency, etc.)
Laboratory tests for monitoring therapy
   • Arterial pH, pCO_2, HCO_3^-, serum electrolytes, every 1–2 hrs until patient is stable
   • Urine electrolytes every 6 hrs
Associated or compensatory metabolic or respiratory disturbances (e.g., hyperventilation or respiratory alkalosis may result in normal pH)

Due To

Type A due to clinically apparent tissue hypoxia, e.g., acute hemorrhage, severe anemia, shock, asphyxia; marathon running, seizures
Type B without clinically apparent tissue hypoxia due to
   • Common disorders (e.g., diabetes mellitus, uremia, liver disease, infections, malignancies, alkaloses).
   • Drugs and toxins (e.g., ethanol, methanol, ethylene glycol, salicylates, metformin).
   • Hereditary enzyme defects (e.g., methylmalonicaciduria, propionicaciduria, defects of fatty acid oxidation, pyruvate-dehydrogenase deficiency, pyruvate-carboxylase deficiency, multiple carboxylase deficiency, glycogen storage disease type I).
   • Others (e.g., short-bowel syndrome).
With a typical clinical picture (acute onset after nausea and vomiting, altered state of consciousness, hyperventilation, high mortality)

- Decreased serum bicarbonate.
- Low serum pH, usually 6.98–7.25.
- Increased serum potassium, often 6–7 mEq/L.
- Serum chloride normal or low with increased AG.
- WBC is increased (occasionally to leukemoid levels).
- Increased serum uric acid is frequent (up to 25 mg/dL in lactic acidosis).
○ • Increased serum phosphorus. Phosphorus/creatinine ratio >3 indicates lactic acidosis either alone or as a component of other metabolic acidosis.
- Increased serum AST, LD, and phosphorus.

See Table 12-3.

Acidosis, Metabolic

○With Increased Anion Gap (AG >15 mEq/L)

Lactic acidosis—most common cause of metabolic acidosis with increased AG (frequently >25 mEq/L) (see previous section)
Renal failure (AG <25 mEq/L)
Ketoacidosis
- Diabetes mellitus (AG frequently >25 mEq/L)
- Associated with alcohol abuse (AG frequently 20–25 mEq/L)
- Starvation (AG usually 5–10 mEq/L)
Drug effects
- Salicylate poisoning (AG frequently 5–10 mEq/L; higher in children)
- Methanol poisoning (AG frequently >20 mEq/L)
- Ethylene glycol poisoning (AG frequently >20 mEq/L)
- Paraldehyde treatment (AG frequently >20 mEq/L)

○With Normal Anion Gap

(Hyperchloremic acidosis)

Decreased serum potassium
- Renal tubular acidosis
    Acquired (e.g., drugs, hypercalcemia)
    Inherited (e.g., cystinosis, Wilson's disease)
- Carbonic anhydrase inhibitors (e.g., acetazolamide, mafenide)
- Increased loss of alkaline body fluids (e.g., diarrhea, loss of pancreatic or biliary fluids)
- Ureteral diversion (e.g., ileal bladder or ureter, ureterosigmoidostomy)
Normal or increased serum potassium
- Hydronephrosis
- Early renal failure
- Administration of HCl (e.g., ammonium chloride)
- Hypoadrenalism (diffuse, zona glomerulosa, or hyporeninemia)
- Renal aldosterone resistance
- Sulfur toxicity
○ *In lactic acidosis the increase in AG is usually greater than the decrease in HCO3–, in contrast to diabetic ketoacidosis in which the increase in AG is identical to the decrease in HCO_3^-.*

♦ Laboratory Findings

Serum pH is decreased (<7.3).
Total plasma CO_2 content is decreased; value <15 mEq/L almost certainly rules out respiratory alkalosis.
Serum potassium is frequently increased; it is decreased in renal tubular acidosis, diarrhea, or carbonic anhydrase inhibition.
Azotemia suggests metabolic acidosis due to renal failure.
Urine is strongly acid (pH = 4.5–5.2) if renal function is normal.
In evaluating acid-base disorders, calculate the AG (see below).

Acidosis, Respiratory

Laboratory findings differ in acute and chronic conditions.

METAB/HERED

Acute

Due to decreased alveolar ventilation impairing CO_2 excretion
- Cardiopulmonary (e.g., pneumonia, pneumothorax, pulmonary edema, foreign-body aspiration, laryngospasm, bronchospasm, mechanical ventilation, cardiac arrest)
- CNS depression (e.g., general anesthesia, drug effects, brain injury, infection)
- Neuromuscular conditions (e.g., Guillain-Barré syndrome, hypokalemia, myasthenic crisis)

○Acidosis is severe (pH 7.05–7.10) but HCO_3^- concentration is only 29–30 mEq/L.
Severe mixed acidosis is common in cardiac arrest when respiratory and circulatory failure cause marked respiratory acidosis and severe lactic acidosis.

Chronic

Due to chronic obstructive or restrictive conditions
- Nerve disease (e.g., poliomyelitis)
- Muscle disease (e.g., myopathy)
- CNS disorder (e.g., brain tumor)
- Restriction of thorax (e.g., musculoskeletal disorders, scleroderma, pickwickian syndrome)
- Pulmonary disease (e.g., prolonged pneumonia, primary alveolar hypoventilation)

Acidosis is not usually severe.
Beware of commonly occurring mixed acid-base disturbances
- Chronic respiratory acidosis with superimposed acute hypercapnia resulting from acute infection, such as bronchitis or pneumonia.
- Superimposed metabolic alkalosis (e.g., due to diuretics or vomiting) may exacerbate the hypercapnia.

Alkalosis, Metabolic

Due To

Loss of acid
- Vomiting, gastric suction, gastrocolic fistula
- Diarrhea in mucoviscidosis (rarely)
- Villous adenoma of colon
- Aciduria secondary to potassium depletion

Excess of base due to
- Administration of absorbable antacids (e.g., sodium bicarbonate; milk-alkali syndrome)
- Administration of salts of weak acids (e.g., sodium lactate, sodium or potassium citrate)
- Some vegetarian diets

Potassium depletion (causing sodium and H^+ to enter cells)
- Gastrointestinal loss (e.g., chronic diarrhea)
- Lack of potassium intake (e.g., anorexia nervosa, administration of IV fluids without potassium supplements for treatment of vomiting or postoperatively)
- Diuresis (e.g., mercurials, thiazides, osmotic diuresis)
- Extracellular volume depletion and chloride depletion
- All forms of mineralocorticoid excess (e.g., primary aldosteronism, Cushing's syndrome, administration of steroids, ingestion of large amounts of licorice)
- Glycogen deposition
- Chronic alkalosis
- Potassium-losing nephropathy

Hypoproteinemia per se may cause a nonrespiratory alkalosis. Decreased albumin of 1 gm/dL causes an average increase in standard bicarbonate of 3.4 mEq/L, an apparent base excess of +3.7 mEq/L, and a decrease in AG of ~3 mEq/L.[1]

♦Laboratory Findings

Serum pH is increased (>7.60 in severe alkalemia).
Total plasma CO_2 is increased (bicarbonate >30 mEq/L).

[1]McAuliffe JJ, et al. Hypoproteinemic alkalosis. *Am J Med* 1986;81:86.

pCO_2 is normal or slightly increased.

Serum pH and bicarbonate are above those predicted by the pCO_2 (by nomogram or Table 12-4).

Hypokalemia is an almost constant feature and is the chief danger in metabolic alkalosis.

Decreased serum chloride is relatively lower than sodium.

BUN may be increased.

Urine pH is >7.0 (≤7.9) if potassium depletion is not severe and concomitant sodium deficiency (e.g., vomiting) is not present. With severe hypokalemia (<2.0 mEq/L), urine may be acid in presence of systemic alkalosis.

○When the urine chloride is low (<10 mEq/L) and the patient responds to chloride treatment, the cause is more likely loss of gastric juice, diuretic therapy, or rapid relief of chronic hypercapnia. Chloride replacement is completed when urine chloride remains >40 mEq/L. When the urine chloride is high (>20 mEq/L) and the patient does not respond to sodium chloride treatment, the cause is more likely hyperadrenalism or severe potassium deficiency.

See Table 12-4.

Alkalosis, Respiratory

(Decreased pCO_2 of <38 mm Hg)

Due To

Hyperventilation
- CNS disorders (e.g., infection, tumor, trauma, cerebrovascular accident [CVA])
- Salicylate intoxication
- Fever
- Bacteremia due to gram-negative organisms
- Liver disease
- Pulmonary disease (e.g., pneumonia, pulmonary emboli, asthma)
- Mechanical overventilation
- Congestive heart failure
- Hypoxia (e.g., decreased barometric pressure, ventilation-perfusion imbalance)
- Anxiety-hyperventilation

Laboratory Findings

Acute hypocapnia—usually only a modest decrease in plasma HCO_3^- concentrations and marked alkalosis

Chronic hypocapnia—usually only a slight alkaline pH (not usually >7.55)

Anion Gap Classification

(Calculated as Na – [Cl + HCO_3]; typically normal = 8–16 mEq/L; if K is included, normal = 10–20 mEq/L; reference interval varies considerably depending on instrumentation.)

Use

Identification of cause of metabolic acidosis

Supplement to laboratory quality control along with its components

Increased In

○Increased "unmeasured" anions
- Organic (e.g., lactic acidosis, ketoacidosis)
- Inorganic (e.g., administration of phosphate, sulfate)
- Protein (e.g., transient hyperalbuminemia)
- Exogenous (e.g., salicylate, formate, nitrate, penicillin, carbenicillin)
- Not completely identified (e.g., hyperosmolar hyperglycemic nonketotic coma, uremia, poisoning by ethylene glycol, methanol, salicylates)
- Artifactual
    Falsely increased serum sodium
    Falsely decreased serum chloride or bicarbonate

- Decreased unmeasured cations (e.g., hypokalemia, hypocalcemia, hypomagnesemia)

○*When AG >12–14 mEq/L, diabetic ketoacidosis is the most common cause, uremic acidosis is the second most common cause, and drug ingestion (e.g., salicylates, methyl alcohol, ethylene glycol, ethyl alcohol) is the third most common cause; lactic acidosis should always be considered when these three causes are ruled out.*

Decreased In

○Decreased unmeasured anion (e.g., hypoalbuminemia is probably most common cause of decreased AG)

○Artifactual
- "Hyperchloremia" in bromide intoxication (if chloride determination by colorimetric method)
- Hyponatremia due to viscous serum
- False decrease in serum sodium; false increase in serum chloride or HCO_3^-

○Increased unmeasured cations
- Hyperkalemia, hypercalcemia, hypermagnesemia
- Increased proteins in multiple myeloma, paraproteinemias, polyclonal gammopathies (these abnormal proteins are positively charged and lower the AG)
- Increased lithium, tris(hydroxymethyl)aminomethane buffer (tromethamine)

○*AG >30 mEq/L almost always indicates organic acidosis even in presence of uremia. AG of 20–29 mEq/L occurs in absence of identified organic acidosis in 25% of patients. AG is rarely >23 mEq/L in chronic renal failure.*

Simultaneous changes in ions may cancel each other out, leaving AG unchanged (e.g., increased chloride and decreased HCO_3^-).

AG may provide a clue to the presence of a mixed rather than simple acid-base disturbance.

Nutritional Deficiencies

Deficiency, Copper

Nutritional Copper Deficiency

Found in patients on parenteral nutrition and in neonates and premature infants and children recovering from severe protein-calorie malnutrition fed iron-fortified milk formula with cane sugar and cottonseed oil.

Anemia not responsive to iron and vitamins

Leukopenia with WBC <5000/cu mm and neutropenia (<1500/cu mm)

♦ Copper administration corrects neutropenia in 3 wks and anemia responds with reticulocytosis.

Decreased copper and ceruloplasmin in plasma and decreased hepatic copper confirm diagnosis.

Kinky-Hair Syndrome

(X-linked recessive error of copper metabolism causing accumulation of excess copper in a low-molecular-weight protein; syndrome of neonatal hypothermia, feeding difficulties, and sometimes prolonged jaundice; at 2–3 mos, seizures and progressive change of hair from normal to steel wool–like texture with light color; striking facial appearance, increasing mental deterioration, infections, failure to thrive, death in early infancy; changes in elastica interna of arteries)

♦ Decreased copper in serum and liver; normal in RBCs

Increased copper in amniotic fluid, cultured fibroblasts, and amniotic cells

Decreased serum ceruloplasmin

Serum Copper Also Decreased In

Nephrosis (ceruloplasmin lost in urine)

Wilson's disease (see p. 250)

Acute leukemia in remission

Some iron deficiency anemias of childhood (that require copper as well as iron therapy)

Kwashiorkor

ACTH and corticosteroid use

Serum Copper Increased In

Anemias
- PA
- Megaloblastic anemia of pregnancy
- Iron-deficiency anemia
- Aplastic anemia

Leukemia, acute and chronic
Infection, acute and chronic
Malignant lymphoma
Biliary cirrhosis
Hemochromatosis
Collagen diseases (including SLE, RA, acute rheumatic fever, GN)
Hypothyroidism
Hyperthyroidism
Frequently associated with increased CRP
Ingestion of oral contraceptives and estrogens
Pregnancy

Deficiency, Niacin (Pellagra)

♦Whole blood niacin level <24 μmol/L
ODecreased excretion of niacin metabolites (nicotinamide) in 6- or 24-hr urine sample
OPlasma tryptophan level markedly decreased

Deficiency, Riboflavin

♦Decreased riboflavin level in plasma, RBCs, WBCs
ORBC glutathione reductase activity coefficient is ≥ 1.20.

Deficiency, Thiamine (Beriberi)

Increased blood pyruvic acid level
♦Decreased thiamine level in blood and urine; becomes normal within 24 hrs after
 therapy begins (thus baseline levels should be established first).
RBC transketolase <8 U (baseline) and addition of thiamine pyrophosphate causes
 >20% increase.
Laboratory findings due to complications (e.g., heart failure)
Laboratory findings due to underlying conditions (e.g., chronic diarrhea, inadequate
 intake, alcoholism)

Deficiency, Vitamin A

♦Decreased plasma level of vitamin A
Elevated carotenoids may cause false low values for vitamin A.
Laboratory findings due to preceding conditions (e.g., malabsorption, alcoholism,
 restricted diet)

Deficiency, Vitamin B$_6$ (Pyridoxine)

♦Decreased pyridoxic acid in urine
♦Decreased serum levels of vitamin B$_6$

Deficiency, Vitamin B$_{12}$ and Folic Acid

See p. 366 and Table 11-11.

Deficiency, Vitamin C (Scurvy)

♦Plasma level of ascorbic acid is decreased—usually 0 in frank scurvy. (Normal =
 0.5–1.5 mg/dL, but lower level does not prove diagnosis.) Ascorbic acid in buffy coat
 (WBC) is decreased—usually absent in clinical scurvy. (Normal is 30 mg/dL.)
Tyrosyl compounds are present in urine (detected by Millon's reagent) in patients with
 scurvy but are absent in normal persons after protein meal or administration of tyrosine.

METAB/HERED

Serum ALP is decreased; serum calcium and phosphorus are normal.
Rumpel-Leede test is positive.
Microscopic hematuria is present in one-third of patients.
Stool may be positive for occult blood.
Laboratory findings due to associated deficiencies (e.g., anemia due to folic acid deficiency)

Deficiency (or Excess), Vitamin D

See Rickets, p. 306 and discussion of excess on p. 606.

1,25-Dihydroxy-vitamin D

Formed from 25-hydroxy-vitamin D by kidney, placenta, granulomas
Use
Differential diagnosis of hypocalcemic disorders
Monitoring of patients with renal osteodystrophy
Increased In
Hyperparathyroidism
Chronic granulomatous disorders
Hypercalcemia associated with lymphoma
Decreased In
Severe vitamin D deficiency
Hypercalcemia of malignancy (except lymphoma)
Tumor-induced osteomalacia
Hypoparathyroidism
Pseudohypoparathyroidism
Renal osteodystrophy
Type I vitamin D–resistant rickets

25-Hydroxy-vitamin D

Use
Evaluation of vitamin D intoxication or deficiency
Increased In
Vitamin D intoxication (distinguishes this from other causes of hypercalcemia)
Decreased In
Rickets
Osteomalacia
Secondary hyperparathyroidism
Malabsorption of vitamin D (e.g., severe liver disease, cholestasis)
Diseases that increase vitamin D metabolism (e.g., tuberculosis, sarcoidosis, primary
    hyperparathyroidism)

Deficiency, Vitamin E

♦ Plasma tocopherol <0.4 mg/dL in adults; <0.15 mg/dL in infants aged 1 mo.
Laboratory findings due to underlying conditions (e.g., malabsorption in adults; diet
    high in polyunsaturated fatty acids in premature infants)

Deficiency, Vitamin K

See p. 476.

Deficiency, Zinc

Due To

Acrodermatitis enteropathica (rare autosomal recessive disease of infancy due to block
    in intestinal absorption of zinc)
Inadequate nutrition (e.g., parenteral alimentation)
Excessive requirements
Decreased absorption or availability
Increased losses

Iatrogenic causes
Plasma zinc levels do not always reflect nutritional status.
Measurement of zinc in hair may be helpful.
Findings of decreased or very excessive urinary zinc excretion may be helpful.
Plasma, RBC, or WBC zinc levels are insensitive markers for zinc status.
Plasma concentrations
- Normal range = 70–120 μg/dL
- Moderate depletion = 40–60 μg/dL
- Severe depletion = 20 μg/dL

Dehydration, Hypertonic

Due To

Loss of water in excess of electrolyte loss (e.g., gastroenteritis with diarrhea, hyper-ventilation, high fever, diabetes insipidus)
Excessive intake of high-solute mixtures (e.g., accidental ingestion, iatrogenic infusion)

○Increased serum sodium to >150 mEq/L
○Metabolic acidosis is almost always present.
Increased blood glucose is common, often >200 mg/dL.
○BUN is increased, often ≥ 60 mg/dL.
♦Serum osmolality is increased.
Hypocalcemia is common and may persist if calcium is not administered.
Urine is concentrated with specific gravity usually >1.020.
Other laboratory findings of dehydration
Rehydration with return of serum sodium to normal should not be completed in <48 hrs because of risk of permanent CNS damage.

Dehydration, Hypotonic

(Usually in children with vomiting and diarrhea treated with oral replacement of tap water)
○Decreased serum sodium, usually <135 mEq/L
Other laboratory findings of dehydration
Urine pH is >7.0 (≤ 7.9) if potassium depletion is not severe and concomitant sodium deficiency (e.g., vomiting) is not present.
○When urine chloride is low (<10–20 mEq/L) and the patient responds to sodium chloride treatment, the cause is more likely loss of gastric juice, diuretic therapy, or relief of chronic hypercapnia.
○When the urine chloride is high (>10–20 mEq/L) and the patient does not respond to sodium chloride treatment, the cause is more likely hyperadrenalism or severe pulmonary deficiency.

Infant Who Fails to Thrive, Laboratory Evaluation

Initial tests
- Pathologic examination of placenta
- CBC (anemia, hemoglobinopathy)
- Urine—reducing substances, ferric chloride test, pH, specific gravity, microscopic examination, colony count and culture
- Stool—occult blood, ova and parasites, pH
- Serum—sodium, potassium, chloride, bicarbonate, creatinine, calcium
More detailed tests
- Sweat chloride and sodium (see section on cystic fibrosis, p. 254)
- Serum TSH and T_4 (hypothyroidism)
- Serum and urine amino acids (aminoacidurias)
- Rectal biopsy
- Serologic tests for congenital infection (rubella, CMV infection, toxoplasmosis, syphilis)
- Duodenal enzyme measurements
- Chromosomal studies (trisomy D, E)

Premature infants (shortened gestation period) should be differentiated from infants whose weight is below that expected for gestational age.

METAB/HERED

Some Causes of Failure to Thrive

	% of Cases
Inadequate caloric intake	87
Maternal deprivation (e.g., caloric restriction, child abuse, emotional disorders)	
Congenital abnormalities (e.g., cleft lip or palate, tracheoesophageal fistula, esophageal webs, macroglossia, achalasia)	
Acquired abnormalities (e.g., esophageal stricture, subdural hematoma, hypoxia, diabetes insipidus)	
Decreased intestinal function	
Abnormal digestion, e.g.,	
Cystic fibrosis	3.0
Trypsin deficiency	
Mono- and disaccharidase deficiencies	
Abnormal absorption, e.g.,	
Celiac syndrome	0.5
Gastroenteritis	
Biliary atresia	
Megacolon	
Giardiasis	
Protein-losing enteropathy	
Increased utilization of calories	
Infant of narcotic-addicted mother	
Prolonged fever (e.g., chronic infections)	
Excessive crying	
Congenital heart disease	
Renal loss of calories	
Aminoaciduria, e.g.,	
Maple syrup disease	0.5
Methylmalonicacidemia	0.5
Chronic renal disease, e.g.,	
Renal tubular acidosis	
Pyelonephritis	
Polycystic disease	
Congenital/acquired nephritis	
Congenital nephrosis	
Nephrogenic diabetes insipidus	
Other	
Anemia	
Fetal-maternal transfusion	
Hemoglobinopathies	
Iron deficiency	
Hypercalcemia	
Hyperparathyroidism	
Vitamin A or D intoxication	
Idiopathic	
Endocrine	
Hypothyroidism	2.5
Hypoadrenalism	
Hyposomatotropism	
Congenital hyperthyroidism	
Metabolic	
Glycogen storage disease	0.5
Galactosemia	
Hypophosphatasia	
Mucopolysaccharidosis	
Rickets	
CNS lesions	
Subdural hematoma	2.5
Intracerebral hemorrhage	
Tumors	
Unknown	

Intrauterine Growth Retardation

(Low-birth-weight infants who are mature by gestational age)

Due To

Chronic hypertension, especially with renal involvement and proteinuria
Chronic renal disease
Severe, long-standing diabetes mellitus
Preeclampsia and eclampsia with underlying chronic vascular disease
Hypoxia, e.g.,
- Cyanotic heart disease
- Pregnancy at high altitudes
- Hemoglobinopathies, especially sickle cell disease

Maternal protein-calorie malnutrition
Placental conditions
- Extensive infarction
- Parabiotic transfusion syndrome
- Hemangioma of placenta or cord
- Abnormal cord insertion

Fetal factors
- Chromosomal abnormalities, especially trisomies of D group and chromosome 18
- Malformations of GI tract that interfere with swallowing
- Chronic intrauterine infections (e.g., rubella, CMV and herpesvirus infection, syphilis, toxoplasmosis)

Unexplained
♦ No specific diagnostic laboratory tests are available.

Malnutrition, Protein-Calorie

Adult Malnutrition and Kwashiorkor

(Occur in patients with inadequate protein intake in presence of low caloric intake or normal caloric intake and increased catabolism [e.g., trauma, severe burns, respiratory or renal failure, nonmalignant GI tract disease]; may develop quickly. Major loss of protein from visceral compartments may impair organ function.)
Decreased serum albumin (2.1–3.0 mg/dL in moderate deficiencies, <2.1 mg/dL in severe deficiencies, 2.8–3.4 mg/dL in mild deficiencies) is a poor marker.
Decreased serum prealbumin (transthyretin) is more sensitive than albumin due to shorter half-life (normal range = 18–36 mg/dL; severe malnutrition is <10.7 mg/dL; moderate malnutrition = 10.7–16 mg/dL; patient is likely to benefit from early therapy). With therapy, increases >1 mg/dL daily. Other proteins with short half-lives that have been suggested as markers are retinol-binding protein and fibronectin. Effective in monitoring growth rate in preterm infants. Also decreased in impaired liver function (e.g., hepatitis, cirrhosis, obstructive jaundice) and some types of amyloidosis.
Decreased serum transferrin (150–200 mg/dL in mild, 100–150 mg/dL in moderate, <100 mg/dL in severe deficiencies) or TIBC. Increase in transferrin due to inflammation decreases diagnostic utility. Direct measurement is preferred because calculation is affected by iron metabolism and laboratory variability. Poor sensitivity in this condition.
All serum complement components except C4 and sometimes C5 are decreased.
Decreased total lymphocyte count evidencing diminished immunologic resistance. (2000–3500/cu mm is normal; <1500/cu mm is indication for further assessment; 800–1200/cu mm is moderate; <800/cu mm is severe; should always be interpreted with total WBC count.)
Diminished delayed hypersensitivity reaction (measured by skin testing)
Normal anthropometric measurements (e.g., creatinine-height index, triceps skinfold, arm circumference measurements)
Clinically, may show pitting edema, ascites, enlarged liver, diarrhea.
○ These laboratory tests all have low sensitivity and specificity or are not easily obtainable.

Marasmus

(Chronic deficiency in total energy intake as in wasting illnesses [e.g., cancer] with protein loss from somatic compartment without necessary losses in visceral component)
Normal serum protein levels
Impaired immune function
Clinically, patient shows severe wasting of skeletal muscle and fat; edema is distinctively absent. May progress to marasmic kwashiorkor.
Laboratory findings due to underlying diseases (e.g., cancer) or complications (e.g., infection)

Monitoring of Nutritional Therapy

Weekly 24-hr urine nitrogen excretion reflects degree of hypermetabolism and correction of deficits.
Increase of serum prealbumin and retinol-binding proteins by 1 mg/dL/day indicates good response. Measure 2–3 times/wk. May precede improvement in albumin levels by 7–10 days.
Somatomedin C has also been suggested for monitoring.
Fluid and electrolyte levels should be corrected.

Nutritional Factors in Young Children, Laboratory Indicators

Protein—BUN <6 mg/dL or urine <8 mg/gm of creatinine suggests recent low protein intake
Serum albumin <3.2 gm/dL suggests low protein intake, but this is a rather insensitive, nonspecific indicator of protein status.
Iron—see p. 360.
Vitamin A—serum carotene <40 μg/dL suggests low intake of carotene. Serum vitamin A <20 μg/dL suggests low stores of vitamin A or may indicate failure of retinol transport out of liver into circulation.
Ascorbic acid—serum ascorbate <0.3 mg/dL suggests recent low intake. Whole blood ascorbate <0.3 mg/dL indicates low intake and reduction in body pool of ascorbic acid. Leukocyte ascorbic acid <20 mg/dL suggests poor nutritional status.
Riboflavin—<250 μg/gm of creatinine in urine suggests low recent intake of riboflavin.
Glutathione reductase–flavin adenine dinucleotide effect expressed as ratio of >1.2:1 suggests poor nutritional status.
Thiamine—<125 μg/gm of creatinine in urine suggests low intake of thiamine. Transketolase–thiamine pyrophosphate effect expressed as a ratio of >1.5:1 suggests poor nutritional status.
Folate—serum folate <6 μg/dL suggests low intake. RBC folate <20 μg/dL or increased excretion of formiminoglutamic acid in urine after histidine load suggests poor nutritional status.
Iodine—<50 μg/gm of creatinine in urine suggests recent low intake of iodine.
Calcium, phosphorus, ALP—rickets (see p. 306).

Total Parenteral Nutrition (TPN), Metabolic Complications

Decreasing serum prealbumin (transthyretin) level after 2 wks of TPN indicates poor prognosis, but increasing or unchanged level indicates anabolism and protein replenishment and suggests probable survival.
Serum cholesterol decreases rapidly during first 2 days, then remains at low level. Apo A decreases 30–50% after long-term TPN but apo B is usually unchanged.
Hyperglycemia (which may cause osmotic diuresis and hyperosmolarity) or hypoglycemia
Serum electrolytes are usually unchanged but sodium may decrease slightly and potassium may increase slightly after fifth day. Changes depend on solution composition and infusion rate. Frequent monitoring is indicated.
Ketosis develops if insufficient calories or low glucose concentration; may indicate onset of infection.
Hyperosmolarity due to TPN infusion
Lactic or hyperchloremic metabolic acidosis develops in some patients.

Serum creatinine and creatinine clearance are not significantly changed.
Serum uric acid decreases markedly after 2–17 day of TPN and returns to pretreatment
level 3–7 days after cessation of TPN.
Abnormal plasma amino acid levels
Deficiency of essential fatty acids (on fat-free TPN), zinc, or copper
Transiently increased serum AST (3–4×), ALT (3–7×), ALP (2×), and GGT.
Direct bilirubin and LD normal or slightly increased. Improve 1 wk after cessation of TPN and return to normal in 1–4 mos.
Serum folate falls 50% if not supplemented.
67% of children show eosinophilia (>140/cu mm) after 9 days of TPN.
Laboratory findings of sepsis (e.g., *Candida*) due to infection of catheter.

Some Guidelines for Monitoring Patients on TPN

Twice weekly: chemistry profile, electrolytes, transthyretin
Weekly: CBC, urinalysis, chemistry and acid-base profiles, iron, zinc, copper, magnesium, triglycerides, ammonia
Every 2 wks: folate, Vitamin B_{12}
Baseline: all of the above tests
Unstable clinical condition may require testing daily or more often.

Nutritional Dwarfism

Serum proteins, amino acids, and BUN are usually normal.
Anemia is not prominent.
Laboratory changes due to underlying condition (e.g., intestinal malabsorption, chronic vomiting, congenital heart disease, chronic infections, chronic renal insufficiency)

Vitamin Reference Ranges (Blood)*

Limited utility because blood levels may not reflect tissue stores.

Vitamin A	
Retinol	360–1200 μg/L
	<20 μg/dL indicates low intake and tissue stores
	20–36 μg/dL indeterminate
Retinyl esters	≤ 1.0 μg/dL
Carotene	48–200 μg/dL
Vitamin C (ascorbic acid)	0.2–2.0 mg/dL
	<0.2 mg/dL represents deficiency
Vitamin D	Indirect estimate by measuring serum ALP, calcium, and phosphorus
Total 25-hydroxy-vitamin D	14–42 ng/mL (winter)
	15–80 ng/mL (summer)
1,25-dihydroxy-vitamin D	15–60 pg/mL
Vitamin E (alpha-tocopherol)	
Children	3.0–15.0 μg/mL
Adults	5.5–17.0 μg/mL
Deficiency	<3.0 μg/mL
Excess	>40 μg/mL
Vitamin B_1 (thiamine)	5.3–7.9 μg/dL
Vitamin B_2 (riboflavin)	3.7–13.7 μg/dL
Vitamin B_{12} (cobalamin)	
Low	<150 pg/mL
Normal	190–900 pg/mL
Unsaturated vitamin B_{12}–binding capacity	870–1800 pg/mL
Folate, serum	≥ 3.5 ng/mL
RBC	
<1 yr	74–995 ng/mL
1–11 yrs	96–362 ng/mL
≥ 12 yrs	180–600 ng/mL

*Values are for serum unless otherwise indicated.

METAB/HERED

Prenatal Screening and Diagnosis[2-5]

(See also Chapter 14, Obstetrical Monitoring of Fetus and Placenta.)

Use

General risk factors
- Maternal age ≥ 35 yrs at delivery
- Abnormal maternal serum AFP, hCG, or unconjugated estriol

Ethnic risk factors
- Sickle cell anemia (presence of sickling; confirmed by Hb electrophoresis)
- Tay-Sachs disease (decreased serum hexosaminidase A)
- Alpha- and beta-thalassemia (decreased MCV; confirmed by Hb electrophoresis)

Specific risk factors
- Rubella, toxoplasmosis, or CMV infection
- Maternal disorder, e.g., diabetes mellitus, PKU
- Teratogen exposure, e.g., radiation, alcohol, isotretinoin, anticonvulsants, lithium
- Previous stillbirth or neonatal death
- Previous child with chromosomal abnormality or structural defect
- Inherited disorders, e.g., cystic fibrosis, metabolic disorders, sex-linked recessive disorders
- Either parent with balanced translocation or structural abnormality

Maternal Serum Sampling

See Table 12-6 and Fig. 12-2.

AFP is increased 4× normal in open neural tube, 7× normal in anencephaly, and in ventral wall defects; associated with exposed fetal-membrane and blood-vessel surfaces.

Maximum serum AFP concentration is between 16–18 wks, but sampling should not be done before 14 or after 20 wks. If both serum and amniotic fluid show increased levels, contamination of amniotic fluid with fetal or maternal blood is ruled out by assay for fetal Hb and acetylcholinesterase. If only maternal serum AFP is increased without demonstrable defect, pregnancy is at increased risk (e.g., premature delivery, low-birth-weight baby, or fetal death).

Decreased AFP and unconjugated estriol in trisomy 21 (Down syndrome) and 18 hCG significantly increased in trisomy 21 (see p. 563).

Amniocentesis

Generally done between 8 and 12 wks of gestation. Risk of fetal loss is ~0.5%. Cell culture takes 5–7 days; activity similar to that in fibroblasts.

Use

Can detect intermediary metabolites of some inborn errors, especially organic acid disorders. AFP is increased ~20× in anencephaly, 7× in open neural tube, and in ventral wall defects associated with exposed fetal-membrane and blood-vessel surfaces. See preceding paragraph.

Chorionic Villus Sampling[5]

Generally done between 8 and 12 wks of gestation; sometimes as early as 6–7 wks. Risk of fetal loss is 0.5–2%.

Contamination with maternal decidua must be avoided for accurate diagnosis based on fetal chromosomes, enzyme assay, or DNA analysis.

---

[2]Wax JR, Blakemore KJ. What can be learned from cordocentesis? *Clin Lab Med* 1992;12:503.
[3]Winchester B, Young E. Prenatal diagnosis of enzyme defects—an update. *Arch Dis Child* 1991;66:451.
[4]D'Alton ME, DeCherney AH. Prenatal diagnosis. *N Engl J Med* 1993;328:114.
[5]Cole HM, ed. Chorionic villus sampling: a reassessment. Diagnostic and therapeutic technology assessment. *JAMA* 1990;263:305.

Table 12-6. Serum Markers in Detection of Various Prenatal Conditions

Condition	AFP	hCG	Unconjugated Estriol	Detection Rate
Anencephaly	4+	—	—	95%
Open spina bifida	3+	—	—	80%
Abdominal wall defects	3+	—	—	75%
Trisomy 21 (Down syndrome)	D	I	D	60%
Trisomy 18	DD	DD	DD	60%
Other chromosomal abnormalities	I/D	I/D	I/D	50%

D = decreased; DD = strongly decreased; I = increased; I/D = increased or decreased.
Source: Wasserman ER. Preventing problem pregnancies. *Advance/Laboratory* Nov 1997:53.

In some patient populations, a negative culture for *Neisseria gonorrhoeae* or HSV may be required.
Associated with ~7% fetal loss similar to amniocentesis (spontaneous rate ~4.5%).
False-positive in 2% of cases compared with 0.3% of cases in amniocentesis.
Most prenatal diagnoses of enzyme defects are now made using this assay.

Indications

Chromosomal examination
- Previous child with chromosomal trisomy
- Mother carrier of X-linked disorder (to determine fetal sex)
- Parent carrier of chromosomal translocation
- Maternal age >35 yrs
Restriction enzyme assay
- Hemoglobinopathy (e.g., thalassemia)
- Lesch-Nyhan syndrome

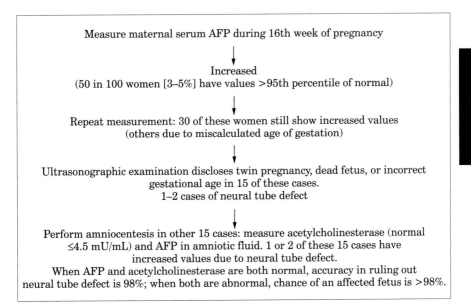

Measure maternal serum AFP during 16th week of pregnancy

↓

Increased
(50 in 100 women [3–5%] have values >95th percentile of normal)

↓

Repeat measurement: 30 of these women still show increased values
(others due to miscalculated age of gestation)

↓

Ultrasonographic examination discloses twin pregnancy, dead fetus, or incorrect
gestational age in 15 of these cases.
1–2 cases of neural tube defect

↓

Perform amniocentesis in other 15 cases: measure acetylcholinesterase (normal
≤4.5 mU/mL) and AFP in amniotic fluid. 1 or 2 of these 15 cases have
increased values due to neural tube defect.
When AFP and acetylcholinesterase are both normal, accuracy in ruling out
neural tube defect is 98%; when both are abnormal, chance of an affected fetus is >98%.

Fig. 12-2. Algorithm for alpha-fetoprotein (AFP) testing in pregnancy (detects virtually all cases of anencephaly and 80% of cases of open spina bifida with very few false-positives).

- Alpha$_1$-antitrypsin deficiency
- PKU

Metabolic assay, e.g.,

- Adenosine deaminase deficiency
- Adrenoleukodystrophy
- Argininosuccinicaciduria
- Citrullinemia
- Cystinosis
- Fabry's disease
- Fanconi's anemia
- Farber's disease
- Gaucher's disease
- GM$_1$ gangliosidosis
- GM$_2$ gangliosidosis (Tay-Sachs disease)
- Homocystinuria
- Krabbe's disease
- Lesch-Nyhan syndrome
- Maple syrup urine disease
- Menkes' syndrome
- Metachromatic leukodystrophy
- Methylmalonicaciduria
- Mucolipidosis II (I-cell disease)
- Mucopolysaccharidosis (Ia, II, III, IV)
- Multiple sulfatase deficiency
- Niemann-Pick disease
- Pompe's disease
- Wolman's disease
- Zellweger syndrome

Fetal Blood Sampling

Generally done at ~15th week but usually also successful between 18th and 23rd wks. Check for maternal serum contamination by determining hCG concentration. Additional risk to fetus of 2%.

Use

Prenatal diagnosis of

- RBC isoimmunization, e.g., Rh, minor antigens
- Alloimmune or autoimmune thrombocytopenia
- Hemoglobinopathies (e.g., thalassemias, sickle cell disorders, spherocytosis, enzyme deficiencies [e.g., G-6-PD])
- Coagulation defects (e.g., factor VIII and IX hemophilias and fetal sex, other factor deficiencies, von Willebrand's disease)
- Immune-deficiency disorders (e.g., SCID, Wiskott-Aldrich syndrome, ataxia-telangiectasia, chronic granulomatous disease, homozygous C3 deficiency, Chédiak-Higashi syndrome)
- Intrauterine infections (detection of specific IgM and increased total IgM, increased WBC and eosinophil count, decreased platelet count, various blood chemistries) (e.g., rubella, toxoplasmosis, varicella, CMV, and parvovirus B19 infection)
- Chromosomal disorders (e.g., mosaicism, fragile X syndrome)
- Metabolic and cytogenetic disorders (e.g., PKU, alpha$_1$-antitrypsin deficiency, cystic fibrosis, Duchenne's muscular dystrophy)
- Other conditions (e.g., familial hypercholesterolemia, hyperphenylalaninemia, adrenoleukodystrophy)
- Fetal acid-base balance and metabolic state

Fetal Biopsy

Use

Liver biopsy for diagnosis of deficiency of long-chain 3-hydroxyacyl–coenzyme A (CoA) dehydrogenase, ornithine transcarbamylase deficiency, atypical PKU due to deficiency of glutamyl transpeptidase cyclohydrolase I, type I primary hyperoxaluria, glycogen storage disease type I.

Skin biopsy (e.g., for certain genetic disorders such as epidermolysis bullosa)

Muscle biopsy for Duchenne's muscular dystrophy

Ultrasonography and Echocardiography

Use

To guide sampling process

To verify gestational age

Karyotyping is done if malformations are found because one-third of these fetuses have a chromosomal disorder.

May be abnormal in trisomy 13, 18, 21, 45, X, and in triploidy.

~50% of major heart, kidney, and bladder abnormalities not detected by maternal serum AFP screening.

Karyotype Analysis

Use

Determine status of chromosomes X, Y, 21, 18, 13

Molecular Diagnosis

Use

Direct detection of gene deletions and mutations and linkage analysis using cultured amniocytes or chorionic villi can make some diagnoses even when gene products are not present (e.g., adult polycystic kidney disease, sickle cell disease, alpha-thalassemia, cystic fibrosis, Gaucher's disease, Duchenne's muscular dystrophy, fragile X syndrome, factor VIII and factor IX deficiencies).

Isolation of Fetal Cells in Maternal Blood

(Usual ratio = 1:1000–1:5000)

Use

Still an investigational procedure but would allow diagnosis by flow cytometry and PCR. PCR can demonstrate Y chromosome in women carrying male fetuses.

Newborn Screening

Chromosome Analysis (Karyotyping)

Use

Suspected autosomal syndromes, e.g.,
    Down syndrome (mongolism)
    Trisomy E, 18
    Trisomy D, 13
    Cri du chat syndrome
Suspected sex-chromosome syndromes, e.g.,
    Klinefelter's syndrome, XXY, XXXY
    Turner's syndrome, XO
    "Superfemale" XXX, XXXX
    "Supermale" XYY
    "Funny-looking kid" syndromes, especially with multiple anomalies including mental retardation and low birth weight
    Possible myelogenous leukemia to demonstrate Ph chromosome
    Ambiguous genitalia
    Infertility (some patients)

Repeated miscarriages
Primary amenorrhea or oligomenorrhea
Mental retardation with sex anomalies
Hypogonadism
Delayed puberty
Abnormal development at puberty
Disturbances of somatic growth

Inherited Disorders that Can Be Identified by Molecular Genetics

Adult polycystic disease
Achondroplasia
Alpha$_1$-antitrypsin deficiency
Canavan's disease
Charcot-Marie-Tooth disease
Congenital adrenal hyperplasia
Cystic fibrosis
Duchenne's and Becker's muscular dystrophies
Familial adenomatous polyposis
Familial hypercholesterolemia
Fragile X syndrome
Galactosemia
Gaucher's disease
Hemophilia A and B
Huntington's disease
Marfan syndrome
Mitochondrial disorders
Myotonic dystrophy
Neurofibromatosis types 1 and 2
Ornithine transcarbamoylase deficiency
PKU
Spinal muscular atrophy
Spinocerebellar ataxia
Sickle cell disease
Tay-Sachs disease
Alpha- and beta-thalassemia

Metabolic Conditions (Inherited), Classification[6]

(Deficient enzyme is shown in parentheses.)
Disorders of carbohydrate metabolism
    Diabetes mellitus
    Pentosuria
    Fructose
      Fructosuria (aldolase B)*
      Fructose-1,6-bisphosphatase deficiency*
    Lactose
     Familial lactose intolerance
    Galactose

Galactosemia (galactose 1-phosphate uridyltransferase)*	PD
Galactokinase deficiency	PD
Glycogen storage diseases*	PD for some
Disorders of amino acid metabolism	
Phenylalanine	
PKU (phenylalanine hydroxylase)	PD
Methionine	
Homocysteinuria (cystathionine synthase)	PD

[6]Cleary MA, Wraith JE. Antenatal diagnosis of inborn errors of metabolism. *Arch Dis Child* 1991;66:816.

Tyrosine
  Tyrosinemia I (fumarylacetoacetate hydrolase)*   PD
  Tyrosinemia II (tyrosine aminotransferase)
Valine, leucine, isoleucine
  Maple syrup urine disease (branched-chain ketoacid   PD
    dehydrogenase)*
Glycine
  Nonketotic hyperglycinemia (glycine cleavage system)*   PD
Lysine
  Hyperlysinemia (aminoadipic semialdehyde synthase)
Proline
  Hyperprolinemia I (proline oxidase)
  Hyperprolinemia II (pyrroline-5-carboxylate dehydrogenase)
  Hyperimidodipeptiduria (prolidase)
Urea cycle disorders
  Citrullinemia (argininosuccinic acid synthetase)*   PD
  Argininemia (arginase)   PD
  Argininosuccinicaciduria (argininosuccinate lyase)*   PD
  Ornithine carbamoyltransferase deficiency*   PD
  N-acetylglutamate synthetase deficiency
  Carbamyl phosphate synthetase deficiency*
Organic acidurias
  Propionate and methylmalonate metabolism
    Propionicacidemia (propionyl–CoA carboxylase)*   PD
    Methylmalonicacidemia (methylmalonyl–CoA mutase,   PD
     adenosylcobalamin synthesis)*
    Multiple carboxylase deficiency (holocarboxylase synthetase,
     biotinidase)
  Pyruvate and lactate metabolism
    LD deficiency
    Pyruvate dehydrogenase deficiency
    Pyruvate carboxylase deficiency*   PD
    Phospho*enol*pyruvate carboxykinase deficiency*
  Branched-chain organic acidemias
    Isovalericacidemia (isovaleryl–CoA dehydrogenase)*   PD
    Mevalonicaciduria (mevalonate)   PD
  Other organic acid disorders
    Alkaptonuria (homogentisic acid oxidase)
    Hyperoxaluria type I, glycolicaciduria (alanine-glyoxylate
     aminotransferase)
    Hyperoxaluria type II, glycericaciduria (glyceric dehydrogenase)
    Glycerol kinase deficiency
    Canavan's disease (aspartoacylase)
  Lysosomal enzyme defects
    Mucopolysaccharidoses   PD
    Mucolipidosis II and III (uridine diphosphate–N-acetyl-   PD
     glucosamine–lysosomal enzyme N-acetylglucosaminyl-L-
     phosphotransferase)
    Glycoproteinoses
     Alpha- and beta-mannosidosis (alpha- and beta-mannosidase)   PD
     Sialidosis types I, II (neuraminidase)   PD
     Fucosidosis (alpha-fucosidase)   PD
  GM_2 gangliosidoses
    Tay-Sachs disease (hexosaminidase A)   PD
    Sandhoff's disease (hexosaminidase A, B)   PD
    GM_2 activator deficiency
  Other lysosomal storage disorders
    Metachromatic leukodystrophy (arylsulfatase A)   PD
    Multiple sulfatase deficiency (multiple lysosomal sulfatases)   PD
    Niemann-Pick disease (sphingomyelinase)*   PD
    Farber's disease (ceramidase)   PD
    Gaucher's disease (cerebroside beta-glucosidase)*   PD

METAB/HERED

Pompe's disease (glycogen storage disease type II) (alpha-1,
4-glucosidase deficiency)   PD
Krabbe's disease (galactocerebrosidase)*   PD
Fabry's disease (alpha-galactosidase)   PD
GM_1 gangliosidosis (beta-galactosidase)*   PD
Wolman's disease (acid lipase)*   PD
Cholesteryl ester storage disease (acid lipase)   PD
Mucolipidosis type IV
Peroxisomal disorders
  Acatalasia (catalase)
  Refsum's disease (phytanic acid hydroxylase)   PD
  Zellweger syndrome (peroxisome biogenesis)*   PD
Purine and pyrimidine metabolism disorders
  Lesch-Nyhan syndrome (hypoxanthine phosphoribosyltransferase)   PD
  Oroticaciduria (uridine 5'-monophosphate synthase)
  Xanthinuria (xanthine oxidase)
Disorders of metal metabolism
  Wilson's disease
  Hemochromatosis
  Menkes' syndrome   PD
Disorders of lipid metabolism (see p. 525, Table 12-7)
Disorders of heme proteins
  Porphyrinurias (see p. 547)   PD for some
  Bilirubin metabolism
    Crigler-Najjar syndromes I and II (uridine diphosphate–
      glucuronyl transferase)
    Gilbert's syndrome (uridine diphosphate–glucuronyl transferase)
    Dubin-Johnson syndrome
    Rotor's syndrome
Membrane transport disorders
  Cystinuria
  Hartnup disease
  Cystinosis   PD
  Hypophosphatemic rickets
Disorders of serum enzymes
  Hypophosphatasia (ALP)   PD
  Hyperphosphatasia
  Alpha$_1$-antitrypsin deficiency
Disorders of plasma proteins
  Analbuminemia
  Agammaglobulinemia
  Atransferrinemia
Disorders of blood
  Coagulation diseases (e.g., hemophilias)   PD
  RBC G-6-PD deficiency   PD
  Hemoglobinopathies and thalassemias   PD
  Hereditary spherocytosis   PD
  Hereditary nonspherocytic hemolytic anemia   PD
Others
  Congenital adrenal hyperplasia
  Menkes' syndrome

PD = Prenatal diagnosis is possible.
*May present in neonate.

○Newborn Screening for Metabolic Disorders

Indications

Screen for disorders that are asymptomatic until irreversible damage has occurred and
for which effective treatment exists.
Population prevalence sufficient to limit false-positive and false-negative results.
High cost/benefit ratio
Adequate follow-up to assure appropriate treatment

Interpretation

PKU (see p. 539)
Neonatal hypothyroidism (see p. 592 and Fig. 13-5)
Galactosemia (see p. 542)
Maple syrup urine disease (see p. 538)
Homocystinuria (see p. 543)
Biotinidase deficiency (one cause of multiple carboxylase deficiency; incidence ~1 in 40,000; ketoacidosis and organic aciduria can develop late)
Sickle cell disease (see p. 434)
Congenital adrenal hyperplasia (see p. 635)
Cystic fibrosis (see p. 254)
Toxoplasmosis (see p. 876)

Nuclear Sexing

Epithelial cells from buccal smear (or vaginal smear, etc.) are stained with cresyl violet and examined microscopically.
A dense body (Barr body) on the nuclear membrane represents one of the X chromosomes and occurs in 30–60% of female somatic cells. The maximum number of Barr bodies is one less than the number of X chromosomes.
If <10% of the cells contain Barr bodies in a patient with female genitalia, karyotyping should be done to delineate probable chromosomal abnormalities.
A normal count does not rule out chromosomal abnormalities.
Two Barr bodies may be found in
- 47 XXX female
- 48 XXXY male (Klinefelter's syndrome)
- 49 XXXYY male (Klinefelter's syndrome)

Three Barr bodies may be found in
- 49 XXXXY male (Klinefelter's syndrome)

Sex Chromosome in Leukocytes

Presence of a "drumstick" nuclear appendage in ~3% of leukocytes in normal females indicates the presence of two X chromosomes in the karyotype. It is not found in males.
It is absent in the XO type of Turner's syndrome.
In Klinefelter's syndrome (XXY) the presence of drumsticks shows a lower incidence than the presence of the extra Barr body. (*Mean lobe counts of neutrophils are also decreased.*)
Incidence of drumsticks is decreased and mean lobe counts are lower in trisomy 21 as well.
Double drumsticks are exceedingly rare and impractical for diagnostic use.

Tests of Lipid Metabolism

See Chapter 5, Coronary Heart Disease, p. 113.
Blood lipid tests should not be performed during stress or acute illness, e.g., recent myocardial infarction, stroke, pregnancy, trauma, weight loss, use of certain drugs; *should not be performed on hospitalized patients until 2–3 mos after illness.*
Abnormal lipid test results should always be confirmed with a new specimen, preferably 1 wk later, before beginning or changing therapy.
Keeping tourniquet in place longer than 3 mins may cause 5% variation in lipid values.

Apolipoproteins, Serum

(Protein component of lipoprotein that regulates their metabolism; each of four major groups consists of a family of two or more immunologically distinct proteins.)

Use

Assess risk of CHD
Classify hyperlipidemias

Apo A is the major protein of HDL; Apo A-I and A-II constitute 90% of total HDL protein in ratio of 3:1.

Apo B is the major protein in LDL; important in regulating cholesterol synthesis and metabolism. Decreased by severe illness and abetalipoproteinemia.

Apo C-I, C-II, and C-III are associated with all lipoproteins except LDL; C-II is important in triglyceride metabolism.

Serum apo A-I and B levels are more highly correlated with severity and extent of coronary artery disease (CAD) than total cholesterol and triglycerides.

Ratio of apo A-I to apo B shows greater sensitivity and specificity for CAD than LDL/HDL cholesterol ratio or HDL cholesterol/triglyceride ratio or any of the individual components.[7]

Because apo B is the only protein in LDL and apo A-I is the major protein constituent of HDL and VLDL, the ratio of apo B to apo A-I reflects the ratio of LDL to HDL and may be a better discriminator of CAD than the individual components, but data on apolipoproteins are still limited.

Cholesterol, HDL (High-Density Lipoprotein), Serum

Intraindividual variation may be ~3.6–12.4%.

Use

Assessment of risk for CAD
Diagnosis of various lipoproteinemias (see below)

Increased In

(>60 mg/dL is negative risk factor for CAD)
Vigorous exercise
Increased clearance of triglyceride (VLDL)
Moderate consumption of alcohol
Insulin treatment
Oral estrogen use
Familial lipid disorders with protection against atherosclerosis (illustrates importance of measuring HDL to evaluate hypercholesterolemia)
- Hyperalphalipoproteinemia (HDL excess)
    1 in 20 adults with mild increased total cholesterol levels (240–300 mg/dL) secondary to increased HDL (>70 mg/dL)
    LDL not increased
    Triglycerides are normal.
    Inherited as simple autosomal dominant trait in families with longevity or may be caused by alcoholism, extensive exposure to chlorinated hydrocarbon pesticides, exogenous estrogen supplementation.
- Hypobetalipoproteinemia (see p. 528)

Decreased In

(<32 mg/dL in men, <38 mg/dL in women)
Is inversely related to risk of CAD. For every 1 mg/dL decrease in HDL, risk for CAD increases by 2–3%.
Secondary causes
- Stress and recent illness (e.g., AMI, stroke, surgery, trauma)
- Starvation; nonfasting sample is 5–10% lower.
- Obesity
- Lack of exercise
- Cigarette smoking
- Diabetes mellitus
- Hypo- and hyperthyroidism

[7]Naito HK. The clinical significance of apolipoprotein measurements. *J Clin Immunoassay* 1986;9:11–20.

- Acute and chronic liver disease
- Nephrosis
- Uremia
- Various chronic anemias and myeloproliferative disorders
- Use of certain drugs (e.g., anabolic steroids, progestins, antihypertensive beta-blockers, thiazides, neomycin, phenothiazines)

Genetic disorders
- Familial hypertriglyceridemia.
- Familial hypoalphalipoproteinemia—common autosomal dominant condition with premature CAD and stroke. One-third of patients with premature CAD may have this disorder.
    HDL <10th percentile (<30 mg/dL in men and <38 mg/dL in women of middle age).
- Homozygous Tangier disease.
- Familial lecithin-cholesterol acetyltransferase deficiency and fish eye disease.
- Nonneuropathic Niemann-Pick disease.
- HDL deficiency with planar xanthomas.
- Apo A-I and apo C-III deficiency variant I and variant II—rare genetic conditions associated with premature CAD and marked HDL deficiency.

Cholesterol, LDL (Low-Density Lipoprotein), Serum

Use

Assess risk and decide treatment for CAD.

Increased In

(Is directly related to risk of CAD)
Familial hypercholesterolemia
Familial combined hyperlipidemia
Diabetes mellitus
Hypothyroidism
Nephrotic syndrome
Chronic renal failure
Diet high in cholesterol and total and saturated fat
Pregnancy
Multiple myeloma, dysgammaglobulinemia
Porphyria
Pregnancy
Wolman's disease
Cholesteryl ester storage disease
Anorexia nervosa
Use of certain drugs (e.g., anabolic steroids, antihypertensive beta-blockers, progestins, carbamazepine)

Decreased In

Severe illness
Abetalipoproteinemia
Oral estrogen use
LDL is measured by ultracentrifugation and by analysis after antibody separation from HDL and VLDL.
LDL can be estimated by the following formula (Friedewald equation):
- LDL = total cholesterol – (HDL cholesterol) – (VLDL).
- VLDL = triglycerides/5.
- Formula underestimates LDL (e.g., in chronic alcoholism), is unsuitable for monitoring, misclassifies 15–40% of patients when triglycerides = 200–400 mg/dL, and fails if fasting triglycerides are >400 mg/dL. Not reliable if type III dyslipidemia is suspected or chylomicrons are present.
Some laboratories also report various ratios.
Total cholesterol/HDL ratio
Low risk	3.3–4.4
Average risk	4.4–7.1

METAB/HERED

Moderate risk	7.1–11.0
High risk	>11.0

Cholesterol (Total), Serum

Use

Monitoring for increased risk factor for CAD
Screening for primary and secondary hyperlipidemias
Monitoring of treatment for hyperlipidemias

Interferences

*Note effect of illness, intraindividual variation, position, season, drug use, etc., when
these values are used to diagnose and treat hyperlipidemias.*
Intraindividual variation may be 4–10% for serum total cholesterol. Repeat cholesterol
values should be within 30 mg/dL. Coefficient of variation should be <3%.
Cholesterol values are up to 8% higher in winter than in summer, 5% lower if patient
bled when sitting than when standing, and 10–15% different when recumbent than
when standing.
Cholesterol values of EDTA plasma can be multiplied by 1.03 to make them comparable to serum values.
Serum cholesterol and HDL can be nonfasting.

Increased In

Hyperlipoproteinemias (see Table 12-7)
• Hyperalphalipoproteinemia
Cholesteryl ester storage disease
Biliary obstruction
• Stone, carcinoma, etc., of duct
• Cholangiolitic cirrhosis
• Biliary cirrhosis
• Cholestasis
von Gierke's disease
Hypothyroidism
Nephrosis (due to chronic nephritis, renal vein thrombosis, amyloidosis, SLE, periar-
teritis, diabetic glomerulosclerosis)
Pancreatic disease
• Diabetes mellitus
• Total pancreatectomy
• Chronic pancreatitis (some patients)
Pregnancy
Drug use (e.g., progestins, anabolic steroids, corticosteroids, some diuretics)
• Methodologic interference (Zlatkis-Zak reaction) (e.g., bromides, iodides, chlor-
promazine, corticosteroids, viomycin, vitamin C, vitamin A)
• 10% of patients on long-term levodopa therapy
• Hepatotoxic effect (e.g., phenytoin sodium)
• Hormonal effect (e.g., corticosteroids, birth control pills, amiodarone)
Total fasting that induces ketosis leads to a rapid increase.
Secondary causes should always be ruled out.

Decreased In

Severe liver cell damage (due to chemicals, drugs, hepatitis)
Hyperthyroidism
Malnutrition (e.g., starvation, neoplasms, uremia, malabsorption in steatorrhea)
Myeloproliferative diseases
Chronic anemia
• PA in relapse
• Hemolytic anemias
• Marked hypochromic anemia
Cortisone and ACTH therapy
Hypobeta- and abetalipoproteinemia
Tangier disease

Infection

Inflammation

Drug use
- Hepatotoxic effect (e.g., allopurinol, tetracyclines, erythromycin, isoniazid, monoamine oxidase inhibitors)
- Synthesis inhibition (e.g., androgens, chlorpropamide, clomiphene, phenformin)
- Diminished synthesis (probable mechanism) (e.g., clofibrate)
- Other mechanisms (e.g., azathioprine, kanamycin, neomycin, oral estrogens, cholestyramine, cortisone and ACTH therapy)
- Methodologic interference (Zlatkis-Zak reaction) (e.g., thiouracil, nitrates)

Cholesterol Decision Levels*

See Figs. 12-3 and 12-4.

	Cholesterol (in mg/dL)			
	LDL	**HDL**	**Total**	**LDL/HDL Ratio**
Desirable level/low risk	<130	>60	<200	0.5–3.0
Borderline level/moderate risk	130–159	35–60	200–239	3.0–6.0
Elevated level/high risk	≥ 160	<35	≥ 240	>6.0

Chylomicrons, Serum

Increased In

Lipoprotein lipase deficiency (autosomal recessive disorder or due to deficient cofactor for lipoprotein lipase) presenting in children with pancreatitis, xanthomas, hepatosplenomegaly

Apo C-II deficiency (rare autosomal recessive disorder due to absence of or defective apo C-II). Accumulation of VLDL and chylomicrons increases risk of pancreatitis.

Type V hyperlipoproteinemia

Lipoprotein Electrophoresis

Use

Identify rare familial disorders (e.g., types I, III, V hyperlipidemias) to anticipate problems in children. Shows a specific abnormal pattern in <2% of Americans (usually type II, IV).

May be indicated if
- Serum triglycerides are >300 mg/dL.
- Fasting serum is lipemic.
- Significant hyperglycemia, impaired glucose tolerance, or glycosuria.
- Increased serum uric acid.
- Strong family history of premature CHD.
- Clinical evidence of CHD or atherosclerosis in patient aged <40.

If lipoprotein electrophoresis is abnormal, tests should be performed to rule out secondary hyperlipidemias (see below).

Lipoproteins, Serum

Decreased In

Abetalipoproteinemia (Bassen-Kornzweig syndrome)

Tangier disease

Hypobetalipoproteinemia

Increased In

Hyperbetalipoproteinemia

Hyperalphalipoproteinemia

*Measure serum total cholesterol, HDL cholesterol, and triglycerides after 12- to 13-hr fast. Average results of two or three tests; if difference of ≥ 30 mg/dL, repeat tests 1–8 wks apart and average results of three tests. Use total cholesterol for initial case finding and classification and monitoring of diet therapy. Do not use age- or sex-specific cholesterol values as decision levels.

Table 12-7. Comparison of Classic Types of Hyperlipoproteinemia

Point of Comparison	Type I (Rarest)	Type II-a (Relatively Common)
Origin	Exogenous hyperlipidemia due to deficient lipoprotein lipase	
Definition	Familial fat-induced hyper-glyceridemia	Hyperbetalipoproteinemia (hypercholesterolemia)
Age	Usually younger than age 10 yrs	
Gross appearance of plasma	On standing: supernatant creamy, infranatant clear	Clear (no cream layer on top)
Serum cholesterol	N or slightly I	Markedly I (300–600 mg/dL)
LDL cholesterol	N	I
HDL cholesterol	N to D	N to D
Apolipoprotein (apo)	I (B-48) I (A-IV) V (C-II)	I (B-100)
Increased lipo-protein	Chylomicrons	LDL
Serum triglycerides	Markedly I (usually >2000 mg/dL)	N
Appearance of lipo-protein components visualized by electrophoresis		
Chylomicron[a]	Marked I	0
Beta-lipoprotein[b]	N or D	I
Pre–beta-lipoprotein[c]	N or D	N
Alpha-lipoprotein[d]		
Other laboratory abnormalities	Glucose tolerance usually N	
Triglyceride-cholesterol ratio	8	1
Lipid changes resembling primary hyperlipidemias		
Diet		
Drugs		Triglyceride-lowering drugs in types III and IV

Type II-b (Relatively Common)	Type III (Relatively Uncommon)	Type IV (Most Common)	Type V (Uncommon)
Overindulgence lipidemia		Endogenous hyperlipidemia	Mixed endogenous and exogenous hyperlipidemia (combined types I and IV)
Combined hyper-lipidemia (mixed hyperlipidemia)	Carbohydrate-induced hyper-glyceridemia with hyper-cholesterolemia. Not known younger than age 25 yrs	Carbohydrate-induced hyper-glyceridemia without hyper-cholesterolemia. Only occasionally seen in children	Combined fat- and carbohydrate-induced hypergly-ceridemia
No cream layer on top; clear to turbid infranatant	Clear, cloudy, or milky	Slightly turbid to cloudy. On standing: unchanged	Markedly turbid. On standing: super-natant, creamy, infranatant milky
Markedly I (300–600 mg/dL)	Markedly I (300–600 mg/dL)	N or slightly I	I (250–500 mg/dL)
I	I	N	N
N to D	N to D	N to D	N to D
I (B-100)	I (E-II). D (E-III). D (E-IV)	V (C-II). I (B-100)	V (C-II). I (B-48). I (B-100)
LDL, VLDL	IDL	VLDL	VLDL, chylomicrons
I ≤ 400 mg/dL	Markedly I (200–1000 mg/dL)	Markedly I (500–1500 mg/dL)	Markedly I (500–1500 mg/dL)
0	0	0	I
I	I, floating beta	N or I	N or I
I	I	I	I
	Hyperglycemia; glu-cose tolerance often abnormal; serum uric acid I	Glucose tolerance often abnormal; serum uric acid often I	Glucose tolerance usually abnormal; serum uric acid usually I
Variable	<2	1–5	>5
Very high cholesterol diet	Same as for type II-a	Caffeine or alcohol before testing	
Same as for type II-a	Triglyceride-lowering drugs in type IV	Cholesterol-lowering drugs, chlorothi-azide, birth control pills, or estrogens	

(*continued*)

METAB/HERED

Table 12-7. (continued)

Point of Comparison	Type I (Rarest)	Type II-a (Relatively Common)
Primary disease		Myxedema, nephrosis, obstructive liver disease, stress, porphyria, anorexia nervosa, idiopathic hyper-calcemia
	[a]Chylomicrons	[c]VLDL
Origin	Gut	Liver
Function	Transport dietary triglycerides	Transport endogenous triglycerides
Electrophoretic mobility	Origin	Pre-beta
Major apolipoproteins	B-48, A-I, C, E	B-100, C, E
Protein	1%	10%
Triglyceride	90%	60%
Cholesterol	5%	15%
Phospholipid	4%	15%

0 = absent; D = decreased; I = increased; N = normal; HDL = high-density lipoprotein; IDL =intermediate-density; LDL = low-density lipoprotein; VLDL = very low density lipoprotein.

Since apo B is the only protein in LDL and apo A-I is the major protein constituent of HDL and VLDL, the ratio of apo-B to apo A-I reflects the ratio of LDL to HDL and may be a better discriminator of coronary artery disease than the individual components; however, data on apolipoproteins are still limited.

Obtain blood only after at least 12–14 hrs' fasting and when patient has been on usual diet for at least 2 wks.

Rule out diabetes, pancreatitis, and hypothyroidism in all groups.

Increased susceptibility to coronary artery disease occurs in types II, III, and IV; accelerated peripheral vascular disease in type III.

Triglycerides, Serum

(80% in VLDL, 15% in LDL)

Classification[8]

Normal	<200 mg/dL
Borderline high	200–400 mg/dL
High	400–1000 mg/dL
Very high	>1000 mg/dL

[8]Summary of the second report of the National Cholesterol Education Program (NCEP) Expert Panel on Detection, Evaluation, and Treatment of High Blood Cholesterol in Adults. *JAMA* 1993;269:3015.

Type II-b (Relatively Common)	Type III (Relatively Uncommon)	Type IV (Most Common)	Type V (Uncommon)
Same as for type II-a	Myxedema, dysgam-maglobulinemia, liver disease	Nephrotic syndrome, hypothyroidism, pregnancy, glycogen storage disease	Myeloma, macroglob-ulinemia, nephrosis
IDL	[b]LDL	[d]HDL	
VLDL	VLDL and IDL	Liver, gut, intravascular metabolism	
Transport cholesteryl esters; LDL precursor	Transport cholesteryl esters	Reverse cholesterol transport	
Beta, pre-beta	Beta	Alpha	
B-100, E	B-100	A-I, A-II, C, E	
15%	20%	50%	
	5%	5%	
35%	50%	20%	
	25%	25%	

Xanthomas appear in types I, II, and III.
Abdominal pain occurs in types I and V.
If dietary or drug treatment has begun, it may not be possible to classify the lipoproteinemia or the classification may be erroneous.
Type II-b is overindulgence hyperlipidemia; shows increased cholesterol and triglycerides, with increased beta and pre-beta; can be distinguished from type III only by detection of abnormal beta-migrating lipoprotein in serum fraction with density >1.006.
Source: Office of Medical Application of Research. National Institutes of Health. Treatment of hyper-triglyceridemia. *JAMA* 1984;251:1196.

Interferences

Diurnal variation causes triglycerides to be lowest in the morning and highest around noon. Intraindividual variation in serum triglycerides is 12–40%; analytical variation is 5–10%.

Increased In

Genetic hyperlipidemias (e.g., lipoprotein lipase deficiency, apo C-II deficiency, familial hypertriglyceridemia, dysbetalipoproteinemia, cholesteryl ester storage disease, Wolman's disease, von Gierke's disease)
Secondary hyperlipidemias (see p. 530)
    Gout
    Pancreatitis
    Acute illness (e.g., AMI [rises to peak in 3 wks and increase may persist for 1 yr]; cold, flu)

METAB/HERED

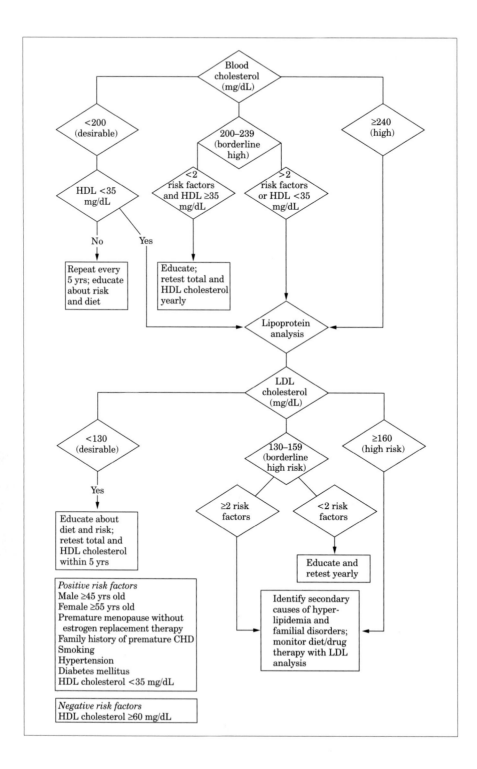

Drug use (e.g., thiazide diuretics, anabolic steroids, cholestyramine, corticosteroids, amiodarone, interferon)
Pregnancy
Concentrations associated with certain disorders
- <250 mg/dL: not associated with any disease state.
- 250–500 mg/dL: associated with peripheral vascular disease; may be a marker for patients with genetic forms of hyperlipoproteinemias who need specific therapy.
- >500 mg/dL: associated with high risk of pancreatitis.
- >1000 mg/dL: associated with hyperlipidemia, especially type I or type V; substantial risk of pancreatitis.
- >5000 mg/dL: associated with eruptive xanthoma, corneal arcus, lipemia retinalis, enlarged liver and spleen.

Decreased In

Abetalipoproteinemia
Malnutrition
Dietary change (within 3 wks)
Recent weight loss
Vigorous exercise (transient)
Drugs (e.g., ascorbic acid, clofibrate, phenformin, asparaginase, metformin, progestins, aminosalicylic acid)
Total and HDL cholesterol levels are similar when fasting or nonfasting but triglycerides should be measured after 12–14 hrs of fasting. Serum levels are 3–5% higher than plasma levels.
Triglyceride levels are not a strong predictor of atherosclerosis or CAD and may not be an independent risk factor. Triglyceride levels are inversely related to HDL cholesterol levels.

Disorders of Lipid Metabolism

Acid Lipase Deficiencies

(Inability to hydrolyze lysosomal triglycerides and cholesteryl esters due to acid lipase deficiency)
♦ Decreased acid lipase in leukocytes or cultured fibroblasts.
Increased serum triglycerides, LDL cholesterol, and cholesteryl esters.

Wolman's Disease

(Rare autosomal recessive deficiency of lysosomal acid lipase activity causing accumulation of cholesterol and triglycerides throughout body tissues and death within first 6 mos)
Prominent anemia develops by 6 wks of age.
Peripheral blood smear shows prominent vacuolation (in nucleus and cytoplasm) of leukocytes.
○Characteristic foam cells in bone marrow resemble those in Niemann-Pick disease.

METAB/HERED

◄ **Fig. 12-3.** Algorithm of recommended testing and treatment of increased serum total and high-density lipoprotein (HDL) cholesterol in adults without evidence of coronary heart disease (CHD). Measure serum total cholesterol, HDL cholesterol, and triglycerides after 12- to 14-hr fast. Average results of two or three tests; if difference of ≥ 30 mg/dL, repeat tests 1–8 wks apart and average results of three tests. Use total cholesterol for initial case finding and classification and monitoring of diet therapy. Do not use age- or sex-specific cholesterol values as decision levels. Always rule out secondary and familial causes. (LDL = low-density lipoprotein.) (Adapted from Adult Treatment Panel II. Report of the Expert Panel on Detection, Evaluation, and Treatment of High Blood Cholesterol in Adults. National Cholesterol Education Program. Bethesda, MD: National Heart, Lung, and Blood Institute, National Institutes of Health, Sep 1993. NIH publication 93-3095.)

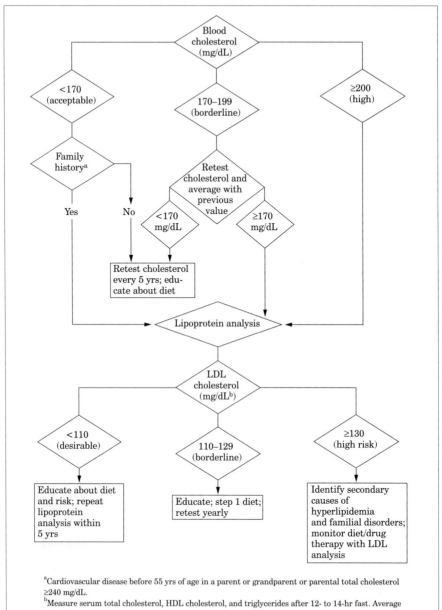

Fig. 12-4. Algorithm of recommended testing and treatment of increased serum cholesterol in children and adolescents. (HDL = high-density lipoprotein; LDL = low-density lipoprotein.) (Adapted from Report of the Expert Panel on Detection, Evaluation, and Treatment of High Blood Cholesterol in Children and Adolescents. National Cholesterol Education Program. Bethesda, MD: National Institutes of Health, Sep 1991. NIH publication 91-2732.)

♦ Abnormal accumulation of cholesteryl esters and triglycerides in tissue biopsy (e.g., liver) establishes the diagnosis; cirrhosis may also be present.

♦ Assay shows absent acid lipase activity in many tissues, including leukocytes and cultured fibroblasts. Heterozygotes have enzyme activity of ~50% of normal in leukocytes or cultured fibroblasts.

♦ Prenatal diagnosis by demonstrating enzyme deficiency in cultured amniocytes.

Laboratory findings due to organ involvement
- Abnormal liver function tests (due to lipid accumulation)
- Malabsorption
- Decreased adrenal cortical function (diffuse calcification on CT scan)

Cholesteryl Ester Storage Disease

(Rare inherited deficiency of lysosomal acid lipase; milder than Wolman's disease)
Pattern similar to that of type II hyperlipidemia
  Increased LDL and decreased HDL cholesterol
Accelerated cardiovascular disease; absent xanthomas; enlarged liver and spleen

Primary Hyperlipidemias

See Table 12-7.

Severe Hypertriglyceridemia (Type I) (Familial Hyperchylomicronemia Syndrome)

(Rare autosomal recessive trait due to deficiency of lipoprotein lipase [LPL] or apo C-II or circulating inhibitor of LPL; marked heterogeneity in causative molecular defects)
Persistent very high triglycerides (>1000 mg/dL) with marked increase in VLDL and chylomicrons. Responds to marked dietary fat restriction.
Patients with apo C-II deficiency cannot activate LPL in vitro. Deficiency of apo C-II is shown by isoelectric focusing or two-dimensional gel electrophoresis of plasma.
Associated with recurrent pancreatitis rather than CAD.
Laboratory changes due to fatty liver (increased serum transaminase)

Familial Hypercholesterolemia (Type II)

(Autosomal dominant disorder)
♦ LDL receptors in fibroblasts or mononuclear blood cells are absent in homozygous patients and 50% of normal levels in heterozygous patients (test performed at specialized labs).
Homozygous—very rare condition (1 per million) in which serum cholesterol is very high (e.g., 600–1000 mg/dL) with corresponding increase (6–8× normal) in LDL. Both parents are heterozygous. Clinical manifestations of increased total cholesterol (xanthomata, corneal arcus, CAD that causes death, usually at <30 yrs).
♦ • Neonatal diagnosis requires finding increased LDL cholesterol in cord blood; serum total cholesterol is unreliable. Because of marked variation in serum total cholesterol levels during first year of life, diagnosis should be deferred until 1 yr of age.
♦ • Prenatal diagnosis of homozygous fetus can be made by estimation of binding sites on fibroblasts cultured from amniotic fluids; useful when both parents are heterozygous.
Heterozygous—increased serum total cholesterol (300–500 mg/dL) and LDL (2–3× normal) with similar change in a parent or first-degree relative; serum triglycerides and VLDL are normal in 90% and slightly increased in 10% of these cases. Gene frequency is 1 in 500 in general population, but 5% in survivors of AMI who are <60 yrs. Premature CAD, tendinous xanthomas, and corneal arcus are often present.
Plasma triglycerides are normal in type II-A but increased in type II-B. This is not the most common cause of phenotype II-A.

Polygenic Hypercholesterolemia (Type II-A)

Persistent total cholesterol elevation (>240 mg/dL) and increased LDL without familial hypercholesterolemia or familial combined hypercholesterolemia.
Premature CAD occurs later in life than with familial combined hyperlipidemia.
Xanthomas are rare.

Familial Combined Hyperlipidemia (Types II-B, IV, V)

(Occurs in 0.5% of general population and 15% of survivors of AMI <60 yrs old)
Any combination of increased LDL and VLDL and chylomicrons may be found; HDL is often low; different family members may have increased serum total cholesterol or triglycerides or both.
Premature CAD occurs later in life (>30 yrs of age) than with familial hypercholesterolemia.
Xanthomas are rare.
Patients are often overweight.

Familial Dysbetalipoproteinemia (Type III)

(Occurs in 1 in 5000 in the population.)
Abnormality of apo E with excess of abnormal lipoprotein (beta mobility–VLDL); total cholesterol >300 mg/dL plus triglycerides >400 mg/dL should suggest this diagnosis. VLDL cholesterol/triglyceride ratio = 0.3.
♦ Diagnosis by combination of ultracentrifugation and isoelectric focusing that shows abnormal apo E pattern.
Tuberous and tendinous xanthomas and palmar and plantar xanthomatous streaks are present.
Atherosclerosis is more common in peripheral than in coronary arteries.

Familial Hypertriglyceridemia (Type IV)

(Autosomal dominant condition present in 1% of general population and 5% of survivors of AMI aged <60 yrs)
Elevated triglycerides (usually 200–500 mg/dL) and VLDL with normal LDL and decreased HDL.
Distinction from familial combined hyperlipidemia is made only by extensive family screening.

Abetalipoproteinemia (Bassen-Kornzweig Syndrome)

(Extremely rare autosomal recessive disorder; should be ruled out in children with fat malabsorption, steatorrhea, failure to thrive, neurologic symptoms, pigmented retinopathy, acanthocytosis)
○Marked decrease in serum triglycerides (<30 mg/dL) with little increase after ingestion of fat, and in total cholesterol (20–50 mg/dL)
○Chylomicrons, LDL, VLDL, and apo B are absent; HDL may be lower than in normal persons.
Plasma lipids are normal in heterozygotes.
○Acanthocytes may be 50–90% of RBCs and are characteristic (see p. 323).
Decreased RBC life span causes anemia that may vary from severe hemolytic anemia to mild compensated anemia.
Low serum levels of carotene and other fat-soluble vitamins (see p. 507).
○Biopsy of small intestine shows characteristic lipid vacuolization; not pathognomonic (occasionally seen in celiac disease, tropical sprue, juvenile nutritional megaloblastic anemia).
Negative sweat test distinguishes this disorder from cystic fibrosis.
Arteriosclerosis is absent.
A variant is normotriglyceridemic abetalipoproteinemia in which patient can secrete apo B-48 but not apo B-100, which results in normal postprandial triglyceride values but marked hypocholesterolemia; associated with mental retardation and vitamin E deficiency.

Hypobetalipoproteinemia

(Autosomal codominant disorder with increased longevity and lower incidence of atherosclerosis; at least one parent shows decreased beta-lipoprotein)
Marked decrease in LDL and LDL/HDL ratio.
Homozygous patients have decreased serum cholesterol (<60 mg/dL) and triglycerides and undetectable or trace amounts of chylomicrons, VLDL, and LDL.
Heterozygotes are asymptomatic and have serum total cholesterol, LDL, and apo B values of 50% of normal (consistent with codominant disorder). May also be caused by

malabsorption of fats, infection, anemia, hepatic necrosis, hyperthyroidism, AMI, acute trauma.

L-Carnitine Deficiency

(Very rare metabolic disorder of fatty acid metabolism [beta oxidation])
Two types
- Myopathic: Deficiency limited to muscle; normal levels in plasma and other tissues. Myoglobinuria in older children or young adults. Biopsy shows lipid deposits. Tissue homogenates do not support normal rates of beta oxidation of long-chain fatty acids unless L-carnitine is added. Serum carnitine is normal or slightly decreased.
- Systemic: More acute clinical picture, presents earlier in life; may mimic Reye's syndrome.
♦ L-carnitine depleted in blood and all tissues.
♦ Tissue contains marked decreased activity of medium-chain acyl-CoA dehydrogenase.
  Hepatic encephalopathy
  Hypoglycemia without ketosis
  Hyperammonemia may be present.
  Serum uric acid may be increased.
  Laboratory findings due to cardiomyopathy

Due To

- Dietary deficiency
- Low renal reabsorption (e.g., Fanconi's syndrome)
- Inborn deficiency of medium-chain acyl-CoA dehydrogenase
- Valproic acid therapy (inducing excretion of valprolycarnitine in urine)
- Excessive loss of free carnitine in urine due to failure of carnitine transport across cells of renal tubule, muscle, and fibroblasts
- Organic acidurias (e.g., methylmalonicaciduria, propionicacidemia)
- Other conditions (e.g., maternal deficiency, prematurity)

Lecithin-Cholesterol Acyltransferase Deficiency (Familial)

(Rare autosomal recessive disorder of adults. Corneal opacities lead to blindness.)
○Serum total cholesterol is normal but cholesteryl esters are virtually absent. Plasma free cholesterol is extremely increased. HDL is low.
Anemia with large RBCs that are frequently target cells
Proteinuria

Lipodystrophy (Total), Congenital

(Rare autosomal recessive disorder characterized by absence of fat in skin and viscera, possibly due to deficiency in number or quality of insulin receptors)
No neonatal laboratory abnormalities
Later in life: marked insulin resistance, glucose intolerance, development of diabetes mellitus (although ketosis is unusual), increased serum triglycerides develop
Laboratory findings due to fatty liver, cirrhosis, acanthosis nigricans
Similar syndromes of leprechaunism, acquired and partial lipodystrophies

Tangier Disease

(Rare autosomal recessive disorder causing defect in metabolism of apo A in which a marked decrease [heterozygous] or absence [homozygous] of HDL is seen)
Plasma levels of apo A-I and A-II are extremely low. In homozygotes, HDL is usually <10 mg/dL and apo A-I is usually <5 mg/dL. In heterozygotes, HDL and apo A-I are ~50% of normal.
Pre–beta-lipoprotein is absent.
Serum total cholesterol (<100 mg/dL), LDL cholesterol, and phospholipid are decreased; triglycerides are normal or increased (100–250 mg/dL).
Deposits of cholesteryl esters in RE cells cause enlarged liver, spleen, and lymph nodes, enlarged orange tonsils, small orange-brown spots in rectal mucosa; premature CAD, mild corneal opacification, and neuropathy may be present in homozygous type.

METAB/HERED

Secondary Hyperlipidemias

Due To

(Many are combined hyperlipidemias)
- Diabetes mellitus*
    Increased VLDL with increased serum triglycerides, low HDL cholesterol; LDL cholesterol may be normal or mildly increased. (Higher triglyceride values correlate with hyperglycemia and poorer control of diabetes; reduced by insulin therapy)
- Hypothyroidism[†]
    Increased LDL and total cholesterol. *Test for hypothyroidism whenever LDL cholesterol is >190 mg/dL.* Rapidly becomes normal with treatment.
    Serum cholesterol is not always increased.
- Nephrotic syndrome*
    Increased serum total cholesterol and LDL cholesterol are usual.
    Increased VLDL and therefore increased serum triglycerides may also occur.
- Other renal disorders (chronic uremia, hemodialysis, after transplantation)[†]
    Increased triglycerides and total cholesterol and low HDL cholesterol may occur.
- Hepatic glycogenoses
    Increased serum lipoprotein is common in any of the forms, but the pattern cannot be used to differentiate the type of glycogen storage disease.
    Predominant increase in VLDL in glucose-6-phosphatase deficiency.
    Predominant increase in LDL in debrancher and phosphorylase deficiencies.
- Obstructive liver disease*
    Increased serum total cholesterol is common until liver failure develops.
    Resistant to conventional drug therapy. The type of lipoproteinemia is variable.
    In intrahepatic biliary atresia, there is often increase in lipoprotein X with marked increase in serum total cholesterol and even more marked increase in serum phospholipids.
- Chronic alcoholism[†]
    Marked increase in VLDL producing type IV or V patterns
- Hyperlipoproteinemia of "affluence" (dietary)*
- Pregnancy*
- Drugs
    Estrogens, steroids, beta-blockers*
    Diuretics, cyclosporine[†]

*Predominantly hypertriglyceridemia.
[†]Predominantly hypercholesterolemia.

Metabolic Errors Associated with Hyperammonemia in Children

Defects in urea cycle—severe hyperammonemia with respiratory alkalosis, e.g.,
- Arginosuccinate synthetase deficiency
- Arginosuccinate lyase deficiency
- Arginase deficiency
- Citrullinemia
- Ornithine transcarbamylase deficiency
- *N*-Acetylglutamate synthetase deficiency
- Carbamoyl phosphate synthetase deficiency

Organic acid defects—mild to moderate hyperammonemia (≤ 500 mg/dL), e.g.,
- Methylmalonicacidemia*
- Isovalericacidemia*
- Multiple carboxylase deficiency*
- Propionicacidemia*
- Glutaricaciduria type II
- Ketothiolase deficiency

Hyperornithinemia
Transient hyperammonemia of newborn
Fatty acid oxidation defect

*Also characterized by lactic acidosis.

Plasma ammonia should be determined in any neonate with unexplained neurologic deterioration or any patient with unexplained encephalopathy or episodic lethargy and vomiting.

Metabolic Errors Causing Acidosis

Amino acid disorders
- Maple syrup urine disease
- Hypervalinemia
- Hyperleucine–isoleucinemia

Organic acid defects
- Isovalericacidemia
- Propionicacidemia
- Methylmalonicacidemia
- Glutaricacidemia
- Combined carboxylase deficiency
- 3-Hydroxy-3-methylglutaricacidemia
- 2-Methyl-3-hydroxybutyricacidemia
- Acyl CoA dehydrogenase deficiencies

Glycogen storage diseases
- Type IA
- Type III

Disorders of Amino Acid Metabolism

See Fig. 12-5, Table 12-9.

Aminoaciduria, Secondary

Due To

Inherited (Generalized)
Cystinosis
Fanconi's syndrome (idiopathic)
Fructose intolerance
Galactosemia
GSD Type I (rare)
Lactose intolerance
Lowe's syndrome
Tyrosinosis
Wilson's disease

Not Inherited (all generalized except as indicated by *, **)
Connective tissue diseases**
Drugs (e.g., deficiency of vitamins B*, C, D; outdated tetracycline, salicylates, steroids, toxic heavy metals)
Endocrine (e.g., hyperparathyroidism**, hyperthyroidism**, neurosecretory tumors*)
Kidney disorders (e.g., nephrotic syndrome, renal transplant reaction)
Liver necrosis
Newborns (normal)
Others

*Cystathionine.
**Hydroxyproline.

Occurs in
- Severe liver disease
- Renal tubular damage due to
    Lysol
    Heavy metals
    Maleic acid

METAB/HERED

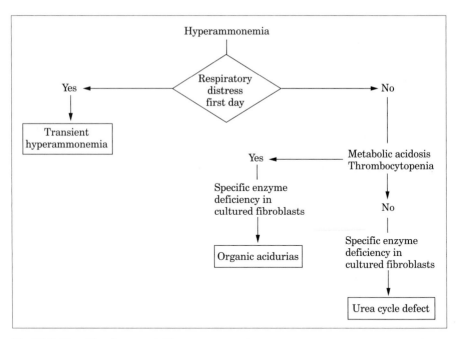

Fig. 12-5. Algorithm for neonatal hyperammonemia.

      Burns
      Galactosemia
      Wilson's disease
      Scurvy
      Rickets
      Fanconi's syndrome (e.g., outdated tetracycline, multiple myeloma, inherited)
    • Neoplasms
      Cystathionine excretion in neuroblastoma of adrenal gland
      Ethanolamine excretion in primary hepatoma

Argininosuccinicaciduria

(Autosomal recessive deficiency of argininosuccinase; brittle hair, absence of metabolic acidosis, and neurologic changes)
○Fasting blood ammonia is normal but level may be markedly increased after eating.
♦Argininosuccinic acid is increased in plasma and urine; may also be increased in CSF.
Because of block in urea cycle, plasma arginine may be decreased and citrulline increased.
Urine orotic acid is increased.
Serum ALP may be increased.
♦Heterozygous carriers show increased argininosuccinic acid in urine and decreased argininosuccinase in RBCs.
♦Prenatal diagnosis by assay of enzyme in cultured amniocytes (*Mycoplasma* contamination may cause a false-negative result) or assay of amniotic fluid for argininosuccinic acid
Neonatal type is usually fatal in infancy. Late-onset type may present at any age triggered by intercurrent infection or stress.

Beta-Aminoisobutyricaciduria

(Familial recessive benign disorder of thymine metabolism)
♦Increased beta-aminoisobutyric acid in urine (50–200 mg/24 hrs)
May also occur in leukemia due to increased breakdown of nucleic acids.

Table 12-8. Summary of Primary Overflow Aminoacidurias (Increased Blood Concentration with Overflow into Urine)

Disease	Increased Blood Amino Acids	Urine Abnormalities*	Other Laboratory Findings
Phenylketonuria	Phenylalanine	Orthohydroxyphenylacetic acid; phenyl-pyruvic, acetic, and lactic acids	Blood tyrosine does not rise after phenyl-alanine load
Maple syrup urine disease			
Severe infantile form	Valine, leucine, isoleucine, alloiso-leucine	Branched-chain ketoacids in great excess; urine has odor of maple syrup	
Intermittent form	Same	Ketoaciduria and urine odor present only during attacks	
Hypervalinemia	Valine		
Homocystinuria	Methionine; homocystine	Homocystine in great excess in urine	Vascular accidents, Marfan-like syndrome, osteoporosis
Tryptophanemia	Tryptophan	Decreased excretion of kynurenine after tryptophan load	
Hyperlysinemia	Lysine	Ornithine, gamma-aminobutyric acid, and ethanolamine in excess	
Congenital lysine intolerance	Lysine, arginine		Ammonia intoxication
Tyrosinosis	Tyrosine; methionine may be markedly increased	p-Hydroxyphenylpyruvic, acetic, and lactic acids; methionine may be prominent	Generalized aminoaciduria, renal glycosuria, renal rickets, cirrhosis, Fanconi's syndrome
Cystathioninuria	Cystathionine slightly increased	Cystathionine (may be >1 gm/day)	Congenital acidosis, thrombocytopenia, pituitary gland abnormalities
Hyperglycinemia			
Severe infantile	Glycine (other amino acids may be elevated)	Acetone	May have ammonia intoxication, ketosis, neutropenia, and osteoporosis
With hypo-oxaluria	Glycine	Decreased oxalate excretion	
Argininosuccinic-aciduria	Argininosuccinic acid (~4 mg/dL); Citrulline	Argininosuccinic acid (2.5–9.0 gm/day); Citrulline	Ammonia intoxication
Citrullinemia	Citrulline; alanine	Citrulline; glutamine	Liver disease, ammonia intoxication; BUN may be low

(continued)

Table 12-8. (continued)

Disease	Increased Blood Amino Acids	Urine Abnormalities*	Other Laboratory Findings
Ornithinemia	Ornithine	Ornithine may be normal	Ammonia intoxication
Histidinemia	Histidine (alanine may also be increased)	Alanine may be increased; imidazole-pyruvic, acetic, and lactic acids	Urocanic acid absent in sweat and urine after oral histidine load
Carnosinuria		Carnosine (20–100 mg/day)	
Hyper-beta-alaninemia	Beta-alanine, GABA	Beta-aminoisobutyric acid, GABA, and taurine in excess	Beta-alanine and GABA increased in CSF
Hyperprolinemia			
Type I	Proline	Hydroxyproline, glycine elevated	Patient may have hereditary nephritis
Type II	Proline	Delta¹-pyrroline 5-carboxylate, hydroxy-proline, glycine elevated	No nephritis
Hydroxyprolinemia	Hydroxyproline	No excretion of delta¹-pyrroline 3-hydroxy-5-carboxylate or gamma-hydroxyglutamic acid after hydroxy-proline load	
Hypophosphatasia	Phosphoethanolamine slightly elevated ($\approx$ 0.4 mg/dL)	Phosphoethanolamine ($\geq$ 150 mg/day)	Bone disease

GABA = gamma-aminobutyric acid.
*In addition to overflow aminoaciduria:
Mental retardation is often present in these patients.
For proper interpretation of aminoaciduria, avoid all drugs and medications for 3–4 days (unless immediate diagnosis is required), since they may cause renal tubular damage with aminoaciduria or may produce confusing spots on chromatograms. Use fresh urine specimens without urinary tract infection or else amino acid pattern may be abnormal. Since aminoaciduria may occur with various acute illnesses, repeat amino acid chromatogram after recovery from acute illness to avoid misdiagnosis. Some aminoacidurias may not be clinically significant (e.g., newborn aminoaciduria, glycinuria, beta-aminoisobutyricaciduria).
Source: Efron MD, Ampola MG. The aminoacidurias. *Pediatr Clin North Am* 1967;14:881.

Table 12-9. Summary of Renal or Gut Transport Aminoacidurias (Blood Amino Acids Are Normal or Low)

Disease	Amino Acids Increased in Urine
Oasthouse urine disease	Methionine (may not be much increased on normal diet but is on high-methionine diet); smaller amounts of valine, leucine, isoleucine, tryosine, and phenylalanine
Hartnup disease	Neutral amino acids (monoamine, monocarboxylic acid) and basic amino acids (methionine, proline, hydroxyproline, and glycine) normal or only slightly increased
Glycinuria (may be harmless; patient may be heterozygous for benign prolinuria; may be associated with many conditions)	Glycine
Severe prolinuria (Joseph's syndrome)	Proline, hydroxyproline, and glycine in great excess (≤ 3 gm/day of proline)
Benign prolinuria	Proline, hydroxyproline, and glycine (≤ 600 mg/day of proline)

Cystine-lysinuria
  Type I (renal calculi)
  Type II
  Type III
	Cystine and dibasic amino acids

Isolated cystinuria (familial hypoparathyroidism, ? incidental)	Cystine

Source: Efron MD, Ampola MG. The aminoacidurias. *Pediatr Clin North Am* 1967;14:881.

Citrullinemia

(Rare autosomal recessive deficiency of argininosuccinate synthetase with metabolic block in citrulline utilization and associated mental retardation)
See Table 12-8.
Genetically heterogeneous (like other disorders of urea cycle) with various clinical pictures and onset from neonatal to adult period
○Massive hyperammonemia (>1000 mg/dL) in neonatal form
♦Markedly increased citrulline levels in blood, CSF, and urine
○Serum levels of glutamine, alanine, and aspartic acid are usually increased; arginine is usually decreased.
Urine orotic acid is increased.
Laboratory findings due to liver disease
♦Deficient enzyme activity can be demonstrated in liver cells and cultured fibroblasts.
♦Prenatal diagnosis by assay of citrulline in amniotic fluid or of enzyme in cultured amniocytes

Cystathioninuria

(Rare autosomal recessive deficiency of cystathionase)
Increased cystathionine in urine

Cystinuria

(Autosomal recessive disorder characterized by failure of amino acid transport; renal tubular reabsorption and intestinal uptake of cystine and dibasic amino acids)

METAB/HERED

◆ Markedly increased cystine in urine (20–30× normal). May also be increased in organic acidemias, hyperuricemia, trisomy 21, hereditary pancreatitis, muscular dystrophy, hemophilia, retinitis pigmentosa.
◆ Confirm diagnosis by identifying increased urinary arginine, lysine, and ornithine in urine after age 6 months.
○ Cystine renal and bladder stones
Laboratory findings due to GU tract infections. *Bacteria can degrade cystine.*

Hartnup Disease

(Autosomal recessive disorder characterized by defect in renal or GI transport of "neutral" amino acids)
◆ Urine contains increased (5–10×) amounts of alanine, threonine, valine, leucine, isoleucine, phenylalanine, tyrosine, tryptamine, histidine.

Histidinemia

(Rare autosomal recessive aminoacidopathy due to deficiency of histidase in liver and skin that causes histidine to be converted to urocanic acid. Incidence is 1 in 14,000–20,000 live births in United States and 1 in 8000 in Japan.)
◆ Plasma histidine is increased to 500–1000 μmol/L (normal = 85–120 μmol/L).
◆ Urine histidine is increased to 0.5–4.0 gm/day (normal <0.5 gm/day). Histidine metabolites (imidazole acetic, imidazole lactic, and imidazole pyruvic acids) are also increased in urine; alanine may be increased.
Urine may show positive Phenistix or ferric chloride test because of imidazole pyruvic acid.
With oral histidine load, no formiminoglutamic acid appears in urine.
Most children show no sequelae; therefore neonatal screening is not performed.
Heterozygote detection is not established yet.

Homocysteinuria/Homocysteinemia[9,10]

(Homocysteine is reduced [sulfhydryl] form and homocystine is oxidized [disulfide] form of homologues cysteine and cystine. Term refers to combined pool of homocystine and homocysteine and their mixed disulfides.)
Is independent risk factor for premature arteriosclerosis of coronary, cerebral, peripheral vessels.

Due To

Autosomal recessive error of methionine metabolism with deficient cystathionine synthetase in liver and brain with inability to catalyze homocysteine to cystathionine.
Incidence of mild form is 5–7% among general population; severe form is rare.

Increased In

Deranged vitamin B_{12} metabolism or block in folate metabolism or deficiency of vitamin B_{12}, folate, or vitamin B_6.
Chronic renal or liver failure, postmenopausal state, drug use (e.g., methotrexate, phenytoin, theophylline, cigarette smoking)
Various neoplastic diseases (e.g., ALL, cancers of breast, ovary, pancreas).

◆ Urine excretion of homocysteine is increased (positive nitroprusside screening test). Urine may also contain increased methionine and other amino acids.
◆ Increased serum homocysteine (up to 250 mg/day; normal = trace or not detected) and methionine (≤ 2000 mg/day; normal is ≤ 30 mg/day); also increased in CSF.
◆ Abnormal homocysteine metabolism may be shown only after methionine-loading test. Blood samples before and at 4- to 8-hr intervals after 100 mg/kg methionine oral load. Normal = transient increase in free and protein-bound homocysteine peaking between 4–8 hrs. Abnormal = plasma homocysteine >2 SD greater than that of normal controls.

[9]Guba SC, Fink LM, Fonseca V. Hyperhomocysteinemia. An emerging and important risk factor for thromboembolic and cardiovascular disease. *Am J Clin Pathol* 1996;105:709.
[10]Welch GN, Loscalzo J. Homocysteine and atherothrombosis. *N Engl J Med* 1998;338:1042.

In homozygous form laboratory findings due to associated clinical conditions
- Mild variable hepatocellular dysfunction
- Mental retardation, Marfan's syndrome, osteoporosis, etc.

Serum methionine levels should be kept at 20–150 μmol/L by low-methionine diet and pyridoxine therapy.

Patients have enzyme activity levels of 0–10% in fibroblasts and lymphocytes; heterozygotes (their parents) have levels <50% of normal.

♦ For neonatal detection, measure methionine in filter paper specimen of blood; confirm by measuring blood and urine amino acids.

♦ Can also measure specific enzyme in cultured fibroblasts.

Hydroxyprolinemia

♦ Increased hydroxyproline in blood

Hyperglycinemia

(Long-chain ketosis [without hypoglycemia] and ketonuria accentuated by leucine ingestion)

Same findings (neutropenia, thrombocytopenia, hypogammaglobulinemia, increased glycine in blood and urine, osteoporosis, hypoglycemia) may occur in propionicacidemia, methylmalonicacidemia, isovalericacidemia, 3-ketothiolase deficiency.

Hyperprolinemia

(Types I and II)
♦ Increased proline in blood
Increased glycine and hydroxyproline in urine

Iminoglycinuria, Familial

(Inherited autosomal defect of renal amino acid transport; may be associated with mental retardation)
Increased urine glycine
Increased urine imino acids (proline, hydroxyproline)

Joseph's Syndrome (Imminoglycinuria)

Asymptomatic malabsorption of proline, hydroxyproline, and glycine)
♦ Urine shows marked increase in proline, hydroxyproline, and glycine.
Heterozygotes may show mild prolinuria.

Lesch-Nyhan Syndrome

(X-linked recessive trait of complete absence of hypoxanthine-guanine phosphoribosyltransferase [HGPRT] that catalyzes hypoxanthine and guanine to their nucleotides, causing accumulation of purines. The syndrome appears in male children, with choreoathetosis, mental retardation, and tendency to self-mutilating, biting, and scratching.)

♦ Increased serum uric acid levels (9–12 mg/dL).
♦ Hyperuricuria
- 3–4 mg of uric acid/mg creatinine
- 40–70 mg of uric acid/kg body weight
- 600–1000 mg/24 hrs in patients weighing ≥ 15 kg
- Marked variation in purine diet causes very little change
- Orange crystals or sand in infants' diapers

♦ Deficient HGPRT in RBCs and fibroblasts; also allows carrier detection and prenatal diagnosis.

Laboratory findings due to secondary gout (tophi after 10 yrs, crystalluria, hematuria, urinary calculi, UTI, gouty arthritis, response to colchine); patients die of renal failure by age 10 yrs unless treated.

Deficiency of HGPRT in RBCs and fibroblasts; also allows carrier detection and prenatal diagnosis.

♦ Deficiency of HGPRT activity detected in cultured fibroblasts (<1.2% of normal) and in RBC hemolysates (0%) establishes the diagnosis; in amniotic cells allows diagnosis in utero. DNA probes allow prenatal diagnosis.
♦ Heterozygotes can be detected by study of individual hair follicles.
♦ Variants with partial deficiency of HGPRT show 0–50% of normal activity in RBC hemolysates and >1.2% in fibroblasts; patients accumulate purines but no orange sand in diapers; no abnormality of CNS or behavior.

L-Glycericaciduria

(Genetic variant of primary hyperoxaluria; autosomal trait that causes disease only when homozygous)
○ Renal calculi composed of calcium oxalate
♦ L-Glyceric acid in urine (not found in normal urine)
○ Increased urinary oxalic acid (3–5× normal)

Maple Syrup Urine Disease (Ketoaciduria)

(Autosomal recessive disorder characterized by deficiency of branched-chain keto acid decarboxylase; incidence is 1 in 216,000 live births; characteristic maple syrup or curry odor in urine, sweat, hair, and cerumen)
♦ Chromatography of urine and plasma show greatly increased urinary excretion of ketoacids of leucine, isoleucine, and valine. Presence of alloisoleucine (stereoisomeric metabolite of isoleucine) is characteristic.
○ Metabolic acidosis and ketoacidosis occur.
○ Ferric chloride test of urine produces green-gray color.
Hypoglycemia is usual.
The disease may be severe or intermittent.
Patient should be monitored by daily urine testing with dinitrophenylhydrazine; because urine levels correlate with plasma levels, plasma levels can be measured once a month if urine is negative or shows only traces. (Control plasma ranges: leucine = 180–700 μmol/L, isoleucine = 70–280 μmol/L, valine = 200–800 μmol/L.)
♦ Measurement of amount of defective enzyme in leukocytes and fibroblasts shows classic form (enzyme level 0–2% of normal), intermittent form (enzyme level 2–8% of normal), and intermediate form (enzyme level 8–16% of normal). Blood levels are normal in intermittent form except during acute episodes caused by infection, surgery, vaccination, or sudden increased intake of protein, which in children resemble classic form. Intermediate form shows persistent elevation of blood amino acids, which can be kept in normal range by maintaining dietary protein at <2 g/kg/day.
♦ Prenatal diagnosis by measurement of enzyme concentration in cells cultured from amniotic fluid.

Methylmalonicaciduria

(Very rare autosomal recessive error of metabolism with neonatal metabolic acidosis and mental and somatic retardation; at least four distinct forms; screening incidence is 1 in 48,000 in infants 3–4 wks of age)
○ Metabolic acidosis
○ Increased methylmalonic acid in urine and plasma
Long-chain ketonuria
Intermittent hyperglycinemia
○ All findings accentuated by high-protein diet or supplemental ingestion of valine or isoleucine.
Hypoglycemia, neutropenia, thrombocytopenia may occur.
Heterozygote detection is not reliable.
♦ Prenatal diagnosis by assay of methylmalonyl-CoA mutase in cultured amniocytes, increased methylcitric or methylmalonic acids in amniotic fluid, or (late in pregnancy) increased methylmalonic acid in maternal urine
Methylmalonicaciduria also occurs in vitamin B$_{12}$ deficiency.

Oasthouse Urine Disease

(Disorder of methionine absorption in gut with distinctive odor of urine)
♦ Increase of various amino acids in blood and also in urine (e.g., phenylalanine, tyrosine, methionine, valine, leucine, isoleucine)

Organic Acidemias

(E.g., methylmalonic, propionic, isovaleric)
Show
- Metabolic acidosis and ketoacidosis.
- Ketonuria.
- Hyperammonemia.
- Hypoglycemia.
- Sweat and urine have odor of sweaty feet.

Ornithine Transcarbamylase Deficiency

(X-linked recessive disorder characterized by deficiency of ornithine transcarbamylase, an enzyme in urea cycle that converts ornithine to citrulline)
○Increased blood ammonia, usually 2–10× normal
○Decreased citrulline in blood
○Increased orotic acid in blood and urine. May also be increased in lysinuric protein intolerance.
○Decreased ornithine transcarbamylase in biopsy of liver.
Ornithine transcarbamylase deficiency can occur after a bacterial or viral infection, thereby causing confusion with Reye's syndrome.
♦ To detect asymptomatic carriers, measurement of urine orotic acid before and 6 hrs after an oral protein loading test may be required for female heterozygotes. Can also be detected by a complementary DNA probe for the ornithine transcarbamylase gene using restriction fragment length polymorphism analysis.
♦ Prenatal diagnosis using restriction fragment length polymorphism analysis for chorionic villus DNA analysis.

Phenylketonuria (PKU)

(Inherited autosomal recessive disorder [due to a variety of mutations on chromosome 12]; absence of phenylalanine hydroxylase activity in liver causes increase in phenylalanine and its metabolites [phenylpyruvic acid, orthohydroxyphenylacetic acid] in blood, urine, and CSF; tyrosine and the derivative catecholamines are deficient. Results in mental retardation. Among whites, 1 in 50 persons is a carrier and 1 in 10,000 is affected with PKU; see Fig. 12-6.)
Unrestricted protein diet
- Normal blood phenylalanine = 2 mg/dL.
♦ • Classic PKU: high blood phenylalanine (usually >30 mg/dL and always >20 mg/dL in infancy) with phenylalanine and its metabolites in urine (incidence is 1 in 14,000); normal or decreased tyrosine concentration.
♦ • Less severe variant form of PKU: blood phenylalanine levels are 15–30 mg/dL and metabolites may appear in urine (incidence is 1 in 15,000).
♦ • Mild persistent hyperphenylalaninemia: blood phenylalanine may be 2–12 mg/dL and metabolites are not found in urine (incidence is 1 in 30,000); diet restriction is not required for this form.
For screening of newborns, urine amounts of phenylpyruvic acid may be insufficient for detection by colorimetric methods when blood level is <15 mg/dL. May not appear in urine until 2–3 wks of age.
Phenylpyruvic acid in urine is significant (gives positive ferric chloride test) but may not be present in some patients.
Preliminary blood screening tests (inhibition assay, fluorometry, paper chromatography) detect levels >4 mg/dL. Screening should be performed after protein-containing feedings have begun.

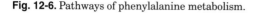

Fig. 12-6. Pathways of phenylalanine metabolism.

♦ When repeat screening test is positive, quantitative blood phenylalanine and tyrosine measurements are performed to confirm phenylalaninemia and exclude transient tyrosinemia of newborn, which is most common cause of positive screening.
   Diagnosis requires serum phenylalanine level ≥ 20 mg/dL. Urine ferric chloride is
   positive and chromatography confirms orthohydroxyphenylacetic acid.
♦ Serial determinations should be performed in untreated borderline cases because
   blood levels may change markedly with time or due to stress and infection.
♦ Diagnosis of PKU may be confirmed by giving 100 mg of ascorbic acid and collecting
   blood and urine 24 hrs later.
False-negative results on Guthrie PKU test for screening newborns may occur if blood
   is collected using capillary tubes and venipuncture rather than applied directly to filter paper, especially if level is within 0.2 mg of cutoff value.
Adjust diet by frequent monitoring of blood phenylalanine (e.g., 10 mg/dL) with consistently negative ferric chloride urine test.
In women with untreated PKU and increased serum phenylalanine, frequency of mental
   retardation, microcephaly, and congenital heart disease in offspring is greatly increased.
♦ Detection of heterozygotes in 75% of families and prenatal diagnosis are now possible using complementary DNA probe.
Laboratory findings due to congenital heart disease in ≤ 15% of PKU patients

Comparison of PKU and Transient Tyrosinemia

	PKU	**Transient Tyrosinemia**
Serum phenylalanine	>15 mg/dL	>4 mg/dL (15–20 mg/dL)
Serum tyrosine	<5 mg/dL (is never increased)	>4 mg/dL (5–20 mg/dL)
Urine orthohydroxy- phenylacetic acid	Present	Absent
Urine	Phenylalanine is >100 μg/mL	Large amounts of tyrosine and its metabolites

Propionicacidemia

**(Rare autosomal recessive disorder with deficiency of propionyl-CoA carboxylase,
   which prevents degradation and therefore causes intolerance of isoleucine,
   valine, threonine, methionine)**
○ Recurrent episodes (often after infections) of massive ketosis, metabolic acidosis,
   hyperammonemia, vomiting, dehydration progressing to coma.
Same picture as hyperglycinemia (see above).
○ Increase plasma and urine glycine
Urine is tested (daily in infants) for ketones (e.g., Acetest reagent strips or tablets) and
   blood is tested for propionic acid to monitor treatment.
Laboratory findings of complications (e.g., sepsis, ventricular hemorrhage)
♦ Prenatal diagnosis is available.
♦ Positive assay of enzyme in cultured fibroblasts can indicate heterozygosity but neg-
   ative assay may not be reliable to indicate absence.

Tyrosinemia

Occurs as both persistent hereditary and transient forms

Tyrosinemia Type I (Tyrosinosis): Persistent Hereditary Form

(Rare autosomal recessive condition due to defect in fumarylacetoacetase; incidence is 1 in 100,000 live births; usually fatal in first year)
♦ Increased blood and urine tyrosine; methionine may also be markedly increased; increased blood phenylalanine may cause positive test when screening for PKU.
○ Urinary excretion of tyrosine metabolites p-hydroxyphenylpyruvic and p-hydroxyphenylacetic acids (detected by chromatography of urine) is increased; may be due to deficiency of enzyme fumarylacetoacetate hydrolase. *May also be increased in myasthenia gravis, liver disease, ascorbic acid deficiency, malignancies.*
♦ Detection of succinylacetone in urine is virtually diagnostic.
Acetic and lactic acids may be increased in urine.
Anemia, thrombocytopenia, and leukopenia are common.
Urine delta-aminolevulinic acid (delta-ALA) may be increased.
Laboratory findings due to Fanconi's syndrome (see pp. 599, 711), hepatic cirrhosis and liver carcinoma are noted.
Dietary restriction of tyrosine, phenylalanine, and methionine can correct biochemical and renal abnormalities but does not reverse or prevent progression of liver disease. Liver transplant can correct biochemical abnormalities.
♦ Prenatal diagnosis by measurement of succinylacetone in amniotic fluid has been used.

Tyrosinemia Type II

(Rare condition due to defect in tyrosine aminotransferase)
♦ Plasma tyrosine is markedly increased (30–50 mg/dL).
Tyrosine is found in urine.
No findings of liver or kidney disease

Transient Tyrosinemia

(E.g., incomplete development of tyrosine-oxidizing system, especially in premature or low-birth-weight infants)
♦ Serum phenylalanine is >4 mg/dL (5–20 mg/dL).
♦ Serum tyrosine is between 10 and 75 mg/dL.
♦ Tyrosine metabolites in urine are ≤ 1 mg/mL (parahydroxyphenyl-lactic and parahydroxyphenylacetic acids can be distinguished from orthohydroxyphenylacetic acid by paper chromatography).
♦ Orthohydroxyphenylacetic acid is absent from urine.
Without administration of ascorbic acid, 25% of premature infants may have increased serum phenylalanine and tyrosine for several weeks (but condition is reversed in 24 hrs after ascorbic acid administration) and increased urine tyrosine and tyrosine derivatives. Rarely seen now because of breast feeding and low-protein formulas.
Similar blood and urine findings that are not reversed by administration of ascorbic acid may occur in untreated galactosemia, tyrosinemia, congenital cirrhosis, and giant-cell hepatitis; jaundice occurs frequently.
Serum serotonin (5-hydroxytryptophan) is decreased.
Urine 5-HIAA excretion is decreased.
Blood levels of phenylalanine deficiency should be monitored frequently during treatment (e.g., twice a week during first 6 mos, once a week during next 6 mos, twice a month up to age 18 mos, once a month thereafter).

Xanthinuria

(Rare autosomal recessive disorder of purine metabolism with deficiency of xanthine oxidase in tissues, which catalyzes conversion of hypoxanthine to xanthine and xanthine to uric acid)
♦ Decreased serum uric acid; <1 mg/dL strongly suggests this diagnosis (see p. 85).
Decreased urine uric acid (usually <30 mg/24 hrs; normal = ≤ 500 mg/24 hrs).
Increased urine and serum levels of xanthine and hypoxanthine
○ Laboratory findings due to urinary xanthine calculi
♦ Enzyme activity <10% of normal in biopsy of liver and jejunal mucosa

META/HERED

Disorders of Carbohydrate Metabolism

Alkaptonuria

(Autosomal recessive disorder in which absence of liver homogentisic acid oxidase causes excretion of homogentisic acid in urine)

Cardinal features are urine changes, scleral pigmentation, lumbosacral spondylitis (Ochronosis). May also cause deformity of aortic valve cusps.

○Presumptive diagnosis by urine that becomes brown-black on standing and reduces Benedict's solution (urine turns brown) and Fehling's solution, but glucose-oxidase methods are negative. Ferric chloride test is positive (urine turns purple-black).

♦Thin-layer chromatography and spectrophotometric assay identify urinary homogentisic acid but are not generally necessary for diagnosis.

♦An oral dose of homogentisic acid is largely recovered in the urine of affected patients but not in that of healthy persons.

Fructose Intolerance, Hereditary

(Severe autosomal recessive disease of infancy due to virtual absence of fructose 1-phosphate aldolase causing fructose 1-phosphate accumulation in liver; clinically resembles galactosemia)

○Fructose in urine of 100–300 mg/dL gives a positive test for reducing substances (Benedict's reagent, Clinitest) but not with glucose oxidase methods (Clinistix, Tes-Tape).

♦Fructose is identified by paper chromatography.

♦Fructose tolerance test shows prolonged elevation of blood fructose and marked decrease in serum glucose that may cause convulsions and coma. Serum phosphorus shows rapid prolonged decrease. Aminoaciduria and proteinuria may occur during test.

Increased serum ALT, AST, bilirubin; cirrhosis may occur.

Asymptomatic carriers have ~50% of enzyme activity.

Fructosuria, Essential

(Benign asymptomatic autosomal recessive disorder due to fructokinase deficiency)

○Large amount of fructose in urine gives a positive test for reducing substances (Benedict's reagent, Clinitest) but not with glucose oxidase methods (Clinistix, Tes-Tape).

♦Fructose is identified by paper chromatography.

♦Fructose tolerance test shows that blood fructose increases to 4× more than in normal persons, blood glucose increases only slightly, and serum phosphorus does not change.

Galactosemia

(Inherited defect in liver and RBCs of galactose 1-phosphate uridyltransferase, which converts galactose to glucose, causing accumulation of galactose 1-phosphate. Rarer variant forms due to galactokinase deficiency and uridine diphosphate–galactose 4-epimerase deficiencies.)

♦Increased blood galactose of ≤ 300 mg/dL (normal is <5 mg/dL).

♦Increased urine galactose of 500–2000 mg/dL (normal is <5 mg/dL). Positive urine reaction with Clinitest but negative with Clinistix and Tes-Tape; may be useful for pediatric screening up to 1 yr of age.

♦Reduced RBC galactose 1-phosphate uridyltransferase establishes diagnosis.

Serum glucose may appear to be elevated in fasting state but falls as galactose increases; hypoglycemia is usual.

Galactose tolerance test is positive but not necessary for diagnosis and may be hazardous because of induced hypoglycemia and hypokalemia.

• Use an oral dose of 35 gm of galactose/sq m of body area.
• Normal: Serum galactose increases to 30–50 mg/dL; returns to normal within 3 hrs.
• Galactosemia: Serum increase is greater, and return to baseline level is delayed.
• Heterozygous carrier: Response is intermediate.
• The test is not specific or sensitive enough for genetic studies.

Albuminuria

General ammoaciduria is identified by chromatography.

Laboratory findings due to complications
- Jaundice (onset at age 4–10 days)
- Liver biopsy—dilated canaliculus filled with bile pigment with surrounding rosette of liver cells
- Severe hemolysis
- Coagulation abnormalities
- Vomiting, diarrhea, failure to thrive
- Hyperchloremic metabolic acidosis
- Cataracts
- Mental and physical retardation
- Decreased immunity (~25% of infants develop *Escherichia coli* sepsis that may cause death)

Findings disappear (but are not reversed) when galactose (e.g., milk) is eliminated from diet. Efficacy of diet is monitored by measuring RBC level of galactose 1-phosphate (desired range <4 mg/dL or <180 μg/gm hemoglobin).

Screening incidence is 1 in 62,000 live births. Cord blood is preferred but this prevents also screening for PKU, because latter test is normal in neonatal cord blood. Filter paper blood may show false-positive results for PKU, tyrosinemia, and homocystinuria. Test is invalidated by exchange transfusion.

♦ Prenatal diagnosis is made by measurement of galactose 1-phosphate uridyltransferase in cell culture from amniotic fluid. Parents show <50% enzyme activity in RBCs.

Lactase Deficiency; Intestinal Deficiency of Sugar-Splitting Enzymes (Milk Allergy; Milk Intolerance; Congenital Familial Lactose Intolerance; Disaccharidase Deficiency)

(Familial disease that often begins in infancy with diarrhea, vomiting, failure to thrive, malabsorption, etc.; patient becomes asymptomatic when lactose is removed from diet)

Oral lactose tolerance test shows a rise in blood sugar of <20 mg/dL in blood drawn at 15, 30, 60, 90 mins (usual dose = 50 gm).

In diabetics, blood sugar may increase >20 mg/dL despite impaired lactose absorption. Test may also be influenced by impaired gastric emptying or small bowel transit.

If test is positive, repeat using glucose and galactose (usually 25 gm each) instead of lactose; subnormal rise indicates a mucosal absorptive defect; normal increase (>25 gm/dL) indicates lactase deficiency only.

♦ Biopsy of small intestine mucosa shows low level of lactase in homogenized tissue. Is used to assess results of other diagnostic tests but is seldom required except to exclude secondary lactase deficiency with histologic studies.

♦ Hydrogen breath test (measured by gas chromatography) is noninvasive, rapid, simple, sensitive, quantitative. Patient expires into a breath-collecting apparatus; complete absorption causes no increase of H_2 formed in colon to be excreted in breath. Malabsorption causes H_2 production by fermentation in colon that is proportional to amount of test dose not absorbed. False-negative test in ~20% of patients due to absence of H_2-producing bacteria in colon or prior antibiotic therapy.

○Lactose in urine amounts to 100–2000 mg/dL. It produces a positive test for reducing sugars (Benedict's reagent, Clinitest) but a negative test with glucose oxidase methods (Tes-Tape, Clinistix).

After ingestion of milk or 50–100 gm of lactose, stools have a pH of 4.5–6.0 (normal pH is >7.0) and are sour and frothy.

Fecal studies are of limited value in adults.

Mannoheptulosuria

Mannoheptulose in urine after consumption of avocados occurs in some persons; not clinically important.

Pentosuria

(Deficiency in L-xylitol dehydrogenase, which catalyzes reduction of xylulose to xylitol in metabolism of glucuronic acid)

♦ Urinary excretion of L-xylulose is increased (1–4 gm/day), and the increase is accentuated by administration of glucuronic acid and glucuronogenic drugs (e.g., aminopyrine, antipyrine, menthol).

METAB/HERED

Table 12-10. Classification of Glycogen Storage Diseases*

Type	Frequency (%)	Clinical Name	Deficient Enzyme
I	20	von Gierke's disease	Liver glucose-6-phosphatase
II	20	Pompe's disease	Lysosomal alpha-1,4-glucosidase
III	30	Forbes' disease	Amylo-1,6-glucosidase (debranched enzyme)
IV	<1	Andersen's disease	Amylo-$[1,4\rightarrow1,6]$-transglucosidase (branched enzyme)
V	5	McArdle syndrome	Muscle phosphorylase
VI	25% for	Hers' disease	Liver phosphorylase
VII	VI + VII	Tarui's disease	Muscle phosphofructokinase
VIII	Very rare	Hug, Huijing	Phosphorylase kinase
X			Muscle phosphoglycerate kinase
XI			Muscle phosphoglycerate mutase
XII			Muscle lactate dehydrogenase

*All are autosomal recessive except type VIII, which is X-linked recessive.

○Urine positive for reducing substances but negative for glucose using glucose oxidase enzymatic strips.
♦Heterozygotes detected by glucuronic acid loading followed by measurement of serum xylulose or assay of reduced nicotinamide-adenine dinucleotide phosphate–L-xylulose dehydrogenase in RBCs.

Differential Diagnosis

Alimentary pentosuria—arabinose or xylose excreted after ingestion of large amount of certain fruits (e.g., plums, cherries, grapes)
Healthy persons—small amounts of D-ribose or trace amounts of ribulose in urine
Muscular dystrophy—small amounts of D-ribose in urine (some patients)

Sucrosuria

Urine specific gravity is very high (≤ 1.07).
Urine tests for reducing substances are negative.
Sucrosuria may follow IV administration of sucrose or the factitious addition of cane sugar to urine.

Glycogen Storage Diseases

See Table 12-10.

Type I Glycogen Storage Disease; Glucose-6-Phosphatase Deficiency (von Gierke's Disease)

(Autosomal recessive disorder characterized by lack of glucose-6-phosphatase in liver and kidney with an incidence of 1 in 200,000 births; may appear in first days or weeks of life)
○Blood glucose is markedly decreased.
○After overnight fast, marked hypoglycemia and increased blood lactate and occasionally pyruvate with severe metabolic acidosis, ketonemia, and ketonuria. *(Recurrent acidosis is most common cause for hospital admission.)*
Blood triglycerides are very high; cholesterol is moderately increased and serum free fatty acids are increased. Results in xanthomas and lipid-laden cells in bone marrow.

Mild anemia is present.

Impaired platelet function may cause bleeding tendency.

Increased serum uric acid, which may cause clinical gout, nephrocalcinosis, proteinuria.

Serum phosphorus and ALP are decreased.

Urinary nonspecific amino acids are increased, without increase in blood amino acids.

Other renal function tests are relatively normal despite kidney enlargement; Fanconi's syndrome is rare.

Liver function test results (other than those related to carbohydrate metabolism) are relatively normal but serum GGT, AST, and ALT may be increased.

Glucose tolerance may be normal or diabetic type; diabetic type is more frequent in older children and adults.

○Functional tests
  • Administer 1 mg of glucagon IV or IM after 8-hr fast. Blood glucose increases 50–60% in 10–20 mins in the normal person. Little or no increase occurs in infants or young children with von Gierke's disease; delayed response may occur in older children and adults.
  • IV administration of glucose precursors (e.g., galactose or fructose) causes no rise in blood glucose in von Gierke's disease (demonstrating block in gluconeogenesis), but normal rise occurs in limit dextrinosis (type III glycogen storage disease).

Biopsy of liver
  • Biochemical studies

♦ Absent or markedly decreased glucose-6-phosphatase on assay of frozen liver provides definitive diagnosis.
      Increased glycogen content (>4% by weight) but normal biochemically and structurally.
      Other enzymes (other glycogen storage diseases) are present in normal amounts.
  • Histologic findings are not diagnostic; vacuolization of hepatic cells and abundant glycogen granules are seen; confirm with Best's stain.

♦ Biopsy of jejunum
  • Intestinal glucose-6-phosphatase is decreased or absent.

Biopsy of muscle shows no abnormality of enzyme activity or glycogen content.

Can be cured by liver transplant.

Type IB Glycogen Storage Disease

(Shows all the clinical and biochemical features of von Gierke's disease except that liver biopsy does not show deficiency of glucose-6-phosphatase)

Patient may have maturation arrest neutropenia; varies from mild to agranulocytosis; usually constant but may be cyclic. Associated increased frequency of staphylococcal and candida infection.

♦ Diagnosis established by finding of impaired function of glucose-6-phosphate activity in granulocytes.

Type II Glycogen Storage Disease; Generalized Glycogenosis; Alpha-1,4-Glucosidase Deficiency (Pompe's Disease)

(Autosomal recessive disease. Classic infantile form [Type IIA] characterized by neurological, cardiac, and muscle involvement, frequent liver enlargement, death within first year; juvenile form [Type IIB] shows muscle disease resembling pseudohypertrophic dystrophy; adult form [Type IIC] characterized by progressive myopathy)

Fasting blood sugar, GTT, glucagon responses, and rises in blood glucose after fructose infusion are normal. No acetonuria is present.

General hematologic findings are normal.

♦ Staining of circulating leukocytes for glycogen shows massive deposition.

♦ Confirm diagnosis by absence of alpha-1,4-glucosidase in muscle and liver biopsy or cultured fibroblasts. Assay in amniotic cell culture allows prenatal diagnosis. Special assay of peripheral leukocytes for diagnosis of heterozygotes.

Type III Glycogen Deposition Disease (Forbes' Disease; Debrancher Deficiency; Limit Dextrinosis)

(Autosomal recessive disease with enlarged liver, retarded growth, chemical changes, and benign course)
Serum CK may be increased.
Mild increase in cholesterol and triglycerides are less marked than in type I disease.
Marked fasting acetonuria (as in starvation).
Fasting hypoglycemia is less severe than in type I disease.
Normal blood lactate; uric acid is usually normal.
Serum AST and ALT are increased in children but normal in adults.
Diabetic type of glucose tolerance curve with associated glucosuria.
Infusions of gluconeogenic precursors (e.g., galactose, fructose) causes a normal hyperglycemic response unlike in type I disease.
○Low fasting blood sugar does not show expected rise after administration of subcutaneous glucagon or epinephrine but does increase 2 hrs after high-carbohydrate meal.
♦Confirm diagnosis by liver and muscle biopsy that show biochemical findings of increased glycogen, abnormal glycogen structure, absence of specific enzyme activity. Normal phosphorylase and glucose-6-phosphatase activity.

Type IV Glycogen Deposition Disease (Andersen's Disease; Brancher Deficiency; Amylopectinosis)

(Extremely rare fatal condition that is due to absence of amylo-[1,4→1.6]-transglucosidase)
Hypoglycemia is not present.
Liver function tests may be altered as in other types of cirrhosis (e.g., slight increase in serum bilirubin, reversed A/G ratio, increased AST, decreased cholesterol). Blood glucose response to epinephrine and glucagon may be flat.
♦Biopsy of liver may show a cirrhotic reaction to the presence of glycogen of abnormal structure, which stains with Best's carmine and periodic acid-Schiff stain, but normal glycogen concentration.
WBC may be increased and Hb may be decreased.

Type V Glycogen Deposition Disease (McArdle's Disease; Myophosphorylase Deficiency)

(Autosomal recessive disease due to absent myophosphorylase in skeletal muscle; patient shows very limited ischemic muscle exercise tolerance despite normal appearance of muscle)
Epinephrine or glucagon causes a normal hyperglycemic response.
Biopsy of muscle is microscopically normal in young; vacuolation and necrosis are seen in later years. Increased glycogen is present.
♦Definitive diagnosis is made by finding of absence of phosphorylase.
○After exercise that quickly causes muscle cramping and weakness, regional blood lactate and pyruvate do not increase (in a normal person they increase 2–5 times). Similar abnormal response occurs in type III disease involving muscle and in types VII, VIII, X.
Myoglobulinuria may occur after strenuous exercise.
○Increased serum muscle enzymes (e.g., LD, CK, aldolase) for several hours after strenuous exercise.

Type VI Glycogen Storage Disease (Hepatic Phosphorylase Deficiency)

Enlarged liver present from birth is associated with hypoglycemia.
Serum cholesterol and triglycerides are mildly increased.
Serum uric acid and lactic acid are normal.
Liver function tests are normal.

Fructose tolerance is normal.
Response to glucagon and epinephrine is variable but tends to be poor.
◆ Diagnosis is based on decreased phosphorylase activity in liver, leukocytes, and RBC hemolysate, but muscle phosphorylase is normal.

Type VII Glycogen Storage Disease (Muscle Phosphofructokinase Deficiency; Tarui's Disease)

(Autosomal recessive disease with deficiency of muscle phosphofructokinase)
Fasting hypoglycemia is marked.
Other members of family may have reduced tolerance to glucose.
◆ RBCs show 50% decrease in phosphofructokinase activity.
◆ Biopsy of muscle shows marked decrease (1–3% of normal) in phosphofructokinase activity.
Clinically identical to type V disease.

Type VIII Glycogen Storage Disease

(Very rare X-linked recessive disease with deficiency of phosphorylase b kinase)
Blood glucose is markedly decreased, causing hypoglycemic seizures and mental retardation.
Glucagon administration causes no increase in blood glucose (see von Gierke's disease, p. 544), but ingestion of food causes a rise in 2–3 hrs.
◆ Biopsy of liver shows marked decrease in glycogen synthetase.

Porphyrias

See Figs. 12-7 and 12-8 and Table 12-11.

Porphyrin Tests of Urine (Fluorometric Methods)
May Be Positive Due To
Drugs that produce fluorescence, e.g.,
  • Acriflavine
  • Ethoxazene
  • Phenazopyridine
  • Sulfamethoxazole
  • Tetracycline
Drugs that may precipitate porphyria, e.g.,
  • Antipyretics
  • Barbiturates
  • Phenylhydrazine
  • Sulfonamides

(1) Congenital Erythropoietic Porphyria

(Extremely rare disorder due to decreased activity of uroporphyrinogen III synthase in RBCs; usual onset in infancy, extreme cutaneous photosensitivity with mutilation, red urine and teeth)
○Ultraviolet fluorescence of urine, teeth, and bones
Variable number of RBCs and marrow normoblasts
Normocytic, normochromic, anicteric hemolytic anemia that tends to be mild; may be associated with hypersplenism, increased reticulocytes and normoblasts.
◆ Urine—marked increase of uroporphyrin I is characteristic; coproporphyrin shows lesser increase. Excretion of porphobilinogen and delta-ALA is normal. Watson-Schwartz test is negative.
◆ RBCs and plasma—marked increase of uroporphyrins; increased coproporphyrin
◆ Stool—marked increase of porphyrins, especially coproporphyrins

METAB/HERED

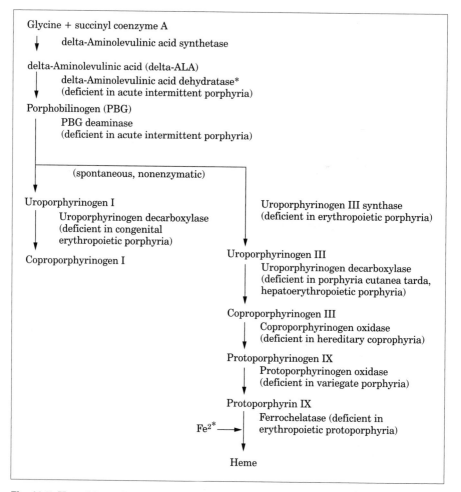

Glycine + succinyl coenzyme A
↓   delta-Aminolevulinic acid synthetase

delta-Aminolevulinic acid (delta-ALA)
↓   delta-Aminolevulinic acid dehydratase*
(deficient in acute intermittent porphyria)

Porphobilinogen (PBG)
PBG deaminase
(deficient in acute intermittent porphyria)

(spontaneous, nonenzymatic)

Uroporphyrinogen I
Uroporphyrinogen decarboxylase
(deficient in congenital
erythropoietic porphyria)

Coproporphyrinogen I

Uroporphyrinogen III synthase
(deficient in erythropoietic porphyria)

Uroporphyrinogen III
Uroporphyrinogen decarboxylase
(deficient in porphyria cutanea tarda,
hepatoerythropoietic porphyria)

Coproporphyrinogen III
Coproporphyrinogen oxidase
(deficient in hereditary coprophyria)

Protoporphyrinogen IX
Protoporphyrinogen oxidase
(deficient in variegate porphyria)

Protoporphyrin IX
Ferrochelatase (deficient in
Fe^{2*} → erythropoietic protoporphyria)

Heme

Fig. 12-7. Heme biosynthesis pathway showing site of enzyme action and disease caused by enzyme deficiency. Accumulation of porphyrins and their precursors preceding the enzyme block are responsible for the clinical and laboratory findings in each syndrome. Porphobilinogen (PBG) and aminolevulinic acid (ALA) cause abdominal pain and neuropsychiatric symptoms. Increased porphyrins (with or without increased PBG or ALA) cause photosensitivity. Thus, deficiencies near the end of the metabolic path cause more photosensitivity and fewer neuropsychiatric findings.
*Lead inhibits formation delta-ALA dehydratase causing accumulation of delta-ALA and inhibits reduction of Fe^3 to Fe^2.

(2) Erythropoietic Protoporphyria

(Relatively common type of porphyria due to deficiency of ferrochelatase activity in bone marrow, reticulocytes, liver, and other cells)
Mild microcytic hypochromic anemia in 20–30% of patients
Laboratory findings due to liver disease (severe in 10% of cases) with increased serum direct bilirubin, AST, ALP (due to intrahepatic cholestasis), and gallstones containing porphyrins may be found.
Urine—porphyrins within normal limits
♦ RBCs—marked increase of free protoporphyrin in symptomatic patients (zinc-chelated form may also be increased in iron-deficiency anemia and lead poisoning

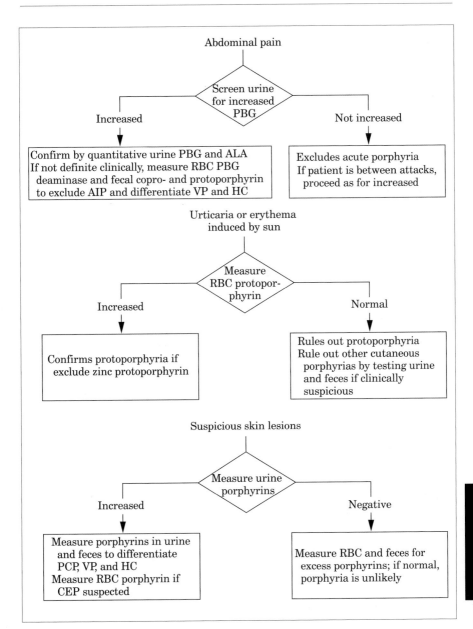

Fig. 12-8. Diagnostic strategy for suspected porphyria according to symptoms. Excess production of porphyrins is associated with cutaneous photosensitivity. Excess production of only porphyrin precursors is associated with neurologic symptoms. Excess production of both is associated with both types of clinical symptoms. (AIP = acute intermittent porphyria; ALA = aminolevulinic acid; CEP = congenital erythropoietic porphyria; HC = hereditary coproporphyria; PBG = porphobilinogen; PCT = porphyria cutanea tarda; VP = variegate porphyria.)

META/HERED

Table 12-11. Comparison of Porphyrias

Type	Enzyme Defect	Inheri-tance	Age at Onset	Fre-quency	Urine
(1) Congenital erythropoietic porphyria	Uroporphyrinogen III cosynthase	AR	Infancy	Very rare	**Uro I**; Watson-Schwartz negative[a]; Copro
(2) Erythropoietic protopor-phyria	Ferrochelatase	AD	Child-hood	Common	Negative
(3) Porphyria cutanea tarda	Uroporphyrinogen decarboxylase	AD	Middle age	Most com-mon type in United States and Europe	**Uro > Copro constant**; PBG not increased; ALA may be slightly increased
(4) Acute inter-mittent porphyria	Porphobilinogen deaminase	AD	Adoles-cence	Uncommon	**ALA[b] and PBG constant; Watson-Schwartz positive**
(5) Variegate porphyria	Protoporphyrino-gen oxidase	AD	Young adult		ALA and PBG during attack[a]
(6) Hereditary copropor-phyria	Coproporphyrino-gen oxidase	AD	Young adult	Rarest	Copro; ALA and PBG during attack[a]
(7) Hepatoery-thropoietic porphyria	Heme synthetase; uroporphyrino-gen decarboxy-lase deficiency more severe than in porphyria cutanea tarda	AR	Early infancy	Rarest	Resembles findings in porphyria cutanea tarda
(8) ALA dehy-drase deficiency	delta-ALA dehydrase	AR		Very rare	**ALA; Copro**

+ through ++++ = present in increasing amounts; – = not present; AD = autosomal dominant;
AR = autosomal recessive; Copro = coproporphyrin; Iso = isocoproporphyrin; PBG = porphobilinogen;
Proto = protoporphyrin; Uro = uroporphyrin.
[a]Present during acute attack; may be absent during remission.
[b]ALA may be increased even more in chronic lead poisoning.
Boldface type indicates body material used for diagnosis.

Feces	RBCs	Comment	Chief Site of Porphyrin Overproduction	Skin Lesions	Neuropsychiatric Symptoms	Liver Disease
Copro	**Uro**; fluorescent under UV light	Hemolytic anemia; red teeth; pink/red urine stain on diapers	Bone marrow	++++	–	–
Proto	**Proto**	Gallstones	Bone marrow; liver variable	++	–	+
Iso > Copro	Negative	Siderosis; precipitated by iron overload, alcoholism	Liver	+	–	+
Negative	Negative	Abdominal pain; SIADH with low sodium and osmolarity	Liver	–	+	–
Proto constant	Negative	Abdominal pain	Liver	+++	+	–
Copro constant	Negative	Abdominal pain	Liver	+	+	–
	Increased zinc-proto		Bone marrow, liver	++++	–	+
Negative	Negative	Acute porphyria symptoms	Liver	–	+	–

METAB/HERED

but nonchelated form is present in protoporphyria). May be normal or slightly increased in asymptomatic carriers. Examination of dilute blood by fluorescent microscopy may show rapidly fading fluorescence in variable part of RBCs.

♦ Stool—protoporphyrin is usually increased in symptomatic patients and in some carriers even when carrier RBC porphyrins are normal.

♦ Three chemical patterns consist of increased free RBCs alone, stool protoporphyrin alone, and both together.

(3) Porphyria Cutanea Tarda

(Most common porphyrin disorder. Inherited form [autosomal dominant] is expressed in ~20% of patients with this gene and is due to deficiency of uroporphyrinogen decarboxylase in liver in toxic/sporadic forms and in all tissues in familial form. Associated with alcoholic liver disease and hepatic siderosis. Acquired form [inhibitor of uroporphyrinogen decarboxylase may be generated in liver] may be due to hepatoma, cirrhosis, chemicals [an epidemic in Turkey was caused by contamination of wheat by hexachlorobenzene]. May be activated by increased ingestion of iron, alcohol, estrogens.)

♦ Urine—marked increase of uroporphyrin (frequently up to 1000–3000 μg/24 hrs; normal is <300 μg) with only slight increase of coproporphyrin and uroporphyrin/coproporphyrin ratio of >7.5 (ratio is <1 in variegate porphyria). In biochemical remission, 24-hr uroporphyrin is <400 μg.

Stool—isocoproporphyrins are present.

Plasma—increased protoporphyrin

♦ Distinguished from variegate porphyria in which fecal protoporphyrins are increased and urine coproporphyrins exceed uroporphyrins during cutaneous symptoms

Serum iron and transferrin saturation are increased in ~50% of cases.

Laboratory findings of underlying liver disease

Liver biopsy shows morphologic changes of underlying disease and fluorescence under ultraviolet light; usually shows iron overload.

Diabetes mellitus in ≤ 33% of patients

Phlebotomy therapy to remove iron is monitored by decreased urine uroporphyrins excretion.

(4) Acute Intermittent Porphyria

Most frequent and severe form of porphyria in United States. Deficiency of porphobilinogen deaminase. Adult onset with acute attacks of various neuropsychiatric and abdominal symptoms. No photosensitivity.

♦ Can be diagnosed in acute or latent states by finding of decreased delta-ALA dehydratase activity and porphobilinogen deaminase activity (~50% of normal) in RBCs (test performed in special laboratories); normal in other porphyrias.

♦ Urine—Diagnostic finding is marked increase of porphobilinogen and, to a lesser extent, of delta-ALA; these decrease during remission but are rarely normal; not increased in silent carriers; also increased in plasma. Watson-Schwartz screening test for porphobilinogen should be confirmed by quantitative test. Coproporphyrin and uroporphyrin may be increased.

♦ RBCs—decreased porphobilinogen activity is used to confirm diagnosis because urine findings may occur during acute attacks of variegate porphyria and hereditary coproporphyria.

Stool—protoporphyrin and coproporphyrin are usually normal.

○ Urine may be of normal color when fresh and become brown, red, or black on standing.

During acute attack, slight leukocytosis, decreased serum sodium (may be marked), chloride, and magnesium, and increased BUN may be seen.

Liver function tests are normal.

Other frequent laboratory abnormalities are increased serum cholesterol, hyperbetalipoproteinemia (type II-a), increased serum iron, abnormal glucose tolerance, increased T_4, and thyroxine-binding globulin (TBG) without hyperthyroidism.

(5) Variegate Porphyria

♦ **Deficiency of protoporphyrinogen oxidase, which also occurs in cultured fibroblasts, liver tissue, peripheral blood lymphocytes. Skin or neurologic manifestations may occur. Precipitated by same factors as acute intermittent porphyria.**

◆ Stool—characteristic change is marked increase of protoporphyrin, which is found during attack, remission, or only with skin manifestations. When stool is normal or borderline, or in asymptomatic patients, increased porphyrins can be demonstrated in bile.

Urine—marked increase of delta-ALA and porphobilinogen during an acute attack; levels are usually normal after acute episode in contrast to acute intermittent porphyria and hereditary coproporphyria.

Blood—porphyrin levels are not increased.

(6) Hereditary Coproporphyria

Deficiency of coproporphyrinogen oxidase. Disease is latent in two-thirds of patients. Precipitated by same factors as acute intermittent porphyria.

◆ Stool—coproporphyrin is always increased, very markedly during an acute attack; also increased in plasma. Protoporphyrin is normal or only slightly increased.

Urine—coproporphyrin may be increased or not; is usually normal during remission. Isolated increase may be secondary to liver, hematologic, neoplastic, and toxic conditions. Increased ALA and porphobilinogen during acute attacks.

◆ RBCs—diminished coproporphyrinogen oxidase is strongly indicative.

◆ Liver—diminished coproporphyrinogen oxidase is diagnostic.

(7) Hepatoerythropoietic Porphyria

◆ **Severe deficiency of uroporphyrinogen decarboxylase (5–10% of normal); 50% of normal in parents.**

◆ Porphyrin abnormalities resemble those in porphyria cutanea tarda but in addition zinc protoporphyrin is increased in RBCs.

Adults usually have mild normochromic anemia; fluorescent normoblasts appear in bone marrow.

Serum GGT and transaminase may be increased. Liver disease may progress to cirrhosis.

Severe skin involvement

(8) ALA Dehydrase Deficiency

◆ **98% deficiency of enzyme; parents had 50% of normal activity.**

Acute porphyria-type symptoms

◆ Urine—increased ALA and coproporphyrin (resembles lead intoxication)

RBC, but not plasma, protoporphyrins are also increased in iron-deficiency anemia and lead intoxication. Screening tests using fluorescence microscopy of RBCs or Wood's lamp viewing of treated whole blood may also be positive in iron-deficiency anemia, lead intoxication, and other dyserythropoietic states. In congenital erythropoietic porphyria, 5–20% of RBCs show fluorescence that lasts up to a minute or more in contrast to erythropoietic protoporphyria in which fluorescence is half that and lasts ~30 secs and in lead poisoning in which almost all RBCs fluoresce for only a few seconds. Fluorescence of hepatocytes occurs in erythropoietic protoporphyria, porphyria cutanea tarda, porphyria variegata, and hereditary coproporphyria.

Laboratory evaluation for porphyrias may include: 24-hr urine for quantitative ALA, porphobilinogen, uroporphyrin, and coproporphyrin (urine should be kept refrigerated as porphyrins deteriorate quickly, especially at room temperature); plasma porphyrin; free RBC protoporphyrin; spot stool quantitative coproporphyrin and protoporphyrin; Watson-Schwartz test to demonstrate porphyrin precursors in urine (Ehrlich's reagent and sodium acetate added to urine; when positive, urine turns cherry red with addition of chloroform); search for evidence of hemolytic anemia, liver disease; fluorescence of appropriate tissues; enzyme activity assay of RBCs, liver tissue, or cultured fibroblasts. Urine delta-ALA and porphobilinogen should be measured during episodes.

Acute episodes (which may include abdominal pain and psychiatric symptoms; hypertension, paresthesias, fever, neuromuscular weakness; seizures are less frequent) are characteristic of acute intermittent porphyria, coproporphyria, and variegate porphyria; may be precipitated by certain drugs (especially barbiturates, alcohol, and sulfonamides; also diphenylhydantoin, chlordiazepoxide, ergots, certain steroids), infection, starvation.

METAB/HERED

Lysosomal Storage Disorders[11]

Disorder	Deficient Enzyme	Major System, Organ, or Tissue Involved
Glycoprotein degradation		
Fucosidosis	Alpha-fucosidase	CNS, high sweat electrolytes
Mannosidosis	Alpha-mannosidase	CNS, mild bone changes, hepatosplenomegaly
Sialidosis (mucolipidosis I)	Alpha-N-acetyl neuraminidase	CNS, bone, liver, spleen
Glycogen storage disease	Alpha-glucosidase	Muscle, heart
Aspartylglycosaminuria	Aspartyl-glucosaminidase	CNS, bone marrow, connective tissue; prominent inclusions in leukocytes
Enzyme localization		
Mucolipidosis II (I-cell disease) (formerly mucopolysaccharidosis VII)	N-Acetylglucosaminyl-phosphor transferase	CNS, bone, connective tissue
Mucolipidosis III (pseudo–Hurler's polydystrophy)	N-Acetylglucosamine-1-transferase	Predominantly joint and connective tissue
Lysosomal efflux		
Cystinosis	?	Kidney
Salla disease	?	CNS

Mucopolysaccharidoses (see Table 12-12)
Sphingolipidoses (see Table 12-13)
Lipidoses
Chédiak-Higashi syndrome (see p. 378)

Cystinosis

(Autosomal recessive lysosomal storage disease due to impaired transport of cystine out of lysosomes; only this one amino acid is accumulated)
Infants (acute nephropathic form)
Fanconi-like syndrome (aminoaciduria, glycosuria, proteinuria, phosphaturia, polyuria)
Metabolic acidosis
Polyuria
Vitamin D–resistant rickets
♦ Diagnosis by finding of high cystine content in leukocytes or cultured fibroblasts
○ Crystalline inclusions in conjunctiva and cornea, and leukocytes, bone marrow, rectal mucosa

Adults (benign disease)
Urinary tract calculi
Cystinuria (cystine crystals in urine; >200 mg of cystine in 24-hr urine specimen)
Asymptomatic cystine crystals also present in eye

Fabry's Disease (Alpha-Galactosidase A Deficiency)

(X-linked recessive disease with deficiency of alpha-galactosidase A that causes skin lesions and accumulation of ceramide in various organs, affecting function [e.g., kidney, heart, lung, brain]. Symptoms due to involvement of these organ systems in infancy and cherry-red spots in macula.)
♦ Prenatal diagnosis by demonstration of enzyme deficiency in cultured amniotic fluid cells
♦ Heterozygote detection by enzyme assay of cultured fibroblasts or individual hair roots or by assay of glycolipid content of urine sediment

[11]Classification adapted from Kornfeld S, Sly WS. Lysosomal storage defects. *Hosp Pract* Aug 15, 1985:71–82.

Gaucher's Disease[12,13]

(Rare autosomal recessive deficiency of beta-glucosidase; most frequent storage disease; may be present in 10,000–20,000 Americans, with highest prevalence in Ashkenazi Jews; gene on chromosome band 1q21)

♦ Measurement of decreased beta-glucosidase activity in leukocytes or fibroblasts is reliable diagnostic method; substantial overlap between heterozygotes and healthy persons.

♦ Diagnostic Gaucher's cells are seen in bone marrow aspiration, needle biopsy, or aspiration of spleen, liver, or lymph nodes examined for thrombocytopenia or unrelated disorder and cause the nonneurologic manifestations.

○ Serum acid phosphatase is increased in most patients (if substrate for test is different from that for prostatic acid phosphatase; i.e., use phenyl phosphate or p-nitrophenyl phosphate instead of glycerophosphate). It may return to normal after splenectomy.

Serum ACE is increased in most patients.

Serum cholesterol and total fats are normal.

Laboratory findings due to involvement of specific organs

- Spleen—hypersplenism occurs with anemia (normocytic normochromic), leukopenia (with relative lymphocytosis; monocytes may be increased), thrombocytopenia without bleeding.
- Bone—serum ALP may be increased.
- Liver—serum AST may be increased.
- CSF—AST may be increased.

Laboratory findings due to increased incidence of lymphoproliferative disorders (e.g., multiple myeloma, CLL).

♦ Prenatal diagnosis by enzymatic determination of cultured amniotic fluid cells. If both parental mutations have been identified at the DNA level, chorionic villus sampling for fetal DNA can be done.

Enzymatic methods do not detect carriers reliably. Molecular methods accurately detect carriers.

♦ Phenotype cannot be predicted from genotype. Common mutations can be detected using PCR and aid in genetic counseling for general risk of transmitting the gene but not specific prognosis for future affected children.

Type 1 (99% of patients): no neurologic involvement

Type 2: fulminating disorder with severe neurologic involvement and death within first 18 mos

Type 3: juvenile form with later onset of neurologic symptoms and milder course with death in early childhood

Bone marrow transplantation is effective therapy but has associated morbidity and mortality. Enzyme replacement therapy usually obviates need for splenectomy.

GM$_1$ Gangliosidosis (Landing's Disease, Systemic Late Infantile Lipidosis)

(Rare autosomal recessive deficiency of acid beta-galactosidase with no racial predilection, characterized by psychomotor deterioration, enlargement of liver and/or spleen, cherry-red macular spots, dysostosis multiplex; infantile, juvenile, and adult forms)

♦ Diagnosis by absence of lysosomal acid beta-galactosidase enzyme in leukocytes, cultured fibroblasts, or brain. Tissue biopsy or culture of marrow or skin fibroblasts shows accumulation of ganglioside GM_1; also can demonstrate GM_1 in brain and viscera and mucopolysaccharides in viscera.

♦ Heterozygote carriers can be detected by enzyme assay in leukocytes.

Vacuolated lymphocytes may be found.

○ Abnormal leukocytic granulations (Alder-Reilly bodies) may be present.

Serum LD, AST, and fructose 1-phosphate aldolase are normal.

○ Foam cell histiocytes (resembling Niemann-Pick cells) may be seen in biopsy from bone marrow, liver, or rectum.

[12]Data from Beutler E. Gaucher's disease. *N Engl J Med* 1991;325:1354.
[13]National Institutes of Health. Gaucher disease: current issues in diagnosis and treatment. Statement presented at: Technology Assessment Conference, Feb 27–Mar 1, 1995.

METAB/HERED

Table 12-12. Classification of Mucopolysaccharidoses

Type of Mucopolysaccharidosis (clinical name)	Deficient Enzyme	Mucopolysaccharide Excreted in Urine	Signs/Symptoms
IH (Hurler's syndrome)	Alpha-L-iduronidase	Dermatan sulfate and heparan sulfate in 7:3 ratio	Progressive mental/physical disability from 1 yr of age; hyperplastic gums; coarse face; stiff joints (clawhands); organomegaly; dwarfing; dysostosis multiplex
IS (Scheie's syndrome)	Alpha-L-iduronidase	Dermatan sulfate and heparan sulfate	Mild form of MPS I; mild or no mental retardation; clawhands; aortic stenosis
IH/S (Hurler-Scheie syndrome)	Alpha-L-iduronidase		Features intermediate between Hurler's and Scheie's syndromes
II (Hunter's syndrome)	Iduronate sulfatase	Dermatan sulfate and heparan sulfate	Dysostosis multiplex; mild to severe mental retardation; no corneal opacity; longer life compared with MPS I
IIIA (Sanfilippo's syndrome, type A)	Heparan N-sulfatase (sulfamidase)	Heparan sulfate	Mild or no connective tissue abnormalities; marked hirsutism; behaviorism progresses to severe mental retardation; no corneal opacity
IIIB (Sanfilippo's syndrome, type B)	Alpha-N-acetylglucosaminidase (alpha-hexosaminidase)	Heparan sulfate	Same as in MPS IIIa
IIIC (Sanfilippo's syndrome, type C)	Acetyl CoA: alpha-glucosaminide N-acetyltransferase	Heparan sulfate	Same as in MPS IIIa

IIID (Sanfilippo's syndrome, type D)	N-Acetylglucosamine-6-sulfatase	Heparan sulfate	Same as in MPS IIIa
IVA (Morquio's syndrome, type A)	N-Acetylgalactosamine-6-sulfatase	Keratan sulfate	Marked skeletal abnormalities; small stature; short neck; prominent lower ribs; normal intellect; coma
IVB (Morquio's syndrome, type B)	Beta-galactosidase	Keratan sulfate	
V	This class is vacant now (formerly was Scheie's syndrome).		
VI (Maroteaux-Lamy syndrome)	N-Acetylgalactosamine-4-sulfatase (aryl-sulfatase B)	Dermatan sulfate	Severe dysostosis multiplex and corneal opacity; retarded growth; normal intellect; cardiac abnormalities; a mild form also occurs
VII (Sly's syndrome)	Beta-glucuronidase	Dermatan sulfate, heparan sulfate, chondroitin 4,6-sulfate	Mild mental retardation; organomegaly; corneal opacity may occur; coarse facies; gingivitis; very heterogeneous clinical appearances

CoA = coenzyme A; MPS = mucopolysaccharidosis.
Notes: All MPSs show metachromatically staining inclusions of mucopolysaccharides in circulating polynuclear leukocytes (Reilly granulations) or lymphocytes, cells of inflammatory exudate, and bone marrow cells (most consistently in clasmatocytes). Detection of deficiency of lysosomal enzyme in cultured fibroblasts establishes the diagnosis and makes prenatal diagnosis possible. Serum can be used for diagnosis in MPS II, IIIB, and VI. Leukocytes can be used for diagnosis in MPS IH, IS, IIIA, IIIC. RBCs can be used for diagnosis in III, IV, VI. Enzyme deficiency is demonstrable in liver in all except V, VII; demonstrable in muscle in all except IH, II. Increased glycogen in affected organs except in IV; glycogen structure is normal except in III, IV. Carrier state detection of IH, III, IV, VI is not reliable due to overlapping with normal persons of enzymatic activity values.
Inheritance in Hunter's syndrome is X-linked recessive; others are autosomal recessive.
Cloudy cornea in IH, IS, IVA, IVB, VI, VII.
Mental retardation in IH, II, IIIA, IIIB, IIIC, IIID, VII.
Hepatosplenomegaly in IH, II, IIIA, IIIB, IIIC, IIID, IVB, VI, VII.
Skeletal defects in all.

Table 12-13. Classification of Sphingolipidosis

Clinical Name	Enzyme Defect Specimen for Assay	Major Lipid Accumulation	Signs/Symptoms
Gaucher's disease	Cerebroside beta-glucosidase in L, F	Glucosyl ceramide	Enlarged spleen and liver; erosion of long bones and pelvis; mental retardation only in infantile form
Niemann-Pick disease	Sphingomyelinase in F, U, S	Sphingomyelin	Enlarged liver and spleen; mental retardation; ~30% have cherry-red spot in retina
Krabbe's disease (globoid cell leukodystrophy)	Cerebroside beta-glucosidase in F, L, A, S	Galactosyl ceramide	X-linked; mental retardation; almost total absence of myelin; globoid bodies in brain white matter; increased CSF protein
Metachromatic leukodystrophy	Arylsulfatase A in L, U, F, S	Sulfatide	Mental retardation; psychological disturbances in adult form
Multiple sulfatase deficiencies	Arylsulfatase A, B, C in F, L	Sulfatide	Resembles metachromatic leukodystrophy; dermatan sulfate and heparan sulfate increased in urine
Ceramide lactoside lipidosis	Beta-galactosidase in L, S	Ceramide lactoside	Slowly progressive brain damage; enlarged liver and spleen

Disease	Enzyme (source)	Accumulated material	Clinical features
Fabry's disease (angio-keratoma corporis diffusum universale)	Alpha-galactosidase in S, L, F, U, T	Trihexosyl ceramide	Skin lesions; loss of renal function; involvement of heart and brain vessels; pain in lower limbs; cherry-red spot in retina
GM₂ gangliosidosis			
Tay-Sachs disease	Hexosaminidase A in S, L, A, F, U, T	Ganglioside GM₂	Mental retardation; cherry-red spot in retina; blindness; muscle weakness
Sandhoff's disease	Hexosaminidase A, B in S, L, A, F, U, T	Ganglioside GM₂ and globoside	Clinical picture same as in Tay-Sachs disease but mild peripheral neuropathy and organomegaly
Landing's disease (GM₁ gangliosidosis)	Lysosomal acid–beta-galactosidase in L, F, U	Ganglioside GM₁	Psychomotor deterioration; cherry-red spot in retina; enlarged liver and spleen; dysostosis multiplex
Farber's lipogranuloma-tosis*	Acid ceramidase in L, F	Ceramide	Granulomas of dermis and viscera; joint disease in infancy
Fucosidosis	Alpha-fucosidase in L	H-isoantigen	
Lactosyl ceramidosis	Neutral beta-galactosidase in F	Lactosyl ceramide	

A = amniocytes; F = fibroblasts; L = leukocytes; S = serum; U = urine; T = tears; CSF = cerebrospinal fluid.
Note: Molecular techniques are now available for diagnosis of Gaucher's, Niemann-Pick, Tay-Sachs, Sandhoff's, Fabry's, and Wolman's diseases and for generalized gangliosidosis.
*Diagnosis confirmed by biopsy of subcutaneous nodules rather than by determination of enzyme activity.

METAB/HERED

559

♦ Prenatal diagnosis by enzyme assay in cultured amniotic fluid cells or by HPLC analysis of galactosyl oligosaccharides in amniotic fluid.

I-Cell Disease (Mucolipidosis II)

(Autosomal recessive disease with defect in recognition and uptake of certain lysosomal enzymes due to deficient activity of *N*-acetylglucosaminylphosphotransferase. Clinical features resemble those of Hurler's syndrome but without corneal changes or increased mucopolysaccharides in urine.)

♦ Deficiency of *N*-acetylglucosaminylphosphotransferase in cultured fibroblasts establishes the diagnosis.
♦ Vacuolation (cytoplasmic inclusions) in lymphocytes, fibroblasts, and liver and kidney cells show positive reaction to Sudan black and acid phosphatase. Lysosomal enzyme activity (hexosaminidase A and B and alpha-galactosidase) is low in these cells but high in serum or culture medium.

Urine mucopolysaccharides are not increased.

♦ Prenatal diagnosis by finding of high levels of multiple acid hydrolases in amniotic fluid or deficiency of them in cultured amniocytes.

Some heterozygotes have abnormal inclusions in fibroblasts. Some heterozygotes have intermediate enzyme levels in leukocytes and cultured fibroblasts.

Krabbe's Disease (Globoid Cell Leukodystrophy; Galactosylceramide Lipidosis)

(Autosomal recessive disorder characterized by deficiency of galactosylceramidase, causing progressive CNS disease from ~3 mos of age and death by ~2 yrs)

♦ Diagnosis by finding of deficiency of this enzyme (5–10% of normal) in leukocytes or cultured fibroblasts
♦ Conjunctival biopsy shows characteristic ballooned Schwann cells.
♦ Brain biopsy (massive infiltration of unique multinucleated inclusion-containing globoid cells in white matter due to accumulation of galactosylceramide; also diffuse loss of myelin, severe astrocytic gliosis)

CSF protein electrophoresis shows increased albumin and alpha globulin and decreased beta and gamma globulin (as in metachromatic leukodystrophy).

♦ Prenatal diagnosis by measurement of enzyme activity in cultured amniotic fluid cells.

Mucolipidosis III (*N*-Acetylglucosaminylphosphotransferase Deficiency; Pseudo–Hurler's Polydystrophy)

(Clinical features resemble those in Hurler's syndrome but without increased mucopolysaccharides in urine.

♦ Autosomal recessive transmission of fundamental defect in recognition or catalysis and uptake of certain lysosomal enzymes due to deficient activity of *N*-acetylglucosamine-1-transferase.
♦ Heterozygotes may have intermediate enzyme levels in leukocytes and cultured fibroblasts.

Mucopolysaccharidoses, Genetic

♦ All mucopolysaccharidoses show metachromatically staining inclusions of mucopolysaccharides in circulating PMNs (Reilly granulations) or lymphocytes, cells of inflammatory exudate, and bone marrow cells (most consistently in clasmatocytes). Mucopolysaccharide is also deposited in various parenchymal cells. Detection of deficiency of lysosomal enzyme in cultured fibroblasts establishes the diagnosis and makes prenatal diagnosis possible. Serum can be used for diagnosis in mucopolysaccharidoses II, IIIB, VI. Leukocytes can be used for diagnosis in mucopolysaccharidoses IH, IS, IIIA, IIIC. RBCs can be used for diagnosis in mucopolysaccharidoses III, IV, VI. Enzyme deficiency is demonstrable in liver in all types except V, VII; demonstrable in muscle in all types except IH, II. Increased glycogen in affected organs except in type IV; glycogen structure is normal except in types III, IV. Carrier state detection of types IH, III, IV, VI is not reliable due to overlap with normal persons in enzymatic activity values.

Inheritance is X-linked recessive in Hunter's syndrome; autosomal recessive in others.

Cloudy cornea in types IH, IS, IVA, IVB, VI, VII.
Mental retardation in types IH, II, IIIA, IIIB, IIIC, IIID, VII.
Hepatosplenomegaly in types IH, II, IIIA, IIIB, IIIC, IIID, IVB, VI, VII.
Skeletal defects in all.

Hurler's Syndrome (Mucopolysaccharidosis IH)

(Most patients die by age 10 yrs.)
♦ Initial diagnosis by quantitative increase of mucopolysaccharide in urine; confirmed by assay of alpha-L-iduronidase in cultured fibroblasts or leukocytes.
Similar enzyme assay detects carriers who have ~50% activity, but the wide range and overlap between normal persons and carriers may make the diagnosis difficult in individual cases.
♦ Prenatal diagnosis by assay of enzyme or mucopolysaccharide in amniocytes.

Hunter's Syndrome (Mucopolysaccharidosis II)

(Clinically similar to Hurler's syndrome but milder and no corneal opacity)
♦ Initial diagnosis by quantitation of total glucosaminoglycans in urine and accumulation of keratan sulfate in tissues is confirmed by enzyme assay in fibroblasts.
♦ Heterozygous female carriers recognized by presence of mucopolysaccharide in fibroblasts or enzyme assay of individual hair roots.
♦ Prenatal diagnosis by enzyme assay of amniotic fluid should be confirmed by assay of cultured cells.
♦ Maternal serum shows increased activity of iduronate sulphate sulfatase with a normal or heterozygous fetus but no increase if fetus has Hunter's syndrome.
Mild and severe subtypes

Sanfilippo's Syndrome Type A (Mucopolysaccharidosis III)

(The four types of Sanfilippo's syndrome cannot be distinguished clinically)
♦ Only mucopolysaccharidosis in which finding only heparan sulfate in urine confirms diagnosis.
♦ Assay of fibroblasts shows deficiency of enzyme in patients and decrease of normal activity in carriers, who also show mucopolysaccharide accumulation.
○ Metachromatic inclusion bodies in lymphocytes are coarser and sparser than in Hurler's syndrome and may be seen in bone marrow cells. Severe cerebral changes with relatively mild changes in other body tissues.

Morquio's Syndrome (Mucopolysaccharidosis IV)

♦ Keratan sulfate is increased in urine (often 2–3× normal).
○ Metachromatic granules may be seen in PMNs.
♦ Diagnosis by enzyme assay in fibroblasts and leukocytes
♦ Prenatal diagnosis by assay of enzymes in cultured amniocytes

Maroteaux-Lamy Syndrome (Mucopolysaccharidosis VI)

○ Metachromatic cytoplasmic inclusions (Alder granules) may be seen in 50% of lymphocytes and 100% of granulocytes, and are more marked than in other mucopolysaccharidoses.
♦ Large amount of dermatan sulfate occurs in urine.
♦ Diagnosis is established by a finding of deficiency of specific enzyme in cultured fibroblasts.
♦ Enzyme assay also allows diagnosis of heterozygotes and prenatal diagnosis.

Other rare diseases due to enzyme deficiencies that resemble these conditions include I-cell disease (mucolipidosis I) and mucolipidosis III and related disorders.

Niemann-Pick Disease

(Sphingomyelin lipidosis)
♦ Diagnosis by demonstration of sphingomyelinase deficiency in cultured fibroblasts or circulating leukocytes

METAB/HERED

○Foamy histiocytes may be found in bone marrow aspiration, liver, spleen, skin, skeletal muscle, and eye and may appear in peripheral blood terminally.

Peripheral blood lymphocytes and monocytes may be vacuolated (2–20% of cells).

WBC is variable.

Rectal biopsy may show changes in ganglion cells of myenteric plexus.

Laboratory findings due to involvement of specific organs

- Anemia is due to hypersplenism or microcytic anemia associated with anisocytosis, poikilocytosis, and elliptocytosis.
- AST may be increased in serum and CSF.
- Enzyme changes in CSF are same as in Tay-Sachs disease, except that LD is normal (see p. 562).

Acid phosphatase is increased (as in Gaucher's disease; see p. 555).

LD is normal in serum and CSF.

Different isoenzyme activities result in different clinical forms.

- Acute infantile form (type A): acute progressive neuropathic loss of motor and intellectual function early in life with death common in infancy. Cherry-red macula is often present.
- Subacute/juvenile forms (types C and D): not neuropathic; later onset.
- Chronic forms (types B and E): similar to acute type but later in onset and not neuropathic.
- Types A and B show primary sphingomyelinase deficiency; type C shows defect in cholesterol esterification (autosomal recessive inheritance).

Oligosaccharidoses with Increased Urinary Oligosaccharides

Sialidosis

I-cell disease (mucolipidosis II)

Fucosidosis

Mannosidosis

Galactosialidosis

Pseudo–Hurler's polydystrophy (mucolipidosis III)

GM_1 gangliosidosis

Aspartylglucosaminuria

Tay-Sachs Disease (GM_2 Gangliosidosis)

(Autosomal recessive trait [chromosome 15] found predominantly in Ashkenazi Jews, French Canadians, and Cajuns characterized in infantile form by appearance of psychomotor deterioration, blindness, cherry-red spot in the macula, and an exaggerated extension response to sound, with death by age 4 yrs; patients with juvenile form die by age 15 yrs; chronic form in adults; macula spot occurs only in infantile form.)

♦ Diagnosis is established by absence of hexosaminidase A activity in serum (also absent in all tissues of body and tears). Accumulation of GM_2 ganglioside in brain is due to deficiency or absence of hexosaminidase A. Electron microscopy shows characteristic cytoplasmic bodies in brain. (In Sandhoff's disease, a variant of Tay-Sachs disease, both hexosaminidase A and B are defective and globoside is accumulated in other tissues as well as brain.)

♦ Heterozygotes can be identified by plasma assay showing 50% decrease in activity of hexosaminidase A; screening should be done before pregnancy, which may cause false-positive results; use of oral contraceptives, diabetes mellitus, and liver disease may also cause false-positive results; in these cases WBCs are used for hexosaminidase A assay.

♦ Prenatal diagnosis using cultured amniotic cells is superior to testing of amniotic fluid or uncultured amniotic cells; false-negative results can occur due to contamination with maternal blood or tissue or bacteria.

♦ PCR for specific DNA mutations in WBCs or fibroblasts is more specific than enzyme assay, and can detect various mutations and predict severity of disease in affected child.

Early marked increase of serum LD and AST is seen; levels return to normal if patient survives 3–4 yrs.

Decrease in serum fructose 1-phosphate aldolase; also decreased in *heterozygotes*

CSF AST parallels serum AST.
Occasional vacuolated lymphocytes are seen.
Liver function tests are normal.
Serum acid phosphatase is normal.

Other Genetic Disorders

Batten Disease (Batten-Spielmeyer-Vogt Disease)

(Autosomal recessive type of juvenile amaurotic idiocy)

♦ Azurophilic hypergranulation of leukocytes occurs in patients and in heterozygous and homozygous members of their families. In Giemsa- and Wright's-stained smears, it resembles toxic granulation but differs by the absence of supravital staining in Batten disease and by normal leukocyte ALP activity (markedly increased in toxic granulation). This granulation occurs in ≥ 15% of neutrophils.

D$_1$ Trisomy (Trisomy 13; Patau's Syndrome)

See Table 12-14.

○In peripheral blood smears, ≤ 80% of PMNs (neutrophils and eosinophils) show an increased number of anomalous nuclear projections (tags, threads, drumsticks, clubs); the nuclear lobulation may appear abnormal (nucleus may look twisted without clear separation of individual lobes, coarse lumpy chromatin, etc.). Present in almost all complete trisomic cases. Nuclear coils of chromatin by electron microscopy.

Fetal hemoglobins may persist longer than normal (i.e., be increased); these include HbF, Bart's, Gower II.

○Decreased AFP in maternal serum and amniotic fluid

Laboratory findings due to multiple congenital abnormalities (including almost pathognomonic tetrad of narrow palpebral fissures and microphthalmos, cleft palate, parieto-occipital scalp defect, polydactyly).

♦ Karyotyping shows numerical abnormality in 80% of cases: 47 XX,+13, or 47 XY,+13. Due to translocations in 20% of cases.

Down Syndrome (Trisomy 21; Mongolism)

See Table 12-14.

♦ Karyotyping shows 47 chromosomes with trisomy 21 in most patients; due to translocation, usually to chromosome 14, to other D group chromosome in <5% of cases. 2% have mosaicism with one cell population trisomic.

Increased leukocyte ALP score.

Leukocytes show decreased incidence of drumsticks (see p. 515) and mean lobe counts.
Serum acid phosphatase may be decreased.

Risk of developing acute lymphocytic or nonlymphocytic leukemia is increased (~1%). Incidence 10–20× greater than in general population.

Congenital AML occurs within several months of birth; always fatal.

Transient leukemoid reaction (WBC ≤ 400,000/cu mm) occurs only with trisomy 21; differentiated from congenital leukemia by bone marrow biopsy including cytogenetic and immunohistochemical studies. ≤ 25% of these Down syndrome infants develop acute megakaryocytic leukemia within 3 yrs.

Increased susceptibility to infection (e.g., hepatitis is common in institutionalized patients, in whom HBsAg was first noted).

Laboratory findings due to associated congenital abnormalities (e.g., GI, GU, cardiovascular systems).

Prenatal Screening and Diagnosis

See Table 12-6 and Fig. 12-2.

Optimal screening combines measurement of hCG, AFP, and unconjugated estriol levels in maternal serum in pregnant patients aged >35 yrs.

Table 12-14. Chromosome Number and Karyotype in Various Clinical Conditions

	Chromosome Number and Karyotype	Incidence
Normal male	46 XY	
Normal female	46 XX	
Suspected autosomal syndromes		
Down syndrome (mongolism; trisomy 21)	47 XX, G+, or 47 XY, G+	1 in 700 live births (2% are 46 count due to translocation and have 10% risk of Down syndrome in subsequent pregnancies; 2% are 46/47 mosaics)
Trisomy D 1	47 XX, D+, or 47 XY, D+	1 in 5000 live births
	Translocations	Rare
	Mosaics	Rare
Trisomy E 18	47 XX, E+, or 47 XY, E+	1 in 3000 live births
	Translocations	Rare
	Mosaics	Rare
Trisomy D 13		
Trisomy 8, 9, 4p, 9p		Rare
Cri du chat syndrome	46 with partial B deletion	1 in 30,000 births
Others (e.g., 4p-, 5p-, 9p-, 13q-)		
Suspected sex chromosome syndromes		
Klinefelter's syndrome	47 XXY	1 in 600 live male births
	48 XXXY	Rare
	48 XXYY	Rare
	49 XXXXY	Rare
	49 XXXYY	Rare
	Mosaics	Infrequent
Turner's syndrome	45 XO	1 in 3000 live female births
	46 XX	Rare
	Mosaics	Infrequent
"Superfemale"	47 XXX	1 in 1000–2000 live female births
	48 XXXX	Rare
	49 XXXXX	Rare
	Mosaics	Rare
"Supermale"	47 XXY	1 in 1000 live male births

Maternal Serum AFP

Interpretation

- Use of maternal serum AFP *alone* is not recommended; should be combined with measurements of hCG and unconjugated estriol when maternal age is >35 yrs; this combination can identify ~60% of cases of Down syndrome with false-positive rate of 6.6%; ultrasonography to verify gestational age (which has profound effect on calculated risk of Down syndrome) reduces false-positive rate to 3.8%.

♦ • *Decreased maternal blood level of AFP in pregnancy is a valuable screening test, but diagnosis should be confirmed by finding of increased levels in amniotic fluid and by ultrasonography* (to rule out missed abortion, molar pregnancy, absent pregnancy), as well as by chromosomal studies to confirm or refute the diagnosis. Lower AFP value makes Down syndrome more likely.
• In midtrimester, usual range is 10–150 ng/mL; is usually reported as multiple of median (MoM) (normal 0.4–2.5 MoM) to minimize interlaboratory variability and correct for patient's race, diabetes mellitus, and gestational age.

Decreased In
Down syndrome (trisomy 21) and trisomy 18
Long-standing death of fetus
Overestimation of gestational age (underestimation of age in amniotic fluid sample)
Choriocarcinoma, hydatidiform mole
Increased maternal weight (does not affect amniotic fluid concentration)
Pseudopregnancy, nonpregnancy
Various drugs (therefore no medications should be taken for at least 12 hrs before test)
Other unknown factors
Women with diabetes mellitus have values 20–40% less than those of nondiabetic women.

Increased In[14,15]
(Should confirm by increase in amniotic fluid)
Twin pregnancy (>4.5 MoM)
Gestational age (for which values must be adjusted)
Race (10–15% higher in blacks) (for which values must be adjusted)
Open neural tube defects (e.g., open spina bifida, anencephaly, encephalocele, myelocele); 80% of severe cases are detected by AFP. Occurs in 2 in 1000 births in the United States. Women with one affected child have 5% chance of giving birth to another; affected families make up 10% of these cases. Optimal screening is in 16th–20th week of gestation. Hydrocephaly. Microcephaly.
Ventral wall defects associated with exposed fetal-membrane and blood-vessel surfaces, e.g.,
• Omphalocele (incidence 1–3 in 10,000)
• Gastroschisis (incidence 1–10 in 10,000)
Hydrops fetalis
Intrauterine death
Fetal-maternal hemorrhage
Esophageal or duodenal atresia
Cystic hygroma
Renal disorders, e.g,
• Congenital proteinuric nephropathies
• Polycystic kidneys
• Renal agenesis
Aplasia cutis
Sacrococcygeal teratoma
Tetralogy of Fallot
Turner's syndrome
Oligohydramnios
Maternal causes (e.g., neoplasm that produces AFP, hepatitis)
Very rare benign hereditary familial elevation of serum AFP

Maternal hCG

(Appears in maternal serum soon after pregnancy and reaches peak by 8–11 wks of gestation, decreases to nadir at 18 wks, and then remains constant to end of pregnancy)
Use
Best *single* marker for Down syndrome screening
Increase of >2.5× MoM at 18–25 wks of gestation detects ~56% of cases. One study that detected 73% of cases had a 4% false-positive rate at that serum level.

[14]Sundaram SG, Goldstein PJ, Manimekalai S, Wenk RE. Alpha-fetoprotein and screening markers of congenital disease. *Clin Lab Med* 1992;12:481.
[15]D'Alton ME, DeCherney AH. Prenatal diagnosis. *N Engl J Med* 1993;328:114.

METAB/HERED

Diagnosis of early pregnancy (see Pregnancy Test, p. 77)
Diagnosis of germ cell tumors and monitoring of treatment effectiveness (see Chapter 14)

Maternal Serum Unconjugated Estriol

(Is of fetal origin from fetal adrenal, liver, and placental function. Begins to appear by seventh to ninth week of gestation.)
Decreased In
Fetal Down syndrome
Low values at 35–36 wks of gestation identify up to one-third of "light for dates" infants.
Interpretation
Value >12 ng/mL rules out postmaturity in cases of prolonged gestation if no other diseases are present (e.g., diabetes mellitus, isoimmunization).
Decreased value detects 45% of cases with a 5.2% false-positive rate.
≤0.6 MoM in 5% of unaffected pregnancies and 26% of Down syndrome cases.
Safe levels indicate fetal well-being.
Increasing serial values rule out prolonged pregnancy and postmaturity.
Constant normal values are consistent with 40–41 wks of gestation.
Declining values are consistent with prolonged gestation.
Low or significantly falling values are seen in fetal distress and postmaturity.

Amniotic Fluid Estriol

Interpretation
Values are not meaningful before 20 wks' gestation (<1.0 μg/dL); gradual increase to 35th week and then rapid increase to 40th week. Each laboratory must establish its own reference ranges.
Decreasing levels are associated with fetal distress, and failure to increase with fetal death.

Human Placental Lactogen

Appears by fifth week of gestation and increases progressively thereafter.
Values correlate better with placental than with fetal weight. Therefore useful to evaluate placental function; sudden decrease in concentration before fetal death. *Use only as adjunct to other tests.*
Useful In
Diabetes mellitus, severe
Hypertension
Postmaturity syndrome
Idiopathic placental failure
Not Useful In
Diabetes mellitus, mild or moderately severe
Rh sensitization disease

Maternal Serum PSA

Recent report of ultrasensitive assay of PSA suggests that second trimester amniotic fluid concentrations are low (normally increases between gestational weeks 11 and 21) and are increased in maternal serum in Down syndrome cases.[16]

Chromosomal Analysis of Amniotic Fluid

Detects ~20% of cases because 80% of Down syndrome infants are born to women <35 yrs old.

Dysautonomia, Familial (Riley-Day Syndrome)

(Autosomal recessive disorder occurring in Ashkenazi Jews; patients show difficulty in swallowing, corneal ulcerations, insensitivity to pain, motor incoordination, excessive sweating, diminished gag reflex, lack of tongue papillae, progressive kyphoscoliosis, pulmonary infections, etc.)

---

[16]Lambert-Messerlian GM, et al. Increased concentrations of prostate-specific antigen in maternal serum from pregnancies affected by fetal Down syndrome. *Clin Chem* 1998;44:205.

Urine VMA (3-methoxy-4-hydroxymandelic acid) may be low, and HVA increased.
Urine VMA may be lower in asymptomatic carriers than in healthy adults.

Fragile X Syndrome of Mental Retardation[17]

(Most common form of inherited mental retardation; due to mutations that increase the size of a specific DNA fragment of the X chromosome [in Xq27.3])
♦ Direct diagnosis by DNA analysis using Southern blot test but PCR is often done simultaneously. Can also be used to establish prenatal diagnosis and to detect asymptomatic carriers. Can distinguish between full mutation, in which 100% of males and ~50% of females are mentally impaired, and premutation, in which only ~3% are impaired.

Mediterranean Fever, Familial (Familial Paroxysmal Peritonitis; "Periodic Disease")

(Autosomal recessive disorder characterized by recurrent polyserositis occurring predominantly in Sephardic Jews, Arabs, and Armenians)
WBC is increased (10,000–20,000/cu mm); eosinophils may be increased during an attack but a return to normal between attacks. ESR is increased during an attack but normal between attacks.
Mild normocytic normochromic anemia is occasionally seen.
Serum glycoprotein is increased in patients and their relatives.
Increased alpha$_2$ globulin and fibrinogen are common.
Amyloid nephropathy that is usually fatal develops in 10–40% of patients; it is not related to frequency or severity of clinical attacks.
♦ PCR amplification of DNA identifies one of three common mutations.

Trisomy 18

(Usually sporadic; due to nondisjunction; associated with increased maternal age)
♦ Decreased AFP, hCG, and unconjugated estriol in maternal serum.
Laboratory findings due to congenital abnormalities (e.g., cardiovascular, GU, GI systems).

METAB/HERED

---

[17]Rousseau F, et al. Direct diagnosis by DNA analysis of the fragile X syndrome of mental retardation. *N Engl J Med* 1991;325:1673.

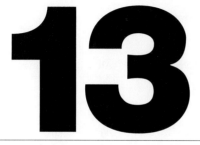

Endocrine Diseases

General Principles in Diagnosis of Endocrine Diseases

Perform stimulatory tests if hypofunction is suspected and suppression tests if hyperfunction is suspected.

Suppression tests suppress normal glands but not autonomous secretion (e.g., functioning neoplasm).

Obtaining multiple or pooled samples of baseline specimens and drawing specimens from indwelling lines are often required to obtain optimal specimens.

Patient preparation is particularly important for hormone studies, the results of which may be markedly affected by many factors such as stress, position, fasting state, time of day, preceding diet, and drug therapy; all of these should be recorded on the laboratory test requisition form and discussed with the laboratory before test ordering.

Appropriate (e.g., frozen) and timely transportation to laboratory and preparation of specimen (e.g., separation of serum may be vital for some tests) are important.

No single test adequately reflects the endocrine status in all conditions.

Tests of Thyroid Function

Thyroid function tests are not indicated for *screening* programs without suspicion of thyroid disease (overall yield ~0.5%; varies from 0% in young men to 1% in women aged >40 yrs). Indicated in certain populations such as newborns (mandatory), those with strong family history of thyroid disease, elderly, women 4–8 wks postpartum, patients with autoimmune diseases (e.g., Addison's disease, type I diabetes mellitus). May be useful in some women aged >40 yrs with nonspecific complaints.

Sensitive TSH complemented by free thyroxine index (FTI) are recommended tests for diagnosis and follow-up of most patients with thyroid disorders (Table 13-1).

Calcitonin

Use

Basal fasting level may be increased in patients with medullary carcinoma of the thyroid even when no mass is palpable in the thyroid. Circadian rhythm with rise to peak after lunchtime. Basal level is normal in approximately one-third of medullary carcinoma cases.

Basal calcitonin levels
- Levels >2000 pg/mL are almost always associated with medullary carcinoma of thyroid, with rare cases due to obvious renal failure or ectopic production of calcitonin.
- Levels of 500–2000 pg/mL generally indicate medullary carcinoma, renal failure, or ectopic production of calcitonin.
- Levels of 100–500 pg/mL should be interpreted cautiously with repeat assays and provocative tests; if these and repeat tests in 1–2 mos are still abnormal, some authors recommend total thyroidectomy.
- Normal basal levels: Males ≤ 19 pg/mL; females ≤ 14 pg/mL.

Calcium infusion and/or pentagastrin injection are used as provocative tests in patients with normal basal levels for whom the index of suspicion is high, e.g., those with a

Table 13-1. Sensitivity and Specificity of Thyroid Function Tests

Patients	Sensitivity			Specificity	
	All	Hyperthyroid	Hypothyroid	All	Nonthyroid Illness
T_4	76	89	61	90	83
Free T_4	82	96	65	94	94
T_3	80	85	74	87	72
Free T_3	73	93	48	90	80
TSH	89–95	86–95	92–94	92–95	85–90

T_3 = triiodothyronine; T_4 = thyroxine; TSH = thyroid-stimulating hormone.
Source: de los Santos ET, Starich GH, Mazzaferri EL. Sensitivity, specificity and cost-effectiveness of the sensitive thyrotropin assay in the diagnosis of thyroid diseases in ambulatory patients. *Arch Intern Med* 1989;149:526.

family history of thyroid carcinoma, a calcified thyroid mass, pheochromocytoma, hyperparathyroidism, hypercalcemia, amyloid-containing metastatic carcinoma of unknown origin, or facial characteristics of the mucosal neuroma syndrome. Normally level should not rise above 0.2 ng/mL. Pentagastrin stimulation is more sensitive than calcium stimulation.

To detect recurrence of medullary carcinoma or metastases after the primary tumor has been removed or to confirm complete removal of the tumor if basal calcitonin has been previously increased.

Increased in Some Patients with

Carcinoma of lung, breast, islet cell, or ovary, and carcinoid due to ectopic production
Hypercalcemia of any cause stimulating calcitonin production
Z-E syndrome
PA
Acute or chronic thyroiditis
Chronic renal failure

Perchlorate Washout Test

Perchlorate is given 2–4 hrs after administration of ^{131}I and RAIU is calculated before and at intervals after perchlorate administration.

Use

Decreased uptake >10% from peak value is positive test indicating an organification defect as the cause of hypothyroidism. Free iodide is present within the thyroid in such patients. Perchlorate blocks the trapping mechanism, causing rapid discharge of iodine so that RAIU within the thyroid diminishes. Normal thyroid gland contains very little inorganic iodine.

Reverse Triiodothyronine (rT₃)

(Hormonally inactive isomer of T₃)

Use

Largely replaced by newer tests
Usually increased in hyperthyroidism and increased serum TBG; often decreased in hypothyroidism but overlaps with normal range.
Has been suggested to distinguish "sick thyroid" patients who are euthyroid (usually normal in euthyroid patients) from true hypothyroid cases, but serum TSH may be more reliable.

Table 13-2. Free Thyroxine (T_4) and Thyroid-Stimulating Hormone (TSH) Levels in Various Conditions

		Sensitive TSH		
		Normal	Low	High
T_4	Normal	Euthyroid	Subclinical/early hyperthyroidism[a] Nonthyroidal illness Drug effects L-dopa Glucocorticoids Excess T_4 therapy for hypothyroidism	Subclinical/early hypothyroidism Nonthyroidal illness Drug effects Iodine, lithium, antithyroid drugs, amiodarone Insufficient T_4 therapy for hypothyroidism
	Low	Secondary hypothyroidism[b] Nonthyroidal illness Drug effects T_3 Phenytoin Androgens Salicylates Carbamazepine Rifampin	Secondary hypothyroidism[b] Drug effects Dopamine[c] Corticosteroids[c] T_3	Primary hypothyroidism Drug effects, e.g., iodine, lithium, antithyroid drugs, amiodarone Insufficient T_4 therapy for hypothyroidism
	High	Nonthyroidal illness Acute and psychiatric illness Abnormal binding (excess TBG, familial dysalbuminemic hyperthyroxinemia, transthyretin-associated hyperthyroxinemia, some monoclonal proteins) Thyroid hormone resistance Drug effects Estrogen Iodine (drugs, contrast media) Thyroxine (factitious)	Nonthyroidal illness Acute psychiatric illness Primary hyperthyroidism[d]	TSH-secreting tumor Thyroid hormone resistance

T_3 = triiodothyronine; T_4 = thyroxine.
[a]Confirm with T_3 suppression test or lack of serum TSH response to TRH.
[b]Pituitary TSH deficiency shows deficient response to exogenous TRH. Hypothalamic TRH deficiency shows normal TSH response but may be prolonged for >30 mins.
[c]Serial monitoring or testing of serum TSH response to TRH may be needed.
[d]95% of cases; serum T_3 needed for diagnosis of T_3 thyrotoxicosis.

Thyroid-Stimulating Hormone Sensitive (Thyrotropin; TSH)

(Hormone secreted by anterior pituitary; third- and fourth-generation assay detection limits are 0.01 mU/L and 0.001 mU/L, respectively)
See Tables 13-2 and 13-3, and Fig. 13-1.
Euthyroid: 0.3–5.0 mU/L

Possible hypothyroid: >5.0 mU/L
Possible hyperthyroid: <0.10 mU/L
Borderline: 0.10–0.29 mU/L

Use

Screening for euthyroidism—normal level in stable ambulatory patient not on interfering drugs excludes thyroid hormone excess or deficiency. Has been recommended as the initial test of thyroid function rather than T_4.

Screening is not recommended for asymptomatic persons without suspicion of thyroid disease or for hospital patients with acute medical or psychiatric illness.

Initial screening and diagnosis for hyperthyroidism (decreased to undetectable levels except in rare TSH-secreting pituitary adenoma) and hypothyroidism

Table 13-3. Thyroid Function Tests in Various Conditions

Condition	TSH	TT_4	FT_4	T_3	Tg	RAIU	Comment
Hypothyroidism							
Primary							
Clinical	I	D	D	D	N/I	D	Increased response to TRH administration
Subclinical	I	N	N	N	N	NA	
Secondary	N/D	D	D	D			No response to TRH administration
Tertiary	N/D	D	D	D			
Nonthyroidal* illness	V	N/D	N/D	D	D		
Hyperthyroidism							
Primary							
Clinical	D	I	I	I	N	I	
Subclinical	D	N	N	N	N	NA	
T_3 thyrotoxicosis	D	N	N	I	N	NA	
TSH-secreting tumor	I	I	I	I	N	NA	
TRH-secreting tumor	I	I	I	I	N	NA	
Factitious							
T_4 ingestion	D	I	I	I	D/N	D	Augmented RAIU response to TSH administration
T_3 ingestion	D	N	N	I	D/N		
Pregnancy	N	I	N	I	I	X	
With hyperthyroidism	N	I	I	I	I	X	
With hypothyroidism	I	I	D	I	I	X	I T_4 and T_3 to normal range
Hereditary increased TBG				I			
Hereditary decreased TBG	N	D	N	D			
Hashimoto's thyroiditis	V	V	V	V		V	Thyroid antibodies; biopsy
Goiter	N	N	N	N	N	A	Biopsy
Thyroid carcinoma	N	N	N	N	I	N	Serum calcitonin I in medullary CA; Tg I in differentiated

(continued)

Table 13-3. (continued)

Condition	TSH	TT$_4$	FT$_4$	T$_3$	Tg	RAIU	Comment
Nephrosis	N	D	D		D	VI	
Drug effects							
Thyroxine	D	I					
Inorganic iodine	I						
Radiopaque contrast media		I	I				
Estrogen; birth control pills		I	N		I		
Testosterone	N	D	N	D	D		D TBH
ACTH and cortico-steroids	N	D	N	D	D		D TBH
Dilantin	VI	D	N	N	D		Tissue resistance to T$_4$
Pituitary only	I	I	I				T$_4$ administration does not suppress TSH
Generalized tissue	VI	VI	VI				

0 = absent; A = abnormal; D = decreased; I = increased; N = normal; NA = not useful; TT$_4$ = total thyroxine; V = variable; VD = variable decrease; VI = variable increase; X = contraindicated.
Underlined test indicates most useful diagnostic change.
*Forms of nonthyroidal illness (euthyroid sick syndrome).

Second-generation or rate assay is required to determine TSH <0.10 mU/L.
Especially useful in early or subclinical hypothyroidism before the patient develops clinical findings, goiter, or abnormalities of other thyroid tests
Differentiation of primary (increased levels) from central (pituitary or hypothalamic) hypothyroidism (decreased levels)
Monitor adequate thyroid hormone replacement therapy in primary hypothyroidism, although T$_4$ may be mildly increased; up to 6–8 wks before TSH becomes normal. Serum TSH suppressed to normal level is the best monitor of dosage of thyroid hormone for treatment of hypothyroidism.
Monitor adequate thyroid hormone therapy to suppress thyroid carcinoma (should suppress to <0.1 mU/L) or goiter or nodules (should suppress to subnormal levels). Third- or fourth-generation assays are required to allow closer titration to balance inhibition of functioning tumor against induced hyperthyroidism.
Help differentiate euthyroid sick syndrome from primary hypothyroid patients. Sensitive TSH is only very slightly depressed in euthyroid sick patients but usually significantly depressed in true thyroid disorder.
Replace TRH stimulation test in hyperthyroidism because most patients with euthyroid TSH level have a normal TSH response and patients with undetectable TSH level almost never respond to TRH stimulation
In very early cases with only marginal elevation, the TRH stimulation test may be preferred.

May Not Be Useful

As a single test to evaluate thyroid status of hospitalized or severely ill patients
To monitor efficacy of thyroid ablation therapy for hyperthyroidism because TSH remains suppressed until T$_4$ declines significantly; T$_4$ or free T$_4$ is test of choice.

Interferences

Dopamine or high doses of glucocorticoids may cause false-normal values in primary hypothyroidism and may suppress TSH in nonthyroid illness.
Presence of RF, human antimouse antibodies, and thyroid hormone autoantibodies may produce spurious results, especially in patients with autoimmune disorders (≤ 10%).

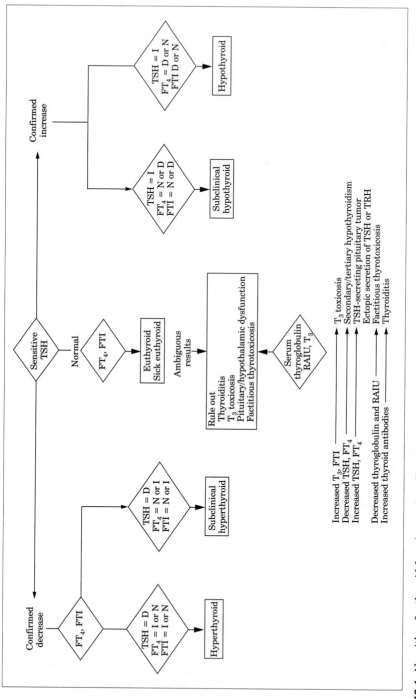

Fig. 13-1. Algorithm for thyroid function testing. (D = decreased; I = increased; N = normal.)

Increased In

Primary untreated hypothyroidism. Increase is proportionate to the degree of hypofunction, varying from 3× normal in mild cases to 100× normal in severe myxedema.
A single determination is usually sufficient to establish the diagnosis.

Patients with hypothyroidism receiving insufficient thyroid hormone replacement therapy

Patients with Hashimoto's thyroiditis, including those with clinical hypothyroidism and
about one-third of those patients who are clinically euthyroid

Use of various drugs (e.g., amphetamine abuse)
- Iodine containing drugs (e.g., iopanoic acid, ipodate, amiodarone)
- Dopamine antagonists (e.g., metoclopramide, domperidone, chlorpromazine,
haloperidol)

Other conditions (test is not clinically useful)
- Iodide-deficiency goiter
- Iodide-induced goiter or lithium treatment
- External neck irradiation
- Post–subtotal thyroidectomy
- Neonatal period

Thyrotoxicosis due to pituitary thyrotroph adenoma or pituitary resistance to thyroid
hormone

Euthyroid sick syndrome, recovery phase

TSH antibodies

Increased in first 2–3 days of life due to postnatal TSH surge

Decreased In

Hyperthyroidism due to
- Toxic multinodular goiter
- Autonomously functioning thyroid adenoma
- Ophthalmopathy of euthyroid Graves' disease
- Treated Graves' disease
- Thyroiditis
- Extrathyroidal thyroid hormone source
- Factitious

Overreplacement of thyroid hormone in treatment of hypothyroidism

Secondary pituitary or hypothalamic hypothyroidism

Euthyroid sick patients

Acute psychiatric illness

Severe dehydration

Drug effect, especially large doses—use free T_4 for evaluation
- Glucocorticoids, dopamine, dopamine agonists (bromocriptine), levodopa, T_4
replacement therapy, apomorphine, pyridoxine; T_4 may be normal or low.
- Antithyroid drug for thyrotoxicosis, especially early in treatment; T_4 may be nor-
mal or low.
- Assay interference, e.g., antibodies to mouse IgG, autoimmune disease.

First trimester of pregnancy

May Be Normal In

Central hypothyroidism

Recent rapid correction of hyperthyroidism or hypothyroidism

Pregnancy

Phenytoin therapy

*In absence of hypothalamic or pituitary disease, normal TSH excludes primary hypothy-
roidism.*

Thyroglobulin (Tg)

**(Cannot compare thyroglobulin values using different assays or assays from dif-
ferent laboratories)**

See Table 13-3.

Use

To assess the presence and possibly the extent of residual, recurrent, or metastatic follicular or papillary thyroid carcinoma after therapy. In patients with these carcinomas treated with total thyroidectomy or radioactive iodine and taking thyroid hormone therapy, Tg is undetectable if functional tumor is absent but detected by sensitive immunoassay if functional tumor is present. Tg correlates with tumor mass, with highest values in patients with metastases to bones and lungs.

Diagnosis of factitious hyperthyroidism. Tg is very low or not detectable in factitious hyperthyroidism and high in all other types of hyperthyroidism (e.g., thyroiditis).

Not recommended for initial diagnosis of thyroid carcinomas.

Do not use in patients with preexisting thyroid disorders.

Predict outcome of therapy for hyperthyroidism; higher remission rates in patients with lower Tg values. Failure to become normal after drug-induced remission suggests relapse after drugs are discontinued.

Diagnosis of thyroid agenesis in newborn

Presence in pleural effusions indicates metastatic differentiated thyroid cancer.

Interferences

Thyroglobulin autoantibodies interferes with the test; patients' serum must always first be screened for these antibodies.

Increased In

Most patients with differentiated thyroid carcinoma but not those with undifferentiated or medullary thyroid carcinomas

Patients with hyperthyroidism; rapid decline after surgical treatment. Gradual decline after radioactive iodine treatment.

Patients with subacute thyroiditis

Some patients with nontoxic nodular goiter

Patients with marked liver insufficiency

Decreased In

Thyroid agenesis in newborn

Thyroid Autoantibody Tests

(Antimicrosomal [also called thyroid peroxidase] and antithyroglobulin autoantibodies)

Use

Positive in almost all cases of Hashimoto's disease and ~80% of Graves' disease. Very high titer is pathognomonic of Hashimoto's thyroiditis but absence does not exclude Hashimoto's thyroiditis. Titer>1 to 1000 occurs virtually only in Graves' disease or Hashimoto's thyroiditis. Significant titer of microsome antibodies indicates Hashimoto's thyroiditis or postpartum thyroid dysfunction.

To distinguish subacute thyroiditis from Hashimoto's thyroiditis, as antibodies are more common in the latter

Hashimoto's thyroiditis is very unlikely cause of hypothyroidism in the absence of microsomal and Tg antibodies.

Significant titer of microsomal and Tg antibodies in euthyroid patient with unilateral exophthalmos suggests the diagnosis of euthyroid Graves' disease.

Occasionally useful to distinguish Graves' disease from toxic multinodular goiter when physical findings are not diagnostic.

Graves' disease with elevated titers of antimicrosomal antibodies should direct surgeon to perform a more limited thyroidectomy to avoid late postthyroidectomy hypothyroidism.

Results of Tg antibody test are less frequently positive than those of microsomal antibody test in autoimmune thyroid disease.

Tg antibodies may interfere with assay for serum Tg.

Thyroid receptor antibody test mainly used in Graves' disease, especially as a predictor of relapse of hyperthyroidism.

Increased In

Occasionally positive in papillary-follicular carcinoma of thyroid, subacute thyroiditis (briefly), lymphocytic (painless) thyroiditis (in ~60% of patients).
Primary thyroid lymphoma often yields very high titers; should suggest need for biopsy in elderly patient with a firm, enlarging thyroid.
Positive in 7% of normal population, reaching peak of 15% in females in sixth decade
Other autoimmune diseases (e.g., PA, RA, SLE, myasthenia gravis)

Thyroid Uptake of Radioactive Iodine (RAIU)

See Table 13-3.
A tracer dose of ^{131}I or ^{123}I is administered orally, and the radioactivity over the thyroid is measured at specific time intervals (e.g., 2–6 hrs and again at 24 hrs). The percentage of administered iodine in the thyroid is an index of thyroid trapping and organification of iodide.
Normal uptake is 9–19% in 1 hr; 7–25% in 6 hrs; 5–30% in 24 hrs. Varies with local iodine intake. 40–70% of administered dose is excreted in urine in 24 hrs. Technetium 99 (^{99}Tc) is a measure of thyroid trapping only.

Use

Detect hyperthyroidism associated with low RAIU, e.g., factitious hyperthyroidism, subacute thyroiditis, struma ovarii
Evaluate use of radioactive iodine therapy
Determine presence of an organification defect in thyroid hormone production
T_3 suppression test. Administration of T_3 causes less suppression of RAIU in the hyperthyroid patient than in the normal person; has been replaced by the TRH stimulation test.

Contraindications: pregnancy, lactation, childhood.

Interferences

Not valid for 2–4 wks after administration of antithyroid drugs, thyroid hormone, or iodides; the effect of organic iodine (e.g., radiographic contrast media) may persist for a much longer time.
Because of widespread dietary use of iodine in the United States, RAIU should not be used to evaluate euthyroid state.
Increased by
• Withdrawal rebound (thyroid hormones, propylthiouracil)
• Increased iodine excretion (e.g., diuretic use, nephrotic syndrome, chronic diarrhea)
• Decreased iodine intake (salt restriction, iodine deficiency)

Increased (>12%) In

Graves' disease (diffuse toxic goiter)
Plummer's disease (toxic multinodular goiter)
Toxic adenoma (uninodular goiter)
Thyroiditis (early Hashimoto's disease; recovery stage of subacute thyroiditis)
TSH excess
• TSH administration
• TSH production by pituitary tumor (TSH >4 μU/mL) or other neoplasm
• Defective thyroid hormone synthesis
Thyrotropin-producing neoplasms (e.g., choriocarcinoma, hydatidiform mole, embryonal carcinoma of testis)

Decreased (<3%) In

Hypothyroidism (tertiary, secondary, late primary)
Thyroiditis (late Hashimoto's; active stage of subacute thyroiditis; RAIU does not usually respond to TSH administration)

ENDOCRINE

Thyroid hormone administration (T_3 or T_4)
- Therapeutic
- Factitious (RAIU is augmented after TSH administration)*

Antithyroid medication
Iodine-induced hyperthyroidism (Jod-Basedow)[†‡]
- Radiographic contrast media, iodine-containing drugs, iodized salt

Graves' disease with iodine excess
Ectopic hypersecreting thyroid tissue
Metastatic functioning thyroid carcinoma*
Struma ovarii*
Use of certain drugs (e.g., calcitonin, thyroglobulin, corticosteroids, dopamine)

*TSH injection causes increase of ≥ 50% of RAIU in normal persons.
[†]TSH injection does not cause a normal increase of ≥ 50% of RAIU.
[‡]Urinary iodine >2000 μg/24 hrs.

Thyroxine (T_4), Free (FT_4)

See Table 13-3.

Use

Gives corrected values in patients in whom total T_4 is altered because of changes in serum proteins or in binding sites, e.g.,
- Pregnancy
- Drug use (e.g., androgens, estrogens, birth control pills, phenytoin [Dilantin])
- Altered levels of serum proteins (e.g., nephrosis)

Monitoring restoration to normal range is only laboratory criterion to estimate appropriate replacement dose of levothyroxine because 6–8 wks are required before TSH reflects these changes.

Increased In

Hyperthyroidism
Hypothyroidism treated with T_4
Euthyroid sick syndrome
Occasional patients with hydatidiform mole or choriocarcinoma with marked hCG elevations may show increased FT_4, suppressed TSH, and blunted TSH response to TRH stimulation. Values return to normal with effective treatment of trophoblastic disease. Severe dehydration (may be >6.0 ng/dL).

Decreased In

Hypothyroidism
Hypothyroidism treated with T_3
Euthyroid sick syndrome

Thyroxine, Total (T_4)

See Tables 13-2 and 13-3, and Fig. 13-1.

Use

Diagnosis of hyperthyroidism

Increased In

Hyperthyroidism
Pregnancy
Drug effects (e.g., estrogens, birth control pills, d-thyroxine, thyroid extract, TSH, amiodarone, heroin, methadone, amphetamines, some radiopaque substances for radiographic studies [ipodate, iopanoic acid])
Euthyroid sick syndrome
Increase in TBG or abnormal T_4-binding prealbumin

Table 13-4. Free Thyroxine Index in Various Conditions

Condition	T_3	T_4	Free Thyroxine Index (T_7) (T_3 Uptake $\times$ T_4)
Normal			
Range	24–36	4–11	96–396
Mean	31	7	217
Hypothyroid	22	3	66
Hyperthyroid	38	12	456
Pregnancy, estrogen use (especially birth control pills)	20	12	240*

*Normal even though T_3 and T_4 alone are abnormal.

- Familial dysalbuminemic hyperthyroxinemia—albumin binds T_4 but not T_3 more avidly than normal, causing changes similar to thyrotoxicosis (total T_4 ~20 μg/dL, normal thyroid-hormone-binding ratio, increased FTI) but patient is not clinically thyrotoxic.
- Serum T_4 >20 μg/dL usually indicates true hyperthyroidism rather than increased TBG.
- May be found in euthyroid patients with increased serum TBG.
- Much higher in first 2 mos of life than in normal adults.

Decreased In

Hypothyroidism
Hypoproteinemia (e.g., nephrosis, cirrhosis)
Use of certain drugs (phenytoin, T_3, testosterone, ACTH, corticosteroids)
Euthyroid sick syndrome
Decrease in TBG

Normal Levels May Be Found in Hyperthyroid Patients with

T_3 thyrotoxicosis
Factitious hyperthyroidism due to T_3 (Cytomel)
Decreased binding capacity due to hypoproteinemia or ingestion of certain drugs (e.g., phenytoin, salicylates)

Interferences

Various drugs

Not Affected by

Mercurial diuretics
Nonthyroidal iodine

Thyroxine Index, Free (FTI; T_7)

American Thyroid Association now recommends the term *thyroid hormone–binding ratios* (THBR).
See Table 13-4.

Use

This index is the calculated product of T_3 resin uptake and serum total T_4. It permits correction of misleading results of T_3 and T_4 determinations caused by conditions that alter the T_4-binding protein concentration (e.g., pregnancy, use of estrogens or birth control pills).

ENDOCRINE

Thyroxine-Binding Globulin (TBG)

Use

Diagnosis of genetic or idiopathic excess TBG

Sometimes used for detection of recurrent or metastatic differentiated thyroid carcinoma, especially follicular type and cases in which patient has had an increased level due to carcinoma.

Differentiation of increased/decreased total T_3 or T_4 concentrations due to changes in TBG from normal free T_3 or T_4. Same purpose as T_3 resin uptake and FTI (see above).

Increased In

Pregnancy

Use of certain drugs (e.g., estrogens, birth control pills, perphenazine [Trilafon], clofibrate, heroin, methadone)

Estrogen-producing tumors

Acute intermittent porphyria

Acute or chronic active hepatitis

Lymphocytic painless subacute thyroiditis

Neonates

Decreased In

Nephrosis and other causes of marked hypoproteinemia such as liver disease, severe illness, stress (T_4-binding-prealbumin also decreased)

Deficiency of TBG, genetic or idiopathic

Acromegaly (T_4-binding-prealbumin also decreased)

Severe acidosis

Use of certain drugs
- Androgens, anabolic steroids
- Glucocorticoids (T_4-binding-prealbumin is increased)

Testosterone-producing tumors

Decreased Binding of T_3 and T_4 Due to Drugs

Salicylates

Phenytoin

Tolbutamide (Orinase), chlorpropamide (Diabinese)

Penicillin, heparin, barbital

An increased TBG is associated with increased serum T_4 and decreased T_3 resin uptake; a converse association exists for decreased TBG.

Thyrotropin-Releasing Hormone (TRH) Stimulation Test[1]

See Fig. 13-2.

Serum TSH is measured before and 20 mins after IV administration of TRH (usually 500 or 200 μg).

Normal response: a significant rise from a basal level of ~1 μU/mL by 8 μU/mL at 20 mins and return to normal by 120 mins. Response is usually greater in women than in men.

Primary hypothyroidism: an exaggerated rise of an already increased TSH level

Secondary (pituitary) hypothyroidism: no rise in the decreased TSH level

Hypothalamic hypothyroidism: low serum T_3 and T_4 and TSH levels, with a TRH response that may be exaggerated or normal or (most characteristically) with a peak delay of 45–60 mins.

Hyperthyroidism: TRH administration does not cause a significant rise in serum TSH in hyperthyroid patients as it does in normal persons; a normal rise (>2 μU/mL) virtually excludes hyperthyroidism. Absent response may also occur in exophthalmic Graves' disease and nodular goiter.

[1]Kolesnick RN, Gershengorn MC. Thyrotropin-releasing hormone and the pituitary. *Am J Med* 1985;79:729.

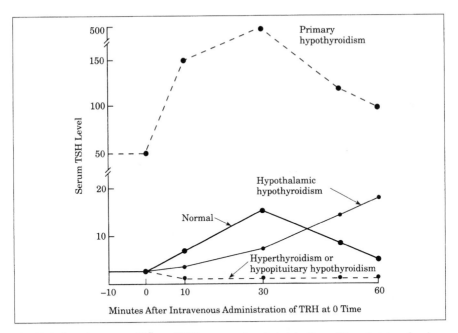

Fig. 13-2. Sample curves of serum TSH response to administration of thyrotropin-releasing hormone (TRH) in various conditions.

Blunted response may occur in uremia, Cushing's syndrome, acromegaly, effect of certain drugs (corticosteroids, levodopa, large amounts of salicylates).

Response may also be suppressed in nonthyroidal conditions (e.g., starvation, renal failure, elevated levels of glucocorticoids, depression, some elderly patients).

The TSH response to TRH is modified by T_4 antithyroid drugs, corticosteroids, estrogens, and levodopa. Response is increased during pregnancy.

Use

Interpretation must be based on clinical studies that exclude the pituitary gland as the site of the disease.

Now largely replaced by TSH.

Confirmation of hyperthyroidism when other test results are equivocal. Lack of response shows adequate therapy in patients receiving thyroid hormones to shrink thyroid nodules and goiters and during long-term treatment of thyroid carcinoma.

Differentiation of two forms (whether or not due to tumor) of thyrotropin-induced hyperthyroidism

May be particularly useful in T_3 toxicosis cases in which the other tests are normal or in patients clinically suspected of hyperthyroidism with borderline serum T_3 levels. TRH stimulation test is superior to the T_3 suppression test of RAIU. Abnormal TSH response to TRH administration does not definitely establish the diagnosis of hyperthyroidism (because autonomous production of normal or slightly increased amounts of thyroid hormones causes pituitary suppression). TRH test may remain abnormal even after successful therapy of Graves' disease.

Hyperthyroid patients in whom associated nonthyroid conditions result in only slight elevation of serum T_4 and T_3

Euthyroid Graves' disease patients presenting with only exophthalmos (unilateral or bilateral). *TRH stimulation test may sometimes be normal in these patients, and T_3 suppression test may be required.*

Elderly patients with or without symptoms of hyperthyroidism may have serum T_4 and T_3 in upper normal range.

Euthyroid sick syndrome (see p. 583). Generally serum TSH is normal with a relatively normal TSH response to TRH.

May help differentiate hypothalamic from pituitary hypothyroidism (see previous section)

	Baseline TSH (μU/mL)	Change in TSH 30 Mins after TRH Administration (μU/mL)
Euthyroidism	<10	>2 (95% of cases)
Hyperthyroidism	<10	<2
Primary hypothyroidism	>10	>2 (exaggerated)
Secondary hypothyroidism	<10	<2
Tertiary hypothyroidism	<10	>2 (delayed or exaggerated or normal)

Triiodothyronine (T$_3$)

See Table 13-3 and Fig. 13-1.

Use

Diagnosing T$_3$ thyrotoxicosis (TSH is suppressed but T$_4$ is normal) or cases in which FT$_4$ is normal in presence of symptoms of hyperthyroidism

Evaluating cases in which FT$_4$ is borderline elevated

Evaluating cases in which overlooking diagnosis of hyperthyroidism is very undesirable (e.g., unexplained atrial fibrillation)

Monitoring the course of hyperthyroidism

Monitoring T$_4$ replacement therapy—is better than T$_4$ or FT$_4$ but TSH is preferred to both.

Predicting outcome of antithyroid drug therapy in patients with Graves' disease

Evaluating amiodarone-induced thyrotoxicosis

Serum T$_3$ parallels FT$_4$; is early indicator of hyperthyroidism but TSH is better.

Good biochemical indicator of severity of thyrotoxicity in hyperthyroidism

Not recommended for diagnosis of hypothyroidism; decreased values have minimal clinical significance.

May decrease by ≤ 25% in healthy older persons, whereas FT$_4$ remains normal.

Free T$_3$ gives corrected values in patients in whom the total T$_3$ is altered because of changes in serum proteins or in binding sites, e.g.,

- Pregnancy
- Drugs (e.g., androgens, estrogens, birth control pills, phenytoin)
- Altered levels of serum proteins (e.g., nephrosis)

Triiodothyronine (T$_3$) Resin Uptake

See Table 13-4.

Use

Measures unoccupied binding sites on TBG. Is not a measure of T$_3$.

Only with simultaneous measurement of serum T$_4$ to calculate T$_7$ to exclude the possibility that an increased T$_4$ is due to an increase in T$_4$-binding globulin. *Measurement of serum T$_3$ concentration should be done by RIA for diagnosis of hyperthyroidism.*

Increased In

See causes of *decreased* serum TBG, p. 580.

Decreased In

See causes of *increased* serum TBG, p. 580.

Normal In

Pregnancy with hyperthyroidism
Nontoxic goiter
Carcinoma of thyroid

Diabetes mellitus
Addison's disease
Anxiety
Use of certain drugs (e.g., mercurials, iodine)

Variable In

Liver disease

Diseases of the Thyroid

See Table 13-3.

Carcinoma of Thyroid

Medullary carcinoma
  • Sporadic (noninherited) accounts for 80% of cases
  • Familial accounts for 20% of cases
      MEN type I (see p. 697).
      Most are MEN type II (see p. 697).
      Familial non-MEN.
♦ Basal serum calcitonin may be increased in patients with medullary carcinoma of the
  thyroid.
♦ Serum Tg levels are increased in most patients with differentiated thyroid carcinoma
  but not in undifferentiated or medullary carcinoma. May not be increased with small
  occult differentiated carcinoma. May be useful to detect presence and possibly extent
  of residual, recurrent, or metastatic differentiated carcinoma. *Increased levels may
  be found in patients with nontoxic nodular goiter; presence of autoantibodies interferes with the test.*
Serum CEA may be increased in medullary carcinoma and may correlate with tumor
  size or extent of disease.
Serum LD, CEA, and Tg may be increased in advanced follicular carcinoma.
Serum T_3, T_4, and TSH are almost always normal in untreated patients. Rarely, evidence of hyperthyroidism may be found with large masses of follicular carcinoma.
Laboratory findings due to associated lesions (e.g., pheochromocytoma and parathyroid
  tumors) (*10–20% of cases of medullary carcinoma of thyroid occur as part of MEN*
  [see p. 697]) and due to production of additional substances (e.g., ACTH, serotonin,
  histaminase) by medullary carcinoma
RAIU is almost always normal.
Radioactive scan of thyroid
♦ Needle biopsy of thyroid nodule

Euthyroid Sick Syndrome (Nonthyroidal Illness)

**(Wide variety of nonthyroidal acute and chronic conditions such as infection, liver
  disease, cancer, starvation, renal failure, heart failure, severe burns, trauma, and
  surgery may be associated with abnormal thyroid function tests in euthyroid
  patients, especially in aged persons; artifactual changes in thyroid tests are not
  included in euthyroid sick syndrome.)**
*No single test is clearly diagnostic, especially in elderly and acutely or severely ill
  patients.*
See Table 13-5.
Initial change in all nonthyroidal illness patients is decreased T_3 with increased rT_3.
  With increasing severity, serum T_4 declines, producing low T_3–low T_4 state.
Increased T_4 syndrome is most common ($\leq$ 20%) in acute psychiatric admissions, espe-
  cially in the presence of certain drugs (e.g., amphetamines, phencyclidine) and in old
  age ($\leq$ 15% of elderly patients); increased values tend to decrease during first 2 wks
  after admission as patient improves. Is rarer in acutely ill patients (e.g., those with
  acute hepatitis).
  • Increased serum T_4, FTI, and T_3.
  • TSH is usually normal in mild to moderate illness.

Table 13-5. Differential Diagnosis of Euthyroid Sick Syndrome

	Euthyroid Sick Syndrome	Primary Hypothyroidism	Primary Hypothyroidism with Concomitant Illness
Serum T_4	N or D	D	D
Serum T_3 uptake	I	D	
Serum T_3	D	N or D	D
T_7 (FTI)	I, N, or D	D	D
Reverse T_3	I	D	D, N, or I
Serum TSH	N	I	I, occasionally N
TSH response to TRH	N or D	I	I

D = decreased; I = increased; N = normal.

Definitely increased T_3 uptake associated with decreased serum T_4 strongly indicates euthyroid sick syndrome, whereas in hypothyroidism T_3 uptake tends to be decreased.

In hypothyroidism with concomitant illness, T_3 uptake tends to increase into normal range but not above normal.

Serum TSH is increased in primary hypothyroidism as the earliest and most specific test; in contrast, basal and TRH-stimulated TSH are typically normal in euthyroid sick syndrome.

Reverse T_3 may be a useful discriminator in many euthyroid sick patients without renal failure, but it is not as useful as serum TSH.

Pituitary hypothyroidism may be difficult to distinguish, since serum TSH is low and not responsive to TRH, which is a common pattern in euthyroid sick patients.

- TRH test often is not useful due to flat TSH response commonly seen in melancholia patients.
- 50% of patients with hyperemesis gravidarum show elevated total and sometimes free T_4 that persist until hyperemesis abates. Patients with symptomatic hyponatremia show transient increase until low sodium is corrected.

Decreased T_4 syndrome
- Occurs in >50% of patients with severe or chronic illness.
- TSH is transiently increased (few days or weeks) during recovery.

Low T_3 syndrome is the most common. Occurs in most illnesses, starvation, and after surgery or trauma. T_3 is decreased in ~70% of hospitalized patients without intrinsic thyroid disease and is normal in 20–30% of hypothyroid patients; therefore T_3 testing is not indicated.
- Increased rT_3
- With progressive illness, tendency is for fall in total T_4 and TBG with increase of free T_4. Thus T_3 uptake increases, and FTI tend to remain normal. A strong correlation is seen between low T_4 ($<3\,\mu g/dL$) and high mortality in hospitalized patients.
- Serum TSH is typically normal or slightly increased; TSH response to TRH is usually normal.

In Neonates

Occurs in ~2.5% of newborns, particularly in association with prematurity, obstetrical or neonatal stress or illness, postmaturity.
- Decreased serum T_4.
- Decreased serum T_3.
- Normal serum TSH.
- By age of 1 mo, serum T_4 is normal in 98% of these infants.
- By age of 4 mos, if T_4 is still decreased, two-thirds of cases are due to genetic TBG deficiency.

Goiter, Neonatal

Due To

Maternal ingestion of iodine (e.g., for thyroid disease, for asthma), propylthiouracil
Inherited hypothyroidism (diminished ability to synthesize thyroid hormones)
Neonatal hyperthyroidism

Dyshormonogenesis
Hemangioma, lymphangioma

Goiter, Simple, Nontoxic Diffuse

No specific laboratory findings

Goiter, Single or Multiple Nodular

See Fig. 13-3.
♦ FNA biopsy produces a definitive diagnosis in 85% of cases of thyroid nodules.
♦ Isotope scanning of thyroid may show decreased ("cold") or increased ("hot") uptake.
Functioning solitary adenoma may produce hyperthyroidism.
In multinodular goiter, TSH is rarely increased; usually is in normal or low-normal range.
T_4, T_3, TBG, thyroglobulin do not differ in benign and malignant cyst fluid.

Hyperthyroidism

See Table 13-3 and Fig. 13-4.

Thyrotoxicosis with Hyperthyroidism

Due To
Thyroid-stimulating immunoglobulins
  Diffuse toxic goiter (Graves' disease—autoimmune disorder due to antibody to TSH
    receptors, causing destruction of thyroid gland)
Autonomous nodules in thyroid (serum TSH is low)
  Toxic adenoma
  Toxic multinodular goiter
Neonatal thyrotoxicosis associated with maternal Graves' disease
Thyrotropin-induced (TRH) hyperthyroidism (serum TSH is increased)
  • With pituitary tumor
  • Without pituitary tumor
Secretion of nonpituitary TSH
  Trophoblastic tissues (neoplasms that secrete hCG which binds to TSH receptors), e.g.,
  • Choriocarcinoma, hydatidiform mole
  • Embryonal carcinoma of testis

Thyrotoxicosis without Hyperthyroidism

Due To
Thyroiditis
  • Hashimoto's
  • Lymphocytic (painless)
  • Subacute granulomatous
Iodide-induced (Jod-Basedow)
Metastatic functioning thyroid carcinoma
Struma ovarii with hyperthyroidism
Factitious
Drug effects (e.g., amiodarone)
In neonate, is usually due to transplacental maternal TSH receptor–stimulating anti-
  bodies that mimic TSH action. May persist for several months.
2% of hospitalized elderly patients have unsuspected hyperthyroidism.

♦ Serum TSH is decreased; is now used by most as initial screening test for thyrotoxicosis because it detects virtually all hyperthyroid patients except the very rare cases
  involving pituitary neoplasms that secrete TSH, ectopic secretion of TSH or TRH,
  resistance to thyroid hormone (pituitary, generalized), and artifact (e.g., autoantibodies to TSH, human antimouse antibodies).
♦ Serum total and free T_4 are increased. With a typical clinical picture of hyperthyroidism, serum T_4 >16 µg/dL confirms the diagnosis. Normal in ~10% of patients but
  TSH is low, suggesting use of both tests to confirm the diagnosis. Severity of hyperthyroidism does not correlate with thyroid hormone levels.

ENDOCRINE

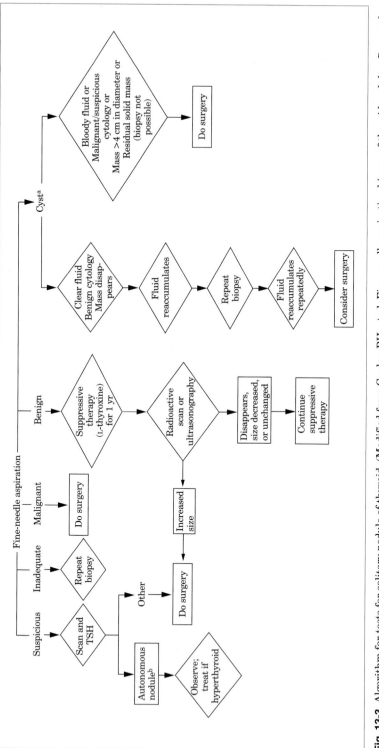

Fig. 13-3. Algorithm for tests for solitary nodule of thyroid. (Modified from Caplan RH, et al. Fine-needle aspiration biopsy of thyroid nodules. *Postgrad Med* 1991;90:183.)

[a]Contrary to common belief, cystic lesions may be malignant.
[b]Autonomous nodules are rarely malignant; thus a "hot" nodule on scan avoids surgery.

♦ Serum T_3 concentration on RIA and T_3 resin uptake are increased in ≤ 85% of patients. T_3 is usually elevated to a greater degree than T_4. Ratio of T_3 to T_4 is >20:1 in T_3-dependent type of Graves' disease.

♦ FTI (serum T_4 concentration × T_3 resin uptake) is a useful initial screening test, because it is not affected by alterations in T_4-binding protein sites. Is increased in ~90% of hyperthyroid patients.

TRH stimulation test—see p. 580.

Serum TBG is normal.

RAIU is increased. It is relatively more affected at 1, 2, or 6 hrs than at 24 hrs. It may be normal with recent iodine ingestion. RAIU is no longer used for diagnosis of hyperthyroidism but should be performed before administration of therapeutic dose of ^{131}I.

Salivary and urinary excretion of radioactive iodine are increased.

○ Technetium pertechnetate (^{99}Tc) uptake parallels hormone production and may be useful when T_4 and TSH results are discordant.

○ Microsomal antibodies are found in moderate to high titers in most patients with Graves' disease; may be helpful in confirming diagnosis in a hyperthyroid patient without ocular findings or a euthyroid patient with eye findings.

○ Other thyroid autoantibodies are thyroid-stimulating immunoglobulins and TSH-binding inhibitory immunoglobulins found only with Graves' disease; sometimes helpful in diagnosis and management. TSH-receptor antibody (formerly called LATS, long-acting thyroid stimulator) is present in 80–100% of untreated Graves' disease patients.

Thyroid suppression test: T_3 administration decreases RAIU in normal persons but not in hyperthyroid persons. Was replaced by TRH stimulation test.

Serum cholesterol is decreased, and total lipids are usually decreased.

Glucose tolerance is decreased with early high peak and early fall. Hyperglycemia and glycosuria are present.

Liver function tests show impairment.

Creatine excretion in urine and creatine tolerance are increased.

Normal serum creatine almost excludes hyperthyroidism.

Serum total and ionized calcium are increased in >10% of patients. Serum phosphorus is high-normal or increased. Parathormone level is decreased. Serum 1,25-dihydroxy-vitamin D is decreased. Urinary and fecal excretion of calcium are increased. Increased serum ALP in 75% of patients (liver and bone origin; only liver ALP in 7%; only bone ALP in 15%). After successful treatment, may continue to increase and not become normal for up to 18 mos.

Serum ferritin is increased.

Hb and TIBC are decreased.

Unusual laboratory manifestations of hyperthyroidism include hypoproteinemia, malabsorption.

Serum ACE is increased.

Laboratory findings due to complications of treatment
- Surgery—hypoparathyroidism (3% of cases), hypothyroidism (30–50% of cases)
- Drugs—agranulocytosis, hepatitis, vasculitis, drug-induced lupus

T_3 toxicosis—causes 5% of cases of hyperthyroidism

Should be suspected in patients with clinical thyrotoxicosis in whom usual laboratory tests are normal (serum T_4, FTI, 24-hr RAIU, TBG, and T_4-binding albumin), but serum T_3 is increased.

RAIU is autonomous (not suppressed by T_3 administration).

TSH may be increased.

Abnormal TRH test (lack of TSH response to TRH)

Factitious Hyperthyroidism

(Self-induced hyperthyroidism by ingestion of T_4 or Cytomel [T_3])

♦ Increased total and free serum T_4 or T_3, depending on which drug is ingested. T_4 may be absent if T_3 is ingested.

♦ Serum Tg is depressed to low-normal level or undetectable unless patient is taking desiccated thyroid extract of Tg; therefore may be useful to distinguish from early or recovery phases of subacute thyroiditis and most causes of hyperthyroidism, in which it is increased.

♦ RAIU is low when all other thyroid function tests indicate hyperthyroidism.

Augmented RAIU after TSH administration, whereas patients with subacute and painless thyroiditis usually do not have any response to TSH administration.

ENDOCRINE

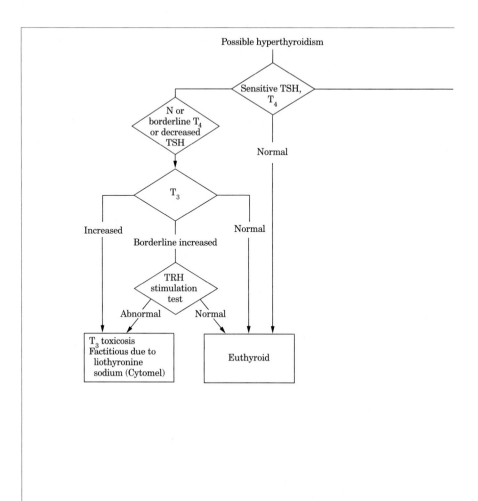

Fig. 13-4. Algorithm for diagnosis of hyperthyroidism. (N = normal.)

Thyroid Storm

(Occurs in operative/perioperative period; fever, symptoms of CNS, GI, and cardio-vascular systems)

Thyroid function test values may be somewhat higher than in uncomplicated thyro-toxicosis but are useless for differentiation.

Transient hyperglycemia is common.

Abnormal liver function tests are common.

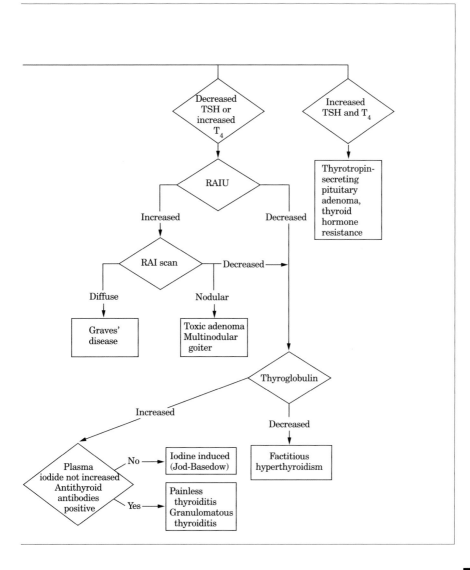

Abnormal serum electrolytes (especially decreased potassium, mild to moderate hyper-
   calcemia) and decreased arterial pCO_2 are common.
Laboratory findings due to associated conditions, especially bacterial infection (increased
   WBC, shift to left; bacteria in urine, sputum, etc.), pulmonary or arterial embolism

Hypothyroidism

See Table 13-6 and Figs. 13-1 and 13-5.

Table 13-6. Laboratory Tests in Differential Diagnosis of Primary
and Secondary Hypothyroidism

Test	Panhypopituitarism	Primary Myxedema
Serum TSH	Decreased	Increased
Serum TSH response to TRH administration	Absent	Normal or exaggerated
Response to administration of thyrotropic hormone	Responds with increase in RAIU	No response
Urine 17–ketosteroids	Absent	Low
Response to insulin	Prompt decrease in blood sugar; fails to return to normal	Usually delayed fall in blood sugar and sometimes delayed return to normal

Due To

Treatment of preceding hyperthyroidism (surgery, drugs, radioiodine)
Irradiation (e.g., treatment of head and neck cancer)
Autoimmune disease, thyroiditis
Pituitary disease (e.g., tumors, granulomas, cysts, vascular disorders)
Hypothalamic disease (e.g., granulomas, TRH deficiency, pituitary-stalk section)
Iodine deficiency
Drugs (e.g., iodides, propylthiouracil, methimazole, phenylbutazone, amiodarone, lithium)
Congenital developmental defects
Organification defect (diagnosis by perchlorate washout test)

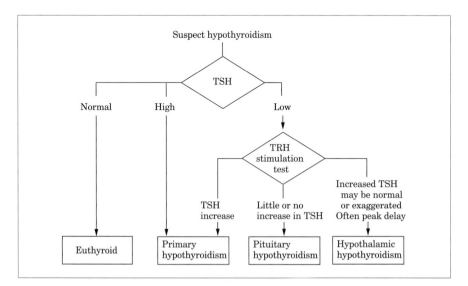

Fig. 13-5. Algorithm for laboratory tests for diagnosis of hypothyroidism. Sensitive thyroid-stimulating hormone (TSH) test is the preferred screening test for thyroid disease in many laboratories. Low TSH obviates need for thyrotropin-releasing hormone (TRH) stimulation test in most patients. Occasionally, decreased T_4, T_3, and FTI are used to confirm increased TSR.

2% of hospitalized elderly patients and 0.5% of patients admitted to psychiatric hospitals or units have unsuspected hypothyroidism.

♦ Serum TSH is increased in proportion to degree of hypofunction; is at least 2× and often 10× normal value. A single determination is usually sufficient to establish the diagnosis. Because increased serum TSH is earliest evidence of hypothyroidism, it should be measured to document subclinical hypothyroidism and begin early therapy in patients with Graves' disease treated with radioactive iodine or surgery or with chronic thyroiditis. TSH is especially useful in cases in which T_4 and FTI are not diagnostic and is essential when the diagnosis of hypothyroidism must be confirmed. Serum TSH should always be measured before treatment for all patients with hypothyroidism to distinguish primary from secondary (pituitary) or tertiary (hypothalamic) types, because the latter two are often associated with secondary adrenal insufficiency, which could be lethal if unrecognized.
  • Increased TSH and decreased FT_4 establishes diagnosis of primary hypothyroidism.
  • Increased TSH and normal FT_4 indicates early stage of primary hypothyroidism.
  • Normal or decreased TSH and decreased FT_4 suggests hypothyroidism secondary to decreased TSH secretion (hypopituitarism).
  • TSH is undetectable or inappropriately low in relation to degree of thyroid hormone deficiency in secondary or tertiary hypothyroidism.
♦ Serum T_4 and FT_4 concentration are decreased; $T_4 > 7$ µg/dL almost certainly excludes hypothyroidism. Measurement of serum FT_4 and TSH together is diagnostic method of choice.
Serum T_3 concentration is decreased (may be normal in 20–30% of hypothyroid patients), and serum T_3 resin uptake is decreased (may be normal in ≤ 50% of hypothyroid patients). T_3 has little role in this diagnosis.
♦ FTI is decreased.
Serum T_3/T_4 ratio is increased.
RAIU is usually decreased; is not helpful in diagnosis. Salivary and urinary excretion of radioactive iodine are decreased.
TSH stimulation (20 U/day for 3 days) increases RAIU to approximately normal (20%) in secondary but not in primary hypothyroidism. Diagnosis of primary hypothyroidism is unlikely if RAIU increases substantially after administration of TSH. Replaced by serum TSH.
A TRH-provocative test shows a normal or delayed TSH response in tertiary, no response in secondary, and exaggerated and prolonged response in primary hypothyroidism. (See Fig. 13-2.)
Serum TBG is normal.
Serum cholesterol is increased (may be useful to follow effect of therapy, especially in children).
Serum myoglobin is significantly increased in 90% of untreated patients with long-term hypothyroidism; inversely proportional to serum T_3 and T_4. Gradual decrease after T_4 therapy begins with return to normal before TSH becomes normal.
Serum total CK and CK-MM are increased.
Increase in serum CK (10–15×), AST (2–6×), LD (2–3×) above upper reference limit in 40–90% of cases.
Glucose tolerance is increased (OGTT results are flat; IV GTT results are normal); fasting blood sugar level is decreased.
Serum calcium is sometimes increased.
Serum ALP is decreased.
Serum carotene is increased.
Normocytic normochromic anemia may occur.
Serum iron and TIBC may be decreased.
Serum sodium is decreased in ~50% of cases.
CSF protein is elevated (100–340 mg/dL) in 25% of cases of myxedema.
Urine 17-KS and 17-OHKS may be increased.
Proteinuria in ~8% of cases.
Adequate levothyroxine treatment results in normal serum T_4 and TSH. When hypothyroidism is due to thyroid failure, the dose is gradually increased, and adequate therapy is indicated when serum T_4 increases to normal and TSH decreases to normal (may take several months). TSH response to TRH also returns to normal if originally abnormal, but this test is generally not necessary. When hypothyroidism

is secondary or tertiary, TSH is not useful and serum T_4 is used to judge adequacy of therapy. When levothyroxine is used for TSH suppression in patients with thyroid cancer, nodular disease, or chronic thyroiditis, the decreased TSH cannot be distinguished from normal levels; therefore levothyroxine dose is increased until serum T_4 is normal and TSH is undetectable, or an abbreviated TRH test is performed with a single TSH measurement 15 mins after injection of TRH—if TSH is undetectable, then TSH secretion is considered adequately suppressed.

Laboratory findings indicative of other autoimmune diseases (e.g., PA and primary adrenocortical insufficiency occur with increased frequency in primary hypothyroidism)

Thyroid hormone status should be reassessed at least yearly in treatment of hypothyroidism.

Laboratory findings due to involvement of other organs (e.g., muscle, heart, ileus, CNS, etc.)

Myxedema Coma

Hypoglycemia, hyponatremia, and findings due to adrenocortical insufficiency may be found.

Serum creatinine may be increased.

Arterial pCO_2 may be increased and pO_2 decreased.

Increased WBC and shift to left may occur.

Hypothyroidism, Neonatal

~2–4% of cases of infantile hypothyroidism are not detected on neonatal screening.

Estimated cost of finding one case of congenital hypothyroidism is ~$10,000. Estimated cost of institutionalization and special education of mental retardation due to late or no therapy is $105,000.

Neonatal screening is usually performed on same filter paper specimen of blood used for PKU screening on third to fifth day of life. *Do not do T_4 or TSH during first few days of life when levels may surge*; e.g., mean cord T_4 of 11–12 μg/dL may increase to 16 μg/dL by 24–36 hrs and then fall. T_3 rises more rapidly. TSH peaks 30 mins after birth. Changes in T_4, T_3, and TSH are less marked in premature infants.

♦ RAIU (^{123}I) scan should be performed on infants with confirmed hypothyroidism to differentiate thyroid agenesis/dysgenesis from dyshormonogenesis.

If mother has autoimmune thyroid disease, infant should be checked for TSH receptor–blocking antibodies, because this type of hypothyroidism cannot be distinguished clinically from thyroid agenesis/dysgenesis and RAIU may be absent. Hypothyroidism is transient.

Due To

Primary Hypothyroidism (Incidence 1 in 3600 to 1 in 4800)

Aplasia and hypoplasia	63%
Ectopic gland	23%
Inborn errors of thyroid hormone synthesis or metabolism	14%

- Increased serum TSH is most sensitive test for primary hypothyroidism.
- Decreased serum T_4.
- Normal or decreased serum T_3.
- Normal serum TBG.
- Increased serum CK.

Deficiency of TBG (Incidence 1 in 8000 to 1 in 12,000)

Hereditary

Drug effect

Hypoproteinemia

- Decreased serum T_4 (e.g., 3.2 μg/dL)
- Normal serum TSH

Secondary Hypothyroidism (Incidence 1 in 50,000 to 1 in 70,000)

Pituitary aplasia, septo-optic dysplasia

Idiopathic hypopituitarism

Hypothalamic disease

Serum TSH is low or not detectable.

Decreased serum T_4

TSH response to TRH differentiates pituitary from hypothalamic cause of hypothyroidism

Normal serum TBG

Transient

Prematurity
Euthyroid sick syndrome
Small size for gestational age
Maternal ingestion of iodides or antithyroid drugs
Idiopathic

Treatment of neonatal hypothyroidism is based on frequent T_4, TSH tests. For example, T_4 should be kept $>10\ \mu g/dL$ during first year, $>8\ \mu g/dL$ during second year, >7 $\mu g/dL$ after that. 10% of congenital hypothyroidism patients may need T_4 of 14–15 $\mu g/dL$ to achieve normal TSH levels.

Pregnancy and Thyroid Function Tests

See Table 13-3.
Thyroid function test values are very different in normal pregnancy.
• Serum TBG is increased.
• Serum T_4 rises from nonpregnant level of 4–8 $\mu g/dL$ to 10–12 $\mu g/dL$ from 12th week of gestation until 6 wks postpartum.
• Serum free T_4 and free T_3 are normal.
• T_3 uptake is decreased; FTI remains normal.
• Increased serum T_3, rT_3.
• TSH is slightly increased by 16th week.
• RAIU is increased but the test is contraindicated.

In hyperthyroidism, both serum T_3 uptake and T_4 are increased, but in the pregnant euthyroid patient or euthyroid patient taking birth control pills or estrogens, T_4 is increased and T_3 uptake is decreased. Hyperthyroidism may be indicated by the failure of T_3 uptake to decrease during pregnancy.

T_3 uptake gradually decreases (as early as 3–6 wks after conception) until the end of the first trimester and then remains relatively constant. It returns to normal 12–13 wks postpartum. Failure to decrease by the eighth to tenth week of pregnancy may indicate threatened abortion (the patient's normal nonpregnancy level should be known).

Maternal hypothyroidism is relatively uncommon because of spontaneous abortion and menstrual irregularities. Most often is iatrogenic or due to Hashimoto's disease. Serum T_4 in the *normal nonpregnancy* range of 4–8 $\mu g/dL$ should suggest hypothyroidism.

Maternal hyperthyroidism: Serum T_4 is increased above the normal range for pregnancy ($>12\ \mu g/dL$) with T_3 uptake increased to normal nonpregnancy range.

Thyroid Hormone, Generalized Tissue Resistance

(Genetic syndrome)

♦ Serum thyroid hormone levels are elevated in presence of nonsuppressed serum TSH with isolated pituitary resistance and show variable degree of thyrotoxicosis. In generalized tissue resistance involving pituitary and peripheral tissues, serum TSH and total and free T_4 show variable increases with or without clinical hypothyroidism.
♦ Elevated thyroid hormone levels are not due to drugs, intercurrent illness or alterations in thyroid hormone transport proteins.
♦ Full replacement doses of thyroid hormone fail to produce expected suppression of TSH and fail to induce appropriate peripheral tissue responses.

Few clinical manifestations; goiter is most common in adults, growth and mental retardation in children. No clinical evidence of hypo- or hyperthyroidism.

Thyroiditis

Hashimoto's Thyroiditis (Chronic Lymphocytic Thyroiditis)

Thyroid function may be normal; occasionally a patient passes through a hyperthyroid stage. 15–20% of patients develop hypothyroidism, but Hashimoto's disease is a very unlikely cause of hypothyroidism in the absence of thyroglobulin and microsomal antibodies.

♦ Test for antimicrosomal antibodies is 99% sensitive and 90% specific. Test for antithyroglobulin antibodies is 36% sensitive and 98% specific and is seldom positive if microsomal antibodies are negative. Thus antimicrosomal antibody alone is sufficient for diagnosis. High titers are pathognomonic.

○Serum TSH is earliest indicator of hypothyroidism; is increased in one-third of persons who are clinically euthyroid and in those with clinical hypothyroidism, many of whom have normal T_4, T_3, and T_7.

Abnormal iodide–perchlorate discharge test exceeding 10% of gland radioactive iodine in 60–80% of cases (indicates an underlying organification defect)

Response to TSH distinguishes primary and secondary hypothyroidism. If thyroid uptake for each lobe is measured separately after TSH, a difference between the lobes may demonstrate lobar thyroiditis when total uptake is apparently normal.

♦ Radioactive iodine scan may show involvement of only a single lobe (more common in younger patients); "salt and pepper" pattern is classical.

RAIU is variable; may be higher than expected in hypothyroidism.

♦ Biopsy of thyroid may be diagnostic.

Lymphocytic (Painless) Thyroiditis; Silent Thyroiditis

This form of hyperthyroidism comprises ≤ 25% of all cases of hyperthyroidism; resolves spontaneously in several weeks to months and is often followed by a transient hypothyroidism during recovery period; common in postpartum period; multiple episodes may occur. Pathologic changes are less severe than in Hashimoto's thyroiditis, but the latter cannot be ruled out in biopsy specimens.

Hyperthyroid phase is briefer in postpartum type (≤ 3 mos) than in sporadic type (≤ 12 mos).
- Increased serum T_4, T_3, T_3 resin uptake, FTI. T_3/T_4 ratio is <20:1. Become normal in 10 days with prednisone therapy.
- RAIU is very low (<3%); not increased after TSH administration.
- Serum TSH is low and fails to respond to TRH.
- Antithyroglobulin antibodies are increased in most patients; antimicrosomal antibodies are increased in ~60% of patients. High titers are rarely in the very high ranges seen in Hashimoto's thyroiditis.
- Nonspecific markers of inflammation are generally normal in contrast to granulomatous thyroiditis. ESR increased in 50% of patients to range of 20–40 mm/hr. WBC and serum proteins are normal.
- Urine iodide level is 2–5× higher than normal (due to leakage of iodinated material from thyroid).

Recovery phase is complete in ~50%.
- Serum T_4 and T_3 fall into normal range, but RAIU and TSH response to TRH remain suppressed.

Hypothyroid phase (occurs in 20–30% of patients; lasts 1–8 mos; most recover completely but a few develop permanent hypothyroidism; recurs in >10% of cases of sporadic type and more often in postpartum type)
- Antithyroid antibody titers are highest during this phase (especially in postpartum patients). Gradually decrease with time; 50% become negative within 6 mos.
- Serum TSH, T_4, and T_3 gradually return to normal.
- RAIU, TRH test begin to normalize toward the end of this phase, and urinary iodide falls to normal levels (50–200 μg/day).

Subacute Granulomatous (de Quervain's) Thyroiditis

(Probably of viral origin)
♦ Biopsy of thyroid confirms diagnosis.

Antithyroglobulin antibodies may be present for up to several months, but the titer is never as high as in Hashimoto's thyroiditis. The level falls with recovery.

ESR is increased.

WBC is normal or decreased.

Four sequential phases may be identified: hyperthyroid, euthyroid, hypothyroid, recovery.

Hyperthyroid phase lasts 1–2 mos.
- Decreased RAIU is the characteristic finding and differentiates it from acute thyroiditis; may be <5% with bilateral involvement; is not increased by TSH administration. It may be >50% for several weeks after recovery.
- Increased total and free T_4; T_3 may be only mildly increased; T_3/T_4 ratio is <20:1.
- Serum TSH is very low and does not respond to TRH.
- ESR is markedly increased.

Euthyroid phase lasts 1–2 wks.
* RAIU remains low.

Hypothyroid phase lasts 2–6 mos.
* TSH increases.

Recovery
* Return of radioactive iodine trapping is the first indication.
* 24-hr RAIU may rise above normal.
* Thyroid hormone levels rise to normal.
* TSH and RAIU fall to normal.

Relapses occur in up to 47% of patients, usually in first year.

Suppurative Thyroiditis, Acute

WBC and PMNs are increased in 75% of cases; absence may indicate anaerobic infection.
ESR is increased.
24-hr RAIU is decreased in <50% of cases.
Thyroid function tests are normal in 80% of cases.
Staphylococcus causes one-third of cases; other organisms include *Streptococcus pyogenes, Streptococcus pneumoniae, Enterobacteriaceae, Haemophilus influenzae, Pseudomonas aeruginosa,* anaerobes. Fungi are rare and principally occur in immunocompromised patients.

Riedel's Chronic Thyroiditis

♦ Biopsy of thyroid confirms diagnosis.
Hypothyroidism when complete thyroid involvement occurs; otherwise normal laboratory findings.

Tests of Parathyroid Function and Calcium/Phosphate Metabolism

Calcitriol (1,25-dihydroxy-vitamin D), Serum

Interpretation

Suppressed during hypercalcemia unless an autonomous source of PTH exists as in hyperparathyroidism. (Normal range <42 pg/mL in hypercalcemic and <76 pg/mL in normocalcemic patients.) Failure to suppress indicates extrarenal production as it is normally secreted only by kidney.

Increased In

Sarcoidosis (synthesized by macrophages within granulomas)
Non-Hodgkin's lymphoma (~15% of cases). Returns to normal after therapy.

Not Increased In

Hyperparathyroidism
Humoral hypercalcemia of malignancy (HHM)

Calcium, Ionized Serum

See p. 45.

Calcium, Total Serum

See p. 46.

Parathyroid Hormone (PTH), Serum

See Fig. 13-6.

ENDOCRINE

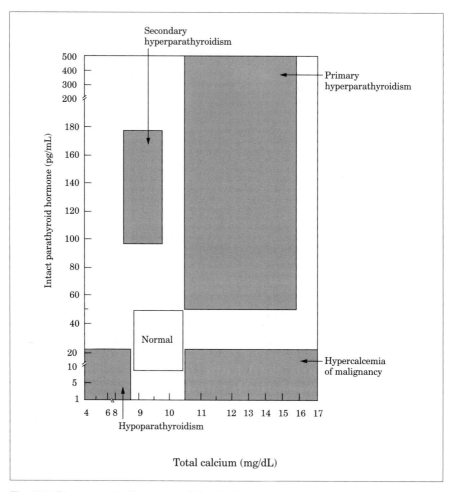

Fig. 13-6. Diagrammatic illustration of distribution of patients according to serum calcium and serum parathyroid hormone (PTH). The values of some patients may lie outside the exact boundaries indicated, and some conditions may overlap. (From *Mayo Laboratories Test Catalog, 1995*. Rochester, MN: Mayo Medical Laboratories, 1995.)

Use

Differential diagnosis of hyper- and hypoparathyroidism.

Very sensitive in detecting PTH suppression by 1,25-dihydroxy-vitamin D; therefore used for monitoring that treatment of chronic renal failure.

Interpretation

Serum calcium should always be measured at same time as PTH.

Immunochemiluminescent method is PTH assay of choice; detects intact PTH and active N-terminal PTH. Sensitivity >90% for hyperparathyroidism. PTH is suppressed (<1 pmol/L) in 95% of cases of HHM unless coexisting parathyroid adenoma is found, which occurs in 4% of HHM cases (especially breast or gastric cancer). Normal in chronic renal failure in which almost all patients have increased C-terminal PTH (inactive) values. PTH >25% above ULN occurs only in hyperparathyroidism (primary or tertiary), post–acute tubular necrosis, or posttransplant hypercalcemia.

Table 13-7. Serum Calcium and PTH in Various Conditions

	PTH Increased	PTH Not Increased
Serum calcium decreased[a]	Secondary hyperparathyroidism (chronic renal disease)	Hypoparathyroidism (surgery, autoimmunity, hormone resistance, magnesium deficiency)
Serum calcium increased[b]	Primary hyperparathyroidism Familial hypocalciuric hypercalcemia Lithium-induced hypercalcemia Some neoplasms (HHM)	Hypercalcemia not due to hyperparathyroidism (e.g., HHM, milk-alkali syndrome, thiazide diuretics, vitamin intoxication, sarcoidosis, hyperthyroidism, immobilization)
Serum calcium normal	Pregnancy Nephrolithiasis Secondary hyperparathyroidism (chronic renal disease)	Normal

HHM = humoral hypercalcemia of malignancy; PTH = parathyroid hormone.
[a]PTH may be normal or increased in hypocalcemic patients due to renal failure, acute pancreatitis, vitamin D deficiency.
[b]PTH may be normal or increased in hypercalcemic patients due to acromegaly, vitamin A intoxication, multiple endocrine neoplasia type IIA, renal tubular acidosis, chronic renal failure.

Some laboratories may assay different parts of PTH molecule. PTH shows diurnal variation with low in morning and peak around midnight (Table 13-7).

Parathyroid Hormone–Related Protein (PTHrP), Serum
Increased (>1.5 pmol/L) In

>90% of cases of HHM
75% of breast cancer patients with hypercalcemia
Some patients with hypercalcemia and hematologic cancers
~10% of cases of cancers without hypercalcemia
Becomes normal when hypercalcemia is corrected by treatment of cancer.
C-terminal PTHrP is increased in renal insufficiency.
May be increased in nonmalignant pheochromocytoma.
Normal lactation
Rarely may be increased in mammary hypertrophy or lymphedema.
~20% of cancer patients with hypercalcemia have only local osteolytic changes but not increased PTHrP.

Not Increased In

Other causes of hypercalcemia (e.g., sarcoidosis, vitamin D intoxication).

Phosphate Clearance

After a diet of 800 mg phosphate/day, determine serum phosphorus and BUN and 12-hr urine phosphorus.
Normal: 6–17 mL/min
Hyperparathyroidism: higher (even with renal dysfunction)
Hypoparathyroidism: lower (e.g., <6 mL/min), even when hypocalcemia has been corrected

Phosphate Deprivation Test

Low-phosphate diet (430 mg phosphate and 700 mg calcium for 3–6 days) causes low serum phosphate and increased serum calcium in persons with hyperparathyroidism but not in normal persons. Formerly used when blood chemistry tests were borderline.

ENDOCRINE

Phosphate, Tubular Reabsorption (TRP)

Use

Diagnosis of hyperparathyroidism. Largely superseded by PTH assay.

After a constant dietary intake of moderate calcium and phosphorus for 3 days, phosphorus and creatinine are determined in fasting blood and 4-hr urine specimens to calculate tubular reabsorption.

$$TRP = 100 \times 1 - \frac{(\text{urine phosphorus} \times \text{serum creatinine})}{(\text{urine creatinine} \times \text{serum phosphorus})}$$

Normal: TRP is >78% on normal diet; higher on low-phosphate diet (430 mg/day).
Hyperparathyroidism: TRP is <74% on normal diet; <85% on low-phosphate diet.

Interferences

False-positive result may occur in uremia, renal tubular disease (some patients), osteomalacia, sarcoidosis.

Phosphorus, Serum

See p. 70.

Diseases of Parathyroid Glands and Calcium, Phosphorus, and Alkaline Phosphatase Metabolism

Humoral Hypercalcemia of Malignancy (HHM)

See Tables 13-8, 13-9, and Figs. 13-6 and 13-7.
♦ Hypercalcemia occurs in patients with cancer (typically squamous, transitional cell, renal, ovarian), 5–20% of whom have no bone metastases compared to patients with widespread bone metastases (myeloma, lymphoma, breast cancer). Both groups have large tumor burden and poor prognosis.
  • Occurs in 20–35% of cases of breast cancer, 10–15% of cases of lung cancer, ~70% of cases of multiple myeloma, rare in lymphoma and leukemia.
  • Rarely may occur in association with benign tumors (e.g., pheochromocytoma, dermoid cyst of ovary) ("humoral hypercalcemia of benignancy").
  • Very high serum calcium (e.g., >14.5 mg/dL) is much more suggestive of HHM than of primary hyperparathyroidism; less marked increase with renal tumors.
♦ Serum PTH is decreased or low normal inappropriate for high serum calcium.
♦ Serum PTHrP is increased (>1.5 pmol/L) in >90% of cases; may be increased when measured by some assay methods (e.g., RIA) but not by others (e.g., IRMA).
○ Serum 1,25-dihydroxy-vitamin D is usually decreased or low normal but increased in T-cell or B-cell lymphoma or Hodgkin's disease. Is increased in hyperparathyroidism.
Urinary cAMP is increased in 90% of cases HHM and of primary hyperparathyroidism; not increased in hypercalcemia due to bone metastases.
Hypercalciuria is much greater than in hyperparathyroidism at any serum calcium level.
Decreased serum chloride
Decreased serum albumin
Alkalosis is present.
Decreased serum phosphorus in >50% of patients
Serum ALP is frequently increased.
Serum proteins are not consistently abnormal.
○ Occult cancer should be ruled out as the cause of hypercalcemia in presence of
  • Hypercalcemia without increased serum PTH together with increased urinary cAMP.
  • Serum ALP >2× ULN.

Table 13-8. Laboratory Findings in Various Diseases of Calcium and Phosphorus Metabolism

Disease	Serum Calcium[a]	Serum Phosphorus	Serum ALP	Urine Calcium[b]	Urine Phosphorus	Serum PTH	Serum 1,25-Dihydroxy-Vitamin D
Primary hyperparathyroidism	I	D (<3 mg/dL in 50%)	I slightly in 50% (N if no bone disease)	I in two-thirds	I	I	I
Humoral hypercalcemia of malignancy	I; frequently marked	D in 50%	Frequently I	I	I	D	D
Familial hypocalciuric hypercalcemia	Mild I	N or slightly D	N	D or low N		I or inappropriately N	Proportional to PTH
Hypoparathyroidism	D	I	N	D	D[c]	D	D
Pseudohypoparathyroidism	D	I	N; occasionally D	D	D[c]	N or I	D
Pseudopseudohypoparathyroidism	N	N	N	N	N	N	
Secondary hyperparathyroidism (renal rickets)	D or N	I	I or N	D or I	D	I	D
Vitamin D excess	I	N	D	I	I	D	I
Rickets and osteomalacia	D or N	D or N	I	D	D	I	D
Osteoporosis	N	N	N	N or I	N		
Polyostotic fibrous dysplasia	N	N	N or I	N	N		
Paget's disease	N	N or I	I	N or I	I		
Metastatic neoplasm to bone	N or I	V	N or I	V	I		
Multiple myeloma	N or I	V	N or I	N or I	N or I		I
Sarcoidosis	N or I	N or I	N or I	I	N		
Fanconi's syndrome or renal loss of fixed base	D or N	D	N or I	I	I		
Histiocytosis X (Letterer-Siwe disease, Hand-Schüller-Christian disease, eosinophilic granuloma)	N	N	N or I	N or I	N		

(continued)

Table 13-8. (continued)

Disease	Serum Calcium[a]	Serum Phosphorus	Serum ALP	Urine Calcium[b]	Urine Phosphorus	Serum PTH	Serum 1,25-Dihydroxy-Vitamin D
Hypercalcemia and excess intake of alkali (Burnett's syndrome)	I	I or N	N	N	N		N
Solitary bone cyst	N	N	N	N	N		N

D = decreased; I = increased; N = normal; V = variable.

[a]Serum calcium. Repeated determinations may be required to demonstrate abnormalities. Serum total protein level should always be known. See also response to cortisone on p. 554.

[b]Urine calcium. Patient should be on a low-calcium diet (e.g., Bauer-Aub).

[c]See Ellsworth-Howard Test, p. 608.

Table 13-9. Comparison of Primary Hyperparathyroidism (HPT) and Humoral Hypercalcemia of Malignancy (HHM)

	HHM	HPT
Etiology	Squamous or large cell carcinoma of bronchus, hypernephroma of kidney, cancer of ovary, colon, others	Primary hyperplasia, adenoma, carcinoma of parathyroids
Serum calcium	Very high: >14 mg/dL in 75% of patients	Moderately high: >14 mg/dL in 25% of patients
	Suppressed by cortisone in 25–50% of patients	Suppressed by cortisone in 50% of cases with and 23% of cases without osteitis fibrosa
Serum PTH	Decreased	Increased
Serum PTHRP	Increased	Not increased
Serum chloride	Low: <99 mEq/L	High: >102 mEq/L
Serum chloride-phosphorus ratio	<30	>33
Serum bicarbonate	Increased or normal	Normal or low
pH	Alkalosis	Acidosis
Serum ALP	Increased in 50% of patients, even without bone disease	Seldom increased unless bone disease is present
Serum phosphorus	Increased, normal, or low	Normal or low
Urine calcium	Often >400 mg/24 hrs	Usually <400 mg/24 hrs
Serum 1,25-dihydroxy-vitamin D	Decreased	Increased
Urine cAMP	Increased in HHM but not due to bone metastases only	Increased in 90% of cases
ESR	Usually increased	Normal
Anemia	May be present	Absent
Serum albumin	Often decreased	Usually normal
Renal stones	Absent	Common
Pancreatitis	Rare	Occurs
Radiographic changes in hand bones	Absent	May be present

- Increased serum phosphorus.
- Serum chloride/phosphorus ratio <30.
- Serum calcium >14.5 mg/dL without florid hyperparathyroidism.
- Urine calcium >500 mg/24 hrs; urine calcium and phosphorus and renal tubular reabsorption of phosphate are not useful in differential diagnosis.
- Anemia, increased ESR.
- Positive cortisone suppression test in absence of osteitis fibrosa; failure to respond is seen in HPT, most cases of HHM, ~50% of cases of multiple myeloma.

Table 13-10. Approximate Sensitivity, Specificity for Hyperparathyroidism (HPT), and Positive and Negative Predictive Values (in %) for the Most Commonly Useful Tests*

	Sensitivity	Specificity	Predictive Value	
			Positive	Negative
Cl >99 mEq/L	98	51	18	99
Cl/P ratio >32	95	53	18	99
Cl/P ratio >28	100	53	15	100
ALP >2× normal	100	53	19	100
PTH >90 μLEq/mL	100	73	29	100
PTH >180 μLEq/mL (>2× normal)	56	100	100	95

*Based on a prevalence of 9.7% of primary hyperparathyroidism in hospitalized hypercalcemic patients.

> *Multiple and repeated tests may be necessary in differential diagnosis of some cases of hypercalcemia.*
> *Primary HPT occurs in up to 10% of patients with HHM as well as in those receiving thiazides or those with other causes of hypercalcemia.*

Hyperparathyroidism (HPT), Primary

See Figs. 13-6 and 13-7 and Tables 13-8 through 13-10.

Due To

- Parathyroid adenoma in 80% of cases.
- Hyperplasia in 15% of cases.
- Parathyroid carcinoma in <5% of cases.
- No laboratory test can differentiate these.
- ~15% of these lesions may be ectopic; these must be sought if biochemical changes are not reversed by surgery.

♦ Increased serum calcium is hallmark of HPT and first step in diagnosis. Ionized calcium is more sensitive than total calcium. Repeated determinations may be required to demonstrate increased levels in HPT. Rapid decrease after excision of adenoma may cause tetany during next few weeks, especially when serum ALP is increased. Drug-induced hypercalcemia (see pp. 45–47) should be reevaluated after discontinuation for 1–2 mos; cessation of thiazides may unmask primary HPT. ≤ 5% of hypercalcemia patients have simultaneous HPT and HHM. Any increased serum calcium must be confirmed by repeat test in fasting state and discontinuance for several days of drugs that may increase serum calcium (e.g., thiazide diuretics). *Serum total protein and albumin must always be measured simultaneously, as marked decrease may cause a decrease in calcium.*

Normal calcium level may occur with coexistence of conditions that decrease serum calcium level (e.g., malabsorption, acute pancreatitis, nephrosis, infarction of parathyroid adenoma); also beware of laboratory error as a cause of "normal" serum calcium. High phosphate intake can abolish increased serum and urine calcium and decreased serum phosphorus; low-phosphate diet unmasks these changes.

♦ Serum PTH level is elevated; a few patients have only high-normal PTH levels. Considerable overlap of serum PTH levels is seen in normal patients and those with HPT. Serum calcium must always be measured concurrently, because PTH in the upper normal range may be inappropriately high in relation to a distinctly increased calcium level, which is consistent with HPT. Blood should always be drawn after 10 a.m. because of circadian rhythm. PTH >2× ULN is almost always due to primary HPT. Failure to detect PTH in the presence of simultaneous hypercalcemia argues against

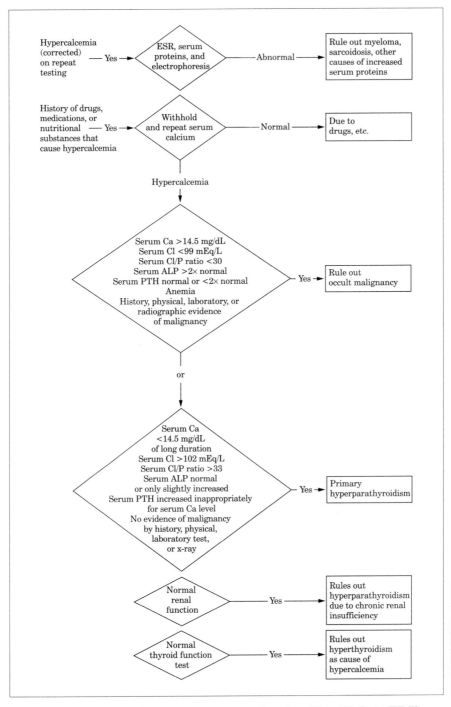

Fig. 13-7. Algorithm for diagnosis of hypercalcemia. (Data from Wong ET, Freier EF. The differential diagnosis of hypercalcemia: an algorithm for more effective use of laboratory tests. *JAMA* 1982;247:75. Johnson KR, Howarth AT. Differential laboratory diagnosis of hypercalcemia. *CRC Crit Rev Clin Lab Sci* 1984;21:51.)

ENDOCRINE

the diagnosis of primary HPT and surgical exploration of the parathyroid glands. In general, nonparathyroid disease causing hypercalcemia (e.g., sarcoidosis, vitamin D intoxication, hyperthyroidism, milk-alkali syndrome, most malignancies) have a normal or low (suppressed) PTH value (see Parathyroid Hormone, Serum, p. 595). Selective catheterization of veins draining the thyroid-parathyroid region for determination of PTH levels may confirm the diagnosis of HPT due to tumor by showing a significant elevation at one site compared to at least one other site. *A low PTH rules out HPT.*

♦ Serum chloride is increased (>102 mEq/L; <99 mEq/L in other types of hypercalcemia). HPT patients tend toward hyperchloremic (non-AG) acidosis, whereas other hypercalcemic patients tend toward alkalosis.

♦ Chloride/phosphorus ratio >33 supports the diagnosis of HPT and ratio <30 contradicts this diagnosis.

○ Serum phosphorus is decreased (<3 mg/dL) in ~50% of cases. It may be normal in the presence of high phosphorus intake or renal damage with secondary phosphate retention. It may be normal in one-half of patients, even without uremia. Low serum phosphorus supports the diagnosis of primary HPT, an increased level supports the diagnosis of nonparathyroid hypercalcemia, but a normal level is not useful.

Serum ALP is of limited value. Normal in 50% of patients with primary HPT and only slightly increased in the rest; infrequently is markedly increased in the presence of bone disease. Level slowly decreases to normal after excision of adenoma. Increase >2× ULN and increased serum LD favors HHM rather than HPT.

Urine calcium is increased (>400 mg on a normal diet; 180 mg on a low-calcium diet) in only 70% of patients with HPT.
• Urine calcium excretion is often >500 mg/24 hrs in malignancy, sarcoidosis, hyperthyroidism.
• Is <200 mg/24 hrs in benign familial hypocalciuric hypercalcemia.
• Lithium-induced hypercalcemia resembles that of familial hypocalciuric hypercalcemia in that both show increased PTH levels and low urine calcium concentrations.

Urine phosphorus is increased except in cases of renal insufficiency or phosphate depletion (especially due to commonly used antacids containing aluminum). Phosphate loading unmasks the increased urine phosphorus of HPT.

Polyuria is present, with low specific gravity.

Cortisone suppression test (e.g., administer hydrocortisone 40 mg 3 times daily for 10 days, then withdraw slowly for 5 days; measure serum calcium at 5, 8, and 10 days). Positive result on suppression test is fall of corrected serum calcium >1.0 mg/dL.
• Test results are positive in 77% of cases with nonparathyroid causes of hypercalcemia (e.g., sarcoidosis, vitamin D intoxication, metastatic carcinoma, multiple myeloma) and in 50% of cases of HPT with osteitis fibrosa.
• Test is negative in HPT without osteitis fibrosa (77% of cases) and therefore is not helpful in this group and in those with familial benign hypercalcemia.

Serum alpha$_2$ and beta$_1$ globulins are slightly increased but return to normal after parathyroidectomy. *Serum protein electrophoresis should be performed in HPT to rule out multiple myeloma and sarcoidosis.*

Serum 1,25-dihydroxy-vitamin D may be elevated in primary HPT and in sarcoidosis (and other granulomatous diseases) but not in HMM; serum 25-hydroxy-vitamin D level may be useful to establish vitamin D intoxication, especially in factitious cases.

Urinary cyclic adenosine monophosphate (cAMP) may be high (>4.0 mmol/L) in >90% of cases of primary HPT and of HHM (not increased in hypercalcemia due to osteolytic metastases) but low in vitamin D intoxication and sarcoidosis. Not usually increased in multiple myeloma or other hematologic malignancies. Drop from an elevated level to normal range within 6 hrs after surgery is said to provide functional confirmation of successful parathyroidectomy. Not widely used because of need for timed samples.

Uric acid is increased in >15% of patients. Uric acid level is not affected by cure of HPT, but a postoperative gout attack may occur. Increased uric acid level favors hypercalcemia due to thiazides, neoplasm, or renal failure rather than HPT.

Increased hydroxyproline in serum and urine may occur with bone disease but is of limited use.

○ Increased ESR is infrequent in HPT (may be due to infection or moderate renal insufficiency). Marked increase occurs in multiple myeloma.

Indirect studies of parathyroid function (e.g., phosphate deprivation, calcium infusion, tubular reabsorption of phosphate) are often borderline, and interpretation is difficult with any significant degree of renal insufficiency (see p. 598).

○*HPT must always be ruled out in the presence of*
- Renal colic and stones or calcification (2–3% have HPT) (see Table 13-7)
- Peptic ulcer (occurs in 15% of patients with HPT)
- Calcific keratitis
- Bone changes (present in 20% of patients with HPT)
- Jaw tumors
- Clinical syndrome of hypercalcemia (nocturia, hyposthenuria, polyuria, abdominal pain, adynamic ileus, constipation, nausea, vomiting) *(present in 20% of patients with HPT; only clue to diagnosis in 10% of patients with HPT)*
- MEN (e.g., islet cell tumor of pancreas, pituitary tumor, pheochromocytoma) (see p. 697)
- Relatives of patients with HPT or "asymptomatic" hypercalcemia
- Mental aberrations

A changing clinical spectrum of HPT has resulted from earlier detection of hypercalcemia by multiphasic screening.
- 50% of cases are asymptomatic (most show only mild elevation of calcium).
- 20% of cases have renal stones.
- 6% of cases show osteitis fibrosa cystica.
- 15% of cases have peptic ulcer.
- Two clinical forms:
  1. Mild form detected by multiphasic screening, progresses slowly, total calcium 10.6–11.5 mg/dL, no bone disease, 30% have renal stones.
  2. Severe form progresses rapidly with higher serum calcium that rises faster, serum phosphate is lower than in mild form, renal stones are less common.

"Asymptomatic" hypercalcemia is detected by routine multiphasic screening in 1–2% of tests.
- 21–38% of hospitalized patients had no documented clinical cause found for hypercalcemia.
- Malignancy caused one-third to two-thirds of hospitalized cases in different series.
- HPT caused 15–50% of cases in different series and is the most common cause in outpatients.

Some patients with asymptomatic primary HPT may be followed medically, but surgery is indicated in presence of serum calcium >11.4 mg/dL or history of any episode of life-threatening hypercalcemia, decreased creatinine clearance (<70% that of age-matched normals), very increased 24-hr urine calcium (>400 mg), presence of kidney stones, or substantially decreased bone mass.

Hyperparathyroidism (HPT), Secondary

(Diffuse hyperplasia of parathyroid glands usually secondary to chronic advanced renal disease)
See Fig. 13-6.
Serum PTH should be monitored to identify autonomous HPT.
Laboratory findings due to underlying causative disease are noted (e.g., renal insufficiency).
◆ Classic findings in renal osteodystrophy are
- Serum calcium is low or normal.
- Serum phosphorus is increased.
- Serum ALP is increased.
- These levels can also be used to monitor response to treatment with calcitriol or alpha-calcidiol.
- Increased serum PTH is suppressed by 1,25-dihydroxy-vitamin D, which can be used to monitor this treatment of chronic renal failure.

Hyperphosphatasemia, Benign Familial

○Rare familial benign persistent increase of serum ALP (usually <5× ULN) in the absence of any known disease. Increase is usually of intestinal or bone (but occasionally of liver) origin.

ENDOCRINE

Mild increase of serum acid phosphatase in some family members does not correlate with increase or type of ALP.

Hyperphosphatasemia, Benign Transient

○Sudden transient increase in serum ALP, often to very high levels, that returns to normal usually within 4 mos. Isoenzymes of bone and liver origin are increased without evidence of liver or bone disease.

Incidental discovery in healthy children, usually <5 yrs old, especially after summer months and after recent weight loss.

Plasma 25-hydroxy-vitamin D is 2× normal for age and time of year.

Occasional slight increase of AST, ALT, and GGT.

Normal serum ALP in family members.

Hyperphosphatasia

(Autosomal recessive syndrome beginning early in life of fragile bones with multiple fractures and deformities, skeletal radiographic changes, increased serum ALP; also referred to as osteoectasia and osteochalasia desmalis familiaris)

♦ Serum ALP is usually chronically increased, sometimes markedly; electrophoresis indicates bone origin. Serum acid phosphatase is also increased. Indicates increased activity of osteoblasts and osteoclasts.

Serum LAP score may also be increased.

Serum calcium is normal or slightly decreased.

Serum phosphorus is normal or increased.

Serum magnesium, proteins, and electrolytes are usually normal.

Uric acid is increased in blood and urine.

Hypervitaminosis D

(Due to ingestion of >500 μg/day in adults or >50 μg/day in infants)
See Table 13-8.

Serum calcium may be increased; preceded by hypercalciuria.

Serum phosphorus is normal

Serum ALP is decreased.

Serum PTH is low or normal.

Urine calcium excretion is increased.

Renal calcinosis may lead to renal insufficiency and uremia.

♦ Serum 25-hydroxy-vitamin D is increased.

Hypocalcemia (Familial), Latent Tetany, and Calcification of Basal Ganglia Syndrome

(Rare clinical syndrome has features resembling those of pseudohypoparathyroidism, pseudopseudohypoparathyroidism, and basal cell nevus syndrome)
Hypocalcemia is not responsive to parathormone administration.

Parathormone administration produces a phosphate diuresis.

Hypocalcemia, Neonatal

Because pH affects ionized calcium values, obtain free-flowing sample anaerobically and seal in capillary tube until analysis.

Age 1–4 wks: serum calcium <7 mg/dL or ionized calcium <4 mg/dL

Age 1–2 days—associated with
- Prematurity and low birth weight occurs in ≤ 30% of infants
- Maternal diabetes found in ≤ 25% of cases
- Birth asphyxia occurs in ≤ 30% of infants

Age 5–10 days—associated with
  • Feeding of cow's milk (increased serum phosphorus and decreased serum calcium)
Rarely associated with
  • Maternal hypercalcemia or HPT
  • Congenital absence of parathyroid glands (see DiGeorge syndrome)
  • Hypoproteinemia (e.g., nephrosis, liver disease)
  • Maternal osteomalacia
  • Renal disease (primary rental tubular defect; decreased GFR causing phosphate retention)
  • Iatrogenic disorders (e.g., citrate administration during exchange transfusions)

○*When tetany syndrome is associated with a normal serum calcium level or is not relieved by administration of calcium, rule out decreased serum magnesium. Hypocalcemia associated with hypomagnesemia does not respond unless hypomagnesemia is treated.*

○*Serum phosphorus is >8 mg/dL when neonatal hypocalcemia is due to high phosphate feeding. BUN is increased when neonatal hypocalcemia is due to severe renal disease.*

Check serum calcium at the following intervals:
  • Infants of diabetic mothers: 6, 12, 24, 48 hrs
  • Infants with intrapartum asphyxia: 1, 3, 6, 12 hrs
  • Premature infants: 12, 24, 48 hrs

Hypocalciuric Hypercalcemia, Familial (Familial Benign Hypercalcemia)

(Rare familial autosomal dominant disorder of chronic lifelong, asymptomatic, non-progressive, mild hypercalcemia due to resistance to action of extracellular calcium on parathyroid gland and kidney; onset before age 10 yrs without renal stones, kidney damage, peptic ulcer; no response to parathyroidectomy; parathyroid glands are histologically normal)

♦ Has many of same biochemical findings as primary HPT, including
  • Mildly increased serum total and ionized calcium.
  • Inappropriately increased (although within normal range) PTH level for hypercalcemia.
  • Serum phosphorus is slightly decreased or normal.
  • Urinary cAMP is increased in about one-third of patients.
♦ Urine calcium excretion is decreased or low normal despite hypercalcemia.
  • ≤ 200 mg/24 hrs in familial hypocalciuric hypercalcemia; calcium/creatinine clearance ratio is usually <0.01 (but usually >0.02 in primary HPT).
  • Up to 300 mg/24 hrs in normal adult males.
  • Increased (often >250 mg/24 hrs) in two-thirds of patients with HPT.
  • Increased (often >500 mg/24 hrs) in patients with malignancies.

Serum magnesium is mildly increased in 50% of patients; this is the only condition in which serum magnesium and calcium are both increased. Urine magnesium excretion is decreased also.

Renal function is maintained with normal creatinine clearance.

Serum 25-hydroxy-vitamin D is normal and 1,25-dihydroxy-vitamin D is proportional to PTH level.

Serum ALP is normal.

No dysfunction of other endocrine glands.

May be family history of hypercalcemia or failed parathyroidectomy attempts.

Hypoparathyroidism

(Rare disorder often detected in childhood; may be autoimmune disorder associated with Addison's disease, diabetes mellitus, hypothyroidism, PA, chronic hepatitis, moniliasis, malabsorption, or hypogonadism)

See Table 13-8 and Fig. 13-6.

♦ Serum calcium is decreased (as low as 5 mg/dL) in presence of low or inappropriately low PTH and normal serum magnesium, which affects PTH secretion and action. Hypocalcemia stimulates PTH secretion in pseudohypoparathyroidism but not in hypoparathyroidism.

○Serum phosphorus is increased (usually 5–6 mg/dL; as high as 12 mg/dL).
Serum ALP is normal or slightly decreased.
Urine calcium is decreased.
Urine phosphorus is decreased. Phosphate clearance is decreased.
Serum PTH is decreased.
♦ Renal resistance to PTH is shown by Ellsworth-Howard test
  • PTH challenge (IV administration of 200 IU of synthetic PTH) causes increased urine phosphate (>10×) and cAMP in normal persons and in primary hypoparathyroidism but little or no increase in urine phosphorus.
  • Increased urine phosphate (<2×) and cAMP in classical type I pseudohypoparathyroidism or pseudopseudohypoparathyroidism.
  • In type II pseudohypoparathyroidism cAMP increases without phosphaturia.
  • Decreased response may occur in basal cell nevus syndrome.
Alkalosis is present.
Serum uric acid is increased.
OGTT results are flat (due to poor absorption).
CSF is normal, even with mental or emotional symptoms or with calcification of basal ganglia.
○Hypoparathyroidism should be ruled out in presence of mental and emotional changes, cataracts, faulty dentition in children, associated changes in skin and nails (e.g., moniliasis is frequent). One-third of these patients may present as "epileptics."
Congenital absence may be associated with thymic aplasia (DiGeorge's syndrome) (see p. 444).

Hypophosphatasia

(Rare [1 in 100,000 live births] autosomal recessive disease of bone mineralization with radiographic changes and at least three different clinical syndromes found in infants [most severe], children, and adults [least severe])
♦ Serum ALP is decreased to ~25% of normal (may vary from 0 ≤ 40% of normal); is not correlated with severity of disease. Due to bone and sometimes liver isoenzymes; normal ALP in intestine and placenta. Is decreased in heterozygotes but the level cannot distinguish patients from carriers.
Serum calcium may be increased in severe cases in newborns.
Serum phosphorus is normal.
♦ Serum and urine levels of phosphoethanolamine are increased (may be increased in asymptomatic heterozygotes and useful for detection).
♦ Treatment with corticosteroids usually causes an increase in serum ALP (but it never attains normal level) with a marked fall in serum calcium; phosphoethanolamine excretion in urine continues to be high.
♦ Prenatal diagnosis by measurement of ALP in cultured amniocytes, but activity in amniotic fluid is unreliable.
Urine hydroxyproline is low; in contrast, it is high in vitamin D–resistant rickets or hyperphosphatasia.

Hypophosphatemia, Primary

(Familial but occasionally sporadic condition of intrinsic renal tubular defect in phosphate resorption)
♦ Serum phosphorus is always decreased in the untreated patient.
Serum calcium is usually normal.
Serum ALP is often increased.
♦ Bone biopsy shows a characteristic pattern of demineralization around osteocyte lacunae.

Milk-Alkali (Burnett's) Syndrome

Increased serum calcium (without hypercalciuria)
Increased serum phosphorus
Mild alkalosis

○ • The previous section should suggest the diagnosis in a patient with peptic ulcer.
Normal serum ALP
Renal insufficiency with azotemia (increased BUN)
Metastatic calcinosis

Pseudohypoparathyroidism

(Heterogeneous group of inherited disorders with renal resistance to PTH action. Patients may be short, stocky with round face, short metacarpals and metatarsals, calvarial thickening, mental retardation.)
♦ Serum calcium, phosphorus, and ALP are the same as in hypoparathyroidism but cannot be corrected by (or respond poorly to) administration of PTH (see description of Ellsworth-Howard test, p. 608).
♦ Serum PTH level is normal or elevated.
♦ Renal resistance to PTH is shown by Ellsworth-Howard test (see previous section).

Pseudopseudohypoparathyroidism

(Clinical anomalies are the same as in pseudohypoparathyroidism.)
Serum and urine calcium, phosphorus, and ALP are normal.
Ellsworth-Howard test (see Hypoparathyroidism, p. 607).

Pseudohypophosphatasia

(Clinical syndrome resembling hypophosphatasia)
Serum ALP is normal.

Tetany with Decreased Tissue Calcium

♦ Tetany associated with normal serum calcium, magnesium, potassium, and carbon dioxide, responds to vitamin D therapy.
♦ Special radioactive calcium studies show decreased tissue calcium pool that returns toward normal with therapy.

Tetany Syndrome Due to Magnesium Deficiency

♦ Serum magnesium is decreased (usually <1 mEq/L).
Serum calcium is normal (slightly decreased in some patients)
Blood pH is normal.
♦ Tetany responds to administration of magnesium but not of calcium.

Tests for Diagnosis of Diabetes Mellitus and Hypoglycemia

C-Peptide, Serum

C-peptide is formed during conversion of proinsulin to insulin; C-peptide serum levels correlate with insulin levels in blood, except in patients with islet cell tumors and possibly in obese patients.

Use

Estimation of insulin levels in the presence of antibodies to exogenous insulin.
Diagnosis of factitious hypoglycemia due to surreptitious administration of insulin, in which high serum insulin levels occur with low C-peptide levels.

Increased In

Insulinoma
Type II diabetes mellitus

ENDOCRINE

Decreased In

Exogenous insulin administration (e.g., factitious hypoglycemia)
Type I diabetes mellitus

Fructosamine, Serum

Measures concentration of nonlabile glycated serum proteins, giving a reliable estimate of mean blood glucose levels during preceding 1–3 wks.
Should primarily be compared with previous values in same patient rather than with reference range.
Reference range in nondiabetic persons: fructosamine = 2.4–3.4 mmol/L; fructosamine:albumin ratio = 54–86 μmol/gm.

Use

To monitor treatment of diabetic patients

Interpretation

Correlates with HbA_{1c} but is not affected by abnormal hemoglobins, HbF, or increased RBC turnover and shows changed glucose levels earlier; is cheaper, faster, less subjective than HbA_{1c}.

Interferences

Changes in fructosamine values correlate with significant changes in serum albumin or protein concentrations. Abnormal values also occur during abnormal protein turnover (e.g., thyroid disease) even though patients are normoglycemic. Obviated by using fructose/albumin ratio.
Dysproteinemias
Increased serum bilirubin may interfere.
Possibly uremia, lipemia, hemolysis, ascorbate.

Glycohemoglobin (Glycated Hemoglobin)

May be reported as HbA_{1c} or as total of A_{1b}, A_{1a}, A_{1c}.
Values may not be comparable using different methodologies and even from different laboratories using same methodology.
Glucose combines with Hb continuously and nearly irreversibly during life span of RBC (120 days); thus glycated Hb is proportional to mean plasma glucose level during previous 6–12 wks.
Glycated Hb predicts risk of progression of diabetic complications.
Glycosylated albumin (half life ~14 days) has been used for monitoring degree of hyperglycemia during previous 1–2 wks when glycated Hb cannot be used. Not yet shown to be related to risk of progression of diabetic complications.

Use

Monitor diabetic patients' compliance with therapeutic regimen and long-term blood glucose level control.
In known diabetics:
- 7% indicates good diabetic control.
- 10% indicates fair diabetic control.
- 13–20% indicates poor diabetic control.
- When mean annual HbA_{1c} is <1.1× ULN, renal and retinal complications are rare, but complications occur in >70% of cases when HbA_{1c} is >1.7 ULN.

Not presently recommended for diagnosis of diabetes mellitus although ~85% sensitivity and specificity each for screening.

Interpretation

Dietary preparation or fasting not required.
Low sensitivity but high specificity compared to OGTT, which has high sensitivity but low specificity in diagnosis of diabetes mellitus.

♦ Increase almost certainly means diabetes mellitus if other factors (see below) are absent (>3 SD above the mean has 99% specificity and ~48% sensitivity), but a normal value does not rule out impaired glucose tolerance. Values less than normal mean are not seen in untreated diabetes.

May rise within 1 wk after rise in blood glucose when therapy is stopped but may not fall for 2–4 wks after blood glucose decrease when therapy is resumed.

Mean blood glucose in first 30 days (days 0–30) before sampling glycated Hb contributes ~50% to final glycated Hb value, whereas mean blood glucose in days 90–120 contributes only ~10%. Time to reach a new steady state is 30–35 days.

When fasting blood glucose = <110 mg/dL, HbA_{1c} is normal in **>96%** of cases.[2]

When fasting blood glucose = 110–125 mg/dL, HbA_{1c} is normal in **>80%** of cases.[2]

When fasting blood glucose = >126 mg/dL, HbA_{1c} is normal in **>60%** of cases.[2]

Normal (A_{1a}, A_{1b}, A_{1c}) = 4–8%

For level of 4–20%, this formula may estimate daily average plasma glucose:

Mean daily plasma glucose (mg/dL) = 10 × (glycohemoglobin level + 4)

1% increase in glycohemoglobin is related to ~30 mg/dL increase in glucose.

Increased In

HbF above normal or 0.5% (e.g., heterozygous or homozygous persistence of HbF, feto-maternal transfusion during pregnancy)
Chronic renal failure with or without hemodialysis
Iron-deficiency anemia
Splenectomy
Increased serum triglycerides
Alcohol
Lead and opiate toxicity
Salicylate treatment

Decreased In

Shortened RBC life span
   Presence of HbS, HbC, HbD
   Hemolytic anemias (e.g., congenital spherocytosis)
   Acute or chronic blood loss
After transfusions
Pregnancy
Ingestion of large amounts (>1 gm/day) of vitamin C or E

Insulin, Plasma

Use

Diagnosis of insulinoma
Not clinically useful for diagnosis of diabetes mellitus

Increased In

Insulinoma. Fasting blood insulin level >50 μU/mL in presence of low or normal blood glucose level. IV tolbutamide or administration of leucine causes rapid rise of blood insulin to very high levels within a few minutes with rapid return to normal.
Factitious hypoglycemia (see p. 623)
Insulin autoimmune syndrome (p. 626)
Untreated obese patients with mild diabetes. The fasting level is often increased.
Patients with acromegaly (especially with active disease) after ingestion of glucose
Reactive hypoglycemia after glucose ingestion, particularly when diabetic type of glucose tolerance curve is present

---

[2]Davidson MB, et al. Relationship between fasting plasma glucose and glycosylated hemoglobin. Potential for false-positive diagnosis of type 2 diabetes using new diagnostic criteria. *JAMA* 1999;281:1203.

ENDOCRINE

Absent In

Severe diabetes mellitus with ketosis and weight loss. In less severe cases, insulin is frequently present but only at lower glucose concentrations.

Normal In

Hypoglycemia associated with nonpancreatic tumors
Idiopathic hypoglycemia of childhood, except after administration of leucine

Insulin/C-Peptide Ratio

Use

To differentiate insulinoma from factitious hypoglycemia due to insulin

Interpretation

<1.0 in molarity units (or >47.17 μg/ng in conventional units)
 • Increased endogenous insulin secretion (e.g., insulinoma, sulfonylurea administration)
 • Renal failure
>1.0 in molarity units (or <47.17 μg/ng in conventional units)
 • Exogenous insulin administration
 • Cirrhosis

Proinsulin

Proinsulin level is normally ≤ 20% of total insulin. Proinsulin is included in the immunoassay of total insulin, and separation requires special technique.

Increased In

Insulinoma. Proinsulin >30% of serum insulin after overnight fast suggests insulinoma.
Factitious hypoglycemia due to sulfonylurea use (see Table 13-14).
Familial hyperproinsulinemia—heterozygous mutation affecting cleavage of proinsulin, leading to secretion of excess amounts of proinsulin.
Non–insulin dependent diabetes mellitus

Interferences

May also be increased in renal disease.

Tolerance Test, Insulin

Administer 0.1 U insulin/kg body weight IV. *Use smaller dose if hypopituitarism is suspected. Always keep IV glucose available to prevent severe reaction.*

Normal

Blood glucose falls to 50% of fasting level within 20–30 mins; returns to fasting level within 90–120 mins.

Increased Tolerance In

Blood glucose falls <25% and returns rapidly to fasting level.
Hypothyroidism
Acromegaly
Cushing's syndrome
Diabetes mellitus (some patients; especially older, obese ones)

Decreased Tolerance In

Increased sensitivity to insulin (excessive fall of blood glucose)
Hypoglycemic irresponsiveness (lack of response by glycogenolysis)
 • Pancreatic islet cell tumor

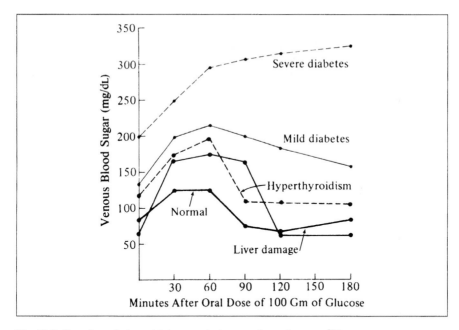

Fig. 13-8. Sample oral glucose tolerance test curves in various conditions.

- Adrenocortical insufficiency
- Adrenocortical insufficiency secondary to hypopituitarism
- Hypothyroidism
- von Gierke's disease (some patients)
- Starvation (depletion of liver glycogen)

Tolerance Test, Insulin Glucose

Administer simultaneously 0.1 U insulin/kg body weight IV and 0.8 gm glucose/kg body
   weight orally.
Insulin-sensitive diabetics show little change in blood sugar.
Insulin-resistant diabetics show a diabetic glucose tolerance curve.
Other changes parallel those in the insulin tolerance test.

Tolerance Test, Oral Glucose (OGTT)[3]

See Fig. 13-8.
Standards for OGTT: Prior diet of >150 gm of carbohydrate daily, no alcohol, and unrestricted activity for 3 days before test. Test in morning after 10–16 hrs of fasting. No
   medication, smoking, or exercise (remain seated) during test. Not to be done during
   recovery from acute illness, emotional stress, surgery, trauma, pregnancy, inactivity
   due to chronic illness; therefore is of limited or no value in hospitalized patients. Certain drugs should be stopped several weeks before the test (e.g., oral diuretics, oral
   contraceptives, phenytoin). Loading dose of glucose consumed within 5 mins: for
   adults = 75 gm, for children = 1.75 gm/kg (of ideal body weight in obese children but
   never >75 gm), for pregnant women = 100 gm. Draw blood at fasting, 30, 60, 90, 120
   mins; 30-min sample offers little additional information but can confirm adequate
   gastric absorption when patient is nauseous.

[3]Data from National Diabetes Data Group, 1978.

Use

OGTT should be reserved principally for patients with "borderline" fasting plasma glucose levels (i.e., fasting range 110–140 mg/dL).

All pregnant women should be tested for gestational diabetes with a 50-gm dose at 24–28 wks of pregnancy; if result is abnormal, OGTT should be performed after pregnancy.

OGTT is not indicated in
- Persistent fasting hyperglycemia (>140 mg/dL).
- Persistent fasting normoglycemia (<110 mg/dL).
- Patients with typical clinical findings of diabetes mellitus and random plasma glucose >200 mg/dL.
- Suspected gestational diabetes.
- Secondary diabetes (e.g., genetic hyperglycemic syndromes, after administration of certain hormones).
- Should never be performed to evaluate reactive hypoglycemia.
- Test is of limited value for diagnosis of diabetes mellitus in children and is rarely indicated for that purpose.

Interpretation

For diagnosis of diabetes mellitus in nonpregnant adults, at least two values of OGTT should be increased (or fasting serum glucose ≥ 140 mg/dL on more than one occasion) and other causes of transient glucose intolerance must be ruled out. See Classification of Diabetes Mellitus and Other Hyperglycemic Disorders, p. 615; Diabetes Mellitus, Gestational, p. 617.

Decreased Tolerance In

Excessive peak
- Increased absorption (normal IV GTT curve) with normal return to fasting level
- Mechanical causes (e.g., gastrectomy, gastroenterostomy)
- Hyperthyroidism
- Excess intake of glucose

Decreased utilization with slow fall to fasting level
- Diabetes mellitus
- Hyperlipidemia, types III, IV, V
- Hemochromatosis
- Steroid effect (Cushing's disease, administration of ACTH or steroids)
- CNS lesions

Decreased formation of glycogen with low fasting levels and subsequent hypoglycemia
- von Gierke's disease
- Severe liver damage
- Hyperthyroidism (normal return to fasting level)
- Increased epinephrine (stress, pheochromocytoma) (normal return to fasting level)
- Pregnancy (normal return to fasting level)

Drugs that may cause increased serum glucose and/or impaired glucose tolerance
- Hormones (e.g., oral contraceptives, thyroid hormone, ACTH or steroids, progestins)
- Antiinflammatory agents (e.g., indomethacin)
- Diuretic and antihypertensive drugs (e.g., thiazides, furosemide, clonidine)
- Neuroactive drugs (e.g., phenothiazines, tricyclics, lithium carbonate, haloperidol, adrenergic agonists)
- Others (e.g., isoniazid, heparin, cimetidine, nicotinic acid)

Increased Tolerance In

Flat peak
- Pancreatic islet cell hyperplasia or tumor
- Poor absorption from GI tract (normal IV GTT curve)
- Intestinal diseases (e.g., steatorrhea, sprue, celiac disease, Whipple's disease)
- Hypothyroidism
- Addison's disease
- Hypoparathyroidism

Late hypoglycemia
- Pancreatic islet cell hyperplasia or tumor

- Hypopituitarism
- Liver disease

See Glucose, p. 58, for effect of drugs.

Difficulty in interpretation has caused abandonment of other GTTs, such as IV GTT, cortisone GTT.

Tolerance Test, Tolbutamide

Administer 1 gm sodium tolbutamide IV within 2 mins. *Always keep IV glucose available to prevent severe reaction.*

Use

Most useful for diagnosis of insulinoma and to rule out functional hyperinsulinism.

Interpretation

In healthy persons, glucose is a more potent stimulus for insulin release than tolbutamide, but the opposite is true in insulinoma, which shows an exaggerated early insulin peak (3–5 mins after injection) with a sustained elevation of insulin and depression of glucose at 150 mins.

The fall in blood sugar is usually more marked in insulinoma than in functional hypoglycemia; more importantly, the blood sugar fails to recover even after 2–3 hrs. A mean serum glucose at 120, 150, and 180 mins after tolbutamide of ≤ 55 mg/dL in lean patients and 62 mg/dL in obese patients has a 95% specificity and >95% sensitivity for insulinoma; this is the most useful test.[4] Other calculations of glucose and insulin levels are less useful.

In functional hypoglycemia, return of blood sugar to normal is usually complete by 90 mins.

Adrenal insufficiency—normal or low curve

Severe liver disease—low curve

Diabetes Mellitus and Other Hyperglycemic and Hypoglycemic Disorders

Beckwith-Wiedemann Syndrome

(Inherited syndrome characterized by various abnormalities [e.g., macroglossia, umbilical hernia, gigantism that may be unilateral, abnormal ear lobe grooves, microcephaly])

Symptomatic hypoglycemia in ≤ 50% of patients, usually within first day, but may occur up to 3 days later; may be severe, difficult to control, and lasts for several months.

Hypocalcemia may occur.

Polycythemia may occur.

Cytogenetic studies are normal.

Classification of Diabetes Mellitus and Other Hyperglycemic Disorders[5]

I. Type I: immune-mediated beta cell destruction diabetes mellitus (formerly called insulin-dependent, juvenile-onset, ketosis-prone, or brittle diabetes mellitus); represents 10–20% of diabetic patients. Autoantibodies are present in 85–90% of cases. Insulin secretion is virtually absent. Plasma C-peptide low or undetectable. Other autoimmune disorders may be present (e.g., Graves' disease, Hashimoto's thyroiditis, Addison's disease, PA). No autoantibodies in 10–15% of cases; strongly inherited.

[4]McMahon MM, O'Brien PC, Service FJ. Diagnostic interpretation of the intravenous tolbutamide test for insulinoma. *Mayo Clin Proc* 1989;64:1481.

[5]Report of the Expert Committee on the Diagnosis and Classification of Diabetes Mellitus. *Diabetes Care* 1997;20:1183.

ENDOCRINE

II. Type 2 (formerly called non–insulin-dependent or adult-onset diabetes mellitus); represents 80–90% of diabetic patients. Varies from predominantly insulin resistance with relative deficiency to predominantly insulin secretory defect with insulin resistance. Relative rather than absolute insulin deficiency. Not due to autoimmunity or other disorders listed below. Plasma insulin may be normal or increased but expected to be higher relative to blood glucose concentration. Ketosis occurs with stress (e.g., infection) but seldom spontaneously. Associated with dyslipidemia, obesity, increasing age, hypertension, family history.

III. Other specific types, e.g.,
1. Genetic defects of beta cell function (e.g., chromosome 12, 7, 20). Formerly referred to as maturity-onset diabetes of the young. Onset of mild hyperglycemia, usually before age 25 yrs, and impaired insulin secretion. Autosomal dominant inheritance.
2. Genetic defects in insulin resistance (e.g., leprechaunism, type A insulin resistance, Rabson-Mendenhall syndrome, lipoatrophic diabetes)
3. Diseases of exocrine pancreas (e.g., pancreatitis, pancreatectomy, neoplasia, cystic fibrosis, hemochromatosis)
4. Endocrine disorders (e.g., Cushing's syndrome, acromegaly, pheochromocytoma, aldosteronoma, hyperthyroidism, glucagonoma)
5. Drug/chemical induced (e.g., glucocorticoids, phenytoin, beta-adrenergic agonists, pentamidine, thiazides, interferon-alpha)
6. Infections (e.g., CMV infection, congenital rubella)
7. Uncommon forms of immune-mediated diabetes (e.g., anti–insulin receptor antibodies, stiff-man syndrome)
8. Other genetic syndromes that may be associated with diabetes mellitus (e.g., Down syndrome, Klinefelter's syndrome, Turner's syndrome, Friedreich's ataxia, Huntington's chorea, Laurence-Moon-Biedl syndrome, porphyria, Prader-Willi syndrome)
9. Gestational diabetes mellitus (see below)

♦ *Criteria for Diagnosis*

Diabetes Mellitus
- Random glucose >200 mg/dL when classical symptoms are seen **or**
- Fasting (>8 hrs) serum glucose ≥ 126 mg/dL **or**
- 2-hr glucose >200 mg/dL after 75-gm glucose load. OGTT not recommended for routine use.
- Must be confirmed on another day by any of the previous tests.
- Fasting blood glucose ≥ 126 mg/dL = provisional diagnosis of diabetes mellitus; must be confirmed as noted previously.
- Diagnosis of "acute metabolic decompensation with hyperglycemia" need not be confirmed on a subsequent day.

Impaired Glucose Tolerance
- Fasting glucose ≥ 110 mg/dL but <126 mg/dL in nonpregnant adult.
- With OGTT, 2-hr value ≥ 140 and <200 mg/dL. Replaces terms *latent* and *chemical* diabetes.

Impaired Fasting Glucose
- Fasting glucose ≥ 110 mg/dL but <126 mg/dL **or**
- With OGTT, 2-hr value ≥ 140 but <200 mg/dL.

In absence of pregnancy, impaired glucose tolerance and impaired fasting glucose are risk factors for future diabetes mellitus and cardiovascular disease; not clinical entities.

Other causes of transient glucose intolerance must be ruled out before an unequivocal diagnosis of diabetes mellitus is made.

Test asymptomatic undiagnosed individuals every 3 yrs over age 45.

Test at younger age if
- HDL cholesterol is ≤ 35 mg/dL or triglyceride is ≥ 250 mg/dL.
- Previous impaired glucose tolerance or impaired fasting glucose.
- Obese.
- Has first-degree relative with diabetes mellitus.
- Member of high-risk ethnic population (e.g., black, Native American, Hispanic).
- Delivered baby weighing >9 pounds.

See sections on diabetic nephrosclerosis, papillary necrosis, GU tract infection, serum lipoproteins, etc.

Table 13-11. Differential Diagnosis of Diabetic Coma

Condition	Serum Glucose (mg/dL)	Serum Ketones (undiluted)	Blood pH	Serum Osmolality (mOsm/kg)	Serum Lactate (mmol/L)	Plasma Insulin
Diabetic ketoacidosis	300–1000	++++	D	300–350	2–3	0–L
Lactic acidosis	100–200	0	D	N–300	≥ 7	L
Alcoholic ketoacidosis	40–200	++++	D	290–310	2–6	L
Hyperosmolar coma	500–2000	0/+	N	320–400	1–2	Some
Hypoglycemia	10–40	0	N	285±6	Low	I

0 = none; + = small amount; up to ++++ = large amount; D = decreased; I = increased; L = low; N = normal.
Normal serum lactate = 0.6–1.1 mmol/L.
Lactic acidosis occurs in one-third of patients with diabetic ketoacidosis.
Hyperosmolar coma and alcoholic ketoacidosis may occur in diabetic ketoacidosis.

Coma, Nonketotic, Hyperosmolar Hyperglycemic

(Due to combination of severe dehydration caused by inadequate fluid intake and insulin deficiency; occurs predominantly in type II diabetes mellitus)
See Tables 13-11 and 13-12.
♦ Blood glucose is very high, often 600–2000 mg/dL, but contrary to expectation in diabetic coma, acidosis and ketosis are minimal and plasma acetone is not found.
♦ Serum osmolality is very high (normal = 280–300 mOsm/L) (see p. 68). In mildly drowsy patients, mean is 320 mOsm/L. At level of 350 mOsm/L, some confusion or some stupor is seen. At level >350 mOsm/L, many patients are in coma. At 400 mOsm/L, most patients are obtunded. State of consciousness does not correlate with height of acidemia.
○ Serum sodium may be increased, normal, or decreased but is disproportionately decreased for degree of dehydration due to marked hyperglycemia (artifactual decrease 1.6 mEq/L for every 100 mg/dL increase of serum glucose).
• Increased sodium with marked hyperglycemia indicates severe dehydration.
Serum potassium may be increased (due to hyperosmolality), low (due to osmotic diuresis with urinary loss), or normal depending on balance of factors.
BUN is increased (70–90 mg/dL) more than in diabetic ketoacidosis.
Laboratory findings due to complications or precipitating factors
• Renal insufficiency in 90% of cases
• Infection (e.g., pneumonia)
• Drugs (e.g., steroids, phenytoin, potassium-wasting diuretics such as thiazides and furosemide, others [propranolol, diazoxide, azathioprine])
• Other medical conditions (e.g., cerebrovascular or cardiovascular accident, subdural hematoma, severe burns, acute pancreatitis, thyrotoxicosis, Cushing's syndrome)
• Glucose overloading or use of concentrated glucose solutions (e.g., hyperalimentation, dialysis, IV infusions in treatment of burns)
• Spontaneous in 5–7% of cases
• Preexisting mild diabetes mellitus type II
• Dehydration
Clinical picture: A middle-aged or older person with diabetes of recent onset or unrecognized diabetes, who shows neurologic symptoms (e.g., convulsions or hemiplegia) and then becomes stuporous or comatose

Diabetes Mellitus, Gestational

Hyperglycemia that develops for the first time during pregnancy; affects ~4% of pregnant women; most have return to normal glucose tolerance after delivery. 60% become diabetic in next 16 yrs.

ENDOCRINE

Table 13-12. Comparison of Diabetic Ketoacidosis and Hyperosmolar Hyperglycemic Nonketotic Coma

	Diabetic Ketoacidosis	Hyperosmolar Hyperglycemic Nonketotic Coma
Laboratory findings		
Serum glucose	Usually <800 mg/dL	>800 mg/dL
Plasma acetone	Positive in diluted plasma	Less positive in undiluted plasma
Serum sodium	Usually low	Normal, I, or low
Serum potassium	Normal, I, or low	Normal or I
Serum HCO_3^-	<10 mEq/L	>16 mEq/L
Anion gap	>12 mEq/L	10–12 mEq/L
Blood pH	<7.35	Normal
Serum osmolality	<330 mOsm/L	>350 mOsm/L
Serum BUN	Not as high	Higher
Blood free fatty acids	>1500 mEq/L	<1000 mEq/L
Clinical findings		
Dehydration	Less	More
Acidosis	More	Less
Coma	Rare	Frequent
Hyperventilation	Yes	No
Age	Younger	Usually elderly
Diabetes type	I—insulin dependent	II—non–insulin dependent
Previous history of diabetes	Almost always	50% of cases
Prodrome	<1 day	Several days
Neurologic findings	Rare	Very common
Cardiovascular or renal disease	15%	85%
Thrombosis	Very rare	Frequent
Mortality	<10%	20–50%

Diagnosis is necessary for short-term identification of increased risk of fetal morbidity (stillbirth, macrosomia, birth trauma, hypoglycemia, hyperbilirubinemia, hypocalcemia, polycythemia).

Screening of all pregnant women should include
- Random (need not be fasting) venous blood glucose 1 hr after ingestion of 50 gm of glucose at 24–28 wks' gestation. Values >140 mg/dL are indication for 3-hr GTT with 100 gm glucose. 1-hr, 50-gm test is abnormal in ~15% of pregnant women, ~14% of whom have abnormal 3-hr OGTT. Sensitivity is ~79%, specificity is ~87%.

◆ Diagnostic Criteria

At least two of the following glucose plasma levels are found on OGTT with 100-gm glucose loading dose:

Fasting   ≥ 105 mg/dL
1 hr   ≥ 190 mg/dL
2 hrs   ≥ 165 mg/dL
3 hrs   ≥ 145 mg/dL

If abnormal results during pregnancy, repeat GTT at first postpartum visit; if GTT is normal, diagnose as diabetes mellitus only during pregnancy, but blood glucose should be tested at every subsequent visit because of increased risk (30% during next 5–10 yrs) of developing diabetes mellitus. If postpartum GTT is abnormal, classify as impaired glucose tolerance, impaired fasting glucose, or diabetes mellitus using above criteria.

Glycosylated Hb and fructosamine are not recommended tests for detection of gestational diabetes.

For management of diabetes mellitus during pregnancy, goal is fasting plasma glucose of 60–110 mg/dL and postprandial levels of <150 mg/dL. Measure serum or 24-hr urine estriol for fetal surveillance. Amniotic fluid lecithin/sphingomyelin ratio, phosphatidylglycerol, shake test, or fluorescence polarization to evaluate fetal pulmonary maturity.

During labor, keep maternal glucose at 80–100 mg/dL; beware of markedly increased insulin sensitivity in immediate postpartum period.

Laboratory Evaluation of Fetus

During third trimester, urinary estriol level is used as indicator of fetoplacental integrity.

> Placental function is also indicated by hCG, human placental lactogen, estradiol, and progesterone levels (see p. 773). Lecithin/sphingomyelin ratio measured on amniotic fluid is used to predict pulmonary maturity.

At time of cesarean section, before opening amniotic sac, obtain sterile sample of amniotic fluid for culture, Gram stain, lecithin/sphingomyelin ratio.

Diabetes Mellitus, Neonatal

Blood glucose is often between 245 and 2300 mg/dL.
Metabolic acidosis of some degree is usually present.
Ketonuria is variable.
Laboratory findings due to dehydration
Laboratory findings due to infection or CNS lesions, which are present in one-third of patients
Has been detected as early as fourth day. Usually is transient.
Increased association with postmaturity, low birth weight, neonatal hypoglycemia, steroid therapy early in neonatal period.

Laboratory Evaluation of Infant

47% risk of hypoglycemia	Check blood glucose at 1, 2, 3, 6, 12, 24, 36, 48 hrs
22% risk of hypocalcemia	Check blood calcium at 6, 12, 24, 48 hrs
34% risk of polycythemia	Check Hct at 1, 24 hrs
19% risk of hyperbilirubinemia	Check serum bilirubin at 24, 48 hrs
Sixfold increased risk of hyaline membrane disease	During first hour of life, examine gastric aspirate with Gram stain for bacteria and PMNs and perform shake test for lecithin/sphingomyelin

ENDOCRINE

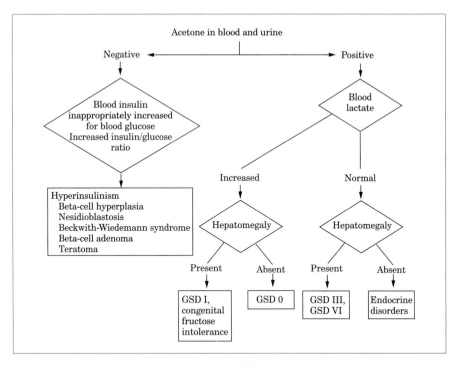

Fig. 13-9. Algorithm for neonatal hypoglycemia. (GSD = glycogen storage disease.)

9% risk of major congenital anomalies (e.g., cardiac, renal) and other problems (e.g., renal vein thrombosis, excess mucus)

Check blood gases for evaluation of ear, nose, and throat, umbilicus, rectum, urine, blood, CSF, gastric aspirate

Glucagonoma

(Arise from alpha cells of pancreatic islets. 60% are malignant.)
Diabetes mellitus
Anemia
♦ Increased serum insulin level is characteristic.
♦ Increased serum level of glucagon. Serum proglucagon is also increased occasionally.
○ Clinical clue is association of dermatitis (necrolytic migratory erythema) with insulin-requiring diabetes.

Hyperglycemia, with Heterogeneous Genetic Diseases

Alström's syndrome
Ataxia-telangiectasia
Diabetes mellitus
Friedreich's ataxia
Hemochromatosis
Herrmann's syndrome
Hyperlipoproteinemias (three different types)
Isolated growth hormone (GH) deficiency
Laurence-Moon-Bardet-Biedl syndrome
Lipoatrophic diabetes
Myotonic dystrophy
Optic atrophy

Prader-Willi syndrome
Refsum's syndrome
Schmidt's syndrome
Werner's syndrome

Hypoglycemia, Classification

See Table 13-13.
♦ Diagnosis requires triad of low blood glucose at the time of spontaneous hypoglycemic
  symptoms and alleviation by administration of glucose that corrects hypoglycemia.
  (Glucose concentration is 15% lower in whole blood than in serum or plasma.)
Reactive (i.e., after eating)
- Alimentary (rapid gastric emptying, e.g., after subtotal gastrectomy, vagotomy)
- Impaired glucose tolerance as in diabetes mellitus (mild maturity onset)
- Functional (idiopathic)
- Rare conditions (e.g., hereditary fructose intolerance, galactosemia, familial fruc-
  tose and galactose intolerance)
Fasting (spontaneous)—almost always indicates organic disease
- Liver—severe parenchymal disease (including sepsis, congestive heart failure,
  Reye's syndrome) or enzyme defect (e.g., glycogen storage diseases, galactosemia)
- Chronic renal insufficiency
- Pancreatic
  Insulinoma (pancreatic islet cell tumor)
  MEN type I
  Pancreatic hyperplasia
- Deficiency of hormones that oppose insulin (e.g., decreased function of thyroid,
  anterior pituitary, or adrenal cortex)
- Postoperative removal of pheochromocytoma
- Large extrapancreatic tumors (65% are intra- or retroperitoneal fibromas or sar-
  comas)
- Certain epithelial tumors (e.g., hepatoma, carcinoid, Wilms' tumor)
- Drugs (including factitious use)
  Insulin
  Sulfonylureas
  Alcohol
  Salicylates
  Pentamidine
  Quinine
  Propranolol (rare)
  Others may potentiate effect of sulfonylurea (e.g., sulfonamides, butazones,
    coumarins, clofibrate)
- Artifactual (high WBC or RBC count, e.g., leukemia or polycythemia)
- Starvation, anorexia nervosa, lactic acidosis, intense exercise
- Insulin antibodies or insulin receptor antibodies
Combined reactive and fasting types
- Insulinoma
- Adrenal insufficiency
- Insulin antibodies or insulin receptor antibodies

Infants

See Fig. 13-9.
Transient (<14 days)
Symptomatic or asymptomatic; occurs in 1–3 in 1000 full-term infants
- Maternal (e.g., diabetes, toxemia, complicated labor or delivery)
- Infant, e.g.,
  Prematurity, small size for gestational age
  Intrauterine malnutrition
  Erythroblastosis
  Secondary, e.g., sepsis, asphyxia, anoxia, cerebral or subdural hemorrhage
  Congenital anomalies
  Iatrogenic, e.g., postoperative complications, abrupt cessation of glucose infu-
    sion, after exchange transfusion, cold injury

ENDOCRINE

Table 13-13. Laboratory Interpretation of 72-Hr Fast for Hypoglycemia

	Glucose (mg/dL)	Insulin (μU/mL)	C-Peptide (mmol/L)	Proinsulin (pmol/L)	Beta-hydroxybutyrate (mmol/L)	Change in Glucose (mg/dL)
Normal[a]	≥ 40	<6	<0.2	<5	>2.7	<25
Insulinoma	≤ 45	≥ 6	≤ 0.2	≥ 5	≤ 2.7	≥ 25
Factitious						
Insulin	≤ 45	≥ 6	<0.2	<5	≤ 2.7	≥ 25
Sulfonylurea[b]	≤ 45	≥ 6	≥ 0.2	≥ 5	≤ 2.7	≥ 25
Insulin-like growth factor	≤ 45	≤ 6	<0.2	<5	≤ 2.7	≥ 25
Not insulin-mediated hypoglycemia	≤ 45	<6	<0.2	<5	>2.7	<25
Eating during 72-hr "fast"[a]	≥ 45	<6	<0.2	<5	≤ 2.7	≥ 25
Nonhypoglycemic syndrome	≥ 40	<6	<0.2	<5	>2.7	<25

[a]Not symptomatic; all others have signs or symptoms.
[b]Sulfonylurea in plasma only if patient has taken this drug. Tolbutamide detection is a separate analysis.
All blood measurements should be performed on the same specimen drawn at start and end of fast and every 6 hrs until plasma glucose is ≤ 60 mg/dL; then every 1–2 hrs.
Terminate when patient has hypoglycemic signs or symptoms *and* plasma glucose is ≤ 45 mg/dL.
Draw specimens for cortisol, growth hormone, glucagon at beginning and end of fast if deficiency of these is suspected.
Diagnosis of reactive hypoglycemia is based on decreased blood glucose at time of signs and symptoms with improvement by eating and a repetitive pattern of occurrence.
Diagnosis should not be based on glucose tolerance test, since 25% of healthy young men may have postprandial glucose <50 mg/dL and 2–3% of subjects may have level <40 mg/dL.
Diagnosis of "nonhypoglycemic syndrome"—normal blood glucose associated with symptoms similar to those in hypoglycemia.
Source: Service FJ. Hypoglycemic disorders. *N Engl J Med* 1995;332:1144.

Persistent

Hyperinsulinism
- Beta cell hyperplasia
- Nesidioblastosis
- Beckwith-Wiedemann syndrome (children also have Wilms' and other embryonal tumors, visceromegaly, macroglossia)
- Beta cell tumor
- Teratoma

Endocrine disorder
- Hypothyroidism
- Congenital adrenal hyperplasia (CAH)
- Anterior pituitary hypofunction
- Decreased glucagon

Hepatic enzyme deficiencies
- Glycogen storage disease types I, III, VI, 0
- Congenital fructose intolerance
- Galactose 1-phosphate deficiency

Maple syrup urine disease
Galactosemia
Hereditary tyrosinemia
Methylmalonic acidemia
Propionicacidemia

Hypoglycemia, Factitious

See Tables 13-13 and 13-14, Fig. 13-10.

Due to Insulin

♦ During hypoglycemic episode, high insulin and low C-peptide levels in serum confirm diagnosis of exogenous insulin administration (diagnostic triad). (Increased endogenous insulin secretion is always associated with increased secretion of C-peptide, which is the part of the proinsulin molecule cleaved off when insulin is secreted and therefore is produced in equimolar amounts with insulin.)

Insulin/glucose ratio >0.3 in serum (normal is <0.3). Increased ratio is also seen in autonomous production due to insulinoma.

♦ Extreme elevations of serum insulin (e.g., >1000 μU/mL) suggest factitious hypoglycemia (fasting levels in patients with insulinoma are rarely >200 μU/mL).

Insulin antibodies appear in 90% of persons injected with beef or pork insulin and 50% of those injected with human insulin for more than a few weeks but are almost never present in persons not taking insulin (rarely occur on an autoimmune basis), although this indicator may be less useful with the future use of more purified and human insulin.

Due to Sulfonylureas

Biochemically indistinguishable from insulinoma (increased serum C-peptide and insulin levels with insulin/C-peptide molar ratio <1.0).

♦ Specific chemical assay can identify the agent in serum or urine.

Due to Tolbutamide

♦ Acidification of urine causes a white precipitate due to formation of carboxytolbutamide.

Hypoglycemia, Leucine-Induced

Symptoms within 30 mins of consumption of high-protein meal or after prolonged fast. May be neonatal or appear later in first year; symptoms become increasingly severe; tends to improve spontaneously by 4–6 yrs of age.

Blood glucose falls >50% within 20–45 mins after oral administration of L-leucine. *Same result in 70% of patients with insulinoma.*

ENDOCRINE

Table 13-14. Comparison of Laboratory Findings in Causes of Hypoglycemia

	Insulinoma	Factitious		Insulin Autoimmune Syndrome
		Exogenous Insulin	Sulfonylurea	
Serum insulin	High; usually <200 µU/mL Occasionally very low because serum has a very high proinsulin level that interferes with the insulin immunoassay	Very high; often up to 2000 µU/mL	High	High
Serum C-peptide	Inappropriate I; parallels serum insulin Insulin infusion suppresses the C-peptide levels in normal case but not in insulinoma	Not I; does not parallel serum insulin	N or L	Disproportionately not as high as serum insulin indicates the possible presence of these antibodies >1.0 in molarity units
Serum insulin/C-peptide ratio during hypoglycemia	>1.0 in molarity units (or <47.17 µU/ng in conventional units)	<1.0 in molarity units		
Insulin antibodies	Absent	Present after using beef or pork insulin for more than a few weeks Species-specific for beef or pork insulin Present in 50% after using human insulin	Absent	Very high levels, fall rapidly
Serum proinsulin (is ≤ 20% of total insulin in normal persons)	I in ~95% of cases	N or L	I	
Other	Fasting provokes hypoglycemia Infusion of fish insulin (not measured by assay for human insulin) does not suppress serum insulin in insulinoma but does in normal persons		Demonstration of sulfonylurea or tolbutamide in urine	Other autoimmune syndromes may be present May be receiving drugs containing sulfhydryl groups

I = increased; N = normal; L = low.

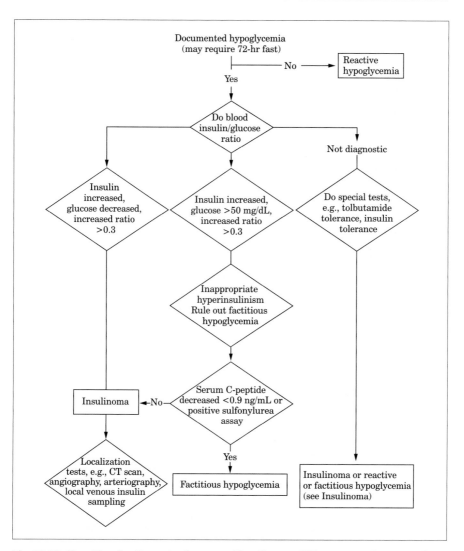

Fig. 13-10. Algorithm for diagnosis of suspected insulinoma. (CT = computed tomography.)

Hypoglycemia, Neonatal

♦ Diagnostic Criteria

Plasma glucose <25 mg/dL in low-birth-weight infants.

Plasma glucose <35 mg/dL in normal-birth-weight infants in first 72 hrs. Plasma glucose <45 mg/dL in normal-birth-weight infants after 72 hrs.

Make diagnosis on basis of two abnormal glucose values, e.g., two plasma levels, one plasma and one CSF level.

- Plasma glucose values are 14% higher than whole blood values.
- Capillary blood samples should be taken from warm heel and transported to laboratory on ice (at room temperature, blood glucose level decreases by 18 mg/dL/hr).
- Determination by measurement of reducing substances may give falsely elevated levels for glucose because in blood of newborns, non–glucose-reducing substances

ENDOCRINE

may range up to 60 mg/dL. Therefore use techniques that measure glucose specifically, e.g., glucose oxidase.
• Bedside glucose monitor utilizing dipsticks should not be used for this diagnosis—is not reliable in the low glucose range.

Due To

Transient symptomatic or asymptomatic hypoglycemia may be associated with delayed feeding, toxemia, perinatal asphyxia, twin birth, hypothermia, or low birth weight, or may be idiopathic. Occurs in 1–3 in 1000 full-term infants.
Hyperinsulinism (e.g., maternal diabetes, erythroblastosis, Beckwith-Wiedemann syndrome, insulinoma, maternal drug therapy or starvation)
Hormone deficiencies (e.g., hypothyroidism, pituitary hypofunction, adrenal insufficiency or unresponsiveness)
Hereditary metabolic disorders
• Galactosemia
• Type I glycogen storage disease
• Amino acid disorders (e.g., tyrosinemia type I)
• Organic acid disorders (e.g., methylmalonicacidemia, propionicacidemia)
• Carnitine deficiency disorders (e.g., carnitine palmityl transferase deficiency)
• Disorders of fat oxidation (e.g., medium-chain acyl-CoA dehydrogenase deficiency)
• Disorders of gluconeogenesis (e.g., pyruvate carboxylase deficiency)
Others
• Iatrogenic (e.g., after exchange transfusion)
• Miscellaneous (e.g., sepsis diarrheal illness, CNS abnormalities, congenital heart disease)

Infants of Diabetic Mothers

Blood glucose is <30 mg/dL in ≤ 50% of infants of diabetic mothers; usually asymptomatic; usually within first hours after birth. Hypocalcemia is common in these cases and occurs at 24–36 hrs after birth.
Glucose levels should be checked every hour for first 6 hrs of life.

Insulin Autoimmune Syndrome

(Cause is unknown but patients may be receiving drugs containing a sulfhydryl group [e.g., pyritinol]. Associated with other autoimmune syndromes [e.g., hyperthyroidism, autoimmune thrombocytopenia with primary biliary cirrhosis]. Appears to be a self-limiting condition.)
Fasting hypoglycemia.
○Elevated serum insulin and C-peptide levels that are discordant (insulin/C-peptide molar ratio >1.0) indicates the possible presence of these antibodies. These elevations are artifactual due to effect of antibody on assay method.
May be difficult to distinguish from factitious hypoglycemia.
♦Extremely high levels of antiinsulin antibodies that rapidly decrease.
Never any prior exposure to exogenous insulin.

Insulinoma

(Tumor of pancreatic islet beta cell origin; most often benign solitary tumor but ~5% are malignant; 5–10% of patients may have MEN type I, see p. 697.)
See Fig. 13-10 and Tables 13-13 and 13-14.
♦*In patients with fasting hypoglycemia, insulinoma should be considered the cause until another diagnosis can be proved.* No single test is certain to be diagnostic; multiple tests may be required.
♦Fasting 24–36 hrs provokes hypoglycemia in 80–90% of these patients; 72 hrs of fasting provokes hypoglycemia in >95% of these patients, especially if punctuated with exercise. Absence of ketonuria implies surreptitious food intake or excess insulin effect (differentiate by blood glucose level). Low serum glucose and high serum insulin establishes the diagnosis, i.e., insulin level is inappropriately elevated for the degree of hypoglycemia (in normal persons, insulin level becomes <5 μU/mL or unde-

tectable). *Serum insulin rarely reaches these high levels in patients with reactive hypoglycemia.* Serum C-peptide is similarly inappropriately elevated, in contrast to factitious hypoglycemia. In women, serum glucose can fall to 20–30 mg/dL during fasting and return to normal without treatment; in men, a fall in serum glucose to <50 mg/dL is considered abnormal.

♦ Serum insulin/C-peptide ratio is <1.0 in molarity units.

♦ Proinsulin level is normally ≤ 20% of total insulin; increased in insulinoma.

♦ Proinsulin >30% of serum insulin after overnight fast suggests insulinoma. (May also be increased in renal disease.) *(Proinsulin is included in the immunoassay of total insulin and separation requires special technique.)*

Serum insulin values are not useful in reactive hypoglycemia but should always be measured in cases of fasting hypoglycemia.

Occasional patients with insulinoma have very low serum insulin levels; their serum shows very high proinsulin level that interferes with the insulin immunoassay, giving falsely low values.

♦ Serum insulin/glucose ratio >0.3 when serum glucose >50 mg/dL indicates inappropriate hyperinsulinism, and this usually indicates insulinoma if factitious hypoglycemia is ruled out. Ratio may be slightly higher (e.g., ≤ 0.35 in obese persons). Has no diagnostic value in insulinoma.

Stimulation tests are not usually necessary and may be dangerous if serum glucose <50 mg/dL. Too many false-positive and false-negative results make these tests unreliable.

• Tolbutamide tolerance test: see p. 615.

• Glucagon stimulation test: Administer 1 mg of glucagon IV during 1–2 mins; measure serum insulin three times at 5-min intervals and then twice at 15-min intervals. Patients with insulinoma show an exaggerated response of serum immunoreactive insulin. Serum insulin >100 μU/mL after glucagon stimulation in a patient with fasting hypoglycemia and inappropriate insulin secretion strongly suggests insulinoma.

• Infusion of exogenous insulin to reduce serum glucose level also suppresses the secretion of insulin and of C-peptide in normal persons but not in patients with insulinoma. C-peptide level usually remains elevated if insulinoma is present (C-peptide is also not suppressed in islet cell hyperplasia and nesidioblastosis) but falls to very low level if beta cell function is normal.

OGTT is useless for diagnosis; results may be normal, flat (in ~20% of healthy persons), or show impaired tolerance.

After overnight fast, reference ranges are

• Serum insulin: 1–25 μU/mL.

• Serum proinsulin: <20% of total measurable insulin.

• Serum C-peptide: 1–2 ng/mL.

• Ratio of insulin to glucose: <0.3 (up to 0.35 in obese persons). During fasting, ratio decreases in healthy persons and increases in insulinoma patients.

Ketoacidosis, Diabetic

See Tables 13-11, 13-12.

♦ Blood glucose is increased (usually >300 mg/dL); range from slightly increased to very high. Very increased glucose (>500–800 mg/dL) suggests nonketotic hyperosmolar hyperglycemia (because glucose levels become very high only when extracellular fluid volume is markedly decreased). Glucose level of <200 mg/dL may occur, especially in alcoholics or pregnant women with insulin-dependent diabetes. Glucose concentration is not related to severity of diabetic ketoacidosis.

♦ Plasma acetone is increased (4+ reaction when plasma is diluted 1:1 with water). (Acetone is usually 3–4× the concentration of acetoacetate but does not contribute to acidosis.) Nitroprusside reagent tests (e.g., Acetest, Ketostix, Chemstrip) react with acetoacetate, not with beta-hydroxybutyrate, weakly with acetone; therefore weak positive reaction with ketone does not rule out ketoacidosis. Beta-hydroxybutyrate/acetoacetate ratio varies from 3:1 in mild cases to 15:1 in severe diabetic ketoacidosis. With correction of diabetic ketoacidosis, conversion of beta-hydroxybutyrate to acetoacetate gives a stronger nitroprusside test reaction; do not mistake this for worsening of diabetic ketoacidosis.

Urine ketone tests are not reliable for diagnosing or monitoring diabetic ketoacidosis. May be positive in ≤ 30% of first morning specimens in pregnancy.

False-positive results reported in presence of some sulfhydryl drugs (e.g., captopril). False-negative results may occur with highly acidic urine, after large doses of ascorbic acid, or when test strips are exposed in air for extended time.

♦ Metabolic acidosis (pH <7.3 and/or bicarbonate <15 mEq/L) is mainly due to beta-hydroxybutyrate and acetoacetate. Some lactic acidosis may exist, especially if shock, sepsis, or tissue necrosis is present; suspect this if pH and AG do not respond to insulin therapy. Whole spectrum of patterns from pure hyperchloremic acidosis to wide-AG acidosis. May be obscured by complicating metabolic alkalosis.

♦ Volume and electrolyte depletion (due to glucose-induced osmotic diuresis)
  • Absence of volume depletion should arouse suspicion of other possibilities (e.g., hypoglycemic coma, other causes of coma).
  • Very low sodium (120 mEq/L) is usually due to hypertriglyceridemia and hyperosmolality although occasionally may be dilutional due to vomiting and water intake. Low in 67%, normal in 26%, increased in 7% of cases. Depleted body stores are not reflected in these initial values, which reflect relative water loss and blood glucose level.
  • Serum potassium is normal in 43%, increased in 39% due to potassium exit from cells secondary to acidosis; initial low potassium in 18% of cases indicates severe depletion.
  • Serum phosphate decreased in 10% of cases, normal in 18%, and increased in 71%; falls with onset of therapy due to loss by osmotic diuresis and cellular uptake. Severe depletion (<0.5 mg/dL) may cause muscle weakness, rhabdomyolysis, impaired cardiac function, etc. Excessive replacement may cause hypocalcemia and hypomagnesemia.
  • Serum magnesium may be decreased in 7% (in prolonged ketoacidosis), normal in 25%, increased in 68% of cases.

Azotemia is present (BUN is usually 25–30 mg/dL); creatinine may be proportionally increased more than BUN due to methodologic interference by acetoacetate.

Serum osmolality is slightly increased (up to 340 mOsm/L).

WBC is increased (often >20,000/cu mm) even without infection; associated with decreased lymphocytes and eosinophils.

Hb, Hct, total protein may be increased due to intravascular volume depletion.

Serum amylase may be increased (may originate from salivary glands rather than pancreas) in ≤ 36% of patients; increase from both sources in 16% of cases.

Serum AST, ALT, LD, and CK are increased in 20–65% of cases, partly due to methodologic interference of acetoacetate in colorimetric methods. CK may be increased due to phosphate depletion and rhabdomyolysis.

Thyroid function tests are not reliable (due to sick thyroid syndrome).

Laboratory findings due to complications in treatment
  • Hypoglycemia
  • Hypokalemia
  • Alkalosis
  • Arterial thrombosis (e.g., organ infarction, limb ischemia)
  • Cerebral edema

Laboratory findings due to precipitating medical problem (e.g., infection, myocardial infarction, vascular disorder, trauma, pregnancy, emotional problem, endocrine disorder; not found in 25% of cases); these should always be sought.

See Acidosis, Metabolic, Acidosis, Lactic, Nonketotic hyperglycemic coma (see p. 617)

Follow-up laboratory tests every 2–4 hrs initially and less often with clinical improvement. Bedside fingerstick glucose test can be performed initially every 30–60 mins to determine rate of fall of glucose and when to add glucose to IV fluids.

ESR may be increased in diabetic patients even in absence of infection and when serum protein is normal, particularly when glycemic control is poor; does not necessarily indicate underlying infection.

Prader-Willi Syndrome

(Mental retardation, muscular hypotonia, obesity, short stature, and hypogonadism associated with diabetes mellitus)

Diabetes mellitus frequently develops in childhood and adolescence but is insulin resistant, responds to oral hypoglycemic drugs, and is not accompanied by acidosis.

Somatostatinoma

(Rare condition)
Diabetes mellitus that improves after resection of the tumor
Hypochlorhydria
Steatorrhea
Occasionally anemia is present.

Tumors of Pancreas (Hormone-Secreting), Primary

Cell Type	Hormone Secreted	Tumor
B cell	Insulin	Insulinoma
D cell	Gastrin	Gastrinoma (see p. 629)
A cell	Glucagon	Glucagonoma (see p. 620)
H cell	VIP	Vipoma (see p. 629)
D cell	Somatostatin	Somatostatinoma (see p. 629)
HPP cell	Human pancreatic poly-peptide (HPP)	HPP-secreting tumor (very rare tumor)

Other rare hormone-secreting tumors have been identified as causing ectopic ACTH syndrome, atypical carcinoid syndrome, SIADH, ectopic hypercalcemia syndrome.

Tumors of Pancreas (Islet Cell), Classification

Insulin-secreting beta cell tumor (may be benign or malignant, primary or metastatic) produces hyperinsulinism with hypoglycemia.
Non–insulin-secreting non–beta cell tumor (benign or malignant, primary or metastatic) may produce several types of syndromes.
• Z-E syndrome.
• Profuse diarrhea with hypokalemia and dehydration.
• Profuse diarrhea with hypokalemia (and sometimes periodic paralysis) may occur as a separate syndrome without peptic ulceration. *(Some patients have histamine-fast achlorhydria.)* Diabetic-type glucose tolerance curves may occur in some patients because of chronic potassium depletion. May be associated with MEN.
• Nonspecific diarrhea.
• Steatorrhea (due to inactivation of pancreatic enzymes by acid pH).

Vipoma

(Secreted by specialized endocrine cells of the amine precursor uptake and decarboxylation system that inhibit gastric acid production and stimulate gastrointestinal secretion of water and electrolytes; most tumors are found in pancreas but ~30% are extrapancreatic, e.g., bronchogenic carcinoma, pheochromocytoma, ganglioneuroblastoma. 60% are malignant.)
♦ Voluminous watery diarrhea (6–10 L/day) with dehydration
Hypokalemia that may be associated with hypokalemic nephropathy
Metabolic acidosis
Hypercalcemia in 50% of cases
Abnormal OGTT
Achlorhydria or hypochlorhydria
♦ Increased plasma VIP >75 pg/mL. RIA may show cross reactivity with other gastrointestinal hormones. (Should be collected in special chilled syringe containing EDTA and a plasma protease inhibitor and frozen immediately after centrifugation.) Specificity is >88% and positive predictive value is 86% (varies among laboratories). Increased values may also occur in patients with cutaneous mastocytoma, severe hepatic failure, or portocaval shunts.

Zollinger-Ellison (Z-E) Syndrome (Gastrinoma)[6]

See Table 13-15.
Due to gastrinomas (non–beta cell tumors often arising in pancreas)

[6]Jensen RT, Fraker DL. Zollinger-Ellison syndrome. Advances in treatment of gastric hypersecretion and the gastrinoma. *JAMA* 1994;271:1429.

Table 13-15. Serum Gastrin Response to Provocative Tests in Hypergastrinemia

Cause	Secretin Injection	Calcium Infusion	Test Meal
Gastrinoma (Z-E syndrome)	I >200 pg/mL (95 pM) over basal	I >400 pg/mL (190 pM) over basal	I <50% over basal or NC
Hypochlorhydric states	I <200 pg/mL, D, or NC	Small I or NC	I <50% over basal or NC
Antral–G cell hyperplasia	I <200 pg/mL	Small I or NC	I >100% over basal
Ordinary duodenal cancer	I<200 pg/mL	Small I	Moderate I
Others (e.g., excluded gastric antrum, gastric outlet obstruction, small intestine resection, thyrotoxicosis)	I <200 pg/mL, D or NC	Small I or NC	I >50% over basal

D = decrease; I = increase; NC = no change.

- *Tumors are multiple* in 28% of patients and may be ectopic (e.g., >50% are in duodenal wall; 9% are extrapancreatic and extraintestinal; selective venous sampling for gastrin may be helpful for localizing tumor).
- *Tumors are malignant* in 62% of patients; 34% of patients have metastases.
- *Diffuse hyperplasia* occurs in 10% of patients.

◆ Increased basal serum gastrin. Fasting serum gastrin >1000 pg/mL and basal acid output >15 mEq/hr with recurrent peptic ulcer is virtually diagnostic. Level of >500 pg/mL (normal <100 pg/mL) is highly suggestive of gastrinoma in absence of achlorhydria or renal failure. Level of <100 pg/mL is unlikely to be gastrinoma. 100–500 pg/mL occurs in ~40% of gastrinoma patients and ~10% of ulcer patients without gastrinoma. If fasting serum gastrin is increased but is <1000 pg/mL, secretin-provocative test and acid secretory rate test should be performed.

◆ IV injection of secretin (1–2 U/kg body weight) is the most sensitive and accurate provocative test. This provokes an increase of serum gastrin ≥ 110 pg/mL within 10 mins. Some ulcer patients may have serum gastrin increase of ≤ 200 pg/mL. Serum gastrin decreases in most nongastrinoma patients. Negative response occurs in ~5% of gastrinoma patients. Selective injection of secretin into gastroduodenal artery causes serum gastrin to increase >50% in 30 secs in hepatic or portal vein blood (both should be sampled). Postoperative fasting serum gastrin and secretin levels are both necessary to determine cure.

Other provocative tests such as IV injection of calcium gluconate (4 mg of calcium/kg) or ingestion of a standard test meal are not as sensitive or specific as secretin test. Response after calcium infusion is positive if serum gastrin is ≥ 395 pg/mL.

◆ There is a large volume of highly acidic gastric juice in the absence of pyloric obstruction. (12-hr nocturnal secretion shows acid of >100 mEq/L and volume of >1500 mL; baseline secretion is >60% of the secretion caused by histamine or betazole stimulation.) It is refractory to vagotomy and subtotal gastrectomy. Hypochlorhydria (basal pH >3) or achlorhydria excludes diagnosis of Z-E syndrome (see Gastric Analysis, p. 159).

◆ Basal acid output is >15 mEq/hr (normal is <10 mEq/hr) in 90% of cases if no previous gastric surgery was done or >5 mEq/hr if previous vagotomy or gastric resection was performed. Ratio of basal acid output to maximal output >0.6 strongly favors gastrinoma, but false-positive and false-negative results are common. If basal acid output determination is not possible, pH >3 excludes Z-E syndrome if patient is not on antisecretory drugs. Fasting serum gastrin >1000 pg/mL and gastric pH

<2.5 almost certainly indicates Z-E syndrome; both should be measured because they may be a poorly correlated in individual patients.

Hypokalemia is frequently associated with chronic severe diarrhea, which may be a clue to this diagnosis.

Serum albumin may be decreased.

Steatorrhea occurs rarely due to low pH produced in intestine.

Laboratory findings due to peptic ulcer (present in 70% of patients) of stomach, duodenum, or proximal jejunum (e.g., perforation, fluid loss, hemorrhage)

○*Clues to Z-E syndrome are ulcers in unusual locations or giant or multiple ulcerations (25% of these patients), rapid or severe recurrence of ulcer after adequate therapy, recurrent ulcer after surgery, prominent gastric folds, gastric acid hypersecretion with hypergastrinemia, family history of peptic ulcer or ulcers with other endocrine disorders, duodenal ulcers without* Helicobacter pylori.

○*MEN type I should be ruled out in all patients with Z-E syndrome, which may be the initial manifestation of MEN type I (see pp. 697). 25% of cases of this syndrome are associated with MEN type I. 40–60% of cases of MEN type I have Z-E syndrome.*

Ultrasonography, angiography, CT scan, and MRI are normal in 50% of patients.

Laboratory Tests for Evaluation of Adrenal-Pituitary Function

Complete 24-hr urine collections may be difficult to obtain in some patients.

Plasma samples are simple to obtain but are altered by diurnal variation, episodic pulsatile secretion, renal and metabolic clearance, stress, protein binding, and effect of drugs. Therefore abnormal screening tests must be confirmed by tests that stimulate or suppress the pituitary-adrenal axis.

Increased function is tested by suppression tests and decreased function is tested by stimulatory tests.

Cortisol measurements have largely replaced other steroid determinations in diagnosis of Cushing's syndrome.

Adrenocorticotropic Hormone (ACTH) Stimulation (Cosyntropin) Test

Use

Differential diagnosis of adrenal insufficiency
Not helpful in diagnosis of Cushing's syndrome.

Rapid Screening Test

Administer 0.25 mg of synthetic ACTH (cosyntropin) IM or IV and measure baseline and 30-, 60-, and 90-min plasma cortisol levels. If response is not normal, perform long test (see below).

Interpretation

Normal: baseline plasma cortisol of >5.0 μg/dL with increase to 2× baseline level ≥ 20 μg/dL is sufficient single criterion of normal adrenal function to preclude need for further workup; 60- and 90-min levels can be omitted. Increase in urine 17-OHKS has also been used.

Addison's disease: ruled out by a positive response.

Hypopituitarism: a slight increase is shown the first day and a greater increase the next day.

Adrenal carcinoma: little or no response; marked increase in urine 17-KS.

Adrenal hyperplasia: shows increase of 3–5× baseline level.

Long Test

Daily infusion of ACTH for 5 days, with before and after measurement of serum cortisol, 24-hr urine measurements for cortisol, 17-OHKS. (Protect possible Addison's disease patient against adrenal crisis with 1 mg of dexamethasone.)

ENDOCRINE

Interpretation

Normal: at least 3× increase with maximum above upper reference value

Complete primary adrenal insufficiency (Addison's disease): no increase in urine steroids or increase of <2 mg/day

Incomplete primary adrenal insufficiency: less than normal increases on all 5 days or slight increase on first 3 days, which may be followed by decrease on days 4 and 5

Secondary adrenal insufficiency (due to pituitary hypofunction): "staircase" response of progressively higher values each day (delayed but normal response)

Adrenal insufficiency due to chronic steroid therapy: may require prolonged ACTH testing to elicit the "staircase" response; may produce increments only in 17-OHKS but not in 17-KS

CAH (21-hydroxylase and 17-hydroxylase deficiency): increase in 17-KGS and 17-KS, little or no change in 17-OHKS

Aldosterone, Plasma

Use

Diagnosis of primary hyperaldosteronism
Differential diagnosis of fluid and electrolyte disorders
Assessment of adrenal aldosterone production

Increased In

Primary aldosteronism
Secondary aldosteronism
Bartter's syndrome
Pregnancy
Very low sodium diet
Urine aldosterone is also increased in nephrosis.

Decreased In

Hyporeninemic hypoaldosteronism
CAH
Congenital deficiency of aldosterone synthetase
Addison's disease
Very high sodium diet

Androstenedione, Serum

(A major adrenal androgen in serum; also produced by testes and ovaries)

Use

Diagnosis of virilism and hirsutism

Increased In

CAH due to 21-hydroxylase deficiency; marked increase is suppressed to normal levels by adequate glucocorticoid therapy. Suppressed level reflects adequacy of therapeutic control. May be better than 17-hydroxyprogesterone for monitoring therapy because it shows minimal diurnal variation, better correlation with urinary 17-KS excretion, and plasma levels are not immediately affected by a dose of glucocorticoid.

Adrenal tumors
Cushing's disease
Polycystic ovarian disease

Decreased In

Addison's disease

Corticotropin-Releasing Hormone (CRH) Stimulation Test[7–9]

1 μg/kg of body weight or 100 μg of CRH is given IV; blood is then drawn at 15-min intervals for 2–3 hrs to measure ACTH and cortisol. ACTH concentration from both inferior petrosal sinuses and peripheral vein is compared after CRH stimulation. For initial test, blood sampling from jugular veins is simpler and less invasive; negative results can be confirmed by petrosal sinus sampling. Use of only peripheral plasma ACTH and cortisol has little value.

Use

Confirm diagnosis of Cushing's disease when patient has positive response to dexa-methasone suppression, CRH administration, or metyrapone stimulation.
Especially useful when high-dose DST is equivocal or when biochemical data indicate a pituitary source but radiographic examination is normal.

Interpretation

Differentiate pituitary and nonpituitary causes of Cushing's syndrome, especially ectopic ACTH production. Ratio of ACTH in jugular and peripheral veins of >2 before and >3 after administration of CRH is diagnostic for Cushing's disease. Pet-rosal sampling sensitivity, specificity, and accuracy approach 100%. Different values obtained from right and left petrosal sinuses suggests side on which tumor is located.
Cushing's syndrome due to pituitary adenoma: positive response is exaggerated increase above baseline of >50% in plasma ACTH and >20% in cortisol concentra-tions. After surgical removal of adenoma, basal concentrations of ACTH and corti-sol are undetectable but response to CRH is normal.
Hypercorticalism of adrenal origin: plasma ACTH is low or undetectable before and after CRH without any cortisol response.
Ectopic ACTH syndrome: no ACTH or cortisol response in ~92% of patients; positive response in ~8% of patients.
Psychiatric states associated with hypercorticalism (e.g., depression, anorexia nervosa, bulimia): in uni- or bipolar depression, both peak and total ACTH response is decreased; only a normal small decrease in cortisol occurs; after recovery response is not distin-guishable from that of normal persons. Similar findings may occur in obsessive-compul-sive disorders and alcoholism. Manic patients have response similar to that of controls.

Dehydroepiandrosterone Sulfate (DHEA-S), Serum

(Produced by androgenic zone of adrenal cortex)

Use

Indicator of adrenal cortical function, especially for differential diagnosis of virilization.
Replaces 17-KS urine excretion with which it correlates; shows no significant diurnal variation, thereby providing rapid test for abnormal androgen secretion.

Increased In

CAH: markedly increased values can be suppressed by dexamethasone. Highest values occur in CAH due to deficiency of 3-beta-hydroxysteroid dehydrogenase (see p. 639).
Adrenal carcinoma: markedly increased levels cannot be suppressed by dexamethasone.
Cushing's syndrome due to bilateral adrenal hyperplasia shows higher values than Cush-ing's syndrome due to benign cortical adenoma, in which values may be normal or low.

[7]Chrousos GP, et al. NIH Conference. Clinical applications of corticotropin-releasing factor. *Ann Intern Med* 1985;102:344.
[8]Kaye TB, Crapo L. The Cushing syndrome: an update on diagnostic tests. *Ann Intern Med* 1990;112:434.
[9]Doppman JL, Oldfield EH, Nieman LK. Bilateral sampling of the internal jugular vein to distin-guish between mechanisms of adrenocorticotropic hormone–dependent Cushing syndrome. *Ann Intern Med* 1998;128:33.

ENDOCRINE

Cushing's disease (pituitary etiology): moderate increase

In hypogonadotropic hypogonadism, DHEA-S is usually normal for chronologic age and high for bone age, in contrast to idiopathic delayed puberty in which DHEA-S is low relative to chronologic age and normal relative to bone age.

First few days of life, especially in sick or premature infants.

Decreased In

Addison's disease
Adrenal hypoplasia

Dexamethasone Suppression of Pituitary ACTH Secretion

Low-Dose Dexamethasone Suppression Test (DST)

0.5 mg of dexamethasone (synthetic glucocorticoid) is given orally every 6 hrs for eight doses; specimen collection as for high-dose test below. A rapid overnight variation for screening uses a single 1-mg dose at 11 p.m. with plasma cortisol collection the next day at 8 a.m. Following in 2 hrs by CRH stimulation improves diagnostic accuracy, sensitivity, and specificity to ~100% in diagnosis of Cushing's syndrome.

Use

Good screening test to rule out Cushing's syndrome and to identify cases for further testing because few (1–2%) false-negative results are seen. Should be reserved primarily for cases with mildly increased urine cortisol or pseudo–Cushing's syndrome.

Interference

False-positive results may occur in acute and chronic illness, alcoholism, depression, and use of certain drugs (e.g., phenytoin, phenobarbital, primidone); estrogens may cause a false-positive overnight DST.

Noncompliance (check by measuring plasma dexamethasone)

Interpretation

Normal response is a fall in urine free cortisol to <25 μg/24 hrs, in plasma cortisol to <5 μg/dL, or in urine 17-OHKS to <4 mg/24 hrs. Fall in urine free cortisol >90% or in 17-OHKS >64% has 100% reported specificity, i.e., normal result excludes hypercorticalism.

Patients with Cushing's syndrome of any cause almost always have abnormal lack of suppressibility. Repeat testing is sometimes needed for accurate diagnosis.

High-Dose DST

2 mg of dexamethasone is given orally every 6 hrs for eight doses; plasma cortisol is measured 6 hrs after last dose and urine free cortisol and 17-OHKS are measured on the second day; baseline specimens are taken for 2 days before test.

Use

The high-dose test is the basic test to differentiate Cushing's disease (in which only relative resistance to glucocorticoid negative feedback is seen) from adrenal tumors or ectopic ACTH production (usually complete resistance).

Interpretation

Cushing's disease (pituitary tumor)
* Suppression of urine free cortisol to <90% of baseline (59% sensitivity, 100% specificity) and urine 17-OHKS to <65% of baseline (72% sensitivity, 94% specificity) strongly differentiates Cushing's disease from ectopic ACTH production, but not all pituitary tumor patients show such marked suppression. Some patients with large ACTH-producing pituitary adenomas have marked resistance to high-dose dexamethasone suppression. In long-standing cases, nodular hyperplasia of adrenal may develop, causing autonomous cortisol production and resistance to DST.

Ectopic ACTH syndrome or nodular adrenal hyperplasia
* No suppression in 80% of cases.

Adrenal adenoma or carcinoma or ectopic ACTH syndrome
* Urinary 17-OHKS and urine and plasma cortisol are not decreased after high or low doses of dexamethasone. Adrenal tumors do not reproducibly suppress.

Patients with psychiatric illness may be resistant.

Interferences

Atypical or false-positive responses may occur due to drugs (e.g., alcohol, estrogens and birth control pills, phenytoin, barbiturates, spironolactone), pregnancy, obesity, acute illness and stress, severe depression.

11-Deoxycortisol (Compound S), Serum

(Present in blood as an intermediate in synthesis of cortisol from 17-hydroxyprogesterone; excretion in urine is included in 17-KGS and Porter-Silber 17-OHKS measurements.)

Use

In metyrapone test (see next section), in which blood level parallels changes in urine 17-OHKS
- In functioning pituitary-adrenal system an increase from <200 ng/dL baseline to >7000 ng/dL is seen 8 hrs after large dose of metyrapone, whereas in nonfunctioning system very little increase in blood level is seen.

Increased In

CAH (11-Beta-Hydroxylase deficiency) (see p. 639)
After metyrapone administration in normal persons

Decreased In

Adrenal insufficiency

Metyrapone Test

Adrenal suppression of pituitary secretion of ACTH is inhibited by administration of 750 mg of metyrapone (which blocks cortisol production, leading to increased ACTH secretion and therefore of 11-deoxycortisol) every 4–6 hrs beginning at midnight; draw baseline plasma levels at 8 a.m. and following 8 a.m.
Do not perform metyrapone test until ACTH test proves that adrenals are sensitive to ACTH.

Use

To distinguish Cushing's disease from ectopic ACTH production
To assess if adrenal insufficiency is secondary to pituitary disease. Some increase in 11-deoxycortisol indicates that some pituitary reserve exists; in primary adrenal insufficiency, no rise occurs.

Interpretation

ACTH deficiency (secondary Addison's disease): see p. 640
Healthy persons and those with pituitary Cushing's disease: basal plasma 11-deoxycortisol increases $\geq 400\times$ or $>10\ \mu g/dL$ if cortisol falls to $<7\ \mu g/dL$ and plasma ACTH rises to >100 ng/L or urine 17-OHKS increases by 70% (71% sensitivity) or to 2.5× the previous baseline concentration or to >10 mg/24 hrs.
Adrenal tumor with excess cortisol production: no increase or fall in urinary 17-OHKS and 17-KS. Test is positive in 100% of cases of adrenal hyperplasia without tumor, 50% of cases of adrenal adenoma, and 25% of cases of adrenal carcinoma.
Ectopic ACTH syndrome: may not be accurate in this condition.

Renin Activity, Plasma (PRA)

See Aldosteronism, p. 643.

Diseases of Adrenal Gland

Adrenal Hyperplasia, Congenital

(Errors of metabolism due to specific deficiencies of enzymes needed for normal steroid synthesis of three main hormone classes [specific abnormalities on short arm of chromosome 6]: mineralocorticoids [17-deoxy pathway], glucocorticoids [17-hydroxy pathway], and sex steroids. All forms have decreased cortisol production; this stimulates compensatory secretion of pituitary ACTH, which causes the adrenal hyperplasia and hypersecretion of other pathways.)

ENDOCRINE

The most common forms are summarized in Table 13-16. The synthetic pathways are shown schematically in Fig. 13-11 to illustrate the altered hormonal levels.

♦ Establish diagnoses by increase in specific precursor steroids in blood or urine, which can be suppressed by administration of glucocorticoids.

♦ Finding of increased 17-hydroxyprogesterone or androstenedione in amniotic fluid permits prenatal diagnosis.

In the United States, occurs in 1 in 80,000–100,000 live births.

CAH should always be ruled out in infants with
• Ambiguous genitalia and presence of nuclear sex chromatin
• Continued vomiting after pyloroplasty
• Siblings affected with CAH
• Salt loss

21-Hydroxylase Deficiency

(>90% of cases of CAH are of this form; three types are recognized)
Severe Deficiency (Salt-Losing) Form

♦ Severe enzyme deficiency not compensated by increased ACTH secretion; cortisol levels are decreased.

♦ Excess production of salt-losing steroids plus inability to secrete aldosterone causes characteristic acute adrenal crisis.

♦ Salt-wasting crisis usually occurs 1–2 wks after birth with hyponatremia, hyperkalemia, acidosis, severe dehydration, and shock.

♦ Increased ACTH causes hypersecretion of androgens and virilization of female external (ambiguous) genitalia but internal genitalia are usually normal. Males do not show abnormal genitals at birth but may show precocious puberty. Both sexes show rapid early growth, but premature closure of epiphyses causes shorter stature.

Moderate Deficiency (Simple Virilizing) Form

Salt-wasting is mild or absent.

♦ Moderate enzyme deficiency compensated by increased ACTH secretion causing cortisol secretion close to normal and marked increase in androgens (characteristic *increase in androstenedione* and, to a lesser extent, testosterone) and cortisol precursors, some of which (progesterone, *17-hydroxyprogesterone*) cause some salt wasting; the latter causes compensatory increase in PRA and increased aldosterone secretion.

♦ Androgen ratio in urine of 11-desoxy-17-KS to 11-oxy-17-KS is ~1:1 (normal adult ratio = 1:4).

Urinary excretion of 17-KS and blood steroid secretion can be suppressed by dexamethasone (1.25 mg/m^2/day for 7 days), *which differentiates CAH from virilizing adrenal tumors.* Urine 17-OHKS levels are normal.

Normal or low cortisol levels show little or no response to ACTH administration.

Karyotyping should be done to establish genetic sex whenever external genitalia are ambiguous.

Mild Deficiency (Attenuated; Late-Onset) Form

At puberty, females show hirsutism and oligomenorrhea; must be differentiated from polycystic ovary syndrome.

♦ Increased 17-hydroxyprogesterone: Extreme increase in salt-wasting form of 21-hydroxylase deficiency (20–500× normal; often >25,000 ng/dL) is usually diagnostic; 24-hr urinary metabolite (pregnanetriol) is also increased. Not as increased in simple virilizing form. In mild deficiency enzyme block is evident only after ACTH stimulation: excessive rise (5–10×) of 17-hydroxyprogesterone 30 or 60 mins after administration of ACTH (cosyntropin) 0.25–1.0 mg IV or 6 hrs after 0.40 mg IV (normal <900 ng/dL; late-onset form >2000 ng/dL; severe form >16,000 ng/dL). Response of exaggerated increase of 17-hydroxyprogesterone is used to identify carriers.

Aldosterone deficiency is also present in salt-wasting form but not in simple virilizing form; increased in both forms.

In nonclassical forms, same biochemical pattern occurs (with lower levels) but symptoms of virilization, abnormal growth and puberty, infertility, etc., may be slight or absent.

17-hydroxyprogesterone and delta-4 levels are used to monitor glucocorticoid therapy by reduction to normal.

♦ Cortisol levels are usually fixed and unresponsive.

♦ Excess adrenal androgen production (e.g., androstenedione, dehydroepiandrosterone [DHEA], testosterone, urinary 17-KS), which is suppressed by glucocorticoids.

Table 13-16. Comparison of Different Forms of Congenital Adrenal Hyperplasia

Enzyme Deficiency	Sexual Ambiguity in Newborn Female	Sexual Ambiguity in Newborn Male	Post-natal Virili-zation	Hyper-tension	Salt-Wasting	Urine Hormone Concentrations				Blood Hormone Concentrations				
						17-KS	17-OH	Preg-nane-triol	Aldo-sterone	17-OHP	Delta-4	DHEA	Testos-terone	Renin
21-Hydroxylase														
Salt-wasting	+	0	+	0	+	II	D	II	D	II	II	N/I	I	II
Simple virilizing	+	0	+	0	0	II	N/D	II	N/I	II	II	N/I	I	N/I
Late-onset	0	0	+	0	0	I	N	I	N/I	I	I	N/I	N/I	N
11-Beta-hydroxylase[a]	+	0	+	+	0	II	II	I	D	I	II	I	I	DD
3-Beta-HSD														
Salt-wasting	+	+	+	0	+	I	DD	N/D	D	N/I	N/I	III	[b]	I
Non-salt-wasting	+	+	+	0	0	I	DD	N/D	N	N/I	N/I	III	[b]	N
Late-onset	0	?	+	0	0	N/I	N	N	N	N/I	N/I	I	N/I	N
17-Alpha-hydroxylase[a]	0	+	0	+	0	DD	DD	DD	D	D	D	D	D	D
Cholesterol desmolase	0	+	0	0	+	DD	DD	DD	DD	D	D	D	D	I

17-OH = 17-hydroxylase; 17-OHP = 17-hydroxyprogesterone; DHEA = dehydroepiandrosterone; I, II = degrees of increased; D, DD = degrees of decreased; 0 = none; + = present.
[a] Increased 17-deoxycortisol (corticosterone) and 11-deoxycortisol (compound B).
[b] N/D in males; N/I in females.

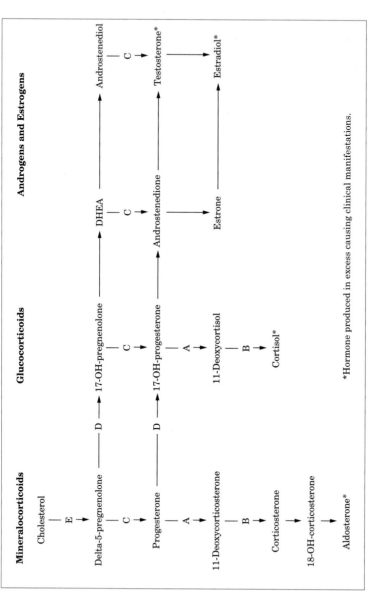

Fig. 13-11. Pathway of adrenal hormone synthesis. Hormones above the level of the deficient enzyme are present in increased amount; those below this level are decreased in amount (see Table 13-16). Shunting to other pathways may occur. Findings depend on completeness of enzyme deficiency, degree of hormone deficiency, or excessive accumulation. (A = 21-hydroxylase; B = 11-hydroxylase; C = 3-beta-hydroxysteroid dehydrogenase; D = 17-hydroxylase; E = 20,22-desmolase; DHEA = dehydroepiandrosterone.)

♦ Genetic testing and prenatal diagnosis are available.
♦ Neonatal screening shows increased 17-hydroxyprogesterone in dried filter paper blood spot.
  • False-positives may occur due to prematurity and low birth weight, illness, and in infants <24 hrs old.

11-Beta-Hydroxylase Deficiency

(Causes <3% of cases of CAH; excess mineralocorticoids cause hypertension, which may not appear until adulthood; excess androgen causes female pseudo-hermaphroditism at birth, postnatal virilism in males and females; males with mild form may have only hypertension or gynecomastia.)
♦ Increased serum deoxycorticosterone causing hypokalemia and suppression of renin and aldosterone.
♦ Increased 11-deoxycortisol and 17-hydroxyprogesterone and increase of their metabolites in urine: tetrahydro-deoxycorticosterone and tetrahydro-11-deoxycortisol.
PRA levels can be used to monitor therapy.
Glucocorticoid therapy returns deoxycorticosterone to normal.

3-Beta-Hydroxysteroid Dehydrogenase Deficiency

(Rare autosomal recessive disorder; complete deficiency causes death)
♦ Impaired secretion with decrease of cortisol, aldosterone, androstenedione, and sex steroids.
♦ Increased plasma 17-hydroxypregnenolone, pregnenolone, DHEA; increased ratio of delta-5 (pregnenolone, 17-hydroxypregnenolone, DHEA) to delta-4 (progesterone, 17-hydroxyprogesterone, delta-4-androstenedione) causing mild virilization.

17-Alpha-Hydroxylase Deficiency

♦ Decreased serum 17-hydroxylated steroids and androgens
♦ Decreased urine 17-KS and 17-OHKS
♦ Increase in serum corticosterone and deoxycorticosterone and their urinary metabolites in urine, causing hypertension, hypokalemia
♦ Decreased aldosterone and PRA
  PRA levels can be used to monitor therapy.

Cholesterol Desmolase Deficiency

(Complete deficiency incompatible with life. Mild condition in females may cause short stature, virilization, irregular menses, infertility. Affected males may show short stature, infertility. Early diagnosis and therapy may prevent this. Ambiguous or female genitalia in male children.)
♦ Virtually no steroids (cortisol, aldosterone, androgens) are produced.
♦ Very low urine 17-OHKS levels are not increased by ACTH stimulation.
♦ Aldosterone is very low in plasma and urine.
♦ Hyponatremia, hyperkalemia, rapid dehydration, shock, and early death if not recognized at birth.

Corticosterone Methyloxidase Deficiency

Type I
  • Hyponatremia and hyperkalemia
♦ • Decreased aldosterone and 18-hydroxycorticosterone
♦ • Increased corticosterone
Type II
♦ • Ratio of urinary metabolites of 18-hydroxycorticosterone to aldosterone is markedly increased (normal is <3.0); is a better marker than 18-hydroxycorticosterone levels.

17-Beta-Hydroxysteroid Dehydrogenase Deficiency

♦ Increased delta-4-testosterone ratios in peripheral and spermatic blood is diagnostic.
During first week of life:
  • Urine total 17-KS may be as high in normal infants as in those with CAH due to maternal steroids. Normally falls to <1 mg/24 hrs during second week of life;

ENDOCRINE

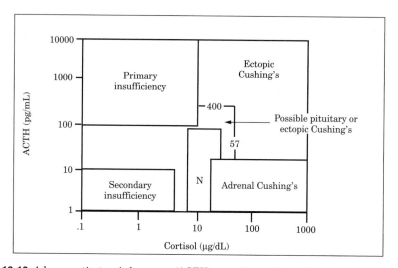

Fig. 13-12. Adrenocorticotropic hormone (ACTH or corticotropin) and cortisol limits that are useful in diagnosis of Cushing's syndrome. This figure shows the corticotropin versus cortisol area ambiguous for the differential diagnosis of pituitary-dependent and ectopic Cushing's syndrome and the area diagnostic for ectopic Cushing's syndrome. (N = normal.) (From Snow K, et al. Biochemical evaluation of adrenal dysfunction. *Mayo Clin Proc* 1992;67:1055, with permission.)

therefore serial determinations should be performed in suspected cases. Level of <1 mg/24 hrs rules out CAH; an increasing level suggests CAH but a decreasing level does not rule out CAH. Is increased in all virilizing forms except lipoid type.
- 17-hydroxyprogesterone is the most valuable test in 21-hydroxylase or 11-hydroxylase deficiency.
- Detectable amounts of pregnanetriol in urine or plasma after first week of life is usually diagnostic of CAH, but in some patients this may not appear until age >1 mo.
- 17-OHKS in urine is not particularly useful in diagnosis of CAH.

Adrenocortical Insufficiency

See Table 13-17 and Fig. 13-12, 13-13.

Acute

- Primary (e.g., Waterhouse-Friderichsen syndrome [hemorrhagic necrosis due to anticoagulant therapy, coagulopathy], antiphospholipid syndrome, sepsis, postoperative state)
- Secondary to pituitary or hypothalamic disorders
- After cessation of prolonged steroid therapy

Dehydration
Azotemia is due to effect of dehydration and shock on renal function.
Serum sodium and chloride are decreased and potassium is increased in some patients.
Hypoglycemia occurs regularly.
Direct eosinophil count is >50/cu mm (<50/cu mm in other kinds of shock).
♦ Blood cortisol is markedly decreased (<5 μg/dL).

Chronic (Addison's Disease)

Due To

Chronic
- Primary
   Granulomas (e.g., TB, sarcoidosis)

Table 13-17. Laboratory Differentiation of Primary and Secondary Adrenal Insufficiency

Test	Primary Adrenal Insufficiency	Adrenal Insufficiency Secondary to Hypopituitarism
Blood ACTH level	Increased	Decreased
Urine 17-KS and 17-OHKS after ACTH stimulation (see p. 631)	No responsive increase	Marked "staircase" response

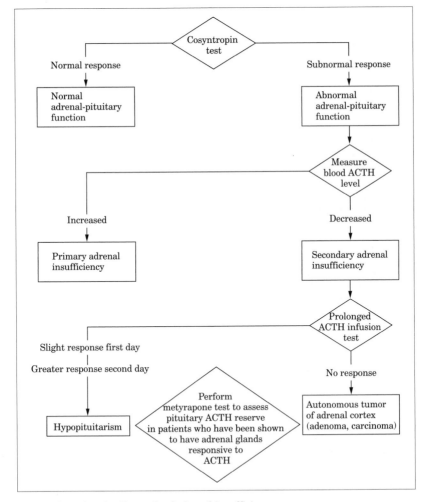

Fig. 13-13. Algorithm for diagnosis of adrenal insufficiency.

ENDOCRINE

Metastatic carcinoma (lung, breast, kidney), lymphoma
Amyloid
Autoimmune adrenalitis: diagnosed by circulating adrenal antibodies; may be associated with other autoimmune conditions (e.g., Hashimoto's thyroiditis, PA)
Systemic fungal infections (e.g., histoplasmosis, cryptococcosis, blastomycosis)
AIDS (e.g., opportunistic infections with CMV, bacteria, protozoa)
Adrenal hypoplasia (neonates)
Adrenoleukodystrophy
- Secondary
Simmonds' disease (idiopathic atrophy of pituitary)
Destruction of pituitary or hypothalamus by granulomas, tumor, etc.

♦ Low serum cortisol and increased ACTH are diagnostic of primary adrenal failure. In primary deficiency both cortisol and aldosterone are deficient, with salt loss causing increased PRA; in secondary deficiency, aldosterone production is maintained but other secondary endocrine deficiencies may appear, e.g., hypothyroidism, hypogonadism.

♦ Increased blood ACTH (200–1600 pg/mL) with wide variation between morning and evening levels in primary adrenal hypofunction but decreased or absent ACTH in pituitary (secondary) hypoadrenalism. Normal value rules out primary but not mild secondary insufficiency. Increased ACTH level is quickly suppressed by replacement therapy.

♦ Decreased ACTH with low cortisol indicates ACTH deficiency.

♦ Decreased blood cortisol ($<5 \mu g/dL$ in 8–10 a.m. specimen) is useful screening test. High or high-normal result excludes both primary and secondary adrenocortical insufficiency. $\leq 3 \mu g/dL$ is said to indicate adrenal insufficiency and obviate need for further testing. Borderline result is indication for ACTH stimulation test.

♦ Long ACTH stimulation test is necessary for diagnosis of secondary adrenal insufficiency (see p. 631).

Metyrapone inhibition test is performed if ACTH test causes some increase in blood cortisol (see p. 635).

Cortisol treatment interferes with all of the above tests and must be discontinued for 24–48 hrs before testing. Dexamethasone interferes with metyrapone test and plasma ACTH levels.

Urine 17-OHKS is absent or markedly decreased.

Urine 17-KS and 17-KGS are markedly decreased.

♦ Antiadrenal antibodies are found in most cases of idiopathic Addison's disease and are said to rule out adrenoleukodystrophy and secondary adrenal insufficiency. Said to have very high sensitivity and specificity, and are predictive of impending or compensated adrenocortical failure. Idiopathic Addison's disease requires ruling out tumor, TB, and other granulomatous diseases of adrenals.

Serum potassium is increased; may be low in secondary adrenal insufficiency.

Serum sodium and chloride are decreased. Sodium-potassium ratio is <30:1.

The Robinson-Power-Kepler water tolerance test and the Cutler-Power-Wilder sodium chloride deprivation test have been replaced by the ACTH stimulation tests, which are more direct and avoid the risk of crisis.

BUN and creatinine may be moderately increased; may be decreased in secondary adrenal insufficiency. Fasting hypoglycemia is present, with a flat oral glucose tolerance curve and insulin hypersensitivity. IV GTT results show a normal peak followed by severe prolonged hypoglycemia.

Neutropenia and relative lymphocytosis are common.

Eosinophilia is present (300/cu mm). (*A total eosinophil count of <50 is evidence against severe adrenocortical hypofunction.*)

Normocytic anemia is slight or moderate but difficult to estimate because of decreased blood volume.

Blood volume is decreased; Hct level is increased (because of water loss).

Laboratory tests for associated conditions
- Primary adrenocortical insufficiency may be caused by CAH (see p. 635) or associated with hypoaldosteronism.
- Secondary (pituitary) insufficiency may be associated with laboratory findings of hypothyroidism (see p. 589), hypogonadism (see p. 672), diabetes insipidus (see p. 689), etc.

Aldosteronism, Primary[10,11]

(Excessive mineralocorticoid hormone secretion causes renal tubules to retain sodium and excrete potassium.)
See Figs. 13-14, 13-15, and 13-16 and Tables 13-18 and 13-19.

Due To

Solitary adrenocortical adenoma (64% of patients)
Idiopathic bilateral adrenal hyperplasia (32% of patients)
Adrenal carcinoma (<5% of patients)
Ectopic production of aldosterone by adrenal embryologic rest within kidney or ovary (rare)
Ectopic production of ACTH or aldosterone by nonadrenal neoplasm (rare)
Glucocorticoid-suppressible hyperaldosteronism (<1% of patients) (see p. 656)

♦ *Classic biochemical abnormalities are*
  • Decreased serum potassium (see Table 13-18).
  • Increased aldosterone production that cannot be suppressed by volume expansion or increased sodium intake (sodium loading).
  • Suppressed PRA.
♦ Hypokalemia (usually <3.0 mEq/L) not related to use of diuretics or laxatives in a hypertensive patient is a strong indicator.
  • Present in 80–90% of cases; is often mild (3.0–3.5 mEq/L). Aldosteronism should be *suspected* in any hypertensive patient with spontaneous or easily provoked hypokalemia. May be normal in cases of shorter duration before classic clinical picture develops (~20% of cases initially).
  • Hypokalemia is usually less in hyperplasia than in adenoma, but considerable overlap occurs.
  • Hypokalemia ≤ 2.7 mEq/L in a hypertensive patient is usually due to primary aldosteronism, especially adenoma.
  • Intermittent hypokalemia or normokalemia may occur, especially in adrenal hyperplasia etiologies.
  • In patients with essential hypertension on diuretic therapy, urine potassium decreases to <30 mEq/L in 2–3 days after cessation of diuretics but continues in primary aldosteronism patients. (This should be checked several times after cessation of diuretic use.)
  • Hypokalemia is alleviated by administration of spironolactone and by sodium restriction but not by potassium replacement therapy. Administration of spironolactone for 3 days increases serum potassium >1.2 mEq/L. It also increases urine sodium and decreases urine potassium. Negative potassium balance reoccurs in 5 days. It increases urinary aldosterone (this is variable in hypertensive and healthy people).
  • Saline infusion causes significant fall in serum potassium. This hypokalemia is a reliable screening test.
  • Hypokalemia is more severe with adenoma than with hyperplasia (normal in ~20% of latter).
  • Hyperkaluria is present even with low potassium intake; values <30 mEq/24 hrs essentially rules out primary aldosteronism. Sodium output is reduced.
○ High normal or increased serum sodium, hypochloremia, and metabolic alkalosis (CO_2 content >25 mEq/L; blood pH tends to increase to >7.42); correlates with severity of potassium depletion. Are clues in all types of primary aldosteronism.
♦ *Suggestive screening* test results are inappropriate kaliuresis, low PRA (<3.0 ng/mL/hr), high plasma aldosterone and aldosterone/PRA ratio (>30) (morning sample, taken with upright posture).
♦ *Confirm diagnosis* by measuring response of aldosterone and PRA excretion to sodium loading and depletion. Discontinue interfering drugs (for ≥ 2 wks).

[10]Blumenfeld JD, et al. Diagnosis and treatment of primary hyperaldosteronism. *Ann Intern Med* 1994;121:877.
[11]Bornstein SR, et al. Adrenocortical tumors: recent advances in basic concepts and clinical management. *Ann Intern Med* 1999;130:759.

ENDOCRINE

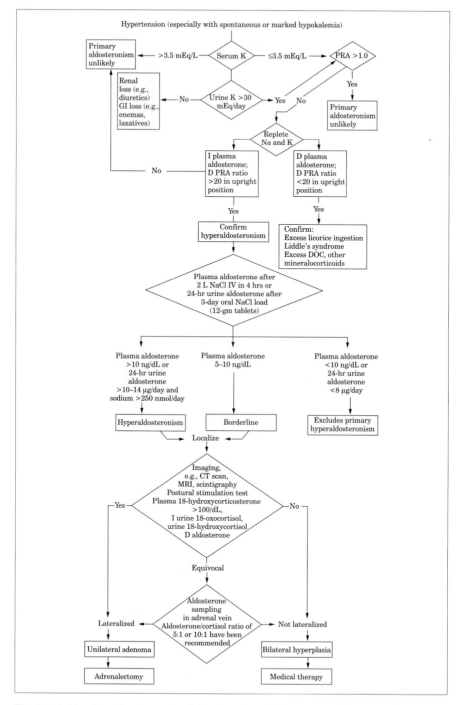

Fig. 13-14. Algorithm for diagnosis of aldosteronism. (CT = computed tomography; D = decreased; DOC = deoxycorticosterone; I = increased; MRI = magnetic resonance imaging.)

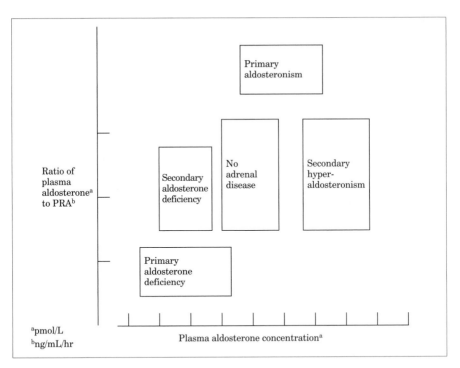

Fig. 13-15. Relationship between plasma aldosterone concentration and ratio of plasma aldosterone to plasma renin activity (PRA) in disorders of mineralocorticoid deficiency or excess.

- Increased plasma (reference range = 30–110 ng/L) and/or urinary aldosterone that is relatively nonsuppressible by salt loading or volume expansion. May be normal in 30% of cases (due to episodic secretion or chronic potassium deficiency, which can suppress aldosterone secretion; therefore must replete potassium before measurement if serum level is <3.0 mEq/L). Plasma aldosterone level of <8.5 ng/dL after morning saline infusion rules out primary aldosteronism. Reference values decline by 30–50% with increasing age. Plasma aldosterone is normal in recumbent hypertensive and nonhypertensive persons without aldosteronism and increases 2–4× after 4 hrs of upright posture; increases ≥ 33% in aldosteronism due to adrenal hyperplasia, but no increase occurs if due to adrenal adenoma.
- Test for increased urinary aldosterone (reference range 2–16 μg/24 hrs) is best initial screening procedure (normal salt intake, no drugs; not detectable on all days). Cannot be reduced by high sodium intake or deoxycorticosterone administration. Therefore high sodium chloride intake (10–12 gm/day) causes 24-hr urine aldosterone level >14 μg/24 hrs and sodium level >250 mEq/24 hrs; urine aldosterone level <14 μg/24 hrs rules out primary aldosteronism except for glucocorticoid-remedial type; 96% sensitivity and 93% specificity.
- Volume expansion (by high salt intake, infusion of 2 L of sodium chloride in 4 hrs, or deoxycorticosterone) suppresses aldosterone level by >50–80% of baseline level in hypertensive patients without primary aldosteronism but not in patients with primary aldosteronism. (Plasma aldosterone level is first increased by having patient in upright position for 2 hrs.) Because plasma aldosterone levels vary from moment to moment, a single specimen may not properly reflect adrenal secretion.
- PRA fails to rise to ≥ 4 ng/mL 90 mins after stimulus of low-sodium diet, furosemide-induced volume contraction, and upright posture.

ENDOCRINE

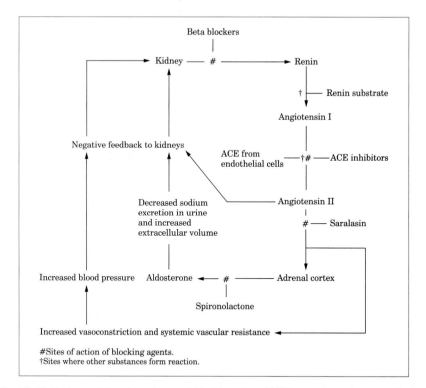

Fig. 13-16. Renin-angiotensin system and blocking sites. (ACE = angiotensin-converting enzyme.)

- Plasma aldosterone/PRA ratio of ≥ 50 at 8 a.m. or in random blood sample after ambulating 2 hrs in patient not on medication is said to indicate primary aldosteronism except in cases of chronic renal insufficiency. Does not distinguish adenoma from hyperplasia.
- ♦ Captopril (ACE inhibitor that blocks angiotensin II production) administered as 25 mg IV at 8 a.m. decreases aldosterone in plasma 2 hrs later in normal persons and those with essential hypertension but remains elevated in patients with primary aldosteronism (Fig. 13-17).

Table 13-18. Differential Diagnosis of Causes of Hypertension and Hypokalemia

Condition	PRA	Aldosterone
Primary hyperaldosteronism	D	I
Cushing's syndrome	D	D
Malignant hypertension	I	I
Renovascular hypertension	I	I
Licorice ingestion	D	D
Exogenous mineralocorticoids (e.g., in nasal spray or for orthostatic hypotension)	D	D
Liddle's syndrome	D	D
Congenital adrenal hyperplasia (11-beta- or 17-alpha-hydroxylase deficiency)	D	D

D = decreased; I = increased; PRA = plasma renin activity.

Table 13-19. Differential Diagnosis of Aldosteronism

Test	Adenoma	Idiopathic Hyperplasia	Adrenal Carcinoma	Glucocorticoid-Remediable Hyperaldosteronism
Hypokalemia	More marked	Less marked	Often profound	Normal
PRA	Suppressed; very low	Less suppressed	Suppressed; very low	Suppressed
Plasma or urine aldosterone	I	I is less marked	Usually very I	Often slightly I
Aldosterone response to postural test	D or not I in 70–80% of cases	I in almost all cases	Often unchanged or random I	D
Excess hormone production	I 18-oxocortisol and 18-hydroxy-cortisol in urine; occasionally cortisol	Only aldosterone and related corticosteroids	Androgen, estrogen, or cortisol often	Aldosterone, 18-oxocortisol, 18-hydroxy-cortisol

I = increased; D = decreased; PRA = plasma renin activity.

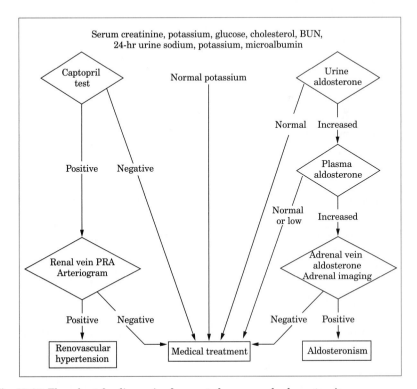

Fig. 13-17. Flow chart for diagnosis of suspected renovascular hypertension.

ENDOCRINE

	Sensitivity (%)	Specificity (%)
Potassium <4.0 mEq/L	100	64
Stimulated renin <2.5 ng/mL/3 hrs	100	88
Suppressed aldosterone >10 ng/dL	98	92
Sequential 1, 2, and 3	98	99

○Basal plasma 18-hydroxycorticosterone level of >100 ng/dL at 8 a.m. supports diagnosis of aldosteronoma.

> Urine is neutral or alkaline (pH >7.0) and not normally responsive to ammonium chloride load.

Its large volume and low specific gravity are not responsive to vasopressin or water restriction (decreased tubular function, especially reabsorption of water).

Plasma cortisol and ACTH are normal.

Urine 17-KS and 17-OHKS are normal.

Serum magnesium falls.

Glucose tolerance is decreased in ≤ 50% of patients.

♦After the diagnosis of aldosteronism is established, *cases due to tumor (treated surgically) should be distinguished from those due to idiopathic hyperplasia (treated medically)* (see Table 13-19 and Fig. 13-14). Aldosterone concentration in adrenal vein plasma is higher on side of adenoma, preferably measured by corticotropin stimulation (90–95% diagnostic accuracy). Cortisol should also be measured to evaluate accuracy of adrenal vein sampling. Adenomas can also be localized by CT, MRI, or scintigraphy with ^{131}I-labeled iodocholesterol after dexamethasone suppression (uptake increased in adenoma and absent in idiopathic cases and usually also in carcinoma). Rarely there is unilateral nodular adrenal hyperplasia similar in function to an adenoma. Patients with adenomas have higher plasma 18-oxocortisol (>15 μg/d) and 18-hydroxycorticosterone (>60 μg/d) concentrations, which decrease on standing; plasma aldosterone also decreases or fails to increase >30% on standing. In patients with bilateral adrenal hyperplasia and normal persons, plasma aldosterone increases with upright position. A small subset of hyperplasia cases mimic adenoma because they are associated with angiotensin-independent aldosterone overproduction and are cured by unilateral adrenalectomy.

PRA

Use

Particularly useful to diagnose curable hypertension (e.g., primary aldosteronism, unilateral renal artery stenosis).

May help to differentiate patients with volume excess (e.g., primary aldosteronism) with low PRA from those with medium to high PRA; if patients in latter group show marked rise in PRA during captopril test, they should be worked up for renovascular hypertension, but patients with little or no rise are not likely to have curable renovascular hypertension.

• Captopril test criteria for renovascular hypertension: stimulated PRA of ≥ 12 μg/L/hr, absolute increase in PRA of ≥ 10 μg/L/hr, increase in PRA of ≥ 150% (or ≥ 400% if baseline PRA is <3 μg/L/hr)

In children with salt-losing form of CAH due to 21-hydroxylase deficiency, severity of disease is related to degree of increase. PRA level may serve as guide to adequate mineralocorticoid replacement therapy.

PRA Is Decreased (<1.5 ng/mL/3 hrs) in

98% of cases of primary aldosteronism. Usually absent or low and can be increased less or not at all by sodium depletion and ambulation in contrast to secondary aldosteronism. PRA may not always be suppressed in primary aldosteronism; repeated testing may be necessary to establish the diagnosis. Normal PRA does not preclude this diagnosis; not a reliable screening test.

Hypertension due to unilateral renal artery stenosis or unilateral renal parenchymal disease

Increased plasma volume due to high-sodium diet, administration of salt-retaining steroids

18–25% of essential hypertensives (low-renin essential hypertension) and 6% of normal controls

Advancing age in both normal and hypertensive patients (decrease of 35% from the third to the eighth decade)

May also be decreased in patients with CAH secondary to 11-hydroxylase or 17-hydroxylase deficiency with oversecretion of other mineralocorticoids

Rarely in Liddle's syndrome and excess licorice ingestion

Use of various drugs (propranolol, clonidine, reserpine; slightly with methyldopa)

Usually cannot be stimulated by salt restriction, diuretics, and upright posture, which deplete plasma volume; therefore measure before and after furosemide administration and 3–4 hrs of ambulation.

Antihypertensive and hypotensive drugs should be discontinued for at least 2 wks before measurement of PRA; spironolactone may cause an increase for up to 6 wks; estrogens may cause an increase for up to 6 mos.

Blood should be drawn in an ice-cold tube and the plasma immediately separated in a refrigerated centrifuge. Renin level should be indexed against 24-hr level of sodium in urine.

PRA May Be Increased In

Secondary aldosteronism (usually very high levels), especially malignant or severe hypertension (see next section)

50–80% of patients with renovascular hypertension (see p. 657). Normal or high PRA is of limited value to diagnose or rule out renal vascular hypertension. Very high PRA is highly predictive but has poor sensitivity. Low PRA using renin-sodium nomogram in untreated patient with normal serum creatinine argues strongly against this diagnosis.[12]

15% of patients with essential hypertension (high-renin hypertension)

Renin-producing tumors of the kidney (see Chapter 14)

Reduced plasma volume due to low-sodium diet, diuretics, hemorrhage, Addison's disease

Some edematous normotensive states (e.g., cirrhosis, nephrosis, congestive heart failure)

Sodium or potassium loss due to GI disease, 10% of patients with chronic renal failure.

Normal pregnancy

Pheochromocytoma

Last half of menstrual cycle (twofold increase)

Erect posture for 4 hrs (twofold increase)

Ambulatory patients compared to bedridden patients

Bartter's syndrome

Use of various drugs (diuretics, ACE inhibitors, vasodilators; sometimes calcium antagonists and alpha-blockers, e.g., diazoxide, estrogens, furosemide, guanethidine, hydralazine, minoxidil, nitroprusside, saralasin, spironolactone, thiazides)

Aldosteronism, Secondary

Due To

Decreased effective blood volume
- Congestive heart failure
- Cirrhosis with ascites (aldosteronism 2000–3000 mg/day)
- Nephrosis
- Sodium depletion

Hyperactivity of renin-angiotensin system
- Renin-producing renal tumor (see Chapter 14)
- Bartter's syndrome (see p. 656)
- Toxemia of pregnancy
- Malignant hypertension
- Renovascular hypertension
- Oral contraceptive drug use

Cushing's Syndrome[13–16]

See Table 13-20 and Figs. 13-12 and 13-18.

[12]Mann SJ, Pickering TG. Detection of renovascular hypertension. State of the art. *Ann Intern Med* 1992;117:845.

[13]Carpenter PC. Cushing's syndrome: update of diagnosis and management. *Mayo Clin Proc* 1986;61:49.

[14]Dunlap NE, Grizzle WE, Siegel AL. Cushing's syndrome. Screening methods in hospitalized patients. *Arch Pathol Lab Med* 1985;109:222.

[15]Orth DN. Cushing's syndrome. *N Engl J Med* 1995;332:791.

[16]Freda PU. Differential diagnosis in Cushing syndrome. Use of CRH. *Medicine* 1995;74:74.

Table 13-20. Comparison of Different Causes of Cushing's Syndrome

	Normal	Pituitary Cushing's	Adrenal Adenoma	Adrenal Carcinoma	Adrenal Hyperplasia	Ectopic ACTH Production	Other Illness
Frequency		70%	9%	8%	Rare	15%	
Free cortisol Urine (μg/24 hr)	<100	>300 establishes diagnosis of Cushing's syndrome if increased					
Plasma (μg/dL)	7–25 at 8 a.m. 2–14 at 4 p.m.	>30 at 8 a.m. and >15 at 4 p.m.					
Low-dose dexamethasone suppression Urine free cortisol	Falls to <25 μg/24 hr	Does not fall to <25 μg/24 hr in Cushing's syndrome due to any cause					False-positive may occur in alcoholism, depression, drug use, etc.
Plasma cortisol	Falls to <5 μg/dL			Not suppressed			
High-dose dexamethasone suppression	Suppressed in >90% of cases		Not suppressed but not reproducible		Not suppressed in 80% of cases		
Plasma ACTH (pg/mL)	60	I or high-normal range Not >200	Decreased or not detectable			>200 in ⅔ cases; 100–200 in ⅓ cases	
CRH stimulation	Rapid I in plasma ACTH and cortisol	ACTH increases	Flat plasma ACTH response to CRH				
ACTH ratio inferior petrosal sinus to peripheral blood		High; enhanced by CRH			Ratio = 1		

ACTH = adrenocoricotropic hormone; CRH = corticotropin-releasing hormone.

Due To

ACTH-dependent (plasma ACTH is increased): 80%
Pituitary (Cushing's *disease*): 85%
- Pituitary tumor: 70–90% (may be part of MEN type I; see p. 697)
- Hyperplasia of pituitary adrenocorticotropic cells (rare)
- Ectopic CRH syndrome: <1%
Ectopic ACTH production: 15%
- Neoplasms (e.g., small-cell carcinoma of lung; carcinoids)
  Oat cell carcinoma: 50%
  Tumors of foregut origin: 35% (e.g., bronchial or thymic carcinoid, medullary thyroid carcinoma, islet cell tumors)
  Pheochromocytoma: 5%
  Others: 10%

ACTH-independent (plasma ACTH is suppressed): 20%
Adrenal (adrenal cause is predominant in children)
- Adenoma: >50%
- Carcinoma: <50%; 65% of patients aged <15 yrs
- Micronodular hyperplasia: ~1%
- Macronodular hyperplasia: <1%
Iatrogenic
- Therapeutic (glucocorticoids or ACTH)
- Illicit use by athletes
- Factitious
Pseudo–Cushing's syndrome
- Major depressive disorder: 1%
- Chronic alcoholism: <1%

♦ Definitive diagnosis or exclusion is made only by laboratory tests, which consist of two parts:
  1. Establish autonomous hypercortisolism and loss of diurnal rhythm.
  2. Determine cause (see Fig. 13-18).
♦ Diagnosis of excessive cortisol production may include measurement of increased plasma cortisol (>30 μg/dL at 8 a.m. and >15 μg/dL at 4 p.m.), measurement of 24-hr urine free cortisol, 17-OHKS, and 17-KS, DST.

Interferences

More than one test may be needed because these are misleading in up to one-third of patients for various reasons:
- Baseline measurements are increased by stress.
- Baseline measurements may vary daily, which makes DST difficult to interpret.
- Some drugs alter ACTH production or interfere with assays.
- Impaired renal function affects measurements.
- Cortisol production is somewhat proportional to obesity or large muscle mass.
- Cortisol production is pulsatile rather than uniform, even in cases of ectopic ACTH production or Cushing's disease.
- Cortisol secretion may not be very increased on every determination.

♦ 24-Hr Urinary Free Cortisol

Use
Screening for
- Cushing's syndrome (increased)
- Adrenal insufficiency (decreased)

Interpretation
Increase is most useful screening test (best expressed as per gram of creatinine, which should vary by <10% daily; if >10% variation, two more 24-hr specimens should be collected). Should be measured in three consecutive 24-hr specimens to ensure proper collection and account for daily variability, even in Cushing's syndrome. Found in 95% of Cushing's syndrome. <100 μg/24 hrs excludes, and >300 μg/24 hrs establishes, the diagnosis of Cushing's syndrome. If values are intermediate, low-dose DST is indicated.

Interferences

False-positives or false-negatives are very rare; is more reliable than blood levels, which
    vary with time of day, require standardized collection, and are secreted in pulsatile
    fashion, making 24-hr urine cortisol preferred test.
Increased values may occur in depression or alcoholism but do not exceed 300 μg/24 hrs.
Alcoholism
Various drugs (e.g., phenytoin, phenobarbital, primidone)
Acute and chronic illnesses
Depression
Not affected by body weight.

◆ Plasma Free Cortisol

Use

Loss of normal diurnal variation for screening for Cushing's syndrome (normal persons
    have highest concentration at 8 a.m. and lowest between 8 p.m. and midnight); this
    diurnal variation disappears early and may be absent or reversed in 70% of Cush-
    ing's syndrome and 18% of patients without Cushing's syndrome (due to depression,
    alcoholism, stress, etc.). Midnight cortisol level >7.5 μg/dL indicates Cushing's syn-
    drome, whereas level <5 μg/dL virtually rules it out.

Interferences

False-negatives are frequent if blood is drawn before 8 p.m. (p.m. blood is commonly
    drawn at 4 p.m. to coincide with hospital employee working hours.)
Because episodic rise and fall occurs in patients with Cushing's disease or ectopic ACTH
    production as well as in normal persons, levels should be measured on at least two
    separate days.
Normal urine-free cortisol and normal diurnal variation in plasma cortisol virtually
    exclude Cushing's syndrome.
To determine the cause of Cushing's syndrome after hypercorticalism has been estab-
    lished, the most useful tests are
    • CRH stimulation test (see p. 633)
    • High-dose DST (see p. 634)
    • Metyrapone test (see p. 635)
    • ACTH stimulation test (see p. 631)
    • DHEA-S concentration (see p. 633)
    • Plasma ACTH concentration (see below)

◆ Basal Plasma ACTH Concentration

◆ Interpretation

Cushing's syndrome due to autonomous cortisol production (e.g., adrenal tumor or
    exogenous steroids): low or undetectable.
Pituitary Cushing's disease: high or high-normal range but rarely >200 pg/mL. Hyper-
    response to CRH. Inferior petrosal sinus sampling (see next paragraph).
Ectopic ACTH syndrome (e.g., carcinoma of lung): very high concentrations with no
    diurnal variation. Two-thirds of patients have high concentrations (>200 pg/mL);
    the other one-third usually have moderately elevated values (100–200 pg/mL); no
    response to CRH. In these cases, difference in ACTH concentrations is measured in
    blood obtained simultaneously from both inferior petrosal sinuses and a peripheral
    vein in basal state and after CRH stimulation; ratio of inferior petrosal sinus value
    to peripheral vein value of ≥ 2 indicates pituitary rather than ectopic source of ACTH;
    has sensitivity of 95% and specificity of 100%. Ratio ≥ 3.0 has 100% sensitivity and
    specificity for pituitary tumor. *New immunoradiometric (IRMA) assay for ACTH is
    more sensitive and specific than RIA method, but some tumors secrete biologically
    active "large" ACTH fragments not detected by IRMA; therefore RIA is preferred for
    initial evaluation of cause.*

Increased In

Primary adrenal insufficiency

Decreased In

Factitious Cushing's syndrome
Secondary adrenal insufficiency

Interferences
ACTH has diurnal variation, episodic secretion, short plasma half-life.

◆ *Urinary Steroid Findings in Different Etiologies of Cushing's Syndrome*
Increased urinary 17-OHKS >4× normal in
- 63% of patients with Cushing's syndrome and 3% of patients without Cushing's syndrome
- 65% of patients with Cushing's syndrome due to ectopic ACTH syndrome
- 3% of patients with Cushing's syndrome due to adrenal hyperplasia without tumor

Urinary 17-OHKS is increased (>10 mg/24 hrs) in virtually all patients with Cushing's syndrome but less useful for screening because increased in 20% of persons without Cushing's syndrome (e.g, obesity, hyperthyroidism).
- Night collection sample is higher than day sample (reverse is true in normal persons).
- ACTH stimulation test produces lowest 17-OHKS in Cushing's syndrome due to adrenal carcinoma and highest 17-OHKS in cases due to adrenal adenoma.

Increased urinary 17-KS
- Cushing's syndrome: may be normal in 35% of patients and increased (>25 mg/24 hrs) in 20% of obese persons without Cushing's syndrome. Not useful unless virilism or marked hirsutism is present.
- Normal or low in 70% of adrenal adenomas (<20 mg/24 hrs) but increased in 90% of adrenal carcinomas; averages 50–60 mg/24 hrs in carcinoma (always >15 mg/24 hrs); >4× normal in 50% of adrenal carcinomas; higher values increase likelihood of diagnosis of adrenal carcinoma and value >100 mg/24 hrs is virtually diagnostic.
- Adrenal carcinoma: most of the increase is usually due to DHEA-S, which is markedly increased; DHEA-S is slightly increased in Cushing's disease and often very low in adrenocortical adenoma (<0.4 mg/dL).
- Adrenal hyperplasia: increased total 17-KS (in 50% of cases) is due to elevation of all of the 17-KS.
- Ectopic ACTH syndrome: increased in 15% of cases.

Isolated urine measurements of 17-KS or 17-OHKS are not recommended as screening tests for Cushing's syndrome. In general, free cortisol is best for screening, 17-OHKS with free cortisol in DSTs, 17-KS to screen for possible adrenal carcinoma or to help differentiate adrenal adenoma from pituitary or ectopic ACTH syndrome causes.
- Increased urinary 17-KGS (>20 mg/24 hrs).

PRA is increased; suppressed activity suggests ectopic ACTH syndrome or adrenal adenoma or carcinoma (causing increased secretion of deoxycorticosterone or aldosterone).
Glucose tolerance is diminished in 75% of cases.
- Glycosuria in 50% of patients.
- Diabetes mellitus in 20% of cases.
- Serum sodium is usually moderately increased.

○Hypokalemic acidosis due to renal tubular loss of potassium chloride is characteristic, but compensatory metabolic alkalosis occurs in ~10% of patients due to attempt to conserve potassium with H^+ exchange. Hypokalemic alkalosis may indicate ectopic ACTH production (e.g., bronchogenic carcinoma). Increased serum sodium and bicarbonate and decreased potassium and chloride is due to increased aldosterone production.
Urine potassium is increased; sodium is decreased.
Hematologic changes:
- WBC is normal or increased.
- Relative lymphopenia is frequent (differential is usually <15% of cells).
- Eosinopenia is frequent (usually <100/cu mm).
- Hct is usually normal; if increased, it indicates an androgenic component.

Changes due to osteoporosis in long-standing cases. Serum and urine calcium may be increased.
Kidney stones occur in 15% of cases.
Serum uric acid may be decreased due to uricosuric effect of adrenal steroids.
Urine creatine is increased due to muscle wasting, which may also cause increased BUN.
Serum gamma globulins may be decreased and alpha$_2$ globulin may be moderately increased.

80% of patients with Cushing's disease have remission after removal of pituitary adenoma; tests of pituitary-adrenal axis may take weeks to months to become normal. Effectiveness of surgery is assessed by plasma cortisol and 24-hr urinary cortisol concentrations in week after surgery.

Pituitary imaging yields false-negative scans because many functional tumors are so small (2–3 mm) and false-positive results because 10–15% of normal persons have nonfunctioning tumors.

Cushing's Syndrome, Factitious

♦ Increased plasma and urinary cortisol
♦ Plasma ACTH is low or undetectable.
♦ These findings may also occur in adrenal Cushing's syndrome. Differentiate by history of ingestion or, in some cases, determination of synthetic steroid analogs by specific plasma assays.

Cushing's Syndrome Due to Adrenal Disease

See Fig. 13-18.
♦ Is suggested by
  • Failure of high-dose DST to cause suppression
  • Very low plasma ACTH level
  • Positive metyrapone test

Adenoma is indicated by low or normal 17-KS with increased 17-OHKS, low DHEA-S
Adrenal carcinoma is suggested by very high 17-KS. Carcinoma cases show hypercorticalism (50%), virilism (20%), or both (10–15%); are nonfunctioning (10–15%). *Virilism favors diagnosis of carcinoma rather than adenoma.*
Nodular adrenal hyperplasia: ACTH levels are variable, unpredictable response to DST; therefore is difficult to distinguish from other adrenal causes.
  • 50% of bilateral micronodular hyperplasia cases occur before age 30 yrs.
  • 50% occur as autosomal dominant disorder associated with blue nevi, pigmented lentigines, myxomas (atrial, skin, mammary), pituitary somatotroph adenomas, testicular and other tumors.
Nonfunctioning adrenal adenoma may be found in 5–10% of healthy persons.

Cushing's Syndrome Due to Ectopic ACTH Production

(By neoplasm, e.g., small-cell carcinoma of lung, thymoma, islet cell tumor of pancreas, medullary carcinoma of thyroid, bronchial carcinoid, pheochromocytoma; occurs in 2% of patients with lung cancer. The primary tumor is often radiologically occult.)
See Table 13-20 and Fig. 13-18.
♦ Plasma ACTH is markedly increased (500–1000 pg/mL) compared to level in pituitary Cushing's disease (≤ 200 pg/mL) but values overlap in 20% of ectopic ACTH cases. Morning basal level in normal persons is 20–100 pg/mL. Extreme increase suggests ectopic rather than pituitary production.
○ Increased plasma and urine free cortisol, which may show marked spontaneous variation; lack of diurnal variation.
♦ Increased ACTH in plasma from inferior petrosal sinus identifies ACTH-producing pituitary adenomas in ~88% of cases; combining with CRH stimulation improves the differentiation of pituitary from ectopic ACTH production (see p. 652).
♦ High-dose dexamethasone suppression does not occur in ectopic ACTH production but does occur in >90% of cases of Cushing's disease.
♦ Use of both DST and CRH stimulation has diagnostic accuracy of 98% in distinguishing Cushing's disease from ectopic ACTH production.
Metyrapone test may not be accurate in distinguishing this condition from Cushing's disease.
Increased urinary 17-OHKS and 17-KS.
Marked hypokalemic alkalosis (due to increased desoxycorticosterone and corticosterone; occurs in ≤ 60% of such patients) rather than metabolic acidosis may suggest this diagnosis.

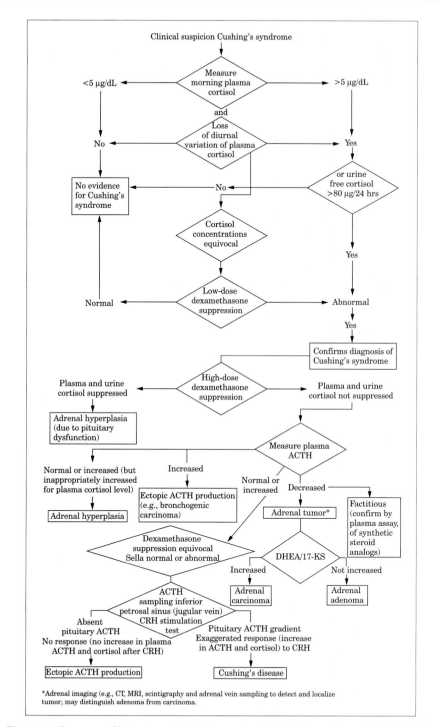

Fig. 13-18. Sequence of laboratory tests in diagnosis of Cushing's syndrome. (>90% of patients with Cushing's syndrome are found to be categorizable using this scheme.) (17-KS = 17 ketosteroids; CRH = corticotropin-releasing hormone; CT = computed tomography; DHEA = dehydroepiandrosterone; I = increased; MRI = magnetic resonance imaging; N = normal.)

Cushing's Syndrome Due to Ectopic CRH Production

(Usually due to bronchial carcinoids; clinically indistinguishable from ectopic ACTH production because most of these tumors also secrete ACTH)
♦ Plasma CRH increased
CRH-stimulated secretion of ACTH suppressed by high doses of dexamethasone may not be present in many cases.

Feminization, Adrenal

(Occurs in adult males with adrenal tumor [usually unilateral carcinoma, occasionally adenoma] that secretes estrogens)
♦ Urinary estrogens are markedly increased.
17-KS is normal or moderately increased and cannot be suppressed by low doses of dexamethasone when due to adrenal tumor.
17-OHKS is normal.
Biopsy of testicle shows atrophy of tubules.

Glucocorticoid Resistance Syndromes

♦ Inability of target tissues to respond to glucocorticoids causes compensatory increase in pituitary corticotropin, which may cause any combination of excess secretion of
  • Adrenal androgens (may result in female masculinization with hirsutism, acne, oligomenorrhea, infertility; precocious puberty; abnormal spermatogenesis)
  • Mineralocorticoid excess (may result in hypokalemic alkalosis, hypertension)
  • Apparently normal glucocorticoid function (patient may be asymptomatic or have chronic fatigue)
No evidence of Cushing's syndrome
  • Plasma cortisol is normal with no loss of diurnal pattern.
  • Urine cortisol and 17-OHKS are normal.
Molecular studies[17]

Hyperaldosteronism, Glucocorticoid Suppressible (Remediable)

(Rare autosomal dominant defect of zona glomerulosa in which beta-methyloxidase produces aldosterone from precursor arising in zona fasciculata)
♦ Usual findings of primary aldosteronism with hypokalemia, increased aldosterone, and suppressed PRA.
♦ Reversal of clinical and laboratory findings (suppression of aldosterone secretion) by dexamethasone for 48 hrs distinguishes this from primary hyperaldosteronism.
♦ Characteristic finding is large amounts of metabolites of 18-oxocortisol in urine.
Anomalous decrease in plasma aldosterone response to posture.
Normal CT and MRI of adrenals.

Hyperaldosteronism, Normotensive, Secondary (Bartter's Syndrome)

(Hypokalemia with renal potassium wasting associated with juxtaglomerular hyperplasia is resistant to antidiuretic hormone [ADH].)
♦ Maintaining normal plasma potassium levels is almost impossible despite therapy (dietary potassium supplement, limiting of sodium intake, drugs such as indomethacin or ibuprofen).
○ Chloride-resistant metabolic alkalosis
♦ Increased PRA is a characteristic feature.
Insensitive to pressor effects of angiotensin II (may occur in patients with prolonged hypokalemia due to any cause)
♦ Increased plasma and urine aldosterone in the absence of edema, hypertension, or hypovolemia.

---

[17]Chrousos GP, Detera-Wadleigh SD, Karl M. Syndromes of glucocorticoid resistance. *Ann Intern Med* 1993;119:1113.

Decreased serum magnesium and increased uric acid frequently occur; often the hypokalemia cannot be corrected without adequate magnesium replacement.

Excretion of large quantities of Na and Cl in urine

Not due to laxatives, diuretics, or GI loss of potassium and chloride

Hypertension, Renovascular[18]

See Fig. 14-5.

Sudden increase in serum creatinine and BUN, especially after onset of ACE-inhibitor therapy. Less common with other antihypertensive therapy.

Hypokalemia (<3.4 mEq/L) in ~15% of patients.

Proteinuria >500 mg/24 hrs usually signifies complete occlusion of a renal artery in a patient with renovascular hypertension.

♦ Captopril test causes

Stimulated peripheral PRA of 12 μg/L(ng/mL)/hr and

Increased peripheral PRA of ≥ 10 μg/L/hr and

Increased peripheral PRA of ≥ 150%, or 400% if baseline value <3 μg/L/hr.

Does not differentiate unilateral and bilateral disease. Less reliable in azotemic patients.

Reported sensitivity and specificity are >72%.

♦ Peripheral PRA (seated patient, drawn in a.m., indexed against sodium excretion) has only 75% sensitivity and 66% specificity but *a low PRA in untreated patients virtually rules out renovascular hypertension.*

♦ PRA is assayed in blood from each renal vein, inferior vena cava, and aorta or renal arteries. The test is considered diagnostic when the concentration from the ischemic kidney is at least 1.5× greater than the concentration from the normal kidney (which is equal to or less than the concentration in the vena cava that serves as the standard) or as increment of PRA between each renal artery and vein. Reported specificity = 80–100%. Reported sensitivity = 62–80%; may be increased by repeating test after captopril administration. This is due to high PRA in the peripheral blood, increase in PRA in the renal vein compared to the renal artery of the affected kidney, and suppression of PRA in the other kidney. Measurement of maximum renin stimulation accentuates the difference between the two kidneys and should always be performed under pretest conditions (avoid antihypertensive, diuretic, and oral contraceptive drugs for at least 1 mo if possible; low-salt diet for 7 days; administer thiazide diuretic for 1–3 days; have patient in upright posture for at least 2 hrs). This is the most useful diagnostic test in renovascular hypertension as judged by surgical results but is not a sufficiently reliable guide to nephrectomy in patients with hypertension due to parenchymal renal disease. *In renovascular hypertension, if renal plasma flow is impaired in the "normal" kidney, surgery often fails to cure the hypertension.* With bilateral renal artery stenosis, most marked change on side with greatest degree of stenosis. Thus of little value in patients with bilateral disease.

Split renal function tests may show disparity between kidneys.

Hypoaldosteronism (Hypofunction of Renin-Angiotensin-Aldosterone System)

Infrequent condition may be due to
- Addison's disease.
- CAH (methyl oxidase, type II defect).
- Autosomal recessive deficiency of aldosterone synthase.
- Prolonged administration of heparin (very rare).
- Removal of unilateral aldosterone-secreting tumor (usually transient).
- Autonomic nervous system dysfunction; aldosterone deficiency causes impaired renal sodium conservation but without hyperkalemia.
- Idiopathic hyporeninism.
- Associated with mild renal insufficiency (especially diabetic nephropathy, some interstitial nephropathies).

ENDOCRINE

[18]Pickering TG. The role of laboratory testing in the diagnosis of renovascular hypertension. *Clin Chem* 1991;37:1831.

Table 13-21. Laboratory Tests in Differential Diagnosis of Benign Pheochromocytoma and Neural Crest Tumors (Neuroblastoma, Ganglioneuroma)

Urinary Levels of	Pheochromocytoma	Neural Crest Tumor (Neuroblastoma, Ganglioneuroma)
Catecholamines	I	I
Vanillylmandelic acid	I	I
Metanephrines	I	I
Dopamine	N*	I
Homovanillic acid	N*	I

I = increased; N = normal.
*I in malignant pheochromocytoma.

Hyperkalemia, hyponatremia, urinary sodium loss, hypovolemia corrected by administration of mineralocorticoids
Mild hyperchloremic metabolic acidosis
♦ Decreased aldosterone and PRA that are not increased by combined diuretic and posture establish the diagnosis.
Normal adrenal glucocorticoid response to ACTH stimulation test
Laboratory findings of associated diseases (e.g., diabetes mellitus, gout, pyelonephritis)

Neuroblastoma, Ganglioneuroma, Ganglioblastoma

See Table 13-21.
♦ Urinary concentrations of catecholamines (norepinephrine, normetanephrine, dopamine, VMA, and HVA) are increased. Excretion of epinephrine is not increased because of rapid catabolism. If only one of these substances is measured, only ~75% of cases are diagnosed. If VMA and HVA or VMA and total catecholamines are measured, 95–100% of cases are diagnosed.
♦ These tests are also useful for differentiating Ewing's tumor from metastatic neuroblastoma of bone and to show response to therapy (surgery, irradiation, or chemotherapy), which should bring return to normal in 1–4 mos. Continued increase indicates need for further treatment.
Cystathionine in urine suggests active disease but absence is not significant because it is not normally present.
Serum neuron-specific enolase may be increased in neuroblastoma; high level is associated with poor prognosis. Ratio of neuron-specific to nonneuronal enolase is reported to improve specificity to >85% for neuroblastoma.
Laboratory findings due to metastases (e.g., tumor in biopsy of marrow, liver, or other sites, anemia, etc.)

Pheochromocytoma

(Tumor of chromaffin cells of sympathetic nervous system; may secrete epinephrine, norepinephrine, dopamine. Occurs in 0.1–0.2% of hypertensive population in the United States. Five percent of patients with pheochromocytoma have normal blood pressure most or all of the time. Sustained hypertension in 50% of cases.)
See Figs. 13-19 and 13-20, and Tables 13-21 and 13-22.
♦ Diagnosis is based on increased blood or urine concentrations of catecholamines (norepinephrine and, to a lesser extent, epinephrine) and their metabolites (normetanephrine and metanephrine), which are usually increased even when patient is asymptomatic and normotensive; rarely are increases found only after a paroxysm. When other studies are negative, a timed urine specimen or plasma concentration for catecholamines and metabolites taken after a typical "spell" may be useful. However, repeated testing may be necessary. Concentrations of >400 pg/dL (normal <100 pg/dL) for epinephrine or >2000 pg/dL (normal <500 pg/dL) for nor-

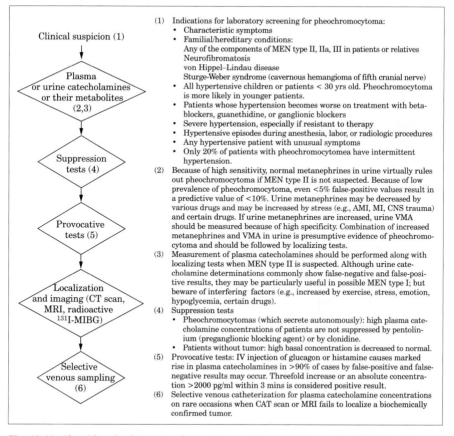

The figure shows a flowchart on the left with the following boxes connected by arrows, and numbered explanations on the right:

Clinical suspicion (1)

↓

Plasma or urine catecholamines or their metabolites (2,3)

↓

Suppression tests (4)

↓

Provocative tests (5)

↓

Localization and imaging (CT scan, MRI, radioactive ^{131}I-MIBG)

↓

Selective venous sampling (6)

(1) Indications for laboratory screening for pheochromocytoma:
  • Characteristic symptoms
  • Familial/hereditary conditions:
    Any of the components of MEN type II, IIa, III in patients or relatives
    Neurofibromatosis
    von Hippel–Lindau disease
    Sturge-Weber syndrome (cavernous hemangioma of fifth cranial nerve)
  • All hypertensive children or patients < 30 yrs old. Pheochromocytoma is more likely in younger patients.
  • Patients whose hypertension becomes worse on treatment with beta-blockers, guanethidine, or ganglionic blockers
  • Severe hypertension, especially if resistant to therapy
  • Hypertensive episodes during anesthesia, labor, or radiologic procedures
  • Any hypertensive patient with unusual symptoms
  • Only 20% of patients with pheochromocytomea have intermittent hypertension.

(2) Because of high sensitivity, normal metanephrines in urine virtually rules out pheochromocytoma if MEN type II is not suspected. Because of low prevalence of pheochromocytoma, even <5% false-positive values result in a predictive value of <10%. Urine metanephrines may be decreased by various drugs and may be increased by stress (e.g., AMI, MI, CNS trauma) and certain drugs. If urine metanephrines are increased, urine VMA should be measured because of high specificity. Combination of increased metanephrines and VMA in urine is presumptive evidence of pheochromocytoma and should be followed by localizing tests.

(3) Measurement of plasma catecholamines should be performed along with localizing tests when MEN type II is suspected. Although urine catecholamine determinations commonly show false-negative and false-positive results, they may be particularly useful in possible MEN type I; but beware of interfering factors (e.g., increased by exercise, stress, emotion, hypoglycemia, certain drugs).

(4) Suppression tests
  • Pheochromocytomas (which secrete autonomously): high plasma catecholamine concentrations of patients are not suppressed by pentolinium (preganglionic blocking agent) or by clonidine.
  • Patients without tumor: high basal concentration is decreased to normal.

(5) Provocative tests: IV injection of glucagon or histamine causes marked rise in plasma catecholamines in >90% of cases by false-positive and false-negative results may occur. Threefold increase or an absolute concentration >2000 pg/ml within 3 mins is considered positive result.

(6) Selective venous catheterization for plasma catecholamine concentrations on rare occasions when CAT scan or MRI fails to localize a biochemically confirmed tumor.

Fig. 13-19. Algorithm for diagnosis of pheochromocytoma. (CAT = computerized axial tomography; CT = computed tomography; ^{131}I-MIBG = metaiodobenzylguanidine labeled with iodine 131; MAO = monoamine oxidase; MEN = multiple endocrine neoplasia; MRI = magnetic resonance imaging; VMA = vanillylmandelic acid.)

epinephrine are considered diagnostic. Concentrations are usually 5–100× normal, although considerable overlap and wide range of normal values are seen. Intermediate values require further workup. Measurement of plasma concentrations is particularly useful to compare paroxysm and basal concentrations and to localize tumors by selective venous sampling. Blood should be drawn in the unstressed supine patient without interfering conditions or drugs. 24-hr urine free norepinephrine has reported sensitivity of 89–100% and specificity of 98%; plasma norepinephrine has sensitivity of 82% and specificity of 95%.[19] In one study, plasma metanephrines were more sensitive than plasma catecholamines or urine metanephrines; normal plasma metanephrines excluded pheochromocytoma.[20]

[19]Duncan MW, Compton P, Lazarus L, Smythe GA. Measurement of norepinephrine and 3,4-dihydroxyphenylglycol in urine and plasma for the diagnosis of pheochromocytoma. *N Engl J Med* 1988;319:136.
[20]Lenders JWM, et al. Plasma metanephrine in the diagnosis of pheochromocytoma. *Ann Intern Med* 1995;123:101.

ENDOCRINE

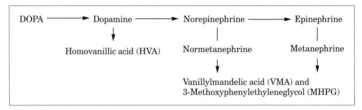

Fig. 13-20. Synthesis and breakdown of catecholamines. Because the hormones are broken down before release, metabolites are present in much larger amounts. When excretion of free catecholamines is greater than that of metabolites, tumor is said to be likely to be very small and difficult to locate.

Another report found 24-hr urine metanephrine values of >0.9 mg to have sensitivity of 100% and positive predictive value of 83%.[21] In a recent series[22] plasma normetanephrine or metanephrine had the highest sensitivity (97%) in patients with familial predispositions; MEN type II patients had high plasma metanephrine concentrations and von Hippel–Lindau disease patients had high plasma concentrations of only normetanephrine.

♦ Secretory Patterns

- Normally: epinephrine is secreted primarily by adrenal medulla and norepinephrine is secreted primarily at sympathetic nerve endings.
- Epinephrine is secreted by tumors, usually of adrenal medulla, and causes characteristic symptoms.
- Norepinephrine is secreted by almost all extra-adrenal tumors and many adrenal tumors; often associated with sustained hypertension and hypermetabolism.
- Dopamine secretion is not associated with hypertension.
- Malignancy: increased dopamine and almost as much norepinephrine with very low epinephrine.
- Part of familial syndrome: more likely to secrete both dopamine and epinephrine.
- Most common: increased norepinephrine predominant with much less epinephrine and dopamine.
- Most patients show increase of two or more catecholamines.
- Less common: equal norepinephrine and epinephrine and some dopamine.
- Predominance of epinephrine suggests tumor in adrenal or organ of Zuckerkandl; rarely bladder or mediastinum.
- Isolated increase of either adrenaline or dopamine is relatively common in normal persons but uncommon in pheochromocytoma patients.
- Repeated urine pattern of secretion is consistent in pheochromocytoma but some normal persons show large changes.
- Presence of HVA is said to suggest malignancy.
- Increased catecholamine concentrations after surgical removal may indicate recurrence of tumor.
- When urine catecholamines are fractionated, both epinephrine and norepinephrine must be measured because some tumors produce only one of these hormones.

♦ Catecholamines, Plasma/Urine

Plasma concentrations may not be increased when secretion is intermittent rather than continuous; for these cases 24-hr urine values are more accurate. Plasma concentrations are useful if 24-hr urine cannot be collected.

---

[21]Peplinski GR, Norton JA. The predictive value of diagnostic tests for pheochromocytoma. *Surgery* 1994;116:1101.
[22]Eisenhofer GE, et al. Plasma normetanephrine and metanephrine for detecting pheochromocytoma in von Hippel–Lindau disease and multiple endocrine neoplasia Type 2. *N Engl J Med* 1999;340:1872.

Table 13-22. Reference Range for Catecholamines and Metabolites

	Urine
Homovanillic acid	2–12 mg/24 hrs
Vanillylmandelic acid	2–7 mg/24 hrs
3-Methoxyphenylethyleneglycol	1.3–4.3 mg/24 hrs
Metanephrines	<1.6 mg/24 hrs
Dopamine	25–525 µg/24 hrs
Norepinephrine	10–64 µg/24 hrs
Epinephrine	0–36 µg/24 hrs
Norepinephrine + epinephrine	<100 µg/24 hrs
	Plasma
Dopamine	<100 pg/mL
Norepinephrine	65–400 pg/mL
Epinephrine	15–55 pg/mL

These data differ depending on source.
Source: Feldman JM. Diagnosis and management of pheochromocytoma. *Hosp Pract* 1989;(Jan 15): 175–198.

Increased In
Pheochromocytoma
Neural crest tumors (neuroblastoma, ganglioneuroma, ganglioblastoma)
Adrenal medullary hyperplasia
Diabetic ketoacidosis (markedly elevated)
AMI (markedly elevated)
Acute CNS disturbance (e.g., infarct, hemorrhage, encephalopathy, tumor)
Progressive muscular dystrophy and myasthenia gravis (some patients)
May also be increased by vigorous exercise before urine collection (<7×)
Stress (emotional, physical, postsurgery)
Hypothyroidism
Thyrotoxicosis
Volume depletion (induced by diuretics)
Renal disease
Heavy alcohol intake
Hypoglycemia
Has also been reported in Guillain-Barré syndrome, acute intermittent porphyria, carcinoid syndrome, acute psychosis

Interferences
False increase may be due to drugs that produce fluorescent urinary products (e.g., tetracyclines, methyldopa (Aldomet), epinephrine and epinephrine-like drugs [nose drops, cough and sinus remedies, bronchodilators, appetite suppressants], large doses of vitamin B complex).
Plasma catecholamines decrease markedly after 5 mins if RBCs are not separated from plasma.
Drugs that destroy catecholamines in bladder urine, e.g., methenamine mandelate
Not all methods include dopamine in determination of urine total catecholamines.
Urine norepinephrine/normetanephrine may be less reliable than VMA or metanephrines in screening for pheochromocytoma due to technical problems; best used to confirm diagnosis (using HPLC) when other tests are equivocal.
Avoid medications for 1 wk before sampling.
Many drugs reported to increase values of catecholamines or metabolites, including alpha$_1$-blockers, aminophylline, amphetamines, ampicillin, beta-blockers, caffeine, chlorpromazine, diazoxide, drug withdrawal (alcohol, clonidine), epinephrine, ephedrine, imipramine, isoproterenol, labetalol, methyldopa, monoamine oxydase inhibitors, nicotine, phenacetin, phenothiazine, quinidine, theophylline, vasodilators (e.g., minoxidil, hydralazine nitroglycerine, sodium nitroprusside), calcium channel blockers (acutely).

ENDOCRINE

Many drugs reported to decrease values of catecholamines or metabolites, including anileridine, aspirin, PAS, alpha$_2$ agonists, bromocriptine, sodium sulfobromoph-thalein (Bromsulphalein), calcium channel blockers (long-term use), cimetidine, clofi-brate, clonidine, chlorpromazine, disulfiram, glyceryl guaiacolate, guanethidine, imipramine, isoproterenol, L-dopa, monoamine oxidase inhibitors, propranolol, mephenesin, methocarbamol, methyldopa, metyrosine, nalidixic acid, penicillin, phenazopyridine, PSP, reserpine, sulfa drugs, thyroxine.

♦ Urine VMA

VMA is the urinary metabolite of both epinephrine and norepinephrine. Excretion is considerably increased in ~90% of patients. Because this analysis is simpler than that for catecholamines, it has been more commonly used, but it is less sensitive than other tests.

Increased In
Pheochromocytoma
Neuroblastoma, ganglioneuroma, ganglioblastoma

Interferences
Beware of false-positive results due to ingestion of certain foods within 72 hrs before the test (e.g., coffee, tea, chocolate, vanilla, some fruits and vegetables, especially bananas) and drugs.
Beware of nonspecific techniques for VMA assay that fail to detect 30% of cases of pheochromocytoma.

♦ Urine Metanephrines

Is reliable screening test as false-negatives = 4% and fewer interferences by drugs and diet are seen than with VMA or catecholamines.
Confirmation by urine catecholamine fraction determinations has been considered an excellent routine to identify pheochromocytoma patients.

Plasma chromogranin A, a marker for pheochromocytoma, has ~50% sensitivity.
Hyperglycemia and glycosuria are found in 50% of patients during an attack.
GTT frequently shows a diabetic type of curve; many patients develop clinical diabetes mellitus.
Thyroid function tests are normal.
Urine changes are secondary to sustained hypertension.
PRA activity is increased.
Relative erythrocytosis sometimes occurs.
Increased incidence of cholelithiasis
Other hormones may be secreted (e.g., serotonin, PTH, calcitonin, ACTH, gastrin, VIP, FSH, insulin). Rarely, can cause Cushing's syndrome and hypercalcemia.
15% of pheochromocytomas are extra-adrenal; 10% are multiple. 10% occur in children, two-thirds of whom are male.
2–10% of adrenal and 20–40% of extra-adrenal pheochromocytomas are malignant.
Familial inheritance in 10–20% of patients; 70% of these are bilateral. Associated with certain neurocutaneous syndromes (e.g., von Hippel-Lindau disease [in ~20% of cases], von Recklinghausen's disease, tuberous sclerosis).
All patients with pheochromocytoma should be screened for other components of MEN type IIa and IIb present in ~4% of cases (see p. 697). Tumors associated with famil-ial syndromes are more likely to be asymptomatic, multiple, and extra-adrenal.

Pseudo–Cushing's Syndrome

Due To

Major depressive disorders: cortisol secretion is abnormal in 80% of these patients but hyper-secretion is usually minimal and transient; disappears with remission of depression.
♦ • Evening nadir in plasma cortisol is preserved; level <5 µg/dL rules out and >7.5 µg/dL indicates Cushing's syndrome.
 • Plasma cortisol is low after administration of dexamethasone and remains low when CRH is given soon after, whereas in Cushing's syndrome, plasma cortisol is not so low after dexamethasone and increases after CRH.

- Insulin-induced hypoglycemia causes increased plasma cortisol but not in chronic Cushing's syndrome.

Chronic alcoholism—abnormal liver function tests; resolves during abstinence as liver function returns to normal.

Pseudoaldosteronism Due to Ingestion of Licorice (Ammonium Glycyrrhizate)

(Excessive ingestion causes hypertension due to sodium retention)
Decreased serum potassium
Decreased aldosterone excretion in urine
Decreased PRA
♦ Urinary glycyrrhetinic acid can be measured by gas chromatography and mass spectrometry.
Unstimulated renin-aldosterone system may be suppressed for ≤ 4 mos after cessation of long-term ingestion of licorice. Effect on electrolyte balance may persist for ≤ 1 wk after cessation.

Pseudohyperaldosteronism (Liddle's Syndrome)

(Rare familial nephropathic disorder [possibly at distal tubule] with clinical manifestations closely resembling those due to aldosterone-producing adrenal adenoma)
Hypokalemia due to renal potassium wasting
Metabolic alkalosis
Hypertension
○ All are corrected by long-term administration of diuretics that act at distal tubule to cause natriuresis and renal potassium retention (e.g., triamterene or amiloride) and by restriction of sodium.
♦ Aldosterone secretion and excretion are greatly reduced and unresponsive to stimulation by ACTH, angiotensin II, or low-sodium diet.
Low plasma renin
Sodium retention

Pseudohypoaldosteronism

♦ Heterogeneous group of disorders due to resistance to aldosterone action with signs and symptoms of aldosterone deficiency, but aldosterone and PRA levels are markedly increased and are resistant to mineralocorticoid therapy.

Tests of Gonadal Function

Chromosome Analysis

See pp. 511–512, 515.
Turner's syndrome (gonadal dysgenesis): usually negative for Barr bodies (see p. 684)
Klinefelter's syndrome: positive for Barr bodies (see p. 681)
Pseudohermaphroditism: chromosomal sex corresponding to gonadal sex

Cytologic Examination of Vaginal Smear (Papanicolaou Smear) for Evaluation of Ovarian Function

Maturation index is the proportion of parabasal, intermediate, and superficial cells in each 100 cells counted.
- Lack of estrogen effect shows predominance of parabasal cells (e.g., maturation index = 100/0/0).
- Low estrogen effect shows predominance of intermediate cells (e.g., maturation index = 10/90/0).

ENDOCRINE

- Increased estrogen effect shows predominance of superficial cells (e.g., maturation index = 0/0/100), as in hormone-producing tumors of ovary, persistent follicular cysts.

Some Patterns of Maturation Index in Different Conditions

	Index
Childhood	
Normal	80/20/0
Cortisone therapy	0/98/2
Childbearing years	
Preovulatory (late follicular) phase	0/40/60
Premenstrual (late luteal) phase	0/70/30
Pregnancy (second month)	0/90/10
Cortisone therapy	0/85/15
Amenorrhea after ovarian irradiation	0/30/70
Surgical oophorectomy	0/80/20–0/90/10
Bilateral oophorectomy and adrenalectomy	0/98/2
Postmenopausal years, early (age 60)	65/30/5
Postmenopausal years, late (age 75)	
Untreated	100/0/0
Moderate estrogen treatment	0/50/50
High-dose estrogen treatment	0/0/100
Years after bilateral oophorectomy	100/0/0
Postadrenalectomy, bilateral	6/94/0

Karyopyknotic index is the percentage of cells with pyknotic nuclei. Increased estrogen effect (e.g., karyopyknotic index $\geq 85\%$) is seen, as in cystic glandular hyperplasia of the endometrium.

Eosinophilic index is the percentage of cells showing eosinophilic cytoplasm; it may also be used as a measure of estrogen effect.

Combined progesterone-estrogen effect: No quantitative cytologic criteria are available. Endometrial biopsy should be used for this purpose.

The pattern may be obscured by cytolysis (e.g., infections, excess bacilli), increased red or white blood cells, excessively thin or thick smears, or drying of smears before fixation (artificial eosinophilic staining).

Estrogens (Total), Serum

(Includes estradiol produced by ovaries and placenta, and smaller amounts by testes and adrenals; estrone and estriol)

Increased In

Granulosa cell tumor of ovary
Theca-cell tumor of ovary
Luteoma of ovary
Pregnancy
Secondary to stimulation by hCG-producing tumors (e.g., teratoma, teratocarcinoma)
Gynecomastia

Decreased In

Primary hypofunction of ovary
- Autoimmune oophoritis is the most common cause. Usually associated with other autoimmune endocrinopathies, e.g., Hashimoto's thyroiditis, Addison's disease, insulin-dependent diabetes mellitus. May cause premature menopause.
- Resistant-ovary syndrome.
- Toxic (e.g., irradiation, chemotherapy).
- Infection (e.g., mumps).
- Tumor (primary or secondary).
- Mechanical (e.g., trauma, torsion, surgical excision).
- Genetic (e.g., Turner's syndrome [see p. 684]).
- Menopause.
Secondary hypofunction of ovary
- Disorders of hypothalamic-pituitary axis

Follicle-Stimulating Hormone (FSH) and Luteinizing Hormone (LH), Serum

(Pituitary gonadotropins)

Use

Differential diagnosis of gonadal disorders
Diagnosis and management of infertility

Increased In

Primary hypogonadism (anorchia, testicular failure, menopause)
Gonadotropin-secreting pituitary tumors
Precocious puberty (secondary to a CNS lesion or idiopathic)
Complete testicular feminization syndrome
Luteal phase of menstrual cycle

Decreased In

Secondary hypogonadism
  • Kallmann's syndrome (inherited autosomal isolated deficiency of hypothalamic gonadotropin-releasing hormone; occurs in both sexes): Found in ~5% of patients with primary amenorrhea. Causes failure of both gametogenic function and sex steroid production (LH and FSH are "normal" or undetectable but rise in response to prolonged gonadotropin-releasing hormone stimulation).
  • Pituitary LH or FSH deficiency.
  • Gonadotropin deficiency.

Müllerian Inhibiting Substance, Serum

(Gonadal hormone produced by prepubertal testes to promote involution of müllerian ducts during normal male sexual differentiation. Detectable in normal boys from birth to puberty, when concentration declines.)

Use

Differentiate anorchia from nonpalpable undescended testes in boys with bilateral cryptorchidism.
Presence indicates testicular integrity in children with intersexual anomalies.
Supplements or replaces measurement of response of serum testosterone to administration of hCG for gonadal evaluation in prepubertal children.

Decreased or Absent In

Anorchia
Negligible concentration in girls until puberty
Female pseudohermaphroditism

Interpretation

In prepubertal children, normal value in boys is sensitive and specific test predictive of testicular tissue (98%) and undetectable value predicts anorchia or ovaries (89%).
Values are better than those for serum testosterone alone; combined with serum testosterone, sensitivity = 62% and specificity = 100% for absence of testes.[23]

Progesterone, Serum

Increased In

Luteal phase of menstrual cycle
Luteal cysts of ovary

ENDOCRINE

---

[23]Lee MM, et al. Measurements of serum müllerian inhibiting substance in the evaluation of children with nonpalpable gonads. *N Engl J Med* 1997;336:1480.

Ovarian tumors (e.g., arrhenoblastoma)
Adrenal tumors

Decreased In

Amenorrhea
Threatened abortion (some patients)
Fetal death
Toxemia of pregnancy
Gonadal agenesis

17-Hydroxycorticosteroids (17-OHKS), Urine

(Derived from cortisol and cortisone. Measure approximately one-half to two-thirds of cortisol and its metabolites.)

Use

Evaluation of adrenocortical function
Screening and diagnostic test of glucocorticoid hypo- or hypersecretory disorders. Often replaced by measurement of urine free cortisol or serum cortisol, which it parallels.

Increased In

Cushing's syndrome
Adrenal tumors
Marked stress (e.g., burns, surgery, infections)
Use of certain drugs (e.g., acetazolamide, chloral hydrate, chlordiazepoxide, chlorpromazine, colchicine, erythromycin, estrogens, etryptamine, glucocorticoids, meprobamate, oleandomycin, paraldehyde, quinine and quinidine, spironolactone)

Decreased In

Addison's disease
ACTH deficiency
Hypothyroidism
Fasting
Use of certain drugs (e.g., high-potency steroids [dexamethasone], narcotics, oral contraceptives, phenothiazines, phenytoin, reserpine)

17-Ketogenic Steroids (17-KGS) (Corticosteroids), Blood and Urine

Use

Evaluation of excessive or deficient glucocorticoid secretion
Evaluation of 21-hydroxylase deficiency type of CAH
Increasingly supplanted by measurements of serum cortisol, urine free cortisol, serum 17-hydroxyprogesterone, urine pregnanetriol

Increased In

Adrenal hyperplasia
Adrenal adenoma
Adrenal carcinoma
ACTH therapy
Stress
Other conditions (e.g., obesity, smoking)
Use of certain drugs (e.g., glucocorticoids, ampicillin)

Decreased In

Addison's disease
Panhypopituitarism

Cessation of corticosteroid therapy
General wasting disease
Use of certain drugs (e.g., estrogens and oral contraceptives, dexamethasone)

17-Ketosteroids (17-KS), Urine

(Metabolites of adrenal and gonadal androgenic steroids)

Use

Indication of adrenal rather than testicular status; two-thirds are of adrenal origin in
men; almost all are of adrenal origin in women.
Diagnosis of ovarian and adrenal tumors. Supplanted by more specific RIA of DHEA
and DHEA-S.
May show daily variation of 100% in same individual.

Increased In

Interstitial cell tumor of testicle
Virilizing ovarian tumors (e.g., adrenal rest tumor, granulosa cell tumor, hilar cell
tumor, Brenner tumor, and, most frequently, arrhenoblastoma); increased in 50% of
patients and normal in 50% of patients
Adrenocortical hyperplasia (causing Cushing's syndrome, adrenogenital syndrome, pre-
cocious puberty)
Adrenocortical adenoma or carcinoma
Severe stress (e.g., burns, surgery, infections); exercise
Pituitary tumor or hyperplasia
ACTH or testosterone administration
Third trimester of pregnancy
Nonspecific chromogens in urine
Use of certain drugs (e.g., ampicillin, cephaloridine, cephalothin, chloramphenicol,
chlorpromazine, cloxacillin, danazol, dexamethasone, erythromycin, ethinamate,
nalidixic acid, oleandomycin, penicillin, phenaglycodol, phenazopyridine, pheno-
thiazines, quinidine, secobarbital, spironolactone)

Decreased In

Primary hypogonadism (e.g., primary ovarian agenesis)
Secondary hypogonadism
Addison's disease
Panhypopituitarism
Nephrosis
Generalized wasting disease
Use of certain drugs (e.g., chlordiazepoxide, estrogens and oral contraceptives, metyrapone,
opiates, phenytoin, probenecid, promazine, reserpine)

Testicle, Biopsy

Use

Infertility workup
Diagnosis of tumor

Interpretation

Normal spermatogenesis and normal endocrine findings in patient with aspermia and
infertility suggests a mechanical obstruction to sperm transport that may be correctable.

Testosterone, Free, Plasma

Use

Evaluation of gonadal hormonal function

ENDOCRINE

Decreased In (Men)

Primary hypogonadism (e.g., orchiectomy)
Secondary hypogonadism (e.g., hypopituitarism)
Testicular feminization
Klinefelter's syndrome levels lower than in normal male but higher than in normal
    female and orchiectomized male
Estrogen therapy
Total testosterone decreased due to decreased sex hormone–binding globulin (e.g., cir-
    rhosis, chronic renal disease)

Increased In

Adrenal virilizing tumor causing premature puberty in boys or masculinization in women
CAH
Idiopathic hirsutism—inconclusive
Stein-Leventhal syndrome—variable; increased when virilization is present.
Ovarian stromal hyperthecosis
Drugs that alter T_4-binding globulins may also affect testosterone-binding globulins;
    however, free testosterone level is not affected.

Gonadal Disorders

Ambiguous Genitalia

(Sexual ambiguity occurs in 1 in 1000 live-born infants.)

Females[24]

Condition	Laboratory Finding
CAH with or without salt losing	See p. 633.
Iatrogenic virilization	No diagnostic test. History of maternal ingestion of virilizing agents (i.e., progestins).
Maternal virilization	Increased androgens in maternal serum
Idiopathic virilization	Normal plasma and urine steroids. 46 XX karyotype. Gonadal biopsy may show Leydig's tissue.
Gonadal dysgenesis	See p. 684. No specific laboratory test. Laparotomy usually shows a streak gonad on one side and testicular tissue on other side. Karyotype may be nondiagnostic (46 XX or 46 XY), multiple mosaic (44 XO/46 XX/47 XXY), or typical (45 XO/46 XY).
True hermaphrodite	No specific laboratory test. Biopsy of gonad shows ovarian follicles and testicular tubules. Karyotype may be 46 XX, 46 XY, or any mosaic included under gonadal dysgenesis. H-Y antigen is present.

Males[24]

Condition	Laboratory Finding
Absent müllerian inhibiting factor	46 XY karyotype. Normal steroid levels. No specific laboratory tests. Testes and uterii inguinali present.
Undescended testes	Normal gonadotropin and hormone levels.
Anorchia	May have low plasma testosterone and very high plasma FSH and LH. Later hCG stimulation is negative.
Leydig's cell agenesis or hypoplasia	Plasma testosterone is very low and fails to

[24]Lippe BM. Ambiguous genitalia and pseudohermaphrodites. *Ped Clin North Am* 1979;26:91.

	rise after hCG stimulation. High LD. Normal FSH. Biopsy of testicle is diagnostic.
Unknown cause for unresponsiveness to androgens	Karyotype 46 XY. Normal testosterone and dihydrotestosterone levels. No specific laboratory test.
Faulty androgen action	46 XY karyotype. Normal testosterone level. *Sex-linked defect type* is diagnosed by in vitro binding study. LH may be high. Dihydrotestosterone level is normal. *Autosomal recessive type* has normal LH and FSH levels. Dihydrotestosterone level is low.
Abnormal testosterone synthesis, no salt loss	Increased 17-KS in urine and low plasma testosterone in one type. Decreased 17-KS in urine in other types.
Abnormal testosterone synthesis, with salt loss	Decreased 17-KS in one type. Increased plasma pregnenolone in other type.
Hypopituitarism	Decreased GH levels. Other tropic hormones may be deficient. Neonatal hypoglycemia is usual.
Microphallus	No specific laboratory test.
Congenital malformations	No specific laboratory test.

Laboratory Differential Diagnosis

Gonads Palpable
Buccal smear chromatin positive and 17-KS normal
- True hermaphroditism
- Klinefelter's syndrome variant

Buccal smear chromatin negative and 17-KS normal
- True hermaphroditism
- Anatomic defect
- Inherited enzyme deficiency syndrome affecting testosterone synthesis, metabolism, or action on target tissues

Buccal smear chromatin negative and 17-KS increased
- CAH (3-beta-hydroxysteroid dehydrogenase deficiency)

Gonads Not Palpable
Buccal smear chromatin positive and 17-KS normal
- True hermaphroditism
- Ovarian tumor (maternal 17-KS increased)
- Maternal exposure to androgens (history)

Buccal smear chromatin positive and 17-KS increased
- CAH
    11-beta-hydroxylase deficiency
    21-hydroxylase deficiency
    3-beta-hydroxysteroid dehydrogenase deficiency

Buccal smear chromatin negative and 17-KS normal
- True hermaphroditism
- Gonadal dysgenesis (45 X/46 XY, 46 XY)

Precautions in Workup of Neonate with Ambiguous Genitalia

Buccal mucosal smear for nuclear sex chromatin determination may show false-negative patterns during first 2 days of life so all chromatin-negative smears should be repeated after the third day. Sex chromatin in >25% of cells from the buccal mucosa indicates presence of at least two X chromosomes. A leukocyte culture for karyotype preparation should begin immediately whenever possible to confirm the sex chromosome constitution. The Y chromosome fluorescence test may also be valuable.

A chromatin-positive newborn is almost always female.

External genitalia are normal in Klinefelter's and most cases of Turner's syndrome.

Amenorrhea/Delayed Menarche (Primary)

See Fig. 13-21.

ENDOCRINE

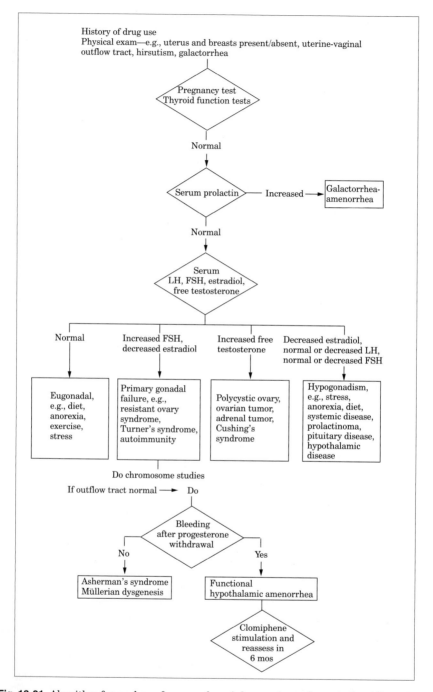

Fig. 13-21. Algorithm for workup of amenorrhea. Asherman's syndrome is the obliteration of endometrial lining by adhesions due to pelvic inflammatory disease, tuberculosis, postabortal or puerperal endometritis, etc. Normal blood steroid levels that do not respond to progesterone administration by bleeding. Müllerian dysgenesis is a congenital deformity or absence of tubes, uterus, or vagina; karyotype and hormone levels are normal. (LH = luteinizing hormone; FSH = follicle-stimulating hormone.)

Due To

Gonadal disorders (60% of all causes)
- Gonadal dysgenesis (75% of gonadal disorders)
    Testicular feminization syndrome (most common form of male hermaphroditism; female phenotype with male 46 XY karyotype, testosterone in male range; testes are present)
- Polycystic ovaries
- Resistant-ovary syndrome

Structural genital tract disorders (35–40% of all causes)
- Imperforate hymen
- Uterine agenesis
- Vaginal agenesis
- Transverse vaginal septum

Pituitary disorders (rare)
- Hypopituitarism
- Adenomas (prolactin secreting)

Hypothalamic disorders (rare)
- Anatomic lesions (e.g., craniopharyngioma)
- Functional disturbance of hypothalamic-pituitary axis (e.g., anorexia nervosa, emotional stress)

Systemic disorders
- Hypothyroidism
- CAH
- Debilitating chronic diseases (e.g., malnutrition, congenital heart disease, renal failure, collagen diseases)

Hormone Profiles

Normal LH, FSH, prolactin, estradiol, testosterone, T_4, and TSH (eugonadal)
- Drugs
- Diet, anorexia
- Exercise
- Stress, illness
- Structural genital tract disorders (see previous section)

Increased LH and normal FSH
- Early pregnancy
- Polycystic ovarian disease (Stein-Leventhal syndrome)
- Ectopic gonadotropin production by neoplasm (e.g., lung, GI tract)

Increased LH and FSH (>30 mIU/mL), decreased estrogen (<50 pg/mL)
- Primary ovarian hypofunction

Normal or low LH and FSH, decreased estrogen
- Hyperprolactinemia (see p. 700)
- Isolated gonadotropin deficiency due to pituitary or hypothalamic impairment.
    Administer clomiphene citrate for 5–10 days; if gonadotropin level increases or menses return, cause is probably hypothalamic.
    Administer hypothalamic LH-releasing factor; normal or exaggerated response in hypothalamic amenorrhea (cause in 80% of patients); smaller or no response in pituitary tumor or dysfunction.

Increased androgen
- Polycystic ovarian disease (testosterone level usually <200 ng/dL)
- Tumor of adrenal or ovary (testosterone level may be >200 ng/dL)
- Testicular feminization
- Use of anabolic steroids (e.g., in athletes)

Androgen Abuse

(By athletes who use synthetic androgens to enhance performance or body building; effects depend on type and dose of drug used.)
♦ When exogenous testosterone is used, urine testosterone/epitestosterone ratio >6:1 is often considered indicative of steroid abuse (normal ratio is ~1:1 in men and women)
♦ Synthetic androgen or its metabolites are identified in urine.

Erythrocytosis may occur.

ENDOCRINE

Serum testosterone may be low.
Decreased or normal LH and FSH
Plasma HDL may be decreased and LDL may be increased.
Platelet counts and platelet aggregation may be increased.
Laboratory findings due to infertility and testicular atrophy

Androgen Deficiency (Hypogonadism)

See Tables 13-23 and 13-24.

Due To

Secondary hypogonadism (hypogonadotropic)
Secondary to pituitary-hypothalamic disorders
- Hyperprolactinemia
- Panhypopituitarism (pituitary or hypothalamus)
    Tumor
    Granulomatous disease
    Hemochromatosis
    Trauma
    Infarction, vasculitis
- Isolated gonadotropin deficiency
    Isolated FSH or LH deficiency
    Idiopathic hypothalamic hypogonadism
    Kallmann's syndrome
- Genetic disorders (e.g., Prader-Willi, Laurence-Moon-Biedl syndromes)
- Systemic (e.g., chronic disease, nutritional deficiency, massive obesity)
- Drugs (e.g., glucocorticoids)
Constitutional (delayed puberty)

♦ Decreased serum testosterone (<100 ng/dL) with low or normal LH and FSH
♦ Decreased gonadotropin-releasing hormone
♦ Administration of gonadotropin-releasing hormone increases serum gonadotropin, testosterone, FSH, and LH

Primary hypogonadism (hypergonadotropic)
Gonadal
- Genetic
    Klinefelter's syndrome
    True hermaphroditism
    Defects in synthesis of androgens due to deficiency of various enzymes (e.g., 20-alpha-hydroxylase, 17,20-desmolase, etc.)
    Agenesis of testicles
    Miscellaneous (e.g., Noonan's syndrome, streak gonads, myotonia dystrophica, cystic fibrosis)
- Acquired (e.g., chemotherapy, irradiation, castration, drugs, alcohol, viral orchitis [especially mumps], cryptorchidism, chronic liver or kidney disease)
Hormonal
- Hormonal insensitivity (e.g., androgen or LH insensitivity)
- Defects in action of androgens (pseudohermaphroditism)
    Complete (testicular feminization)
    Incomplete
        Type I (defects in testosterone receptors)
        Type II (5-alpha-reductase deficiency)

Climacteric, Male

○ Decreased testosterone level in blood (<300 ng/mL) and urine (<100 μg/24 hrs)
○ Urinary gonadotropin level is elevated. (Gonadotropin is decreased when low testosterone level is due to pituitary tumor, gout, or diabetes.)

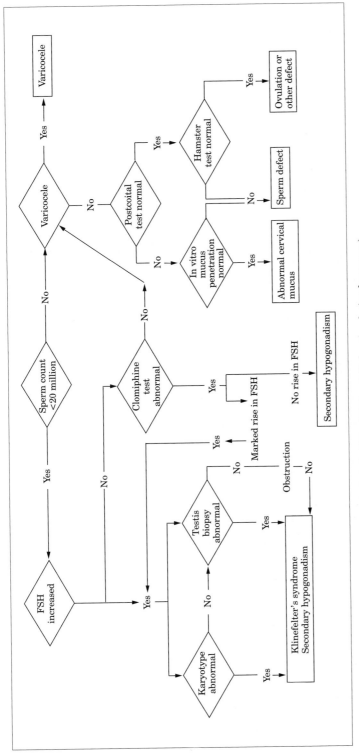

Fig. 13-22. Algorithm for evaluation of nonazoospermic infertility. (FSH = follicle-stimulating hormone.)

Table 13-23. Laboratory Differentiation of Primary and Secondary (to Pituitary Defect) Hypogonadism

Test	Primary Hypogonadism	Hypogonadism Secondary to Pituitary Defect
Level of FSH and gonadotropin in urine	High	Low
After administration of gonadotropins		
17-KS excretion	Does not increase	Increases
Clinical evidence of hypogonadism	Does not subside	Subsides with Increased sperm count Increased estrogenic effect in Papanicolaou smear

17-KS = 17-ketosteroid; FSH = follicle-stimulating hormone.

Corpus Luteum Deficiency

(Corpus luteum produces insufficient progesterone for development of endometrium receptive for pregnancy.)

Due To

Any condition that interferes with follicle growth and development
- Severe systemic illness including liver, kidney, or heart dysfunction
- Hyperprolactinemia
- X-chromosome abnormalities
- Polycystic ovarian disease or other causes of inadequate FSH level early in cycle
- Deficient LH receptors on corpus luteum cells
- Inadequate LH level or deficient ovulatory surge

Findings of endometrial biopsy on 26th day of cycle show less development than those of biopsy on menstrual day.
♦ Serum progesterone measured on three different days during midluteal phase totals <15 ng/mL and random level is <5 ng/mL.

Germinal Aplasia

♦ Biopsy of testicle shows that Sertoli's and Leydig's cells are intact and germinal cells are absent.
○ Azoospermia
○ Buccal smears are normal (negative for Barr bodies).
○ Chromosomal pattern is normal.
Urinary gonadotropin is normal.
Urinary pituitary gonadotropin is increased.
17-KS is decreased.

Table 13-24. Serum Hormone Levels in Various Types of Androgen Deficiency

Disorder	FSH	LH	Testosterone
Primary testicular disease	I	I	D
Secondary to pituitary-hypothalamic disorders[a]	D	D	D
Testosterone resistance[b]	N to I	I to N	I to N
Isolated germinal cell disease	I to N	N	N

D = decreased; FSH = follicle-stimulating hormone; I = increased; LH = luteinizing hormone; N = normal.
[a]Decreased (less than twofold) or absent response of FSH and LH to administration of clomiphene (100 mg/day for 7–10 days) confirms pituitary-hypothalamic cause.
[b]Testosterone-receptor defects are the most common cause of testosterone resistance; characteristic pattern is increased serum testosterone and LH.

Gynecomastia

See Fig. 13-23.

Due To

Neonatality
Puberty (25%)
Drugs (10–20%) (e.g., spironolactone, estrogens, cimetidine)
Cirrhosis or malnutrition (8%)
Testicular tumors (3%) (e.g., Leydig's cell, Sertoli's cell, germ cell tumors containing trophoblastic tissue)
Ectopic production of hCG by tumors (e.g., lung, liver, kidney)
Primary gonadism (8%)
Secondary gonadism (2%)
Hyperthyroidism (1.5%)
Renal disease (1%)
Klinefelter's syndrome
Feminizing adrenal cortical tumors
Idiopathic (25%)
Conditions usually associated with ambiguous genitalia or deficient virilization
- Androgen-insensitivity syndromes
- True hermaphroditism
- Enzymatic defects of testosterone production

Hirsutism

See Fig. 13-24.

Due To

Ovarian
- Polycystic ovary syndrome
- Hyperthecosis syndrome
- Tumors (e.g., arrhenoblastoma, gonadoblastoma, dysgerminoma; Brenner cell, granulosa-theca cell, lipoid cell tumors)

Adrenal
- Adenoma, carcinoma
- Cushing's syndrome
- CAH (21-hydroxylase deficiency, 11-hydroxylase deficiency, 3-beta-hydroxysteroid dehydrogenase deficiency)

Drugs (e.g., anabolic steroids, androgens)
Idiopathic (e.g., increased 5-alpha-reductase activity)

Infertility

See Figs. 13-22, 13-25, and 13-26.
85% of couples conceive after 12 mos of unprotected intercourse.
Remaining 15% warrant investigation for infertility.

Due To

Male factors (identified in ~40% of couples) (see Fig. 13-25)
- Testicular abnormalities (e.g., cryptorchidism, torsion, trauma, infection, varicocele)
- Coital factors (e.g., impotence)
- Toxins (e.g., anabolic steroids, marijuana, alcohol, medications [cyclosporine, spironolactone, cimetidine, nitrofurantoin])
- Others, e.g.,
    Sperm antibodies (numerous assay methods)
        Clinical significance of serum antibodies in men and women is controversial.
        Present in 10% of infertile men
        Present in infertile women in cervical mucus in 25% and in serum in 13%
    Irradiation

ENDOCRINE

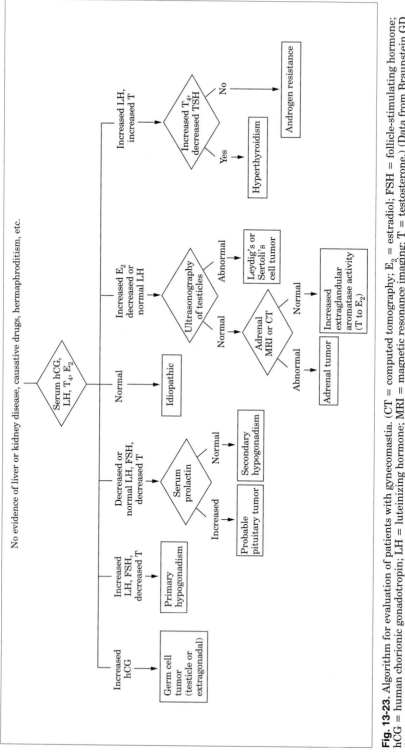

Fig. 13-23. Algorithm for evaluation of patients with gynecomastia. (CT = computed tomography; E₂ = estradiol; FSH = follicle-stimulating hormone; hCG = human chorionic gonadotropin; LH = luteinizing hormone; MRI = magnetic resonance imaging; T = testosterone.) (Data from Braunstein GD. Gynecomastia. *N Engl J Med* 1993;328:490.)

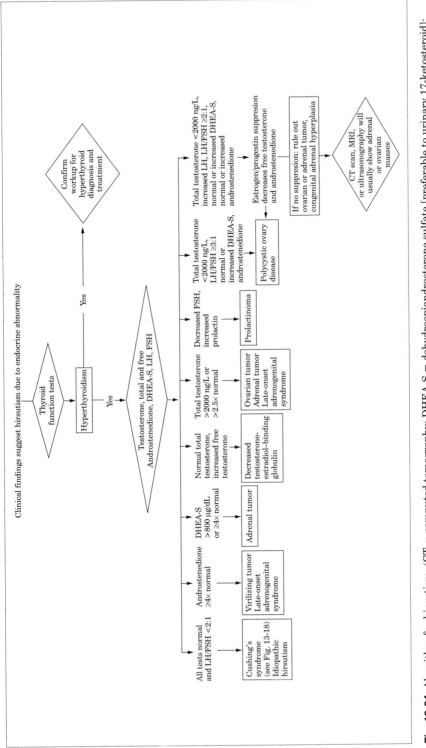

Fig. 13-24. Algorithm for hirsutism. (CT = computed tomography; DHEA-S = dehydroepiandrosterone sulfate [preferable to urinary 17-ketosteroid]; FSH = follicle-stimulating hormone; LH = luteinizing hormone; MRI = magnetic resonance imaging.)

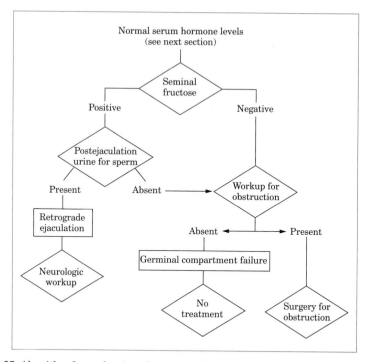

Fig. 13-25. Algorithm for evaluation of azoospermia.

       Hyperthermia
       Heavy metals, e.g., lead, cadmium, manganese
       Pesticides
- Hypothalamic/pituitary disorders (e.g., hyperprolactinemia, deficiency of gonado-tropin-releasing hormone)
- Chromosome abnormalities (e.g., Klinefelter's syndrome, Down syndrome)

Female factors (identified in ~40% of couples) (see Fig. 13-22)
- Uterine factors
       Cervical (e.g., decreased cervical mucus quality or quantity, sperm antibodies)
       Uterine (e.g., endometriosis)
       Tube (e.g., salpingitis)
- Hypothalamic/pituitary disorders (e.g., hyperprolactinemia)
- Disorders of ovulation (e.g., polycystic ovaries)
- Chromosome abnormalities (e.g., Turner's syndrome)
- Others (e.g., irradiation)

Combined male and female or unidentified factors in 20%.

Semen Analysis[25–27]

Use
Infertility studies
Absence of sperm to confirm vasectomy
DNA test to confirm rape assailant

[25]Adams JE. Infertility in men: diagnosis and treatment. *ASCP Check Sample CC 87-9 (CC-187).* 1987;27:1.

[26]Rothmann SA, Morgan BW. Laboratory diagnosis in andrology. *Cleve Clin J Med* 1989;(Nov-Dec):805.

[27]Ferrara F, et al. Automation of human sperm cell analysis by flow cytometry. *Clin Chem* 1997;43:801.

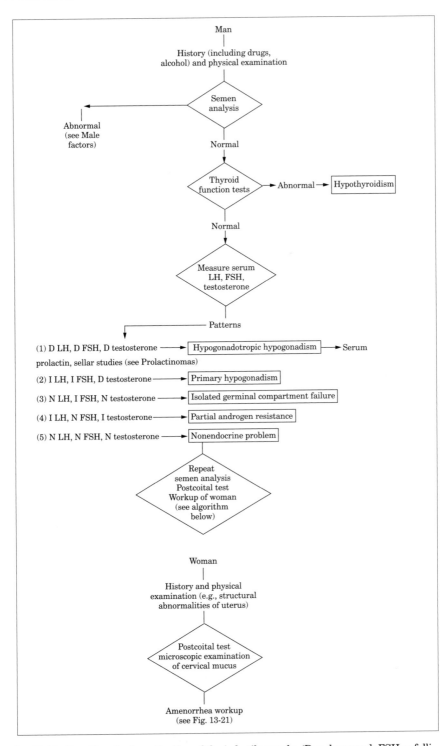

Fig. 13-26. Algorithm for investigation of the infertile couple. (D = decreased; FSH = folli-cle-stimulating hormone; I = increased; LH = luteinizing hormone; N = normal.) (Male portion of figure from Swerdloff RS. Infertility in the male. *Ann Intern Med* 1985;103:906.)

ENDOCRINE

Reference Ranges

Volume	>2 mL
pH	7.2–8.0
Color	Translucent, gray-white, or opalescent
Liquefaction	<30 mins
Viability	>65%
Motility	>50% viable sperm with forward progression
	Progressive motility 3+ to 4+
Sperm density (count)	>20 million/mL
Morphology	>30% normal forms
Total motile functional sperm	>40 million
(= volume × % motility × sperm density × % normal morphology)	
RBCs	0–5/HPF
WBCs	0–5/HPF ($<10^6$/mL)
Crystals	None
Clumping	None
Mixed antiglobulin reaction	Negative
Bovine cervical mucus penetration	>30 mm
Cultures for bacteria (*Ureaplasma*, *Chlamydia*)	No pathogens
Antisperm antibodies	Negative

Sterile males usually show
- Volume of <3 mL
- <20 million sperm/mL; only a count <5 million sperm/mL seems to reduce chance for pregnancy
- <25% motility

Abnormal motility or morphology can occur with normal sperm counts but are usually seen with decreased counts. Abnormal forms indicate impaired spermatogenesis. Decreased motility may reflect defects in cilia structure elsewhere (in respiratory and reproductive tracts). Agglutination may indicate antisperm antibodies (which can be measured but relationship to infertility is not established).
- Normal morphology is >60% normal oval forms, <6% tapered forms, <0.5% immature forms, <8% amorphous forms. Tapered forms and spermatids are often increased in infertility associated with varicocele.

Inflammatory cells may indicate infection of GU tract.

Absent fructose (normally produced by seminal vesicles) may indicate absence or obstruction of vas deferens and seminal vesicles. Azoospermia, normal semen fructose, and normal serum FSH suggest obstruction proximal to entry of ejaculatory ducts.

Large numbers of sperm in postejaculation urine in these patients suggests retrograde ejaculation.

Repeated semen analysis (specimens collected 7 days apart) are necessary to characterize average spermatogenesis.

Specimens should not be collected within 24 hrs of, or >5–7 days later than, previous ejaculation. Should be received in laboratory within 1 hr.

≤40% variability between different semen samples

Comparison of split ejaculate specimens is useful in patients with abnormal semen analysis associated with a high volume; specimens may show marked differences.

Antisperm antibodies (may test male serum or seminal fluid or female serum or cervical mucus) may occur in
- Testicular trauma (even minor)
- Almost all vasectomized patients
- Viral orchitis (permanent)
- Bacterial infections of GU tract (usually transient)

Cervical mucus penetration test measures greatest distance traveled by an individual sperm from a small aliquot of semen incubated 90 mins in a capillary tube of bovine cervical mucus. 68% of infertile men had penetration scores <20 mm whereas 79% of fertile men had scores >30 mm.

Hamster egg penetration assay: hamster oocytes enzymatically treated to remove outer layers of egg (which prevent cross-species fertilization) are incubated with human sperm selected for their motile ability. Penetration rates of <15% (number of eggs penetrated) indicate reduced fertility. May also be reported as number of sperm pen-

etrations per egg (normal = ≥ 5). Positive test results indicate ability of sperm to propel itself to oocyte, bind to oocyte, and penetrate oocyte.
After vasectomy, spermatozoa are present for some time. To confirm efficacy, two centrifuged specimens properly collected 1 mo apart should be sperm free and fructose should be absent.

Klinefelter's Syndrome

(Patients have 2 or more X chromosomes)
Azoospermia
♦ Plasma LH and FSH are increased; high FSH is best demarcator between normal men and those with Klinefelter's syndrome.
Urinary gonadotropin level is elevated.
Plasma testosterone levels are decreased to normal.
Buccal smears are helpful if positive for Barr bodies but a negative result does not rule out mosaicism. If negative, chromosome analysis should be performed, but in 70% of patients mosaic pattern may occur only in testes, so that chromosomal analysis of testicular cells is required for definite diagnosis.
♦ Abnormal chromosomal pattern. XY males have an extra X; 47 XXY is the classic type; 10% of patients have the mosaic form (46 XY/47 XXY); may have additional X (e.g., XXXY, XXXXY).
Biopsy of testicle shows atrophy, with hyalinized tubules lined only by Sertoli's cells, clumped Leydig's cells, and absent spermatogenesis.
Laboratory findings due to associated conditions, e.g., breast cancer, diabetes mellitus, thyroid dysfunction.

Menopause (Female Climacteric)

♦ Serum estradiol <5 ng/dL and FSH >40 mU/mL confirms primary ovarian failure; progesterone is <0.5 ng/mL.
Urinary estrogens are decreased.
Urinary 17-KS are decreased.
Plasma and urinary gonadotropin are increased.
Vaginal cytology shows menopausal pattern (see p. 663).

Ovarian Insufficiency, Secondary

Due To

Deficient estrogen production, e.g., diseases of the pituitary or hypothalamus (see separate sections)
Normal or increased estrogen production, e.g., ovarian tumors, functional cysts of ovary that suppress LH and FSH secretion
Disorders of adrenal function (increased production of cortisol or androgens) or thyroid function.

♦ Urinary gonadotropin is decreased or absent.
♦ Plasma LH is <0.5 mU/mL.

Ovarian Tumors

Feminizing Ovarian Tumors

(E.g., granulosa cell tumor, thecoma, luteoma)
○Pap smear of vagina and endometrial biopsy show high estrogen effect and no progestational activity; no signs of ovulation during reproductive phase.
○Urinary FSH is decreased (inhibited by increased estrogen).
Urine 17-KS and 17-OHKS are normal.
○Pregnanediol is absent.

Masculinizing Ovarian Tumors

(E.g., arrhenoblastoma, hilar cell tumors, adrenal rest tumors)
♦ Androgen-secreting tumor of ovary or adrenal gland is highly likely if serum total testosterone is >200 ng/dL or DHEA-S is >800 µg/dL. Localization may require androgen measurement in blood from adrenal and ovarian veins.

○Pap smear of vagina shows decreased estrogen effect.
○Endometrial biopsy shows moderate atrophy of endometrium.
Urine FSH (gonadotropins) is low.
♦ Urine 17-KS level is normal or may be slightly increased in arrhenoblastoma. Level
may be markedly increased in adrenal tumors of ovary ("masculinovoblastoma").
The higher the urine 17-KS level, the greater the likelihood of adrenocortical carcinoma; value of >100 mg/24 hrs is virtually diagnostic. Level may be moderately
increased in Leydig's cell tumors.
♦ *In arrhenoblastoma an increased amount of androsterone, testosterone, etc., may be
excreted in urine even though the 17-KS level is not much increased. Normal or
slightly increased urine 17-KS level in association with plasma testosterone in male
range is almost certainly due to ovarian tumor.*
*In adrenal cell tumors of ovary, laboratory findings may be the same as in hyperfunc-
tion of adrenal cortex with Cushing's syndrome, etc.*
*In some cases no endocrine effects are seen from these tumors. Some cases of arrhenoblas-
toma with masculinization also show evidence of increased estrogen formation.*

Struma Ovarii

♦ ~5–10% of cases are hormone producing. Classic findings of hyperthyroidism may
occur. These tumors take up radioactive iodine. *(Simple follicle cysts may also take
up radioactive iodine.)*

Primary Chorionepithelioma of Ovary

♦ Urinary chorionic gonadotropins are markedly increased.
Estrogen and progesterone secretion may be much increased.

Nonfunctioning Ovarian Tumors

Only effect may be hypogonadism due to replacement of functioning ovarian parenchyma.

♦ Tumor Markers

See p. 901.
Serum CA-125 is useful for
- Postoperative monitoring for persistent or recurrent disease; poorer prognosis
if elevated 3–6 wks after surgery. Lower levels in patients with no residual
tumor or <2 cm of residual tumor. But a negative test does not exclude residual disease.
- Rising level during chemotherapy is associated with tumor progression and fall
to normal is associated with response. Remains elevated in stable or progressive
disease.
- Rising level may be indication for second-look operation even in presence of normal clinical examination. Specificity = 99%, sensitivity = 46%, positive predictive
value = 97% for second-look cases.
- Higher levels are seen in less differentiated tumors (grade 2 and 3) and in serous
cystadenocarcinoma. Not increased in mucinous adenocarcinoma.
- Sequential determinations are more useful than a single test because levels in
benign disease do not show significant change but progressive rise occurs in malignant disease.
- Rising level may precede clinical evidence of recurrence by up to 11 mos.
- Not used for screening because it is negative in 20% of cases at time of diagnosis;
normal level does not exclude tumor; greater elevation roughly related to poorer
survival.
- CA-125 is positive in 80% of cases of common epithelial tumors, 50% of early-stage
disease, 0.6% of healthy women older than age 50 yrs.
Beta-hCG is positive in almost all cases of choriocarcinoma, 10–30% of cases of semi-
nomas, and 5–35% of cases of dysgerminoma. See Trophoblastic Neoplasms section.
AFP is present in 80–90% of cases of endodermal sinus tumors or immature teratomas.
CEA is present in 50–70% of cases of serous carcinoma. CA-125/CEA ratio is much higher
in serous carcinoma (>10 and often >100) than in carcinomas of breast, lung, colon,
or pancreas (usually <10), which may also cause increased levels of these markers.

Germe Cell Tumors of the Ovary

Tumor	AFP*	hCG*
Seminoma	–	+
Seminoma with syncytiotrophoblastic giant cells (STGC)	–	+
Embryonal carcinoma	+	–
Embryonal carcinoma with STGC	+	+
Yolk sac tumor	+	–
Yolk sac tumor with STGC	+	+
Choriocarcinoma	–	+
Mature teratoma	–	–

*See Chapter 16.
When both markers are positive, both should be assayed after therapy, as recurrence or metastases may be reflected by increase of only one marker.

Stein-Leventhal Syndrome (Polycystic Ovarian Disease)

♦ Serum increased ~3× normal (>35 mU/mL) in ~60% of patients in association with normal or slightly low FSH level. Abnormally high LH/FSH ratio (>2) is more consistently abnormal than is either measurement alone. Ratio ≥ 2 is considered highly suggestive; ratio ≥ 3 is considered diagnostic.

♦ Increased serum LH, LH/FSH ratio of >2, and mild increase of ovarian androgen level are sufficient for diagnosis in presence of the symptoms and clinical signs. *Because of erratic daily fluctuations of LH and androgens, obtaining daily plasma specimens for 3–5 days may be necessary.*

♦ Plasma free testosterone is increased ≤ 200 μg/dL in 40–60% of cases (>200 μg/dL usually indicates an androgen-producing tumor); not suppressed by dexamethasone.

♦ Plasma androstenedione (DHEA) is increased in ≤ 50% of cases.

♦ Serum 3-alpha-androstanediol glucuronide (metabolite of dihydrotestosterone) is markedly increased in this and in idiopathic hirsutism.

Synthetic estrogens and progestins (as in oral contraceptives) for 21 days, with before and after measurement of free testosterone and androstenedione:

• Free testosterone and androstenedione decrease by 50% or become normal in LH-dependent hyperandrogenism, e.g., polycystic ovaries.

• No suppression occurs in patients with ovarian tumors or adrenal disorders.

• Change in free testosterone accounts for estrogen-caused increase in sex hormone–binding globulin, which could result in unchanged or increased total testosterone level.

♦ ~85% of these patients have one or more abnormalities of serum LH/FSH ratio, testosterone, or androstenedione. Hyperandrogenism does not differentiate condition from CAH but CAH is more likely if LH/FSH ratio is <2:1 and ovaries are normal in size.

Urinary 17-KS are somewhat increased (higher values occur in congenital virilizing adrenal hyperplasia and hyperadrenalism due to Cushing's syndrome). (Measurement of DHEA-S is preferable to evaluate adrenal disease.) Dexamethasone administration (0.5 mg four times a day for 5–7 days) causes partial suppression in cases of ovarian origin, but complete suppression suggests adrenal origin (e.g., late-onset CAH). Administration of gonadotropin increases urinary 17-KS.

Biopsy of ovary is consistent with increased androgen effect but is not specific; ovarian visualization and biopsy are not routine part of diagnosis.

Plasma cortisol, urinary 17-OHKS, and 17-KGS are normal.

Plasma prolactin is increased in ~30% of patients.

Hyperinsulinemia occurs for unknown reason; correlates with degree of increased androgens.

10–13% of these patients have partial 21-hydroxylase defects.

○ If testosterone is >2 ng/mL or DHEA is >7000 ng/mL, ovarian or adrenal tumor should be ruled out.

Laboratory tests may be helpful in defining pathogenesis, following course of treatment, or ruling out adrenal or ovarian tumors.

Increased serum LH with normal or decreased FSH may occur in simple obesity, hyperthyroidism, liver disease.

Testicular Tumors

Tumor	Serum Tumor Marker
Seminoma	hCG increased in ~10% AFP not increased in pure seminoma without teratomatous component
Embryonal carcinoma	hCG or AFP or both increased in 90%
Yolk sac tumor	AFP increased in 100%
Choriocarcinoma (pure)	hCG increased in 100%
Teratoma	hCG or AFP or both increased in 50%
Mixed tumor	hCG and AFP increased in 90%

♦ Increased serum hCG (>1–2 ng/mL or >5–10 mU/mL) is found in 40–60% of patients with metastatic nonseminomatous tumors and in 15–20% of patients with apparently pure metastatic seminoma. In the latter case, immunochemical staining of paraffin-embedded tumor should be performed, because isolated syncytiotrophoblastic cells may show the hormone but are not by themselves evidence of choriocarcinoma.

♦ Increased serum AFP (>20 ng/mL) is found in ≤ 70% of patients with metastatic nonseminomatous tumors (embryonal carcinoma and yolk sac tumors).

♦ Both markers should always be measured simultaneously. 40% of patients with nonseminomatous tumors have increase of only one marker. 90% of patients with testicular tumors are positive for AFP or hCG or both; these are valuable for gauging efficacy of chemotherapy. 30% of patients receiving intensive chemotherapy apparently have a complete clinical remission; AFP levels may remain increased, although lower than pretreatment levels.

20–30% of patients have false-negative results preoperatively despite tumor (usually microscopic) in the retroperitoneal lymph nodes. Therefore, lymphadenectomy should not be omitted simply because marker levels are normal.

Serum markers for AFP and beta-hCG may be increased in conditions other than testicular cancer. See Chapter 16. False-positive increase is rare.

♦ The most important use is for follow-up after surgery or chemotherapy. Failure of increased preoperative levels to fall after surgery suggests metastatic disease and the need for chemotherapy. Rise of levels that had previously declined to normal suggests recurrent tumor even with no other evidence of disease. Serum half-life of AFP = 5–7 days and of hCG = 30 hrs.

Negative marker findings are not useful for differential diagnosis of scrotal mass, but elevated levels indicate testicular cancer.

Serum LD is a third marker; not specific for testicular cancer but also appears to be an independent prognostic factor for advanced germ cell tumors. Increased in ~60% of nonseminomatous germ cell tumors and 80% of seminomatous germ cell tumors.

Turner's Syndrome (Ovarian Dysgenesis)

♦ Diagnosis is based on karyotype analysis (see p. 668). Chromosomal pattern includes wide spectrum of abnormalities, e.g., 45 chromosomes (monosomy X with XO; or, if XX, one X is abnormal; or XO mosaic), various deletions of part of an X chromosome. Female is phenotypic. Prenatal diagnosis by chorionic villus sampling or amniocentesis.

Barr body test is negative (male) in 80% of patients.

Because of the frequency with which 45 X cells are admixed with 46 XX cells, the diagnosis (i.e., 45 X karyotype) cannot be excluded by either buccal smear or chromosome analysis alone.

♦ Biopsy of ovary shows connective tissue stroma with rare follicular structure.

Vaginal smear and endometrial biopsy are atrophic.

Increased FSH, LH, and gonadotropins.

17-KS and 17-OHKS are normal.

ACTH is normal.

Glucose intolerance is common, with mild insulin resistance.

Serum cholesterol is frequently increased.

Laboratory findings due to increased prevalence of associated conditions, e.g.,
• Hashimoto's thyroiditis (10–30%)
• Bicuspid aortic valves (≤ 50%)
• Coarctation of aorta (≤ 20%)

- Horseshoe kidneys
- Pyelonephritis due to anomalous obstruction of ureteropelvic junction
- Hypertension
- Frequent otitis media

~60% of patients with primary amenorrhea have Turner's syndrome or sometimes testicular feminization. 90% never menstruate. ~10% menstruate for a few years and then present as cases of secondary amenorrhea.

Turner's Syndrome in the Male

- ♦ Biopsy of testicle reveals dysgenetic tubules with few or no germ cells.
- ♦ Chromosomal pattern: 46 chromosomes (XY pattern with very defective Y that is equivalent to XO).

Laboratory Tests for Diagnosis of Disorders of the Pituitary and Hypothalamus

Arginine Vasopressin (Antidiuretic Hormone [ADH])

Use

Diagnosis of central diabetes insipidus and of SIADH, and differentiation from nephrogenic diabetes insipidus
Differential diagnosis of hyponatremias

Increased in Serum

SIADH (inappropriately increased for degree of plasma osmolality)
Ectopic ADH syndrome
Use of certain drugs (e.g., chlorpropamide, phenothiazine, carbamazepine [Tegretol])
Nephrogenic diabetes insipidus (normal for degree of plasma osmolality)

Decreased in Serum

Central diabetes insipidus

In Urine

Central diabetes insipidus: low arginine vasopressin and osmolality
Nephrogenic diabetes insipidus: high arginine vasopressin and low osmolality
SIADH: normal arginine vasopressin relative to osmolality

Growth Hormone (GH)

Use

Differential diagnosis of short stature, slow growth
Evaluation of pituitary function

Increased In

Acromegaly and gigantism due to certain pituitary adenomas
Laron dwarfism (GH resistance; GH–binding protein cannot be detected)
Renal failure
Uncontrolled diabetes mellitus
Use of certain drugs (e.g., estrogens, oral contraceptives, tranquilizers, antidepressants)
Starvation
2 hrs after sleep

Decreased In

Hypothalamic defect causes most cases (e.g., tumors, infection, diseases such as hemochromatosis, perinatal insult such as birth trauma)

ENDOCRINE

Hypopituitarism (e.g., familial isolated GH deficiency, tumors, infection, granulomas, trauma, irradiation)
Dwarfism
Corticosteroid therapy
Obesity
Low levels must be measured after stimulation (e.g., with insulin, arginine)

Growth Hormone–Releasing Hormone

(Hypothalamic secretion stimulates pituitary to release GH)

Increased In

1% of cases of acromegaly due to production of GH–releasing hormone by hypothalamus or ectopic secretion by neoplasms (e.g., pancreatic islet, carcinoid of thymus or bronchus, neuroendocrine tumors)

Normal In

Most cases of acromegaly due to pituitary tumors.

Prolactin

See Prolactinoma, p. 700.

Somatomedin C

(Insulin-like growth factor I, which mediates most growth-promoting effects of GH)

Use

Diagnosis of acromegaly and pituitary deficiency; preferable to GH because it is constant after eating and during the day
Screening of other growth disorders
Assessment of nutritional status
Monitoring of effectiveness of nutritional repletion. Is more sensitive indicator than prealbumin, transferrin index, or retinol-binding protein.

Increased In

Acromegaly and gigantism
Pregnancy (2–3× nonpregnancy values)

Decreased In

Pituitary deficiency
Laron dwarfism
Anorexia or malnutrition
Acute illness
Hepatic failure
Hypothyroidism
Diabetes mellitus
Normal aging

Diseases of the Pituitary and Hypothalamus

Acromegaly and Gigantism

- ◆ Serum somatomedin C (insulin-like growth factor I) is uniformly increased in untreated cases; is more precise and cost-effective screening than serum GH because GH levels fluctuate and have short serum half-life (22 mins).
- ◆ Autonomous serum GH is increased. (Avoid stress before and during venipuncture because stress stimulates secretion of GH; several random measurements should be performed.) Annual random blood GH levels, FTI, and ACTH are used for treatment follow-up.

- Fasting levels >5 ng/mL in men or >10 ng/mL in women are suggestive but not diagnostic of acromegaly.
- ♦ Most patients show a fall of <50% or even an increase 60–90 mins after glucose administration (50–100 gm orally), whereas normal subjects show almost complete suppression of GH (or to <5 ng/mL) by induced hyperglycemia. This is the most reliable test. Failure to suppress GH to <2 ng/mL after oral glucose load is essential to diagnosis.
- ♦ If borderline response to hyperglycemia, perform TRH test. (500 μg TRH IV causes transient increase [>50% over basal levels] of GH in 15–30 mins in acromegaly patients but has little effect in normal persons.)
- ♦ GH–releasing hormone excess secretion (e.g., ectopic source such as pancreatic tumor or carcinoid causes <1% of acromegaly cases). Thus GH–releasing hormone should be measured in all patients with acromegaly.
- ♦ All patients with acromegaly should have baseline serum prolactin measured because ≤ 40% of these adenomas may secrete both prolactin and GH.

IV ACTH administration may cause excessive increase in urine 17-KS but normal 17-OHKS excretion.

Glucose tolerance is impaired in most patients. Mild diabetes mellitus that is insulin resistant is found in <15% of patients.

Adrenal virilism and increased urine 17-KS are common in women.

Urine 17-KS, 17-KGS, and gonadotropins are usually normal or may be slightly changed but level not diagnostically useful.

Hypogonadism develops in ≤ 50% of cases.

Rare associated endocrinopathies are hyperthyroidism, HPT, pheochromocytoma, insulinoma.

In inactive cases, all secondary laboratory findings may be normal.

In late stage, panhypopituitarism may develop.

Serum phosphorus is increased for age of patient in 40% of cases.

Serum ALP may be increased.

Urine calcium is increased.

Urine hydroxyproline is increased.

Biopsy of costochondral junction evidences active bone growth.

CBC and ESR are normal.

- ♦ After successful surgery—basal plasma GH <5 ng/mL, should decrease to ≤ 2 ng/mL after glucose administration and level of insulin-like growth factor I should become normal.

Due To

Excess GH secretion
- Pituitary adenomas, hyperplasia, or carcinoma
- Ectopic pituitary tumor (sphenoid or parapharyngeal sinus)
- Ectopic hormone production (e.g., tumor of pancreas, lung, ovary, breast)

Excess secretion of GH–releasing hormone
- Hypothalamic tumor (e.g., hamartoma, ganglioneuroma)
- Ectopic hormone production (e.g., carcinoid of bronchus, GI tract, pancreas; pancreatic islet cell tumor, small cell carcinoma of lung, adrenal adenoma, pheochromocytoma)

Other Causes of Tall Stature in Children

Klinefelter's syndrome (see p. 681)

Marfan syndrome (inherited disorder with thin limbs, malformation of eyes and ears, medionecrosis of aorta, cardiac valve deformities, hypotonia, kyphoscoliosis)

Beckwith-Wiedemann syndrome (hypoglycemia, omphalocele, macrosomia, macroglossia)

Untreated CAH (see pp. 635)

Precocious secretion of androgens or estrogens

Obesity

Anorexia Nervosa

No diagnostic or typical laboratory profile; diagnosis by exclusion. Findings may be compensatory regulatory changes secondary to nutritional deprivation rather than primary hypothalamic dysfunction.

ESR is low.

Vomiting may cause hypokalemic acidosis.

Prerenal azotemia with increased BUN and serum creatinine

Decreased serum glucose, sodium, magnesium

Renal calculi

Laboratory findings of euthyroid sick syndrome

Basal GH levels may be increased as in other forms of protein-calorie malnutrition; response to stimulation tests is usually normal.

Increased plasma somatomedin C

Plasma prolactin level is normal.

Plasma LH and FSH may be low with impaired response to LH-releasing hormone.

Decreased serum estradiol

Decreased serum testosterone

Adrenal function abnormalities may be found (e.g., normal or increased plasma corti-coids, absence of diurnal variation of glucocorticoids, hyperresponse to ACTH test, incomplete suppression by dexamethasone, intact or excessive response to metyrapone, low 17-KS and 17-KGS in urine; no adrenal insufficiency)

Atrophic vaginal smear

Increased serum carotene (>250 mg/dL) in ~60% of cases and increased cholesterol

Anemia is unusual; leukopenia; thrombocytopenia.

With marked loss of body weight, serum protein, potassium, and phosphorus may be decreased.

Vitamin deficiencies are rare.

Carcinoid Syndrome[28]

See Table 13-25.

(The syndrome in malignant carcinoids [argentaffinomas] includes flushing, diarrhea, bronchospasm, endocardial fibrosis, arthropathy, glucose intolerance, hypotension.)

Liver metastases are present in 95% of cases with syndrome except when lung and ovary are primary sites, but laboratory tests are not reliable indicators and serum ALP is frequently normal despite extensive metastases.

♦ Urinary level of 5-HIAA (a metabolite of serotonin) is increased in 75% of cases (>9 mg/24 hrs in patients without malabsorption or >30 mg/24 hrs with malabsorption; normal is <6 mg/24 hrs), usually when tumor is far advanced (with large liver metastases often 300–1000 mg/day), but may not be increased despite massive metastases. Sensitivity = 73%. Useful in diagnosis in only 5–7% of patients with a carcinoid tumor but in ~45% of those with liver metastases. Disease extent and prognosis correlate generally with urine 5-HIAA excretion; becomes normal after successful surgery. If urine HIAA is normal, check blood level of serotonin or a precursor, 5-hydroxytryptophan. Urine HIAA may be decreased in renal insufficiency.

Increased In

Whipple's disease

Nontropical sprue

Small increases may occur in pregnancy, ovulation, after surgical stress.

Consumption of various foods (e.g., pineapples, kiwis, bananas, eggplants, plums, tomatoes, avocados, plantains, walnuts, pecans, hickory nuts, coffee)

Use of certain drugs (e.g., acetanilid, acetaminophen, acetophenetidin, caffeine, glyceryl guaiacolate, heparin, L-dopa, mephenesin, methocarbamol, phenothiazine derivatives, Lugol's solution, reserpine, salicylates)

Decreased In

Use of certain drugs (e.g., chlorpromazine, promazine, imipramine, isoniazid, monoamine oxidase inhibitors, methenamine, methyldopa, phenothiazines, promethazine)

♦ Serum and urine serotonin may be increased (>0.4 μg/mL) in 20% of cases but without increased urine 5-HIAA.

♦ Platelet serotonin and urine serotonin are increased in 64% of cases.

Increased plasma chromogranin A predicts adverse prognosis.

---

[28]Kulke MH, Mayer RJ. Carcinoid tumors. *N Engl J Med* 1999;340:858.

Table 13-25. Carcinoid Tumors of GI Tract

Tumor Site[a]	Frequency	Origin	Comment
Bronchus	32%	Foregut	Serotonin production low
Stomach[b]	3.8%		Mainly produces serotonin precursor (5-hydroxytryptophan)
Duodenum	2.1%		Increased urine 5-hydroxyindole acetic acid (5-HIAA)
Pancreas	<5%		May metastasize to bone
			Intense symptoms
Appendix	7.6%	Midgut	Mainly produces serotonin
Ileum	17%		Urine 5-HIAA normal or slightly increased
Jejunum	2.3%		Classical symptoms
Cecum	5%		Rarely metastasizes to bone
Rectum	10.1%	Hindgut	Rarely produces serotonin or precursor
Transverse, descending, and sigmoid colon	6.3%		Rarely metastasizes to bone
Other (e.g., thymus, ovary, kidney, breast)	12.5%		

≤ 25% of cases have other malignancies.
[a]85% occur in GI tract, 10% in bronchi/lungs, 5% in thymus, ovary, kidney, breast, other. Cause 55% of GI tract endocrine tumors. ≤ 25% of cases have other malignancies.
[b]≤ 75% of gastric carcinoids are associated with chronic atrophic gastritis type A, are often multiple, and are not associated with carcinoid syndrome. 5–10% of gastric carcinoids are associated with Zollinger-Ellison syndrome and multiple endocrine neoplasia type I, may be multiple, and are not associated with carcinoid syndrome. 15–25% of gastric carcinoids are sporadic and frequently metastasize and are associated with atypical carcinoid syndrome.

Some tumors can produce various functionally active substances (e.g., histamine, ACTH, somatostatin, gastrin, catecholamines, prostaglandins, kinins) causing different paraneoplastic syndromes. Most are clinically silent because of small amounts secreted and rapid inactivation.

VMA and catecholamine levels in urine are normal.

Laboratory findings due to other aspects of carcinoid syndrome (may include pulmonary valvular stenosis, tricuspid valvular insufficiency, heart failure, liver metastases, electrolyte disturbances)

Nonfunctioning tumors can be diagnosed only by histological examination.

Some patients may have decreased serum albumin and pellagra (due to diversion of tryptophan to synthesis of serotonin).

Diabetes Insipidus

See Table 13-26.

Due To

Central (pituitary)
Nephrogenic
Psychogenic
High-set osmoreceptor

Diabetes Insipidus, Central

See Table 13-26.

Table 13-26. Comparison of Different Types of Diabetes Insipidus

	After Dehydration[a]				
	Urine Specific Gravity	Urine Osmolality (mOsm/kg)	Plasma Osmolality (mOsm/kg)	After Pitressin,[b] Urine Osmolality (% change)	Plasma Vasopressin (pg/mL)
Normal	≥ 1.015	700–1400	288–291	No change (<5%)	1.3–4.1
Central diabetes insipidus (complete)	<1.010	50–200	310–320	Doubles (>100%)[c]	<1.1
Central diabetes insipidus (partial)	1.010– 1.015	250–500	295–305	Increases (9–67%)[c]	
Nephrogenic diabetes insipidus	<1.010	100–200	310–320	No change[d]	12–13 (>2.7 in high Ca/ low K type)
High-set osmo-receptor dia-betes insipidus	≥ 1.015	700–1400	300–305	No change	
Primary (psy-chogenic) polydipsia		700–1200		No change after medullary wash-out; normal increase after high-sodium diet	3.0–7.5

[a]Dehydration test: No fluid intake for 4–18 hrs, measure urine osmolality and/or specific gravity hourly, weigh patient (or urine) frequently to avoid loss of >3% of body weight (*if >3% of body weight, measure plasma and urine osmolality, and terminate test to avoid hypotension*). If three successive hourly urine osmolality determinations indicate no further change (i.e., a plateau has been reached), administer 5 U vasopressin (Pitressin) subcutaneously, and 60 mins later, measure urine osmolality.
[b]1 hr after subcutaneous injection of 5 U of aqueous Pitressin.
[c]Useful to distinguish partial from complete central diabetes insipidus.
[d]Therefore differs from diabetes insipidus.
Plasma vasopressin levels must always be interpreted relative to plasma osmolality.

Due To

Primary
- Idiopathic (now accounts for <50% of cases)
- Heredity (~1% of cases)

Secondary
- Supra- and intrasellar tumors
    - Neoplasms (suprasellar and intrasellar
        - Primary (e.g., craniopharyngioma, cyst)
        - Metastatic (e.g., carcinoma of breast, lung; leukemias)
- Histiocytosis (eosinophilic granuloma is most common)
    - Hand-Schüller-Christian disease
- Granulomatous lesions (e.g., sarcoidosis, TB, syphilis, Wegener's granulomatosis)
- Trauma, with or without basal skull fracture; neurosurgical procedures
- Vascular lesions (e.g., aneurysms, thrombosis, sickle cell disease, Sheehan's syndrome
- Infections (e.g., meningitis, encephalitis, Guillain-Barré syndrome, CMV infection)
- Autoimmune disorders
- Others (e.g., hypoxemic encephalopathy)

♦ Urine is inappropriately dilute (low specific gravity [usually <1.005] and osmolality [50–200 mOsm/kg]) in presence of increased serum osmolality (295 mOsm/kg) and increased or normal serum sodium.

Large urine volume (4–15 L/24 hrs) is characteristic.

Table 13-27. Comparison of Hyponatremia Due to Various Causes

Cause	Urine Sodium	Urine Osmolarity	BUN
Hypervolemic (e.g., congestive heart failure, cirrhosis, nephrotic syndrome)			
Early	D (usually <10–15 mEq/L)	I (usually >350–400 mOsm/L)	N
Late	D with isotonic urine is ominous finding	(>200 mmol/kg)	I disproportionate to creatinine
Hypovolemic			
Extrarenal	D (<10 mEq/L)	I (>400 mOsm/L)	N
Gastrointestinal			
Skin (burns, sweat)			
Third space			
Renal			
Diuretic (most common)	I (>20 mEq/L)	Isotonic to plasma	Usually I
Chronic renal disease (especially interstitial)		If severe volume contraction, 300–450 mOsm/kg	
Mineralocorticoid deficiency			
Normovolemic			
SIADH (almost always) (see p. 702)	I (>20 mmol/L)	I (>200 mmol/kg)	Often D (<8–10 mg/dL)
Reset osmostat (see p. 692)	V	V	N or D

D = decreased; I = increased; SIADH = syndrome of inappropriate antidiuretic hormone secretion; V = variable.

♦ Plasma vasopressin level is decreased.
♦ Dehydration test fails to increase urine specific gravity or osmolality, and serum osmolality remains elevated. After administration of vasopressin, urine osmolality increases by 50%.
Partial central diabetes insipidus shows intermediate values between complete central and normal.
See Tables 13-26 and 13-27.

Diabetes Insipidus, Nephrogenic

See Table 13-26.

Due To

Chronic renal failure (e.g., GN, pyelonephritis, gout, analgesic nephropathy, polycystic kidneys, nephrosclerosis)
Other tubulointerstitial diseases (e.g., polycystic kidneys, medullary sponge disease, sickle cell disease or trait, amyloidosis)
Diuretic phase of acute tubular necrosis
After renal transplant or relief of urinary tract obstruction
Hypergammaglobulinemia (e.g., multiple myeloma, amyloidosis, Sjögren's syndrome)
Drugs (e.g., lithium, demeclocycline, amphotericin, propoxyphene, methoxyflurane, vincristine)
Prolonged potassium depletion and hypokalemia (condition is reversed by restoring potassium level to normal)

ENDOCRINE

Prolonged hypercalciuria, usually with hypercalcemia (condition is reversed by restoring calcium level to normal)

Hereditary renal tubular unresponsiveness to vasopressin due to X-linked genetic defect; severe form occurs in males; family history of this condition is frequent.

Primary hyperaldosteronism

Pregnancy

♦ Laboratory findings are the same as in hypophyseal (central) diabetes insipidus except that in nephrogenic type
  • Plasma vasopressin level is normal or increased.
  • Dehydration test does not cause urine osmolality to increase above plasma osmolality.
  • Dehydration test causes the plasma vasopressin level to increase.
  • Urine osmolality does not increase with subsequent injection of vasopressin.

Diabetes Insipidus Due to High-Set Osmoreceptor

(Rare entity in which the set point for stimulating release of ADH is ≥ 300 mOsm/kg instead of the normal 285 mOsm/kg level)

See Table 13-26.

As plasma osmolality increases, patient becomes thirsty and drinks fluids, thereby diluting the plasma before it reaches the higher set level to stimulate release of ADH, initiating cycle of polyuria and polydipsia. If thirst center is also impaired, patient develops essential hypernatremia (see p. 693).

♦ Plasma osmolality after dehydration is significantly higher than in normal state.

♦ Urine osmolality does not increase after administration of vasopressin.

Growth Hormone (GH) Deficiency

May be isolated deficiency with dwarfism or may be associated with TSH deficiency, with ACTH deficiency, or with TSH and ACTH deficiencies. GH deficiency is usually due to deficiency of hypothalamic GH–releasing hormone.

♦ Serum GH basal levels are decreased (<1.0 ng/mL). Use pooled or average of three samples. Stimulation tests have greater sensitivity. Increased basal or random serum level excludes this diagnosis but low levels do not distinguish normal persons from those with GH deficiency.

♦ Stimulation (functional) tests
  • Draw serum at 0, 30, 60, 90, and 120 mins.
  • Administration of insulin (regular crystalline, IV, 0.05 to 0.3 U/kg body weight) should normally produce at least 2× increase in serum GH level and 3× increase in serum prolactin level at 60-min peak. This is the most reliable challenge for GH secretion.
  • Administration of levodopa (500 mg orally) should normally produce at least 2× increase in serum GH level at 60-min peak.
  • Administration of arginine (0.5 gm/kg body weight as 5% solution IV over 30 mins) should normally produce at least 3× increase in serum GH and at least 2× increase in serum prolactin level at 30- to 60-min peak.
  • Failure to produce these minimal responses indicates a lesion of pituitary or hypothalamus but does not differentiate between them.
  • A normal response is at least 10 ng/mL peak value; 5–10 ng/mL is indeterminate, ≤ 5 ng/mL is subnormal. (A normal value rules out GH deficiency; in some laboratories the normal level is ≥ 7 ng/mL.)
  • Approximately one-fourth of patients with normal GH secretory capacity are unable to secrete GH in response to provocative tests indicated above, at any given time. Therefore, at least two of these tests should be used to confirm diagnosis of GH deficiency.
  • Nonpituitary factors that impair GH response include obesity, primary hypothyroidism, thyrotoxicosis, primary hypogonadism, Kallmann's syndrome, Cushing's syndrome, use of various drugs (e.g., alpha-adrenergic antagonists, beta-adrenergic antagonists, serotonin antagonists, dopamine antagonists). Impaired GH response may even occur in presence of elevated GH basal level.

- *Normal response may also occur in patients with partial deficiency.*
- GH response is normal or exaggerated in growth failure due to resistance to GH (Laron dwarfism) or resistance to somatomedins (African pygmies).
- Glucagon and clonidine have also been used.

Decreased fasting blood sugar (<50 mg/dL) is frequent; responds to GH therapy. Serum phosphorus and ALP are decreased in prepubertal children but normal in adult-onset cases.

♦ Serum prolactin baseline level is low and does not rise appropriately after TRH administration or other stimulation. In hypothalamic disease, basal prolactin level is increased and response may be normal or blunted.

Laboratory findings due to involvement of other endocrines
- TSH deficiency (see Sensitive Thyroid-Stimulating Hormone, p. 571; TRH stimulation test, p. 580, Hypothyroidism, p. 589; and Table 14-3).
- ACTH deficiency (see tests of adrenal function, p. 631).
- Gonadotropins are decreased or absent from urine in postpubertal patients (but increased levels occur in primary hypogonadism).

Hypernatremia, "Essential"

(Due to hypothalamic lesions [e.g., infiltration of histiocytes, neoplasm] that cause impaired osmotic regulation but intact volume regulation of ADH secretion.)
See Fig. 13-27.

♦ Serum sodium shows sustained but fluctuating elevations, corrected by administration of ADH but not corrected by fluid administration.

♦ Serum osmolality is increased.

Serum creatinine, BUN, and creatinine clearance are normal.

There is spontaneous excretion of random specimens of urine, which may be very concentrated or very dilute and opposite to plasma osmolality.

Hyponatremias

See Table 13-27 and Fig. 13-28.

Due To

Isotonic (spurious—occurs with flame photometer but not with ion-selective electrode technology)
- Hyperlipidemia (plasma looks milky) "falsely" lowers serum sodium; measured serum osmolality exceeds calculated serum osmolality.

  Calculated serum osmolality = $2 \times Na + (serum\ glucose/18) + (BUN/2.8)$

- Hyperproteinemia (e.g., myeloma, macroglobulinemia)

Hypertonic
- Hyperglycemia (each increase of blood sugar of 100 mg/dL decreases serum sodium by 1.7 mEq/L)
- Excess mannitol treatment

Hypotonic
- Hypervolemic, usually with clinical edema
    With low urine sodium (<10 mEq/L) may be due to congestive heart failure, cirrhosis with ascites, nephrotic syndrome
    With high urine sodium (>20 mEq/L) may be due to acute tubular necrosis or end-stage chronic renal failure in which sodium and water intake exceeds excretion. Serum uric acid and BUN tend to be increased.

Hypovolemic
- Urine sodium <10 mEq/L. Due to extrarenal loss of sodium (e.g., GI tract, fistulas, pancreatitis, exercise, sweating, burns).
- Urine sodium >20 mEq/L. Due to renal loss of sodium (e.g., diuretics such as furosemide or osmotic diuresis due to glucose or urea, diabetic ketoacidosis, renal tubular acidosis, salt-losing nephritis, adrenal insufficiency, hyporeninemia, hypoaldosteronism).

Normovolemic—usually no edema is present.

ENDOCRINE

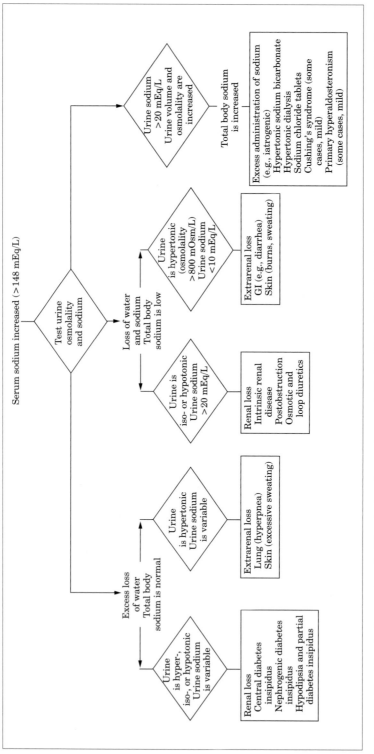

Fig. 13-27. Algorithm for hypernatremia. (Hypotonic urine—urine osmolality is <800 mOsm/L; isotonic urine—urine osmolality is between 800 mOsm/L and plasma osmolality; hypertonic urine—urine osmolality >800 mOsm/L.)

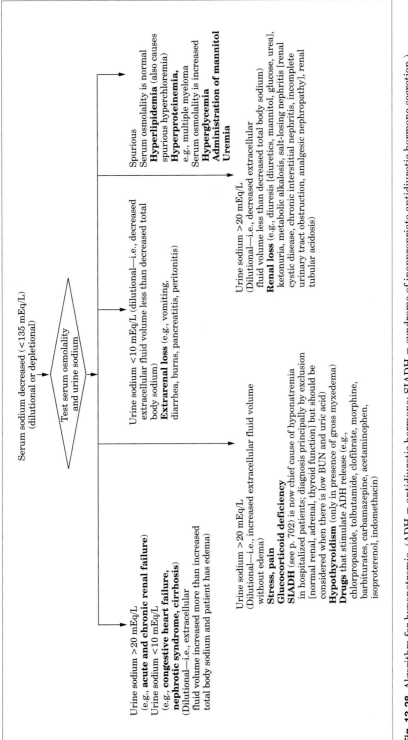

Serum sodium decreased (<135 mEq/L) (dilutional or depletional)

Test serum osmolality and urine sodium

Urine sodium >20 mEq/L (e.g., **acute and chronic renal failure**)
Urine sodium <10 mEq/L (e.g., **congestive heart failure, nephrotic syndrome, cirrhosis**)
(Dilutional—i.e., extracellular fluid volume increased more than increased total body sodium and patient has edema)

Urine sodium >20 mEq/L (Dilutional—i.e., increased extracellular fluid volume without edema)
Stress, pain
Glucocorticoid deficiency
SIADH (see p. 702) is now chief cause of hyponatremia in hospitalized patients; diagnosis principally by exclusion [normal renal, adrenal, thyroid function] but should be considered when there is low BUN and uric acid)
Hypothyroidism (only in presence of gross myxedema)
Drugs that stimulate ADH release (e.g., chlorpropamide, tolbutamide, clofibrate, morphine, barbiturates, carbamazepine, acetaminophen, isoproterenol, indomethacin)

Urine sodium <10 mEq/L (dilutional—i.e., decreased extracellular fluid volume less than decreased total body sodium)
Extrarenal loss (e.g., vomiting, diarrhea, burns, pancreatitis, peritonitis)

Urine sodium >20 mEq/L (Dilutional—i.e., decreased extracellular fluid volume less than decreased total body sodium)
Renal loss (e.g., diuresis [diuretics, mannitol, glucose, urea], ketonuria, metabolic alkalosis, salt-losing nephritis [renal cystic disease, chronic interstitial nephritis, incomplete urinary tract obstruction, analgesic nephropathy], renal tubular acidosis)

Spurious
Serum osmolality is normal
Hyperlipidemia (also causes spurious hyperchloremia)
Hyperproteinemia, e.g., multiple myeloma
Serum osmolality is increased
Hyperglycemia
Administration of mannitol
Uremia

Fig. 13-28. Algorithm for hyponatremia. (ADH = antidiuretic hormone; SIADH = syndrome of inappropriate antidiuretic hormone secretion.)

- Large amounts of sodium appear in urine (>20 mEq/L). May be due to SIADH, hypothyroidism, hypopituitarism, low-reset osmostat syndrome, physical or emotional stress, potassium depletion, renal failure, water poisoning, certain drugs (e.g., ADH analogs, amitriptyline, carbamazepine, chlorpropamide, cyclophosphamide, diuretics, haloperidol, thioridazine, vincristine).

Hyponatremic patients with BUN <10 mg/dL and uric acid <3.0 mg/dL should be considered to have SIADH or reset osmostat until proved otherwise.

"Pseudohyponatremia"—see above. Serum osmolality is normal.

Hypopituitarism

Due To

Pituitary disease
- Neoplasms (e.g., craniopharyngioma, chromophobe adenoma, eosinophilic adenoma, meningioma, metastatic tumor [especially breast, lung]); prolactin-secreting tumor is the most common pituitary neoplasm.
- Infiltrative diseases
  Granulomatous lesions (e.g., sarcoidosis, Hand-Schüller-Christian syndrome, histiocytosis X)
  Infection (e.g., TB, mycoses)
  Hemochromatosis
  Autoimmune inflammation
- Hemorrhage
  Pituitary necrosis secondary to postpartum hemorrhage (Sheehan's syndrome)
  Hemorrhage into pituitary tumor
- Infarction (e.g., sickle cell disease, cavernous sinus thrombosis)
- Miscellaneous
  Head trauma
  Internal carotid artery aneurysm
  Empty sella syndrome
- Idiopathic
  Isolated hormone deficiency (e.g., GH, ACTH, TSH, gonadotropin)
  Multiple hormone deficiency
- Iatrogenic (e.g., hypophysectomy, irradiation, section of stalk)
- Familial pituitary deficiency (deficient hormone production or production of abnormal hormone)
- Partial GH deficiency (some forms of "constitutional short stature" with delayed onset of adolescence)

Hypothalamic disease (see p. 697)
End-organ resistance to GH (normal or increased serum GH with low somatomedin level)
- Laron dwarfs (somatomedin levels are often undetectable and fail to rise when GH is administered).

♦ *Serum somatomedin C levels are 5–15% of normal in most hypopituitary dwarfs and 4–12 times normal in all active acromegaly patients.*
♦ Endocrinologic findings: diagnosis is based on low serum level of target organ hormone and of the corresponding pituitary-stimulating hormone, e.g.,
  - Hypogonadism
    Men: low sperm count, low serum testosterone, inappropriately low serum LH and FSH
    Women: low serum estradiol, inappropriately low serum LH and FSH
  - Hypothyroidism
    Low serum T_4 and FTI, inappropriately low serum thyrotropin
  - Hypocorticalism:
    Low serum cortisol and ACTH
    Low serum GH unresponsive to provocative tests
    Low serum prolactin unresponsive to provocative tests. Usually occurs late in course of hypopituitarism except in Sheehan's syndrome, in which it may be the earliest manifestation. Rarely or never due to hypothalamic disease.

See sections on secondary insufficiency of gonads, thyroid, adrenals. Only one (usually gonadal first) or all of these may be involved.

♦ *Dynamic tests are usually needed to detect partial deficiencies.*
See Diabetes Insipidus, Central, p. 689.

Hypothalamus, Diseases

Due To

Neoplasms (primary or metastatic cancer, craniopharyngioma) (most frequent cause)
Inflammation (e.g., TB, encephalitis)
Head trauma (e.g., basal skull fractures, gunshot wounds)
Granulomas (e.g., histiocytosis X, sarcoidosis)
Releasing-hormone deficiency, genetic or idiopathic
Irradiation for childhood cancer

Manifestations

Sexual abnormalities are the most frequent manifestations of hypothalamic disease.
Precocious puberty
Hypogonadism (frequently as part of Fröhlich's syndrome)
Diabetes insipidus is a frequent but not an early manifestation of hypothalamic disease.
Hypopituitarism—differentiate primary hypopituitarism from this secondary form of
hypopituitarism by appropriate stimulation tests.

Multiple Endocrine Neoplasia (MEN Syndrome)[29]

MEN Type I (Wermer's Syndrome)

♦ **(Triad of parathyroid, pancreatic islet cell, and anterior pituitary tumors)**
○Hyperparathyroidism (due to involvement of all four glands) in >88% of patients; is
usual presenting feature; associated renal and bone disease are infrequent. 15% of
cases of HPT have MEN; frequently multicentric. 10% of parathyroid tumor patients
have relatives with MEN.
○Pancreatic endocrine tumors in ~60% of patients; most are functional; usually multiple.
  • Gastrinomas with Z-E syndrome occur in ~50% of cases and ~50% are malignant.
    50% of cases of Z-E syndrome have MEN type I.
  • Insulinomas (beta cells) in ~25% of MEN type I patients; usually benign; multiple
    foci are common.
  • Glucagonomas (alpha cells) syndrome of distinctive rash, diabetes mellitus, ane-
    mia, weight loss.
  • Vipomas occur less often.
○Pituitary adenomas in 40–50% of cases
  • ~25% are prolactinomas.
  • ~15% are eosinophilic adenomas causing acromegaly.
  • ~5% are basophilic adenomas causing Cushing's syndrome.
  • ~10% are nonfunctional adenomas causing hypopituitarism due to space-occupy-
    ing effect.
○Tumors possible related to MEN type I
  • Adrenal cortical adenomas or hyperplasia are incidental and nonfunctioning in
    ~10%, functioning in ~5% of cases. Adrenal medulla is not involved.
  • Thyroid disease in ~20% of cases including benign and malignant tumors, colloid
    goiter, thyrotoxicosis, Hashimoto's disease.
  • Uncommon lesions include carcinoids (~16%), schwannomas, multiple lipomas,
    gastric polyps, testicular tumors.

MEN Type II (or IIa) (Sipple's Syndrome)

○Medullary thyroid carcinoma in >90% of cases is usually multicentric and preceded
by C-cell hyperplasia (thereby differing from sporadic type). Produces calcitonin and
sometimes ACTH or serotonin. Calcitonin response to IV pentagastrin stimulation

ENDOCRINE

---

[29]National Institutes of Health Conference. Multiple endocrine neoplasia type I: clinical and genetic
topics. *Ann Intern Med* 1998;129:484.

has >90% sensitivity and specificity. 25% of these carcinomas occur as part of MEN type II. May be asymptomatic but lethal.

○Pheochromocytoma in 10–50% of cases; usually bilateral, often multiple, and may be extra-adrenal. 10% of pheochromocytomas occur as part of MEN.

○Hyperparathyroidism in ~20% of cases; due to hyperplasia in 84% and adenoma in 16%; occurs late in disease; may occur without medullary thyroid carcinoma.

♦ DNA analysis detected carriers of the gene before biochemical manifestations (100% sensitivity and specificity).[30]

MEN Type III (or IIb)

(Features in common with MEN type II but is a separate genetic syndrome)
○Medullary thyroid carcinoma in 75% of cases.
○Pheochromocytoma in 33% of cases.
Hyperparathyroidism is rare (<5% of cases).
○Other lesions:
  • Multiple mucosal gangliomas in >95% of cases appear early in life.
  • Marfan syndrome habitus, hypertrophy of corneal nerves, ganglioneuromas of GI tract, characteristic retinal changes and facial appearance are frequent.
○*All first-order relatives of MEN patients should have appropriate serial testing.*

Nonendocrine Neoplasms, Causing Endocrine Syndromes

(Tumors secrete proteins, polypeptides, or glycoproteins that have hormonal activity.)
♦ Diagnosed by measuring arteriovenous gradient of hormone across tumor bed or between tumor and nontumor tissue; confirm by in vitro demonstration of hormone production by tumor cells and by resolution of endocrine syndrome after successful removal of tumor.

♦ Cushing's syndrome: increased blood ACTH level (>200 pg/mL), inability to suppress with high-dose DST (except in bronchial carcinoids), loss of diurnal variation of cortisol levels (usually >40 μg/dL). Therefore cannot be distinguished from excessive pituitary secretion of ACTH by use of DST. Typically malignant disease causing ectopic ACTH production has acute effects on adrenal glands manifested predominantly by excess mineralocorticoid production with hypokalemia and hypertension. May sometimes require selective venous catheterization to measure ACTH levels or in vitro hybridization assay to demonstrate ACTH-encoding messenger RNA to establish the diagnosis. Patients with lung cancer may have elevated ACTH levels without Cushing's syndrome.

Due To

  • Bronchogenic oat cell carcinoma (causes ~50% of cases) and carcinoid
  • Thymoma
  • Hepatoma
  • Carcinoma of ovary
  • Also medullary carcinoma of thyroid, islet cell tumor of pancreas, etc. Hypercalcemia simulating HPT (see Humoral Hypercalcemia of Malignancy, p. 598; and Table 13-7)
  • Renal carcinoma
  • Squamous cell and large-cell carcinoma of respiratory tract
  • Carcinoma of breast (occurs in 15% of patients with bone metastases)
  • Malignant lymphoma, myeloma, etc.
  • Cancer of ovary, pancreas, etc.
SIADH (see p. 702)
  • Especially with oat cell carcinoma of lung
♦ Hypoglycemia: serum insulin is low in presence of fasting hypoglycemia. Not associated with decreased serum phosphorus as in insulin-induced hypoglycemia.
  • Bronchogenic carcinoma
  • Carcinoma of adrenal cortex (6% of patients)

---

[30]Lips CJM, et al. Clinical screening as compared with DNA analysis in families with multiple endocrine neoplasia type 2A. *N Engl J Med* 1994;331:828.

- Hepatoma (23% of patients)
- Retroperitoneal fibrosarcoma (most frequently)

Thyrotoxicosis: signs and symptoms are rare, but laboratory findings are present.
- Tumors of GI tract, hematopoietic tumors, pulmonary tumors, etc.
- Trophoblastic tumors in women
- Choriocarcinoma of testis

Struma ovarii

Precocious puberty in boys
- Hepatoma

Acromegaly
- Pancreatic tumors producing GH or GH-releasing factor in presence of normal sella; increased GH not suppressed by glucose.
- Carcinoid.

Erythrocytosis (due to erythropoietin production) (see p. 381)
- Carcinoma of kidney, liver
- Fibromyoma of uterus
- Cerebellar hemangioblastoma

See also Carcinoid Syndrome (p. 688), Precocious Puberty, Syndrome of Inappropriate Secretion of Antidiuretic Hormone (p. 702).

Pineal Tumors

Boys—precocious puberty in 30% of patients
Girls—delayed pubescence
Diabetes insipidus occurs occasionally.

Pituitary Tumors

♦ Findings due to increased production of hormones or effect of growing mass.
Most common tumors are
- Prolactin-secreting tumors comprise ~30% of all pituitary tumors (see Prolactinomas, p. 700)
- GH-secreting tumors (see Acromegaly and Gigantism)
- ACTH-secreting tumors (see Cushing's Syndrome)
- Nonfunctioning adenomas, which may produce findings of intracranial mass, especially with visual changes, and hypopituitarism (sometimes with impaired hypothalamic function)

Microadenomas (<10 mm in size) may be present in 10–20% of the population by autopsy and radiographic studies ("incidentaloma") but tumors >10 mm in size are quite rare.

Polydipsia, Psychogenic

(Excessive intake of water causes loss of medullary sodium and urea to renal venous blood and abnormally reduced tonicity of renal medulla.)

See Table 13-26.

○Should be suspected when large volumes of very dilute urine occur with plasma osmolality that is only slightly decreased or low normal.

Test dose of vasopressin often shows failure to concentrate urine, simulating nephrogenic diabetes insipidus. However, the test is normal when performed after restoration of normal hypertonicity of renal medulla by a period of high sodium and low water intake.

Fluid deprivation test is least reliable in differentiating this from partial central diabetes insipidus; e.g., some increase in urine osmolality after dehydration with an inconclusive (~10%) further increase after vasopressin may be due to either condition.

Polyglandular Syndromes, Autoimmune

Type I

♦ Requires two or more of the following: hypoparathyroidism, Addison's disease, chronic mucocutaneous candidiasis (all three are present in approximately one-third

Table 13-28. Comparison of Polyglandular Syndromes Types I and II

	Prevalence (%)	
	Type I	Type II
Hypoparathyroidism	90	Rare
Adrenal insufficiency	60	100
Autoimmune thyroid disease	12[a]	70[b]
Insulin-dependent diabetes mellitus	≤ 4	50
Gonadal failure	17–45	5–50
Mucocutaneous candidiasis	75	Rare
Alopecia	20	Rare
Pernicious anemia	16	1
Malabsorption	25	Rare
Vitiligo	4	4
Chronic active hepatitis	9–13	Rare
Onset	Youth/infancy	Adulthood
Human leukocyte antigen associations	None	B8, DR3, DR4
Autosomal	Recessive	Dominant
Family members affected	Only siblings	Multiple generations

[a]Primary myxedema or Hashimoto's thyroiditis.
[b]Hypo- and hyperthyroidism are equally prevalent.
Sources: Whitley RJ. Polyglandular autoimmune syndromes: disorders affecting multiple endocrine glands. *Am Assoc Clin Chem Endocrinol* 1994;12:39; and Baker JR. Autoimmune endocrine disease. *JAMA* 1997;278:1931.

of patients). Patient may also have associated immune disorders, e.g., autoimmune hypothyroidism. Gonadal failure and chronic hepatitis may also occur.

Type II (Schmidt's Syndrome)

♦ Autoimmune thyroiditis or insulin-dependent diabetes (15% of all patients with insulin-dependent diabetes mellitus have type II) with Addison's disease. Interval between onset of endocrinopathies may be up to 20 yrs. Gonadal failure may sometimes occur. (For comparison of types I and II, see Table 13-28.)

Type III

♦ Autoimmune thyroid disease with two other autoimmune disorders, including insulin-dependent diabetes mellitus, PA, or a non-endocrine-organ–specific autoimmune disorder (e.g., myasthenia gravis) but without Addison's disease.

Prolactinomas

Serum Prolactin Reference Values

Normal <25 ng/mL in females; lower in males and children.
Gradual increase from birth until adolescence
13- to 15-yr-old boys: 2.5× adult levels
13- to 15-yr-old girls: 3× adult levels
Serum samples should be collected under basal conditions with minimal stress and by pooling three blood samples collected at 20-min intervals for one assay; all drugs should be discontinued for at least 2 wks before testing.

Interpretation

40–85 ng/mL: seen in craniopharyngioma, hypothyroidism, effect of drugs
50 ng/mL: 25% chance of a pituitary tumor

100 ng/mL: 50% chance of a pituitary tumor

<200 ng/mL with a macroadenoma, particularly with extrasellar extension, is most likely due to compression of pituitary stalk rather than prolactinoma.

200–300 ng/mL: nearly 100% chance of a pituitary tumor; >200 ng/mL may indicate a macroadenoma rather than microadenoma and tumor usually is visible on CT or MRI, but CT or MRI is normal in ≤ 20% of microadenomas.

High levels may be seen with simultaneous multiple additive factors that usually cause lesser increases (e.g., chronic renal failure plus use of methyldopa)

♦ Immediate postoperative level of <7.0 ng/mL indicates long-term cure but higher levels are associated with recurrence.

♦ Repeated serum levels in late morning or early afternoon that are increased 3–5× normal in men or nonlactating women are usually considered diagnostic of pituitary adenoma or rarely of hypothalamic disease or pituitary stalk section or hypothyroidism. One elevated level is not adequate for diagnosis. Level normally increases sharply during sleep; higher in morning than afternoon.

Increased Serum Prolactin In

Amenorrhea/galactorrhea
- 10–25% of women with galactorrhea and normal menses
- 10–15% of women with amenorrhea without galactorrhea
- 75% of women with both galactorrhea and amenorrhea/oligomenorrhea
- Causes 15–30% of cases of amenorrhea in young women

Pituitary lesions (e.g., prolactinoma, section of pituitary stalk, empty sella syndrome, 20–40% of patients with acromegaly, up to 80% of patients with chromophobe adenomas)

Hypothalamic lesions (e.g., sarcoidosis, eosinophilic granuloma, histiocytosis X, TB, glioma, craniopharyngioma)

Other endocrine diseases
- ~20% of cases of hypothyroidism (second most common cause of hyperprolactinemia). *Therefore serum TSH and T_4 should always be measured.*
- Addison's disease
- Polycystic ovaries

Glucocorticoid excess—normal or moderately elevated prolactin

Ectopic production of prolactin (e.g., bronchogenic carcinoma, renal cell carcinoma, ovarian teratomas, acute myeloid leukemia)

Children with sexual precocity—may be increased into pubertal range

Neurogenic causes (e.g., nursing and breast stimulation, spinal cord lesions, chest wall lesions such as herpes zoster)

Stress (e.g., surgery, hypoglycemia, vigorous exercise)

Pregnancy (increases to 8–20× normal by delivery, returns to normal in 2–4 wks postpartum unless nursing occurs)

Lactation

Chronic renal failure (20–40% of cases; becomes normal after successful renal transplant but not hemodialysis)

Liver failure (due to decreased prolactin clearance)

Idiopathic causes (some probably represent early cases of microadenoma too small to be detected by CAT scan)

Interferences

Drugs—*most common cause*; usually subsides a few weeks after cessation of using drug; these elevations are usually <100 ng/mL
- Neuroleptics (e.g., phenothiazines, thioxanthenes, butyrophenones)
- Antipsychotic drugs (e.g., Compazine, chlorpromazine [Thorazine], trifluoperazine hydrochloride [Stelazine], thioridazine hydrochloride (Mellaril), haloperidol lactate [Haldol])
- Dopamine antagonists (e.g., metoclopramide, sulpiride)
- Opiates (morphine, methadone)
- Reserpine
- Alpha-methyldopa (Aldomet)
- Estrogens and oral contraceptives
- TRH
- Amphetamines
- Isoniazid

Serum Prolactin May Be Decreased In

Hypopituitarism
- Postpartum pituitary necrosis (Sheehan's syndrome)
- Idiopathic hypogonadotropic hypogonadism

Use of certain drugs
- Dopamine agonists
- Ergot derivatives (bromocriptine mesylate, lergotrile mesylate, lisuride hydrogen maleate)
- Levodopa, apomorphine, clonidine

Interpretation

♦ Normal value in child with growth retardation virtually rules out hypopituitarism but a low value is not diagnostic. Single blood value may be more reliable than multiple measurements of GH in diagnosis of active acromegaly.

♦ TRH stimulation of patients with increased prolactin not due to pituitary tumors usually doubles serum prolactin level to peak of >12 ng/mL in 15–30 mins, but most patients with prolactinomas do not respond to TRH stimulation (response <2× baseline level). Enhanced responsiveness in hypothyroidism and blunted prolactin rise in chronic renal failure. Unresponsiveness to TRH (<2× baseline level) also occurs in panhypopituitarism. Measurement of multiple basal prolactin levels has replaced stimulation tests for diagnosis of prolactinoma.

Microscopic examination of breast discharge shows numerous fat globules; if not seen, rule out intraductal breast carcinoma or infection.

Normal or decreased serum FSH, LH, and testosterone may occur in men.

Women may also present with hirsutism, infertility. Men may present with decreased libido, impotence, oligospermia, low serum testosterone levels, and sometimes galactorrhea.

Hypothyroidism

Acute fasting and chronic protein-calorie deprivation (when GH often rises)

Syndrome of Inappropriate Secretion of Antidiuretic Hormone (SIADH)

(Syndrome of continuing release of vasopressin in presence of low plasma osmolality; kidney responds normally to arginine vasopressin.)

Due To

CNS disease of all types (e.g., neoplastic, degenerative, infective, traumatic, vascular, psychogenic)

Advanced endocrinopathies (e.g., myxedema, ACTH deficiency, adrenal insufficiency)

Neoplasms (most commonly oat cell carcinoma of lung; adenocarcinoma of lung, carcinoma of pancreas, carcinoma of duodenum, lymphoma), some of which show ectopic production of ADH

Pulmonary diseases (e.g., cancer, pulmonary emboli, TB, pneumonia, chronic infections, lung abscess, aspergillosis)

Miscellaneous (e.g., acute intermittent porphyria, postoperative state)

Idiopathic causes

Various drugs
- Oral hypoglycemic agents (chlorpropamide, tolbutamide, phenformin, metformin)
- Antineoplastic agents (vincristine, cyclophosphamide)
- Diuretics (chlorothiazide)
- Sedatives, analgesics (morphine, barbiturates, acetaminophen)
- Psychotropic drugs (amitriptyline, phenothiazines)
- Miscellaneous (clofibrate, isoproterenol, nicotine)

Cause should be established because some causes are curable with resolution of SIADH. Cortisol deficiency and hypothyroidism should always be excluded.

♦ Dilutional hyponatremia with appropriately decreased osmolality (usually <280 mOsm/kg) when urine is not at maximum dilution; this is basis for diagnosis in patient with no evidence of cardiac, liver, kidney, adrenal, pituitary, or thyroid disease, or hypovolemia and not on drug therapy (especially diuretics).

♦ Increased urine sodium (>20 mmol/L; >30 mmol/day) with inappropriately high urine osmolality (>500 mOsm/kg) is essential for diagnosis because it excludes hypovolemia as the cause of hyponatremia (in absence of abnormal renal function or causative drugs)

♦ Increased urine osmolality higher than serum osmolality

Normal serum potassium, CO_2, BUN, and creatinine

Decreased serum chloride

Decreased AG

Decreased uric acid (due to dilution)

Increase in plasma vasopressin that is inappropriate for the degree of plasma osmolality is not helpful in diagnosis because most causes of true hyponatremia are associated with detectable or increased vasopressin. (See Arginine Vasopressin, p. 685.)

Clinical and biochemical response to fluid restriction but not to administration of isotonic or hypertonic saline

Thyroid-Stimulating Hormone (TSH)–Secreting Pituitary Adenomas

(Rare type of adenoma that causes hyperthyroidism)

♦ Laboratory findings of hyperthyroidism except serum TSH is increased and does not increase in response to TRH stimulation or does not decrease in response to suppressive doses of thyroid hormone.

♦ Increased molar ratio of alpha subunit of TSH to whole TSH.

○ Secretion of other hormones (e.g., prolactin, GH) occurs in about one-third of these cases.

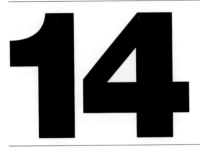

Genitourinary Diseases

Renal Function Tests

See Urea Nitrogen (p. 83), Creatinine (p. 55), Blood Urea Nitrogen/Creatinine Ratio (p. 44).

Biopsy, Renal

Should be preceded by
- Confirmation that two kidneys are present
- Confirmation that no renal infection is present (urine Gram stain)
- Confirmation that no bleeding disorder is present (CBC, PT, aPTT, possibly BT)

Examination should include histology (stained by hematoxylin and eosin, trichrome, PAS, silver; other stains [e.g., for amyloid] when indicated), immunofluorescence (with antisera specific for IgG, IgA, IgM, C1q, C3, C4, fibrinogen, albumin, kappa and lambda light chains), and electron microscopy (e.g., necessary for diagnosis of Alport's syndrome, thin basement membrane nephritis).

Contraindicated In

Solitary kidney
Large renal cyst
Renal artery aneurysm
Renal neoplasm
Acute pyelonephritis
Hemorrhagic diathesis
Uncontrolled hypertension

Indicated In

Acute renal allograft dysfunction
- Primary nonfunction for >10–14 days
- Unexplained deterioration of graft function
- Unexplained proteinuria (usually months to years later; may indicate recurrent or new glomerular disease)
- Before beginning antilymphocyte therapy to prove diagnosis of rejection

Nephritic syndrome (acute onset of hematuria, RBC casts, proteinuria, hypertension, declining renal function) for differential diagnosis (postinfectious or membranoproliferative GN, anti–glomerular membrane disease, IgA nephropathy, Henoch-Schönlein purpura, SLE, vasculitides) or assess disease severity.

Nephrotic syndrome (see p. 733). Usually due to minimal-change disease in children; biopsy only if no response to corticosteroids.

Nonnephrotic proteinuria with progressive disease

Not Indicated In

End-stage renal disease because of presence of small scarred kidneys unless question of risk of recurrence (e.g., primarily glomerular diseases)

Nonnephrotic proteinuria (<3.5 gm/day) because prognosis is good and indications for therapy are rare.

Asymptomatic hematuria without proteinuria, decreased renal function or hypertension (e.g., due to IgA nephropathy, hereditary nephritis, thin basement membrane disease, isolated vascular C3 deposition) because no effective treatment exists.

Concentration Test, Urine

Fluid deprivation may be contraindicated in heart disease or early renal failure.

Interpretation

Normal: urine specific gravity is ≥ 1.025.
With decreased renal function, specific gravity is <1.020.
As renal impairment becomes more severe, specific gravity approaches 1.010.
Sensitive for early loss of renal function, but a normal finding does not necessarily rule out active kidney disease.

Interferences

Unreliable in the presence of any severe water and electrolyte imbalance (e.g., adrenal cortical insufficiency, edema formation), consumption of low-protein or low-salt diet, chronic liver disease, pregnancy, lack of patient cooperation

Concentration Test, Vasopressin (Pitressin)

May be used in the presence of edema or ascites. Contraindicated in coronary artery disease and pregnancy.

Interpretation

Same as for the urine concentration test.
Normal: specific gravity should reach ≥ 1.020.
In diabetes insipidus (see p. 689), urine specific gravity becomes normal after vasopressin administration but not after fluid restriction.

Dilution Test, Urine

Water loading may be contraindicated in kidney and heart disease.

Interpretation (Normal)

Urine volume is >80% of ingested amount (1200 mL).
Specific gravity is 1.003 in at least one specimen.
With decreased renal function, a smaller volume of urine is noted.
Specific gravity may not fall below 1.010.
Loss of dilution ability occurs later than loss of concentrating ability.

Glomerular Filtration Rate (GFR)

GFR is measured with urea clearance, creatinine clearance, or inulin clearance.

Use

The creatinine clearance test, particularly serial measurements, is the most reliable test of renal function; is independent of rate of urine flow. After baseline urine creatinine has been obtained, serum creatinine levels can be used to calculate clearance. Creatinine clearance overestimates GFR when GFR is <5–10% of normal; in these cases value should be averaged with urea clearance, which underestimates GFR. Is excreted by tubules as well as filtered by glomeruli and therefore may overestimate GFR, but is widely used and best measurement of GFR in most clinical instances. Low concentration of creatinine in serum of infants and young children makes laboratory test difficult and inaccurate.

Interpretation

GFR decreases ~1%/yr after age 40.

Elderly patients with a normal serum creatinine and diminished muscle mass may have a 30% decrease in GFR.

Usually good correlation is seen between urine concentrating function and GFR. A normal GFR in association with impaired concentrating ability may be found in sickle cell anemia, diabetes insipidus, nephronophthisis, and various acquired disorders (e.g., pyelonephritis, potassium deficiency, hypercalciuria).

Impairment may be more severe than indicated by laboratory studies if signs and symptoms are more disabling.

Normal Clearances

(Corrected to 1.73 sq m body surface area)

Endogenous Creatinine

Age (yrs)	Mean Creatinine Clearance (mL/min/1.73 sq m body surface area)
0–1	72
1	45
2	55
3	60
4	71
5	73
6	64
7	67
8	72
9	83
10	89
11	92
12	109
13–14	86

	Males	Females[1]
20–29	94–140	72–110
30–39	59–137	71–121
40–49	76–120	50–102
50–59	67–109	50–102
60–69	54–98	45–75
70–79	49–79	37–61
80–89	30–60	27–55
90–99	26–44	26–42

Inulin*	Males	110–150 mL/min
	Females	105–132 mL/min
Urea†	Maximum	60–100 mL/min
	Standard	40–65 mL/min

*Normal inulin clearance = 25–30 mL/min during first few days of life; 50–60 mL/min by end of first month. Adult values by 12–18 mos. Considerable individual variation makes interpretation difficult unless level is clearly abnormal. Is best determinant of GFR but requires continuous infusion to maintain adequate blood concentration during test.

†Urea clearance: marked variability in contributing factors (e.g., BUN, diet, urine flow) makes interpretation difficult and limits usefulness in most clinical situations.

Creatinine clearance decreases ~8 mL/min/1.73 m^2/decade after age 30.

Estimate of creatinine clearance from single serum creatinine clearance value may be required for prompt therapy of nephrotoxic drug reaction or because of difficulty of accurate 24-hr urine collection. This estimate may be calculated by the following formulas or by the nomogram (Fig. 14-1).

[1]Kampmann J, et al. Rapid evaluation of creatinine clearance. *Acta Med Scand* 1974;196:517.

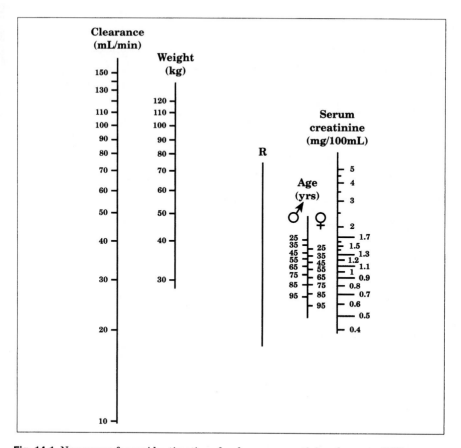

Fig. 14-1. Nomogram for rapid estimation of endogenous creatinine clearance. With a straightedge, join weight to age. Keep straightedge at crossing point of line marked "R." Then move the right-hand side of the straightedge to the appropriate serum creatinine value and read the patient's clearance from the left side of the nomogram. (From Appel GB, Neu HC. Antimicrobial agents in patients with renal disease. *Med Times* 1977;105:116.)

To *estimate* GFR from serum creatinine, this equation may be used, but it may be accurate only in patients with chronic renal failure who have stable renal function and are not massively obese or edematous:

GFR = [(140 – age in yrs) × (weight in kg)]/(72 × serum creatinine)

(Values for women are 85% of predicted)

Creatinine clearance (mL/min/1.73 sq m) = [(9.8 – 0.8) × (age – 20)]/serum creatinine

(Values for women are 90% of predicted)
See Table 14-1.

Osmolality, Urine

Measurement of urine osmolality during water restriction is an accurate, sensitive test of decreased renal function.

Table 14-1. Laboratory Guide to Evaluation of Renal Impairment

Condition	Renal Clearance of Endogenous Creatinine* (Glomerular Filtration Rate)	Urinary Excretion of IV PSP in 15 Mins (Renal Tubular Transport Mechanisms)
Normal	Men: 130–200 L/24 hrs (90–139 mL/min)	≥ 25%
	Women: 115–180 L/24 hrs (80–125 mL/min)	
Slight impairment	75–90 L/24 hrs (52.0–62.5 mL/min)	15–25%
Mild impairment	60–75 L/24 hrs (42–52 mL/min)	10–15%
Moderate impairment	40–60 L/24 hrs (28–42 mL/min)	5–10%
Marked impairment	<40 L/24 hrs (<28 mL/min)	<5%

IV = intravenous; PSP = phenolsulfonphthalein.
*Creatinine clearance is normally less in women than in men, and it usually decreases with age, starting at 20 yrs of age.

Interpretation

Normal: concentration of >800 mOsm/kg
Minimal impairment of renal concentrating ability: 600–800 mOsm/kg
Moderate impairment: 400–600 mOsm/kg
Severe impairment: <400 mOsm/kg
Urine osmolality may be impaired when other tests are normal (Fishberg concentration test, BUN, PSP excretion, creatinine clearance, IV pyelogram); may be especially useful in diabetes mellitus, essential hypertension, silent pyelonephritis.
Measurement of serum osmolality and calculation of urine/serum ratio (normal >3) may also be helpful.
See Diabetes Insipidus, p. 689.

Phenolsulfonphthalein (PSP) Excretion Test

Test is hazardous in severe renal insufficiency or heart failure because adequate prior hydration is required to obtain sufficient urine volume.

Use

Detect slight to moderate decrease in renal function. It is not useful in chronic azotemia with fixed specific gravity (serum creatinine and creatinine clearance are more useful in these cases).

Interferences

Use of small urine volumes magnifies errors.
Test is distorted by presence of residual bladder urine, abnormal drainage sites (e.g., fistulas), and interfering substances (e.g., hematuria).
Hepatic disease may lead to falsely elevated values (because 20% of the dye is normally removed by the liver).
False-positive results may also occur in multiple myeloma (because of excessive protein binding) and in hypoalbuminemia.
Certain drugs may interfere with PSP excretion (e.g., salicylates, penicillin, some diuretic and uricosuric drugs, and some radiographic contrast media).
False-positive results have been reported with kaolin, magnesium, methylene blue, nicotine acid, quinacrine (mepacrine), quinidine, quinine.

Interpretation

Normal: >25% in urine in 15 mins; 55–75% in 2 hrs

The 15-min PSP excretion correlates with the GFR; a normal 15-min value indicates normal GFR. Progressive decrease of 15-min value is proportional to decreased GFR (e.g., 15% PSP excretion in 15 mins approximates a 45% GFR). If the GFR is normal, the PSP test indicates renal blood flow or tubular function; better tests are available for measuring these two functions, and the PSP test is now rarely used.

Increased dye excretion in later time periods compared to the initial 15-min period suggests increased residual urine due to obstructive uropathy or incomplete bladder emptying; the latter can be ruled out by placement of indwelling catheter during the test.

PSP that is normal with increased BUN and serum creatinine and decreased GFR suggests acute GN. PSP parallels these parameters in most chronic renal diseases.

Renal Function Tests, Other

Measurement of Effective Plasma Flow (RPF) and Tubular Function

Para-aminohippurate

Males	560–800 mL/min
Females	500–700 mL/min
Diodrast	600–800 mL/min
Filtration fraction = GFR/RPF	
Males	17–21%
Females	17–23%
Maximal Diodrast excretory capacity, TmD	
Males	43–59 mg/min
Females	33–51 mg/min

Interpretation

Urea clearance is normal until >50% of renal parenchyma is inactivated. With renal insufficiency, the clearance test parallels the parenchymal destruction.

Urinary acidification is impaired in chronic renal disease with azotemia. It is decreased without parallel impairment of GFR in renal tubular acidosis, some cases of Fanconi's syndrome, and some cases of acquired nephrocalcinosis.

Proximal tubular malfunction is indicated by urinary excretion of substances normally reabsorbed by tubules: in renal glycosuria (blood glucose <180 mg/dL as in Fanconi's syndrome, heavy metal poisoning), aminoaciduria, phosphaturia.

Serum creatinine and BUN are not useful in discovering early renal insufficiency because they do not become abnormal until 50% of renal function has been lost.

Serum creatinine increase occurs in 10–20% of patients taking aminoglycosides and up to 20% of patients taking penicillins (especially methicillin).

Split Renal Function Tests

Interpretation

Affected kidney shows decreased urine volume and sodium excretion and decreased urine concentration of creatinine, inulin, or para-aminohippurate.

Use

Aid in diagnosis of renal artery stenosis

Not useful in presence of GU tract obstruction (e.g., in men older than age 50)

Kidney Diseases

See Table 14-2.

Abscess, Perinephric

Laboratory findings due to underlying or primary diseases

- Hematogenous from distant foci (e.g., furuncles, infected tonsils) usually due to staphylococci and occasionally streptococci
- Direct extension from kidney infection (e.g., pyelonephritis, pyonephrosis) due to gram-negative rods and occasionally tubercle bacilli
- Infected perirenal hematoma (e.g., due to trauma, tumor, polyarteritis nodosa) due to various organisms

Urine changes due to underlying disease
- Urine may be normal and sterile. *Do acid-fast smear and culture for tubercle bacilli.*

Increased PMNs

Increased ESR

Positive blood culture (some patients)

Abscess, Renal

(Due to metastatic infection not related to previous renal disease)

Urine
- Trace of albumin
- Few RBCs (may have transient gross hematuria at onset)
- No WBCs
◆ • Very many organisms in stained sediment

WBC high (may be >30,000/cu mm)

Acidosis, Renal Tubular

(Inadequate H⁺ secretion; glomerular function is either normal or relatively less impaired; four different types)

Type 2 (Proximal)

◆ Low plasma bicarbonate concentration with hyperchloremic acidosis

◆ Alkaline urine that becomes acid if extracellular bicarbonate level is decreased below the patient's maximum reabsorptive limit

Normal urine pH in the absence of bicarbonate in the urine

◆ IV $NaHCO_3$ ($\leq$ 1.0 mEq/kg/hr) causes rapid increase in urine pH even though plasma HCO_3^- has increased, but it is still less than normal (24–26 mEq/L).

Due To

Most commonly due to increased excretion of monoclonal Ig light chains in multiple myeloma or use of carbonic anhydrase inhibitor (e.g., acetazolamide for glaucoma) in adults, and cystinosis or idiopathic cause in children.

Primary (defect in bicarbonate reabsorption)
- Usually occurs in males.
- Only clinical manifestation is retarded growth; renal and metabolic complications are absent.
- Good prognosis with clinical response to alkali therapy, which is usually not permanently required.

Secondary
- Idiopathic or secondary Fanconi's syndrome (cystinosis, Lowe's syndrome [X-linked recessive disorder with congenital cataracts, neurologic involvement], tyrosinemia, glycogen storage disease, Wilson's disease, hereditary fructose intolerance, heavy-metal intoxication, toxic effects of drugs such as outdated tetracycline)
- Vitamin D–deficient rickets
- Medullary cystic disease
- After renal transplantation
- Nephrotic syndrome, multiple myeloma, renal amyloidosis

Type 1 (Distal 1)

(Collecting ducts do not secrete sufficient H⁺ to form ammonium or secreted H⁺ backleaks out of collecting tubule lumen)

◆ Hyperchloremic acidosis, low plasma bicarbonate concentration; should be suspected in any patient with metabolic acidosis with normal AG and inappropriately high urine pH (>5.3 in adults, >5.6 in children). Incomplete type 1 renal tubular acidosis should be suspected with normal plasma bicarbonate concen-

Table 14-2. Urinary Findings in Various Diseases

Disease	Volume	Specific Gravity	Protein[a]	RBCs[b]	WBCs and Epithelial Cells[b]	Casts[c, d]	Comment
Normal	600–2500	1.003–1.030	0 (0.05 gm)	0-occ. (0–0.130)	0–0.65	0-occ. (2000/24 hrs)	
Acute febrile states	D	I	Trace to +			Few	
Orthostatic proteinuria	N	N	I (≤ 1 gm)	N (0–0.130)	0–3	V; H & G	Normal when recumbent; abnormalities after upright posture
Glomerulonephritis							
Acute	D	I	2–4+ (0.5–5.0)	1–4+ (1–1000)	1–400	2–4+; H & G; *RBC, epithelial, mixed RBC & epithelial*	Gross hematuria or "smoky" urine
Latent			(0.1–2.0)	(1–100)	1–20	*RBC,* H & G	
Nephrosis ("nephrotic stage")	D	I	4+ (4–40)	0–few (0.5–50.0)	20–1000	*Epithelial, fatty, waxy;* H & G	Fat-laden epithelial cells, anisotropic fat in epithelial cells and casts
Terminal	I or D	D; fixed	1–2+ (2–7)	Trace–1+ (0.5–10.0)	1–50	1–3+ *broad, waxy,* H & G, epithelial	
Pyelonephritis							
Acute	N	N	0–2+ (0.5–2.0)	Few (0–1)	20–2000	*WBC,* H & G, *bacteria*	Bacteria, many WBCs in clumps
Chronic	N or D	N or D	2–4+ (0–5)	Few (0–1)	0.5–50.0	Same as acute; often few or none	Same as acute; findings may be intermittent
Renal TB			(0.1–3.0)	(1–20)	1–50	*WBC,* H & G	Tubercle bacilli

			Protein[a]		Cells[b]	Casts[c],[d]	
Disseminated lupus erythematosus	V	N or D	1-4+ (0.5-20.0)	1-4+ (1-100)	1-100	1-4+ RBC, *fatty, waxy*; H & G	
Toxemia of pregnancy	D	I	3-4+ (0.5-10.0)	0-1+ (0-1)	1-5	3-4+ H & G	
Malignant hypertension	V	D; fixed	1-2+ (1-10)	Trace-1+ (1-100)	1-200	1-2+ H & G, RBC, fatty	Increasing uremia with minimal or marked protein-uria and hematuria
Benign hypertension	N or I	N or D	0-1+	0-trace (1-5)		0-1+ H & G	
Congestive heart failure	D	I	1-2+	0-1+		1+ H & G	
Intercapillary glomerulosclerosis (Kimmelstiel-Wilson syndrome)			1-4+ (2-20)	(0-1)	1-30	Epithelial, fatty, H & G	Frequently associated: pyelonephritis and nephrosclerosis
Lower nephron nephrosis							
Acute	D	I		1-4+	1-4+	RBC; H & G, epithelial	
Diuretic	I		0.5-10.0	(0-1)	1-100	Broad, waxy, epithelial, H & G	

D = decreased; H & G = hyaline and granular casts; I = increased; occ. = occasionally; N = normal; V = variable.

[a]Protein: quantitative values in ( ) given as gm/24 hrs.

[b]Quantitative values given in ( ) as cells × 10^6/24 hrs.

[c]Casts require examination of fresh or preserved urine and acid pH.

[d]Italics denote most important or diagnostic finding.

713

tration, urine pH persistently >5.3 and calcium stone disease or positive family history.
♦ Alkaline urine (pH 6.5–7.0) that persists at any level of plasma bicarbonate.
♦ Ammonium loading test (ammonium chloride, 0.1 gm/kg) shows inability to acidify urine below pH 6.5 and depressed rates of excretion of titratable acid and ammonium.
No other tubular defects
Often presents with complications (e.g., nephrocalcinosis, interstitial nephritis renal calculi, rickets, and osteomalacia) as well as growth retardation
Occurs predominantly in females (70%)
Due To
Most commonly due to autoimmune disorders (e.g., Sjögren's syndrome) or hypercalciuria in adults; hereditary form in children.
Hypokalemic or Normokalemic Type
Primary (inability of tubular cell to secrete enough H^+)
Secondary
- Increased serum globulins (especially gamma) (e.g., SLE, Sjögren's syndrome, Hodgkin's disease, sarcoidosis, chronic active hepatitis, cryoglobulinemia)
- Pyelonephritis
- Medullary sponge kidney
- Ureterosigmoidostomy
- Hereditary insensitivity to ADH (vasopressin)
- Various renal diseases (e.g., hypercalcemia, potassium-losing disorders, medullary cystic disease, polyarteritis nodosa, amyloidosis, Sjögren's syndrome)
- Various genetically transmitted disorders (e.g., Ehlers-Danlos syndrome, Fabry's disease, hereditary elliptocytosis)
- Starvation, malnutrition
- Hyperthyroidism
- Hyperparathyroidism
- Vitamin D intoxication
Hyperkalemic Type (due to impaired sodium reabsorption in cortical collecting tubules)
- Hypoaldosteronism
- Obstructive nephropathy
- SLE
- Sickle cell nephropathy
- Cyclosporine toxicity
An incomplete or mixed tubular acidosis may be seen in obstructive uropathy and in hereditary fructose intolerance.
Type 4 (Aldosteronism)
Consists of a variety of conditions characterized by
- Mild to moderate renal impairment.
- Hyperchloremic acidosis.
- *Hyper*kalemia.
- Acid urine pH.
- Reduced ammonium secretion.
- Frequently, tendency to lose sodium in urine.
- Decreased mineralocorticoid secretion in some patients due to isolated hypoaldosteronism; others have decreased tubular response to aldosterone.

Amyloidosis of Kidney, Primary or Secondary

♦ Persistent proteinuria that varies from mild, with or without hematuria, to severe, with nephrotic syndrome
Vasopressin-resistant polyuria is present if the medulla alone is involved (rare).
See Amyloidosis (p. 890).

Arteriovenous Fistula, Renal

Hematuria
Laboratory findings due to congestive heart failure and hypertension

Azotemia Due to Cardiac Failure

May also occur in other functional forms of acute renal failure, e.g., hepatorenal syndrome, volume contraction.
Parallels the degree of heart failure
Serum creatinine rarely is >4 mg/dL even when BUN is >100 mg/dL in pure prerenal azotemia.
Urine is hypertonic (increased osmolality) with low sodium concentration (<10 mEq/L).
Protein excretion is frequently increased but rarely >2 gm/24 hrs.
Urine sediment may contain granular or hyaline casts, but cellular or pigmented casts are conspicuously absent.
In contrast, in *acute tubular necrosis,* which may complicate cardiac failure or may be due to cardiogenic shock or excessive use of diuretics or vasodilators (see p. 749):
• Urine osmolality approaches that of plasma.
• Urine sodium is usually high (40–80 mEq/L).
• Urine sediment contains many renal tubular cells and casts and many narrow (often pigmented) casts.

Berger's Disease (IgA Nephropathy)

(A focal proliferative GN; immunologic mediation; probably the most common form of GN)
○Persistent or intermittent microscopic hematuria with episodes of painless gross hematuria and minimal proteinuria, often associated with (rather than following by 4–10 days) infection of any type.
○Plasma IgA increased in ≤ 50% of patients.
Progression to renal failure in 5–25 yrs in 20–40% of cases
♦ Diagnosis is based on renal biopsy with immunofluorescence showing predominant mesangial IgA, IgG, and C3.
May be associated with celiac disease, dermatitis herpetiformis, some liver diseases.
May be related to Henoch-Schönlein purpura.

Calculi, Renal

(Autopsy incidence = 1.12%; cause of death = 0.38%)
Calcium oxalate alone or with phosphate is the constituent of kidney stones in 75% of patients in the United States. (See Fig. 14-2.)
• Idiopathic hypercalciuria in ~50% of patients. (See Table 14-3.)
• Primary hyperparathyroidism in ~5% of patients with nephrolithiasis; 50–75% of hyperparathyroidism patients have renal calculi.
• 20–30% of patients have
   Bone diseases—destructive (e.g., metastatic tumor) or osteoporosis (e.g., immobilization, Paget's disease, Cushing's syndrome)
   Milk-alkali (Burnett's) syndrome
   Hypervitaminosis D
   Sarcoidosis
   Renal tubular acidosis, type 1 (hypercalciuria, highly alkaline urine, serum calcium usually normal)
   Hyperthyroidism
   Other
Oxalate is present in 65% of stones, but hyperoxaluria is a relatively rare cause of these calculi and may be due to:
• Primary hyperoxaluria (see pp. 726–727)
• Secondary hyperoxaluria (see p. 726)
Struvite stones (staghorn calculi) (magnesium, ammonia, calcium, phosphate) are present in 10–15% of cases. Occur only when urine pH is high due to infection with urea-splitting bacteria, particularly *Proteus* spp. (but *Klebsiella, Pseudomonas, Serratia, Enterobacter* should be ruled out), and in patients with persistently alkaline urine.
Cystine stones (present in 1–2% of cases) form when urine contains >300 mg/day of cystine in congenital familial cystinuria. Cystine-only stones form only in homozygotes. Tend to have bilateral obstructive staghorn calculi with associated renal fail-

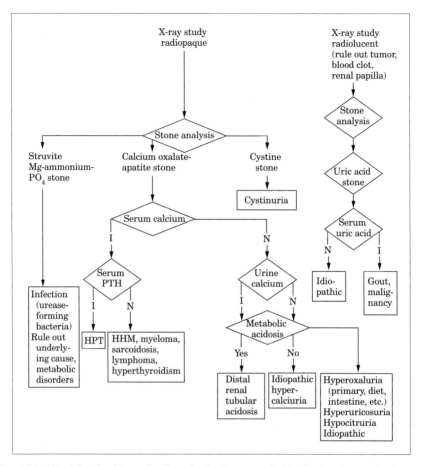

Fig. 14-2. Algorithm for diagnosis of renal calculi, as revealed by flank pain, renal colic, hematuria, fever, and urinalysis findings. (HHM = humeral hypercalcemia of malignancy; HPT = hyperparathyroidism; I = increased; N = normal; PTH = parathyroid hormone.)

ure. Urine shows cystine crystals. Cyanide-nitroprusside test is positive. Heterozygotes form stones with little or no cystine.

Uric acid is present in 5% of stones.

- Gout: 25% of patients with primary gout and 40% of patients with marrow-proliferative disorders have calculi.
- Urine is more acid than normal, often <5.5 (e.g., patients with chronic diarrhea, ileostomy).
- >50% of patients with urinary calculi have normal serum and urine uric acid levels.

Xanthine is present in children with inborn error of metabolism.

Hereditary glycinuria is a rare familial disorder associated with renal calculi.

In Children

Infections account for 13–40% of stones

Hypercalciuria is most common noninfectious cause (especially idiopathic but also due to distal renal tubular acidosis and therapy with furosemide, prednisone, or ACTH)

Oxaluria accounts for 3–13% of stones.

Uric acid stones comprise 4% of stones.

Table 14-3. Comparison of Types of Idiopathic Hypercalciuria

	Resorptive	**Absorptive**	**Renal**
Due to	Primary hyper-parathyroidism	Primary increase in intestinal absorption; autosomal dominant	Abnormal renal tubular reabsorption
Frequency	Least common	Most common	1/10 as common as absorptive type
2-hr urine after fasting			
Calcium	30 mg	<20 mg	Increased
Calcium/creatinine ratio	>0.15	<0.15	>0.15

Cystinuria is found in 5–7% of children with stones.
Hypocitraturia is found in 10% of children with stones.

Anatomic abnormalities
Microscopic hematuria is found in 80% of patients.
In renal colic, hematuria and proteinuria are present, and WBC is increased due to associated infection.
Crystalluria is diagnostically useful when cystine crystals (occur only in homozygous or heterozygous cysteinuria) or struvite crystals are present. Calcium oxalate, phosphate, and uric acid should arouse suspicion about possible cause of stones but they may occur in normal urines.

Dialysis for End-Stage Renal Disease, Laboratory Tests for Management[2]

See Table 14-4.

Conditions to Evaluate Routinely

Azotemia (A)
Residual renal function (A)
Electrolyte and mineral balance (A)
Liver function tests (B)
Renal osteodystrophy (osteomalacia) (C)
Anemia (D)
Coagulation disorders (E)
  A. Weekly creatinine and BUN; monthly serum calcium, potassium, chloride, bicarbonate, phosphorus; semiannual tests for residual renal functions, including 24-hr urine volume
  B. Monthly liver function tests (serum total protein, albumin, LD, ALP, AST), HBsAg (if seronegative) or annually if antibodies present after HBV vaccination.
  C. Monthly serum calcium and phosphorus and quarterly serum parathormone for detecting secondary hyperparathyroidism
  D. Monthly CBC; CBC or Hct with each dialysis
  E. Clotting time with each dialysis; weekly PT if on coumadin

[2]National Center for Health Services Research and Health Care Technology Assessment Reports 1986, No. 5. U.S. Department of Health and Human Services, Public Health Service.

Table 14-4. Chief Causes of Chronic Insufficiency in Patients Presenting for Dialysis

Glomerulonephritis	44%
Diabetic nephropathy	15%
Nephrosclerosis and renal vascular disease	12%
Congenital or hereditary disease (including polycystic kidney)	10%
Chronic pyelonephritis	6%
Others and unknown	15%

Conditions to Evaluate Nonroutinely

(See appropriate separate sections.)
- Bleeding or clotting disorders.
- Heart disease.
- Bone disease.
- Hepatitis.
- Symptomatic endocrine problems.
- Neuropathies.
- Acute complications associated with dialysis.
- Aluminum toxicity as cause of encephalopathy, vitamin D–resistant osteodystrophy, and iron-resistant anemia. Histochemical staining of bone biopsy (if serum level >100 μg/L) or atomic absorption of serum (level >200 μg/L is toxic; level >100 μg/L should be viewed with concern; level of 60–100 μg/L appears to cause no problem). Serum assay every 6–12 mos or every 3 mos, especially in pediatric patients; serum level may not reflect tissue content.
- Iron overload (due to frequent transfusions); assay serum ferritin every 3 mos.
- Specific conditions (e.g., renal tumors, diabetes mellitus).

Endocarditis (Bacterial), Renal Changes

Three types of pathologic changes are seen: diffuse subacute GN, focal embolic GN, microscopic or gross infarcts of kidney.
Laboratory findings due to bacterial endocarditis (see p. 114)
Albuminuria is almost invariably present, even when no renal lesions are found.
Hematuria (usually microscopic, sometimes gross) is usual at some stage of the disease, but repeated examinations may be required.
Renal insufficiency is frequent (15% of cases during active stage; 40% of fatal cases).
- BUN is increased (usually 25–75 mg/dL).
- Renal concentrating ability is decreased.

Glomerulonephritis (GN), Chronic

Due To

Poststreptococcal GN	1–2% of cases progress to chronic GN
Rapidly progressive GN	90% of cases progress to chronic GN
Membranous GN	50% of cases progress to chronic GN
Focal glomerulosclerosis	50–80% of cases progress to chronic GN
Membranoproliferative GN	50% of cases progress to chronic GN
IgA nephropathy	30–50% of cases progress to chronic GN

Various Clinical Courses

Early death after marked proteinuria, hematuria, oliguria, progressive increasing uremia, anemia
Intermittent or continuous or incidental proteinuria, hematuria with slight or absent azotemia, and normal renal function tests (may develop into late renal failure or may subside)
Exacerbation of chronic nephritis (with accentuation of proteinuria, hematuria, and decreased renal function) shortly after streptococcal URI

Nephrotic syndrome

○*Compared to pyelonephritis, chronic GN shows lipid droplets and epithelial and RBC casts in urine, more marked proteinuria (>2–3 gm/day), poorer prognosis for equivalent amount of azotemia.*

Glomerulonephritis, Classification[3]

See Tables 14-5 and 14-6 and Fig. 14-3.
Antibody mediated
- Anti–glomerular basement membrane diseases
    Goodpasture's syndrome
    Anti–glomerular basement membrane GN
    Alport's disease
    After renal transplantation
- Immune complex-mediated diseases
    IgA nephropathy
    Henoch-Schönlein purpura
    SLE
    Acute postinfectious GN
    Membranoproliferative GN
    Membranous GN
    Fibrillary GN
Cell-mediated
- Wegener's granulomatosis
- Polyarteritis
- Churg-Strauss syndrome
- ANCA-positive GN
- Scleroderma

Glomerulonephritis, Focal Proliferative

Attacks of hematuria usually occur at height of URI (bacterial or viral).
Prognosis is usually good, especially in children, but progressive nephritis causing renal failure is more common in adults.
Serum IgA is often increased.
Azotemia is usually absent.
Proteinuria is slight or absent.

Glomerulonephritis, Membranoproliferative

Clinical course may be active, or periods of remission may occur; 50% of patients have chronic renal insufficiency in 10 yrs.
○Marked proteinuria and nephrotic type of syndrome is found in 70% of patients.
○Normal serum C4 but prolonged or permanent depression of C3 is found in 60–80% of patients; clinical course is not related to serum complement levels.
♦Renal biopsy and immunofluorescent antibody findings.
GFR is <80 mL/min/1.73 sq m in two-thirds of patients

Glomerulonephritis, Poststreptococcal, Acute

See Table 14-5.
♦Evidence of infection with group A beta-hemolytic *Streptococcus* by
- Culture of throat
- Serologic findings indicative of recent streptococcal infection
    ASOT of >250 Todd units (increased in 80% of patients). Rise begins 10–14 days after infection, peaks in 4–6 wks, declines in next 4–6 mos. Usually develops 7–21 days after a beta-hemolytic streptococcal infection. Titer unreliable after *Streptococcus* pyoderma. *Increased in ~20% of cases of membranoproliferative GN. Early use of penicillin prevents rise of ASOT in either condition.*
    Antihyaluronidase

---

[3]Ambrus JL, Sridhar NR. Immunologic aspects of renal disease. *JAMA* 1997;278:1938.

Table 14-5. Classification of Glomerulonephritis

Glomerular Disorder	Situations in Which May Be Found	Hematuria (% of cases)		Proteinuria (% of cases)		Renal Function Decreased	Comment
		Micro Present	RBC Casts Present	1–3 gm Present	>3 gm Present		
IgA nephropathy (Berger's disease)	Focal proliferative GN	100	50	75	25	25% or NS; N in 75%	
IgM mesangial nephropathy		50	Rare	50	50	>75% or NS	
Acute GN secondary to infection (focal GN)	SBE, bacterial pneumonia, viral infections, infection of implanted devices	100	50	75	25	100%	
Crescentic (rapidly progressive) GN							
Anti-GBM	Goodpasture's syndrome in % of patients	100	50	50	50	100%	90% have HLA-DR2 antigen.
Immune complex	SLE, mixed cryoglobulinemia, Henoch-Schönlein purpura	100	50	50	50	100%	
Non-immune complex	Wegener's granulomatosis, polyarteritis						See Chapter 16.
GN and vasculitis	Wegener's granulomatosis, Henoch-Schönlein purpura, mixed cryoglobulinemia; Goodpasture's syndrome may occur	100	50	50	50	100%	

SLE						
Mesangial		15		10	N	Most frequent type in SLE.
Focal proliferative		50		25	N or D	
Membranous		50		85	N or D	
Diffuse proliferative (<25% of SLE patients)		75		75	Usually D; uremia develops in 50–75%	
Minimal-change disease	Lipid nephrosis, nil disease	20		100	N	85% respond to steroid therapy. Most common cause of NS in children.
Focal sclerosis		75	25	75	Usually D	Frequent cause of NS.
Membranous nephropathy	Usually idiopathic; occasionally due to heavy-metal toxicity (e.g., gold, mercury), persistent hepatitis B infection, other viruses (e.g., measles, varicella, Coxsackie), other infections (e.g., malaria, syphilis, leprosy, schistosomiasis), neoplasias (e.g., colon carcinoma, lymphoma, leukemia), sarcoidosis, SLE, others	50	25	75	N early; D late	Frequent cause of NS. Strong association with HLA-DR3. Spontaneous remission in 25–50%. Persistent proteinuria without progression in 25%. Progressive glomerular sclerosis causing renal failure in 50%. Common in adults; uncommon in children.

(continued)

Table 14-5. (continued)

Glomerular Disorder	Situations in Which May Be Found	Hematuria (% of cases)		Proteinuria (% of cases)		Renal Function Decreased	Comment
		Micro RBCs Present	RBC Casts Present	1–3 gm Present	>3 gm Present		
Membranoproliferative GN							
Type I (idiopathic)	SBE, essential cryoglobulinemia, Henoch-Schönlein purpura, SLE, sickle cell disease, hepatitis and cirrhosis, C2 deficiency, alpha$_1$-antitrypsin deficiency; infected shunts (*Staphylococcus, Corynebacterium*)	75	25	50	50	Usually D; NS at onset in 75%	Renal failure within 5 yrs common in adults but may be delayed 10–20 yrs. Persistent, marked proteinuria is poor prognostic sign. Renal vein thrombosis may occur.
Type II (idiopathic)	Infection with streptococci, pneumococci, *Candida*, lipodystrophy						

D = decreased; GBM = glomerular basement membrane; N = normal; NS = nephrotic syndrome; SBE = subacute endocarditis.
Goodpasture's syndrome occurs in <5% of cases of GN.
Source: Border WA, Glassock RJ. Progress in treating glomerulonephritis. *Drug Therapy* 1981;(Apr):97. Miller TR, et al. Urinary diagnostic indices in acute renal failure: a prospective study. *Ann Intern Med* 1978;89:47. Oken DE. On the differential diagnosis of acute renal failure. *Am J Med* 1981;71(Dec):916.

Table 14-6. Serum Complement in Acute Nephritis

Disorder	Approximate Percentage of Cases
Depressed Serum C3 or Hemolytic Complement Levels	
Systemic disease	
SLE (focal)	75
SLE (diffuse)	90
Subacute bacterial endocarditis	90
"Shunt" nephritis	90
Cryoglobulinemia	85
Renal disease	
Acute poststreptococcal glomerulonephritis	90
Membranoproliferative glomerulonephritis	
Type I	50–80
Type II	80–90
Normal Serum Complement Level	
Systemic disease	
Polyarteritis nodosa	
Wegener's granulomatosis	
Hypersensitivity vasculitis	
Henoch-Schönlein purpura	
Goodpasture's syndrome	
Visceral abscess	
Renal disease	
IgG-IgA nephropathy	
Idiopathic rapidly progressive glomerulonephritis	
Anti–glomerular basement membrane disease	
Immune complex disease	
Negative immunofluorescence findings	

      Anti–desoxyribonuclease-beta
      Antistreptokinase
      Anti–diphosphopyridine nucleotidase
      Anti–nicotinamide adenine dinucleotidase, etc.
- Combined use of serologic tests establishes recent streptococcal infection in virtually all cases.
♦ Urine
- Hematuria—gross or only microscopic. Microscopic hematuria may occur during the initial febrile URI and then reappear with nephritis in 1–2 wks. It lasts 2–12 mos; usual duration is 2 mos.
- RBC casts show glomerular origin of hematuria.
- WBC casts and WBCs show inflammatory nature of lesion.
- Granular and epithelial cell casts are present.
- Fatty casts and lipid droplets occur several weeks later; not related to hyperlipemia.
- Proteinuria is usually <2 gm/day (but may be ≤ 6–8 gm/day). May disappear although RBC casts and RBCs still occur.
- Decreased urinary aldosterone occurs in the presence of edema.
- Oliguria is frequent.
GFR usually shows greater decrease than renal blood flow; therefore filtration factor is decreased.
PSP excretion is normal in cases of mild to moderate severity; increases with progression of disease.

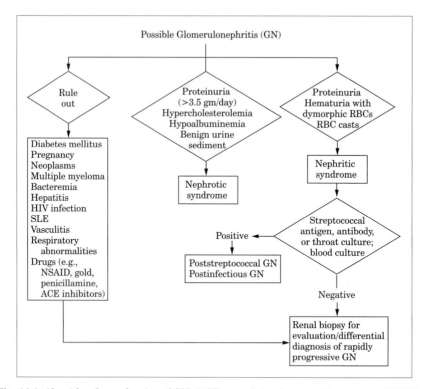

Fig. 14-3. Algorithm for evaluation of GN. (ACE = angiotensin-converting enzyme; NSAID = nonsteroidal antiinflammatory drug; SLE = systemic lupus erythematosus.)

Blood
- Azotemia is found in ~50% of patients.
- ESR is increased.
- Leukocytosis with increased PMNs.
- Mild anemia is seen, especially when edema is present (may be due to hemodilution, bone marrow depression, or increased destruction of RBCs).
- Serum proteins are normal, or nonspecific decrease of albumin and increase of alpha$_2$ and sometimes of beta and gamma globulins are noted.
- Serum cholesterol may be increased.
- Serum C3 and total hemolytic complement fall 24 hrs before onset of hematuria and return to normal within ~8 wks when hematuria subsides. If C3 is low for >8 wks, consider lupus nephritis or membranoproliferative GN.
- Antihuman kidney antibodies are present in serum in 50% of patients.
♦ Renal biopsy shows characteristic findings with electron microscopy and immunofluorescence.
Chronic renal insufficiency reported in ≤ 20% of patients.
○Azotemia with high urine specific gravity and normal PSP excretion usually means acute GN.

Glomerulonephritis, Rapidly Progressive (Nonstreptococcal)

Preceded by systemic diseases in many patients
- Infections
- Poststreptococcal GN
- Infective endocarditis

- Sepsis
- Hepatitis B, C

Preceded by multisystem diseases
- SLE
- Goodpasture's syndrome
- Necrotizing vasculitis
- Polyarteritis nodosa
- Wegener's granulomatosis
- Henoch-Schönlein purpura
- Cryoglobulinemia

No cultural or serologic (e.g., ASOT) evidence of recent streptococcus infection

○Oliguria is present with urine volume often <400 mL/day.

○Hematuria is often gross.

○RBCs, WBCs, and casts are present in urine.

○Proteinuria is usually >3 gm/day.

○Renal function declines rapidly. Azotemia is usually marked, with BUN >80 mg/dL and serum creatinine >10 mg/dL (in poststreptococcal type, BUN is usually 30–100 mg/dL and serum creatinine 1.5–4.0 mg/dL).

○Serum complement levels are normal.

♦Renal biopsy and immunofluorescent antibody findings

Prognosis is poorer than for poststreptococcal GN

Gout, Kidney Disorders In

Kidney stones occur in 25% of patients with gout; may occur in absence of arthritis.

Early renal damage is indicated by decreased renal concentrating ability, mild proteinuria, and decreased PSP excretion.

Later renal damage is shown by slowly progressive azotemia with slight albuminuria and slight or no abnormalities of urine sediment.

Arteriolar nephrosclerosis and pyelonephritis are usually associated.

Renal disease causes death in ≤ 50% of patients with gout.

The suggestion has been made that acute uric acid nephropathy may be differentiated from other forms of acute renal failure if ratio of urine urate to urine creatinine is >1.0 in an adult (many children under age 10 yrs have ratio >1.0).

Hemolytic-Uremic Syndrome

See Purpura, Thrombotic Thrombocytopenic, p. 480.

Hepatorenal Syndrome

Oliguria is marked (urine volume is <500 mL/day).

Progressive azotemia (serum creatinine >2.5 mg/dL)

Urine sodium is decreased to almost absent (<10 mEq/L; often 1–2 mEq/L).

Concentrated urine with high specific gravity and urine/plasma osmolality ratio >1.0.

Urine is acid; small amount of protein (<500 mg/day), few hyaline and granular casts, few RBCs (<50/HPF) may be found.

○Urine indices resemble those of prerenal azotemia and contrast with acute tubular necrosis, in which urine has low fixed specific gravity and high sodium content and a characteristic sediment may be found (see Table 14-7).

○Usually appears in patients with laboratory findings of decompensated cirrhosis with moderate to marked ascites, especially after fluid loss (e.g., GI hemorrhage, diarrhea, forced diuresis).

Hyponatremia, hyperkalemia, hepatic encephalopathy, coma may be present.

Must be differentiated from renal failure due to toxins, drugs (e.g., NSAIDs, acetaminophen, carbon tetrachloride); infection; acute tubular necrosis; obstructive nephropathy.

Horseshoe Kidneys

Laboratory findings due to complications
- Renal calculi
- Pyelonephritis
- Hematuria

Table 14-7. Comparison of Three Types of Renal Insufficiency

Laboratory Tests	Prerenal Azotemia	Hepatorenal Syndrome	Acute Renal Failure
Urine sodium (mEq/L)	<10	<10	>30 (may be less with sepsis)
Urine/plasma creatinine	>30:1	>30:1	<20:1
Urine osmolality	⊢────── At least 100 mOsm > plasma ──────⊣ osmolality		Same as plasma osmolality
Urine sediment	Normal	Not remarkable	Cell debris, casts
Response to plasma expansion	Good	Absent	Variable

Hypercalciuria, Idiopathic

See Table 14-3.
♦ Increased excretion of urinary calcium of >350 mg/24 hrs on diet containing 600–800 mg/day.
  • >4 mg/kg (either sex)
  • >140 mg/gm of urinary creatinine is most useful criterion in short or obese patients.
Normal blood calcium levels
Serum 1,25-dihydroxy-vitamin D_3 levels are usually high.
♦ Diagnosis requires exclusion of all other causes of hypercalciuria (see p. 88); may be familial. Occurs in ~40% of patients who form calcium renal stones. Occurs in 5–10% of general population.
Three types of hypercalciuria, as shown by findings from 2-hr urine collection after fasting
  • Renal: calcium/creatinine ratio >0.15. Hypercalciuria persists despite absent dietary calcium in intestine after fasting. One-tenth as common as absorptive type. Due to abnormality of renal tubular reabsorption.
  • Absorptive: <20 mg calcium or calcium/creatinine ratio <0.15. 24-hr urine level falls to <200 mg/24 hrs after ingestion of low-calcium diet (400 mg/day) for 3–4 days. Almost always due to primary increase in intestinal calcium absorption. Probably autosomal dominant. Is most common type.
  • Resorptive (nonabsorptive): >30 mg calcium or calcium/creatinine ratio >0.15. Due to primary hyperparathyroidism.
  • Indeterminate: calcium is 20–30 mg/2-hr urine.

Hyperoxaluria

Secondary

Due To
Increased oxalate in diet (e.g., green leafy vegetables, chocolate, tea)
Ingestion of oxalate precursors (e.g., ascorbic acid, ethylene glycol)
Methoxyflurane anesthesia
Primary diseases of ileum with malabsorption (e.g., bypass surgery, Crohn's disease, pancreatitis) causing increased absorption of dietary oxalate
Urinary oxalate is usually 50–100 mg/24 hrs.

Primary

Types 1 and 2
(Rare autosomal recessive inherited disorders of glyoxylate metabolism causing recurrent calcium oxalate renal lithiasis, nephrocalcinosis, and uremia)
♦ Urinary oxalate is usually >100 mg/24 hrs unless renal function is diminished.

Oxalosis, Primary

(Rare autosomal recessive disease due to deficient liver enzyme)
♦ Increased serum and urinary oxalic acid
Increased urinary glycolic and glyoxylic acid
Calcium oxalate renal calculi and nephrocalcinosis with extrarenal deposition of calcium oxalate in skin joints, bone, retina.
Uremia causes death.
Manifestations of hyperoxaluria are the same, but extrarenal calcium oxalate deposits are absent.
♦ Characterizing alanine: glyoxylate aminotransferase in liver tissue

Infarction of Kidney

Microscopic or gross hematuria is usual.
Proteinuria ($\leq 4+$) and pyuria may occur.
BUN is normal unless other renal disease is present.
Urine may show no protein or abnormal sediment unless emboli reach glomeruli.
WBC, AST, ALT are increased if area of infarction is large; peak by second day; return to normal by fifth day.
Serum and urine LD may be increased markedly. Increased serum LD is the most sensitive enzyme abnormality.
CRP and serum LD peak on third day; return to normal by tenth day.
Changes in serum enzyme levels, WBC, CRP, ESR are similar in terms of timing to those in myocardial infarction.
PRA may rise on second day, peak on ~11th day, and remain elevated for more than 1 mo.
Increased serum ALP (from vascular endothelium) occurs in approximately one-third of cases and is the least discriminating enzyme abnormality.
Laboratory findings due to infarction of other organs (e.g., brain, heart, retina, mesentery)
♦ Atheromatous emboli cause eosinophilia (>350 eosinophils/cu mm) in ~80% of cases, eosinophiluria, increased ESR. Renal biopsy is specific for this diagnosis.

Due To

Renal artery embolism (e.g., atrial fibrillation, after myocardial infarction, myxoma, paradoxical embolism)
Dissecting aneurysm of aorta or renal artery
Renal artery vasculitis (e.g., polyarteritis nodosa)
Renal artery thrombosis (e.g., atherosclerosis, hypercoagulability, angioplasty or catheterization, trauma)

Kimmelstiel-Wilson Syndrome (Diabetic Intercapillary Glomerulosclerosis)

See Table 14-8.
(Recognized after diabetes mellitus has been present for years. Occasionally is associated only with prediabetes. Incidence of end-stage renal disease is nearly 30% in insulin-dependent diabetes mellitus and 4–20% in non–insulin-dependent diabetes mellitus.)
♦ Defined as persistent proteinuria in absence of other renal disease. (Normal sedentary male should excrete <200 mg/dL.) Proteinuria may be earliest clinical clue and may be marked (often >5 gm/day). Nephrotic syndrome may be associated. Periodic protein testing of urine should be part of routine treatment of all diabetics. Dipstick assay detects 200–300 mg/dL.
Microalbuminuria is persistent proteinuria below level of detection by routine dipstick testing but above normal (≥ 30–300 mg/24 hrs or 20–200 μg/min). Albumin/creatinine ratio of >30 mg/gm predicts overnight excretion rate of >30 μg/min. Albuminuria of ≤ 0.3 gm/day is detectable only by sensitive assays; measure by EIA, RIA, nephelometry, or electrophoresis if routine dipstick testing is negative. Can now be detected by new dipstick (Clinitek Microalbumin. Bayer Diagnostics, Tarrytown, NY.)

Table 14-8. Evolution of Renal Disease in Insulin-Dependent Diabetes Mellitus (IDDM)

Stage	Time of Onset	Laboratory Findings*	Morphologic Findings	% of Cases that Progress
Early	At time of diagnosis	I GFR	Kidney size I	100
Renal lesions; no clinical signs	2–3 yrs after diagnosis	I GFR; albuminuria cannot be detected	I thickness of glomerular and tubular capillary basement membrane; glomerulosclerosis	35–40
Incipient nephropathy	7–15 yrs after diagnosis	Albuminuria 0.03–0.3 gm/day. N or sl I GFR; beginning to decline	Glomerulosclerosis progressing	80–100
Clinical diabetic nephropathy	10–30 yrs after diagnosis	Albuminuria > 0.3 gm/day. N or sl D GFR; steady fall	Glomerulosclerosis widespread	>75
End-stage renal disease	20–40 yrs after diagnosis	GFR <10 mL/min; serum creatinine ≥ 10 mg/dL		

D = decreased; I = increased; N = normal; sl = slightly.
*When albuminuria is 0.075–0.1 gm/day in IDDM, significant renal disease is present and albuminuria will progress to clinical nephropathy. GFR declines ~10 mL/min/yr after nephropathy is established.
Source: Selby JV, et al. The natural history and epidemiology of diabetic nephropathy. *JAMA* 1990;263:1954.

Interferences

Do not test urine during periods of exercise or prolonged upright posture; in presence of hematuria, blood contamination, or GU tract infection; or in glass containers (albumin adheres to glass).
False-positive results may occur if pH is ≥ 8, temperature is $>77°F$, or Tamm-Horsfall protein occurs.

Interpretation

♦ Diagnosed when protein present in two or more urine samples collected over 6-mo period.
  • Present in ~25% of patients with type I disease and 36% of patients with type II disease who have negative dipstick test. In insulin-dependent diabetes, microalbuminuria is 82% sensitive, highly specific (96%), and has 75% positive predictive value for subsequent overt nephropathy; lower values in non–insulin-dependent diabetes. Compared to normal results, microalbuminuria is associated with longer duration of diabetes, poorer glycemic control, higher blood pressure, development of more advanced retinopathy and neuropathy, development of overt nephropathy and subsequent renal failure, increased vascular damage, and risk for cardiovascular disease.

	Normal	Microalbuminuria*	Advanced Nephropathy
Albumin concentration			
Albumin/creatinine ratio (μg/mL)	<0.01	0.02–0.2	>0.2
Volume 1000 mL/day	<15	30	>30
Volume 1500 mg/day	<10	20	>20
Albumin excretion rate			
μg/min	<10	20–200	>200
mg/day	<15	30–300[†]	>300[‡]

*Amounts defined in consensus statement of American Diabetes Association.
[†]Albuminuria of ≥ 300 mg/day.
[‡]Creatinine clearance of <70 mL/min/1.73 sq m of body surface area.

Urine shows many hyaline and granular casts and double refractile fat bodies.
Hematuria is rare.
Serum protein is decreased.
Azotemia develops gradually after several years of proteinuria.
♦ Biopsy of kidney is diagnostic.
Laboratory findings are those due to frequently associated GU tract infection.
See sections on diabetes mellitus, acidosis, papillary necrosis, UTI, diabetic neuropathy.

Lupus Erythematosus, Systemic (SLE), Nephritis

See Table 14-9.
Renal involvement occurs in two-thirds of patients with SLE.
Nephritis of SLE may occur as acute, latent, or chronic GN, nephrosis, or asymptomatic albuminuria or hematuria. Histology may be mesangial, focal or diffuse proliferative, or membranous GN.
Urine findings are as in chronic active GN. Azotemia or marked proteinuria usually indicates death in 1–3 yrs.
Laboratory findings of SLE may disappear during active nephritis, nephrosis, or uremia.
♦ Examination of needle biopsy specimen should always include immunofluorescence and electron microscopy as well as light microscopy. May show normal or minimal disease, mesangial lesions, focal proliferative GN, diffuse proliferative GN, or membranous GN.
Laboratory findings due to drug therapy
  • Prednisone
  • Cytotoxic drugs (e.g., azathioprine, cyclophosphamide)
    Leukopenia—nadir WBC kept at 1500–4000/cu mm
    Infection (e.g., herpes zoster, opportunistic organisms)
    Gonadal toxicity
    Hemorrhagic cystitis
    Neoplasia

Table 14-9. Comparison of Clinical and Morphologic Types of Systemic Lupus
Erythematosus Nephritis

	Mesangial Changes (% of patients)	Focal Proliferative GN (% of patients)	Diffuse Proliferative GN (% of patients)	Membranous GN (% of patients)
% of total patients	39	27	16	18
Hematuria, pyuria	13	53	78	50
Proteinuria	36	67	89	100
Nephrotic syndrome	0	27	56	90
Azotemia	13	20	22	10
Decreased complement	54	77	100	75
Increased anti-DNA	45	75	80	33
Decreased complement and increased anti-DNA	36	63	80	33
Hypertension	22	40	56	50
Prognosis	Better	Worse	Worse	Better

Source: Appel GB. The course of management of lupus nephritis. *Intern Med* 1981;2:82.

Myeloma Kidney

Renal function is impaired in ≤ 50% of patients with increased BUN and creatinine;
usually there is loss of renal concentrating ability. Uric acid is increased in 60% of
patients, but uric acid stones and gout are rare.

Renal failure is usually present when Bence Jones protein in blood is markedly
increased. May also be due to hypercalcemia.

○Proteinuria is very frequent and is due to albumin and globulins in urine; Bence Jones
proteinuria may be intermittent. Bence Jones protein occurs in <50% of myeloma
patients but in almost all patients with renal failure due to myeloma kidney. Casts
may be present.

Severe anemia out of proportion to azotemia.

Occasional changes due to altered renal tubular function
- Renal glycosuria, aminoaciduria, renal potassium wasting
- Renal loss of phosphate with decreased serum phosphorus and increased serum ALP
- Nephrogenic diabetes insipidus
- Oliguria or anuria with acute renal failure may be precipitated by dehydration.

○*Hyperchloremia or hyperbicarbonatemia with normal or low serum sodium values
reduces AG and should suggest myeloma in an appropriate clinical setting.*

○Changes due to associated amyloidosis (see p. 890). Changes due to associated hypercalcemia.

♦ See Myeloma, Multiple, p. 420.

Nephritis, Hereditary

Classified into two types
- Angiokeratoma corporis diffusum (familial condition of abnormal glycolipid deposition in glomerular epithelial cells, nervous system, heart, etc.)
    Proteinuria begins in second decade.
    Urine may contain lipid globules and foam cells.
    Uremia occurs by fourth or fifth decade.
- Familial autosomal dominant disease associated with nerve deafness and lens
defects (Alport's syndrome) is rare. Renal disease is progressive.
    Hematuria, gross or microscopic, is common; more marked after occurrence of
    unrelated infection. Other laboratory findings are the same as in other types
    of nephritis.

Nephritis, Interstitial, Acute

(Typical clinical triad of fever, rash, and eosinophilia in patient in acute renal failure)

Due To

Recent exposure to a causative drug in ≤ 45% of cases
>   Especially antibiotics, diuretics, NSAIDs, miscellaneous drugs (e.g., allopurinol, street drugs)

After infections
>   Especially A beta-hemolytic streptococcal infection, diphtheria, brucellosis, leptospirosis, IM, toxoplasmosis, Rocky Mountain spotted fever, measles

Metabolic disorders (e.g., calcium, oxalate, uric acid)
Infiltrative diseases (e.g., sarcoid, Sjögren's syndrome, lymphoma, leukemia)
Idiopathic

Blood
◆ • Eosinophilia (in 60–100% of patients) with increased blood IgE.
  • Increased WBC, neutrophils, and bands.
  • Anemia with Hb as low as 6.5 gm/dL; no evidence of hemolysis or iron deficiency; negative indirect Coombs' test; normal bone marrow. Anemia resolves when renal function becomes normal.
  • ESR is increased.
  • Serum IgG is usually increased; serum complement is normal.
  • Varying degrees of renal insufficiency with increased BUN and creatinine, hyponatremia, hyperchloremic metabolic acidosis, decreased serum albumin.
Urine
  • May be oliguric or nonoliguric.
  • Urinary indices are similar to those seen in acute tubular necrosis.
◆ • Eosinophiluria reported in ≤ 100% of patients.
  • Microscopic hematuria.
  • Proteinuria is usually mild to moderate, <1.0 gm/sq m/24 hrs, unless nephrotic syndrome is present.
  • Sterile pyuria is minimal or absent.
  • Casts are uncommon.
  • Low osmolality and specific gravity.
  • Glycosuria without hyperglycemia and reduced phosphate tubular reabsorption may occur.
Enlarged, poorly functioning kidneys may be demonstrated by IV pyelogram, ultrasonography, or renal scan.
Nephrotic syndrome may occur.
◆ Biopsy of kidney establishes the diagnosis and usually shows more severe disease than indicated by urinalysis and renal studies.

Nephritis, Interstitial, Chronic

Due to infections
  • Pyelonephritis (see p. 736)
Not due to infections
  • Analgesic abuse (see Phenacetin, Long-Term Excessive Ingestion, p. 933)
  • Diabetes mellitus (see Kimmelstiel-Wilson Syndrome, p. 727)
  • Drugs
>   Allergic response (e.g., antibiotics, diuretics, phenytoin, cimetidine, NSAID)
>   Toxic (e.g., cyclosporine, lithium, cisplatin, amphotericin B)

  • Toxic substances
>   Exogenous (e.g., lead, mercury, cadmium)
>   Endogenous, e.g.,
>>   Uric acid (see Gout, Kidney Disorders in, p. 725)
>>   Hypercalcemic nephropathy, nephrocalcinosis (see p.732)
>>   Oxalate (see p. 726)

  • Irradiation nephritis (see below)
  • Sarcoidosis
  • Others

♦ Diagnosis is usually by exclusion. Renal biopsy may be helpful in undiagnosed cases.
May be associated with metabolic acidosis and hyperkalemia out of proportion to degree
of renal insufficiency, decreased urine concentrating capacity, and renal salt wasting.

Nephritis, Irradiation

(Exposure [of one or both kidneys] to >2300 rads for 6 wks or less)
Latent period is >6 mos.
Slight proteinuria is present.
Hematuria and oliguria are absent.
Refractory anemia is present.
Progressive uremia is found; may be reversible later.
♦ Renal biopsy

Nephropathy, Hypercalcemic

Diffuse nephrocalcinosis is the result of prolonged increase in serum and urine calcium
(due to hyperparathyroidism, sarcoidosis, vitamin D intoxication, multiple myeloma,
carcinomatosis, milk-alkali syndrome, etc.).
Urine is normal or contains RBCs, WBCs, WBC casts; proteinuria is usually slight or absent.
Early findings are decreased renal concentrating ability and polyuria.
Later findings are decreased GFR, decreased renal blood flow, azotemia.
Renal insufficiency is insidious and slowly progressive; it may sometimes be reversed
by correcting hypercalcemia.

Nephropathy, Sickle Cell

Gross and microscopic hematuria are common.
Early decrease of renal concentrating ability is evident even with normal BUN, GFR,
and renal plasma flow; it occurs in sickle cell trait as well as sickle cell anemia, but
chronic renal failure occurs only with SS (4.2% of patients) or SC (2.4% of patients).
The decrease is temporarily reversed by transfusion in children but not in adults.
Renal tubular acidosis may produce severe hypokalemia.

Nephropathy, Tubulointerstitial

Three basic patterns of functional disturbance depending on site of injury: proximal
tubular acidosis, distal tubular acidosis, medullary injury (reduced ability to concentrate urine, causing nephrogenic diabetes insipidus in most severe form)

Due To

Bacterial infection (e.g., acute and chronic pyelonephritis)
Drugs (e.g., acute interstitial nephritis [see p. 230], analgesic nephropathy)
Immune disorders (e.g., acute interstitial nephritis, transplant rejection, disorders asso-
ciated with GN, Sjögren's syndrome)
Metabolic disorders (e.g., urate, hypercalcemic, hypokalemic, oxalate nephropathies)
Heavy metals (e.g., lead, cadmium)
Physical factors (e.g., obstructive uropathy, irradiation nephritis)
Neoplasia (e.g., myeloma kidney, infiltration in leukemia and lymphoma)
Hereditary renal diseases (e.g., medullary cystic disease, familial interstitial nephritis,
Alport's syndrome)
Miscellaneous conditions (e.g., granulomatous diseases [sarcoidosis, TB, leprosy],
Balkan nephropathy)

Nephrosclerosis

"Benign" nephrosclerosis (essential hypertension)
  • Urine contains little or no protein or microscopic abnormalities.
  • 10% of patients develop marked renal insufficiency.
"Accelerated" nephrosclerosis (malignant hypertension)
  • Syndrome may occur in the course of benign nephrosclerosis, GN, unilateral renal
artery occlusion, or hypertension due to any cause.
  • Increasing uremia is associated with minimal or marked proteinuria and hematuria.

Nephrotic Syndrome

Characterized By

♦ Marked proteinuria: >3.5 gm/1.73 sq m of body surface/day—usually >4.5 gm/day
♦ Hyperlipidemia: increased serum cholesterol (free and esters)—usually >350 mg/dL. (Low or normal serum cholesterol occurs with poor nutrition and suggests poor prognosis.) Increased serum triglycerides, phospholipids, neutral fats, low-density betalipoproteins, and total lipids
♦ Decreased serum albumin (usually <2.5 gm/dL) and total protein
♦ Serum alpha$_2$ and beta globulins are markedly increased, gamma globulin is decreased, alpha$_1$ is normal or decreased. If gamma globulin is increased, rule out systemic disease (e.g., SLE).
♦ Urine containing doubly refractive fat bodies seen by polarizing microscopy; many granular and epithelial cell casts.

Hematuria: present in 50% of patients but is usually minimal and not part of syndrome.
Azotemia: may be present but not part of syndrome.
Changes secondary to proteinuria and hypoalbuminemia (e.g., decreased serum calcium, decreased serum ceruloplasmin, increased fibrinogen)
Increased ESR due to increased fibrinogen
Serum C3 complement is normal in idiopathic lipoid nephrosis but decreased when underlying GN is present.
Changes due to primary disease
Laboratory findings due to
• Increased susceptibility to infection (especially pneumococcal peritonitis) during periods of edema
• Hypercoagulability with thromboembolism; abnormalities in coagulation factors, clotting inhibitors, fibrinolytic system, platelet function have been described. Associated renal vein thrombosis has been reported in ~35% of patients (≤ 40% of these have pulmonary emboli), especially that due to membranous nephropathy, membranoproliferative GN, rapidly progressive GN.
♦ Renal biopsy
Minimal-change disease—fused epithelial podocytes by electron microscopy

Due To

Relative Frequency (%) of Primary Glomerular Diseases Underlying Nephrotic Syndrome in Children and Adults[4]

Disease	Children	Adults	
		<60 yrs	>60 yrs
Minimal-change disease	76	20	20
Focal segmental glomerulosclerosis	8	15	2
Membranous GN	7	40	39
Membranoproliferative GN	4	7	0
Other diseases	5	18	39

Renal (causes 95% of cases in children, 60% in adults)
Primary glomerular disease (>50% of patients), e.g.,
• Membranous GN: ~65% have spontaneous complete or partial remission of proteinuria and ~15% develop end-stage renal disease.
• Membranoproliferative GN.
• Other proliferative GN (e.g., focal, IgA nephropathy, pure mesangial): accounts for 10% of cases in children, 23% of cases in adults.
• Rapidly progressive GN.
• Minimal-change disease (formerly called *lipoid nephrosis* or *nil lesion*; may be associated with Hodgkin's disease and non-Hodgkin's lymphoma).
• Focal segmental glomerulosclerosis.
Systemic (most common)
• Diabetic glomerulosclerosis (cause in 15% of adult patients—most common cause of nephrotic proteinuria)
• SLE (cause in 20% of adult patients)
• Amyloidosis (primary and secondary)

[4]Orth SR, Ritz E. The nephrotic syndrome. *N Engl J Med* 1998;338:1202.

Systemic (less common)
- Henoch-Schönlein purpura
- Multiple myeloma
- Goodpasture's syndrome (rare)
- Berger's disease
- Polyarteritis (rare)
- Takayasu's syndrome
- Sarcoidosis
- Sjögren's syndrome
- Wegener's granulomatosis (rare)
- Dermatitis herpetiformis
- Cryoglobulinemia

Venous obstruction
- Obstruction of inferior vena cava (thrombosis, tumor)
- Constrictive pericarditis
- Tricuspid stenosis
- Congestive heart failure

Infections
- Bacterial (poststreptococcal GN, bacterial endocarditis, syphilis, leprosy, etc.)
- Viral (HBV, HCV; also HIV and CMV infections, IM, varicella)
- Protozoal (quartan malaria)
- Parasitic (schistosomiasis, filariasis, toxoplasmosis)

Allergic reactions (e.g., serum sickness, bee sting)

Neoplasm associated in 10% of adults and 15% of those aged >60 yrs (e.g., Hodgkin's disease; carcinoma of colon, lung, stomach, and other sites; lymphomas and leukemia; paraproteinemia [multiple myeloma, light chain nephropathy]). *In adult with minimal-change nephrotic syndrome without evident cause, first rule out Hodgkin's disease. With membranous lesion, carcinoma may be more likely.*

Toxin exposure (e.g., heavy metals, heroin, captopril, probenecid, NSAIDs, penicillamine, mephenytoin, ampicillin, anticonvulsants, chlorpropamide, lithium, rifampin, interferon alfa). Heroin may cause focal segmental glomerulosclerosis and progressive renal insufficiency.

Hereditary/familial disorders (e.g., Alport's syndrome, Fabry's disease, sickle cell disease). In atypical familial nephrotic syndrome, course is benign; more than one sibling is involved.

Miscellaneous conditions
- Preeclampsia
- Chronic allograft rejection

Other causes

Urine immunoelectrophoresis should always be performed to rule out myeloma and renal primary (AL) amyloidosis.

Obstructive Uropathy

Partial obstruction of both kidneys may cause
- O • Increasing azotemia with normal or increased urinary output (due to decreased renal concentrating ability).
- O • Inexplicable wide variations in BUN and urine volume in patients with azotemia. In PSP test, PSP excretion is less in first 15-min period than in any later period. Considerable PSP excretion occurs after the 2-hr test period.
- • In unilateral obstruction, BUN usually remains normal unless underlying renal disease is present.
- • Laboratory findings due to superimposed infection or underlying disease.

Laboratory findings due to underlying disease
- • Obstruction of bladder (e.g., benign prostatic hypertrophy, carcinoma of prostate or bladder, urethral stricture, neurogenic bladder dysfunction [multiple sclerosis, diabetic neuropathy])
- • Obstruction of both ureters (e.g., infiltrating neoplasm [especially of uterine cervix], bilateral calculi, congenital anomalies, retroperitoneal fibrosis)

If ureter is obstructed for >4 mos, functional recovery is unlikely. When obstruction is relieved, most functional recovery takes place in 2–3 wks; then continued improvement occurs for several months.

Papillary Necrosis, Kidney

Hematuria
Sudden diminution in renal function; occasionally oliguria or anuria with acute renal failure
Findings of associated diseases
- Diabetes mellitus
- Urinary tract obstruction/infection
- Chronic overuse of analgesics (e.g., phenacetin)
- Sickle cell anemia

Polyarteritis Nodosa

See p. 127
Renal involvement occurs in 75% of patients.
Azotemia is often absent or only mild and slowly progressive.
Albuminuria is always present.
Hematuria (gross or microscopic) is very common. Fat bodies are frequently present in urine sediment.
There may be findings of acute GN with remission or early death from renal failure.
Always rule out polyarteritis in any case of GN, renal failure, or hypertension that shows unexplained eosinophilia, increased WBC, or laboratory evidence of involvement of other organ systems.

Polycystic Kidney Diseases

Occurs in numerous forms, e.g.,
1. Autosomal dominant form is usually slowly progressive and asymptomatic until patient is >50 yrs old; accounts for ~10% of transplant or dialysis cases.
2. Autosomal recessive form is usually more severe and becomes manifest earlier with fewer patients surviving as adults.
3. Acquired form is often seen in cases of progressive renal failure due to diabetes mellitus or GN, especially after dialysis.

Polyuria is common.
Hematuria may be gross and episodic or an incidental microscopical finding (50% of patients).
Proteinuria occurs in approximately one-third of patients and is mild (<1 gm/24 hrs).
Renal calculi may be associated (≤ 30% of patients with autosomal dominant polycystic kidney disease).
Superimposed UTI is frequent (33% of patients).
Renal failure affects 45% of patients by age 60 years. Death occurs within 5 yrs after BUN rises to 50 mg/dL (33% of patients).
Death usually occurs in early infancy or in middle age when superimposed nephrosclerosis of aging or pyelonephritis has exhausted renal reserve.
Laboratory findings in autosomal dominant polycystic kidney disease due to
- Cysts that may occur in liver, ovary, pancreas, spleen, and CNS
- Associated intracranial aneurysms, which cause cerebral hemorrhage and death in 10% of patients

Hypertension (affects 30% of children; affects ≤ 60% of adults before onset of renal insufficiency and >80% with end-stage renal failure).
Increased incidence of gout in patients with polycystic kidneys
Polycythemia may occur due to production of erythropoietin.
Anemia of renal failure is less severe than that in other forms of kidney disease.
♦ Prenatal diagnosis is possible using DNA obtained by amniocentesis or chorionic villus sampling.
Young adults negative by ultrasonography do not have autosomal dominant polycystic kidney disease.

4. Familial nephronophthisis-medullary cystic disease—group of disorders whose mode of inheritance may be autosomal dominant, autosomal regressive, or sporadic.
- Anemia is often severe and out of proportion to degree of renal failure.
- Urinalysis shows minimal or no proteinuria; presence of RBCs, WBCs, casts, or bacteria is rare.
- Impaired urine concentrating capacity with polyuria.
- Salt-losing syndrome and tubular acidosis are prominent in children.

Table 14-10. Sensitivity, Specificity, and Predictive Values of Tests in Predicting Bacteriuria (10^5 colonies/mL)

Test	Sensitivity (%)	Specificity (%)	Predictive Value (%) of	
			Positive Test	Negative Test
>5 WBC/HPF	80	83	46	96
>10 WBC/HPF	63	90	53	93
Nitrite	69	90	57	94
Leukocyte esterase	71	85	47	94
Nitrite + leukocyte esterase (either positive)	86	86	54	97

- May cause ~20% of cases of chronic renal failure in children and adolescents.
- Death from renal insufficiency may take many years.
- Associated nonrenal abnormalities (e.g., eye, bone, liver) in patients with autosomal recessive disease.

5. Medullary sponge kidney
- Findings due to complications, e.g., calculi in ≤ 50% of patients; infection; hematuria.
- Disease is asymptomatic, not progressive.

6. Renal cysts associated with other inherited conditions, e.g., tuberous sclerosis, von Hippel–Lindau disease.

Purpura, Allergic (Henoch-Schönlein), Renal Disease In

Urine is abnormal in 50% of patients, but renal biopsy is abnormal in most (usually a focal proliferative GN).

Clinical picture varies from minimal urinary abnormalities to severe, rapidly progressive nephritis that is indistinguishable from GN. Nephrotic syndrome may occur. Chronic course with remissions and exacerbations, and permanent renal damage may occur. Serum complement is normal.

Platelet count is normal.

Pyelonephritis

♦ Tests for Bacteriuria and Pyuria

See Table 14-10.
Use
Diagnosis of UTI and determination of antibiotic sensitivity of causative organism.
Interferences
When urine is allowed to remain at room temperature, the number of bacteria doubles every 30–45 mins.

Falsely low colony counts if there is a high rate of urinary flow, low urine specific gravity, low urine pH; if antibacterial drugs have been administered; or if inappropriate culture techniques have been used (e.g., tubercle bacilli, *Mycoplasma*, *Ureaplasma urealyticum*, *Chlamydia trachomatis*, anaerobes).

High doses of vitamin C may cause false-negative test for nitrite on dipstick.

Trichomonas may cause a positive leukocyte esterase reaction.
Interpretation
Dipstick test for pyuria (measures leukocyte esterase of neutrophil granules; does not detect lymphocytes) has negative predictive value of >90% and positive predictive value of 50% for bacterial infection. For dipstick detection of WBC, sensitivity = 100% for >50 WBCs/HPF, 90% for 21–50 WBCs, 60% for 12–20 WBCs, 44% for 6–12 WBCs. For detection of bacteria, sensitivity = 73% for "large" numbers of bacteria, 46% for "moderate" numbers.[5] The combination of positive esterase and nitrate strip tests

[5]Propp DA, et al. Reliability of a urine dipstick in emergency department patients. *Ann Emerg Med* 1989;18:560.

is sufficient indication for colony count to identify bacteriuria. Dipstick test of first-catch urine is a cost-effective way to detect asymptomatic urethritis (*Chlamydia, Neisseria*) in males.

Direct microscopic examination of uncentrifuged urine, either unstained or Gram stained, that shows one PMN or one organism/HPF has sensitivity of 85% and specificity of 60% for bacteriuria. It may yield >10% false-positive results. Uncentrifuged urine showing one organism/oil-immersion field (threshold of detection for microscopy) correlates with count ≥ 10,000 colonies/mL. Gram staining of cytospin specimen has >90% sensitivity and >80% specificity for ≥ 10^5/mL. With pyuria and bacteriuria, Gram staining to differentiate gram-positive cocci (e.g., enterococci or staphylococci) from gram-negative bacilli indicates appropriate immediate initial therapy. ≤ 50% of patients with chronic UTI and asymptomatic bacteriuria may not show significant numbers of WBCs on urine microscopic examination; however, pyuria is associated with bacteriuria in ~90% of cases. The finding of both bacteria and WBCs has a higher predictive value than either finding alone. The presence of large numbers of squamous epithelial cells may indicate a specimen that contains greater numbers of bacteria from the vagina or the perineum rather than from the urinary tract. High ratio of WBC to epithelial cells suggests infection. Bacteriuria and pyuria are often intermittent; in the chronic atrophic stage of pyelonephritis, they are often absent. In acute pyelonephritis, marked pyuria and bacteriuria are almost always present; hematuria and proteinuria may also be present during first few days. WBC casts are very suggestive of pyelonephritis. Glitter cells may be seen.

A colony count should be performed under the following conditions: a midstream, clean-catch, first morning specimen is submitted in a sterilized container; the specimen is refrigerated until the colony count is performed; periurethral area has first been thoroughly cleaned with soap. Transport tubes have an inhibitory effect and should be used. Suprapubic sterile needle aspiration is the most reliable sampling technique, and the presence of any organisms on culture of such a specimen is virtually diagnostic of UTI (97% sensitivity); it is the only acceptable method in infants, as urine collection bags have a very high false-positive rate; compared to urethral catheterization of adults, the method is more accurate, simpler, and less traumatic.

- Count of >100,000 bacteria/mL indicates active infection (>85% sensitivity).
- Count of <10,000/mL in the absence of therapy largely rules out bacteriuria.
- Count of 10,000–100,000/mL should be repeated and specimen should be cultured.
- Count of <100,000/mL with clinical findings of acute pyelonephritis with no obvious explanation, such as recent use of antibiotics, suggests urinary tract obstruction or perinephric abscess.

A culture should be performed for identification of the organism and determination of antibiotic sensitivity when these screening tests are positive. This antibiogram is useful in subsequently identifying the same organism in relapsing infections.

- If culture shows a common gram-positive saprophyte, it should be repeated because the second culture is often negative.
- Causative bacteria are usually enteric organisms; <10% are gram-positive cocci (see Table 16-1).
- Positive significant single culture or finding of a predominant organism should be considered positive in symptomatic patients (95% reliable) and repeat culture is unnecessary.
- A finding of three or more species with none being predominant (i.e., >80% of the growth) almost always represents specimen contamination and culture should be repeated; however, true mixed infections may occur after instrumentation or with chronic infection.
- *Presence of* Pseudomonas *or* Proteus *may indicate that the patient has an anatomic abnormality. If organism other than* Escherichia coli *is found, patient probably has chronic pyelonephritis, even if this is the first clinical episode of infection.*
- In women, >80% of UTIs are due to *E. coli* and a smaller percentage are due to *Staphylococcus saprophyticus*; UTIs are less often due to other aerobic gram-negative bacilli. In men, gram-negative bacilli cause ~75% of UTIs, but *E. coli* causes only ~25% of infections in men and <50% of infections in boys.
- Other common gram-negative bacilli are *Proteus* and *Providencia* spp. Gram-positive organisms (especially enterococci and coagulase-negative staphylococci) cause ~20% of infections in men and boys but *S. saprophyticus* infection is rare. Infection due to *Gardnerella vaginalis* is found in <3% of men with bacteriuria.

- If *Candida* organisms are isolated, should rule out contaminated specimen, diabetes mellitus, papillary necrosis, indwelling catheter, broad-spectrum antibiotic exposure, immunosuppressive chemotherapy, malignancy, malnutrition.
- Presence of "sterile" (i.e., pyogenic infection is absent) pyuria ($\geq$ 10 WBCs/HPF in centrifuged urine) and absence of bacilli ($<$1 bacillus in multiple oil-immersion fields or 20–40 bacteria/HPF in centrifuged sediments) should cast doubt on diagnosis of untreated bacterial UTI and may occur in renal TB, chemical inflammation, mechanical inflammation (e.g., due to calculi, instrumentation), early acute GN before appearance of hematuria or proteinuria, polycystic kidney disease, papillary necrosis, chronic prostatitis, interstitial cystitis, transplant rejection, sarcoidosis, GU tract neoplasm, uric acid and hypercalcemic nephropathy, lithium and heavy metal toxicity, extreme dehydration, hyperchloremic renal acidosis, genital herpes, nonbacterial gastroenteritis, and respiratory tract infections, and after administration of oral polio vaccine; may persist for several months after transurethral prostatectomy.
- *When urine cultures are persistently negative in the presence of other evidence of pyelonephritis, specific search should be made for tubercle bacilli.*

○With pyuria and bacteriuria, persistent alkaline pH may indicate infection with urea-splitting organism (e.g., *Proteus*, or less often *Pseudomonas* or *Klebsiella*), suggesting a calculus.

Bacteria should be cleared from urine within 48 hrs of initiation of antibiotic therapy; persistence indicates need to change antibiotic treatment or to search for another explanation.

Asymptomatic bacteriuria occurs in $\leq$ 15% of pregnant women. Routine urinalysis is done on first prenatal visit because 20–40% of untreated patients with positive cultures develop acute pyelonephritis during pregnancy (occurs in only 1% of women with negative cultures). Persistent or recurrent infection may be due to stones or obstruction. Colony count of $>10^5$/mL of a single organism found on culture of midstream specimen indicates significant bacteriuria.

Bacteriuria may be found in
- $\leq$ 15% of patients who are pregnant
- 15% of patients with diabetes mellitus
- 20% of patients with cystocele
- ~50% of patients with dysuria
- 70% of patients with prostatic obstruction
- $\leq$ 5% of patients during catheterization
- 95% of patients (untreated) who have an indwelling catheter for >4 days
- Should be sought in elderly patients with altered mental status and in infants with failure to thrive, persistent fever, or lethargy

♦Acute pyelonephritis shows two consecutive colony counts of $\geq$ 100,000 organisms/mL with or without upper GU tract symptoms (flank pain, fever, costovertebral angle tenderness, fever, chills, nausea, vomiting, leukocytosis).

♦Acute urethral syndrome and acute cystitis show colony count of $\geq$ 100 organisms/mL and lower GU tract symptoms (dysuria, frequency, urgency, suprapubic pain). Urine dipstick test for WBC (leukocyte esterase) detects 8–10 WBC/HPF. Pyuria is rarely present unless bacterial count is >10,000/mL.

Bacteriuria identified in specimens obtained by suprapubic aspiration, cystoscopy, and nephrostomy and in a setting of renal transplant accompanied by a positive dipstick test suggests infection; a negative dipstick test suggests colonization.

♦Catheterization for <30 days or intermittent catheterization: criterion for bacteriuria is $\geq$ 100 organisms/mL; >95% of patients progress to >100,000 organisms/mL within days. Multiple organisms are common.

♦Catheterization for >30 days: mixed infections with >100,000 organisms/mL occur in >75% of cases. Organisms constantly change, with new ones appearing approximately every ~2 wks.

Dye tests (bacterial reduction of nitrate to nitrite; tetrazolium reduction) do not detect 10–50% of infections. Bacteria show great variability in rate of dye reduction; some important bacteria do not reduce dye at all; e.g., coliforms are more likely to be detected than enterococci. If overnight urine specimen is impossible to obtain, then urine should incubate in patient's bladder for $\geq$ 4 hrs.

Decreased glucose in urine (<2 mg/dL) in properly collected first morning urine (no food or fluid intake after 10 p.m., no urination during night) correlates well with colony count.

Positive result on test for antibody-coated bacteria (using fluorescein-conjugated anti-human globulin) is said to indicate bacteria of renal origin and to be 81% predictive of

Table 14-11. Some Renal Indices in Three Types of Postischemic Acute Renal Failure

Postischemic Time	Type A[a]		Type B[b]		Type C[c]
	1 hr	3 days	7 days	12 days	21 days
Urine flow rate (mL/min)	2.2–4.4	1.4–2.0	1.3–1.9	1.4–1.6	0.4–0.8
Inulin clear (mL/min/ 1.73 sq m)	18–28	27–33	10–14	26–32	3–7
U/P inulin	10–18	12–20	9–11	18–26	6–8
U/P osmolality	1.1–1.2	1.3–1.4	1.03–1.09	1.2–1.4	0.96–1.04
FE_{Na} (%)	8.8–17.2	0.6–1.0	4.6–5.6	0.8–2.0	4.6–11.6

U/P = urine/plasma ratio; FE_{Na} = fractional excretion of sodium.
[a]Isolated renal ischemic insult (e.g., suprarenal aortic clamping for 15–90 mins for repair of abdominal aneurysm) with preoperative (volume expansion and mannitol administration) and postoperative (furosemide and dopamine infusion) treatment. When >50 mins, acute renal failure is likely to occur.
[b]More severe and sustained partial renal ischemia (e.g., cardiopulmonary bypass for several days). When >160 mins, acute renal failure is likely to occur. Recovery after 2–3 wks. Values given are those that occur during nadir.
[c]Protracted acute renal failure (e.g., type B or C with additional or prolonged renal ischemia as in rupture of aortic aneurysm) is fatal in >50% of patients.
Source: Myers BD, Moran SM. Hemodynamically mediated acute renal failure. *N Engl J Med* 1986;314:97.

upper GU tract infection, but result is negative in lower tract infection. False-positives may occur with heavy proteinuria, prostatitis, or contamination with vaginal or rectal bacteria. False-negatives may occur early in infection. Test is less reliable for children and adults with neurogenic bladder. Test is not recommended for routine use.

Albuminuria is usually <2 gm/24 hrs (≤ 2+ qualitative); this finding therefore helps to differentiate pyelonephritis from glomerular disease, in which albuminuria is usually >2 gm/24 hrs; may be undetectable in a very dilute urine associated with fixed specific gravity.

Beta$_2$ microglobulin is increased in 24-hr urine specimen in pyelonephritis (due to tubular damage) but not in cystitis.

LD-4 and LD-5 are increased in urine in renal medullary damage (pyelonephritis); less useful than beta$_2$ microglobulin to distinguish upper from lower urinary tract damage.

Hyperchloremic acidosis (due to impaired renal acid excretion and bicarbonate reabsorption) occurs more often in chronic pyelonephritis than in GN.

Decreased concentrating ability occurs relatively early in chronic renal infection but not in bladder infections. Persistent dilute urine (low specific gravity or osmolarity) suggests renal rather than bladder infection if patient is not forcing fluid. Not a sensitive or specific test because of overlapping values, even though it is more marked in bilateral than unilateral infection and concentrating ability increases with cure.

Renal blood flow and GFR show parallel decrease proportional to progress of renal disease. Comparison of function in right and left kidneys shows more disparity in pyelonephritis than in diffuse renal disease (e.g., nephrosclerosis, GN).

Fluctuation in renal insufficiency (e.g., due to recurrent infection, dehydration) with considerable recovery is more marked and frequent in pyelonephritis than in other renal diseases.

24-hr creatinine clearance decreases before BUN and blood creatinine rise.

Laboratory findings of associated diseases, e.g., diabetes mellitus, urinary tract obstruction (stone, tumor, etc.), neurogenic bladder dysfunction. UTI in infant <1 yr old is associated with an underlying GU tract anomaly in 55% of males and 35% of females.

Laboratory findings due to sequelae (e.g., papillary necrosis, bacteremia)

"Cured" patient should be followed with routine periodic urinalysis and colony count for at least 2 yrs because asymptomatic recurrence of bacteriuria is common.

Renal Failure, Acute

♦ Serum creatinine increased by ≥ 0.5 mg/dL or >50% over baseline value, or 50% decrease in creatinine clearance or decreased renal function resulting in need for dialysis.

See Tables 14-7, 14-11, and 14-12, and Fig. 14-4.

Table 14-12. Urinary Diagnostic Indices in Acute Renal Failure

	Prerenal Azotemia	Postrenal (Acute Obstructive)	Acute GN and Vasculitis	Acute Interstitial Nephritis	Acute Tubular Necrosis Oliguric	Nonoliguric	Renal Vascular Occlusion Arterial	Venous
Urine volume (mL/24 hrs)	~500*	Usually <500; fluctuates from day to day	<500	V	<350	1000–2000	V; Anuria if bilateral/complete	V
Urine specific gravity	H (>1.015)				L; <1.010			
Urine osmolality (mOsm/ kg H$_2$O)	>500	V; usually <500	<500	V	<350	350	V	V
Urine sodium (mEq/L)	L; <20	H; >40	L; usually <20	V	>40	V	V	V
U/P osmolality	>1.5	<1.2			<1.2	<1.2		
U/P urea nitrogen	>8	Usually >8	>8		<3	<8		
U/P creatinine	>40	<20	>40		<20	<20		
Renal failure index	<1 (90% of cases)	>2 (95% of cases)	<1		>2 (95% of cases)	>3		
FENa	<1 (≤ 94% of cases)	>1	<1	V	>1	>1	V	V

BUN:creatinine ratio	>20:1	>20:1	>20:1	<20:1	<20:1	<20:1	<20:1	<20:1
Urine sediment	Hyaline casts	N; RBCs, WBCs, crystals may be present	RBCs, RBC casts	WBCs, WBC casts, eosinophils	Granular casts, renal tubular epithelial cells, cell debris, pigment, crystals	Nephrotoxin	V	V
Comments	Decreased renal perfusion	Evidence of GU tract obstruction	Biopsy findings classify disease	Eosinophilia; thrombocytopenia	Renal hypo-perfusion; nephrotoxin		Aortic injury; athero-matous emboli	Renal vein occlusion with nephrotic syndrome

H = high; L = low; N = normal; U/P = urine/plasma ratio; V = variable.

*Polyuria may be present.

Sources: Andreoli TE, et al., eds. *Cecil essentials of medicine*, 2nd ed. Philadelphia: WB Saunders, 1990:212; Okun DE. On the differential diagnosis of acute renal failure. *Am J Med* 1981;71:916; Schrier RW. Acute renal failure: pathogenesis, diagnosis, and management. *Hosp Pract* 1981;(Mar):93; and Miller TR, et al. Urinary diagnostic indices in acute renal failure: a prospective study. *Ann Intern Med* 1978;89:47.

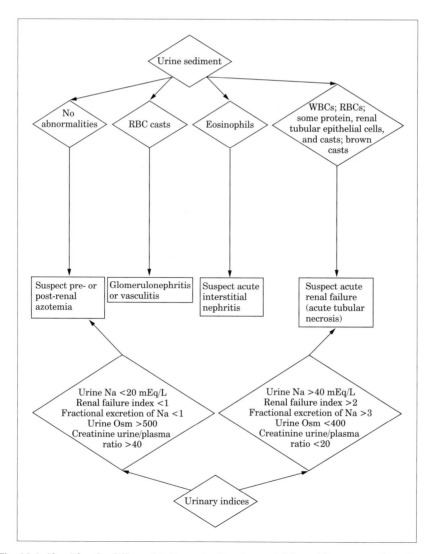

Fig. 14-4. Algorithm for differential diagnosis of acute renal failure. (Osm = osmolarity.) (Data from Schrier DW. Acute renal failure: pathogenesis, diagnosis, and management. *Hosp Pract* 1981;[March]:93.)

Due To

Prerenal (causes ~40% of hospital-acquired and ~70% of community-acquired cases)
- Hypotension (e.g., shock, sepsis, drug effects)
- Volume contraction (e.g., hemorrhage, dehydration, burns)
- Severe heart failure (e.g., myocardial infarction, cardiac tamponade, pulmonary emboli)
- Hepatorenal syndrome
- Drugs (e.g., cyclosporine, amphotericin B)
- Combinations of insults (e.g., NSAID treatment in presence of congestive heart failure, aminoglycoside exposure in patient with sepsis, use of radiocontrast agents in patients receiving ACE inhibitors)

- Occlusion of renal artery or vein (e.g., due to thrombosis, embolism, severe arteriosclerotic stenosis, dissecting aneurysm)

Renal
- Acute tubular necrosis (see p. 749), e.g.,
    Acute interstitial nephritis (see p. 731) causes ~10% of cases.
        Drugs (e.g., methicillin)
        Infection
        Cancer (e.g., lymphoma, leukemia)
        Other (e.g., sarcoidosis)
    Prolonged ischemia due to prerenal events causes ~50% of cases.
    Toxic agents cause ~35% of cases.
        Heavy metals (e.g., lead, mercury, cisplatin, arsenic, cadmium, bismuth)
        Organic solvents (e.g., carbon tetrachloride, ethylene glycol)
        Antibiotics (e.g., aminoglycosides [often nonoliguric], tetracyclines, penicillins, amphotericin)
        Radiographic contrast media (especially in diabetic persons or those with preexisting renal insufficiency); tends to be oliguric.
        Pesticides, fungicides
        Others (e.g., phenylbutazone, phenytoin, calcium)
        Pigment induced (e.g., Hb, myoglobin)
        Intratubular obstruction (e.g., myeloma light chains; crystals such as uric acid, calcium oxalate, acyclovir, sulfonamide, methotrexate)
- GN, e.g., causes ~5% of cases.
    Acute poststreptococcal
    Rapidly progressive
    SLE
    SBE
    Henoch-Schönlein purpura
    Goodpasture's syndrome
    Malignant hypertension
    Hemolytic-uremic syndrome
    TTP
    Drug-related vasculitis
- Large-vessel disease, e.g.,
    Bilateral renal vein occlusion (thrombosis, tumor infiltration)
    Renal artery occlusion (embolism, thrombosis, stenosis, aortic dissection, trauma to renal arteries)
- Small-vessel disease (e.g., malignant hypertension, vasculitis, sickle cell anemia, hemolytic-uremic syndrome, toxemia of pregnancy, scleroderma, atheroembolism, hypercalcemia, transplant rejection)

Postrenal
- Bladder obstruction (e.g., benign prostatic hypertrophy, carcinoma, urethral stricture)
- Bilateral obstruction of ureters or renal pelves (e.g., carcinoma, calculi, papillary necrosis, blood clots)

60% of cases of acute renal failure occur during or immediately after surgery, most often with cardiac or aneurysm surgery.

10% of cases are associated with obstetric problems.

30% of cases are associated with medical conditions, usually due to nephrotoxins or renal ischemic mechanisms.

Often, combined mechanisms are involved (e.g., crushing injury with myoglobinemia plus shock, shock plus intravascular hemolysis from transfusion reaction or bacteremia)

Early Stage

♦ Urine is scant in volume (often <50 mL/day) for ≤ 2 wks; anuria for >24 hrs is unusual. Usually bloody. Specific gravity may be high because RBCs and protein are present. Urine sodium concentration is usually >50 mEq/L.

♦ BUN rises ≤ 20 mg/dL/day in transfusion reaction. It rises ≤ 50 mg/dL/day in overwhelming infection of severe crushing injuries.

♦ Serum creatinine is increased.

Serum uric acid is often increased; may be >20 mg/dL in some types (e.g., rhabdomyolysis)

Hypocalcemia may occur.
ODisproportionately increased serum phosphorus and creatinine indicate tissue necrosis.
Serum amylase and lipase may be increased without evidence of pancreatitis.
Metabolic acidosis is present.
WBC is increased even without infection.

Second Week

♦ Urine becomes clear several days after onset of acute renal failure, and a small daily increase in volume occurs. Daily volume of 400 mL indicates onset of tubular recovery. Daily volume of 1000 mL occurs in several days or ≤ 2 wks. RBCs and large hematin casts are present. Protein is slight or absent.
♦ Azotemia increases. BUN continues to rise for several days after onset of diuresis.
Metabolic acidosis increases.
Serum potassium is increased (because of tissue injury, failure of urinary excretion, acidosis, dehydration, etc.). ECG changes are always found when serum potassium is >9 mEq/L but are rarely found when it is <7 mEq/L.
Serum sodium is often decreased, with increased extracellular fluid volume.
Anemia usually appears during second week.
Bleeding tendency is frequent, with decreased platelets, abnormal prothrombin consumption, etc.

Diuretic Stage

High urinary potassium excretion may cause decreased serum potassium level.
Urine sodium concentration is 50–75 mEq/L.
Serum sodium and chloride may increase because of dehydration from high diuresis if replacement of water is inadequate.
Hypercalcemia may occur in some patients with muscle damage.
Azotemia disappears 1–3 wks after onset of diuresis.

Later Findings

Anemia may persist for weeks or months.
Pyelonephritis may first occur during this stage.
Renal blood flow and GFR do not usually become completely normal.
Recovery from renal cortical necrosis complicating pregnancy may be followed by renal calcification, contraction of kidneys, and death from malignant hypertension in 1–2 yrs.

Laboratory Findings Due to Complications

Infections develop in 30–70% of patients.
GI bleeding occurs in 10–30% of patients.
Anemia (Hct = 20–30%)
Cardiovascular complications (e.g., pericarditis, heart failure, arrhythmias, hypertension)
Suspect urinary tract obstruction, bilateral renal vascular thrombi or emboli, cortical necrosis, or acute GN if complete anuria occurs for >48 hrs.
Suspect cortical necrosis if proteinuria is >3–4 gm/L, BUN does not fall, and diuresis does not occur.
Suspect urinary tract obstruction if recurrent oliguria and increasing azotemia occur during period of diuresis.

Urinary Diagnostic Indices in Acute Renal Failure

See Table 14-12 and Fig. 14-5.
Urinary sodium levels between 20 and 40 mEq/L may be found in all forms of acute renal failure.

$$\text{Fractional excretion of sodium } (FE_{Na}) = 100 \times \frac{\text{(urine sodium/plasma sodium)}}{\text{(urine creatinine/plasma creatinine)}}$$

Is an index of renal ability to conserve sodium and represents percentage of filtered sodium to reach the urine. Is considered the most reliable test to distinguish prerenal azotemia from acute tubular necrosis with oliguria.

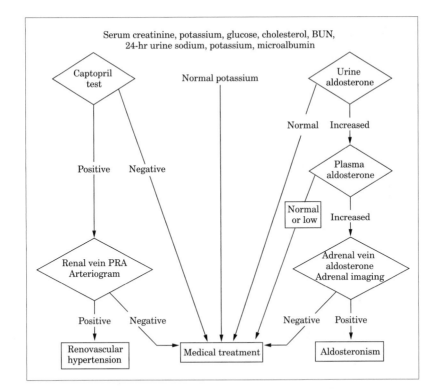

Fig. 14-5. Algorithm for diagnosis of suspected renovascular hypertension.

Some causes of FE_{Na} <1%
- Prerenal azotemia
- Acute GN
- Early acute urinary tract obstruction (first few hours)
- Early sepsis
- Some cases of acute tubular necrosis due to radiographic contrast material or myoglobinuria due to rhabdomyolysis
- 10% of cases of nonoliguric acute tubular necrosis

Some causes of FE_{Na} >1% (injured tubules)
- 90% of cases of acute tubular necrosis
- Later urinary tract obstruction (days to months)
- Diuretic administration
- Preexisting chronic renal failure
- Diuresis due to mannitol, glycosuria, or bicarbonaturia

Renal failure index = urine sodium/(urine creatinine/plasma creatinine); measures sodium conservation and concentrating ability.

Use
Indices (especially renal failure index and FE_{Na}) are chiefly of value in *oliguric* patients for the early differentiation of prerenal azotemia from acute tubular necrosis.

Indices are not useful for diagnosis of presence or absence of obstruction in cases of acute renal failure.

Interpretation
Values ≤ 1 for renal failure index and FE_{Na} strongly suggest prerenal azotemia and values ≥ 3 strongly suggest acute tubular necrosis with confidence level of 90%; values of 1–3 are less definitive but usually indicate tubular necrosis; values for nonoliguric

acute renal failure frequently are intermediate between those for prerenal azotemia and oliguric renal failure.

Values are usually >1 in cases of urinary obstruction or acute interstitial nephritis; values are usually <1 in acute GN.

Diagnostic indices for patients with reversible acute obstructive uropathy often resemble indices for patients with acute tubular necrosis or prerenal azotemia; indices for patients with obstructive uropathy depend on duration of obstruction and severity of azotemia.

Differences between prerenal azotemia and acute tubular necrosis as measured by these indices are particularly blurred in elderly patients as well as those with hypertensive or diabetic nephrosclerosis or other chronic parenchymal renal diseases.

These diagnostic indices are often intermediate in value, and considerable overlapping of values is frequent, especially at time of initial evaluation. Even the total profile may not be useful in the individual case.

Interferences

Specimens used to compute urinary indices should be obtained before onset of treatment if possible; several therapies may make results uninterpretable, especially administration of dopamine, mannitol or other diuretics. Glucose and radiographic contrast material in urine may also interfere with indices. A timed 12- or 24-hr urine specimen need not be obtained, because in the patient with acute renal failure urine sodium or osmolality cannot vary significantly from hour to hour; a random specimen is sufficient.

Urine Sediment in Acute Renal Failure

Renal tubular cells (or cellular casts) and pigmented granular casts indicate acute tubular necrosis; present in ~80% of patients; urine sodium is >20 mEq/L.

Sediment may be normal in cases with prerenal or postrenal causes with minimal or absent proteinuria.

Eosinophils may be found in acute interstitial nephritis; increased WBCs and WBC casts; minimal proteinuria.

RBC casts indicate GN, vasculitis, or microembolic disease; increased RBCs and moderate proteinuria.

RBCs indicate presence of blood from lower GU tract or from glomerulus.

Myoglobin casts indicate myoglobinuria.

WBCs in hyaline casts indicate renal parenchymal infection rather than lower GU tract infection.

In a patient with two functioning kidneys, obstruction of only one ureter should cause serum creatinine to rise ~50% to 2 mg/dL; acute renal failure that is postrenal with creatinine level of >2 mg/dL suggests that obstruction is bilateral or patient has only one functioning kidney.

Total anuria for more than 2 days is uncommon in acute tubular necrosis and should suggest other possibilities (e.g., ruptured bladder, GU tract obstruction, micro- or large-vessel disease, renal cortical necrosis, GN, allergic interstitial nephritis).

Renal Failure, Chronic

♦ Chronic renal insufficiency is defined as serum creatinine = 1.5–3.0 mg/dL.
♦ Chronic renal failure is defined as serum creatinine >3.0 mg/dL.
♦ BUN and serum creatinine are increased and renal function tests are impaired.

Creatinine clearance
>30 mL/min/1.73 sq m	Usually asymptomatic
<30 mL/min/1.73 sq m	Usually symptomatic
<15 mL/min/1.73 sq m	Metabolic disturbances requiring intervention
<5 mL/min/1.73 sq m	End-stage renal disease requiring dialysis and transplantation

♦ Loss of renal concentrating ability (nocturia, polyuria, polydipsia) is an early manifestation of progressive renal functional impairment. Specific gravity is usually same as that of glomerular filtrate.
♦ Abnormal urinalysis is usually the first finding. Variable abnormalities include proteinuria, hematuria, pyuria, and granular and cellular casts, and may be found in asymptomatic patients.

Hypotonic urine unresponsive to vasopressin may occur in
- Obstructive uropathy
- Chronic pyelonephritis
- Nephrocalcinosis
- Amyloidosis
- Familial nephrogenic diabetes insipidus

Serum sodium is decreased (because of tubular damage with loss in urine, vomiting, diarrhea, diet restriction, etc.). The decrease is indicated by increased urine sodium levels (>5–10 mEq sodium/L). It may occur in any renal disease, especially when polyuria is marked, but is more common with obstructive uropathy, chronic pyelonephritis, and interstitial nephritis than with chronic GN.

Serum potassium is increased (because of dietary sodium restriction and increased potassium ingestion, acidosis, impaired potassium excretion, oliguria, tissue breakdown). Decreased serum potassium with increased loss in urine (>15–20 mEq/L) occurs in primary aldosteronism and may also occur in malignant hypertension, tubular acidosis, Fanconi's syndrome, nephrocalcinosis, diuresis during recovery from tubular necrosis.

Acidosis is present (due to renal failure to secrete acid as NH_4^+ and to reabsorb filtered bicarbonate, and to decreased production of tubular bicarbonate).

Serum calcium is decreased (because of decreased calcium absorption in intestine, increased serum phosphorus, decreased serum albumin, etc.). Decreased renal production of calcitriol. Tetany is rare. Secondary parathyroid hyperplasia may occur, but hypercalcemia is not found.

Serum phosphorus increases when creatinine clearance falls to ~25 mL/min.

Serum ALP may be normal or may be increased with renal osteodystrophy.

Serum magnesium increases when GFR falls to <30 mL/min.

Increase in serum uric acid is usually <10 mg/dL. Secondary gout is rare. If clinical gout and family history of gout are present or if serum uric acid level is >10 mg/dL, rule out primary gout nephropathy.

Increased serum amylase occurs frequently; baseline level should be obtained in dialysis patients to evaluate episodes of abdominal pain, because these patients have an increased incidence of pancreatitis.

Serum CK and cTnT may be increased; a subset of uremic patients have a persistently increased CK-MB fraction without evidence of cardiac disease.

Increased serum triglycerides, cholesterol, and VLDL (prebeta) are common as renal failure progresses.

Serum homocysteine is often increased; correlated with cardiovascular complications.

Blood organic acids, phenols, indoles, certain amino acids, etc., are increased.

Normochromic normocytic anemia is usually proportionate to the degree of azotemia. Responds to erythropoietin. Burr cells or schistocytes are common.

Bleeding tendency is evident. There may be decreased platelets, increased capillary fragility, abnormal prothrombin consumption (possible platelet defect), normal BT and clotting time.

GI hemorrhage from ulcers anywhere in GI tract may be severe.

Laboratory findings due to uremic pericarditis, pleuritis, and pancreatitis are noted. (BUN is usually >100 mg/dL).

Laboratory findings due to uremic meningitis are noted (~50% of these patients have increased CSF protein or leukocytes; protein may be reduced by hemodialysis; pleocytosis is not related to degree of azotemia).

Serum albumin and total protein are decreased. When edema is seen without hypoproteinemia or heart failure, rule out acute GN, toxemia of pregnancy, excess fluid intake in oliguria during acute tubular necrosis or terminal renal failure.

Chronic Renal Failure with Normal Urine May Occur In

Nephrosclerosis (e.g., aging, hypertension)
Renal tubular acidosis
Interstitial nephritis
Hypercalcemia
Potassium deficiency
Uric acid nephropathy
Obstruction (including retroperitoneal fibrosis)

Scleroderma, Renal Disease In

Renal involvement occurs in two-thirds of patients; one-third die of renal failure.
Proteinuria may be minimal and is usually <2 gm/day; this may be the only finding for a long period.
Azotemia usually signals death within a few months.
Terminal oliguria or anuria may occur.

Stenosis, Renal Artery

See Fig. 14-5.
Mild proteinuria occurs often.
BUN and creatinine may show recent increase.
PRA in peripheral vein is increased and may cause hypokalemic metabolic alkalosis (see p. 643).
Urine sodium concentration may be low.
○Asymmetrical renal function or size (e.g., scan, ultrasonography, pyelogram).
○IV pyelogram, arteriography, MRI, Doppler ultrasonography of renal arteries may support diagnosis.
Late-onset (age >55 yrs) or early-onset (age <20 yrs) hypertension is often severe; stenosis is >70%.

Thrombosis, Renal Vein

Hematuria
Microscopic pyuria
Proteinuria and decreased creatinine clearance show marked variability from day to day.
Postprandial glycosuria
Nephrotic syndrome (see p. 733)
Hyperchloremic acidosis (renal tubular acidosis)
Hyperosmolarity
Oliguria and uremic death if infarction is extensive
Anemia is common.
Platelet count may be decreased.
Increased fibrin degradation products in blood may be >3× normal limits (DIC).
Laboratory findings due to thromboembolic disease elsewhere (e.g., pulmonary)
Laboratory findings due to underlying causative conditions (e.g., nephrotic syndrome, hypernephroma, metastatic cancer, trauma, amyloidosis, diabetic glomerulosclerosis, hypertension, papillary necrosis, DIC, sickle cell disease, polycythemia, heart failure, etc.)

Transplantation of Kidney

Laboratory Criteria

Donor: Three successive urinalyses and cultures must be negative.
Donor and recipient must show
• ABO and Rh blood group compatibility
• Leukoagglutinin compatibility
• Platelet agglutinin compatibility

Rejection

Total urine output is decreased.
Proteinuria is increased.
Cellular or granular casts appear.
Urine osmolality is decreased.
BUN and creatinine increase.
Hyperchloremic renal tubular acidosis may be an early sign of rejection or indicate smoldering rejection activity.
Renal clearance values decrease.
Iodohippurate sodium I-131 renogram is altered.
♦Biopsy of kidney shows a characteristic microscopic appearance allowing definitive diagnosis.

♦ Sequential measurement of subsets of activated T cells by flow cytometry is useful for diagnosing rejection and monitoring reversibility of rejection.

Tuberculosis (TB), Renal

○ Should be ruled out in cases of unexplained albuminuria, pyuria, microhematuria with negative cultures for pyogenic bacteria, especially in presence of TB elsewhere
♦ Urine culture for TB
♦ Guinea pig inoculation
See Tuberculosis, p. 823, for general findings.

Tubular Necrosis, Acute

See Table 14-12.

Due To

Nonoliguric form (one-third to two-thirds of all cases of acute tubular necrosis) is usually due to nephrotoxic agents. Mortality is ~25%.
Oliguric form is usually due to ischemic events (e.g., renovascular occlusion, bilateral cortical necrosis), rapidly progressive GN, obstructive uropathy. Mortality is ~50%.
Usually multiple causes (e.g., hypotension, sepsis, nephrotoxic drugs, radiographic contrast material, volume depletion).

Sudden progressive increase in BUN and serum creatinine with ratio of <20:1.
In patients with oliguric type who have not had recent diuretic therapy, urine osmolality is <350 mOsm/kg H_2O, and spot sodium is >20 mEq/L.
Urine sodium usually is >40 mEq/L but may be <20 mEq/L in nonoliguric patients.
FE_{Na} is usually >1% in both oliguric and nonoliguric patients.

Tubulointerstitial Rather than Glomerulovascular Disease, Laboratory Findings

Minimal or absent proteinuria
Moderate polyuria
Hyperchloremic metabolic acidosis
Severe sodium wasting
Disproportionate hyperkalemia
Mild or absent hypertension

Tumors of Kidney

Carcinoma of Renal Pelvis and Ureter

Hematuria is present.
Renal calculi are associated.
UTI is associated.
♦ Cytologic examination of urinary sediment for malignant cells is necessary.

Renal Cell Carcinoma

○ Even in the absence of the classic loin pain, flank mass, and hematuria, renal cell carcinoma should be ruled out in the presence of the following *unexplained* (paraneoplastic) laboratory findings, which are associated with a poorer prognosis.
  • Abnormal liver function tests (in absence of metastases to liver) found in 40% of these patients, e.g., increased serum ALP, increased serum AST, prolonged PT, altered serum protein values (decreased albumin, increased alpha$_2$ globulin)
  • Hypercalcemia
  • Polycythemia
  • Thrombocytosis
  • Leukemoid reaction
  • Refractory anemia and increased ESR
  • Amyloidosis
  • Cushing's syndrome

- Salt-losing syndrome
- Increased serum ferritin (due to hemorrhage within tumor)
- von Hippel-Lindau disease
♦ • Exfoliative cytology of urine for tumor cells
- Test for increased urine enzyme concentration
- Radioisotope scan of kidney

Needle biopsy is not recommended.

Renin-Producing Renal Tumors

(Hemangiopericytomas of juxtaglomerular apparatus; Wilms' tumor; rarely lung cancer)
♦ PRA is increased, with levels significantly higher in renal vein from affected side.
○ PRA responds to changes in posture but not to changes in sodium intake.
♦ PRA maintains circadian rhythm despite marked elevation.
○ Secondary aldosteronism is evident, with hypokalemia, etc. (see p. 647).
Laboratory changes (and hypertension) are reversed by removal of tumor.

Leukoplakia of Renal Pelvis

♦ Cell block or Pap smear of urine shows keratin or keratinized squamous cells.

Nonrenal Genitourinary Diseases

Bladder, Carcinoma

Hematuria may be gross or only microscopic.
♦ Biopsy of tumor confirms the diagnosis.
♦ Cytologic examination of urine for tumor cells is useful for grades II, III, and IV carcinoma but not for grade I, for which it has a high false-positive rate. Positive cytology with negative cystoscopy correlates with eventual development of transitional cancer. It may be of value in screening dye workers in chemical industry.

	Sensitivity*	
	First Urine Specimen	**Third Urine Specimen**
Grade I	None	20% (many false-positives)
Grade II	30%	80%
Grade III	65%	85%
Grade IV	92%	98%

*False-positives may occur due to atypia in chronic cystitis, calculi, irradiation, chemotherapy (e.g., busulfan [Myleran]).

♦ Flow cytometry of urine quantitatively measures DNA content or ploidy; cells with normal DNA content are diploid and cells with abnormal DNA content are aneuploid; aneuploidy is found only in neoplastic cells although diploidy is found in both normal and neoplastic cells. Aneuploidy is early indicator of neoplasia and may be present before microscopic evidence of tumor is found. Sensitivity for bladder cancer is 78%; specificity for nonneoplastic disease is 2%.
♦ Measurement of bladder tumor antigen (BTA) in urine is a recent qualitative latex agglutination test for bladder cancer that detects basement membrane proteins (due to degradation); can be done before, or at time of, cystoscopy. Reported sensitivity of 40% compared to 17% for cytologic examination of voided urine in patients with cancer diagnosed by cystoscopy. Specificity = 96% in healthy persons with no GU complaints and 82% if some GU tract disease is present. Positive predictive value for monitoring = 71% if prevalence is 20%. With tumors of low stage and grade (stage Ta, grades I and II), BTA sensitivity = 30% and sensitivity of cytologic examination of voided urine = 19%. Positive results for BTA may occur within 14 days of prostate biopsy or resection and may be seen in the presence of renal or bladder calculi, symptomatic sexually transmitted disease (STD), and other GU tract cancers (e.g., penis, ovary, endometrium, cervix). BTA and cytologic examination may predict relapse of cancer before cystoscopy.
♦ NMP22 measures nuclear mitotic apparatus protein in urine, a component of the nuclear matrix. Value >10 U/mL has reported sensitivity of 70% and specificity of 79%. 86% of patients with a value <10 U/mL had no bladder cancer.

FDP test identifies fibrinogen and fibrin degradation products in urine; high levels are associated with bladder malignancy.

BTA, NMP22, and FDP tests are approved by FDA *only* to detect recurrence of bladder cancer, in conjunction with cystoscopy.

Urinary LD level may be useful in screening studies to identify asymptomatic patients with neoplasm of GU tract (e.g., occupational exposure).

Laboratory findings due to complications stemming from infection or from obstruction of ureter

Laboratory findings due to preexisting conditions (e.g., schistosomiasis, stone, or infection)

Cystitis, Eosinophilic

Urinalysis may show proteinuria, microscopic hematuria, pyuria; eosinophiluria is rare. (See p. 92.)

Eosinophilia is diagnostically useful if present; is unusual.

♦ Diagnosis is established by bladder biopsy.

Epididymitis

Due To

Chlamydiae cause 50% of acute cases in men <35 yrs old.

Gonococci cause most of the remaining cases.

Occasionally due to
* *Mycobacterium tuberculosis* (only 35% of patients have history of previous TB)
* *Coccidioides immitis*
* *Blastomyces*
* Idiopathic

Pyuria

Evidence of urethritis (see Fig. 14-6) or aspirate or biopsy material for appropriate organisms

Laboratory findings due to complications (e.g., abscess formation, infarction of testicle)

Patient should be tested for other STDs.

Fibrosis, Retroperitoneal

Due To

Primary (70% of cases)
* Angiomatous lymphoid hamartoma

Secondary (30% of cases)
* Infection
* Trauma
* Connective tissue disease
* Aortic aneurysm
* Irradiation
* Drugs (e.g., methysergide; also methyldopa, ergotamine, phenacetin, hydralazine, propranolol)

ESR is increased.

Anemia is present.

Leukocytosis is present.

Occasionally eosinophilia occurs.

Serum protein and A/G ratio are normal; if the person is chronically ill, total protein may be decreased. Gamma globulins may be increased.

Laboratory findings due to ureteral obstruction

Postvasectomy Status

Sperm Count

May fall to low levels after three or four ejaculations and then rise abruptly before falling again.

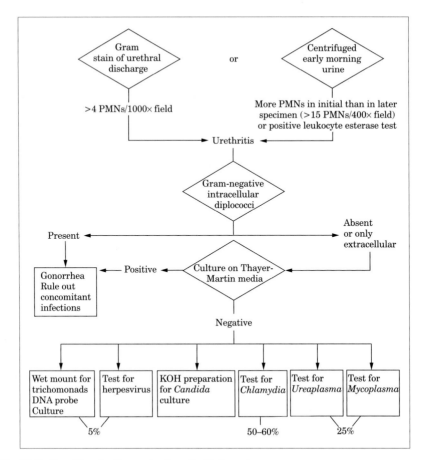

Fig. 14-6. Algorithm for diagnosis of urethritis in males.

15–20 ejaculations may be required before sperm count reaches 0.

25–50 HPFs are examined microscopically (e.g., phase contrast) for motile and non-motile sperm. If none seen, examine sediment after centrifugation.

♦ Two consecutive azoospermic specimens 6–10 wks after surgery, 1 mo apart, are recommended before dispensing with contraception.

Reanastomosis of the vas deferens may occur.

Priapism

Due To

Sickle cell disease
Leukemia
Polycythemia
Carcinoma metastatic to penis
Pelvic thrombophlebitis
Retroperitoneal bleeding
Penile trauma
Prostatitis
Spinal cord injury or anesthesia

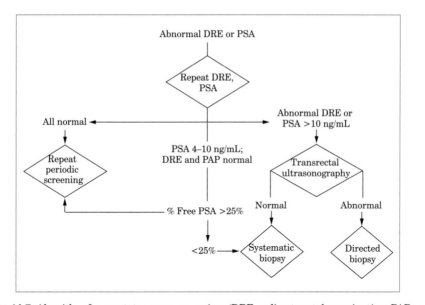

Fig. 14-7. Algorithm for prostate cancer screening. (DRE = direct rectal examination; PAP = prostatic acid phosphatase.)

CNS infection (e.g., syphilis, TB)

Drugs (e.g., antihypertensives, hydralazine, testosterone, phenothiazine, heparin, ethanol, marijuana)

Treatment of impotence by penile drug injection (e.g., papaverine, prostaglandin, phentolamine)

Unknown causes

Prostate Carcinoma

♦ Serum Prostate-Specific Antigen (PSA)

(Glycoprotein found in prostate acinar cells; reference range <4 ng/mL; increases with age [reference range ≤ 6.5 ng/mL older than age 70]; higher in black than white men)

See Fig. 14-7.

Use

Monitor response to total prostatectomy (failure to decline at least to normal range indicates residual prostatic tissue or metastases; increasing levels indicate recurrent disease) or radiation therapy for cancer.

Now approved for screening by FDA but is controversial because

- Increased in 25–46% of patients with benign prostatic hypertrophy.
- Value >10 ng/mL occurs in 2% of cases of benign prostatic hypertrophy and 44% of cases of cancer.
- PSA is not sufficiently specific (59–69%) or sensitive to be used alone for screening. PSA is <4.0 ng/mL for ~45% of confined cancers and 25% of unconfined cancers.
- Detects only ~2% of cancers in screening of healthy asymptomatic men. Cases detected by PSA and by digital rectal examination may not be the same ones.
- Cost-benefit of early diagnosis and treatment of prostate carcinoma is questionable because it is not likely to cause symptoms or affect survival in 30% of men aged >50 yrs.
- Not recommended without digital rectal examination.

Staging of patients with prostate carcinoma.

Superior to and replaces prostatic acid phosphatase for routine monitoring at each stage of disease. PSA is more sensitive but less specific than prostatic acid phosphatase. Useful in advanced cancer in which PSA is increased, whereas prostatic acid phosphatase is normal in >20% of cases.

Interpretation

Monitoring

Successful radiation or antiandrogen therapy reduces PSA in patients with residual disease. Increasing levels after treatment indicate relapse, often many months before clinical symptoms occur.

Failure of radiation therapy to decrease PSA to <1 ng/mL means substantial likelihood of recurrence; some reports suggest that a value of <0.5 ng/mL predicts long-term disease-free status.

With successful radiation therapy, PSA may not return to normal or baseline for 2–6 mos.

After removal of all tumor, PSA may not return to normal or baseline for >2 wks. PSA ≥ 0.2 ng/mL indicates recurrence.

Doubling time
- Occurs in 4 to >33 mos in ~67% of patients before treatment.
- Correlates with recurrence of disease after radiation therapy.
- After radical prostatectomy, doubling time reflects aggressiveness of original cancer.

Diagnosis

In patients with cancers diagnosed by careful pathologic examination, 80% had a normal PSA; of those with tumor volumes of 0.5–1.9 cc, 50% had a normal PSA.[6]

Percentage of Patients with Prostate Cancer

	Total PSA (ng/mL)			
	0–2	2–4	4–10	>10
Digital rectal examination negative	1	15	25	>50
Digital rectal examination positive	5	20	45	>75

PSA of >100 ng/mL predicts bone metastases with >90% accuracy, >66% sensitivity, 96% specificity, 73% positive predictive value. Bone metastases are rare with PSA of <10 ng/mL.

PSA density (quotient of serum PSA to prostate gland volume by transrectal ultrasonography) may help to distinguish benign prostatic hypertrophy and cancer, especially when PSA is 4.0–10.0 ng/mL; low PSA density is unlikely to indicate cancer but increased density (>0.15) is more likely to represent cancer. Additional data are needed.

PSA velocity (rate of change): more rapid rate of increase (>0.75 ng/mL/yr) in early cancer may distinguish carcinoma from benign prostatic hypertrophy (reported sensitivity = 90%, specificity = 100%). Requires up to three measurements over 2-yr period. Is not useful for staging. Additional data are needed.

Ambulatory values are higher than sedentary values, which may decrease by ≤ 50% (mean = 18%).

Different assays yield different values.

♦ Increased In

(Transient increases return to normal in 2–6 wks)

Prostate diseases
- Cancer
- Prostatitis   5–7×
- Benign prostatic hypertrophy
- Prostatic ischemia
- Acute urinary retention   5–7×

Manipulations
- Prostatic massage   ≤ 2×
- Cystoscopy   4×
- Needle biopsy   >50×
- Transurethral resection   >50×

[6]Babaian R. PSA and prostate cancer. First Annual CIBA Corning Symposium, 1994.

- Digital rectal examination increases PSA significantly if initial value is >20 ng/mL and is not a confusing factor in falsely elevating PSA.
- Radiation therapy
- Indwelling catheter
- Vigorous bicycle exercise   ≤ 2–3× several days
  Treadmill stress test   No change
  Drugs (e.g., testosterone)
  Physiologic fluctuations   ≤ 30%

     • PSA has no circadian rhythm, but 6–7% variation can occur between specimens collected on same day.

Analytic factors
- Different assays yield different values.
- Antibody cross reactivity.
- High-titer heterophile antibodies.

Other diseases/organs. Small amounts are found in
- Other cancers (sweat and salivary glands, breast, colon, lung, ovary)
- Skene's glands of female urethra
- Full-term placenta
- Acute renal failure
- AMI

Decreased In
Ejaculation within 24–48 hrs
Castration
Use of antiandrogen drugs
Radiation therapy
Prostatectomy
PSA falls 17% in 3 days for patient lying in hospital bed.
Artifactual (e.g., improper specimen collection; very high initial PSA levels)

♦ Increased Serum Prostatic Acid Phosphatase (PAP) Activity

Use
Identify local extension or distant metastases from prostate carcinoma. Increased in 60–75% of patients with bone metastases, 20% of patients with extension into periprostatic soft tissue but without bone involvement, 5% of patients with carcinoma confined to gland. Occasionally remains low despite active metastases.

Monitor response to treatment. Increased PAP shows pronounced fall in activity within 3–4 days after castration or within 2 wks after estrogen therapy is begun; may return to normal or remain slightly elevated; failure to fall corresponds to failure of clinical response, which occurs in 10% of patients. Increased PAP should return to normal 1 wk after surgery or radiation therapy for carcinoma palpable on rectal examination; failure to do so suggests the presence of metastatic lesions.

Interpretation
Most patients with invasive carcinoma show a significant increase in PAP after massage or palpation; this rarely occurs in patients with normal prostate, benign prostatic hypertrophy, or in situ carcinoma, or in patients with prostate carcinoma who are receiving hormone treatment.

PAP measured by immunoassay is nearly always increased in cases of palpable prostatic carcinoma. Specificity is >94% but may be normal in poorly differentiated or androgen-insensitive prostate carcinomas. More frequently increased with advancing stage and grade of cancer and in presence of lymph node or bone metastases. If PAP assay is elevated in presence of a negative biopsy, the biopsy should be repeated. If PAP is elevated and PSA is normal, the diagnosis lies elsewhere; rule out disseminated malignancy, myeloproliferative or chronic infectious disease. Not increased in nonprostate diseases listed below.

May be increased in ≤ 8% of prostate carcinoma patients with normal PSA.

Increased In
Prostate carcinoma
Infarction of the prostate (sometimes to high levels)
Operative trauma, instrumentation of the prostate, or prostatic massage may cause transient increase.

Gaucher's disease (only when certain substrates are used in the analysis)

Excessive destruction of platelets, as in ITP with megakaryocytes in bone marrow

Thromboembolism, hemolytic crises (e.g., sickle cell disease) due to hemolysis (only when certain substrates are used in the laboratory analysis); is said to occur often.

Leukemic reticuloendotheliosis (hairy) cells using a specific assay

In the absence of prostatic disease, occurs occasionally in

- Partial translocation trisomy 21
- Diseases of bone
- Advanced Paget's disease
- Metastatic carcinoma of bone
- Multiple myeloma (some patients)
- Hyperparathyroidism
- Various liver diseases (slight)
    Hepatitis
    Obstructive jaundice
    Laënnec's cirrhosis
- Acute renal impairment (not related to degree of azotemia)
- Other diseases of the RE system with liver or bone involvement (e.g., Niemann-Pick disease)
- In vitro hemolysis

Decreased In

Not clinically significant

Serum ALP is increased in 90% of patients with bone metastases. Increases with favorable response to estrogen therapy or castration and reaches peak in 3 mos, then declines. Recurrence of bone metastases causes new increase in ALP.

Anemia is present.

♦ Carcinoma cells may appear in bone marrow aspirates.

♦ Molecular analysis (PCR based on tissue-specific RNA) can detect 1 cell in $>10^6$ peripheral nucleated blood cells. Research technique at present.

Fibrinolysins are found in 12% of patients with metastatic prostatic cancer; occur only with extensive metastases and are usually associated with hemorrhagic manifestations; they show fibrinogen deficiency and prolonged PT.

UTI and hematuria occur late.

♦ Needle biopsy of prostate confirms diagnosis.

Cytologic examination of prostatic fluid is not generally useful.

Prostatic Hypertrophy, Benign (BPH)

Serum PSA may be increased in 55–83% of patients (may be >10 ng/mL in 3–21%), confusing use of PSA for screening for prostate cancer. Is more common cause of increased PSA than prostate carcinoma. PSA returns to reference range after resection.

Finasteride treatment causes a median decrease of ~50% in PSA.

Laboratory findings due to urinary tract obstruction and secondary infection.

Prostatitis

Bacterial form is most frequently due to

- *E. coli*
- *Proteus mirabilis*
- *Pseudomonas*
- *Klebsiella*
- *Streptococcus faecalis*
- *Staphylococcus aureus*

Acute Prostatitis

♦ WBCs in centrifuged sediment of last portion of voided specimen.

♦ Urine usually yields positive results on colony count and culture.

Blood cultures should be done.

Chronic Bacterial Prostatitis

♦ To differentiate from urethritis, compare specimens from initial urine, midstream urine, prostatic secretions (by prostatic massage), and first urine after prostatic massage. All show a greater colony count (usually by 10×) compared to the first urine specimen, but the finding is the reverse in urethritis.

Laboratory findings due to associated or complicating conditions (e.g., epididymitis)

Chronic Nonbacterial Prostatitis

Much more common than chronic bacterial prostatitis.

♦ Prostatic fluid usually shows >10 WBC/HPF with negative cultures of urine and prostatic fluid; no response to antibiotic therapy.

May be due to organisms that are difficult to culture (e.g., *Ureaplasma*, *Chlamydia*, trichomonads, CMV, or herpes virus) or to treatment.

Serum PSA may be increased, causing confusion in the screening for prostate cancer.

Sexually Transmitted Diseases (STDs) (Including Urethritis)

See Fig. 14-6.

Due To

Bacteria

* *Neisseria gonorrhoeae*
* *Treponema pallidum*
* *Mycoplasma hominis*
* *Calymmatobacterium granulomatis*
* *Campylobacter fetus*
* *Streptococcus* group B (?)
* *C. trachomatis*
* *Ureaplasma urealyticum*
* *Haemophilus ducreyi*
* *Shigella* spp.
* *Gardnerella vaginalis* (?)

Viruses

* HIV
* HAV and HBV
* Papillomavirus (genital wart)
* HSV
* CMV
* Molluscum contagiosum virus

Protozoa

* *Trichomonas vaginalis*
* *Giardia lamblia*
* *Entamoeba histolytica*

Ectoparasites

* Crab louse
* Scabies mite

♦ Urethritis is diagnosed if smear of urethral discharge shows >4 PMNs/1000× field.

♦ In absence of urethral discharge,

* First-void urine specimen showing >10 WBC/HPF or positive leukocyte esterase test.
* Early morning urine specimen is collected in three sequential containers. The initial 10-mL specimen is centrifuged and compared to the rest of the sample. If the first specimen shows more PMNs (>15 PMNs/400× field) than the later sample, urethritis is diagnosed. If equal numbers of PMNs are present in both specimens, the inflammation is higher up in the GU tract. If no PMNs are present, urethritis is unlikely. Sediment of the first specimen should also be examined for *T. vaginalis*.

♦ Gram stain shows gram-negative intracellular diplococci in >95% of cases of gonorrhea (see p. 803). When only some extracellular diplococci are seen, subsequent cultures are positive for *N. gonorrhoeae* in <15% of patients.

♦ In males, a positive Gram-stained smear establishes the diagnosis of gonorrhea and a culture is not necessary, but in females, a positive smear should be confirmed by culture on appropriate media (i.e., Gram stain preparations are highly sensitive and specific in males but not in females).

Chlamydia and *Ureaplasma* cannot be identified in Gram stain preparations, and cultures must be done at specialized laboratories.

When Gram staining and cultures for gonorrhea yield negative results, the presumptive diagnosis is nongonococcal urethritis, and *C. trachomatis* causes ~50% of such cases. This is the most frequent venereal disease and is estimated to be more than twice as frequent as gonorrhea (see p. 797).

In venereal disease clinics, ≤ 50% of males with gonococcal urethritis have concomitant *C. trachomatis* present. *Chlamydiae* are responsible for 70% of postgonococcal urethritis. In venereal disease clinics, *C. trachomatis* can be cultured from 25–50% of females.

In sexually active men with no symptoms or laboratory findings of urethritis, chlamydial infection is found in <3%.

In sexually active young men, acute epididymitis is almost always due to STD; 10% of cases are due to gonorrhea; 50–80% are due to *C. trachomatis* infection in heterosexuals but *E. coli* infection is a more common cause in homosexual men and men aged >35 yrs. Laboratory findings of urethritis are usually present even if patient is asymptomatic.

Women infected with *C. trachomatis* show infection of urethra (50% of cases), rectum (25% of cases), and cervix (75% of cases). Present in <50% of women with cervical gonococcal infection.

Sexually active women with symptoms of lower UTI and pyuria (>15 WBCs/HPF) but sterile urine cultures probably have chlamydial infection. If coliforms or staphylococci are found, bacterial cystitis is likely even when bacterial count is <100,000/mL.

U. urealyticum probably causes 20–30% of cases of urethritis in males.

M. hominis may cause pyelonephritis (5% of cases), pelvic inflammatory disease (10% of cases), and postpartum febrile complications (10% of cases). *U. urealyticum* and *M. hominis* are usually diagnosed by culture; DNA probes are less sensitive. Serologic methods are not widely used for various reasons (lack of specificity, complexity, etc.); diagnosis requires 4× rise in IgG titer; increased IgM titer may be reliable in urethritis or salpingitis.

Candida albicans, T. vaginalis, herpes simplex, and CMV probably cause 10–15% of cases of nongonococcal urethritis.

Laboratory findings of complications
- Prostatitis (20% of patients)
- Epididymitis (<3% of patients)
- Urethral stricture (<5% of patients)
- Reiter's syndrome (2% of patients)
- Cervicitis, cervical erosion, cytologic atypia on Pap smear, salpingitis
- Sterility
- Acute proctitis

Obstetric/Gynecologic Diseases

Abortion, Septic

Due To

Mixed aerobic and anaerobic gram-negative and gram-positive bacteria, e.g.,
  E. coli
  Bacteroides fragilis
  Enterococcus
  Beta-hemolytic *Streptococcus*
  Clostridium perfringens and *Clostridium tetani*

Laboratory findings due to sequelae (e.g., endometritis, parametritis, salpingo-oophoritis, uterine perforation, peritonitis, septic thrombophlebitis, septicemia)

Laboratory findings due to complications
- Renal failure
- DIC
- Septic shock

Abruptio Placentae

(Premature separation of normally implanted placenta after 20th week of gestation; occurs in ~1 in 120 deliveries; causes 15% of third-trimester stillbirths.)

♦ No diagnostic laboratory findings

Laboratory findings due to
- Hypovolemic shock
- Acute renal failure
- DIC (is most common cause of DIC in pregnancy)

Amniotic Fluid Embolism

Laboratory findings due to pulmonary embolism (see Chapter 6)
♦ Identification in maternal lung tissue
  • Morphologic identification of fetal products (e.g., fat from vernix caseosa, mucin derived from meconium)
  • Immunohistochemical identification of fetal isoantigen A[30] and mucin-type glycoprotein derived from meconium and amniotic fluid

Delivery, Preterm

(Gestational age <37 wks/259 days; premature infant weighs <2500 gm.)
Fetal fibronectin in cervical secretions of >50 ng/mL (by immunoassay) identifies women who deliver before term with sensitivity of 60–93% and specificity of 52–85%; positive predictive value = 25% and negative predictive value = 96% in different studies.[7]
Laboratory findings due to associated conditions, e.g., hyaline membrane disease, intraventricular hemorrhage
See Amniotic Fluid to Monitor Fetal Lung Maturity, p. 770.

Infection, Intra-Amniotic

Due To

Bacteria (in congenital pneumonia and chorioamnionitis, two-thirds of causative organisms are gram-negative). Most common organisms are *G. vaginalis*, *C. albicans*, group B *Streptococcus*, diphtheroids. Most dangerous are *E. coli* and group B *Streptococcus*. 20% of intra-amniotic infections cause two-thirds of cases of maternal or neonatal bacteremia.
Virus (e.g., rubella virus, CMV, HSV, HSV)

Bacterial Infection

♦ Amniotic fluid glucose level of ≤ 5 mg/dL has positive predictive value of 90% but level of 10 mg/dL has positive predictive value of 52%; level of >20 mg/dL is 98% predictive of negative culture. Level of 6–20 mg/dL is not helpful in ruling out infection.
♦ Gram staining is highly specific; sensitivity of only 50–79%.
WBC may be increased; >50 WBC/cu mm predicts clinical infection.
♦ Amniotic fluid culture may demonstrate causative bacteria.
Maternal PMNs and shift to left may be seen.
Increase in maternal serum CRP may precede clinical findings by 12 hrs.
Presence in amniotic fluid of acetic, propionic, butyric, and succinic acids produced by bacteria (assayed by gas-liquid chromatography) is said to be >94% sensitive and specific for infection.
Serologic tests for viruses
♦ Histologic examination of fetal membranes establishes diagnosis.

Menstruation, Altered Laboratory Test Results During

Platelet count is decreased by 50–70%; returns to normal by fourth day.
Hb is unchanged.
Fibrinogen is increased.
Serum cholesterol may increase just before menstruation.
Urine volume, sodium, and chloride decrease premenstrually and increase postmenstrually (diuresis).
Urine protein may increase during premenstrual phase.
Urine porphyrins increase.
Urine estrogens decrease to lowest level 2–3 days after onset.

Pelvic Inflammatory Disease

(See also Sexually Transmitted Diseases, p. 757.)

[7]Pitkin RM. Obstetrics and gynecology. *JAMA* 1996;275:1829.

Includes

Urethritis; see p. 757.
Cervicitis
    Cervical Gram staining shows >10 PMNs/HPF (1000×) in nonmenstruating women
    Tests for appropriate organism
    Culture
    Direct antigen test (e.g., *Chlamydia*)
Vulvovaginitis (see p. 766)
Pelvic abscess—usually due to multiple (three or more) organisms, aerobic (e.g., *Strep-tococcus*, *E. coli*), and anaerobic (e.g., *Peptococcus*, *Bacteroides*) organisms. *Chlamydia* and *N. gonorrhoeae* recovered from cervix in one-third of cases.
Perihepatitis (Fitz-Hugh–Curtis syndrome); see discussion of *C. trachomatis*, Chapter 15.
Laboratory findings due to complications, e.g., infertility, ectopic pregnancy, premature birth, neonatal conjunctivitis, infant pneumonia, septicemia, septic shock, peritonitis, pelvic thrombophlebitis

Due To

C. trachomatis (see Chapter 15). *Pelvic inflammatory disease due to* C. trachomatis *causes less leukocytosis, fever, less severe symptoms than that due to* N. gonorrhoeae.
N. gonorrhoeae infection is found in 8% of acute cases (see Chapter 15).
Anaerobic bacteria
Coliform bacilli
Actinomyces israelii
M. hominis (see Chapter 15)
Many cases are polymicrobial.
See causes of vulvovaginitis (following section).
Human papillomavirus infection (HPV)—suspected in presence of koilocytic changes on Pap smear or cervical biopsy. Low-risk types (e.g., 6, 11) are commonly associated with viral condyloma or mild cervical dysplasia (cervical intraepithelial neoplasia type I) that do not usually progress to invasive disease. High-risk types (e.g., 16, 18, 31, 33, 35) are often associated with moderate dysplasia (cervical intraepithelial neoplasia type II) and severe dysplasia or carcinoma in situ (cervical intraepithelial neoplasia type III), and are present in most patients with cervical cancer. Found in 1–4% of routine screening Pap smears and ≤ 16% of women in STD clinics.
♦ May be confirmed by antigen detection staining of tissue or DNA hybridization. Commercial kit detects HPV types 6, 11, 16, 18, 31, 33, 35 in endocervical or urethral swabs or tissues by nucleic acid hybridization. Southern blot hybridization detects HPV DNA in ~90% of cases of genital warts and 70–95% of cases of in situ and invasive carcinoma of cervix. HPV also found in 6% of unselected men by DNA studies of cell scrapings from penis.
    • Culture is not available.
    • At present, serologic tests (ELISA) are not clinically useful.
Genital TB—usually tubal via hematogenous spread from primary site in lung.
♦ • Culture of menstrual fluid is most reliable diagnostic procedure.
    • >10 WBC/HPF (1000×) without microscopic bacteriuria; hematuria and proteinuria are very unusual.
    • Pap smear may show cytoplasmic inclusion bodies in metaplastic squamous cells of cervix, which have low sensitivity, specificity, and positive predictive values of 10–40%.
HSV—see Chapter 15.

Placenta Previa

(Occurs in 1 in 200 deliveries.)
Laboratory findings due to painless vaginal hemorrhage
Laboratory findings due to associated factors (e.g., syphilis, Rh disease, multiple gestations, fetal anomalies, prematurity)
Maintain maternal Hct at ≥ 35% by administration of iron or folate, or blood transfusion.
Avoid preterm delivery and hyaline membrane disease of infant by amniocentesis to determine lung maturity (see p. 770).

Pregnancy, Altered Laboratory Test Results During

(By term unless otherwise specified)

RBC, Hb, and Hct decrease ~15%.

RBC volume increases 20%, but plasma volume increases 45%.

WBC increases 66%.

ESR increases markedly during pregnancy, making this a useless diagnostic test during pregnancy.

Serum iron decreases 40% in patients not on iron therapy.

Serum transferrin increases 40% and percent saturation decreases ≤ 70%.

Serum total protein decreases 1 gm/dL during first trimester; remains at that level.

Serum albumin decreases 0.5 gm/dL during first trimester; decreases 0.75 gm/dL by term.

Serum alpha$_1$ globulin increases 0.1 gm/dL.

Serum alpha$_2$ globulin increases 0.1 gm/dL.

Serum beta globulin increases 0.3 gm/dL.

Serum ceruloplasmin increases 70%.

Fasting blood glucose decreases 5–10 mg/dL by end of first trimester.

Renal function changes are difficult to assess because they are based on body surface area and because of changes in plasma volume during pregnancy.

BUN and creatinine decrease 25%, especially during first half of pregnancy. *BUN of 18 mg/dL and creatinine of 1.2 mg/dL definitely represent increased (abnormal) levels in pregnancy, although these levels are normal in nonpregnant women.*

Serum uric acid decreases 35% in first trimester; returns to normal by term.

Serum cholesterol increases 30–50%.

Serum triglycerides increase 100–200%.

Serum phospholipid increases 40–60%.

Serum CK decreases 15% by 20 wks; increases at beginning of labor to peak at 24 hrs postpartum, then gradually returns to normal. CK-MB is detected at onset of labor in ~75% of patients with peak level at 24 hrs postpartum, then returns to normal. Serum LD and AST remain low.

In cases of threatened abortion during first 20 wks of pregnancy, progressive increase in serum diamine oxidase is usually associated with continuation of pregnancy.

Serum ALP progressively increases (200–300%) during the last trimester of normal pregnancy due to increase in heat-stable isoenzyme from the placenta.

Serum LAP may be moderately increased throughout pregnancy.

Serum lipase decreases 50%.

Serum pseudocholinesterase decreases 30%.

Serum calcium decreases 10%.

Serum magnesium decreases 10%.

Serum osmolality decreases 10 mOsm/kg during first trimester.

Serum vitamin B$_{12}$ level decreases 20%.

Serum folate decreases 50% or more. Overlap of decreased and normal range of values often makes this test useless in diagnosis of megaloblastic anemia of pregnancy.

Serum T$_3$ uptake is decreased and T$_4$ is increased. T$_7$ (T$_3$ × T$_4$) is normal. TBG is increased. (See Pregnancy and Thyroid Function Tests, p. 593.)

Serum aldosterone is increased.

No changes are found in serum levels of sodium, potassium, chloride, phosphorus, amylase, AST, ALT, LD, acid phosphatase, alpha-hydroxybutyrate dehydrogenase.

Occasionally cold agglutinin test results may be positive and osmotic fragility increased.

Urine volume may increase ≤ 25% in last trimester.

Proteinuria is common (present in ~20% of patients).

Glycosuria is common with decreased glucose tolerance.

Lactosuria should not be confused with glucose in urine.

Urine porphyrins may be increased.

Gonadotropins (hCG) are increased (see Pregnancy Test, p. 762).

Urine estrogens increase from 6 mos to term (≤ 100 μg/24 hrs)

Urine 17-KS levels rise to ULN at term.

Pregnancy, Ectopic (Tubal)

See Fig. 14-8.

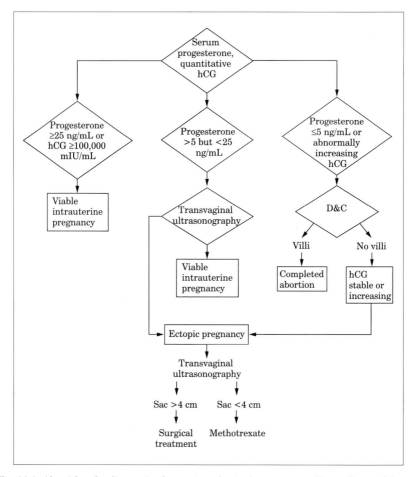

Fig. 14-8. Algorithm for diagnosis of unruptured ectopic pregnancy. (From Carson SA, Buster JE. *N Engl J Med* 1993;329:1174, with permission.)

♦ Serum beta-subunit hCG assay (pregnancy test) is positive in ~95% of patients; sensitivity of assay is <10 mU/mL; detects pregnancy 2 days earlier than urine test. Newest urine assays (sensitivity = 20–25 mU/mL) can detect hCG as early as 24–26 days after last menses. By 28 days after last menses, urine hCG is usually >200 mU/mL and monoclonal antibody urine tests are positive. Qualitative test confirms pregnancy in 30 mins.
   • hCG normally peaks at ~100,000 mU/mL near end of first trimester; then declines to 10,000 mU/mL to end of pregnancy.
   • hCG titer doubles every 2–3.5 days during first 40 days of normal pregnancy (at least two measurements 48–72 hrs apart are needed to calculate this); an abnormally slow increase in hCG (<66% in 48 hrs) indicates ectopic pregnancy (80% sensitivity, 91% specificity) or abnormal intrauterine pregnancy in ~75% of cases.
   • hCG of >6500 mU/mL (equivalent to level at ~6 wks' gestation) without visualization of an intrauterine gestational sac by transabdominal sonography favors ectopic pregnancy, because at this titer an intrauterine pregnancy should be visualized.
   • hCG of <6000 mU/mL without a sac indicates unknown diagnosis; absent gestational sac at this hCG concentration is associated with ectopic pregnancy in >85% of cases.

- hCG of <6000 mU with a sac suggests either ectopic pregnancy or an early normal/abnormal pregnancy.
- Improved ultrasonographic instruments may change upper limits of hCG to ~1500 mU/mL for nonvisualization of sac. Sac can be detected earlier by transvaginal sonography, at a stage that is reported to correspond to an hCG level of ~750 mU/mL.
- Decrease in hCG of ≥ 15% 12 hrs after curettage is diagnostic of completed abortion, but increase or no change in hCG indicates ectopic pregnancy.

Serum hCG level is used to monitor methotrexate treatment of ectopic pregnancy (testing is done weekly until hCG is undetectable).

♦ Serum progesterone should be measured to screen all patients at risk for ectopic pregnancy at time of first positive pregnancy test. Level ≥ 25 ng/mL is said to indicate normal intrauterine pregnancy (sensitivity = 98%) and level ≤ 5 ng/mL confirms nonviable fetus (100% sensitivity), so that diagnostic uterine curettage can be used to distinguish ectopic pregnancy from spontaneous intrauterine abortion.

WBC may be increased; usually returns to normal in 24 hrs. Persistent increase may indicate recurrent bleeding. 50% of patients have normal WBC; 75% of patients have WBC of <15,000/cu mm. Persistent WBC of >20,000/cu mm may indicate pelvic inflammatory disease.

Anemia depends on degree of blood loss; often precedes the tubal pregnancy in impoverished populations. Progressive anemia may indicate continuing bleeding into hematoma. Absorption of blood from hematoma may cause increased serum bilirubin.

Culdocentesis fluid with Hct >15% indicates significant intraperitoneal hemorrhage.

♦ Dilatation and curettage shows decidual changes without chorionic villi.

Pregnancy, Multiple

Increased maternal serum AFP
Laboratory findings due to associated conditions (e.g., polyhydramnios)

Pregnancy, Prolonged

(>294 days/42 wks' gestation)

Amniotic fluid L/S ratio is <2 in 6% of cases. High ratio (~4) can occur before 42 wks' gestation. Thus L/S ratio not useful for this diagnosis.

Progressively falling rather than rising estriol (E_3) level is usually found.

Squalene (derived from fetal sebaceous glands) is markedly increased in amniotic fluid after 39 wks.

Squalene/cholesterol ratio in amniotic fluid
<0.40 before 40 wks
>0.40 after 40 wks
>1.0 after 42 wks

Pregnancy, Toxemia of

Preeclampsia

(Hypertension, proteinuria, edema after 20th week of pregnancy)

♦ Proteinuria varies from a trace to very marked (≤ 800 mg/dL, equivalent to 15–20 gm/day). >15 mg/dL may indicate early toxemia.
- In mild preeclampsia proteinuria of >300 mg is found in at least two random clean-catch urine specimens collected 6 hrs apart but level is <2 gm/24 hrs.
- In severe preeclampsia significant proteinuria of ≥ 500 mg/24 hrs (2+ on dipstick) is seen.
- Proteinuria of ≥ 5 gm/24 hrs correlates with 3–4+ on dipstick.

♦ Oliguria—urine output <400 mL/24 hrs.

Thrombocytopenia and abnormal liver function tests may be present.

RBCs and RBC casts are not abundant; hyaline and granular casts are present. BUN, renal concentrating ability, and PSP excretion are normal unless the disease is severe or a prior renal lesion is present. *(BUN usually decreases during normal pregnancy because of increase in GFR.)*

Serum uric acid is increased (decreased renal clearance of urate) in 70% of patients in absence of treatment with thiazides, which can produce hyperuricemia independent of any disease.

Serum total protein and albumin commonly are markedly decreased.

Multiple clotting deficiencies may occur in severe cases. Lupus anticoagulant, antiphospholipid antibodies may be present.

Evidence of microangiopathic hemolysis, abnormal liver function tests, falling platelet count (HELLP syndrome) occurs in 4–12% of cases.

♦ Biopsy of kidney can establish diagnosis; rules out primary renal disease or hypertensive vascular disease.

Weekly creatinine clearance to follow renal function.

Eclampsia

♦ Is indicated by occurrence of generalized seizures.

~20% of women develop eclampsia with only mild hypertension and often without proteinuria or edema.

Amniocentesis to determine fetal maturity if induction of labor is required.

Usefulness of monitoring maternal estriols, human placental lactogen, and other components is questionable.

Laboratory findings due to complications, e.g., cerebral hemorrhage, pulmonary edema, renal cortical necrosis

Magnesium sulfate treatment requires urine output of ≥ 100 mL/4 hrs. Therapeutic magnesium range = 4–7 mEq/L. Toxicity begins at 7–10 mEq/L; respiratory depression begins at 10–15 mEq/L; cardiac arrest begins at 30 mEq/L.

Beware of associated or underlying conditions (e.g., hydatidiform mole, twin pregnancy, prior renal disease, diabetes mellitus, nonimmune hydrops fetalis).

Premenstrual Syndrome

No specific laboratory findings.

Rape/Sexual Assault

Acid Phosphatase in Vaginal Fluid

♦ Because of high level of acid phosphatase in prostatic fluid, presence indicates recent sexual intercourse.

For diagnosis of sexual assault, rape, or recent sexual intercourse
* Normal level is <10 U/L in noncoital women.
* Level of ≥ 50 U/sample is "semen positive."
   Increased in 100% of women immediately after intercourse
   Increased in 83% of women 8 hrs after intercourse
   Increased in 40% of women 24 hrs after intercourse
   Increased in 11% of women 72 hrs after intercourse

Low levels do not exclude recent intercourse; variable duration for hours to days after intercourse.

In cases of possible rape, in addition to smears for sperm, specimens for identification of organisms causing STDs (e.g., *Trichomonas vaginalis*, *Gonococcus*) should also be taken.

Semen specimens should be obtained for special genetic identification studies. Contact local police authorities in medical-legal cases for information on appropriate specimen types, handling, and identification.

Motile sperm in vaginal fluid may be useful in estimating time between intercourse and examination.
* Motile sperm in vaginal fluid—usually indicates an interval of <8 hrs.
* Can be seen in approximately one-third of women within 6 hrs.
* Can be seen in 20% of women between 7 and 24 hrs.
* In menstruating women, average period of motility is ~4 hrs.
* Motile sperm are not seen in two-thirds of women examined within 6 hrs.
* Sperm motility in anal or oral cavity is reduced; presence indicates interval of only a few hours.

Ruptured Membranes, Detection of

♦ Diagnosis based on finding that fluid from posterior fornix is amniotic fluid rather than urine.

- Detection of fetal isoform of fibronectin (by immunoassay) in vaginal secretions indicates presence of amniotic fluid. Is 5–10× greater in amniotic fluid than in maternal plasma; not present in normal vaginal secretions or urine.
- Other methods for detecting amniotic fluid in the vagina include pooling, ferning, Nitrazine pH paper, ultrasonography, and dye injection, which are either difficult to interpret, invasive, or expensive.
    - Fern test is most reliable test (>96% accuracy) (fluid air-dried on a glass slide shows a characteristic fernlike pattern microscopically)
    - Microscopic detection of fat-laden fetal squamous epithelial cells (Nile blue sulfate stain)
    - Reagent strip test showing pH of ≥ 7 (normal vaginal pH = 4.5–5.5) and protein level of ≥ 100 mg/dL indicate presence of amniotic fluid.

	Sensitivity	Specificity
pH alone	85%	83%
Protein alone	90%	87%
Either or both	95%	91%

Blood, meconium, renal disease, infection interfere with accuracy.

To detect premature rupture of membranes in any trimester, measure hCG level in saline washings of vaginal fornix. hCG levels of >50 mU/mL reportedly indicate rupture with high sensitivity, specificity, and positive predictive value.[8]

Measurement of AFP level in vaginal secretions is unreliable. Same concentration in amniotic fluid and maternal plasma in third trimester.

Uterine Cancer

Cancer of Cervix

See Human Papillomavirus, Chapter 15.

◆ Pap Smear

Use

Routine screening of asymptomatic women to detect carcinoma of cervix or various atypias
Also used to monitor response to therapy for carcinoma, infections, etc.
Occasionally detects carcinoma from other sites (e.g., endometrium, ovary, tube).
Often detects presence of various previously undiagnosed infectious agents (e.g., *T. vaginalis*, HSV, human papillomavirus, *Candida*, etc.). (See p. 767.)
Estimation of hormonal status
Occasionally useful in chromosome studies
In cases of atypia of undetermined significance, positive testing for HPV DNA may help identify patients with high-grade squamous intraepithelial lesions.

Interferences

(False-negative in ~5–10% of cases)
Sparse cells—100 abnormal cells is threshold for reliable screening; usual Pap smear contains 50,000 to 300,000 cells.
Sampling problems (poor fixation or staining), mislabeling, floating cells, obscured cells due to exudate, blood, degeneration, drying, etc. Malignant cells may not be present if smear is repeated too soon after previous abnormal smear.
Certain tumor types are less readily diagnosed (e.g., adenocarcinoma, lymphoma, sarcoma, verrucous carcinoma).
Human error in interpreting cells that are difficult to classify; <3% of preventable cervical cancer are due to misread smears.

Interpretation

Routine screening in the general population may yield positive results for ~6 of every 1000 women tested (prevalence); only 7% of these lesions are invasive. The prevalence is greatest in the following groups:
- Women aged 21–35 yrs, with peak in 31st to 35th year
- Black and Puerto Rican women
- Women who use birth control pills rather than diaphragm for contraception
- Women with early onset or long duration of sexual activity

---

[8]Anai T, et al. Vaginal fluid hCG levels for detecting premature rupture of membranes. *Obstet Gynecol* 1997;89:261.

- *Vaginal pool Pap smear has an accuracy rate of ~80% in detecting carcinoma of the cervix. Smears from a combination of vaginal pool, exocervical scrapings, and endocervical scrapings have an accuracy rate of 95%.*
- *After an initial abnormal smear, the follow-up smear taken in the next few weeks or months may not always be abnormal; no clear explanation exists for this finding.*
- ◆*Biopsy shows important lesions of the cervix in some of these patients. Therefore an abnormal initial smear requires further investigation of the cervix regardless of subsequent cytologic reports.*

Laboratory findings due to
- Obstruction of ureters with pyelonephritis, azotemia, etc.
- General effects of cancer

◆ Cancer of Uterine Body

◆ Pap smear of vagina/cervix is positive in ≤ 70% of patients with endometrial adenocarcinoma; a false-negative result occurs in 30% of patients. Therefore a negative Pap smear does not rule out carcinoma.

◆ Pap smear from aspiration of endometrial cavity is positive in 95% of patients.

◆ Endometrial biopsy may be helpful, but a negative result does not rule out carcinoma. Diagnostic curettage is the only way to rule out carcinoma of the endometrium.

Trophoblastic Neoplasms

Hydatidiform mole—5% progress to choriocarcinoma.
- Complete mole—normal amount of DNA that is all of paternal origin. 75–85% of cases are homozygous 46 XX (fertilization of an anucleate ovum); rest are heterozygous, mostly 46 XY with a few 46 XX (fertilization of empty ovum by two separate sperm).
- Partial mole—paternal and maternal DNA present but overabundance of paternal DNA. Fertilization of oocyte by two spermatozoa causes triploid 69 XYY, 68 XXY, 69 XXY karyotypes in two-thirds of cases; rest have diploid karyotype (46 XX or 46 XY). beta-hCG is not usually very increased and spontaneously regresses in >95% of cases requiring chemotherapy.
- hCG level is important in identifying the 15–20% of hydatidiform moles that persist after curettage.
- Increased incidence of preeclampsia.

Choriocarcinoma—50% are preceded by molar pregnancy, 25% by term pregnancy, 25% by abortion or ectopic pregnancy. Beta-hCG level corresponds to tumor burden.

◆ hCG level is used for diagnosis and management of both benign and malignant types.
- Persistently elevated or slowly declining level indicate persistent trophoblastic disease and the need for systemic therapy for invasive mole or choriocarcinoma.
- Amount of hCG produced correlates with amount of trophoblastic tissue.
- After evacuation of the uterus, hCG is negative by 40 days in 75% of cases. Of women who have positive test results at 56 days, 50% have trophoblastic disease.
- Repeat test every 1–2 wks with clinical examination. Disease remits in 80% of cases without further treatment.
- Plateau or rise of titer indicates persistent disease. Chemotherapy is indicated if disease persists or metastasizes.
- Repeat negative titer should be rechecked every 3 mos for 1–2 yrs. Initial serum titer of >40,000 mU/mL indicates high-risk patient.
- Frequent follow-up titers are indicated after radiation therapy with titers measured every 6 mos for life.

◆ Measurement of hCG in CSF (ratio of serum/CSF <60:1) is used in diagnosis of brain metastases.

Laboratory findings due to treatment (e.g., hemorrhage, infection, perforation of uterus, irradiation, chemotherapy)

◆ Diagnosis by histologic examination of tissue removed by curettage

Rh D-negative patients should receive Rh Ig at the time of evacuation.

Vulvovaginitis

Laboratory confirmation is necessary for reliable diagnosis.
See Table 14-13.

Table 14-13. Comparison of Various Causes of Vaginitis

Condition	pH	Saline Mount	10% KOH Mount	Culture	Amine Test
Normal	4.0–4.5	PMN/EC <1; rods dominant; 3+ squames	–		–
Bacterial vaginosis	>4.5	Clue cells; PMN/ED <1; D rods; I coccobacilli	–	No value.	>70% +
Vulvovaginal candidiasis	4.0–4.5	PMN/EC <1; hyphae in ~40%; rods dominant; 3+ squames	Hyphae in 70%	If wet mount is –.	–
Trichomoniasis	5.0–6.0	Motile trichomonads in ~60%; 4+ PMNs; mixed flora	–	Use if wet mount is –.	Often +
Atrophic vaginitis	>6.0	1–2+ PMNs; I cocci and coliforms; D rods; parabasal cells	–		–

+ = positive; – = negative; D = decreased; I = increased; PMN/EC = ratio of PMNs to epithelial cells.

Due To

♦ **Fungi**, especially *C. albicans* (causes 20–25% of cases)
  • Normal vaginal pH (4.0–4.5).
  • Wet mount in potassium hydroxide or Gram stain of vaginal fluid may not detect 15% of cases.
  • May be seen on Pap smears.
  • Culture on Nickerson's or Sabouraud's medium is most sensitive; is needed for definitive identification.
  • Sexual transmission plays a very minor role.
  • Underlying conditions may be present, especially uncontrolled diabetes mellitus, use of antibiotics, use of vaginal sponges or intrauterine devices.
♦ *T. vaginalis*
  • Wet-mount preparation of freshly examined vaginal fluid. Sensitivity = 50–70% compared with culture; requires 10^4 organisms/mL; specificity is almost 100%.
  • Frequently an incidental finding in routine urinalysis.
  • Frequently found in routine Pap smears. Sensitivity is ~70%, specificity is ~95%, positive predictive value is 75%, negative predictive value is 38%. The organism is often not identified but may be associated with characteristic concomitant cytologic changes. Not recommended for screening.
  • Increased PMNs are present.
  • pH is increased.
  • Culture is the gold standard.
  • DNA probe test kit allows prompt results; excellent method. *Douching within 24 hrs decreases sensitivity of tests.* Do not test during first few days of menstrual cycle.
  • Occasionally detected in material from male urethra in cases of nonspecific urethritis. Found in ≤ 40% of male sexual partners of infected women. Prostatic fluid usually contains few organisms.

Serologic tests are not useful.
♦ **Bacterial vaginosis:** polymicrobial infection due to increase in anaerobic organisms, including *G. vaginalis* and/or *Mobiluncus*, and concomitant decrease in lactobacilli.
Diagnosis based on ≥ 3 of the following:
- Vaginal pH >4.5 (using pH indicator paper) in >80% of these cases (found in one-third of normal women)
- Wet mount of vaginal discharge shows curved rods; "clue cells" (>20% of vaginal squamous cells coated with small coccobacilli) found in 90% of these cases.
- Positive culture on HB or chocolate agar for *G. vaginalis* in 95% of clinical cases but not recommended for diagnosis or test of cure because may also be found in 40–50% of asymptomatic women with no signs of infection.
- DNA probe kit allows prompt results.
- Gram stain and Pap smear may also suggest this diagnosis: gram-negative curved rods and decreased to absent gram-positive rods resembling lactobacilli.

Local cause is most common (e.g., endocrine factors, poor hygiene, pinworms, scabies, foreign body, irritants [e.g., soaps, perfumes, spermicides], hypersensitivity reaction [e.g., to antimycotic creams, latex condoms]).

Atrophic vaginitis
Increased pH (5.0 to 7.0)
Wet smear shows increased PMNs and parabasal epithelial cells
Mixed nonspecific gram-negative rods with decreased lactobacilli
Vaginal cytology shows atrophic pattern.

Desquamative inflammatory vaginitis
Purulent discharge
Increased pH
Gram stain shows absent gram-positive bacilli replaced by gram-positive cocci
Massive vaginal cell exfoliation with increased number of parabasal cells

Other organisms
N. gonorrhoeae (see p. 803)
Chlamydia (see p. 797)
Group A *Streptococcus*
S. aureus with toxic shock syndrome
Idiopathic associated with HIV infection

Other causes, e.g.,
Collagen vascular disease, Behçet's syndrome, pemphigus, lichen planus
Multiple causes may be present and should be sought in each case.

Obstetric Monitoring of the Fetus and Placenta

Amniotic Fluid (Amniocentesis)

Use

Determination of increased bilirubin level in severe Rh disease (see Hemolytic Disease of the Newborn, p. 389)
Determination of L/S ratio to estimate fetal lung maturity (see below).
Gram stain for organisms and WBC for diagnosis of amnionitis.
Diagnosis of congenital anomalies (e.g., Down syndrome, neural tube defect).
Prenatal diagnosis of genetic disorders, e.g.,
Wilms' tumor may be associated with deletion of chromosome 11, aniridia, and other malformations (e.g., overgrowth of one side or parts of one side of body); testing may be indicated when other children in family have Wilms' tumor. Chromosome studies and renal investigation are also indicated in presence of aniridia in newborn because Wilms' tumor is often curable.
See Chorionic Villus Sampling, Chapter 12, p. 508
Assessment of intrauterine growth retardation
Assessment of postdate pregnancies (>40 wks)
Evaluation of other conditions (e.g., fetal death)
May contain abnormal metabolites (e.g., excess methylcitrate in propionicacidemia) or enzyme activity (e.g., *N*-acetyl-D-hexosaminidase A activity in Tay-Sachs disease) but usually tissue culture of amniotic fluid cells is used with analysis for specific deficient enzyme.

Volume

At 38 wks, normal range = 200–1500 mL, average = 1000 mL; progressive decrease thereafter.

Decreased (Oligohydramnios) In
Fetal anomalies
Renal agenesis (including Potter's syndrome)
Fetal obstructive uropathies
Postmaturity syndrome
Placental insufficiency (e.g., preeclampsia)
Donor-twin transfusion syndrome

Increased (Hydramnios) In
Idiopathic (35%)
Maternal diabetes (25%)
Hemolytic disease of the newborn (10%)
Multiple pregnancy (10%)
Congenital malformations (20%)
  • CNS malformation with exposed meninges
  • Anencephaly, hydrocephaly, microcephaly
  • Mongolism
  • Volvulus with atresia or congenital bands of upper jejunum or with common mesentery and herniation of liver
  • Tracheoesophageal fistula with esophageal atresia
  • Pyloric stenosis, duodenal atresia
  • Imperforate anus
  • Cleft palate
  • Congenital heart disease
  • Disease of GU tract
  • Deformity of limbs
  • Agenesis of ears

Color

May be milky or turbid (due to vernix caseosa and squamous debris) until centrifugation, which should yield a clear supernatant that is colorless to light straw color.
Yellow
  • Usually due to bilirubin (normal maximum occurs at 20–28th wks); may be increased with fetal RBC hemolysis (e.g., hemolytic disease of the newborn); increase correlates with fetal condition and prognosis.
  • May also occur from fetal ascitic fluid, amniotic cysts, maternal urine (accidental puncture of mother's bladder).
  • Yellow-brown color may be due to traces of meconium.
Green (may be with brown or black hue) is due to biliverdin from meconium, which may indicate fetal distress.
Red to brown is usually due to RBCs or Hb. Special staining (Kleihauer-Betke) or electrophoresis distinguishes fetal Hb from maternal blood due to trauma; or flow cytometry.
Bright red indicates recent intrauterine hemorrhage or hemolysis; may be port wine color in abruptio placentae.
Brown may be due to oxidized Hb from degenerated RBCs.
Brown-black may be due to fetal maceration.

Amniotic Fluid, Maternal and Fetal Serum, Normal Values[9]

	Amniotic Fluid	Maternal Serum	Fetal Serum
Glucose (mg/dL)	10.7 (5.2)	66.6 (8.7)	48.7 (10.4)
Creatinine (mg/dL)	2.4 (0.3)	1.1 (0.2)	1.1 (0.3)
Urea (mg/dL)	33.9 (11.7)	17.1 (8.7)	16.5 (8.14)

[9]Castelazo-Ayala L, Karchmer S, Shor-Pinsker V. The biochemistry of amniotic fluid during normal pregnancy. Correlation with maternal and fetal blood. In: Hodari AA, Mariona F, eds. *Physiological biochemistry of the fetus. Proceedings of the international symposium.* Springfield, IL: Charles C Thomas Publisher, 1972:32–53.

Uric acid (mg/dL)	7.5 (0.3)	3.1 (0.8)	2.6 (0.9)
Total protein (gm/dL)	0.28 (0.3)	6.5 (0.6)	5.8 (0.7)
Albumin (%)	65.2 (4.8)	46.4 (3.1)	60.8 (4.8)
A/G ratio	1.9 (0.7)	0.8 (0.1)	1.5 (0.3)
Total cholesterol (mg/dL)	42.8 (3.2)	258.6 (47.2)	83.5 (39.7)
Triglycerides (mg/dL)	19.3 (9.4)	153.7 (51.4)	16.1 (10.7)
LD (U/mL)	112.3 (64.8)	199.5 (46.4)	328.2 (114.0)
Aldolase (U/mL)	10.1 (7.5)	9.5 (7.0)	23.2 (9.4)

Values are mean values. Numbers in parentheses represent 1 SD.

Amniotic Fluid, Normal Chemical Components[10]

	Second Trimester	**At Term**
Uric acid	3.7 mg/dL	9.9 mg/dL (due to increased muscle mass and increased urinary output of fetus)
Creatinine	0.9 mg/dL	2.0 mg/dL (due to increased muscle mass of fetus)
Total protein	0.6 gm/dL	0.3 gm/dL
Albumin	0.4 gm/dL	0.95 gm/dL
AST	17 U/dL	40 U/dL
ALP	25 U/dL	80 U/dL (≤ 350 U in some cases)

Levels of glucose, bilirubin, urea nitrogen, calcium, phosphorus, cholesterol, LD do not change significantly during gestation.

Amniotic Fluid, Tests to Monitor Fetal Lung Maturity[11–13]

Use

Determination of fetal maturity to predict likelihood of RDS and to determine when it is safe to interrupt gestation because of threat to fetus (e.g., erythroblastosis fetalis) or mother (e.g., toxemia, hypertension).

Incidence of RDS by 37 wks' gestation is <1%. Thus no fetal lung maturity testing is done after 37 wks' gestation except in cases of poorly controlled maternal diabetes.

At 34 wks' gestation, risk of RDS is 20% and increases to 60% at 29 wks. Thus most difficult decision time is 34–37 wks' gestation.

♦ L/S Ratio (determined by thin-layer chromatography)

The single most accurate test of fetal maturity

L/S ratio	(Some laboratories use these values)	Lung Maturity
<1	<2.0	Very immature lungs (up to 30th week of gestation); severe RDS is expected; many weeks may be required to reach lung maturity; do not resample before 2 wks.
1.0–1.49		Immature lungs; moderate to severe RDS is expected; lung maturity may be reached in 2 wks; resample in 1 wk.
1.5–1.9	2.0–3.0	Lungs on threshold of maturity (within 14 days); mild to moderate RDS may occur. Test should be repeated in 1 wk.
≥ 2	>3.0	Mature lungs (35th week of gestation); RDS is not expected. 80–85% sensitivity and specificity.

[10]Tsuda T, Bloch D, Wolf PL. An automated profile of amniotic fluid. *Lab Med* 1971;32:6.

[11]Dubin SB. Assessment of fetal lung maturity. Practice parameter. *Am J Clin Pathol* 1998;110:723.

[12]Dito WR, Patrick CW, Shelly J. *Clinical pathologic correlations in amniotic fluid.* Chicago: American Society of Clinical Pathologists, 1975.

[13]Natelson S, Scommegna A, Epstein MB, Eds. *Amniotic fluid. Physiology, biochemistry, and clinical chemistry.* New York: John Wiley and Sons, 1974.

| Abundant lecithin with trace or no sphingo- myelin | Postmature lungs |

Definite exceptions to prediction of pulmonary maturity when L/S ratio is >2.0
- Infant of diabetic mother (L/S ratio of >2.0 has been frequently seen in cases in which RDS developed)
- Erythroblastosis fetalis

Possible exceptions
- Intrauterine growth retardation
- Toxemia of pregnancy
- Hydrops fetalis
- Placental disease
- Abruptio placentae

In twin pregnancies, L/S ratio must be determined on fluid from each amniotic sac.

◆ Foam (Shake) Test

Reliable, simple bedside method providing qualitative expression of L/S ratio that gives prompt results. Commercial kit said to have sensitivity of 87%, specificity of 97%.

Interferences (L/S Ratio and Foam Tests)

Contamination of amniotic fluid with meconium, blood, vernix caseosa, or vaginal mucus makes L/S determinations unreliable (fluid should be leukocyte esterase–negative using urine dipstick). Whole-blood L/S ratio is ~1.5.

Collection in siliconized tubes.

Dilution due to oligo- or polyhydramnios may make foam test unreliable.

Interpretation

Although an L/S ratio of >2 and a positive foam test indicate pulmonary maturity and absence of RDS in >95% of cases, a ratio of <2 and a negative foam test have a high false-negative rate in predicting RDS and therefore are unreliable.

If amniotic fluid is not available, L/S ratio or foam test can be done on gastric aspirate from infant during first 6 hrs of life if no milk has been given and the trachea is not occluded by intubation. Tracheal fluid or hypopharyngeal secretion can also be used.

Other Tests

◆ Phosphatidylglycerol content of >2% (0.5 μg/mL by new immunoagglutination kit) and phosphatidylinositol content of >15% in amniotic fluid indicate fetal lung maturity; they are not affected by contamination of amniotic fluid, maternal diabetes mellitus, or hemolytic disease of the newborn and are thus more sensitive measures than L/S ratio, although more laborious to perform (commercial rapid slide agglutination test is now available). Absence of both indicates high risk of RDS for at least 3–4 wks. Phosphatidylglycerol does not appear in amniotic fluid until after 36 wks' gestation; therefore absence has poor predictive value for RDS. If these values and L/S ratio are available, little is added by other measurements. However, the total profile of tests provides the most reliable results.

○ Measurement of optical absorbance at 650 nm to evaluate amniotic fluid turbidity; maturity criterion is a value of ≥ 0.1. Interference by blood, meconium, dilution due to oligo- or polyhydramnios. Corresponds to the gross pearly opalescence of mature amniotic fluid and to a count of lamellar bodies (derived from fetal lung) using automated platelet counter.

○ Nile blue sulfate staining of amniotic fluid differentiates fetal squamous cells from anucleated fat cells. Finding of >50% fat cells indicates mature fetus (40 wks) and also correlates with occurrence of RDS. Low counts should be interpreted with caution and correlated with other findings. *Maternal diabetes may cause spurious elevation of fat cell count.*

◆ Creatinine level of ≥ 2 mg/dL represents muscle mass of fetus and the presence of 1 million functioning glomeruli, and corresponds to pregnancy of ≥ 37 wks in >90%

of cases. Values of 1.6–2.0 mg/dL are considered equivocal. Value of <1.6 mg/dL indicates fetal weight of <2500 gms and <37 wks' gestation. May be decreased in mature but low-birth-weight infants. May be spuriously increased by hypertensive disorders of pregnancy (e.g., preeclampsia) and maternal renal disease; therefore maternal serum creatinine should also be determined. Ratio of maternal serum creatinine to amniotic creatinine ≥ 3 suggests gestational age of ~36 wks in 97% of cases. Urea and uric acid levels show more fluctuation and therefore are less useful than creatinine level.

○Bilirubin virtually disappears by 36 wks of gestation. May be increased due to maternal hyperbilirubinemia (e.g., hepatitis, hemolytic anemia, cholestasis) or to administration of drugs (e.g., phenothiazines), which makes the test useless. Meconium results in positive interference. Oligohydramnios may cause false-positive results and polyhydramnios may cause false-negative results.

♦Osmolarity of <250 mOsm/L indicates term pregnancy.

♦Lamellar bodies in amniotic fluid can be counted as platelets in electronic cell counter. A count of <30,000/μL has sensitivity of 100%, specificity of 64%, and negative predictive value of 100% as an indicator of lung maturity. At a count of 10,000/μL, specificity = 95%, sensitivity = 75%, and negative predictive value = 96%.[14]

These tests are valid indicators of fetal maturity (low false-positive rates) but less reliable indicators of immaturity (appreciable false-negative rates). In general, multiple tests give more reliable results than any single test.

GGT/ALP ratio of >2.0 in amniotic fluid has been reported to indicate pulmonary maturity.

Amniotic Fluid and Urine Differences

	Amniotic Fluid	Urine
Specific gravity	1.025	1.005–1.030
pH	Neutral or alkaline	Usually acid
Protein	Significant quantity	Absent
Urea	Similar to plasma	High
Bilirubin	May be present	Absent
Chloride	Moderate to high	Low to high
Creatinine	Similar to plasma	High
Uric acid	Similar to plasma	High
ALP	High	Low
Ascorbic acid	Low	Low to high

Fetal Death in Utero

♦Amniotic fluid may be brown with markedly increased CK level.

Intrauterine fetal death has been said to be reliably indicated by increased CK (usually >200 sigma U/mL; normal is <3 sigma U/mL).

DIC may occur, especially if gestation is >16 wks and dead fetus is retained for ≥ 4 wks.

Fibronectin, Fetal

(Secreted by chorionic trophoblast throughout pregnancy. Measured by ELISA or rapid test using cervicovaginal sample.)

Use

Indicator of risk of preterm labor/birth (level of >50 ng/mL).

Interpretation

Normally absent from cervicovaginal fluid after 20 wks. Normally present in early pregnancy and within 1–2 wks of onset of labor at term.

For high-risk patients, sensitivity = 70%, specificity = 75%.

---

[14]Dalence CR, et al. Amniotic fluid lamellar body count: a rapid and reliable fetal lung maturity test. *Obstet Gynecol* 1995;86:235.

GU

Hormones

Maternal Urine Estriol

Use

Reflects both placental and fetal adrenal cortex function and fetal liver function. Monitoring is usually begun at 34 wks but may begin at 28 wks in high-risk pregnancy (e.g., severe maternal hypertension, intrauterine growth retardation).

Interpretation

Reliable evaluation requires *serial* (rather than isolated) determinations (at least twice a week) to detect an abrupt fall. A decrease of ≥ 50% is generally considered significant, but level may be affected by variable maternal renal function.

24-hr urine level of estriol normally shows a progressive increase during gestation. *May show a 25% variation from day to day in an individual patient. Therefore two values in same direction are needed.*

>12 mg/24 hrs at term indicates a healthy neonate.

4–12 mg/24 hrs or decrease of >50% indicates infant in jeopardy.

<4 mg/24 hrs indicates fetal death or severe jeopardy.

Decrease Due To

Fetus

Intrauterine death

Fetal abnormalities (e.g., anencephaly, adrenal hypoplasia)

Placenta

Sulfatase deficiency

Infarcts

Placental dysfunction

Hydatidiform mole

Mother

Use of oral antibiotics (values may be two-thirds of normal)

Renal disease

Liver disease

Corticosteroid administration (values may be 50% of normal)

Incomplete urine collection

Laboratory

Mandelamine in urine (prevents bacterial splitting or reabsorption of estriol)

Plasma Progesterone and Urinary Pregnanediol (Its Chief Metabolite)

Increase progressively during pregnancy.

Reflect only adequate placental function but not fetal status.

Sexually Transmitted Diseases, Prenatal Screening

All pregnant women at first prenatal visit should have

Rapid plasma reagin test for syphilis

HBsAg test for HBV infection

Pap smear if not done in preceding year

HIV test should be offered

High-risk women should have

Test for *N. gonorrhoeae* at first prenatal visit and repeat test during third trimester

Test for *C. trachomatis* in third trimester

Neonatal Monitoring

Bacterial Infection in Neonates and Young Infants

◦Gram staining of gastric aspirate should be performed within 6 hrs of birth for any infant at risk of infection. Presence of PMNs and bacteria is suspicious for infection. Amniotic fluid Gram staining, culture, and tests for lung maturity in prenatal period may also indicate risk of infection.

ESR increase (normal value is <15 mm/hr on first day) is suspicious for infection but beware of false-positive results (e.g., DIC, Coombs'-positive hemolytic disease and Rh disease, clot in tube). CRP test has also been used.

Findings of total WBC of <5000/cu mm, total neutrophil count of <1000/cu mm, or >20% bands are consistent with infection. Decreased WBC may also occur with toxemia and increased WBC may also be associated with maternal use of glucocorticoids.

♦ Detection of bacterial antigen is most sensitive and specific test; urine, CSF, amniotic fluid, and blood (least desirable) can be used.

♦ Cultures of blood, CSF, and urine (do all three) and of tracheal aspirate. Do not use heel stick specimen for blood culture. Urine should be obtained by bladder tap or catheter.

♦ Abnormal urinalysis or CSF examination; but these are often normal in presence of infection.

♦ Gram stain preparation of buffy coat of spun Hct may show bacteria.

Platelet count of <100,000/cu mm.

Laboratory findings due to site of infection, e.g.,
- Pneumonia.
- Umbilical cord—staphylococci, gram-negative organisms.
- UTI—often same organism as in mother. Gram staining of unspun urine may identify organism. Colony count of >10,000/cu mm of one organism is diagnostic in bladder tap urine.
- Skin—staphylococci.
- Bone—staphylococci, group B streptococci, gram-negative organisms, gonococci, *Candida.*
- Joint—gonococci, gram-negative organisms, staphylococci, *Haemophilus influenzae.*
- GI tract—enteropathogenic *E. coli, Salmonella, Pseudomonas, Klebsiella, Enterobacter, Proteus, S. aureus, C. fetus,* viruses; *Shigella* is rare.
- Otitis media—*S. aureus,* gram-negative enteric bacteria.
- Indwelling catheter sites—*Candida,* staphylococci.
- Sepsis may be present with or without any of the following: group B streptococci, *E. coli, Listeria monocytogenes, Staphylococcus epidermidis,* anaerobes (including *Clostridium* and *B. fragilis*).
- Viral and parasitic infections—see p. 879.

Chromosome Analysis (Karyotyping), Indications

See p. 511.

High-Risk Infants, Recommended Laboratory Tests

(Approximately 3 infants per 100 deliveries; e.g., low-birth-weight infants, high-birth-weight infants, postmaturity infants, infants of high-risk mothers [those with toxemia, diabetes, drug addiction, cardiac or pulmonary disease], cases involving polyhydramnios, oligohydramnios, cesarean section delivery, infection, other major illnesses such as hepatitis, thyrotoxicosis)

Same tests as in newborn nursery

BUN

pH, pO_2, pCO_2

Neonatal Intensive Care, Recommended Laboratory Tests

(Approximately 3 infants per 1000 deliveries)

Same tests as for high-risk infants

Platelet count

PT

Blood total protein, phosphorus, magnesium

pH, Fetal Blood

When fetal scalp blood is acidotic, maternal acidosis should be differentiated from fetal acidosis, because maternal acidosis does not have the same serious implications. Base deficit and blood pH measurements are shown in Table 14-14. Fetal pH is usually ~0.04 units below maternal pH. pH of >7.25 is normal during labor; pH of 7.20–7.25 is worrisome, and another determination should be done promptly; pH of ≤ 7.20 suggests significant fetal hypoxia and need for prompt delivery.

Table 14-14. Base Deficit and Blood pH Measurements

	Maternal pH (mean)	Fetal pH (mean)	Base Deficit (mEq/L)
Normal mother and fetus	7.42	7.25	7.0
Normal mother and acidotic fetus	7.42	7.25	2.6
Acidotic mother and vigorous fetus	7.36	7.15	4.8

- After age of 3 hrs, sample of capillary blood from infant's warmed heel correlates well with arterial blood samples in measurements of acid-base status.
- In uncomplicated pregnancy umbilical cord blood pH has normal lower limit of 7.15. *Blood pH is the only objective measure available at delivery by which a diagnosis of asphyxia can be made.*
- In general, mean blood pH of 7.27 in the newborn is associated with an Apgar score of ≥ 7. Mean blood pH of 7.22 is associated with an Apgar score of ≤ 6. Fetal acid-base status is a valuable index of fetal asphyxia or oxygenation; should be evaluated with other evidence of fetal distress. Fetal blood pH provides best correlation with fetal outcome. In almost 20% of infants, the fetal acid-base status may be misleading (e.g., due to fetal scalp edema, contamination with amniotic fluid).

False Normal

(Normal blood pH but depressed infant function)

Due To
Medications administered
Obstetric manipulation (e.g., difficult forceps delivery)
Precipitous delivery
Prematurity (especially weight of <1000 gm with noncompliant lungs)
Congenital anomalies preventing normal onset of good lung function at birth (e.g., laryngeal web, choanal atresia, hypoplastic lungs associated with diaphragmatic hernia, edematous cyst of lung)
Aspiration syndromes
Previous episodes of asphyxia with resuscitation
Intrauterine infection

False Abnormal

Maternal acidosis is usual cause

Malformations, Congenital

2–3% of infants of >20 wks' gestational age have serious congenital malformations. Recognizable factors are present in ~50% of cases (e.g., genetic disorders, drugs, maternal conditions [e.g., diabetes mellitus])
Chromosomal analysis with banding (sterile tissues may include blood, skin, spleen, thymus, gonad) when multiple anomalies or other indications are present
Autopsy, photographs, bone radiography of infants in cases of stillbirth or neonatal death
TORCH (*Toxoplasma*, others, rubella, CMV, HSV) titers in presence of congenital heart defects, microcephaly, macrocephaly, cataracts, hepatomegaly, growth retardation
Most common sex chromosome abnormalities (e.g., 47 XXY, 47 XYY, 47 XXX) cannot be identified by physical examination.

Recurrent Risk of Some Common Birth Defects in Subsequent Pregnancies

Single mutant gene
    Autosomal dominant (e.g., Melnick-Needles syndrome, Holt-Oram syndrome)   50%
    Autosomal recessive (e.g., infantile polycystic kidney disease)   25%

Chromosomal abnormality (e.g., trisomy 21 or Down syndrome)	1%
Multifactorial inheritance (e.g., anencephaly-meningomyelocele, cleft lip, clubfoot, hypospadias, ventricular septal defect)	2–7%

Nuclear Sexing

See p. 515.

Evaluation of Sex Chromosome in Leukocytes

See p. 515.

Neonatal Screening

Disorder	Incidence
PKU	1:14,000
Iminoglycinuria	1:10,000
Cystinuria	1:15,000
Histidinemia	1:22,000
Hartnup disease	1:18,000
Genetic mucopolysaccharidoses	1:25,000
Galactosemia	1:62,000
Argininosuccinicacidemia	1:100,000
Cystathioninemia	1:100,000
Hyperglycinemia (nonketotic)	1:150,000
Fanconi's syndrome (renal)	1:150,000
Propionicacidemia	<1:300,000
Hyperlysinemia	<1:300,000
Hyperornithinemia	<1:300,000
Hyperprolinemia	<1:300,000
Maple syrup urine disease	1:224,000
Homocystinuria	1:230,000
Tyrosinemia	<1:500,000
Hypothyroidism	1:3600–1:4800
Cystic fibrosis of pancreas	1:2400 in United States and Western Europe
	1:90,000 in native Hawaiians
CAH (90% of cases are of	1:67,000 in Maryland
21-hydroxylase type)	1:490 in Yupik people of Alaska

Various genetic metabolic diseases are so often associated with certain clinical and laboratory findings that such clues should alert the physician to rule out these diseases.

Some Clinical Clues to Metabolic Diseases

- History of unexplained neonatal deaths in the family
- Mental retardation
- Coarse facial features, gargoylism
- Extensive candidal dermatosis
- Hypopigmentation
- Trichorrhexis nodosa
- Self-mutilation
- Renal stones
- Osteoporosis, osteomalacia, rickets

Such findings begin after an interval of good health.

They progress in absence of CNS disease, infection, or other acquired or congenital conditions and in spite of usual therapy, but improve after peritoneal dialysis or exchange transfusion.

Some Clinical Clues to Metabolic Diseases in Infants

- Neonatal jaundice, liver enlargement, failure to thrive, poor feeding, weight loss, vomiting, diarrhea, dehydration, lethargy, unusual color or odor to sweat or urine
- Overwhelming neonatal illness (e.g., organic acidemias)
- Sepsis

GU

- Coma
- Seizures
- Chronic hiccups
- Hypotonia
- Minor malformations
- Extensive monilial dermatosis
- History of early death in siblings

Conditions Associated with a Specific Urine Odor

Condition	Odor
Maple syrup urine disease	Maple syrup, burned sugar
Oasthouse disease	Brewery
Methylmalonic-, propionic-, and isovalericacidemia	Sweaty feet
Butyric/hexanoicacidemia	Sweaty feet
Tyrosinemia	Cabbage, fish
Trimethylaminuria	Stale fish
Hypermethioninemia	Rancid butter, rotten cabbage
PKU	Musty
Ketosis	Sweet
3-Oxothiolase deficiency	Sweet
3-Methylcrotonyl-CoA carboxylase deficiency	Cat urine
Hawkinsinuria	Swimming pool

Conditions Associated with a Positive Test for Reducing Substances in Urine

Condition	Involved Compound
Diabetes mellitus	Glucose
Essential fructosuria	Fructose
Fanconi's syndrome	Glucose
Galactokinase deficiency	Galactose
Galactosemia	Galactose
Hereditary fructose intolerance	Fructose
Pentosuria	Xylulose
Renal glycosuria	Glucose
Severe liver disease with secondary galactose intolerance	Galactose
Lactase insufficiency	Lactose
Alkaptonuria	Homogentisic acid
PKU, tyrosinemia	Phenolic compounds

Conditions Associated with a Positive Ferric Chloride Reaction in Urine

Condition	Color
PKU	Green
Tyrosinemia	Green, fading rapidly
Maple syrup urine disease	Gray-green
Oasthouse urine disease	Purple
Histidinemia	Blue-green
Alkaptonuria	Dark brown
Diabetic ketoacidosis	Cherry red
Melanoma	Black
Pheochromocytoma	Blue-green
Formiminotransferase deficiency	Gray-green
Drug intoxication (salicylates, phenothiazines, aminosalicylic acid)	Purple, red-brown, or green
Conjugated hyperbilirubinemia	Green

Conditions Associated with Crystalluria

Condition	Type of Crystal
Cystine storage disease	Cystine*
Cystinuria	Cystine*

Tyrosinemia   Tyrosine[†]
Xanthinuria   Xanthine
Orotic aciduria   Orotic acid

Cystine crystals are also found in WBCs, cornea, and rectal mucosa.
[†]*Cystine and tyrosine crystals are also found in marrow.*

Urinary calculi in older children
- Hyperuricemias
- Cystinuria
- Oxalosis
- Xanthinuria
- Deficiency of adenine phosphoribosyltransferase

Hypoglycemia
- Galactosemia
- Fructosemia
- Glycogen storage disease
- Glycerol tolerance
- Maple syrup urine disease
- Propionicacidemia
- Methylmalonicacidemia
- Tyrosinemia

Metabolic acidosis
- Galactosemia
- Hereditary fructose intolerance
- Glycogen storage disease
- Hyperalaninemic lactic acidosis
- Maple syrup urine disease
- Organic acidemias; rule out tubular acidosis

Ketosis
- Galactosemia
- Hereditary fructose intolerance
- Maple syrup urine disease
- Organic acidemias

Massive ketosis, especially in the presence of severe vomiting, is otherwise rare in neonates, even in juvenile diabetes.

Hyperammonemia
- Organic acidemias (infants usually have neutropenia, thrombocytopenia for first 12 mos of life, anemia for first month of life)
- Hyperammonemia syndromes

Increased serum indirect bilirubin
- Inborn errors of RBC metabolism, e.g., pyruvate-kinase deficiency or G-6-PD deficiency
- Crigler-Najjar syndrome
- Gilbert's syndrome
- Hypothyroidism

Increased serum direct bilirubin
- Rotor's syndrome
- Dubin-Johnson syndrome
- Galactosemia
- Hereditary fructose intolerance
- Alpha$_1$-antitrypsin deficiency

Coarse facial features
- Lysomal storage diseases, e.g., Hurler's syndrome
- Lipidoses, e.g., Gaucher's disease

Hepatomegaly is prominent in
- Lysomal storage diseases, e.g., mucopolysaccharidosis, mucolipidoses, glycoprotein storage diseases, gangliosidosis
- Lipidoses, e.g., Gaucher's disease, Niemann-Pick disease, Wolman's disease
- Disorders of carbohydrate metabolism, e.g., galactosemia, hereditary fructose intolerance, glycogen storage diseases
- Tyrosinemia
- Alpha$_1$-antitrypsin deficiency

GU

Feeding difficulties and vomiting are associated with many metabolic diseases but are most prominent with
- Protein intolerance, e.g., organic acidemias or hyperammonemia syndromes
- Carbohydrate intolerance, e.g., hereditary fructose intolerance
- Adrenogenital syndrome

Seizures
- Glycogen storage disease (hypoglycemia)
- Galactosemia
- Fructose intolerance
- Maple syrup urine disease
- Congenital lactic acidosis
- Vitamin D–resistant rickets
- Organic acidemias
- Urea cycle disorders
- Hyperglycemia
- Pyridoxine dependency

Premature Infants, Initial Management

Blood gases (pO_2, pCO_2, and pH) as often as indicated by baby's color, condition, and respiratory symptoms

Blood glucose at birth, 0.5, 1, 2, and 12 hrs to screen for hypoglycemia

Blood calcium measured on cord blood and after baby has become stable, especially if acidosis has occurred

Red Blood Cell Count, Nucleated

>10 nucleated RBCs is highly suggestive of fetal ischemic encephalopathy.[15]

Well-Baby Newborn, Recommended Routine Laboratory Tests

Hct, WBC, and differential

Urinalysis

Standard bacteriologic tests

Cord blood should be saved for 2 wks
- Blood type and hold until or if needed and Coombs' tests if mother is Rh negative or if jaundice develops by 24 hrs
- Serologic test for syphilis and for HBV if mother not tested antepartum
- Possible screening for *Toxoplasma* or viral infection if requested

Microchemistries: direct and total bilirubin, glucose, sodium, potassium, chloride, calcium

PKU and thyroid function tests (e.g., T_4 or TSH) for screening on day of discharge or follow-up at age 4 days.

[15]Phelan JP. Nucleated red blood cells: a marker for fetal asphyxia? *Am J Obstet Gynecol* 1995;173:1380.

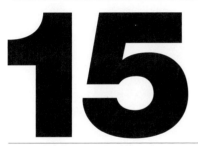

Infectious Diseases

Laboratory Tests for Infectious Diseases

Antibody Detection Tests

Bacteria

Bartonella henselae
Bordetella pertussis
Borrelia spp. (relapsing fever)
Borrelia burgdorferi (Lyme disease)
Brucella spp.
Clostridium botulinum toxin
Clostridium tetani toxin
Corynebacterium diphtheriae toxin
Escherichia coli O157 toxin
Francisella tularensis
Haemophilus influenzae type b
Helicobacter pylori
Legionella pneumophila
Leptospira spp.
Salmonella typhi
Treponema pallidum
Yersinia pestis

Viruses

Adenovirus
Colorado tick fever virus
Coronavirus
Coxsackieviruses A and B
Cytomegalovirus
Dengue virus
Eastern and Western equine encephalitis viruses
Echovirus
Epstein-Barr virus
Hantavirus
Hepatitis A, B, C, D viruses
Herpes simplex virus
Human herpesvirus (HHV) 6
Human immunodeficiency viruses (HIV) 1 and 2
Human T-lymphotropic viruses (HTLV)-1 and -2
Influenza A and B viruses
Lymphocytic choriomeningitis virus
Mumps virus
Parainfluenza virus
Parvovirus B19
Poliovirus
Reovirus

Respiratory syncytial virus
Rubella virus
Rubeola virus
St. Louis encephalitis virus
Varicella-zoster virus

Chlamydiae/Mycoplasmas

Chlamydia spp.
Mycoplasma pneumonia

Rickettsiae

Coxiella burnetii (Q fever)
Ehrlichia chaffeensis (ehrlichiosis)
Rickettsia typhi (murine typhus)
Rickettsia rickettsii (Rocky Mountain spotted fever)
Rickettsia tsutsugamushi (scrub typhus)

Fungi

Aspergillus spp.
Blastomyces dermatitidis
Candida spp.
Coccidioides immitis
Cryptococcus neoformans
Histoplasma capsulatum
Penicillium marneffei
Sporothrix schenckii
Zygomycetes

Parasites

Babesia microti
Echinococcus spp.
Entamoeba histolytica
Fasciola hepatica
Filariae
Giardia lamblia
Leishmania spp.
Paragonimus westermani
Plasmodium spp.
Schistosoma spp.
Strongyloides stercoralis
Taenia solium (cysticercosis)
Toxocara canis
Toxoplasma gondii
Trichinella spiralis
Trypanosoma cruzi

Antigen Detection Tests

Provide rapid, specific, reliable detection of certain bacterial antigens in virtually any body fluid obtained from the patient (CSF, serum, urine, joint). In bacterial meningitis, CSF is best specimen; urine is occasionally useful in establishing diagnosis; serum is usually not helpful. Sensitivity may be improved by testing serum and urine and CSF. Are especially valuable when patient has received antibiotics before cultures and Gram stain preparations are done and whenever smear and culture are negative. Unlike with cultures, results can be obtained within a few hours. Is most useful for identification of *H. influenzae* type b, *Streptococcus pneumoniae*, *Neisseria meningitidis* (groups A and C), group B *Streptococcus*. A negative test, however, does not unequivocally exclude infection due to that organism. Larger amounts of antigen correlate with more complications and poorer prognosis. *Cross reaction and nonspecific precipitation may occur with some antisera.*

For all of these tests, false-positives may occur due to the presence of a number of different organisms. False-negatives can occur early in disease; repeat specimens are often useful. Do not use grossly lipemic or hemolyzed specimens, which may give inaccurate results.

CIE is now largely replaced by latex agglutination. Other sensitive immunologic tests for rapid detection of specific antigens include coagglutination of *Staphylococcus aureus*, immunofluorescence, ELISA.

Other Organisms Detected Include

Bacteria
Bacillus anthracis
Bartonella henselae
Bordetella pertussis
Borrelia spp. (relapsing fever)
Borrelia burgdorferi (Lyme disease)
Brucella spp.
Chlamydia trachomatis
Clostridium difficile toxins A and B
Francisella tularensis
Klebsiella pneumoniae
Legionella spp.
Listeria monocytogenes in CSF
Mycobacterium tuberculosis
Neisseria gonorrhoeae
Pseudomonas aeruginosa
Staphylococcus aureus in pleural fluid
Trophermyma whippleii (Whipple's disease)
Yersinia pestis

Viruses
Adenovirus
Colorado tick fever virus
Coronavirus
Epstein-Barr virus
Hepatitis B, C viruses
Herpes simplex virus
Human papillomavirus
Human immunodeficiency virus 1
Human T-lymphotropic viruses 1 and 2
Influenza A virus
Virus of Jakob-Creutzfeldt disease
Parainfluenza virus
Parvovirus B19
Respiratory syncytial virus
Rotavirus
Varicella-zoster virus

Fungi
Candida spp.
Cryptococcus neoformans (meningitis) in CSF, urine, or serum
Pneumocystis carinii (pneumonitis)

Parasites
Cryptosporidium parvum
Entamoeba histolytica, especially in liver abscess material
Giardia lamblia
Taenia solium (cysticercosis)
Toxoplasma gondii
Trichinella spiralis

Bactericidal Titer, Serum

That dilution of serum able to kill >99.9% of the original bacterial inoculum in 18–24 hrs when patient is on antibiotic therapy (usually for bacterial endocarditis; has also been recommended for patients with osteomyelitis, septic arthritis, and empyema; patients receiving multiple antimicrobials; and immunosuppressed patients with sepsis). CSF or urine, instead of serum, has been used for bacterial meningitis and GU

INFECTIOUS

Table 15-1. Etiology of Bacteremia

Organism	% of Cases	Predisposing Factors
Staphylococcus epidermidis	34	Contaminated IV catheters, heart valve prostheses, shunts
Escherichia coli	22	GU indwelling catheters and instruments, perforated bowel, septic abortion
Staphylococcus aureus	15	Abscess, decubitus ulcer, osteomyelitis, staphylococcal pneumonia
Pseudomonas species	6	Burns, immunosuppressive chemotherapy
Alpha *Streptococcus*	6	Dental procedures, gum disease
Streptococcus pneumoniae	6	Alcoholism, chronic obstructive pulmonary disease, pneumococcal pneumonia
Bacteroides species	3.5	Trauma, GI or GU tract disease
Haemophilus influenzae	3	*H. influenzae* nasopharyngitis
Candida species	1.5	Burns, immunosuppressive chemotherapy, parenteral alimentation
Streptococcus pyogenes	1.4	Streptococcal pharyngitis/tonsillitis
Clostridium species	1.4	Septic abortion, biliary tract disease/surgery
Salmonella species	0.8	Contaminated food/water

One-third of staphylococcal bacteremias are primary; predisposing factors are decreased immune defenses (e.g., diabetes mellitus, neoplasms, steroid therapy, hemodialysis).

tract infections. Generally correlates with in vitro broth concentration that kills microorganism. Can also be used to determine serum inhibitory activity. Assays effect of antimicrobial level. Method is not standardized. Requires three days. Many doubt clinical value of test.

Beta-Lactamase Testing

(Iodometric, acidimetric, chromogenic cephalosporin methodologies)
Positive test
- Predicts resistance to penicillin, ampicillin, and amoxicillin among *Haemophilus* spp, *N. gonorrhoeae,* and *Moraxella catarrhalis.*
- Predicts resistance to penicillin and acylamino-, carboxy-, and ureidopenicillins among staphylococci and enterococci.

Cultures, Blood

See Table 15-1.
Perform as soon as possible after onset of chills or fever.
Perform before antimicrobial therapy is started.
Use resin-assisted blood cultures if patient is already on antimicrobial therapy.
Take two or three specimens for culture at least 30–60 mins apart if possible; shorter time interval if urgent need to begin therapy.
Take two or three cultures per septic episode or per 24-hr period.
Draw 20–30 mL of blood per culture.
Do not draw blood from IV catheter unless no vein sites are available or from umbilical artery catheter in infants.
Special methods should be used if suspected organisms are fungi or mycobacteria; routine methods yield negative results in 66% of cases of disseminated mycotic disease.
Use strict aseptic technique; contamination rate should be <3%/month.
Suspect contamination in the following cases:
- Only one of several cultures is positive (90% of cases).
- Type of organism.

True infection is almost always present if organisms are streptococci (nonviridans group), aerobic and facultative gram-negative rods, anaerobic cocci and gram-negative rods, yeasts (possible exception is *Candida tropicalis*).

Common contaminants are *Staphylococcus epidermidis, Bacillus* spp., *Propionibacterium acnes, Corynebacterium* spp., *Clostridium perfringens*, viridans streptococci, *C. tropicalis*.

Drug Monitoring, Therapeutic

See Table 19-1, p. 954.

Use

In cases in which margin between therapeutic and toxic concentrations is narrow, e.g., aminoglycosides, vancomycin.
Patients with renal failure.

Infectious Disease Indicators, Nonspecific

Acute-phase reactants (see pp. 50, 55)
Limulus lysate assay detects trace amounts of endotoxin from all gram-negative bacteria (including *E. coli, N. meningitidis, H. influenzae*). Presence in CSF is sensitive indicator of gram-negative bacterial meningitis, but rapid clearance from blood makes serum test unreliable. (See p. 270.)

Molecular Biology

(Techniques include nucleic acid amplification, DNA sequencing and typing, direct molecular probe [in situ hybridization], nucleic acid quantitation.)

Use

Cases requiring increased sensitivity and specificity of identification
Cases requiring faster report turnaround time (e.g., *M. tuberculosis*)
Confirmation of culture
Fastidious transport may not be required.
Identification of organisms that are nonviable or cannot be cultured (e.g., HBV, HCV, HPV, *Ehrlichia, T. whippleii*, parvovirus, astroviruses, caliciviruses)
Identification of fastidious, slow-growing organisms (e.g., *M. tuberculosis, Mycoplasma pneumoniae, Legionella pneumophila*, some pathogenic fungi)
Identification of organisms that are dangerous to culture (e.g., *F. tularensis*, HIV, *Brucella* spp., hemorrhagic fever viruses, *C. immitis, C. burnetii*)
Identification of previously unknown infectious agents
Identification of organisms present in small numbers (e.g., CMV in transplanted organs, HSV in CSF in encephalitis, HIV in antibody-negative patients) or in small-volume specimens (e.g., analysis of intraocular fluid for HSV, CMV, EBV, herpes virus, VZV; or forensic samples)
Density of amplifiable DNA correlates with microbial density (e.g., *Plasmodium vivax, B. burgdorferi, Chlamydia trachomatis*, HSV)
Monitoring of disease progression or initiation or modification of therapy (e.g., measure HIV viral load)
Drug susceptibility testing (e.g., detect resistance genes or mutations as in methicillin-resistant *Staphylococcus*)
Differentiation of antigenically similar organisms (e.g., HPV types 16 and 18 compared to types 6 and 11, which are associated with cervical cancer)
Molecular epidemiology and infection control (identify source of disease outbreak in hospital or community)
Disease diagnosis by characterization of genetic materials without direct identification of infectious agent (e.g., toxins of *Clostridium difficile* and *E. coli* O157:H7, staphylococcal toxic shock syndrome, staphylococcal enterotoxins, streptococcal pyogenic exotoxins)
Determination of virulence of antimicrobial resistance genes

Determination of relationship of organisms to neoplasms (e.g., relation of HHV-8 to Kaposi's sarcoma)

Other Organisms That Can Be Detected by Molecular Biology Techniques

(This list will certainly expand rapidly.)
Bacteria
Bordetella pertussis
Borrelia burgdorferi (Lyme disease)
Mycobacterium avium-intracellulare
Mycobacterium leprae
Neisseria gonorrhoeae
Neisseria meningitidis
Treponema pallidum
Viruses
Enteroviruses
Hepatitis A virus
Human T-lymphotropic viruses (HTLV)-1 and -2
Parainfluenza virus
Rhinovirus
Rotavirus
Rubella virus
Chlamydiae/Mycoplasmas
Chlamydia trachomatis
Mycoplasma hominis
Mycoplasma pneumoniae
Parasites
Babesia microti and *Babesia divergens*
Babesia-like organisms (*Pyroplasmas*)
Filariae (*Wuchereria bancrofti, Brugia malayi, Loa loa, Onchocerca volvulus*)
Histoplasma capsulatum
Leishmania donovani and *Leishmania braziliensis*
Plasmodium falciparum, Plasmodium malariae, and *Plasmodium vivax*
Toxoplasma gondii
Trypanosoma cruzi and *Trypanosoma brucei*
Fungi
Aspergillus spp.
Blastomyces dermatitidis
Candida spp.
Cryptococcus neoformans
Pneumocystis carinii
Staphylococcal *mec*A gene by PCR

Infectious Diseases

See Table 15-2.

Bacteria

Anaerobic Bacterial Infections

Frequently several anaerobic organisms are present simultaneously and are often associated with aerobic bacteria as well. If cultures from suspicious sites are reported as negative, the culturing for anaerobic organisms has not been performed properly.

Mixed aerobic-anaerobic infections are often successfully treated by suppressing only the anaerobes.

The most common anaerobic organisms cultured are *Bacteroides* and *Clostridia* spp. and streptococci.

The most commonly associated aerobic bacteria are the gram-negative enteric bacteria (*E. coli, Klebsiella, Proteus, Pseudomonas*, enterococci).

Table 15-2. Organisms Commonly Present in Various Sites

Site	Normal Flora	Pathogens
External ear	*Staphylococcus epidermidis* Alpha-hemolytic streptococci Aerobic corynebacteria *Enterobacteriaceae* spp. *Corynebacterium acnes* *Candida* spp. *Bacillus* spp.	*Pseudomonas* spp. *Staphylococcus aureus* Coliform bacilli Alpha-hemolytic streptococci *Proteus* spp. *Streptococcus pneumoniae* *Corynebacterium diphtheriae* *Aspergillus* spp. *Candida* spp. VZV HSV Papovavirus Molluscum contagiosum
Middle ear	Sterile	**Acute Otitis Media** *H. influenzae* *Streptococcus pneumoniae* *Moraxella catarrhalis* Beta-hemolytic streptococci Respiratory syncytial virus (RSV) Influenza viruses Enteroviruses Adenoviruses **Chronic Otitis Media** *Staphylococcus aureus* *Proteus* spp. *Pseudomonas* spp. Other gram-negative bacilli Alpha-hemolytic streptococci RSV Influenza virus
Nasal passages	*Staphylococcus epidermidis* *Staphylococcus aureus* Diphtheroids *Streptococcus pneumoniae* Alpha-hemolytic streptococci Nonpathogenic *Neisseria* spp. Aerobic corynebacteria	**Acute Sinusitis** *Staphylococcus aureus* *Streptococcus pneumoniae* *Klebsiella-Enterobacter* spp. Alpha-hemolytic streptococci Beta-hemolytic streptococci *Moraxella catarrhalis* **Chronic Sinusitis** *Staphylococcus aureus* Alpha-hemolytic streptococci *Streptococcus pneumoniae* Beta-hemolytic streptococci *Mucor, Aspergillus* spp. (especially in diabetics)
Pharynx and tonsils	Alpha-hemolytic streptococci *Neisseria* spp. *Staphylococcus epidermidis* *Staphylococcus aureus* (small numbers)	Beta-hemolytic streptococci *Corynebacterium diphtheriae* *Bordetella pertussis* *Neisseria meningitidis* *H. influenzae*

(*continued*)

INFECTIOUS

Table 15-2. (continued)

Site	Normal Flora	Pathogens
	Streptococcus pneumoniae	*Staphylococcus aureus*
	Nonhemolytic (gamma) streptococci	*Candida albicans*
		Respiratory viruses
	Diphtheroids	*Mycoplasma pneumoniae*
	Coliforms	*Neisseria gonorrhoeae*
	Beta-hemolytic streptococci (not Group A)	*Chlamydia pneumoniae*
	Actinomyces israelii	
	Haemophilus spp.	
	Marked predominance of one organism may be clinically significant even if it is a normal inhabitant.	
Epiglottis		*H. influenzae*
Larynx		Respiratory viruses
		Corynebacterium diphtheriae
		EBV (Infectious mononucleosis)
		Candida albicans
Bronchioli		RSV
Bronchi		*Mycoplasma pneumoniae*
		Viruses (e.g., influenza, rhinovirus, coronavirus, adenovirus)
		Corynebacterium diphtheriae
		Streptococcus pneumoniae
Lungs		Bacteria
		Pseudomonas aeruginosa
		E. coli
		Klebsiella pneumoniae
		Serratia marcescens
		Enterobacter spp.
		Staphylococcus aureus
		Proteus mirabilis
		Streptococcus pneumoniae
		H. influenzae
		Bordetella pertussis
		Mycoplasma pneumoniae
		Chlamydia pneumoniae
		Chlamydia psittaci
		Legionella pneumophila
		Pneumocystis carinii
		Tubercle bacilli
		Francisella tularensis
		Yersinia pestis
		Fungi (e.g., *Histoplasma, Coccidioides* in particular; *Blastomyces* spp., *Aspergillus* spp.)
		Viruses (e.g., influenza, parainfluenza, adenoviruses, RSV, echovirus, coxsackievirus, reovirus, CMV, viruses of exanthems, HSV, hantavirus)

Site	Normal Flora	Pathogens
		Rickettsiae (e.g., typhus, *Coxiella burnetii*)
		Protozoans (e.g., *Toxoplasma*, *Pneumocystis carinii*)
Gastrointestinal tract		
Mouth	Alpha-hemolytic streptococci	*Candida albicans*
	Enterococci	*Borrelia vincentii* with *Fusobacterium fusiforme*
	Lactobacilli	
	Staphylococci	
	Fusobacteria	
	Bacteroides spp.	
	Diphtheroids	
	Neisseria spp. (except *Neisseria gonorrhoeae*)	
Esophagus		*Candida albicans*
		CMV
		HSV
Stomach	Sterile	*Helicobacter pylori*
Small intestine	Sterile in one-third	*Campylobacter jejuni*
	Scant bacteria in two-thirds	*Helicobacter pylori*
	E. coli	
	Klebsiella-Enterobacter	
	Enterococci	
	Alpha-hemolytic streptococci	
	Staphylococcus epidermidis	
	Diphtheroids	
Colon	Abundant bacteria	Enteropathogenic *E. coli*
	Bacteroides spp.	*Candida albicans*
	E. coli	*Aeromonas* spp.
	Klebsiella-Enterobacter	*Salmonella* spp.
	Paracolons	*Shigella* spp.
	Proteus spp.	*Campylobacter jejuni*
	Enterococci (group D streptococci)	*Yersinia enterocolitica*
	Yeasts	*Staphylococcus aureus*
		Clostridium difficile
		Vibrio cholerae
		Vibrio parahaemolyticus
		Amebae and parasites
		Viruses (e.g., rotavirus, CMV, HSV, Norwalk)
Rectum		*Chlamydia* spp.
		Neisseria gonorrhoeae
		Treponema pallidum
		Lymphogranuloma venereum
		Enterobius vermicularis (anus)
Gallbladder	Sterile	*E. coli*
		Enterococci
		Klebsiella-Enterobacter-Serratia

(continued)

INFECTIOUS

Table 15-2. (continued)

Site	Normal Flora	Pathogens

		Occasionally
		  Coliforms
		  Proteus spp.
		  Pseudomonas spp.
		  Salmonella spp.

Blood	Sterile	*Staphylococci epidermidis*
		Staphylococci aureus
		E. coli
		Enterococci
		Pseudomonas spp.
		Alpha- and beta-hemolytic
		  streptococci
		Streptococcus pneumoniae
		H. influenzae
		Clostridium perfringens
		Proteus spp.
		Bacteroides and related
		  anaerobes
		Neisseria meningitidis
		Brucella spp.
		Pasteurella tularensis
		Listeria monocytogenes
		Achromobacter (Herellea) spp.
		Streptobacillus moniliformis
		Leptospira spp.
		Vibrio fetus
		Salmonella spp.
		Opportunistic fungi
		  Candida spp.
		  Nocardia spp.
		  Blastomyces dermatitidis
		  Histoplasma capsulatum

Eye	Usually sterile
	Occasionally small numbers
	  of diphtheroids and
	  coagulase-negative
	  staphylococci
		Staphylococcus aureus
		Haemophilus spp.
		Streptococcus pneumoniae
		Neisseria gonorrhoeae
		Alpha- and beta-hemolytic
		  streptococci
		Achromobacter (Herellea) spp.
		Coliform bacilli
		Pseudomonas aeruginosa
		Other enteric bacilli
		Morax-Axenfeld bacillus
		Bacillus subtilis (occasionally)
		Chlamydia spp.

Spinal fluid	Sterile	*H. influenzae* *Neisseria meningitidis* *Streptococcus pneumoniae* *M. tuberculosis*

Site	Normal Flora	Pathogens
		Staphylococci, streptococci
		Cryptococcus neoformans
		Coliform bacilli
		Pseudomonas and *Proteus* spp.
		Bacteroides spp.
		Listeria monocytogenes
		Leptospira
		Treponema
		Borrelia burgdorferi
		Viruses (e.g., coxsackie A and B, echovirus, HSV, mumps, HIV, VZV, lymphocytic, chorio-meningitis, CMV, adenovirus)
		Fungi (e.g., *Histoplasma capsulatum, Cryptococcus neoformans, Coccidioides immitis*)
		Free amoebas (e.g., *Naegleria, Acanthamoeba*)
Urethra, male	*Staphylococcus aureus*	*Neisseria gonorrhoeae*
	Staphylococcus epidermidis	*Chlamydia* spp.
	Enterococci	*Ureaplasma urealyticum*
	Diphtheroids	Enterococci
	Achromobacter wolffi (Mima)	*Gardnerella vaginalis*
	Bacillus subtilis	Beta-hemolytic streptococci (usually group B)
		Anaerobic and micro-aerophilic streptococci
		Bacteroides spp.
		Haemophilus ducreyi
		E. coli and *Klebsiella-Enterobacter*
		Staphylococcus aureus
Urethra, female, and vagina	Lactobacillus (large numbers)	Yeasts and *Candida albicans*
	Coli-aerogenes	*Clostridium perfringens*
	Staphylococci	*Listeria monocytogenes*
	Streptococci (aerobic and anaerobic)	*Gardnerella vaginalis*
		Trichomonas vaginalis
	Candida albicans	*Neisseria gonorrhoeae*
	Bacteroides sp.	*Chlamydia* spp.
	Achromobacter wolffi (Mima)	(See also Urethra, male.)
		Ureaplasma urealyticum
Prostate	Sterile	*Streptococcus faecalis*
		Staphylococcus epidermidis
		E. coli
		Proteus mirabilis
		Pseudomonas spp.
		Klebsiella spp.
		Anaerobic and microanaerophilic streptococci (alpha, beta, gamma types)
		Bacteroides spp.

(continued)

Table 15-2. (continued)

Site	Normal Flora	Pathogens
		Enterococci
		Beta-hemolytic streptococci (usually group B)
		Staphylococci
		Proteus spp.
		Clostridium perfringens
		E. coli and *Klebsiella-Enterobacter-Serratia*
		Listeria monocytogenes
Urine	Staphylococci, coagulase negative	*E. coli*
	Diphtheroids	*Klebsiella-Enterobacter-Serratia*
	Coliform bacilli	*Proteus* spp.
	Enterococci	*Pseudomonas* spp.
	Proteus spp.	Enterococci
	Lactobacilli	Staphylococci, coagulase positive and negative
	Alpha- and beta-hemolytic streptococci	*Providencia* spp.
		Morganella morganii
		Alcaligenes spp.
		Achromobacter (Herellea) spp.
		Candida albicans
		Beta-hemolytic streptococci
		Neisseria gonorrhoeae
		Mycobacterium tuberculosis
		Salmonella and *Shigella* spp.
Wound		*Staphylococcus aureus*
		Staphylococcus epidermidis
		Coliform bacilli
		Pseudomonas spp.
		Enterococci
		Streptococcus pyogenes
		Clostridium spp.
		Bacteroides spp.; other gram-negative rods
		Proteus spp.
		Achromobacter (Herellea) spp.
		Serratia spp.
Pleura	Sterile	*Staphylococcus aureus*
		Staphylococcus epidermidis
		Streptococcus pneumoniae
		H. influenzae
		Mycobacterium tuberculosis
		Anaerobic streptococci
		Streptococcus pyogenes
		E. coli
		Klebsiella pneumoniae
		Actinomyces spp.
		Nocardia spp.

Site	Normal Flora	Pathogens
Pericardium	Sterile	*Staphylococcus aureus*
		Streptococcus pneumoniae
		Enterobacteriaceae
		Pseudomonas spp.
		H. influenzae
		Neisseria meningitidis
		Streptococcus spp.
		Anaerobic bacteria
		Coccidioides immitis
		Actinomyces spp.
		Candida spp.
Peritoneum	Sterile	*E. coli*
		Enterococci
		Streptococcus pneumoniae
		Bacteroides spp.; other gram-negative rods
		Anaerobic streptococci
		Clostridium spp.
		Staphylococcus epidermidis
		Staphylococcus aureus
		Pseudomonas spp.
		Alpha-hemolytic streptococci
		Klebsiella pneumoniae
Bones	Sterile	**Acute Hematogenous**
		Staphylococcus aureus
		H. influenzae
		Streptococci (groups A and B)
		Neisseria gonorrhoeae
		Gram-negative bacilli (e.g., *Pseudomonas aeruginosa, Serratia marcescens, E. coli*)
		Mycobacterium tuberculosis
		Salmonella spp. in sickle cell disease
		Contiguous
		Anaerobic bacteria (e.g., *bacteroides*, fusobacteria, anaerobic cocci)
Joints	Sterile	*Staphylococcus aureus*
		Staphylococcus epidermidis
		Beta-hemolytic streptococci
		Streptococcus pneumoniae
		H. influenzae
		Klebsiella pneumoniae
		Gram-negative pathogens in newborns
		Salmonella spp. in sickle cell disease
		Neisseria gonorrhoeae
		Mycobacterium tuberculosis

(continued)

INFECTIOUS

Table 15-2. (continued)

Site	Normal Flora	Pathogens
		Mycobacterium kansasii
		Mycobacterium intracellulare
		Borrelia burgdorferi
		Viruses (e.g., mumps, rubella, HBV, parvovirus B 19)
		Fungi (e.g., *Candida, Sporothrix schenckii, Coccidioides immitis, Blastomyces dermatitidis*)
Skin	*Staphylococcus aureus* *Staphylococcus epidermidis*	*Staphylococcus aureus* (impetigo, folliculitis, furunculosis)
		Group A streptococcus (impetigo, erysipelas)
		Corynebacterium diphtheriae
		Bacillus anthracis
		Francisella tularensis
		Mycobacterium ulcerans
		Mycobacterium marinum
		Anaerobic bacteria
		Viruses (e.g., papillomavirus, varicella-simplex, HSV, molluscum contagiosum)
		Fungi (e.g., *Trichophyton, Microsporum, Epidermophyton, Actinomyces, Nocardia*)

○Anaerobic organisms should be sought especially in cultures from intraabdominal infections (e.g., bowel perforations, acute appendicitis, biliary tract disease), obstetric and gynecologic infections (e.g., pelvic abscess, Bartholin's gland abscess, and postpartum, postabortion, posthysterectomy infections), chest infections (e.g., bronchiectasis, lung abscess, necrotizing pneumonia), UTIs, soft tissue infections; anaerobes account for <5% of endocarditis cases (especially streptococci), 10% of cases of bacteremia.

○*Bacteremia due to anaerobic organisms is characterized by high incidence of jaundice, septic thrombophlebitis, and metastatic abscesses; the GI tract and the female pelvis are the usual portals of entry (in aerobic bacteremia, the GU tract is the most common portal of entry).*

Anthrax[1]

(Due to anthrax bacillus)
♦ Identification of gram-positive bacillus in material by Gram stain and culture from site of involvement.
- Pleural fluid from patients with pulmonary/mediastinal disease.
- Stool, vomitus, ascitic fluid (clear or purulent) from patients with intestinal disease.
- Blood from patients with bacteremia; culture almost always positive.
- Fluid from cutaneous lesions less useful diagnostically because test has only <65% sensitivity.
- Bloody CSF in meningitis.

[1]Dixon TS, Meselson M, Guillemin J, Hanna PC. Anthrax. *N Engl J Med* 1999;341:815.

♦ Serology
  • ELISA showing 4× increase in antibody titer against capsular antigens or exotoxin is diagnostic of past infection or vaccination.
  • Indirect microhemagglutination is similar.
  • In systemic infection, antibodies cannot be detected until late in course, which may be too late for treatment.
  • In treated infection, no increase in antitoxin antibody occurs.
♦ PCR methods for detection may soon become available.
♦ Anthraxin skin test is available to diagnose acute and previous cases of anthrax; 82% sensitivity 1–3 days after onset. Suitable for rapid diagnosis of acute cases and retrospective diagnosis.
WBC and ESR normal in mild cases; increased in severe cases.

Bacteroides Infection

This is usually a component of mixed infection with coliform bacteria, aerobic and anaerobic streptococci or staphylococci.
Local suppuration or systemic infection is secondary to disease of the female genital tract, intestinal tract, or tonsillar region.
Laboratory findings due to complications (e.g., thrombophlebitis, endocarditis, metastatic abscesses of lung, liver, brain, joint)
Laboratory findings due to underlying conditions (e.g., recent surgery, cancer, arteriosclerosis, diabetes mellitus, alcoholism, prior antibiotic treatment, and steroid, immunosuppressive, or cytotoxic therapy)

Bartonellosis

(Due to tiny fastidious gram-negative bacilli of genus *Bartonella*)
Cat-Scratch Disease
(Due to *Bartonella* [formerly *Rochalimaea*] *henselae* [causes ~85% of cases] and *Afipia felis* [causes ~15% of cases])
♦ Serologic tests: sensitivity = 84%, specificity = ~95%
  • EIA for detection of IgG antibodies to *B. henselae*; sensitivity; may be higher if test for IgM or paired sera are used.
  • IFA for *B. henselae* (≥ 1:64).
  • Antibodies react in serologic tests for *Chlamydia* and *Coxiella*.
♦ Organisms can be isolated from blood using special cultures and occasionally from tissue lesions. Usually impractical because bacilli are slow-growing, fastidious, poorly staining.
♦ PCR can detect organisms in blood, CSF, and tissue.
○ Histologic appearance of excised lymph node suggests this diagnosis and rules out other lesions; culture is often sterile. Organisms may be demonstrated by special stains and electron microscopy.
Skin tests are no longer used; low sensitivity.
ESR is usually increased.
WBC is usually normal but occasionally is increased ≤ 13,000/cu mm; eosinophils may be increased.
○ Blood cultures from infected cats may be positive for prolonged periods. Widely distributed among pet cats; transmitted by cat flea.
Laboratory findings due to organ involvement, e.g.,
  • Liver (e.g., increased serum GGT and ALP), peliosis in 25% of patients
  • Endocarditis
  • CNS (brain abscess, aseptic meningitis)

Bartonella (formerly *Rochalimaea*) *quintana* Infection
(Causes trench fever, cutaneous bacillary angiomatosis, and endocarditis)
♦ Blood culture may be positive in cases with bacteremia. Should be suspected in endocarditis when blood culture is negative. Reported to cause ~3% of cases of endocarditis.
♦ Species identification by direct immunofluorescence of isolate and DNA hybridization studies and analysis of restriction-fragment-length polymorphisms.
♦ Demonstration of *B. quintana* in heart valves or lymph nodes by Gram stain and identification by immunofluorescence and immunohistochemistry.
♦ Increased serologic IgG titer against *B. quintana*. Frequently cross-reacts with *Chlamydia* spp.

Oroya Fever
(Due to *Bartonella bacilliformis*; sand fly is vector.)
◆ Blood smears may show bacilli in ≤ 90% of RBCs (with Giemsa stain); they are also present in monocytes. Bacteria are also present in phagocytes of RE system.
◆ Blood culture is positive. (Use special enriched media.)
○ Sudden, very marked anemia is found.
Beware of secondary Salmonella *infection.*

Verruga Peruana
(Vascular proliferative phase of Oroya fever)
◆ Blood smears and blood cultures are positive for bacilli.
Moderate anemia is found.

Botulism

(Due to *Clostridium botulinum*)
CSF is normal.
Usual laboratory tests are not abnormal or useful.
◆ Diagnosis is made by injecting suspected food, serum, and stool intraperitoneally into mice, which die in 24 hrs unless protected with specific antiserum.
◆ Diagnosis of wound botulism by anaerobic culture of wound exudate or tissue sample in addition to serum toxin assay.

Brucellosis

(Due to *Brucella melitensis, Brucella suis,* and *Brucella abortus*)
◆ Serologic tests
  • Agglutination reaction becomes positive during second to third week of illness; 90% of patients have titers of ≥ 1:160. Rising titer is of diagnostic significance. False-negative results are rare. False-positive test results may occur with tularemia or cholera, with cholera vaccination, or after brucellin skin test. In chronic localized brucellosis, titers may be negative or ≤ 1:200. They may remain positive long after infection has been cured. Antibodies due to *Brucella canis* are not detected with the usual antigens; *B. canis* antigen must be used.
  • EIA is method of choice to detect specific IgM and IgG antibodies. Opsonophagocytic test and complement fixation (CF) test are not generally useful.
◆ Multiple blood cultures are more likely to be positive with high agglutination titer. (*B. abortus* requires 10% carbon dioxide for culture.)
◆ Bone marrow culture is occasionally positive when blood culture is negative. It may show microscopic granulomas.
○ Biopsy of tissue may show nonspecific granulomas suggesting a diagnosis of brucellosis. Tissue may be used for culture.
WBC is usually <10,000/cu mm, with a relative lymphocytosis. Decreased WBC occurs in one-third of patients.
ESR is increased in <25% of patients and usually in nonlocalized type of brucellosis.
Anemia appears in <10% of patients and usually with localized type of disease.
Liver function tests may be abnormal.

Campylobacteriosis

(Usually due to *Campylobacter jejuni*; few cases due to *Campylobacter coli* and *Campylobacter fetus*)
Clinical Types
Disseminated Form without Diarrhea
Meningitis—occurs in infants less than 2 mos old, usually premature or with congenital CNS defects; 50% mortality.
Pediatric bacteremia—rare disorder, usually secondary to malnutrition or diarrhea; patients usually recover.
Disseminated adult infection—patients commonly have predisposing conditions (e.g., immunosuppression, malignancy, cardiovascular, endocrine disease, etc.).
◆ • Blood culture is positive in 90% of cases.
◆ • IHA shows antibody titers of 1:1600–1:6400 in acute phase and 1:40–1:320 6 mos after cure.

Gastroenteritis

Most common bacterial cause in developed countries
- ♦ Stool culture using microaerophilic incubation and selective media
- ♦ Microscopic examination of stool shows "seagull" organisms. Few to moderate number of WBCs.

Stools become negative in 3–6 wks even without therapy, but 5–10% of patients have organisms in stool for a year or longer.

Blood culture positive in <1% of cases.

CF and EIA have good sensitivity and specificity and are used epidemiologically. High EIA titer may indicate recent or ongoing infection.

Chancroid

(Due to *Haemophilus ducreyi*)

○ Biopsy of genital ulcer or regional lymph node is helpful.
- ♦ Gram stain of smear from genital ulcer shows bacteria.
- ♦ Gram stain preparations and cultures of lymph node aspirate are usually negative; only after rupture is culture likely to be positive. Culture requires special media not widely available; sensitivity is ≤ 80%; limited practical value.

Serologic tests are not presently available. PCR test may become available.

Syphilis, AIDS, HSV infection, and granuloma inguinale should be ruled out in cases of ulcerative genital lesions (see separate sections).

Chlamydial Infections

(Obligate intracellular organism requires tissue culture but classified as a bacterium because contains both DNA and RNA.)

See Table 15-3.
- ♦ Serologic tests
  - Not useful for superficial infections; 4× rise in antibody titer between acute and convalescent sera may be useful in diagnosis of invasive and systemic infections, e.g., infantile pneumonia, pelvic inflammatory disease, lymphogranuloma venereum.
  - Microimmunofluorescence is not widely available; CF is used as alternative. Primarily used for diagnosis of lymphogranuloma venereum and psittacosis. Not useful for definitive diagnosis in most oculogenital infections.
  - In neonates, antibody may be derived from mother rather than due to neonatal infection. The only syndrome in which serologic tests are method of choice is neonatal pneumonia, in which high IgM levels should be diagnostic.

Genital Tract Infection

(Due to *C. trachomatis*; at least 10 major immunotypes)

See discussion of nonspecific urethritis, p. 757. Incidence of chlamydial cervicitis and urethritis is 10× greater than incidence of *N. gonorrhoeae* infection. 50% of patients with the latter have concomitant chlamydia infection. Most *C. trachomatis* genital infections are asymptomatic.
- ♦ Isolation in cell culture (obligate intracellular pathogen) is the most sensitive (≤ 90%) and specific (~100%) test but is technically difficult and test may not be easily available. Remains the gold standard. Culture requires sample of infected epithelial cells rather than discharges, urine, or semen. Longest turnaround time (2–3 days). Culture should be performed in cases of suspected sexual assault or abuse or when diagnosis is in dispute. Urethral culture increases the diagnostic sensitivity of a single endocervical culture by up to 20%.
- ♦ Serologic tests
  - Antigen detection provides high sensitivity and specificity by EIA of secretions (>79% and >95%, respectively) or staining of smears by direct immunofluorescence (>90% and >95%, respectively) in symptomatic patients or high-prevalence groups; positive and negative predictive values are >80% and >90% for EIA and >87% and >98% for direct immunofluorescence.
- ♦ Identification of intracytoplasmic inclusions by Giemsa or immunofluorescent staining of scrapings from genital lesions to detect elementary bodies within epithelial cells has low sensitivity but high specificity. Has been replaced by immunologic procedures.

Table 15-3. Methods for Diagnosis of Chlamydial Infections

Method	Application	Sensitivity/Specificity
Culture	All chlamydial infections; suspected sexual assault or abuse	Gold standard; most valuable $\leq 80\%$ sensitivity
Cytology	Inclusion conjunctivitis, trachoma.	~95% sensitivity
Serology	Invasive infection (pneumonia, psittacosis, lymphogranuloma venereum). Not for genital or superficial eye infections.	
Complement fixation	*Chlamydia psittaci* infection; not for infantile pneumonia.	
Microimmuno-fluorescence	Infantile pneumonia (IgM).	
Antigen detection		
Direct fluorescent antibody	Specimens from GU tract, conjunctiva, rectum, nasopharynx.	~75% sensitivity, 95% specificity
Enzyme immuno-assay	Specimens from GU tract, conjunctiva.	81% sensitivity, 99% specificity from endo-cervix; rapid turnaround
Nucleic acid hybrid-ization probes	Specimens from GU tract specimen.	Very high sensitivity and specificity
Amplification (PCR or ligase chain reaction)	Specimens from GU tract.	$\leq 100\%$ sensitivity and specificity

Note: Positive nonculture results should be verified by culture or another nonculture technology.

Diagnosis should be sought and tests performed for
- All symptomatic patients (e.g., those with acute urethritis, mucopurulent cervicitis, endometritis, pelvic inflammatory disease, acute proctitis, etc.).
- Asymptomatic women.
    Those in various high-risk groups
    Those with abnormal vaginal Pap smear
    IV drug abusers
    Pregnant women, specifically screening in cases of premature labor
    Those with high-risk sexual partners
- Tests should be performed on men in appropriate groups if resources permit; otherwise treat empirically.

Reiter's syndrome—*C. trachomatis* has been isolated from the urethra in $\leq 60\%$ of men with Reiter's syndrome, but tetracycline therapy does not change the clinical course, and causative role is speculative. (See p. 318.)

Acute proctitis—see pp. 195, 803.

Mucopurulent cervicitis—cervical material shows >10 PMNs/HPF (1000×) in non-menstruating women; positive culture or direct antigen test.

Acute urethral syndrome in women—pyuria with bacteriuria, positive culture or direct antigen test on specimen from cervix or urethra.

Pelvic inflammatory disease—findings of mucopurulent cervicitis, acute urethral syndrome; endometrial specimen may show positive culture or direct antigen test and endometritis on biopsy.

Perihepatitis—may show findings of pelvic inflammatory disease and high titer of IgM (44% of cases) or IgG antibody to *C. trachomatis*.

Increased WBC and ESR in <20% of patients.

Adult form of inclusion conjunctivitis is associated with genital tract infections.
- ◆ • Typical intracytoplasmic inclusions in epithelial cells on Giemsa-stained smears from conjunctival scrapings are found in 50% of cases. Immunofluorescent staining of inclusions has sensitivity of 70–95% and specificity of 98% for conjunctival lesions (sensitivity <50% in genital lesions). Inflammatory response shows both neutrophils and mononuclear cells, whereas viral conjunctivitis shows predominantly lymphocytes and allergic conjunctivitis shows predominantly eosinophils. Immunofluorescent stains are commercially available and significantly increase sensitivity.
- ◆ • Tissue culture of *Chlamydia* is the most sensitive and specific test and positive cultures are usually detectable within 48 hrs. Requires special techniques and may not be locally available.
- ◆ • Detection of antigen in secretions by EIA or direct immunofluorescent staining of smears.

Distinctive Pneumonia Syndrome of Infants
(Afebrile, chronic diffuse lung involvement, slight eosinophilia, distinctive cough)
The major cause of pneumonia before age 6 mos with incidence of 8 in 1000 live births.

Ophthalmia Neonatorum
Occurs in 18–50% of infants of mothers with genital infection (usually cervicitis); fathers often have urethritis.

Trachoma
(Due to *C. trachomatis* serotypes A, B, and C)
- ◆ Typical cytoplasmic inclusion bodies are in epithelial cells scraped from conjunctiva of upper eyelid (Giemsa stain).
- ◆ Preferred method of diagnosis is by presence of serum IgM or rise in IgG (EIA); is more sensitive than CF, which should no longer be used. Presence of IgM in infants with pneumonia is diagnostic of pneumonia due to *Chlamydia*.
- ◆ Detection of *Chlamydia* antigen (EIA, DFA) is becoming increasingly useful.
Secondary bacterial infection is common.

Psittacosis
(Due to *Chlamydia psittaci*)
- ◆ With compatible clinical illness, diagnosis is *confirmed* by
  - • Culture from respiratory secretions *or*
  - • Antibody increase ≥ 4× (to ≥ 1:32) by CF or microimmunofluorescence in paired specimens 2 wks apart *or*
  - • IgM detected by microimmunofluorescence titer of ≥ 1:16
- ◆ With compatible clinical illness, diagnosis is *probable* by
  - • Single antibody titer by CF or microimmunofluorescence of ≥ 1:32
Positive CF test in early stage is presumptive; is usually also positive with other *Chlamydia* species and sometimes with other infections (e.g., brucellosis, Q fever). Rise titer (≥ 4×) between acute and convalescent sera is diagnostic but not species specific. Microimmunofluorescence is species specific.
- ◆ Detection of IgM or rising IgG titer (EIA, IFA) indicates recent infection; IgM can be present for 4 wks after infection. May cross-react with *C. trachomatis* and lymphogranuloma venereum (LGV).
Tetracycline treatment can delay or diminish antibody response.
- ◆ Culture of sputum, pleural fluid, or clotted blood may be positive during acute illness before antimicrobial treatment; culture performed by few laboratories.
Cold agglutination test is negative.
Albuminuria is common.
Sputum smear shows normal flora.
WBC may be normal or decreased in acute phase and increases during convalescence.
ESR is increased or frequently is normal.

Respiratory Illness
(Due to *Chlamydia pneumoniae*)
Causes pharyngitis, tonsillitis, sinusitis, pneumonia similar clinically to *Mycoplasma* infection

Lymphogranuloma Venereum
(Due to serotypes L1, L2, L3 of *C. trachomatis*)
- ◆ High (≥ 1:32) or increasing (4×) CF titers or conversion of negative to positive results may indicate recent infection; also present in psittacosis.
  - • Fall in titer suggests therapeutic success in acute stage. Persistent negative results in the presence of disease are rare.

♦Detection of antibody by microimmunofluorescence

○Biopsy of regional lymph node shows stellate abscesses.

○Serum globulin is increased with reversed A/G ratio during period of activity.

Biologically false-positive reaction for syphilis that becomes negative in a few weeks appears in 20% of patients. If titer increases, beware of concomitant syphilitic infection.

WBC is normal or increased by <20,000/cu mm. Relative lymphocytosis or monocytosis may be seen.

ESR is increased.

Slight anemia may be present.

Cholera

(Due to *Vibrio comma*)

♦Stool culture is positive.

♦Identification by immunofluorescence, dark-field microscopy, and phase-contrast microscopy of motile vibrios in stool that are immobilized by specific antisera allows rapid specific diagnosis.

♦Serologic tests

- EIA for antitoxin antibodies shows ≥ 4× increase in titer in paired sera. Increases by 12 days; increase may persist for months. Does not occur due to vaccination. May cross-react with some *E. coli* enterotoxins. Not positive with nontoxigenic strains of *Vibrio cholerae*.
- Direct agglutination and vibriocidal antibody tests show ≥ 4× rise in titer in >90% of patients; vaccination also elicits vibriocidal antibodies. Agglutination detects nontoxigenic strains.

Laboratory findings due to marked loss of fluid and electrolytes

- Loss of sodium, chloride, and potassium
- Hypovolemic shock
- Metabolic acidosis
- Uremia

Infections Due to Other *Vibrio* Species

(Short, curved, gram-negative bacilli; at least 10 species are pathogenic for humans; often difficult to classify; most are found in marine or estuarine water.)

Causes three types of infection.

Gastroenteritis Infection

Contracted from eating uncooked seafood, especially oysters or clams. Some forms (e.g., due to *Vibrio vulnificus*) may rapidly progress to bacteremia with 50% fatality rate. Due to *V. cholerae*, others (e.g., *Vibrio vulnificus, Vibrio alginolyticus, Vibrio fluvialis, Vibrio parahaemolyticus*)

Wound Infection

Usually associated with seawater (e.g., contracted while fishing or swimming). 20% mortality rate. Often rapidly progress to bacteremia. Superficial localized type of wound infection of eyes, ears, skin due to *V. alginolyticus*.

Systemic Infections

Occurs in presence of preexisting disease (e.g., due to *V. vulnificus, V. hollisae*)

V. vulnificus septicemia occurs most often (75% of cases) in patients with iron overload (e.g., hemochromatosis, thalassemia major, cirrhosis).

Clostridial Gas Gangrene, Cellulitis, and Puerperal Sepsis

(Due to *Clostridium perfringens, Clostridium septicum, Clostridium novyi*, etc.)

WBC is increased (15,000 to >40,000/cu mm).

Platelets are decreased in 50% of patients.

In postabortion sepsis, sudden severe hemolytic anemia is common.

Hemoglobulinemia, hemoglobinuria, increased serum bilirubin, spherocytosis, increased osmotic and mechanical fragility, etc., may be associated.

Protein and casts are often present in urine.

Renal insufficiency may progress to uremia.

♦Smears of material from appropriate sites show gram-positive rods, but spores are not usually seen and other bacteria are often also present.

♦Anaerobic culture of material from appropriate site is positive. *Clostridia are frequent contaminants of wounds caused by other agents. Other bacteria may cause gas formation within tissues.*

Coliform Bacteria Infections

(*Escherichia coli, Enterobacter-Klebsiella* group, paracolon group)
Bacteremia

Secondary to infection elsewhere; occasionally due to transfusion of contaminated blood

Secondary to debilitated condition in 20% of patients (e.g., malignant lymphoma, irradiation or administration of anticancer drugs, steroid therapy, cirrhosis, diabetes mellitus)

Early diagnosis and treatment reduces mortality.

Polymicrobial in 6–21% of cases. Higher mortality than when due to one organism. Most common sources are GI tract and intravascular site. Most often mixed gram-negative; occasionally gram-negative and gram-positive; mixed gram-positive organisms are infrequent.

Shock due to infection with gram-negative bacteria occurs in 20–40% of patients.
- Increased serum potassium.
- Decreased serum sodium.
- Metabolic acidosis.
- Increased serum amylase (decreased renal perfusion)
- Renal findings due to shock (e.g., oliguria, proteinuria, azotemia, acute tubular necrosis). Renal insufficiency in sepsis without shock may be due to GN, interstitial nephritis, bacterial endocarditis, etc. (see appropriate separate chapters).
- Hematologic findings: leukocytosis with shift to left, Döhle's bodies, toxic granules, eosinopenia. DIC occurs in 10% of cases, usually associated with shock.
- ARDS with hypoxemia; tachypnea (an early sign) is usually associated with respiratory alkalosis; metabolic acidosis is much less common and occurrence is usually late.
- GI manifestations: stress ulcers of stomach with or without bleeding; mild cholestatic jaundice with increased bilirubin (up to 10 mg/dL), mildly increased ALP, and increased AST may occur several days before positive findings on blood cultures or clinical recognition of infection.
- Hypoglycemia is relatively uncommon; hyperglycemia in diabetics may be early clue to infection.
- Infection is most frequently from GU tract, GI tract, uterus, lung (in that order).
- *E. coli* is the most frequent organism; it causes the lowest mortality (45%) and the lowest incidence of shock. *P. aeruginosa* infection has the highest mortality (85%). *Klebsiella-Enterobacter*, paracolon bacilli, and *Proteus mirabilis* infections are intermediate, with 70% mortality.

GU Tract Infection
(75% of cases due to *E. coli*)
Wound Infections, Abscesses, etc.

Sepsis Neonatorum
(Bacterial infection during the first 30 days of life with primary involvement of blood and, frequently, meninges)

◆ Positive blood culture—*E. coli* and *Klebsiella-Enterobacter* cause ~75% of cases. Group B and group D streptococci and *L. monocytogenes* cause most of the other cases. May also be caused by a large variety of other bacteria. *Incidence of contaminated blood cultures is high in newborns. Negative blood culture does not rule out this condition; cultures should be taken from umbilical stump, skin lesions, mucous membranes, urine.*

◆ Positive culture of CSF occurs frequently. *No WBC increase may be seen early in the course of the disease.*

WBC is variable; leukopenia is often associated with a high mortality.

Anemia and decreased platelets may be present.

Laboratory findings due to involvement of other organs (e.g., kidney, with albumin, cells, or casts increased in urine; liver, with increased direct or indirect bilirubin)

Gastroenteritis

Verotoxin-producing *E. coli*—associated with two separate diseases.
- Hemolytic-uremic syndrome and hemorrhagic colitis
- O157:H7 (primarily from undercooked beef; also raw milk, apple cider, roast beef; especially in elderly and children). Most common cause of renal failure in children.

◆ Specific enteropathogenic strains identified by genetic probes (especially O157:H7 serotype). Is an important cause of hemolytic-uremic syndrome in children and TTP in adults.

Enterotoxigenic *E. coli*—toxins cause cholera-like secretory diarrhea in Third-World countries.

Enteroinvasive *E. coli*—causes inflammation of colon; resembles bacillary dysentery.

Enteropathogenic *E. coli*—diarrhea in infants and children

Infections of Intestinal Tract and Biliary Tree

E.g., appendicitis, cholecystitis

Pneumonia

(1% of primary bacterial pneumonias due to *Klebsiella* [Friedländer's bacilli], especially in alcoholics.)

WBC is often normal or decreased.

♦ Sputum is very persistent, brown or red ("currant jelly"). Smear shows encapsulated gram-negative bacilli. (*Gram stain of sputum in lobar pneumonia allows prompt diagnosis of this organism and appropriate therapy.*) Bacterial culture confirms diagnosis. Bacteremia in 25% of cases of *Klebsiella* pneumonia.

Laboratory findings due to complications (lung abscess, empyema) or underlying diseases

Rarely, chronic lung infection due to Klebsiella simulates tuberculosis.

Colitis, Pseudomembranous

(Antibiotic-associated diarrhea and colitis due to *Clostridium difficile* toxins A and B)

♦ Toxin detected in stool in >95% of patients with pseudomembranous colitis but may also be found in some asymptomatic patients or those with uncomplicated diarrhea.
  • EIA has sensitivity of 72–84%.
  • Tissue culture assay is 10% more sensitive.

Fecal leukocytes in stool (see p. 165)

Recent antibiotic exposure (especially to cephalosporin) followed in >6 days by onset of diarrhea (often semiformed stool).[2]

Diphtheria

(Due to *Corynebacterium diphtheriae*)

♦ Smear from involved area stained with methylene blue is positive in >75% of patients.

♦ Culture from involved area is positive within 12 hrs on Loeffler coagulated serum medium (more slowly on blood agar) (toxin-producing strain). *If antibiotic therapy has been given earlier, culture may be negative or organisms may take several days to grow.* Penicillin G eliminates *C. diphtheriae* within 12 hrs; without therapy, organisms usually disappear after 2–4 wks.

♦ Fluorescent antibody staining of material from involved area provides more rapid diagnosis, with a higher percentage of positive results.

WBC is increased (≤ 15,000/cu mm). If >25,000/cu mm are found, a concomitant infection (e.g., hemolytic streptococcal) is probably present.

Albumin and casts are frequently present in urine; blood is rarely found.

Moderate anemia is common.

Decreased serum glucose occurs frequently.

Laboratory findings of peripheral neuritis are present in 10% of patients, usually during second to sixth week. Increased CSF protein, which may be prolonged.

Laboratory findings of myocarditis (which occurs in up to two-thirds of patients)

Serologic tests (EIA) are used for epidemiologic studies or to assess immune function by comparing pre- and postimmunization sera. Toxoid antibody by EIA of ≥ 0.1 U/mL indicates immunity and eliminates need for antitoxin; titers decrease with age. Cannot be used for diagnosis.

Dysentery, Bacillary

(Due to *Shigella* spp.)

♦ Stool culture is positive in >75% of patients. Rectal swab test can also be used.

Microscopy of stool shows mucus, RBCs, and WBCs.

Serologic tests are not useful. EIA and PCR techniques are not available.

WBC is normal.

Blood cultures are negative.

---

[2]Manabe YC, et al. *Clostridium difficile* colitis: an efficient clinical approach to diagnosis. *Ann Intern Med* 1995;123:835.

Laboratory findings due to complications
- Marked loss of fluid and electrolytes (hyponatremia, hypokalemia, hypoproteine-mia, hypoglycemia).
- Intestinal bleeding.
- Relapse in 10% of untreated patients.
- Carrier state.
- Acute arthritis—especially in untreated disease due to *Shigella shigae* (culture of joint fluid negative).
- Hemolytic-uremic syndrome may occur in severe infections.

Glanders

(Due to *Malleomyces mallei*)
♦ Culture or animal inoculation of infected material from appropriate sites is performed.
○ Agglutination and CF tests are positive in chronic disease.
WBC is variable.

Gonococcal Infections
Genital Infection
(See also Sexually Transmitted Diseases, pp. 757.)
♦ Gram stain of smear from involved site, especially urethra, prostatic secretions, cervix, site of pelvic inflammatory disease. Consider smear positive only if *intracellular* gram-negative diplococci are found; presence of extracellular gram-negative diplococci is considered equivocal, correlates poorly with culture results, and should always be confirmed with culture. Smear is positive in only 50% of asymptomatic patients; culture should always be performed for asymptomatic patients. *Smear may become negative within hours of antibiotic therapy.* In women, positive results on Gram stain preparation has sensitivity of 45–65% for specimen obtained from endocervical canal and 16% for specimen from urethra with >90% specificity; smears from vagina, anal canal, and pharynx are not recommended. Gram stain of specimen from urethra has sensitivity and specificity of >95% in symptomatic men, and sensitivity of 69% and specificity of 86% in asymptomatic men; Gram stain of specimen from anal canal has sensitivity of 57% and specificity of >87%.
♦ Bacterial culture (*use special media such as Thayer-Martin*) should always be taken at the same time (before beginning antibiotic therapy). In ~2% of male patients, Gram stain of urethral exudate is negative when a simultaneous culture of the same material is positive.
♦ Fluorescent antibody test on smear of suspected material
♦ Detection of antigen (EIA) in centrifuged sediment of urine has sensitivity of >80% and specificity of >97%. Antigen detection is sensitive and specific for urethral infection in men but less sensitive than culture in women. Present methods are useful for screening high-risk patients when distant from the laboratory and should be considered presumptive. Confirm with culture if there are medicolegal implications.
♦ DNA probe tests appear to be highly sensitive and specific but have not yet been sufficiently evaluated; present recommended use is to confirm cultures, especially in low-risk patients.
Coexistent *C. trachomatis* infection is present in 20–60% of cases.
Beware of concomitant inapparent venereal infection, which may be suppressed but not adequately treated by antibiotic therapy of gonorrhea.
Proctitis
Is symptomatic in ~5% of cases (see also pp. 195, 798).
Gram-stained smears are not sufficiently reliable because of presence of nonpathogenic *Neisseria* species; not recommended unless mucopurulent exudate is present.
♦ Bacterial culture on special media (e.g., Thayer-Martin) is required for confirmation; avoid fecal contamination.
Rectal biopsy shows mild and nonspecific inflammation. In a few cases, Gram stain of tissue section may reveal small numbers of gram-negative intracellular diplococci after prolonged examination.
♦ *Rectal gonorrhea accompanies genital gonorrhea in 20–50% of women and is found without genital gonorrhea in 6–10% of infected women. Therefore rectal cultures for Gonococcus should be taken in all suspected cases of gonorrhea.*

Oropharyngeal Infection
Is present in 10% of women and 20% of homosexual men.
♦ Bacterial cultures are required for diagnosis; Gram-stained smears are not suffi-
ciently reliable because of presence of nonpathogenic *Neisseria* species.

Arthritis
Synovial fluid (see Table 10-4, p. 309).
  • Variable; may contain few WBCs or be purulent.
♦ • Gonococci identified in approximately one-third of patients.
Gonococcal CF test for differential diagnosis of other types of arthritis
  • Not a reliable test in urethritis but may rarely be helpful in arthritis, prostatitis,
    and epididymitis. Becomes positive at least 2–6 wks after onset of infection,
    remains positive for 3 mos after cure. If test is negative, it should be repeated; two
    negative tests help to rule out *Gonococcus* infection. False-positive test may occur
    after *Gonococcus* vaccine has been used. Test is of limited value and is seldom used.
Associated nonbacterial ophthalmitis in ≤ 20% of patients

Ophthalmitis of the Newborn

Acute Bacterial Endocarditis
Toxic hepatitis is common.
Gonococcus is the most common bacteria infecting tricuspid or pulmonic valves.

Bacteremia
Resembles meningococcemia; occurs in 1–3% of patients. CNS and cardiac infection
occur in 1% of these cases. Only 40% of blood cultures are positive. Gram stain of skin
lesions may be useful.

Peritonitis and Perihepatitis after Spread from Pelvic Inflammatory Disease
♦ Cultures should always be done on specimens from contacts of known cases of gonorrhea, for suspected extragenital gonorrhea, and to evaluate cure. Cultures for test of
cure should be from all sites cultured before therapy and from both endocervix and anal
canal in women 3–4 days after treatment; if pharynx culture was positive, at least 2 post-
therapy cultures should be taken from this site due to difficulty in eradicating bacteria
from the pharynx.

Granuloma Inguinale

(Due to gram-negative intracellular bacterium *Calymmatobacterium granulomatis*)
♦ Wright- or Giemsa-stained smears of lesions show intracytoplasmic Donovan bodies
in large mononuclear cells in acute stage; they may be present in chronic stages.
♦ Biopsy of lesion shows suggestive histologic pattern and is usually positive for Dono-
van bodies in acute stage; they may also be seen on crush preparation.
Cultures are not useful for routine diagnosis as organisms cannot be cultured on stan-
dard media.
No serologic tests are available.
Serologic tests and dark-field examination for syphilis are negative unless concomitant
infection is present.

Helicobacter pylori Infections[3]

**(Due to spiral urease-producing microaerophilic gram-negative rod formerly clas-
sified as *Campylobacter pylori*)**
H. pylori gastritis is found in ≤ 95% of persons with duodenal ulcer (except in Z-E syndrome due to neoplasia), 80% of those with non–NSAID-induced gastric ulcer, 60% of
persons with gastric cancer. Found in >50% of persons over age 50; 1 in 6 infected
persons eventually develops peptic ulcer disease. Questionable association with nonul-
cer dyspepsia. Lifetime risk of gastric carcinoma is 1–3%; lymphoma is less frequent.
♦ Endoscopic antral biopsy for histology, culture, urease test, PCR.
  • Histologic demonstration of the organism. Superficial chronic active gastritis is
    almost characteristic of *H. pylori* infection even if organism is not identified, and
    absence excludes infection (sensitivity = 95%; specificity = 80%).

---

[3]Fennerty MB. A review of tests for the diagnosis of *Helicobacter pylori* infection. *Lab Med*
1998;29:561.

- Kit for rapid urease test uses gastric biopsy specimens (urease converts urea in kit to ammonia, changing pH indicator color) (sensitivity and specificity = 90–95%).
- Culture of antral biopsy specimen (sensitivity = >90%, specificity = 100%). Can be used to determine antibiotic resistance.

♦ Nonendoscopic (noninvasive) tests

- Serologic tests for IgG antibodies to *H. pylori* (now available in rapid kit form) by ELISA (sensitivity and specificity <95%) indicate infection unless antibiotic therapy has been given. Titer slowly decreases; cannot be used for 46 mos to determine cure. Does not distinguish current and past infection. IgA and IgM testing are not recommended.
- Antigen in stool (rapid EIA test) detects active infection.
- Urease breath tests using oral ^{14}C- or ^{13}C-labeled urea (radiolabeled C measured in breath before and after ingestion is produced in presence of *H. pylori* urease). Can determine if infection is active and ascertain if therapy has been successful. Represents global sample of gastric mucosa. Test of choice to determine cure in patients with complicated ulcers or recurrent symptoms. Should wait 5–10 mins before collection to avoid false-positive results due to mouth flora.
- Tests for antibodies in saliva and urine are inferior to serum tests.
- Tests presently used in research settings are PCR of antral biopsy, gastric juice and saliva, detection of IgG in saliva, measurement of serum ^{13}C-bicarbonate after ingestion of ^{13}C-labeled urea, stool culture, fecal antigen.

Except for serology assays, tests may be falsely negative if patient has taken antibiotics, bismuth, or proton-pump inhibitors recently.

All of these tests have >90% sensitivity and ≤ 100% specificity.

Routine monitoring for eradication after therapy is not presently recommended unless symptoms recur or ulcer is complicated.

Haemophilus influenzae Infections

Strains	Type of Infection
Type B	
Encapsulated	Meningitis, bacteremia, pneumonia, otitis, epiglottitis, cellulitis
	Occurs mainly in children
Non–type B	
Nonencapsulated	Bronchitis, sinusitis, otitis
	Bacteremia and meningitis are rare
	Occurs in children and adults
Types A, C, D, E, F	
Encapsulated	Similar to nonencapsulated; less common

Increased WBC (15,000–30,000/cu mm) and PMNs

♦ Positive blood culture in ~50% of patients with meningitis

♦ Latex agglutination test can detect type B bacterial capsular antigen in CSF and urine. Has replaced CIE due to ease, speed, and high specificity (see Chapter 9, p. 282).

Presence of non–B strain (especially unencapsulated) in CSF may indicate immunodeficiency or defect in meninges.

Infants aged <1 yr commonly have empyema, bacteremia, and meningitis concomitantly; therefore CSF should always be examined in infants with empyema.

Legionnaire's Disease

(Due to *Legionella pneumophila*, a gram-negative bacillus that is a facultative aerobic, intracellular, opportunistic pathogen widely disseminated in the environment; at least 12 serogroups are known.)

♦ Optimal diagnosis combines culture, detection of antigen and DFA or PCR of sputum, BAL fluid, or pleural fluid, and detection of antigen in urine.

♦ Organism may be cultured in 3–7 days on special media from pleural fluid, lung biopsy specimen, transtracheal or bronchial aspirate, blood; isolate can then be identified only by special tests (e.g., DFA).

♦ DFA may demonstrate the organism in sputum, pleural fluid, or lung, or other tissue within 2–3 days of onset of clinical disease; is extremely useful for rapid specific diagnosis (sensitivity = ~70%). May be negative with few organisms present in early or mild cases or after erythromycin treatment. Hence negative test is of little value and does not substitute for culture. Specificity is >88% compared to culture or serologic tests.

♦ Urinary antigen assay is 90% sensitive and 100% specific; antigen can be detected for weeks after acute illness. Detects only serogroup 1, which accounts for large majority of cases.

♦ PCR can detect *Legionella* in urine, serum, BAL fluid. Used on clinical specimens or culture material; reported sensitivity = 74% and specificity = 100%. Detects all species; rapid. Negative result does not exclude diagnosis.

♦ IFA (allows detection of IgM versus IgG antibody), ELISA

Titers of <1:64 are considered negative. Single titers of 1:64–1:256 suggest prior infection at undetermined time. Single IFA titer of >1:256 is strong presumptive evidence. Antibody titers (IFA, ELISA or agglutination) show fourfold increase to 1:128 in two-thirds of patients in 3 wks and in all patients in 6 wks and such a finding is evidence of recent infection; most useful for retrospective diagnosis or epidemiologic study but too late for clinical use.

Gram stain of sputum shows few to moderate number of PMNs; bacteria are not seen because *Legionella* stains poorly in clinical specimens.

○ Pleural effusion may be bilateral in ≤ 50% of patients; usually small exudates; culture and test for antigen (as in urine) should be performed.

WBC = 10,000–20,000/cu mm in 75% of cases; leukopenia is a bad prognostic sign.

Mild to moderate increase of serum AST, ALP, LD, or bilirubin is found in ~50% of patients. Hypoalbuminemia of <2.5 gm/dL.

○ Decreased serum phosphorus and sodium occurs in ~50% of patients.

○ Diagnosis should be suspected in pneumonia patients with decreased serum phosphorus, abnormal liver function tests, and bradycardia.

Proteinuria occurs in ~50% of patients; microscopic hematuria.

Renal failure and DIC are unusual complications.

CSF is normal.

Leprosy (Hansen's Disease)

(Due to *Mycobacterium leprae*)

♦ Acid-fast bacilli are found in smear or tissue biopsy from nasal scrapings or lepromatous lesions. Acid-fast diphtheroids are not infrequently found in nasal septum smears or scrapings in normal persons, and *M. leprae* is not found here in two-thirds of early lepromatous cases. Therefore nasal smear may have very limited diagnostic value. Bacilli may show a typical granulation and fragmentation that precede the clinical improvement due to sulfone therapy. Larger, more nodular lesions are more likely to be positive. During lepra reactions, enormous numbers of bacilli may be present in skin lesions and may be found in peripheral blood smears. Bacilli are usually very difficult to find in skin lesions of tuberculoid leprosy.

○ Histologic pattern of the lesions is used for classification of type of leprosy.

Laboratory findings due to complications

○ • Amyloidosis occurs in 40% of patients in the United States.
   • Other diseases (e.g., TB, malaria, parasitic infestation) may be present.
   • Sterility due to orchitis is very frequent.

○ False-positive serologic test for syphilis occurs in ≤ 40% of patients.

Mild anemia. Sulfone therapy frequently causes anemia, which indicates that dosage change is needed.

ESR is increased.

Serum albumin is decreased, and serum globulin is increased.

Serum cholesterol is slightly decreased.

Serum calcium is slightly decreased.

Leptospirosis

(Most frequently due to *Leptospira icterohaemorrhagiae*, *Leptospira canicola*, and *Leptospira pomona*)

♦ Blood and CSF cultures may be positive during first 10 days of disease in ≤ 90% of patients.

♦ Urine culture may be positive after first week and only intermittently; culture is difficult because of contamination and low pH. Culture is rarely positive after the fourth week.

♦ Serologic tests
   • ELISA to detect IgM may be positive in 4–5 days. An increasing titer ($\geq 4\times$ in 2 wks) is diagnostic.
   • Microscopic agglutination test shows $4\times$ increase between acute and convalescent sera. Probable positive result is titer of $\geq 200{:}1$. Is standard for serologic diagnosis but difficult to perform and not widely available (refer to Centers for Disease Control and Prevention via state health departments).
   • CF has been used for screening; may become positive in 10–21 days; positive results should be confirmed by agglutination because of cross reaction with HAV, CMV, scrub typhus, and *Mycoplasma* antibodies.
♦ PCR can quickly establish diagnosis. Useful for epidemiologic studies.
Normochromic anemia is present.
WBC may be normal or $\leq 40{,}000$/cu mm.
ESR is increased.
Urine is abnormal in 75% of patients: proteinuria, WBCs, RBCs, casts.
○ Liver function tests are abnormal in 50% of patients.
   • Increased serum bilirubin, ALP, reversed A/G ratio.
   • Increased AST and ALT, but average levels are not as high as in hepatitis.
○ *Increased CK in one-third of patients during first week may help to differentiate condition from hepatitis.*
○ CSF is abnormal in cases with meningeal involvement (less than two-thirds of patients).
   • Increased cells (≤ 500/cu mm), chiefly mononuclear type.
   • Increased protein (≤ 80 mg/dL).
   • Glucose and chloride normal.
   • Organisms are not found in CSF.
Dark-field examination of body fluids is not helpful.
Laboratory findings due to complications (e.g., renal failure, hemorrhage)

Listeriosis

(Due to *Listeria monocytogenes*)
May occur during pregnancy, especially in third trimester, and may cause amnionitis, septic abortion, bacteremic flulike syndrome, etc. Usually asymptomatic or mild during pregnancy. Infection of adult nonpregnant patients is associated with debilitated or immunocompromised condition. No screening test available.
♦ Neonatal infection from maternal infection
   • Meningitis
      Purulent CSF with 100–10,000 WBCs/cu mm; 70% show preponderance of PMNs; protein is usually increased; glucose is normal in 60% of cases. Gram stain is positive in <20% of cases but cultures are usually positive. Negative Gram stain and monocytic response may lead to misdiagnosis as viral infection, syphilis, Lyme disease, TB, etc. Positive blood cultures in 60–75% of cases. CNS involvement without meningitis is based on blood cultures, as <50% of CSF cultures are positive.
   • Granulomatosis infantisepticum: abscesses or granulomas of viscera may occur (e.g., endophthalmitis, septic arthritis, osteomyelitis, liver abscess, pleuropulmonary infection).
   • Increased WBC and other evidence of infection.
   • Gram stain of meconium may show gram-positive bacilli. *This test should be done whenever mother is febrile before or at onset of labor.*
♦ Diagnosis requires isolation of organism from a normally sterile site (e.g., blood).
♦ Isolation of pure culture from food may require days to weeks. Monoclonal antibodies or nucleic acid hybridizations do not require pure culture; they identify the genus but are not specific for *L. monocytogenes*.
♦ Serologic tests
   • CF showing $\geq 4\times$ rise in titer after absorption of reactive sera with *S. aureus* to remove cross-reacting agglutinins. Titer of <1:8 has high predictive value.
   • EIA for specific antibodies, antigen detection in CSF are under development.
Laboratory findings due to bacteremia, endocarditis (in presence of underlying cardiac lesion), skin infection, etc.
Epidemic cases are usually food borne. Food role in sporadic cases is unknown. Foodborne organism present in feces of some healthy persons.

Lyme Disease

(Due to *Borrelia burgdorferi*; primary tick vector is *Ixodes dammini* in northeast United States and *Ixodes pacificus* in western United States.)

Stage 1: ~1 wk (varies from 3 to 33 days) after tick bite; nonspecific febrile "viral syndrome"; ≤ 85% of patients have characteristic erythema migrans rash. Serologic test is not helpful or necessary because it is only 40–60% sensitive at this stage and diagnosis is not ruled out by a negative test. Early antibiotic treatment often prevents antibody response. Antibiotic therapy is critical to prevent long-term involvement of various organs.

Stage 2: 4 wks after tick bite, 10% of patients develop cardiac involvement (causes most deaths); 15% have neurologic findings (triad of aseptic meningitis, Bell's palsy, and peripheral neuropathy is very suggestive).

Stage 3: 6 wks to several years after tick bite; occurs in 60% of untreated cases, principally as arthritis, frequently mistaken as juvenile RA.

Reinfection causing recurrence of clinical disease is recognized.

♦ Diagnostic Criteria

Isolation of organism from clinical specimen *or*

Diagnostic titers of IgG and IgM in serum or CSF *or*

Significant change in serum titers of IgG or IgM in paired acute- and convalescent-phase sera.

Serologic Tests

Recommended protocol is ELISA (sensitivity = 89%, specificity = 72%) or IFA, which should be confirmed by Western blot (immunoblot). Assays for IgM, IgG, or both.

Interpretation

Serologic tests should be ordered *only* to support clinical diagnosis; not for screening of persons with nonspecific symptoms. Is generally not clinically useful if pretest probability is <0.20 or >0.80. If probability is <0.20, positive ELISA is more likely to be false-positive than true-positive. If probability is >0.20, positive ELISA rules in diagnosis of Lyme disease.

A positive serological test does not necessarily indicate current infection or establish the diagnosis and a negative serological test, especially within 2 wks of onset of symptoms, should not be the only basis for excluding diagnosis.

Specific IgM antibodies usually appear 2–4 wks after erythema migrans, peak after 3–6 wks of illness, decline to normal after 4–6 mos; positive in only 40–60% of stage 1 cases. In some patients, IgM remains elevated for many months or reappears late in illness, which predicts continued infection. IgM titer of ≥ 1:200 is considered positive. IgM titer of 1:100 is considered indeterminate. IgM of <1:100 is considered negative. A negative test within 2 wks of onset of symptoms does not rule out infection.

IgG titers rise more slowly (appear ~4–8 wks after rash), peak after 4–6 mos, may remain high for months or years, even with successful antibiotic therapy. Almost all patients with complications of stages 2 and 3 have positive IgG on first specimen. A single increased IgG titer indicates only previous exposure but not timing of infection or cause of current symptoms. IgG titer of ≥ 1:800 is considered positive, titer of 1:200–1:400 is indeterminate, titer of <1:100 is considered negative.

Paired acute and convalescent sera at 4–6 wk intervals showing conversion or significant rise in titer indicate infection and are principally useful in evaluating ill patients who have no known tick bite or rash who have been in an area where the disease is endemic.

Interferences (ELISA)

Presence of RF may cause false-positive result for IgM.

False-positive IgG in high titers may be due to antibodies from spirochetal diseases (syphilis, relapsing fever, yaws, pinta); low titers may be found in patients with infectious mononucleosis, hepatitis B, autoimmune diseases (e.g., SLE, RA), periodontal disease, ehrlichia, rickettsia, or other bacterial infections (e.g., *H. pylori*), and in 5–15% of normal persons in areas of endemic disease.

Low concordance between results using different test kits.

Western blot test is more sensitive and specific than ELISA and is used to distinguish true-positive and false-positive ELISA results, to confirm an indeterminate ELISA result, or to evaluate an undiagnosed antibiotic-treated patient, and is the present gold standard; positive results on Western blot test indicate past or current infection. However, Western blot results may not become positive until the patient has been ill for many months; when Western blot results are negative, test should be repeated in 2–4 wks if Lyme disease is strongly suspected. Test is expensive, limited in availability, technically difficult, and not standardized, and there are many cross-reacting antibodies.

True seronegativity is uncommon with disseminated or chronic Lyme disease. Serologic tests cannot judge therapeutic efficacy or provide test of cure (unlike the VDRL test for syphilis). Absence of titer does not rule out Lyme disease.

♦ Antigen detection in urine, blood, and tissue and use of PCR to identify specific DNA in blood, CSF, joint fluid, skin biopsy, urine. Reported sensitivity = 35%, specificity = 100%; not yet widely evaluated.

♦ Culture may take several weeks; organism is infrequently found even when special stains are used in known positive tissues. Low yield except in biopsy of erythema migrans lesions (60–80% sensitivity), which is rarely necessary.

T-cell proliferative assay needs further evaluation.

Organism is not detected in peripheral smears.

Laboratory findings due to organ involvement

- Neurologic: 80% of patients with meningitis may show increased lymphocytes (up to 450/cu mm), increased protein and IgG, oligoclonal bands. May have encephalitis (tends to involve white matter), myelitis, radiculitis, cranial or peripheral neuritis in various combinations.
    - ♦ Intrathecal antibody may be demonstrated by higher titer in CSF than in serum. IgG and IgM may be present in CSF but not in serum. Almost all of these patients have positive serologic tests.
- Arthritis: joint fluid may show increased WBC (up to 34,000/cu mm), PMNs (≤ 96%), and protein (up to 6.6 gm/dL).
    - ♦ Lyme antibodies in fluid differentiates this from other arthritides.
- Diffuse fasciitis with eosinophilia

Nonspecific findings of mild increase in ESR, lymphopenia, cryoglobulinemia, mild increase in AST, increased serum IgM, etc.

Fluorescent treponemal antibody absorption test (FTA-ABS) may be positive but nontreponemal tests (VDRL, rapid plasma reagin) should be nonreactive.

Morphologic changes in tissues are not specific.

Coinfection with *Babesia* may occur.[4,5]

Melioidosis

(Due to *Pseudomonas pseudomallei*)

♦ Culture or animal inoculation of infected material (e.g., pus, urine, blood, sputum) from appropriate sites is performed.

♦ Serologic tests

- EIA for IgG antibodies is >90% sensitive and specific; EIA for IgM is 92% sensitive for active disease and can be used to monitor therapy.
- Agglutination test results are positive in chronic disease; infection can be inactive for many years. Results may be negative in fulminant septicemic form.

WBC is normal or increased.

Infection is occasionally transmitted among narcotic addicts using needles in common.

Meningococcal Infections

Clinical syndromes

- Meningococcemia.
- Meningitis (see p. 282)—CSF must be examined in all suspected cases of meningococcal disease; >90% of adults with meningococcal infections have meningitis.
- Waterhouse-Friderichsen syndrome occurs in 3–4% of cases (see p. 640).

♦ Gram-stained smears of body fluids

- Tissue fluid from skin lesions

[4]Tugwell P, et al. Laboratory evaluation in the diagnosis of Lyme disease. *Ann Intern Med* 1997;127:1109.
[5]Brown SL, et al. Lyme disease test kits: potential for misdiagnosis. *FDA Medical Bulletin* 1999;Summer/3.

- Buffy coat of blood
- CSF
- Nasopharynx
♦ Culture (use chocolate agar incubated in 10% carbon dioxide)—blood, CSF, specimens from skin lesions, nasopharynx, other sites of infection; may take ≤ 1 wk to grow.
♦ Latex agglutination and counterimmune electrophoresis (see p. 783)
♦ Only microbiological methods are specific; other findings are nonspecific.
CSF (see Table 9-1, p. 264)
- Markedly increased WBC (2500–10,000/cu mm), almost all PMNs.
- Increased protein (50–1500 mg/dL).
- Decreased glucose (0–45 mg/dL).
♦ • Positive smear and culture. Gram stain results are diagnostic in 50–70% of patients with positive cultures. Pyogenic meningitis in which bacteria cannot be found in smear is more likely to be due to *Meningococcus* than to other bacteria.
♦ • Detection of antigen by EIA has >80% sensitivity and >95% specificity; is especially useful if antibiotic therapy has begun before CSF is obtained.
Increased WBC (12,000–40,000/cu mm)
Urine—may show albumin, RBCs; occasional glycosuria
Laboratory findings due to complications (e.g., DIC, myocarditis) and sequelae (e.g., subdural effusion)
Laboratory findings of predisposing conditions such as asplenic condition (e.g., sickle cell anemia) or IgM immunodeficiency

Mima-Herellea Infections

♦ Bacteria are isolated from appropriate sites (e.g., blood, CSF, sputum).
Often associated with IV catheters or cutdowns

Moraxella (Branhamella) Catarrhalis Infections

(Formerly *Micrococcus catarrhalis* and *Neisseria catarrhalis*)

Acute Purulent Tracheobronchitis and Pneumonia

○ Sputum shows many WBCs and intracellular gram-negative diplococci.
Increased WBC (~15,000/cu mm)
May also cause bacteremia (usually with pneumonia), otitis media, sinusitis.

Mycoplasma pneumoniae Pneumonia

(Epidemics every 4 to 6 yrs; also endemic and sporadic)
Serologic tests
♦ • IgM (EIA) increases in 1 wk, begins to decrease in 4–6 mos, and may persist ≤ 1 yr; sensitivity = 75–80%, specificity = 80–90%. May also be associated with other infections, neoplastic and connective tissue diseases. IgG indicates previous exposure. Presence of IgM (>1:64) or 4× rise in IgG indicates recent infection. Are preferred tests; both should be performed in acute-phase and convalescent-phase (2–4 wks) sera.
- 4× increase in CF titer occurs in ~50% of patients; increase begins in 7–9 days, peaks at 3–4 wks, may last for 4–6 mos, then gradual fall is seen for 2–3 yrs. If only a convalescent serum is available, a titer of ≥ 1:32 is suggestive of diagnosis of *M. pneumoniae* infection. False-positive result may occur in acute inflammatory diseases (e.g., bacterial meningitis, pancreatitis).
♦ • Antigen detection by immunoblotting, RNA detection by hybridization, and PCR are not routinely available. Detection by PCR may not indicate current disease; serologic tests should be used to distinguish acute from persistent infections.
- Increased cold hemagglutination occurs late in course in 35–75% of patients (≤ 90% in severe illness); becomes positive at approximately seventh day, rises to peak at 4 wks, then declines rapidly and usually is negative by 4 mos. Specificity <50%. May be present in other conditions (see pp. 42–43). Not very helpful diagnostically.
♦ Culture of organism by special techniques may require 7–10 days. Sensitivity is >90%; specificity is 50–90%. Isolates need DNA probe for speciation. Difficult to interpret as may persist in throat after infection.

WBC is slightly increased (in 25% of patients) or is normal.
ESR is increased in 65% of patients.
M. hominis may cause pyelonephritis, PID, and postpartum febrile complications (see
p. 759). *Mycoplasma* infection should also be considered in the differential diagnosis
of acute arthritis, hemolytic anemia, various dermatologic disorders, myocardial or
cerebral disease, and severe bilateral pneumonia.

Pasteurella Multocida Infections

♦ Gram stain and culture of bacteria from appropriate sites (e.g., blood, skin, CSF).
WBC is increased.

Pertussis (Whooping Cough)

(Due to *Bordetella pertussis/Bordetella parapertussis*)
○Marked increase in WBC (≤ 100,000/cu mm; usually 12,000–25,000/cu mm) and ≤ 90%
mature lymphocytes
♦ Positive cultures from nasopharynx or cough plate differentiate organisms; 20% of
cases show positive cultures. Cultures may be positive only during catarrhal and early
paroxysmal stage.
Negative blood cultures
♦ Serologic tests
  • Presence of serum IgM and IgG (EIA) establishes diagnosis from first sample in
    75% of cases; paired sera are needed before 6 mos of age. IgM may persist for
    months after infection or vaccination.
  • Direct agglutination test (correlates with IgG) usually requires paired acute- and
    convalescent-phase sera taken 2–4 wks apart; persists after illness; insensitive in
    infants <6 mos old.
  • Detection of antigen on nasopharyngeal smears or serum by DFA or CIE is avail-
    able; poor diagnostic sensitivity.
♦ Laboratory diagnosis requires that both paired sera and culture be positive.

Plague

(Due to *Yersinia pestis*)
♦ Identify bacteria by smear, culture, fluorescent antibody technique, or animal inoculation
of suspected material from appropriate site (e.g., lymph node aspirate, blood, sputum).
Serum hemagglutination antibodies are present.
WBC is increased (20,000–40,000/cu mm), with increased PMNs.

Pneumococcal Infections

(Due to *Streptococcus pneumoniae*)
Pneumonia
Increased WBC (usually 12,000–25,000/cu mm) with shift to the left; normal or low
WBC in overwhelming infection, in aged patients, or with other causative organisms
(e.g., Klebsiella)
♦ Blood culture positive for pneumococci in 25% of untreated patients during first 3–4 days.
♦ Gram stain of sputum—many PMNs, many gram-positive cocci in pairs and singly;
direct *Pneumococcus* typing using Neufeld's capsular swelling method rarely done now.
♦ Pleural effusion in ~15% of patients
Laboratory findings due to complications (endocarditis, meningitis, peritonitis, arthri-
tis, empyema, etc.)
Endocarditis
See p. 114.
Meningitis
Is the most common cause of meningitis in adults and children > 4 yrs old. See p. 283,
Table 9-3. Laboratory findings due to associated or underlying conditions (pneumo-
coccal pneumonia, endocarditis, otitis, sinusitis, multiple myeloma)
Peritonitis
Positive blood culture
Increased WBC

♦Ascitic fluid—identification of organisms by Gram stain and culture; see pp. 166–169.

○*Increased susceptibility to* Pneumococcus *infection in hyposplenism (e.g., post-splenectomy, sickle cell disease, congenital abnormalities of spleen, children with nephrotic syndrome)*

Proteus Infections

Proteus infections usually follow other bacterial infections.
* Indolent skin ulcers (decubital, varicose ulcers)
* Burns
* Otitis media, mastoiditis
* Urinary tract infection
* Bacteremia

Characteristic spreading growth on culture plate may obscure associated bacteria because Proteus *infection frequently is part of mixed infection; antibiotic sensitivity testing may not be possible.*

Pseudomonas Infections

Occur in various sites.
Associated with
Replacement of normal bacterial flora or initial pathogen because of antibiotic therapy (e.g., in urinary tract, ear, lung)

Burns

Debilitated condition of patient (e.g., premature infants, the aged, patients with leukemia)

♦Bacteremia is most common in patients with acute leukemia; usually acquired in hospital.

   Overall mortality ~40%.

* Laboratory findings due to associated factors (e.g., shock and pneumonia each occur in one-third of patients).
* Shock, pneumonia, persistent neutropenia are each associated with poorer prognosis.
* Positive blood culture is usually (80% of cases) only one time.

Decreased WBC during bacteremia in patients with leukemia or burns is more frequently due to Pseudomonas *than to other gram-negative rods.*

Relapsing Fever
(Endemic due to *Borrelia hermsii* transmitted by *Ornithodoros* tick or epidemic due to *Borrelia recurrentis* transmitted by human body louse)

♦Identification of organism by
* Wright, Giemsa, or acridine orange stain of peripheral blood smear or buffy coat or dark-field or phase-contrast microscopy of plasma wet mounts (platelet fraction) during febrile episode have sensitivity of >70%.
* Intraperitoneal injection of rats.
* Culture on special medium is most specific but is not widely performed.

♦Serologic tests
* 4× rise in titer between acute- and convalescent-phase sera.
* IFA using monoclonal antibody has been reported.
* Biological false-positive serologic test for syphilis in ≤ 25% of patients.

Increased WBC (10,000–15,000/cu mm); moderately increased ESR; thrombocytopenia

Protein and mononuclear cells sometimes increased in CSF

Laboratory findings due to complications (e.g., hemorrhage, rupture of spleen, secondary infection)

Salmonella Infections

Typhoid Fever
(Due to *Salmonella typhi*)

♦Diagnosis is based on culture.
* Blood cultures are positive during first 10 days of fever in 90% of patients and during relapse; cultures are positive for <30% after third week.

- Stool cultures are positive after tenth day, with increasing frequency up to fourth or fifth week, in <50% of cases. Positive stool culture after 4 mos indicates a carrier; occurs in 3% of cases.
- Urine culture is positive during second to third week in 25% of patients, even if blood culture is negative.

Serologic criteria for diagnosis of ≥ 4× increase in O titer in unvaccinated patients in nonendemic areas is rarely useful. Serologic diagnosis is unreliable and Widal's test has been largely abandoned for these reasons:

- Positive Widal's test may occur because of typhoid vaccination or previous typhoid infection; nonspecific febrile disease may cause this titer to increase (anamnestic reaction). False-positive may occur in autoimmune diseases.
- Early treatment with chloramphenicol or ampicillin may cause titer to remain negative or low.
- Increase in O titer may reflect infection with any organism in the group D salmonellae (e.g., *Salmonella enteritidis, Salmonella panama*) and not just *Salmonella typhi*.
- Because of differences in commercially manufactured antigens, a 2× to 4× difference may be seen in O titers on the same sample of serum tested with antigens of different manufacturers.
- Measurement of H titer is very variable and may show nonspecific response to other infections; it is therefore of little value in diagnosis of typhoid fever.
- >10% of cases in endemic areas are seronegative.
- EIA and DNA probes continue to be developed.

WBC is decreased—4000–6000/cu mm during first 2 wks, 3000–5000/cu mm during next 2 wks; ≥ 10,000/cu mm suggests perforation or suppuration.

Decreased ESR is found.

Normocytic anemia is frequent; with bleeding, anemia becomes hypochromic and microcytic.

Laboratory findings due to complications

- Increased serum LD, ALP, and AST are frequent; increased CK occurs in some patients.
- Intestinal hemorrhage is occult in 20% of patients, gross in 10%; it occurs usually during second or third week. It is less frequent in treated patients.
- Intestinal perforation occurs in 3% of untreated patients.
- Relapse occurs in ≤ 20% of patients, usually 1–2 wks after defervescence.
  Blood culture becomes positive again.
  Widal's test titers are unchanged.
- Secondary suppurative lesions (e.g., pneumonia, parotitis, furunculosis) are found.
- Abnormal liver function tests (e.g., serum bilirubin, AST) occur in ~25% of patients as an incidental finding. Hepatitis is the chief clinical feature in ~5% of patients.

Enteritis
♦Stool culture remains positive for 1–4 wks, occasionally longer.
WBC is normal.

Paratyphoid Fever
(Usually due to *Salmonella paratyphi* A or B or to *Salmonella choleraesuis*)
♦Cultures of blood and stool and decreased WBC show same values as indicated in preceding section.

Bacteremia
Especially due to *S. choleraesuis*
♦Blood cultures are intermittently positive.
Stool cultures are negative.
WBC is normal. It increases (≤ 25,000/cu mm) with development of focal lesions (e.g., pneumonia, meningitis, pyelonephritis, osteomyelitis).

Local Infections
Meningitis, especially in infants
Local abscesses with or without preceding bacteremia or enteritis
One-third of patients are predisposed by underlying disease (e.g., malignant lymphoma, SLE). Nontyphoid strains are recognized with increasing frequency as causes of opportunistic infection in AIDS. Patients with GI salmonellosis at risk for AIDS should be treated with antibiotics even in absence of bacteremia.
Bacteremia and osteomyelitis are more common in patients with sickle hemoglobinopathy. Bacteremia is more common in patients with acute hemolytic Bartonella infection.

Agglutination tests on sera from acute and convalescent cases are often not useful unless present in high titer (>1:560) or rising titer is shown.

Staphylococcal Infections

Pneumonia
Often secondary to measles, influenza, mucoviscidosis, debilitating diseases such as leukemia and collagen diseases, or to prolonged treatment with broad-spectrum antibiotics
- WBC is increased (usually >15,000/cu mm).
♦ • Sputum contains very many PMNs with intracellular gram-positive cocci.
♦ • Bacteremia occurs in <20% of patients.

Acute Osteomyelitis
Due to hematogenous dissemination
♦ • Bacteremia occurs in >50% of early cases.
- WBC is increased.
- Anemia develops.
○ • Secondary amyloidosis occurs in long-standing chronic osteomyelitis.

Endocarditis
Occurs in valves without preceding rheumatic disease and showing little or no previous damage; causes rapid severe damage to valve, producing acute clinical course of mechanical heart failure (rupture of chordae tendineae, perforation of valve, valvular insufficiency) plus results of acute severe infection
- Metastatic abscesses occur in various organs.
- Anemia develops rapidly.
- WBC is increased (12,000–20,000/cu mm); occasionally is normal or decreased.
- *From 1–13% of cases of bacterial endocarditis are due to coagulase-negative* Staphylococcus albus; *bacterial endocarditis due to* S. albus *is found after cardiac surgery in one-third of patients and without preceding surgery in two-thirds of patients.*
- Bacteremia is common.
♦ • Teichoic acid antibodies are found in titer of ≥ 1:4 in approximately two-thirds of patients with *S. aureus* endocarditis or bacteremia with metastatic infection, approximately one-half of patients with nonbacteremic staphylococcal infections. May be found in ~10% of patients with other infections or in normal persons. Titer of ≥ 1:4 is said to suggest current or recent serious staphylococcal infection; positive result without suppuration at primary site of infection suggests endocarditis or metastatic infection. May also be useful when cultures are negative because of prior antibiotic therapy or when deep-tissue infection is inaccessible to culturing (e.g., osteomyelitis, abscesses of brain, liver, etc.). Major value is to determine length of treatment of bacteremia, because lack of rise of titer during 14 days of therapy makes it unlikely that undetected metastatic seeding has occurred.

Food Poisoning
Due to enterotoxin
♦ Culture of staphylococci from suspected food (especially custard and milk products and meats)

Necrotizing Enterocolitis of Infancy
As seen in Hirschsprung's disease

Impetigo
Especially in infants between ages of 3 wks and 6 mos

Meningitis
See p. 282.

Streptobacillus moniliformis Infections (Rat-Bite Fever, Haverhill Fever)

♦ Isolation of bacteria from appropriate sites (e.g., blood, pus, joint fluid) during acute febrile stage
Previous slide agglutination test is no longer available because of performance limitations.

Streptococcal Infections

(Uncommon in children younger than age 2 yrs)

Classification of Streptococci

Group	Name	
None	*S. pneumoniae*	See Pneumococcal Infections, p. 811.
None	Viridans streptococci	Show alpha hemolysis. Cause SBE (see p. 114).
A	*S. pyogenes*	Show beta hemolysis. Cause scarlet fever, URI. Are the most frequent type of streptococci causing otitis media, mastoiditis, sinusitis, meningitis, cerebral sinus thrombosis, pneumonia, empyema, pericarditis, bacteremia, suppurative arthritis, puerperal sepsis, lymphangitis, lymphadenitis, erysipelas, cellulitis, impetigo (in older children, is often mixed infection with staphylococci that overgrow the culture plate).

♦ Throat swab analysis for direct antigen for group A streptococci has specificity of >97% and sensitivity of 64–100% depending on criteria; allows identification within minutes. (Take two swabs: if first is positive, treat as streptococcal pharyngitis; if first is negative, use second swab for routine culture method.) Positive result means patient has streptococcal pharyngitis or is carrier.

♦ Streptococci appear in smears and cultures from appropriate sites.

♦ Blood culture may be positive.

WBC is usually increased (14,000/cu mm) early in scarlet fever and URI. It becomes normal by end of first week. (If still increased, look for complication, e.g., otitis.) Is often more markedly increased (≤ 20,000–30,000/cu mm) with infection at other sites.

Increased eosinophils appear during convalescence, especially with scarlet fever.

Urine may show transient slight albumin, RBCs, casts, without sequelae.

ASOT (see pp. 38, 128)

Acute GN follows streptococcal infection after latent period of 1–2 wks; preceding infection may be pharyngeal or of the skin. Latent period before onset of acute rheumatic fever is 2–4 wks; preceding infection is pharyngeal but rarely of the skin.

See sections on rheumatic fever, p. 128 and acute GN, p. 719.

Group	Name	
B	*S. agalactiae*	Especially affects neonates (sepsis, meningitis, puerperal sepsis) and the elderly. Most are nosocomial. Involves devitalized soft tissues, decubiti, pneumonia, GU tract, chorioamnionitis, postpartum endometritis

♦ Antigen detection in CSF or urine is useful for rapid diagnosis in neonates with meningitis or bacteremia with >90% sensitivity and specificity.

Group	Name	
C	*S. equisimilis* and *S. zooepidemicus*	Colonize <3% of normal persons. Cause pharyngitis (which may be followed by GN); occasional cases of bacteremia, endocarditis, meningitis, puerperal sepsis, pneumonia.
D	*Enterococcus faecalis* and *S. bovis*	Both are important causes of endocarditis. *(Half of adults with* S. bovis *endocarditis have anatomic lesion of colon, e.g., carcinoma, polyp, adenoma.)* S. bovis *rarely causes other infection.* E. faecalis *causes infections of GU tract and peritoneal cavity, pneumonia in elderly persons, infection of damaged tissues (e.g., decubiti, burns, diabetic tissues), polymicrobial bacteremia
F	*S. milleri*, others	
G	No name	Comprise 5–10% of streptococci in blood cultures. Cause polymicrobial bacteremia, bacteremia with no known primary focus, major underlying diseases, serious infection of compromised skin and soft tissue (e.g., irradiated, edematous). Clinically indistinguishable from *S. pyogenes* infection. Can increase ASOT and cause GN.

INFECTIOUS

Anaerobic streptococci	Associated with coliform bacilli, clostridia, bacteroides in compound fractures and soft tissue wounds, puerperal and postabortion sepsis, visceral abscesses (e.g., lung, liver, brain).
	Associated with *S. aureus* in gangrenous postoperative abdominal incision.
	Without associated bacteria in burrowing skin and subcutaneous infection.

Syphilis

(Due to *Treponema pallidum*)
See Tables 15-4, 15-5, 15-6 and Figs. 15-1, 15-2, 15-3.
Primary Syphilis
♦ *Direct immunofluorescent staining of smears from lesion has essentially replaced dark-field examination* and allows properly prepared specimens to be mailed to the laboratory.
♦ If immunofluorescent examination of genital lesion is negative, regional lymph node aspirate may be used.
　　Is particularly useful for oral lesions. *Immunofluorescent assay is negative if the patient has received recent therapy with penicillin or other treponemicidal drugs.*
♦ Serologic test shows rising titer with or without positive immunofluorescent examination. VDRL does not become positive until 7–10 days after appearance of chancre.
♦ Biopsy of suspected lesion for histologic examination using silver stain or DFA for *Treponema* may be useful in certain seronegative cases (e.g., HIV infections).
Secondary Syphilis
♦ Dark-field examination of mucocutaneous lesions is positive.
♦ Serologic tests are almost always positive in high titer (>1:32).
Prozone reaction may cause false-negative test.
Latent Syphilis
♦ A positive serologic test is the only diagnostic method.
Congenital Syphilis
♦ Immunofluorescent examination of mucocutaneous lesions or scraping from moist umbilical cord is positive.
♦ Serologic tests are positive and show rising (4×) or very high titer or a stable titer at age 3 mos. *The test may be positive because of maternal antibodies when congenital syphilitic infection is not present.* Rising titer in infant or titer higher than mother's establishes diagnosis of congenital syphilis. If mother has been adequately treated, infant's titer falls steadily to nonreactive level in 3 mos. If mother acquires syphilis late in pregnancy, infant may be seronegative and clinically normal at birth and then manifest syphilis 1–2 mos later.
Only the quantitative VDRL is recommended for the diagnosis of congenital syphilis (performed serially to detect rise or fall in titers).
Nearly all infants born of mothers with primary and secondary syphilis have congenital infection; 50% are clinically symptomatic.
At delivery, use maternal blood rather than cord blood for screening because of false-positive reactions (due to Wharton's jelly) and false-negative reactions (due to infection acquired late in pregnancy).
Late Syphilis
CNS
♦ • VDRL on CSF is highly specific but lacks sensitivity (20–60%); therefore should be used to rule in, not rule out, neurosyphilis. VDRL cannot be used to follow response to therapy. Other serologic tests should not be used on CSF.
♦ • PCR has been used to detect treponemal DNA in CSF in patients with syphilis who were not previously treated; has sensitivity 59%, specificity of 97%, positive predictive value of 91%, negative predictive value of 83%.
Meningitis
　• ≤ 2000 lymphocytes/cu mm
♦ • Positive serologic test in blood and CSF
Meningovascular disease
　• Increased cell count (≤ 100 mononuclear cells/cu mm) in 60% of cases
　• Increased protein (up to 260 mg/dL) in 66% of cases; increased gamma globulin in 75% of cases

Table 15-4. Stages of Syphilis

Stage	Symptom	Time After Exposure	Laboratory Changes	Response to Treatment		
				VDRL	FTA-ABS/MHA-TP	
Primary	Chancre	Average 3 wks (11–90 days)	Dark-field positive Serologic tests often negative Rising VDRL and FTA-ABS titers	Remains negative	Remains negative	
	Lymph nodes	Average 4 wks	Dark-field positive Rising antibody titers	Usually becomes negative within 6 mos	After seroconversion, usually remains positive indefinitely without regard for stage of disease or adequacy of treatment	
Secondary		6–20 wks	Dark-field positive Peak antibody titers CSF abnormal in 25–50% of patients without CNS findings Increased serum ALP (due to pericholangitis) in 20% Proteinuria	Usually becomes negative within 12–24 mos		
Latent		Early: 3–12 mos Late: >12 mos	CSF VDRL negative Serum treponemal test positive Falling VDRL titers			
Late (tertiary)	Neurosyphilis (asymptomatic)	Usually >4 yrs	CSF: VDRL positive or increased cells and protein Serum treponemal test positive; nontreponemal test positive or negative Without treatment, CNS disease occurs within 10 yrs in 20% of patients			
Late (tertiary)	Symptomatic	>4 yrs	Same as asymptomatic Treatment does not reverse nontreponemal test in 25–75% of patients	Usually remains positive indefinitely with gradually declining titer		

FTA-ABS = fluorescent treponemal antibody absorption test; MHA-TP = microhemagglutination assay for *Treponema pallidum.*

INFECTIOUS

Table 15-5. Sensitivity and Specificity of Serologic Tests for Untreated Syphilis at Different Stages (%)

Test	Sensitivity				Specificity
	Primary	Secondary	Late	Latent	
VDRL	78	97	71	92	98
MHA-TP	76	100	94	97	99
FTA-ABS	85	99	95	95	97

FTA-ABS = fluorescent treponemal antibody absorption test; MHA-TP = microhemagglutination assay for *Treponema pallidum*.

♦ • Positive serologic test in blood and CSF
  • Laboratory findings due to cerebrovascular thrombosis
Tabes dorsalis
  • Early—increased cell count and protein.
  • Positive serologic test in blood and CSF (titer may be low).
  • Increased gamma globulin is less marked than in general paresis.
  • Late—~25% of patients may have normal CSF and negative serologic tests in blood and CSF.
General paresis (CSF always abnormal in untreated patients)
  • Increased cell count of ≤ 175 mononuclear cells/cu mm.
  • Increased protein of ≤ 100 mg/dL with marked increase in gamma globulin.
♦ • Positive serologic test (titer usually high).
  • CSF cell count should return to normal within 3 mos after therapy; otherwise retreatment is indicated.
♦ Asymptomatic CNS lues
  • May have negative blood and positive CSF serologic test.
  • Increased cell count and protein are index of activity.
♦ Cardiovascular syphilis—VDRL is usually reactive but titer is often low.
♦ Gummatous lesions—VDRL is almost always reactive, usually in high titer.
Involvement of other organs, e.g., liver
♦ Biopsy of skin, lymph node, larynx, testes, etc.
Adequately treated primary and secondary syphilis usually show decreasing titer and become serologically nonreactive in ~9 and 12 mos, respectively; 2% of patients remain positive for several years. Therapy causes a negative reagin test in 75% of patients with early latent syphilis in 5 yrs, but <25% of patients with late syphilis become nonreactive, although titers may fall steadily over a long period.

Table 15-6. Serologic Tests for Syphilis in Various Conditions

Diagnosis	Nontreponemal Test	FTA-ABS
Syphilis—any stage, treated or untreated	+	+
Congenital syphilis	+	+
Yaws, pinta, bejel	+	+
Untreated early primary or late syphilis	–	+
Adequately treated syphilis	–	+
Lyme disease	–	+
Rare false + FTA-ABS (<1%)	–	+
False + nontreponemal test	+	–
Very early syphilis	–	–
No syphilis	–	–
Syphilis in HIV-infected patient (occasionally)	–	–

FTA-ABS = fluorescent treponemal antibody absorption test.

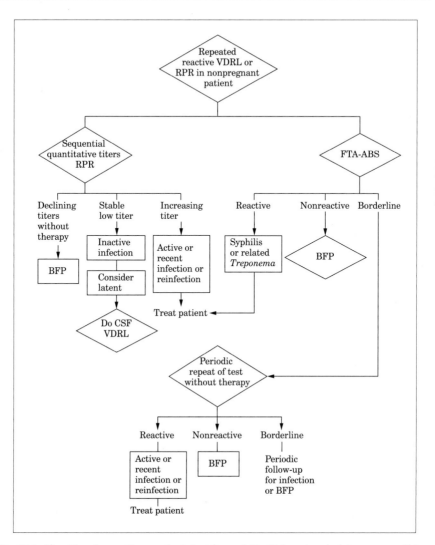

Fig. 15-1. Algorithm for positive serologic test for syphilis. Rule out underlying causes of biological false-positive (BFP) results. (FTA-ABS = fluorescent treponemal antibody absorption test; RPR = rapid plasma reagin test.)

Serologic Tests for Syphilis
Nontreponemal Tests (e.g., VDRL, rapid plasma reagin test, automated reagin test)
(Detect IgG and IgM antibodies to a cardiolipin-lecithin-cholesterol antigen)

Use and Interpretation
Routine screening of asymptomatic persons. Simple, convenient; frequent local requirement for premarital and prenatal serology. False-positive rate of 1–2% in pregnant women.

Diagnosis of symptomatic infection. Does not become positive until 7–10 days after appearance of chancre.

- High titer (>1:16) usually indicates active disease.
- Low titer (≤ 1:8) indicates biological false-positive test in 90% of cases or occasionally due to late or late latent syphilis.

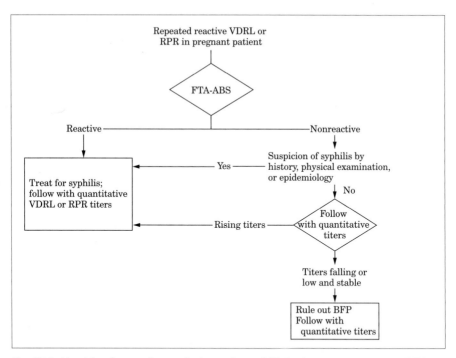

Fig. 15-2. Algorithm for reactive serologic test for syphilis in the pregnant patient. (BFP = biological false-positive results; FTA-ABS = fluorescent treponemal antibody absorption test; RPR = rapid plasma reagin test.)

Following of titers to determine effect of therapy. Quantitation of VDRL should always be performed before initiation of treatment.
- 4× decrease in titer indicates response to therapy. Treatment of primary syphilis usually causes progressive decline (2-tube at 6 mos, 3-tube at 12 mos, 4-tube at 24 mos) to negative VDRL within 2 yrs. Treatment of secondary syphilis usually causes 3-tube decline at 6 mos and 4-tube decline at 12 mos. In early latent

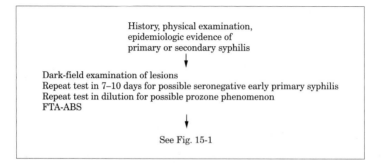

Fig. 15-3. Algorithm for nonreactive serologic test for syphilis in the nonpregnant patient. (FTA-ABS = fluorescent treponemal antibody absorption test.)

syphilis 2-tube decline may not be seen until 12 mos. In secondary, late, or latent syphilis, low titers persist in ~50% of cases after 2 yrs despite fall in titer; this does not indicate treatment failure or reinfection, and these patients are likely to remain positive even if retreated. Titer response is unpredictable in late and latent syphilis. First infections are more likely to serorevert than repeat infections. Falling titer indicates response to treatment. Adequate treatment of primary and secondary syphilis should cause a 4× decline in titer by fourth month and 8× decline by eighth month. Treatment of early syphilis usually results in little or no reaction after 1 yr.
- Rising titer (4×) indicates relapse, reinfection, or treatment failure and need for retreatment.

Differentiation of congenital syphilis from passive transfer of maternal antibodies

Serial titers should be measured; rising titer during 6 mo period of infancy is diagnostic of congenital syphilis because passively transferred antibodies should not be detected after 3 mos. Because infection may occur as early as ninth week of gestation, women at high risk should be tested during first and again during third trimester. Cord blood should not be used because false-positive and false-negative results can occur. In early congenital syphilis, treatment causes VDRL to become nonreactive, but after age 2 yrs, titer decreases slowly but may never become nonreactive.

Interferences
May be nonreactive in early primary, late latent, and late syphilis (~25% of cases)

VDRL may be nonreactive in undiluted serum in presence of an actual high titer (prozone phenomenon) in 1% of patients with secondary syphilis.

Reactive and weakly reactive tests should always be confirmed with FTA-ABS. Sera from one-third of patients only weakly reactive on VDRL test are reactive with more sensitive test.

≤ 20% of reactive screening tests may have biological false-positive results. In two-thirds of these cases, titer is low (<1:8) and reverts to normal within 6 mos.

Short-term false-positive test results (<6 mos' duration) may occur in
- Various acute viral illnesses (e.g., infectious mononucleosis, hepatitis, measles)
- *M. pneumoniae* infection
- *Chlamydia* infection
- Malaria
- Some immunizations
- Pregnancy (rare)

Long-term false-positive test results (>6 mos' duration) may occur in the following cases.
- 50% of patients are shown to have syphilis or other treponemal infections.
- 25% have serious underlying disease (e.g., collagen vascular diseases, leprosy, malignancy).
- Biological false-positive results occur in 20–25% of IV drug users.
- >20% of patients with biological false-positive results also show positive tests for RA, ANA, antithyroid antibodies, cryoglobulins, elevated serum gamma globulins; they may show ITP, autoimmune hemolytic anemia, antiphospholipid syndrome, Sjögren's syndrome, AIDS, thyroiditis.
- ≤ 10% of patients older than age 70 years may show biological false-positive results.
- Patients taking some antihypertensive drugs.

Treponemal Tests
Use and Interpretation
Confirmation of results of nontreponemal tests that conflict with clinical findings (i.e., to distinguish true-positive from false-positive results on nontreponemal tests)

Diagnosis of late syphilis when nontreponemal tests may be negative.

Not to be used for screening.

Are qualitative tests that cannot be used to monitor efficacy of treatment. Are less likely to become negative due to treatment than are nontreponemal tests.

Nonreactive test results generally indicate no past or present infection unless disease is treated in early primary stage, in which case 10–25% of tests yield nonreactive results 2–3 yrs later. 1% of cases are false-positive (same percentage as for nontreponemal tests).

Passively transferred antibodies disappear from noninfected infant in 6–8 mos but persist in cases of congenital syphilis.

Interferences

Positive in presence of antibodies of related treponematoses (e.g., yaws, pinta, bejel). Once antibodies develop, may thereafter remain positive despite therapy. (This is the mechanism for one type of biological false-positive result.)

If therapy is given before antibodies develop, these tests may never be positive.

Treponema pallidum Immobilization Test

Replaced by these tests:

- **MHA-TP** (microhemagglutination assay for *T. pallidum*) and **HATTS** (hemagglutination treponemal test)

    Sensitized or unsensitized cells may occasionally be reactive with sera from drug addicts and patients with SLE, autoimmune diseases, viral infections, or leprosy.

    Compares well with FTA-ABS in sensitivity and specificity as a confirmatory test with fewer false-positive reactions but is less sensitive in early primary syphilis

FTA-ABS IgG

Use

Most sensitive and specific test

More sensitive than MHA-TP in primary syphilis; parallels findings in other stages

If late syphilis of any type is suspected, always do FTA-ABS, even if VDRL is nonreactive.

Test of choice for confirmation of diagnosis (e.g., biological false-positive)

Titers not correlated with clinical activity

Remains positive indefinitely in ~95% of patients, reflecting previous infection any time in past except for early primary syphilis

Not used to document adequacy of treatment, as remains positive for 2 yrs after adequate therapy in 80% of cases of seropositive early syphilis; thus a positive test does not separate active from inactive disease.

Beaded pattern is common in collagen diseases (e.g., SLE) but is considered negative for syphilis.

No longer recommended for early detection of congenital syphilis in infants because of passive transfer of IgG across placenta; for this, FTA-ABS IgM is used, which has 35% false-negative and 10% false-positive rate.

Tetanus

(Due to *Clostridium tetani*)

WBC, urine, CSF are normal.

Identification of organism in local wound is difficult and not usually helpful.

Serologic tests (EIA) are used to assess immunity and to evaluate immune function by assay of pre- and postimmunization sera. Antibody level of ≥ 0.1 U/mL is protective. Cannot be used for diagnosis.

Toxic Shock Syndrome

(Due to toxin-producing strains of *Staphylococcus aureus* or group A streptococci. Fever, rash, shock, and involvement of at least four organ systems are characteristic.)

Anemia is normocytic, normochromic, nonhemolytic, moderate, progressive and may persist for ≤ 1 mo after onset of illness; resolves without treatment; occurs in ~50% of cases.

ESR may be normal or very high.

Moderate leukocytosis with predominance of immature granulocytes in 70% of cases and toxic granulation. Usually increases for several days and then rapidly returns to normal.

Thrombocytopenia* (<100,000/cu mm) in ~25% of cases and DIC causing hemorrhage are not significant clinical problems.

Decreased serum albumin,* total and ionized calcium,* phosphorus

Hypokalemia, hyponatremia, and metabolic acidosis frequently accompany vomiting and diarrhea.*

Sterile pyuria* in 80% of cases, proteinuria, and RBCs resolve within 2 wks.

Increased PT and PTT in two-thirds of patients.

Increased serum bilirubin, AST, LD, CK, BUN, and creatinine to 2× ULN are found in ~60% of cases on approximately the seventh day of illness, at which time clinical improvement begins to occur and these values rapidly become normal.

No evidence of other infection (bacterial, viral, rickettsial), drug reaction, or autoimmune disorder.

○Organisms need not be isolated to fulfill criteria for diagnosis.

*Abnormalities usually become normal by fifth day of illness.

Toxic Shock Syndrome Due to Streptococcal and Staphylococcal Toxins

	Streptococcal	Staphylococcal
Usually associated with	Invasive tissue infection	Use of tampons in healthy menstruating women
	Bacteremia (60%)	No
	Pneumonia, peritonitis, osteomyelitis, myometritis	Rarely
	Focal soft tissue necrosis (e.g., cellulitis, fasciitis)	Not usually
Culture	*S. pyogens* (usually)	*S. aureus*
Serologic tests	Positive for DNase B and streptococcal toxins	

Tuberculosis (TB)

♦Acid-fast stained smears and cultures of concentrates of suspected material from involved sites (e.g., sputum, effusions, urine, CSF, pus) should be performed on multiple specimens. Reported sensitivity of smear compared to culture is 22–78%; analyzing multiple sputum smears more than doubles sensitivity. Acid-fast smears are highly specific but do not differentiate from other mycobacteria species. 10^4 acid-fast bacilli/mL of sputum are required for detection on smear. When sputum is not available or smears are negative, can use gastric aspirates (especially in children), specimens obtained from bronchoscopy (especially useful for endobronchial lesions) with bronchial washings, lavage, brushings or transbronchial biopsy, pleural fluid, or biopsy. Fluorochrome stain is faster and more sensitive for screening than Ziehl-Neelsen stain.

♦Culture on conventional solid media (e.g., Löwenstein-Jensen) is required for conventional biochemical tests and nucleic acid probes. Therefore should be inoculated and BACTEC radiometric method should be used. 80–85% sensitivity in detecting all cases. Culture essential for drug susceptibility testing, detection of non-TB mycobacteria, epidemiologic studies, identification of specimen cross contamination.

♦Molecular techniques show sensitivity higher than ~88%, specificity higher than ~95%.
- Direct detection of specific mycobacterial DNA by PCR has greater sensitivity than Ziehl-Neelsen staining; can detect ~10 bacilli/specimen.
- Same-day detection is possible.
- Mycobacterial genus and species are identified by DNA probes.
- Can identify strains resistant to multiple drugs.
- May identify some newly infected persons before tuberculin conversion.
- Nucleic acid probes in cultures are almost 100% sensitive and specific except for *Mycobacterium kansasii*, with identification in 8 days.

♦Gas-liquid or high-performance liquid chromatography measure characteristic fatty acids; identifies 90% of mycobacteria rapidly.

○Characteristic histologic pattern appears in random biopsy of lymph node, liver, bone marrow (especially in miliary dissemination), or other involved sites (e.g., bronchus, pleura).

WBC is usually normal. Granulocytic leukemoid reaction may occur in miliary disease. Active disseminated disease is suggested by more monocytes (10–20%) than lymphocytes (5–10%) in peripheral smear.

ESR is normal in localized disease; increased in disseminated or advanced disease. It is not used as index of activity.

Moderate anemia may be present in advanced disease.

○Urine—rule out renal TB in presence of hematuria (gross or microscopic) or pyuria with negative cultures for pyogenic bacteria. Routine urine cultures positive in ~7% of TB patients with normal urinalysis and no GU symptoms.

Laboratory findings due to extrapulmonary TB
- Tuberculous meningitis
  CSF shows
  ◆ Acid-fast smear (positive in 20% of cases) and culture (positive in 75% of cases) from pellicle; detection by PCR is more sensitive.
  100–1000 WBC/cu mm (mostly lymphocytes)
  Increased protein (slight in early stages but continues to increase; >300 mg/dL associated with advanced disease; much higher levels when block of CSF occurs.
  Decreased glucose (<50% of blood glucose)
  Decreased chloride is not useful in diagnosis
  Increased tryptophan
  Serum sodium may be decreased (110–125 mEq/L) especially in elderly; may also occur in overwhelming tuberculous infection.
  Detection of anti-BCG-IgC by ELISA or of antbody-secreting cells by solid immunospot assay has been reported recently.
  ◆ Detection of mycobacterial antigen and antibody by ELISA provides rapid identification.
  ≤ 33% of cases have miliary TB
- Miliary TB
  ◆ Sputum smears and cultures positive in 30–60% of patients
  ◆ Culture from liver, marrow, urine may be positive.
- Tuberculoma
- Tuberculous pleural or pericardial effusions (see p. 149)
  Pleural effusions occur in ≤ 5% of all TB patients, >15% of patients with extrapulmonary TB, and >20% of TB patients with negative sputum smears.
  Fluid is an exudate with increased protein (>3 gm/dL) and increased lymphocytes.
  ◆ Acid-fast stained smears are rarely positive.
  ◆ Pleural fluid culture is positive in 25% of patients.
  ◆ Tissue biopsy for histology and culture is usually needed for diagnosis.
  ◆ Sputum is positive on culture in ~25% of patients.
- Lymph nodes
  ◆ Culture is important to rule out infection due to other mycobacteria (atypical or anonymous; e.g., *M. avium-intracellulare* in AIDS).
◆ • Bone marrow is positive in 30–70% of patients with miliary TB.
◆ • Liver biopsy shows granulomas in 50–90% of cases with ~10% positive for acid-fast bacillus.
◆ • Positive smear of tissue for acid-fast bacillus by direct microscopy requires ~1000–10,000 mycobacteria/gm of tissue.
Laboratory findings due to complications (see appropriate separate sections), e.g.,
○ • Amyloidosis
○ • Addison's disease
Laboratory findings due to underlying diseases (e.g., diabetes mellitus, sickle cell anemia, AIDS)
In AIDS, *Mycobacterium avium* and *M. avium-intracellulare* are the major problem (present in 20–60% of AIDS cases at autopsy) but *M. tuberculosis* is also increased. >50% of active TB in late AIDS cases is extrapulmonary.
◆ Persistent prolonged bacteremia is characteristic; blood culture is sensitive means of diagnosis.
◆ Direct examination of Kinyoun carbolfuchsin stain preparation of buffy coat smear may be helpful; marrow cultures are frequently positive. Blood culture is positive in <20% of AIDS patients with CD4 count of >100/μL but in ≤ 50% of cases with CD4 count of <100/μL. May involve lymph nodes, spleen, liver, GI tract, lung, and brain.
All patients with TB should be tested for HIV coinfection.

Environmental Mycobacteria
(Soil and water are reservoir for these organisms, in contrast to *M. tuberculosis*, which is an obligate human pathogen)

	Diagnosis	**Comment**
Pulmonary disease		
Common		
M. kansasii	Positive culture, absence	Rarely a contaminant
M. avium-intracellulare	of other causal agents, compatible clinical picture	

M. chelonae	Lung biopsy may be needed	
Rare		
M. xenopi		
M. szulgai		
M. fortuitum		
M. simiae		
AIDS-associated		
M. avium-intracellulare	May be found in many sites (e.g., lymph nodes, blood, marrow, liver, spleen, GI tract)	Disseminated infection in ~50% of AIDS cases relatively late; CD4 count usually <100/cu mm
		Most common bacterial infection in AIDS
Lymphadenitis	Histologic examination of tissue	
Common		
M. avium-intracellulare		95% involve unilateral
M. scrofulaceum		cervical nodes; most common in children 2–5 yrs old
Rare		
M. kansasii		
M. fortuitum		
M. chelonae		
Cutaneous	Culture of skin biopsy	
Common		
M. marinum	Incubate culture at low temperature (28–30°C)	Swimming pool granu-loma
M. fortuitum	Culture skin biopsy	Postsurgical or environmental wound contamination
M. chelonae		
Rare		
M. avium complex		
M. kansasii		
M. smegmatis		
M. haemophilum		

INFECTIOUS

Tularemia

(Due to *Francisella tularensis*)

Clinical types
- Typhoidal (18% of cases)
- Ulceroglandular (60% of cases)
- Glandular (15% of cases)
- Oropharyngeal (7% of cases)
- Rarely oculoglandular (1% of cases), pneumonic, gastrointestinal, endocardial, meningeal, osteomyelitic, etc.

♦ Serologic tests
- EIA showing increased specific IgM and rising IgG titer is diagnostic; is more sensitive than agglutination; may persist for years.

♦ Culture and animal inoculation (positive with ≥ 5 organisms) of suspected material from appropriate site are performed. (Positive blood culture is rare; regional lymph node and mucocutaneous lesions are usually positive.)

WBC is usually normal.

ESR may be increased in severe typhoidal forms; it is normal in other types.

Serum AST is commonly elevated.

♦ Biopsy of involved lymph node shows a characteristic histologic picture.

Yersinia enterocolitica Infections

(Facultative anaerobic gram-negative coccoid bacillus; transmitted primarily by ingestion of contaminated food, milk, and water)

Stool may contain WBCs and RBCs; gross blood in ≤ 25% of cases.

♦ Stool culture requires special techniques; should be interpreted cautiously because of possibility of low-virulence environmental strains not related to human disease; serotyping may be useful to distinguish these.

♦ Serologic tests

• Tube agglutination, ELISA, RIA increase 1 wk after onset of symptoms and peak in second week. Titer of ≥ 1:200 present in most cases but 4× increases are rare. Titer of ≥ 1:128 at time of complications is presumptive evidence of yersiniosis. May be useful for retrospective diagnosis in patients with reactive arthritis.

• Limitations

Antibodies may be detected for years after infection.

Cross reactions may occur with *B. abortus, Rickettsia* spp., *Salmonella* spp., *Morganella morganii.*

Titers of ≥ 1:32 are present in ≥ 1.5% of healthy persons with no previous history of infection.

Laboratory findings due to focal infection in many extraintestinal sites without detectable bacteremia (e.g., pharyngitis, lymphadenitis, liver and spleen abscesses, endocarditis)

Laboratory findings due to reactive disease (e.g., arthropathy, erythema nodosum, Reiter's syndrome, myocarditis, GN)

Viruses

Diagnosis of Viral Infections

♦ Serologic evidence of recent infection may be based on the following.

• Seroconversion from negative to positive results is conclusive evidence of recent infection if appropriate test method is used but results are usually obtained too late to be useful in treating a particular episode.

• ≥ 4× rise in antibody titer in paired serum samples collected 2–4 wks apart is usually diagnostic. Some exceptions are anamnestic reactions, cross reactions to related antigens; some specific exceptions exist (e.g., high CMV antibody titers in influenza A or *M. pneumoniae* infections).

• Single serum specimens that show specific IgM antibody within the first few weeks of infection (e.g., EBV, CMV, VZV, rubella virus, coxsackieviruses) are useful.

• Various exceptions must be remembered:

Some may recur with reactivation or reinfection (e.g., herpesvirus, CMV, EBV, VZV)

Some may persist for ≥ 6 mos (e.g., CMV, rubella virus)

Heterotypic response of one virus antibody to another infection (e.g., CMV and EBV) may occur.

• False-positive results are frequent for sera that contain RF. *Spurious results may also occur in other conditions (e.g., bacterial endocarditis, chronic liver disease, TB and other chronic infections, sarcoidosis) and in some healthy persons.*

• False-negative results may occur in immunocompromised patients, neonates, infants.

For diagnosis of congenital infection, serial sera from mother and infant should be submitted.

• Level of passive antibody in infants acquired transplacentally decreases markedly in 2–3 mos; unchanged or increasing titer indicates active infection, but maternal HIV antibodies may persist for ≤ 18 mos in infant.

• Specific IgM in neonatal blood or cord blood can be used to diagnose congenital infection because mother's IgM does not cross placenta.

• Single maternal serum sample negative for IgG may be useful to exclude that particular congenital infection in neonate (e.g., rubella, CMV infection).

• Positive IgG titer that does not rise indicates previous exposure and often immunity. Tests to determine immune status may be used for viruses of rubella (in women of childbearing age), CMV (in women of childbearing age working in high-risk environments, e.g., hemodialysis, transplant units, pediatric and nursery units), measles and mumps (IFA indicate prior infection), chickenpox (VZV).

• Preferred to culture in cases in which virus does not grow well in cell culture (e.g., rubella virus, EBV) or is too hazardous to handle.

Paired sera should always be submitted for diagnosis of viral disease; acute-phase serum should be obtained as early as possible in clinical course; convalescent-phase serum is usually obtained 2–4 wks later. When the first specimen is submitted, the clinician would be wise to notify the laboratory that a convalescent-phase specimen will be sent subsequently.

♦ Direct identification of virus or viral antigens in patient tissues by
  • Cytopathology of inclusion bodies (e.g., CMV, VZV, herpes virus, measles; smudge cells for adenovirus, respiratory syncytial cell for RSV infection) has sensitivity of ~50%; therefore virus identification should be further confirmed by immunofluorescent and immunoenzyme specific antibody staining. Isolation of virus is >4× more sensitive than finding CMV inclusion bodies in urine.
  • Electron microscopic identification of viral antigen in patient tissues (e.g., brain biopsy for HSV particles in encephalitis, Jakob-Creutzfeldt virus) or specimens (e.g., urine for CMV in congenital infection of infants; feces for rotaviruses, Norwalk agents, adenoviruses, coronaviruses, caliciviruses; vesicle fluid for HSV and poxviruses). Is often enhanced by other techniques (e.g., antibody binding).
  • Direct detection of viral antigens
      Immunofluorescent staining, DFA and IFA
      EIA—commercial kits for RSV, rotavirus, adenovirus, influenza A, HSV
      Agglutination kits for rotavirus
  • Standard viral tube culture showing typical cytopathologic changes is the gold standard for proving etiology but may require 10 days to weeks. Shell viral cultures confirmed with fluorescent monoclonal antibodies can provide results in 1–2 days. Sensitive for CMV and HSV but less successful for RSV and parainfluenza. Prompt inoculation and appropriate media are needed. Infection by some viruses (e.g., herpesvirus, adenovirus, CMV) may not indicate disease, whereas presence of others does indicate disease (e.g., influenza, parainfluenza, RSV).
      Other constraints are:
      Some viruses cannot be cultured and require other techniques, as in most cases of viral gastroenteritis (e.g., rotavirus in stool requires electron microscopy or antigen detection).
      Finding of enterovirus in stool supports diagnosis but does not prove it is the cause of present illness (e.g., aseptic meningitis, myopericarditis).
      Some viruses can be shed for months in asymptomatic persons (e.g., adenoviruses, HSV, CMV) but this is unusual for other viruses (e.g., measles, mumps, influenza, parainfluenza viruses, RSV)
  • Appropriate source of specimen, e.g.,
      Throat swabs (HSV, enterovirus and adenovirus), nasopharyngeal swabs (RSV, parainfluenza), and nasal swabs (rhinovirus)
      Urine—CMV, mumps virus, adenovirus. Sensitivity is increased by using several specimens. Useful in mumps encephalitis when other sites are negative.
      Rectal swabs and stool—stools are generally more useful; see previous.
      Blood—serum for enteroviruses; leukocytes for CMV and arborvirus.
      Tissue—lung (CMV, influenza, adenovirus) and brain (HSV) are the most productive.
      BAL or brushings
      Also CSF, skin vesicles, eye in appropriate cases
  • Direct nucleic acid probe system available for diagnosis of papillomavirus.
  • Amplification techniques are being commercially developed. PCR of blood leukocytes is useful for ruling out CMV infection.
Some specific serologic disease or organ system panels are the following:
  • CNS
      HSV; mumps virus; western equine encephalitis, eastern equine encephalitis, St. Louis encephalitis, and California encephalitis viruses; enteroviruses; EBV.
  • Respiratory
      RSV—nasopharyngeal washings; sensitivity for fluorescent antibodies = 80–100%, for EIA = 70–100%, for centrifugation-enhanced cultures = 70–92%.
      Influenza A and B—culture is most sensitive but takes >4 days. Fluorescent antibodies and EIA are very specific; reported sensitivities = 39–100%.
      Parainfluenza—conventional tube cell culture. Reported sensitivity = 49–94% for fluorescent antibodies.
      Adenovirus—conventional tube cell culture. Fluorescent antibodies and EIA are very specific but sensitivity is poor.
      M. pneumoniae, Chlamydia (RSV and parainfluenza virus only in children)

Table 15-7. Correlation of CD4 Count and Disease in HIV Infection

CD4 Count (per cu mm)	Disease
500–800	Aggressive bacterial, respiratory, skin, enteric infections
>500	Kaposi's sarcoma
200–500	Weight loss, fever, sweats
	Hairy leukoplakia
	Candida (oral, esophageal)
	TB reactivation
<200	Pneumocystosis
	Mycobacterium avium-intracellulare
	Cryptococcosis
	Dementia
<50	Toxoplasmosis
	CMV
	Death

Source: Shelhamer JH, et al. Respiratory disease in the immunosuppressed patient: NIH Conference. *Ann Intern Med* 1992;117:415.

- Exanthems
    Measles—conventional and centrifugation-enhanced shell viral assay, monoclonal antibody, IFA detection of infected cells.
    Rubella—centrifugation-enhanced shell viral assay with fluorescent antibody staining; rarely requested.
    Also HSV and VZV if vesicular
- Mumps—rarely requested. Culture of urine confirmed with fluorescent antibody staining.
- Myocarditis and pericarditis—group B coxsackievirus types 1 through 5, influenza A and B

Acquired Immunodeficiency Syndrome (AIDS)

(Due to human RNA retrovirus subfamily of lentiviruses, human immunodeficiency virus type [HIV-I], formerly called human T-cell lymphotropic virus HTLV-III)
See Tables 15-7 and 15-8, and Figs. 15-4 through 15-7 and appropriate separate section for diseases or tests referred to below.
♦ **Laboratory evidence of HIV infection (any of the following)**
Repeated reactive screening test for HIV antibody (e.g., EIA) confirmed by Western blot or IFA
Positive test for HIV serum antigen

Table 15-8. 1993 Revised Classification System for HIV Infection and Expanded AIDS Surveillance Case Definition for Adolescents and Adults (≥ 13 Yrs)

CD4+ T-Cell Categories		Clinical Categories		
Number	%	A	B	C
(1) ≥ 500/cu mm	≥ 29	A1	B1	C1
(2) 200–499/cu mm	14–28	A2	B2	C2
(3) <200/cu mm	<14	A3	B3	C3

Notes: Groups A3, B3, C3 with CD4+ T-cell counts <200/cu mm are reported as AIDS. Groups C1, C2, C3 with AIDS-indicator conditions are reported as AIDS. T-cell count <200/cu mm is an AIDS indicator. The lowest accurate CD4+ T-cell count is used for classification; need not be the most recent count.

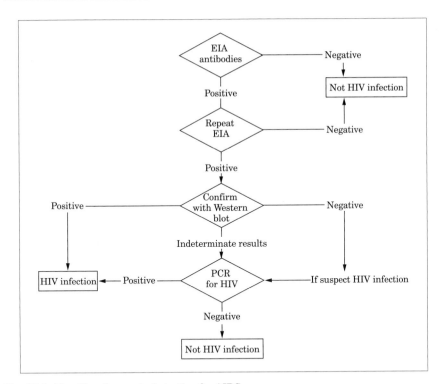

Fig. 15-4. Algorithm for serologic testing for AIDS.

Positive HIV culture confirmed by both reverse transcriptase detection and a specific HIV antigen test or in situ hybridization using nucleic acid probe. Not a standard diagnostic test because it is expensive, time consuming, and potentially dangerous; may be useful in unusual cases. Positive in 100% of cases in late stages but in 20–60% of early asymptomatic cases.

Positive result on any other highly specific test for HIV (e.g., nucleic acid probe of peripheral blood lymphocytes)

Child <15 mos old whose mother had HIV infection during perinatal period with repeated reactive screening test, plus increased serum Ig levels and at least one of the following abnormal immunologic tests: reduced absolute lymphocyte count, depressed CD4 (helper T cells) lymphocyte count, or decreased CD4/CD8 (helper/suppressor) ratio if subsequent confirmatory antibody tests are positive.

Neonatal infection
- IgG antibodies cross placenta during third trimester; all infants born to HIV-1–infected women are HIV-1 seropositive for ≤ 18 mos. Passive transfer of maternal HIV antibody makes serologic tests difficult to interpret in infants.
- Diagnostic testing should be done by age 48 hrs (40% sensitivity), and at 14 days, 1–2 mos, and 3–6 mos.
- HIV DNA PCR is preferred testing method during infancy.
- ≤ 40% of infants born to HIV-infected women acquire HIV infection.
- ≤ 30% of infected infants are HIV-positive at birth (DNA PCR), which suggests in utero infection, whereas ≤ 75% are HIV-negative at birth but positive after 7 days, which suggests intrapartum infection. >90% of infected infants are HIV-positive at 14 days.
- Diagnosis of vertical HIV infection is indicated if one blood specimen is positive by culture and a separate blood specimen is positive by DNA PCR or culture, or (if infant is >28 days old) by plasma p24 antigen assay.

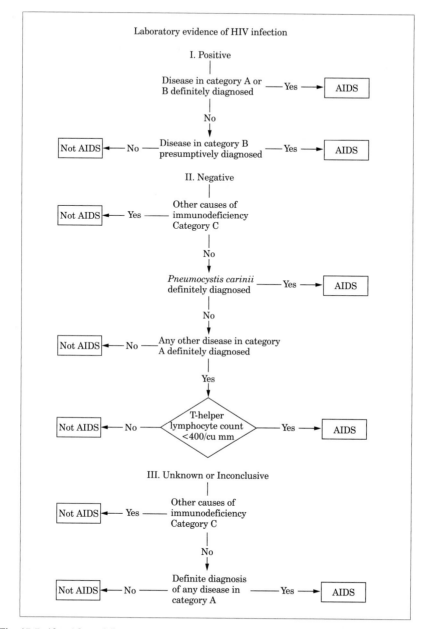

Fig. 15-5. Algorithm of Centers for Disease Control and Prevention (CDC) definition of acquired immunodeficiency syndrome (AIDS). I, II, and III refer to criteria on pp. 838–839. (Adapted from Leads from MMWR: Revision of the CDC surveillance case definition for acquired immunodeficiency syndrome: *JAMA* 1987;258:1143.)

- Increased risk of vertical HIV-1 transmission if maternal CD4 T-cell count is low, HIV-1 RNA level is high, and there is prolonged rupture of membranes. Positive predictive value is 55% in neonates and 83% in infants >30 days old, but the probability of HIV infection is <3% if PCR is negative; thus positive DNA PCR must be interpreted cautiously in neonates, but negative results are informative.

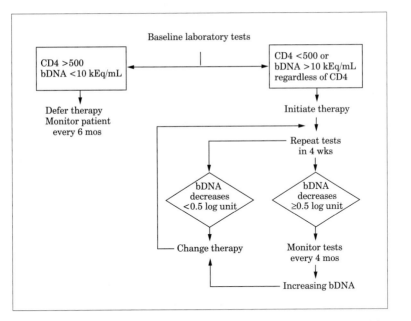

Fig. 15-6. Laboratory tests to assist therapy decisions in AIDS. (bDNA = branched deoxyribonucleic acid.) (From *Signals*. Emeryville, CA: Chiron Reference Testing Laboratory, 1966 March.)

- HIV-1 infection is excluded if DNA PCR is negative after 6 mos.
- Most infected neonates have related symptoms within 1 yr and ~50% have AIDS by 5 yrs; therefore early diagnosis and therapy is essential.
- HIV-1 DNA may still be detected in peripheral blood mononuclear cells in treated children with undetectable HIV-1 RNA, and normal humoral and cellular immune function.
- HIV RNA may prove more sensitive than DNA PCR for early diagnosis of HIV infection in infants.
- HIV culture also has high sensitivity but results may take 2–4 wks.
- p24 antigen tests have high specificity but less sensitivity than other tests. Not recommended as sole test for infants <1 mo old due to possibility of false-positive results.
- HIV infection is diagnosed if two virologic tests on separate blood samples yield positive results.
- HIV is excluded if results are negative on two or more virologic tests performed at >1 mo and >4 mos or on two or more IgG antibody tests performed 1 mo apart after age 6 mos if no clinical evidence of HIV infection or hypogammaglobulinemia exists.[6–8]

Antibody to Human Immunodeficiency Virus Type 1 (HIV-1)

HIV appears in plasma and circulating mononuclear cells 1 to several weeks after infection; HIV antibodies usually appear in 1–4 mos and, rarely >12 mos, after infection; found in >95% of patients within 6 mos. HIV DNA has been detected in cryopreserved lymphocytes as much as 3 yrs before seroconversion. In experiments with HIV vaccine, two-thirds of healthy adults became positive for HIV antibody by EIA and

[6]Luzuriaga K, Sullivan JL. DNA polymerase chain reaction for the diagnosis of vertical HIV infection [Editorial]. *JAMA* 1996;275:1360.
[7]Luzuriaga K, Sullivan JL. Prevention and treatment of pediatric HIV infection. *JAMA* 1998;280:17.
[8]Guidelines for the use of antiretroviral agents in pediatric HIV infection. Centers for Disease Control and Prevention, 1998; 47; No. RR-4.

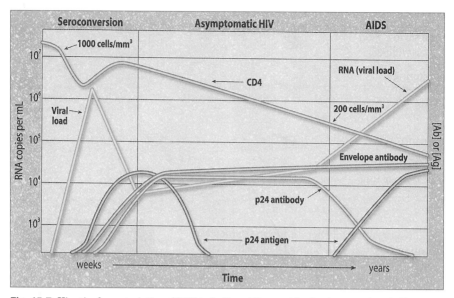

Fig. 15-7. Kinetic characteristics of HIV infection. (Ab = antibody; Ag = antigen.) (From Constantine NT. Quantifying viremia. *Clin Lab News* 1997;[Nov], with permission of AACC, Washington, D.C.)

Western blot test during the first 12 mos. Antigens decline and disappear, and viral isolation from blood becomes more difficult as antibodies arise. 80% of patients are asymptomatic and 20% may have nondescript illness with low fever, rash, diarrhea. In late-stage AIDS, HIV is usually easily recovered from blood and CSF. Mean time from infection to symptoms is >8 yrs.

HIV antibody develops in all patients infected with this virus and is taken as evidence of past or present infection outside of perinatal and neonatal periods. Presence of antibody does not cause immunity, however, because virus can be cultured from antibody-positive individuals for years. Thus, antibody-positive persons can transmit the virus to others. Reversion to antibody-negative status is said to occur rarely. Anti–HIV IgG can cross placenta and enter fetal circulation; thus if mother is negative, neonate will be negative. If mother is HIV-positive, neonate with positive HIV test should be classified as indeterminate and clinical and serologic follow-up should be performed. If infant becomes HIV-negative by 15 mos, infant probably does not have AIDS. Can confirm HIV infection during first months only by culture or DNA, RNA, or p24 antigen detection; these tests have ~50% sensitivity at birth; ~95% sensitivity by age 3–6 mos. Diagnosis is presumptive if results of one of these tests are positive and confirmed if results of one are positive on repeat assay. If test results are positive at birth, in utero infection is considered to have occurred. If negative test result at first week is followed by positive test result, infection is considered to be intrapartum.

♦ Recommended screening test is EIA, which has a sensitivity and specificity of >99%. False-positive or false-negative rate is <2%. When results of EIA test is positive or uncertain, repeat positive EIA result must be confirmed using Western blot test or IFA, which are more specific but less sensitive and less standardized than EIA. If EIA result is negative, Western blot test is usually not done, and this blood may be used for transfusion if donor does not belong to a high-risk group; incidence of HIV antibody in donated blood in the United States is ~0.22% by EIA and 0.1% by Western blot. If EIA is positive and results are confirmed by Western blot test or IFA, the individual has been infected with HIV. If EIA is positive and Western blot test is negative, the patient's blood should not be used for transfusion, although the diagnosis of AIDS is not confirmed. If EIA is positive and Western blot and/or IFA results are equivocal, HIV infection status is unknown and Western blot test should be repeated on a subsequent specimen in 4–6 mos; this person should not be used as a blood donor. Western blot test is considered the gold standard for confirmation of HIV tests but is technically demanding. PCR for HIV is used to confirm indeterminate Western blot test results or negative results for persons suspected of infection.

Third-generation EIA detects IgM and IgA as well as IgG, allowing earlier diagnosis; rapid turnaround is possible in <2 hrs.

False-Positive EIA Results May Be Due To
Administration of influenza vaccine up to 3 mos before test

Administration of immune globulin (e.g., for HBV) manufactured before 1985 within ~6 wks of testing from products (antibody is present but gamma globulin cannot transmit the AIDS virus)

Presence of HLA-DR antibodies in multigravida women

Presence of RF

Autoimmune disorders

Hemodialysis

Hypergammaglobulinemia, e.g., multiple myeloma

Positive RPR test

Hemophilia

Alcoholic hepatitis

Unknown causes

Degree of test reactivity is important. In population with low HIV prevalence, high reactivity of specimens has a positive predictive value of >86%, but low or moderate reactivity has a positive predictive value of <2%. In high-risk population, moderate or high reactivity has a positive predictive value of >95%.

Positive EIA results mean that each positive test has been repeatedly positive in duplicate on the same serum specimen.

EIA May Also Be Positive In
Subclinical infections that are asymptomatic

Active carriers of viral antigen

Persons with immunity

False-Negative EIA or Western Blot Test Results May Be Due To
Advanced AIDS disease (but other evidence of AIDS is usually present)

Early infection before antibodies are detectable. *This donated blood may transmit HIV.* Early reports suggest that 6–20% of HIV-infected persons may be seronegative.

True rate of false-negatives is unknown, but there are a few reports of positive virus cultures in asymptomatic seronegative persons.

Some unusual HIV-1 subtypes (e.g., subtype O) may yield negative results on screening tests.

False-Positive Western Blot Test Results May Be Due To
HLA antibodies

Presence of antibody to another human retrovirus

Poorly understood cross reaction with other non–virus-derived proteins in healthy persons

Connective tissue disorders

Polyclonal gammopathies

Hyperbilirubinemia

False-positive results occur in ≤ 4.8% of low-risk blood donors compared to RNA PCR.

Indeterminate Western Blot Test Results May Be Due To
Recent HIV infection; test usually becomes unequivocally positive in 6 wks to 6 mos.

Condition of advanced immunodeficiency in AIDS patients because of loss of antibodies

HIV Virus Culture
Use
Confirm diagnosis of AIDS when serologic tests are inconclusive.

Only a positive result is conclusive. False-negative results may occur.

Only used in a research setting.

Quantitative HIV RNA Assay
(Measures viral load)
Use
Diagnosis
- Initial evaluation of newly diagnosed HIV infection. Is earliest marker of HIV infection; may be detected 2 wks after infection is established before antibody production begins.
- Newer tests are reported to measure as few as 50 copies/mL of plasma.

- Patients with syndrome consistent with acute HIV infection.
- Confirmation of indeterminate Western blot test results.
- Differentiation between HIV-1 and HIV-2.
- During latent periods.
- High-risk seronegative patients.
- Neonates born to HIV-seropositive mothers.

Guideline for treatment
- Is best measure of effective therapy.
- Should decline within days of effective therapy to 1% of initial level within 2 wks to nadir below detectable levels within ~8 wks. With very high levels decline may take ~16 wks.
- Goal is sustained decrease.
- Rebound after suppression may indicate presence of drug-resistant variants in compliant patients.
- Begin therapy in chronically HIV-infected patients.
    When HIV RNA level is >10,000 copies/mL or branched DNA level (RT-PCR) is >20,000 copies/mL even if CD4 count is <500
    When CD4 count is >500, even if RNA is <10,000 or branched DNA is <20,000 copies/mL
- Before initiating or changing therapy (on two occasions) and at intervals thereafter (e.g., 4 wks, 3–4 mos).
- Do not use during or within 4 wks after successful treatment of intercurrent infection, resolution of symptomatic illness, or immunization.
- Change in clinical status or decline in CD4 cell count.
- Gauge response to therapy and long-term outcome during antiviral therapy or during latent periods.
- Predictive value improves when combined with CD4 cell counts performed at same time.
- Patients with higher viral loads are likely to benefit from antiretroviral treatment.
- Surrogate marker for drug resistance.

Monitoring of disease progression
- Initial peak during primary infection, then rapid decline (≤ 3 log copies) of titer to steady state within 6–12 mos after seroconversion, lasting months or years.
- Viral load at 6–12 mos predicts long-term progression to AIDS.
    <1000 copies/mL—9% had AIDS after 8 yrs
    1000–5551 copies/mL—33% had AIDS after 8 yrs
    5552–19,760 copies/mL—38% had AIDS after 8 yrs
    >19,761 copies/mL—63% had AIDS after 8 yrs
- Any child with >100,000 copies/mL is at high risk of death.

Interpretation
Only changes of >3× (or 0.5 log unit) in adults and >5× (or 0.7 log unit) at age <2 yrs are significant because of biological variation within same person.
Values are not interchangeable between assays; may be a twofold or greater difference; same assay should be used for same patient or new baseline should be established if change is made from one assay to another.
HIV-infected persons with viral load below detectable limits should be considered infectious.
HIV replication may be continuing in various tissues.[9,10]

Interferences
Prone to contamination, which causes false-positive reactions
Some degradation occurs during storage and delay in processing.

Branched DNA by Signal Amplification
Use
Quantitative measurement of HIV viral load; avoids risk of contamination using PCR.
Interpretation
Monitor progression of disease. Earlier and more accurate prediction than CD4$^+$ cell count.
    Long-term nonprogressors have low levels of virus (<10 kEq/mL) (kilo equivalent = 1000 molecules of HIV-1 RNA).

---

[9]Guidelines for the medical management of HIV/AIDS. New Jersey State Department of Health; 1997 Sep.
[10]*MMWR*. Centers for Disease Control and Prevention; 1998; 47; No. RR-4, RR-5.

Monitor response to treatment; antiviral drugs reduce viral load.

Interferences

Improper specimen collection or handling (e.g., plasma should be separated within 4 hrs and promptly frozen) may cause acute degradation of HIV-1 RNA.

Intercurrent infection, illness, or vaccination may cause immune stimulation; therapeutic decisions should be based on long-term trends.

Other Tests for HIV-1

(Approved by FDA)

Antigen Assay (for p24 Antigen in Blood)

Is very specific but low sensitivity in asymptomatic seropositive persons.

Use

Detection of early HIV infection before seroconversion, especially in high-risk persons

Diagnosis of HIV infection in infants born of seropositive mothers

Monitoring of antiviral drug therapy in AIDS and AIDS-related complex; less reliable than HIV RNA and not clinically useful.

Differentiation of AIDS from primary immunodeficiency syndrome in HIV-1–negative children.

Staging of disease in persons with indeterminate confirmatory antibody results.

Home-Collection HIV Blood Test Kit

Patient can mail test card containing three drops of blood from finger prick.

Reported sensitivity and specificity comparable to those of blood ELISA

Results available in 3–7 days.

Allows for anonymity.

Reactive result must be confirmed by Western blot test.

Single-Use Diagnostic System

Subjective qualitative test using serum or plasma

Rapid test results within 30 mins.

Reported sensitivity and specificity comparable to those of blood ELISA.

Urine Test for HIV Antibodies

When EIA screening and supplemental Western blot test are used, has reported sensitivity of >99% and specificity of 100%.

Assay for only the gp160 band in contrast to blood assay, which requires presence of two out of three protein bands associated with HIV to be considered positive.

Reported very high sensitivity and specificity

Uses random urine sample; noninfectious, stable at room temperature.

Fewer indeterminate results than with serum Western blot test.

May be positive when serum is HIV-negative.

EIA Test Kit to Test for HIV Antibody in Oral Mucosal Transudate

Material collected from lower gums and cheek *(not saliva)* is noninvasive.

Used in patients ≥ 13 yrs old.

Collection must be supervised by physician.

Not affected by oral disease, recent dental treatment, smoking.

Reported sensitivity and specificity comparable to those of blood ELISA

Results available in 3 days.

Reactive result must be confirmed by Western blot test.

No occupational exposure

HIV-2 is a recently described virus that causes a disease not distinguishable from AIDS in Africans and small numbers of Europeans and South Americans. Current screening tests for HIV-1 do not consistently and reliably detect antibody due to HIV-2 infection. All donated blood must be tested for HIV-2 as well as HIV-1.

Laboratory Evidence against HIV Infection

Nonreactive screening test for serum HIV antibody without positive results on any other laboratory test for HIV infection (e.g., antibody, antigen, culture).

Inconclusive Laboratory Evidence (either item below)

Repeatedly reactive screening test for serum HIV antibody (e.g., EIA) followed by a negative or inconclusive test result (e.g., on Western blot test, IFA) without positive result for serum antigen or culture.

In child <15 mos old whose mother had HIV infection during perinatal period, repeatedly reactive HIV antibody screening test, even if positive results are obtained on supplemental test, but without additional evidence of immunodeficiency and without positive result for serum antigen or culture.

Other Laboratory Findings in AIDS

○Most valuable tests for evaluation of immune status, which is essential for care of HIV infections, are CD4 and CD8 T-cell counts.

- Should be obtained immediately after positive virologic test and then every 3 mos in children.
- Vaccination or mild intercurrent illness can cause transient decrease of CD4 cell number and percentage.
- Lymphopenia largely due to progressive decrease in CD4 and increased CD8 (flow cytometry). (Normal range of CD8 lymphocytes = 200–800/cu mm; each laboratory should establish its own normal range.) Normal CD4/CD8 ratio is 2.0; AIDS patients have reversed ratio of <1.0; sensitivity is ~85% but specificity is low because ratio of 1.0–2.0 may be seen in other diseases, particularly infections with EBV, HSV, and CMV. Antiretroviral therapy is recommended if CD4 count is <500/cu mm and prophylaxis against *Pneumocystis pneumonia* is recommended if CD4 count is <200/cu mm. CD8 count is relatively labile and may diminish the value of the CD4 count alone. Lymphopenia is found in 50% of patients with Kaposi's sarcoma and almost all patients with opportunistic infections. Total B cell and natural killer cell counts are usually normal.
- Infected infants with CD4 count of <1900/cu mm and CD8 count of >850/cu mm have more rapid disease progression.
- CD4 counts may change ≤ 30% without change in clinical status due to biological and methodologic variation. Therefore trends over time should be monitored, rather than change results on one specific test.

Hypoalbuminemia
Leukopenia, anemia, idiopathic thrombocytopenia are common; thrombocytosis also occurs.
Increased serum transaminase
Complement C3 and C4 levels are usually normal.
Decreased T-cell function evidenced
- In vivo by
    Decreased delayed-type hypersensitivity (skin test reactivity)
    Opportunistic infections
    Neoplasms
- In vitro by various tests that are not routinely available
Other serologic findings (not used in clinical diagnosis): increased levels of
- Acid-labile interferon alpha (previously known in patients with autoimmune disease; found in 63% of homosexual AIDS patients and 29% without AIDS) (more studies are needed to determine value as screening test)
- Thymosin alpha$_1$ (found in <1% of normal persons, 70–80% of AIDS patients, and 60–70% of patients with chronic reactive lymphadenopathy syndrome)
- Level of beta$_2$-microglobulins appears to correlate with clinical course of HIV infection (also increased in patients with hepatitis, kidney diseases, B-cell malignancies such as multiple myeloma)
- Circulating immune complexes
Laboratory findings due to coexisting infection
- HBcAg is positive in >90% of AIDS patients and 80% of patients with lymphadenopathy syndrome. Rate of hepatitis B is 10–30 times that of general population in United States.
- EBV and human T-cell leukemia virus
Laboratory findings due to involvement of organ systems
- Pneumonia
    Parasites (*P. carinii, T. gondii*)
    Viruses (CMV, HSV)
    Fungi (*C. neoformans, H. capsulatum, C. immitis, Candida* species)
    Bacteria (*M. tuberculosis* and *M. avium-intracellulare* [culture of blood and marrow may be positive], *S. pneumoniae, H. influenzae, S. aureus, Legionella* species, *Nocardia asteroides*)
    Others (lymphoma, Kaposi's sarcoma, lymphocytic interstitial pneumonitis)
- Nervous system (see Chapter 9)
    Dementia (subacute encephalitis) occurs in >50% of cases.

> Aseptic meningitis
> Meningitis due to various organisms (*C. neoformans, T. gondii*)
> Myelopathy
> Peripheral neuropathy
> CNS lymphoma
> CSF should be examined for syphilis routinely in all patients with AIDS. AIDS causes treatment failures, relapses after treatment, and increased incidence of early neurosyphilis. AIDS also alters serologic response to spirochete.
- Gastrointestinal system
  > Oropharyngeal candidiasis
  > Cryptosporidiosis
  > *M. avium-intracellulare* infection causing diarrhea, or malabsorption or hepatitis
  > CMV esophagitis or colitis or hepatitis
  > Isosporosis causing diarrhea
- Nephropathy—resembles nephrotic syndrome with rapid progress to end-stage renal disease and very poor prognosis; death usually occurs within 6 mos even with dialysis. Acute renal failure may be due to drugs, sepsis, etc. May also occur in asymptomatic carriers or AIDS-related complex. Patients may also have acute tubular necrosis, chronic tubulointerstitial nephritis, nephrocalcinosis, heroin nephropathy.
- Neoplasms
  > Kaposi's sarcoma—$\geq$ 50% probability of occurrence within 10 yrs in men infected with both HIV and HHV-8
  > Non-Hodgkin's B-cell lymphoma—rapid course, poor prognosis, frequent extranodal and CNS involvement
  > Hodgkin's disease, stage III/IV—mixed cellularity, nodular sclerosis
  > Possible HIV association (T-cell non-Hodgkin's lymphomas, cervical dysplasia/neoplasia, pediatric smooth muscle tumors)
- Lymph node aspirate[11]
  > Mycobacterial infection in 17% of cases
  > Lymphoid hyperplasia in 50%
  > Non-Hodgkin's lymphoma in 20%
  > Kaposi's sarcoma in 10%
  > Occasional cases of Hodgkin's disease, squamous cell and other carcinomas
- Other
  > Infectious mononucleosis–like syndrome (rash, pharyngitis, enlarged spleen, etc.) may occur during initial viremia period with hematologic picture of infectious mononucleosis but serologic tests for EBV and CMV are negative; meningeal signs with CSF pleocytosis may occur. Most patients are asymptomatic during initial HIV viremia.
- Because of diminished immune function, AIDS patients
  > With syphilis with positive VDRL results may have negative FTA-ABS results, have accelerated course, and be refractory to standard therapy.
  > Have high rates of *Salmonella* infection.
  > Have lower seroconversion rates and shorter duration of protection after HBV vaccination.

Laboratory findings due to treatment
- Anemia, leukopenia, thrombocytopenia
- Altered liver and renal function tests
- Increase in MCV often occurs with zidovudine therapy and is useful to confirm patient compliance
- Severe hemolysis may occur in G-6-PD deficiency after exposure to Trimethoprim-Sulfamethoxazole (TMP-SMZ)

Laboratory findings that should heighten suspicion in patients at risk:
- Lymphopenia
- Positive serologic test for syphilis
- Increased ESR
- Increased serum LD

[11]Bottles K, McPhaul I, Volberding P. Fine-needle aspiration biopsy of patients with the acquired immunodeficiency syndrome (AIDS): experience in an outpatient clinic. *Ann Intern Med* 1988;108:42.

- Low serum cholesterol
- Indicator diseases

In the absence of laboratory evidence of HIV infection, any of these known causes of immunodeficiency disqualify the indicator disease:

- High-dose or long-term corticosteroid or other immunosuppressive/ cytotoxic therapy within 3 mos of onset of indicator disease
- Genetic (congenital) immunodeficiency syndrome or an acquired syndrome atypical of HIV infection (e.g., with hypogammaglobulinemia)
- Any of the following diseases diagnosed <3 mos after diagnosis of indicator disease: Hodgkin's disease, non-Hodgkin's lymphoma (other than primary brain lymphoma), lymphocytic leukemia, multiple myeloma, any other cancer of lymphoreticular or histiocytic tissue, angioimmunoblastic lymphadenopathy

Indicator diseases that are considered evidence of AIDS when laboratory evidence of AIDS is present in a **child aged <13 yrs**: multiple or recurrent bacterial infections, septicemia, pneumonia, meningitis, bone or joint infection, abscess of internal organ or body cavity, due to *Haemophilus*, *Streptococcus* (including pneumococcus) or other pyogenic bacteria.

Recommended for HIV blood testing are

- Persons with a history of identifiable risks (e.g., IV drug users, prostitutes, homosexual or bisexual men, persons with infected sex partners) or have sexual partners with such risks
- All patients with TB
- Inmates of correctional institutions
- Persons who may have an STD, TB, hepatitis B or C, or non-A, non-B hepatitis
- Persons who received transfusions of blood or blood products (e.g., factor VIII) between 1978 and 1985 but not including immune serum globulin or albumin
- Persons who are planning marriage
- Women of childbearing age
- Patients admitted to hospitals
- Those who consider themselves at risk
- Donors of blood, organs, sperm

A repeat positive test result requires the blood donor facility to inform the donor.

Approximately 22–50% of persons positive for HIV antibody developed AIDS by 5 yrs and 50–70% by 10 yrs.

Prediction of which seropositive persons will develop AIDS or show clinical symptoms is not possible. Antibody-positive persons are potentially infectious.

Increased serum gamma globulins early in course of HIV infection, especially IgG and also IgA; slight IgM increase may occur; associated with opportunistic infection.

Clinical Category (A)

- Asymptomatic patients with none of the disorders of Category (B) or (C)
- Documented HIV infection and ≥1 of the following
Asymptomatic HIV infection

Persistent generalized lymphadenopathy

Acute HIV infection.

Clinical Category (B)

- Symptomatic patients with none of the disorders of Category (A) or (C) with conditions due to HIV infection or defect in cell-mediated immunity or where clinical course or management is complicated by HIV infection.
- Examples of conditions include (but are not limited to):
Bacillary angiomatosis; Candidiasis, oropharyngeal (thrush); Candidiasis, vulvo vaginal; frequent, persistent, or poorly responsive to therapy. Cervical dysplasia, moderate or severe or carcinoma in situ. Constitutional symptoms e.g., fever or diarrhea for >1 mo. Hairy leukoplakia, oral. Herpes zoster of >1 dermatome or at least 2 episodes. Idiopathic thrombocytopenic purpura. Listeriosis. PID, especially if with tubo-ovarian abscess. Peripheral neuropathy.

Clinical Category (C)–AIDS-indicator conditions

Candidiasis of trachea, bronchi, lungs or esophagus. Cervical cancer, invasive.* Coccidioidomycosis, extrapulmonary or disseminated. Cryptococcosis, extrapulmonary. Cryptosporidiosis, intestinal for >1 mo. CMV other than liver, spleen or lymph nodes. CMV retinitis with loss of vision. Encephalopathy, HIV related. Herpes simplex ulcer for >1 mo or bronchitis, pneumonitis, esophagitis. Histoplasmosis, disseminated or extrapulmonary. Isosporiasis, intestinal for >1 mo. Kaposi's sarcoma. Lymphoma, Burkitt's or immunoblastic or primary of brain. Mycobacterium tuberculosis, any site.* Mycobacterium, any species, disseminated or extrapulmonary. Pneumoncystis carinii pneumonia. Pneumonia, recurrent (more than 1 episode in a year).* Progressive multifocal leukoencephalopathy. Salmonella septicemia, recurrent. Toxoplasmosis of brain. Wasting syndrome due to HIV.

* = Added to list since 1991.

AIDS-Related Complex (Chronic Lymphadenopathy Syndrome)

♦ Defined as lymphadenopathy lasting for >3 mos involving more than two extrainguinal sites in homosexual men without other illness or drug use known to cause lymphadenopathy. Lymph node biopsy shows reactive hyperplasia.

CD4⁺ T-Lymphocytopenia, Idiopathic[12]

♦ Low CD4⁺ T-cell count (usually <300/cu mm) and level of <20% on one or more occasions; counts are stable rather than progressive depletion.
♦ HIV-1, HIV-2, HTLV-I, HTLV-II are not identified by serologic, immunologic, or virologic studies; no other obvious causes of immunosuppression can be identified.
Immunoglobulins are normal or slightly decreased, unlike in AIDS.
Opportunistic infections may be present.
Syndrome not present in sex partners, household contacts, or blood donors; other epidemiologic and clinical differences from AIDS.

Antibody to Human T-Lymphotropic Virus Type I (HTLV-I)
HTLV-I is a retrovirus but not closely related to HIV. HTLV-I does not cause depletion of helper T lymphocytes and is not generally associated with immunosuppression. HTLV-I does not cause AIDS, and presence of antibody does not imply HIV infection or risk of AIDS. HTLV-I and HIV antigens do not cross-react. HTLV infection and positive serology are lifelong.
Positive screening test (ELISA) is recommended for screening for whole blood and cellular components and should be confirmed by more specific tests (Western blot; if indeterminate then radioimmune precipitation). Sensitivity and specificity of ELISA is >97%. Source plasma need not be screened for HTLV-I. Repeatedly positive donors should be permanently deferred and counseled against donating blood, sharing needles, breast feeding, etc. Neither the screening tests nor more specific tests distinguish between antibodies to HTLV-I and HTLV-II (a closely related human retrovirus). HTLV-II has been isolated from patients with hairy cell leukemia but has not been proved to cause any disease.
Seroconversion occurs in 63% of recipients of blood transfusions containing cells but not plasma fractions, 25% of breast-fed infants of seropositive mothers, and fewer non–breast-fed infants. Smaller percentage in sexual partners.
Viral culture and PCR for research use only
May Be Positive In
Adult T-cell leukemia/lymphoma (see p. 406). Risk of disease estimated at 2–4% after infection for 20 yrs.
Degenerative neurologic disease called tropical spastic paraparesis in Caribbean and HTLV-I–associated myelopathy in Japan. Latent period of clinical disease is ~4 yrs after blood transfusion.
In United States in female prostitutes, recipients of multiple blood transfusions, up to 49% of IV drug users. Rare in homosexual men, patients in STD clinics; nonexistent in hemophiliacs. 0.025% incidence in random blood donors.
In Caribbean islands, found in 5% of general population and 15% of older persons.
In Japan, found in up to 15% of general population and 30% of older persons.

Retroviral Syndrome, Acute

(Syndrome of fever, malaise, lymphadenopathy, skin rash occurring in first few weeks after HIV infection)
Antibody test is not yet positive.
Nucleic acid testing is needed to detect HIV.

[12]Fauci AS. CD4⁺ T-lymphocytopenia without HIV infection—no lights, no camera, just facts. *N Engl J Med* 1993;328:429.

Chickenpox (Varicella-Zoster) and Herpes Zoster (Shingles)

(Shingles is reactivation of latent VZV.)

◆ Demonstration of DNA sequences by PCR is 88% sensitive in stained smears and 97% sensitive in unstained smears.

○ Microscopic demonstration of epithelial giant cells with intranuclear inclusion in fluid or base of vesicle (Tzanck smear) has 75% sensitivity. Also positive in herpes simplex.

◆ Demonstration of VZV antigen by immunofluorescent staining in material from a lesion is diagnostic of acute infection; is more sensitive than culture (in contrast to HSV and CMV infections), especially with crusted lesions. Allows prompt diagnosis.

◆ Isolation of VZV by culture of vesicle fluid or scrapings of lesion; is insensitive (44%), may take up to 2 wks.

◆ Serologic tests (ELISA, CF) to confirm prior infection and immunity; often not helpful in acute infection because antibody increases late. Antibody may not prevent clinical infection, especially in immunocompromised persons. Heterotypic rise in antibodies is very frequent in primary HSV infection. Useful for diagnosis of fetal infection. Presence in CSF is diagnostic of aseptic meningitis due to VZV even without presence of skin lesions.

  • ELISA titers of IgG and IgM usually appear within 5 days of varicella rash; IgM disappears in weeks to months but IgG persists for indeterminate time. Significant titer increase is diagnostic. Sensitivity = 87–96%; specificity = 82–99%. 20× more sensitive than CF.

  • CF usually appears at 7–10 days and peaks 2–3 wks after varicella rash; becomes undetectable in several months in >50% of patients; appears 1–2 days after herpes zoster. Least sensitive test; not reliable to determine immunity. Not reliable in childhood leukemia. Acute and convalescent sera with ≥ 4× increase in CF titer is diagnostic of acute infection.

  • Latex agglutination test is sensitive, commercially available, rapid, simple to perform.

  • IFA, RIA, IHA tests are not suitable for use in general laboratories.

WBC is normal; may increase with secondary bacterial infection.

○ 40% of herpes zoster patients show increased cells (<300 mononuclear cells/cu mm) in CSF.

  • Culture is rarely positive in HSV encephalitis; PCR-based detection is useful. ≤ 40% of bone marrow transplant recipients develop infection or reactivation.

Choriomeningitis, Lymphocytic

○ CSF

  • Cell count is increased (100–3000 lymphocytes/cu mm, occasionally <30,000).

  • Protein is normal or slightly increased.

  • Glucose is usually normal.

◆ Serologic tests

  • IgM (IFA) may be detected in serum and CSF within first week of illness.

  • IgG (IFA) may appear very early (therefore sera should be drawn early), making 4× increase in titer difficult to detect; slowly declines over months.

  • Increasing CF antibody titer between acute and convalescent sera (2–3 wks). Disappears in a few months.

  • Neutralizing antibodies appear in 1–2 mos, last for many years; therefore useful to document past infection.

Viral isolation by animal inoculation is not routinely performed.

WBC is slightly decreased at first; normal with onset of meningitis.

ESR is usually normal.

Thrombocytopenia develops during first week.

Colorado Tick Fever

(Due to an orbivirus)

◆ Serologic tests show an increase in antibodies (EIA, IFA, CF, and neutralizing) between acute- and convalescent-phase sera. EIA and IFA titers are larger and appear earlier, often within 10 days, and persist for life. IFA for IgG is 90% sensitive and IFA for IgM is 66% sensitive. CF antibodies last only a few months, so presence of CF suggests recent infection.

◆ DFA method can demonstrate antigen in peripheral RBCs in 40% of cases 8 wks after onset and sometimes for up to 6 mos. During first week 50% of cases show false-negative results.

♦ Virus isolation is the most reliable test.
♦ Blood may be inoculated into suckling mice.
WBC is decreased (2000–4000/cu mm). The number of PMNs is decreased, but with shift to the left.

Coxsackievirus and Echovirus Infections

(These include epidemic pleurodynia, grippe, meningitis, myocarditis, herpangina.)
Laboratory findings are not specific.
CSF
  • Cell count of ≤ 500/cu mm, occasionally ≤ 2000/cu mm; predominantly PMNs at first, then predominantly lymphocytes.
  • Protein may increase by ≤ 100 mg/dL.
  • Glucose is normal.
WBC varies but is usually normal.
Serologic tests may show increasing titer of neutralizing or CF antibodies between acute- and convalescent-phase sera. Are generally not clinically helpful because of many serotypes and extensive cross reaction with other enteroviruses. With coxsackievirus A or B infection, CF antibodies are often increased in acute phase, making 4× rise in titer difficult to demonstrate.
  ♦ Culture is required for certain syndromes (e.g., chronic meningoencephalitis with agammaglobulinemia may show echovirus 11 in CSF).

Cytomegalic Virus (CMV) Inclusion Disease

(Member of herpesvirus family)
Confirmation of diagnosis is important for diagnosis of opportunistic infection in immunosuppressed patients.
  ♦ • Sampling of BAL fluid for diagnosis of interstitial pneumonitis in immunocompromised patients through shell culture and monoclonal antibody testing is more sensitive than routine cytology and can be combined with nucleic acid hybridization assay or routine cell culture.
  ♦ • GI tract disease is confirmed by biopsy findings showing presence of typical inclusions, immunologic stain for CMV antigen, or in situ DNA probe for CMV DNA.
  ♦ Counseling of pregnant women who may have been exposed
  • Intrauterine CMV infection due to infection of mother during pregnancy causes obvious CMV inclusion disease in 10–15% of infants at birth; many affected infants die soon after birth and others may require lifelong institutionalization. Fetal infection in ~20% of these (≤ 2 in 1000 births). In 5 yrs, 25% have sequelae (e.g., CNS effects, chorioretinitis).
  • Special culture techniques using urine specimens give earlier results in congenital CMV infection than in infection in other populations; within first 2 wks, is most sensitive and specific means for diagnosis of congenital CMV infection.
  • PCR to detect CMV is rapid, sensitive, specific.
  • CMV IgM antibodies (>1:32) are found in approximately two-thirds of infants infected in utero; presence in single infant serum specimen is diagnostic. Amniotic fluid viral culture is sensitive and specific indicator of intrauterine CMV infection.
  • Finding of intranuclear inclusions in epithelial cells in urine sediment and liver biopsy is diagnostic; more useful in infants than adults.
  • Negative finding of CMV IgG in mother and child excludes CMV infection.
  ♦ Congenital infection
  • Isolation in standard cell culture (shows cytopathic effects in 3–7 days) of urine, saliva, or tissue within first 21 days of life is gold standard for diagnosis of intrauterine infection. After 21 days, perinatal infection cannot be ruled out.
  • Shell viral assay—see following.
  • Maximum sensitivity when both culture systems are used.
  • Detection of CMV IgM by EIA (94% specificity, 69% sensitivity) or RIA (100% specificity, 89% sensitivity), but EIA is more convenient. Should be confirmed by culture.
  • Electron microscopy of urine has ~66% sensitivity. Cannot distinguish CMV from other herpesviruses.
  • Microscopic examination of tissue showing intranuclear inclusions and giant cell formation in stillborn infants.

- PCR assay for CMV DNA in urine, CSF, serum has excellent sensitivity and specificity.

○Screening and diagnosis in blood transfusion and organ transplant patients
- CMV infection occurs in >50% of bone marrow transplant patients, usually in 1–3 mos. CMV pneumonia causes significant mortality in allogeneic bone marrow transplant patients. Seronegative patients should be given CMV seronegative blood products. Filtration to reduce leukocytes to <10^6/U may prevent transmission by transfusion of unscreened blood.

○Syndrome of heterophil-negative infectious mononucleosis in immunologically competent adults characterized by
- Hematologic and hepatic test findings identical with those in heterophil-positive infectious mononucleosis due to EBV (see p. 842). CMV causes two-thirds of all heterophil-negative mononucleosis-like illness in patients over age 14 yrs.
- Immunologic findings.
  Increased cold agglutinin titer (same as in heterophil-positive patients)
  Cryoglobulinemia is common (mixed IgG-IgM).
  Increased RF (cold reactive more common than warm reactive)
  Positive result on direct Coombs' test is common.
  Polyclonal hypergammaglobulinemia is common.
  False-positive results on serologic test for syphilis in <3% of cases
  ANAs (speckled pattern) commonly present transiently

◆Serologic tests
- Latex agglutination to detect CMV antibody is rapid assay with sensitivity of 98%; useful for blood and organ donor screening; negative tests are confirmed by EIA. ~50% of adults in North America are seropositive for CMV antibodies; in urban areas incidence may be >80%.
- Presence of CMV IgM within 1–2 wks allows rapid diagnosis of primary infection using a single test during acute illness (>1:32); titer of <1:16 may persist for 12 mos in 24% of patients. Only IgG appears during reactivation. IgM in adults indicates acute infection, reinfection (within past 3–4 mos), or reactivation; IgM in newborns indicates in utero infection as IgM does not cross placenta.
- 4× increase in serial CMV IgG antibody titer in 2–4 wks in primary infection but only occasionally in reactivation or reinfection limits value in adults.
- CMV antigenemia test kit is said to have 83% sensitivity and 89% specificity.

◆Confirmatory tests for CMV
- Isolation of virus in standard cell culture.
- Active CMV infection is most accurately diagnosed by rapid tissue culture (shell viral) with DFA staining, which permits detection in urine, blood, secretions, and tissues in <36 hrs. CMV antigen can be detected in infected cell cultures within hours. Because virus may be shed in absence of disease for up to 2 yrs after primary infection, results must be interpreted carefully. Peripheral blood leukocytes are frequently positive for CMV in immunocompromised patients and those with CMV mononucleosis and indicates viremia. Virus may be isolated in cell culture in 7–21 days.
- Identification of CMV inclusion bodies or CMV antigen in infected tissue (e.g., BAL fluid) by IFA is more rapid but less sensitive than culture. CMV immediate early antigen can be detected by IFA before cytopathic findings are positive.
- Nucleic acid hybridization and PCR techniques have high sensitivity and specificity.
Hemolytic anemia with icterus and thrombocytopenic purpura in infants
Laboratory changes due to involvement of liver, kidney, brain
- Encephalitis found in 16% of HIV-infected patients; 85% of cases are infected with HIV.
  PCR sensitivity = 79%, specificity = 95%.
  Viral cultures of CSF are usually negative.
  Other techniques include detection of pp65 antigen in CSF WBCs, CMV DNA in CSF, in situ hybridization of CSF WBCs, increased CMV antibody CSF/serum ratio.
Laboratory findings due to predisposing or underlying conditions (e.g., AIDS, malignant lymphoma, leukemia, refractory anemia, after renal transplant) or after receiving many transfusions of fresh blood; may be associated with infection by other opportunistic pathogens in adults.
- Disseminated CMV disease occurs in immunosuppressed patients (e.g., retinitis-induced blindness occurs in 10–45% of AIDS patients).

Dengue

(Due to arbovirus of Flavivirus genus)
♦ Serologic tests
* IgM-specific antibodies (ELISA) appear by third afebrile day, last 30–60 days, then decline but may persist for long periods. Cross reaction with other viruses may occur (e.g., St. Louis encephalitis, Japanese encephalitis viruses).
* Acute- and convalescent-phase sera show increasing titer.
* Viral cell culture and IFA.
* PCR and nucleic acid hybridization.

WBC decreased (2000–5000/cu mm) with toxic granulation of leukocytes in early stage; often increased during convalescence
Children commonly have decreased platelets.

Encephalitides, Arboviral

(Includes LaCrosse, eastern and western equine, and St. Louis encephalitis)
CSF findings (see Table 9-1, p. 264).
♦ Serologic tests for arboviruses
* Antibody-capture ELISA detects IgM early in single specimen in serum and CSF; becomes positive in <1 wk and lasts a few weeks; persists ≤ 8 mos in 29% of St. Louis encephalitis cases.
* Paired sera testing for IgG (EIA, IFA, neutralization, hemagglutination) showing 4× increase in titer can confirm diagnosis but has poor specificity. CF is unpredictable for routine diagnosis.

Marked decrease occurs in WBC with relative lymphocytosis.

Encephalomyelitis (Viral and Postinfectious)

CSF
* Early (first 2–3 days)
    Cell count is usually increased (≤ 100/cu mm), mostly PMNs (higher total count and more PMNs in infants).
    Protein is usually normal.
    Glucose and chloride are normal.
* Later (after third day)
    Increased cell count is >90% lymphocytes.
    Protein gradually increases after first week (≤ 100 mg/dL).
    Glucose and chloride remain normal.

Serologic tests for specific virus identification and additional laboratory tests; see separate sections for each agent and disease (e.g., CMV, mumps, measles, rabies, psittacosis, poliomyelitis, coxsackievirus and echovirus, lymphocytic choriomeningitis, equine encephalomyelitis, etc.)

Epstein-Barr Virus (EBV) Infections

(Human herpesvirus-4 of DNA viruses; infects B lymphocytes and epithelial cells; long lasting, generally latent, frequent reactivation is common.)
Infectious Mononucleosis
♦ Diagnostic criteria are
* Compatible clinical syndrome.
* Hematologic findings of absolute (>4500/cu mm) and relative (≥ 50%) lymphocytosis in >70% of cases and ≥ 10% (often ≤ 70%) characteristically atypical lymphocytes. <10% atypical lymphocytes are found in other viral diseases and conditions (e.g., rubella, roseola, mumps, acute viral hepatitis, toxoplasmosis, CMV infection, acute HIV infection, drug reactions). Automated cell counters may not identify atypical lymphocytes.
* Serologic findings. See Heterophil Agglutination (Paul-Bunnell Test).

Leukopenia and granulocytopenia are evident during first week. Later, WBC is increased (usually 10,000–20,000/cu mm) because of increased lymphocytes; peak changes occur in 7–10 days; may persist for 1–2 mos. Increased number of bands and >5% eosinophilia are frequent.
○ Evidence of mild hepatitis (e.g., increased serum transaminases, increased urine urobilinogen) is very frequent at some stage but may be transient. Increased serum

Table 15-9. Sample Titers in Heterophil Agglutination

Presumptive Test	After Guinea Pig Kidney Absorption	After Beef RBC Absorption	Interpretation of Diagnosis of Infectious Mononucleosis
1:224	1:112	0	+
1:224	1:56	0	+
1:224	1:28	0	+
1:224	1:14 or less	0	−
1:224	1:56	1:56	−
1:224	0	1:112	−
1:56	1:56–1:7	0	+
1:56	1:56	1:28	−
1:28	1:28–1:7	0	+

bilirubin in ≤ 30% of adults and <9% of children. Bilirubin/enzyme dissociation (serum bilirubin normal or <2 mg/dL with moderate increase of ALP, GGT, AST, ALT) occurs in 75% of cases. If no liver function abnormalities can be found, another diagnosis should be sought.
♦ EBV can be confirmed in liver biopsy by in situ hybridization or PCR.
Serologic test for syphilis, RA test, and ANA may show transient false-positive results.
Occasional RBCs and albumin are seen in urine.
Mild thrombocytopenia is seen in ~50% of early cases, and platelet dysfunction is frequent.
Hemolytic anemia is rare.

♦ **Heterophil Agglutination (Paul-Bunnell Test)**
(Agglutination of sheep RBCs by serum of patients with infectious mononucleosis due to EBV)
Commercial slide agglutination ("spot") tests are now performed as the usual initial test and tube dilution tests are done only if necessary for confirmation; sensitivity is ≤ 92%, specificity is >96%, except for children <4 yrs old, for whom slide test is less sensitive. False-positive slide test results may occur in leukemia, malignant lymphoma, malaria, rubella, serum hepatitis, and pancreatic carcinoma, and may be present for years in some persons with no known explanation. False-positive results in ~2% and false-negative results in ~5–7% of adults.
Titers of ≤ 1:56 may occur in normal persons and in patients with other illnesses.
A titer of ≥ 1:224 is presumptive evidence of infectious mononucleosis but may also be caused by recent injection of horse serum or horse immune serum. Therefore a differential absorption test should be performed using guinea pig kidney and beef cell antigens. See Table 15-9.
Guinea pig absorption will not reduce the titer in infectious mononucleosis to <25% of the original value; most commonly the titer is not reduced by more than one or two tube dilutions. If >90% of the agglutination is removed by guinea pig adsorption, the test is considered negative.
Beef red cell absorption takes most (90%) or all of the sheep agglutinations and does reduce the titer in infectious mononucleosis; failure to reduce the titer is evidence against a diagnosis of infectious mononucleosis.
Heterophil agglutination is positive in 60% of young adults by 2 wks and in 90% by 4 wks after onset of clinical infectious mononucleosis; thus may be negative when positive hematologic and clinical findings are present, and a second heterophil agglutination test performed 1–2 wks later may be positive. Heterophil agglutination results may have become negative even though some residual hematologic findings are still present. Low titers may persist for a year.
When horse RBCs are used for the test, results may still be positive up to 12 mos after the acute illness in up to 75% of cases.

Heterophil antibodies are found in only 30% of children <2 yrs old, 75% of children 2–4 yrs old, and >90% of older children with infectious mononucleosis.

False-positive test results are very rare and occur with relatively low titers. A resurgence of heterophil antibody titer may occur in response to other infections (e.g., viral URI). Occasionally positive in other diseases (e.g., lymphoma, hepatitis, autoimmune disease [e.g., RA], rubella).

Is not specific for EBV. Titer does not cross-react with or correlate with antibodies for EBV; neither correlates with severity of illness. Not useful for evaluating chronic disease.

Heterophil agglutination test is almost never positive in Japanese patients with infectious mononucleosis for unknown reasons.

Heterophil-negative infectious mononucleosis-like disorder may occur in 10% of patients (mostly young children) with clinical syndrome due to toxoplasmosis, viral infections, CMV infection, hepatitis, rubella, and acute HIV infection. When heterophil agglutination results are negative, diagnosis must be confirmed by identification of EBV-specific antibodies.

Chronic Mononucleosis Syndrome
(Three types are described; many question the existence of this syndrome.)

♦ • True chronic mononucleosis is caused by EBV in >90% of cases; typical clinical picture with positive heterophil and serologic evidence of primary EBV infection but patient does not recover for many months or years; may be related to immunodeficiency. Caused by CMV (see p. 840) in 5–7% of cases and by *T. gondii* in <1% of cases. Less common causes include AIDS, HSV-2, varicella, viral hepatitis, adenovirus, rubella, certain drugs (e.g., PAS, phenytoin, sulfasalazine, dapsone).

• Severe chronic active EBV infection (very rare) with very high EBV antibody titers and persistent serious disease (e.g., pancytopenia, agranulocytosis, chronic hepatitis, pneumonia); may coexist with true chronic mononucleosis.

• "Chronic mononucleosis"—rare distinct entity marked by pancytopenia, chronic lymphadenopathy, interstitial pneumonitis, no preceding acute mononucleosis, fatigue, fever, for >6 mos. Heterophil is positive in ~10% of cases. No definitive diagnostic laboratory tests. Usually not more than three of the following are present in a patient:

Leukopenia (3000–5000/cu mm) with monocytosis (7–15%), relative lymphocytosis (>40%), atypical lymphocytes (1–20%).
Low ESR (<4 mm/hr)
Mild increase in serum AST and ALT
Reduction in immunoglobulins
Low levels of circulating immune complexes
Increased CD4/CD8 ratio
EBV serology
IgG–viral capsid antigen (VCA) and early antigen (EA) antibody present
IgM-VCA not detectable
Epstein-Barr nuclear antigen (EBNA)–antibody <1:5

♦ Serologic Tests for EBV

EBV antibody tests are rarely required because 90% of cases are heterophil positive and false-positive results are rare, and because illness is usually self-limited and relatively mild. May be useful in atypical or very severe cases with negative heterophil tests, especially in young children or immunocompromised patients. (See Table 15-10 and Fig. 15-8.)

IgG-VCA indicates past infection and immunity. May be present early in illness, usually before clinical symptoms are present, detected at onset in 100% of cases; only 20% show 4× increase in titer after visiting a doctor. Decreases during convalescence but detectable for many years after illness; therefore not helpful in establishing diagnosis of infectious mononucleosis.

IgM-VCA detected at onset in 100% of cases, high titers present in serum 1–6 wks after onset of illness, starts to fall by third week and usually disappear in 1–6 mos; sera are often taken too late for IgM-VCA to be detected. Is almost always present in active EBV infection and thus most sensitive and specific to confirm acute infectious mononucleosis. May be positive in other herpesvirus infections (especially CMV); therefore confirmation with IgG and EBNA assays is recommended.

Table 15-10. Serologic Antibody Patterns in Epstein-Barr Virus (EBV) Infection

	Susceptible (No Past Infection)	Primary EBV (Acute Infection)	Convalescent (3 mos)	Prior (Past Infection)	Reactivated (Chronic Infection)
VCA-IgM	–	+	±	–	–
VCA-IgG	–	+	+	+	+
EA-D	–	+*	+*	–	+*
EA-R					
EBNA	–	–	+	+	+

EA-D = early antigen complex, diffuse component; EA-R = early antigen complex, restricted component; EBNA = Epstein-Barr–associated nuclear antigen; VCA = viral capsid antigen.
+ indicated titer of >1:5.
*Titer is <1:5 in 80% of patients.

Early antigen anti-D titers rise later in course of infectious mononucleosis (3–4 wks after onset; increase is transient) than VCA-antibody and disappear with recovery; combined with IgG-VCA, suggests recent EBV infection; found in only 70% of patients with infectious mononucleosis due to EBV. High titers are found in nasopharyngeal carcinoma.

Early antigen anti-R antibodies rarely occur in primary EBV infection, appear 2 wks to months after onset, may persist for a year; found more often in atypical or protracted cases. No clinical significance; high titers are found in chronic active EBV infection or Burkitt's lymphoma.

EBNAs are the last antibodies to appear, are rare in acute phase; rise during convalescence (3–12 mos) and are found a few weeks after onset of clinical illness; persist for many years after illness. Absence when IgM-VCA and anti-D are present implies recent infection. Appearance early in illness excludes primary EBV infection. Appearance after previous negative test evidences recent EBV infection. ELISA kits detect EBNA IgG and IgM simultaneously; IgM > IgG indicates acute infection but IgG > IgM indicates previous exposure to EBV. Absent EBNA and presence of VCA indicates acute infection.

Acute primary EBV infection is indicated by one or more of the following serologic findings:
- IgM-VCA that is found early and later declines
- High titer (≥ 1:320) or ≥ 4× rise in IgG-VCA titer during the illness
- Transient rise in early antigen anti-D titer (≥ 1:10)
- Early IgG-VCA without EBNA and later appearance of EBNA

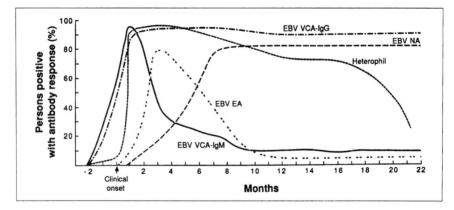

Fig. 15-8. Percentage of persons with positive antibody response to Epstein-Barr virus (EBV) at specified time intervals. (EA = early antigen; NA = nuclear antigen; VCA = viral capsid antigen [Ortho Diagnostic Systems, Raritan, NJ].)

Acute or primary EBV infection is excluded when IgG-VCA and EBNA titers are unchanged in acute- and convalescent-phase serum samples.

Current or recent infection is indicated by IgM anti-VCA or IgM/IgG early antigen with low or absent EBNA antibodies.

Persistence of early antigen and IgG-VCA in high titer indicates chronic EBV infection.

50% of persons have antibodies to EBV by age 5 yrs, 90% by age 20, >95% by mid-20s.

EBNA is often absent in immunosuppressed patients. Early antigen-D and early antigen-R may be increased with no change in VCA.

EBV is associated with Burkitt's lymphoma and B-cell lymphoma in immunosuppressed patients (e.g., AIDS patients, organ transplant recipients) and with poorly differentiated nasopharyngeal carcinoma. In both, anti-VCA titers are increased 8–10×.
- *Anti–early antigen-R titer is high and correlated with tumor burden in Burkitt's lymphoma.*
- *Anti–early antigen-D titer is high and correlated with tumor burden nasopharyngeal carcinoma.*
- Severe, often fatal mononucleosis occurs in patients with X-linked lymphoproliferative syndrome; predisposes to subsequent lymphoma.
- May be implicated in some cases of Hodgkin's disease and some cases of aplastic anemia.

Erythema Infectiosum (Fifth Disease)

(Due to parvovirus B19)
♦ Indirect EIA for IgG has sensitivity of 94% and specificity of 86%. Persists for several years. Present in 10% of children <5 yrs old and 50% of adults. Indicates previous infection and immunity. IgM is detected within 3 days after symptoms, peaks in ~1 mo, undetectable after 2–3 mos but may last for 6 mos.

IgG	IgM	Interpretation
–	–	No exposure/immunity
+	–	Past infection and immunity
–	+	Recent infection
+	+	Recent infection

Detection by electron microscopy is difficult and expensive.

WBC is normal. Some patients have slight increase in eosinophils.

Laboratory findings due to sequelae
- Pure erythrocyte aplasia and persistent infection in patients with underlying hemolytic anemias (sickle cell disease, hereditary spherocytosis, pyruvate kinase deficiency, beta-thalassemia) and immunosuppressed hosts.
- Fetal hydrops or spontaneous abortion during pregnancy.
- Acute arthritis.
- Chronic infection may cause severe anemia in immunocompromised persons.

Intrauterine infection is uncommon.
- Fetal anemia may occur without permanent damage.
- Intranuclear inclusions in erythroid precursors.
- Fetal mortality is ~9%.
- Causes ~25% of cases of nonimmune hydrops fetalis.
- Congenital malformations are rare.

♦ Diagnosis by
- Specific IgM present in cord blood.
- IgG seroconversion; high concentrations of IgG persist for >1 yr.
- In situ DNA hybridization or PCR applied to maternal or fetal blood or amniotic fluid.

Exanthema Subitum (Roseola Infantum)

(Due to human herpesvirus 6)
WBC is increased during fever, then decreased during rash, with relative lymphocytosis.

HHV-6 (a newly recognized virus) can be isolated from these patients (and also from some patients with HIV-1, HIV-2, and HTLV-I and patients with some lymphoproliferative disorders in which it may be a cofactor).

Infection with HHV-6 (variant B) occurs in 30–60% of bone marrow and organ transplant patients. May cause marrow suppression (varies from transient to fatal aplas-

tic anemia), encephalitis, interstitial pneumonitis, susceptibility to other viral infections (e.g., EBV, CMV, RSV, adenovirus).
♦ Tissue cell cultures show specific cytopathic effects (requires 5–21 days).
♦ Rapid shell viral (early antigen) assay can detect infection within 72 hrs. Sensitivity of 86% and specificity of 100% reported in marrow and liver transplant patients.
♦ PCR to detect HHV-6 DNA in blood cells has limited value in diagnosing active infections, although in latent infections blood monocytes contain <10 HHV-6 genomes/10^6 cells.
♦ Antibody titer to HHV-6 rises in convalescent-phase serum 3 wks after onset of exanthema subitum. Seroprevalence in healthy adults is >90%. Useful to detect latent infection or seroprevalence but may not be reliable indicator of reactivation.
♦ Immunohistochemical stains can detect HHV-6 in tissues.

Gastroenteritis (Infections of GI Tract)

See p. 181.

Hemorrhagic Epidemic Fevers

(Due to hantavirus, a genus in family Bunyaviridae)
Hemorrhagic Fever with Renal Syndrome
Laboratory findings due to renal damage
• Proteinuria
• Oliguria with azotemia and hemoconcentration and abnormal electrolyte concentrations
• *Return of normal tubular function may take 4–6 wks.*
WBC is increased, with shift to the left.
Coagulopathy
• Platelet count is decreased (<100,000/cu mm) in 50% of patients.
• PT and aPTT may be increased.
• DIC may occur.
Increased serum LD and decreased albumin and total protein.
Hantavirus Pulmonary Syndrome
(Recently described in Southwestern United States; causes rapidly progressive noncardiac pulmonary edema. Primarily carried by deer mice. Mortality is >55%.)
♦ Immunohistochemical staining can identify hantaviral antigens in formalin-fixed tissues.
♦ Rapid test using Western blot and recombinant antigens detects IgG and IgM antibodies. Positive tests are confirmed by ELISA at CDC.
CDC is distributing ELISA assays to state laboratories to detect IgG and IgM.
CBC shows thrombocytopenia, hemoconcentration, presence of immunoblasts.
Other viral hemorrhagic fevers (e.g., in Philippines, Thailand, Singapore, Argentina, Bolivia, Crimea, Omsk, Kyasanur forest) show much less severe renal damage, and WBC is normal (Philippines, Thailand) or decreased.

Hepatitis

See Chapter 8, e.g., p. 223.

Herpes Simplex

(Due to HSV)
♦ Cell culture of vesicles or ulcers is reference method, and confirmation by staining with specific monoclonal antibodies establishes the diagnosis; is most sensitive (83%) and specific method; may take up to 7 days but usually available within 4 days. Cultures from crusted lesions and from recurrent late disease are much less sensitive. Immune assay studies confirm that isolate is HSV and differentiate HSV-1 and HSV-2.
♦ Antigen detection (EIA or direct fluorescence) in clinical specimen (e.g., skin vesicles) is more rapid (1–4 hrs) and as sensitive (70–94%) as culture in asymptomatic persons, and is significantly more sensitive and specific than Tzanck test or direct electron microscopy. Specificity is >92%. Distinguishes HSV-1 and HSV-2 and permits rapid diagnosis.
♦ DNA identification by PCR identifies HSV in tissue or cell samples, is sensitive, specific, rapid but not commercially available.
♦ Direct cytologic examination of scrapings of lesions (Wright-Giemsa stain) show multinucleated giant cells with intranuclear inclusions (Tzanck smear). Skin vesicles yield

a positive smear in 66% and a positive viral culture in 100% of cases; pustules yield a positive smear in 50% and a positive viral culture in 70% of cases; crusted ulcers yield a positive smear in 15% and a positive viral culture in 34% of cases. Permits rapid diagnosis. Does not differentiate HSV-1, HSV-2, and VZV. Occasionally smears from pemphigus or contact dermatitis lesions have been called positive. ("Positive smear" refers to presence of multinucleated giant cells not necessarily showing inclusions.) May also be identified in routine Pap smear of cervix by multinucleated cells showing typical intranuclear inclusions and halo. Direct electron microscopy can also be used. Other microscopy-based tests include IFA and immunoperoxidase test, which approach sensitivity of viral isolation. Negative test does not rule out this diagnosis.
Serologic tests are much less useful than detection of antigen in infected tissue (e.g., brain) by culture, microscopy, or immunoassay. Not useful clinically except rarely in primary genital herpes.
  • Primary infections show seroconversion or a ≥ 4× increase in titer of CF, EIA (IgG or IgM), and neutralizing antibodies in convalescent-phase compared with acute-phase sera.
  • In recurrent infections, a high titer is present in acute-phase sera and thus is rarely useful (5% of patients). May help in retrospect.
  • EIA, HAI, RIA, latex agglutination methods may also be used.
  • False-positive IgM may occur in presence of RF.
  • CF does not distinguish HSV-1 and HSV-2.
  • Western blot test is accurate for subtyping.
Presence of IgG does not indicate reinfection, recurrent infection, or immunity. Presence or absence in newborn is not related to severity of CNS infection. IgM can be demonstrated for weeks after primary infection. Treatment status (e.g., use of acyclovir) should be known as it may affect titers.
  • Specificity of positive tests should be checked by assay for VZV antibody.
  • Type-specific serologies include neutralization tests and Western blot assay.
♦ Findings of encephalitis if this complication occurs. High-titer serologic tests in CSF may be useful to establish the diagnosis. Antigen detection in CSF is not reliable. CSF viral culture may be useful in diagnosis of congenital infection. Causes 5% of cases of aseptic meningitis.
WBC is normal.
♦ For neonatal infection
  • Virus isolation by culture of buffy coat of blood is most reliable method; can be done within 24–48 hrs, often before IgM can be detected.
  • Specific IgM antibodies can be detected within 2 wks of onset of infection. Seroconversion or increasing IgG/IgM titers.

Human Papillomavirus Infections

(Due to subgroup of papovaviruses; >60 distinct types)
Causes genital warts, condyloma acuminatum (especially HPV-6 and 11), and cervical dysplasia and carcinoma (especially HPV-16, 18, others). May also cause juvenile laryngeal papillomatosis.
See Pelvic Inflammatory Disease, p. 759.

Measles (Rubeola)

WBC shows slight increase at onset, then falls to ~5000/cu mm with increased lymphocyte count. Increased WBC with shift to the left suggests bacterial complication (e.g., otitis media, pneumonia, appendicitis).
Mild thrombocytopenia in early stage.
Wright staining of sputum or nasal scrapings shows measles multinucleated giant cells, especially during prodrome and early rash.
♦ Pap stain of urine sediment after appearance of rash shows intracellular inclusion bodies; more specific is fluorescent antibody demonstration of measles antigen in urine sediment cells.
♦ Viral serologic tests
  • Within 6 days after onset of rash, antibodies are found in >80% of cases (HAI, EIA, IFA, CF; HAI is most sensitive). Maximum titers are reached in 2–3 wks. Paired sera show significant increases in titer. IgM is used for diagnosis of recent infection and IgG for screening for immunity. False-positive IgM may occur due to RF.

- Serum IgM (IFA, EIA) is detectable with onset of rash and usually persists for 4 wks; 50% of cases become negative by 4 mos (beginning by 2 mos). Presence of IgM or ≥ 4× rise in IgG indicates recent infection. Presence of IgG generally indicates previous exposure and present immunity.

Measles encephalitis: WBCs are markedly increased. CSF may show slightly increased protein and ≤ 500 mononuclear cells/cu mm. ≤ 10% of all measles patients have a significant increase in cells in CSF.

Postmeasles encephalitis is an autoimmune disorder; virus is not detected in brain.

Persistent CNS infection causes subacute sclerosing panencephalitis (progressive fatal illness in children 5–14 yrs old). Diagnosed by presence of IgM or ≥ 4× rise in IgG titers in CSF.

Measles may cause remission in children with nephrosis.

Mumps

Uncomplicated salivary adenitis
- WBC and ESR are normal; WBC may be decreased, with relative lymphocytosis.
- Serum and urine amylase are increased during first week of parotitis; therefore increase does not always indicate pancreatitis.
- Serum lipase is normal.
♦ • Serologic tests
  Serum IgG and IgM should be measured as early as possible and again in 10–14 days (EIA, IFA). ≥ 4× rise in IgG (88% sensitivity) or presence of IgM indicates recent infection. IgM (EIA) is present by day 2 in 70% of patients and by day 5 in 100% patients; may last >5 mos in 50% of patients. Presence of IgG indicates immunity due to past infection or vaccination. Have largely replaced serum neutralization, CF, and HAI tests, which become positive later and are much less sensitive.

Laboratory findings due to complications of mumps
- Orchitis (in 20% of postpubertal males but rare in children)—WBC is increased with shift to the left. ESR is increased. Sperm are decreased or absent after bilateral atrophy.
- Ovaries—involved in 5% of adult females.
- Pancreatitis (pp. 258–260)—much less frequent in children. Serum amylase and lipase are increased. Patient may have hyperglycemia and glycosuria.
- Meningitis or meningoencephalitis (p. 264)—aseptic meningitis occurs in 4–6% of clinical cases of mumps; causes >10% of cases of aseptic meningitis. Clinical mumps may be absent in 20–60% of patients. The disease may be clinically identical with mild paralytic poliomyelitis. WBC is usually normal. Serum amylase may be increased even if no abdominal symptoms are present. CSF contains 0–2000 mononuclear cells/cu mm.
♦ Simultaneous serum and CSF specimens show increased mumps IgG antibody index (in 83% of patients) and increased mumps IgM antibody index (in ~67% of patients with IgM in CSF). Oligoclonal Ig in CSF in 90% of cases. Virus can be isolated from CSF. PCR has been reported to provide rapid diagnosis.

Thyroiditis, myocarditis, arthritis, etc.

Phlebotomus Fever (Sandfly Fever)

Decreased WBC and lymphocytes with shift to the left of PMNs are most marked when fever ends.

CSF is normal.

Liver function tests are normal.

Urine is normal.

Poliomyelitis

CSF
- Cell count is usually 25–500/cu mm; rarely, is normal or ≤ 2000/cu mm. At first, most are PMNs; after several days, most are lymphocytes.
- Protein may be normal at first; increased by second week (usually 50–200 mg/dL); normal by sixth week.

- Glucose is usually normal.
- AST is always increased but does not correlate with serum AST; reaches peak in 1 wk and returns to normal by 4 wks; level of AST does not correlate with severity of paralysis.
- *CSF findings are not diagnostic but may occur in many CNS diseases due to viruses (e.g., coxsackievirus infection, mumps, herpes) or bacteria (e.g., pertussis, scarlet fever), other infections (e.g., leptospirosis, trichinosis, syphilis), CNS tumors, multiple sclerosis, etc.*

Blood shows early moderate increase in WBCs ($\leq$ 15,000/cu mm) and PMNs; normal within 1 wk.

Laboratory findings of associated lesions (e.g., myocarditis) or complications (e.g., secondary bacterial infection, stone formation in GU tract, alterations in water and electrolyte balance due to continuous artificial respiration)

Increased AST in 50% of patients is due to the associated hepatitis.

Serologic tests may show $\geq$ 4× increase in titer of CF antibody types 1, 2, and 3 between acute- and convalescent-phase sera (after 3 wks), but titer may have already reached peak at time of hospitalization. Not useful to determine immune status, for which neutralization test is useful. EIA, immunofluorescence, and neutralization tests have also been used.

♦ Virus may be cultured from stool up to early convalescence (done by CDC).

Rabies (Hydrophobia)

(Due to bite of rabid animal; in United States, skunks [62% of cases], bats [12%], raccoons [7%], cattle [6%], cats [4%], dogs [3%]; in Africa and Asia, dog rabies is endemic.)

Immediate notification of state and local health departments is required for prompt, expert evaluation of patient and suspected animal.

Tissue and fluids should be tested at state departments of health or CDC.

♦ Microscopic examination of brain tissue sections or imprint smears of rabid animal shows Negri bodies (intracytoplasmic inclusions) in ~80% of cases. Rabid animal dies within 7–10 days. Demonstration of Negri bodies (50–80% sensitivity) has largely been supplanted by following tests.

♦ Direct detection of virus in brain smears by fluorescein-labeled antibodies has sensitivity and specificity of >96%.

♦ Brain tissue of suspected animal is inoculated into brain of white mouse, which is later examined by immunofluorescent antibody sections. >96% sensitivity and specificity.

♦ IFA staining of corneal smears (only in research laboratories) is positive in ~50% of cases; skin and buccal mucosa biopsies, and brain biopsy material can also be used for diagnosis during clinical phase.

♦ Positive CF or neutralizing antibody in CSF is conclusive evidence of infection; serum antibodies usually require rising titer for accurate diagnosis. Antibody does not appear until >8 days (50% of cases) after onset of clinical symptoms, which may be months after exposure and is sometimes delayed or absent; almost all patients have antibodies by 15 days. Antibody appears 1–8 days later in CSF than in serum; does not occur due to immunization.

♦ PCR may be positive on nuchal skin biopsy, saliva, tears, CSF. Viral RNA can indicate variant associated with various animal sources.

♦ Viral culture from brain or saliva may be positive and can sometimes be reported in 48 hrs.

Intradermal prophylactic immunization may not be adequate and should be checked with serologic tests. Preferred is rapid fluorescent focus inhibition neutralization test.

CSF is usually normal or shows a slight increase in protein and an increased number of mononuclear cells (usually <100/cu mm).

WBC is increased (20,000–30,000/cu mm), with increased PMNs and large mononuclear cells.

Urine shows hyaline casts; reaction for albumin, sugar, and acetone may be positive.

Rubella (German Measles)

(Identifying exposure to rubella infection and verifying immunity in pregnant women is important because infection in the first trimester of pregnancy is associated

with congenital abnormalities, abortion, or stillbirth in ~30% of patients; during
first month up to 80% of patients show this association.)
♦ To determine antenatal immunity, test for IgG (EIA, HAI); IgM should also be tested
  if rubella is present in the community. IgG titer of >1:10 confirms immunity. Up to
  one-third of persons show no detectable IgG 10 yrs after vaccination. 25–50% of cases
  are subclinical.
♦ IgM is detected 11–25 days after onset of rash in all patients and may persist for up
  to 1 yr; detected 15–25 days after vaccination in 60–80% of cases. In congenital infection IgM can be detected at birth and persists for ≤ 6 mos in 90–97% of infants. During first 6 mos of life, IgM is the best test for congenital or recent infection. After age
  7 mos, persistence of IgG is assessed by HAI and EIA. IgG appears 15–25 days after
  infection and >25–50 days after vaccination. Absence of IgG in infant excludes congenital infection.
Low levels of IgM may occur in infectious mononucleosis; cross reaction may occur with
  parvovirus IgM. Some pregnant women with IgM antibodies to rubella may also have
  IgM to CMV, varicella-zoster, and measles virus.
♦ With rubella rash, diagnosis is established if acute-phase sample titer is >1:10 or if
  convalescent-phase serum taken 7 days after rash shows increase in titer.
♦ Even if no rash develops in a patient exposed to rubella, convalescent-phase serum
  taken 14–28 days after exposure that shows ≥ 4× increase in titer compared to the
  earlier sample indicates rubella infection.
♦ Reinfection (occurs occasionally but usually asymptomatic) can be suspected if
  serum samples drawn ≥ 2 wks apart show ≥ 4× increase in IgG titer and IgM does
  not develop.
♦ Rubella virus isolated from amniotic fluid indicates congenital infection.

Smallpox (Variola)

♦ Microscopic findings of cytoplasmic elementary bodies (Guarnieri's bodies) in scrap-
  ings from base of skin lesions
♦ Fluorescent antibody staining of virus from skin lesion
♦ Viral serologic tests
  • Increased titer of neutralizing antibody in acute- and convalescent-phase (2–3 wks
    later) sera
  • Rapid technique using vesicular fluid in hemagglutination, precipitation, or CF tests
WBC decreased during prodrome, increased during pustular rash.

Upper Respiratory Viral Infections

Due to Respiratory Syncytial Virus (RSV)
(Major cause of bronchiolitis and pneumonia in infants and young children)
♦ Serologic tests
  • Direct detection of antigen in clinical specimens by EIA or fluorescent antibody
    testing has high sensitivity and specificity and is test of choice.
  • Presence of serum IgM or ≥ 4× increase in IgG (EIA) indicates recent infection.
♦ Viral culture requires 4–6 days.
ESR and WBC may be increased in children.
Pharyngeal smears may reveal many epithelial cells that contain cytoplasmic inclusion
  bodies.

Due to Adenovirus
**(May cause at least six clinical syndromes involving pharynx, conjunctiva, and pneu-
  monitis; also has been associated with acute hemorrhagic cystitis, infant diar-
  rhea, genital ulcers and urethritis, CNS disease)**
♦ Serologic tests
  • EIA and immunofluorescent tests have variable sensitivity but are rapid and accurate.
♦ Cell culture can take 10–20 days. Centrifugation culture can take 2–5 days.
♦ Direct electron microscopy has been useful for diagnosis of gastroenteritis in children.
WBC is slightly decreased after ~7 days.
ESR is increased.

Due to Rhinoviruses
♦ EIA provides simple rapid diagnosis.
WBC may be slightly increased.
ESR is increased in ~5% of patients.

Due to Parainfluenza Virus

♦ Type-specific diagnosis requires recovery of virus in tissue culture.
Serologic tests
• EIA is more sensitive but less specific than CF. Not useful for routine clinical studies.
WBC is variable at first; later becomes normal or decreased.

Due to Influenza A, B

WBC is usually normal (5000–10,000/cu mm) with relative lymphocytosis.
• Leukopenia occurs in 50% of the patients. WBC >15,000/cu mm suggests secondary bacterial infection.
♦ Serologic tests
• EIA and direct immunofluorescence detection of antigen in ciliated epithelial cells from nasopharyngeal swab is now available for rapid diagnosis. Has replaced following tests.
• Presence of IgM or ≥ 4× increase in IgG (EIA, IFA) indicates recent infection. IgM peaks at 2 wks and IgG at 4–7 wks. IgG indicates past exposure and immunity.
• CF and HAI may show 4× increase in sera taken during acute phase and 2–3 wks later.

Vaccinia

(Vaccine-virus skin infection due to vaccination against smallpox)
○ Guarnieri's bodies (cytoplasmic inclusions) in skin lesions
Laboratory findings due to complications
• Progressive vaccinia. Rule out malignant lymphoma, chronic lymphatic leukemia, neoplasms, hypogammaglobulinemia, and dysgammaglobulinemia
• Superimposed infection (e.g., tetanus)
• Postvaccinal encephalitis

Yellow Fever

Decreased WBC is most marked by sixth day, associated with decrease in both leukocytes and lymphocytes.
Proteinuria occurs in severe cases.
Laboratory findings are those due to GI hemorrhage, which is frequent; associated oliguria and anuria may be present.
○ Liver function tests are abnormal, but serum bilirubin is only slightly increased.
○ Biopsy of liver for histologic examination
♦ Serum is positive by mouse intracerebral inoculation on or before the fifth day; serum during convalescence protects mice.

Rickettsiae

♦ IFA or ELISA detection of rickettsial-specific IgG and IgM. ELISA is more sensitive and specific for IgM and is now the test of choice; specimens taken at 3- to 4-day intervals show seroconversion.
♦ CF or agglutination tests are positive in most cases when group-specific and type-specific rickettsial antigens are used. These tests permit differentiation of various rickettsial diseases. No test is available for trench fever. Rising titer during convalescence is the most important criterion. Early antibiotic therapy may delay appearance of antibodies for an additional 1–4 wks, and titers may not be as high as when treatment is begun later. Low titers of CF antibodies may persist for years. CF is less sensitive than IFA.
Weil-Felix reaction has poor sensitivity and specificity and has been replaced by ELISA.
Guinea pig inoculation—scrotal reaction after intraperitoneal injection of blood into male guinea pig. Test is not often used at present.
• Marked in Rocky Mountain spotted fever and endemic typhus
• Moderate in Boutonneuse fever
• Slight in epidemic typhus and Brill-Zinsser disease
• Negative in scrub typhus, Q fever, trench fever, and rickettsialpox
♦ Microscopic examination of organisms after animal inoculation; test is not often used.
In less severe cases, blood findings are not distinctive.
In severe cases, the following changes are found:
• Early in disease WBC is decreased and lymphocytes are increased (usually 4000–6000/cu mm; as low as 1200/cu mm in early scrub typhus). Later WBC

increases to 10,000–15,000/cu mm with shift to the left and toxic granulation. If count is higher, rule out secondary bacterial infection or hemorrhage.
- Mild normochromic normocytic anemia (as low as Hb = 9 gm/dL) appears around tenth day.
- Decreased platelet count (<150,000/cu mm) is frequent.
- ESR is increased.
- Total protein and serum albumin are decreased.
- Serum sodium is frequently decreased.
- BUN may be increased (prerenal). Urine may show slight increase in albumin, hematuria, granular casts.
- CSF is normal despite symptoms of meningitis.
- Blood cultures for bacteria are negative (to rule out other tick-borne diseases, e.g., tularemia).

Laboratory findings due to specific organ involvement (e.g., pneumonitis, hepatitis) or due to complications (e.g., secondary bacterial infection, hemorrhage)

Acute GN occurs in 78% of patients with epidemic typhus, 50% of patients with Rocky Mountain spotted fever, and 30% of patients with scrub typhus.

Ehrlichiosis

(Two recently discovered tick-borne obligate intracellular rickettsial-like coc-cobacillus diseases with clinical picture similar to that of Rocky Mountain spot-ted fever or Lyme disease)

Human granulocytic ehrlichiosis due to *Ehrlichia equi* transmitted by tick (*Ixodes scapularis*)

Human monocytic ehrlichiosis due to *E. chaffeensis* transmitted most often by Lone Star tick (*Amblyomma americanum*).

♦ PCR positive for *Ehrlichia* DNA or recombinant DNA in serum or CSF in acute stage.
♦ Indirect IFA showing ≥ 4× change in specific IgG titer suggests recent infection. Is often useful only in retrospect. Peak titer of 1:160 during acute or convalescent phases. Antibodies may persist for >1 yr in ≤ 50% of patients. Some cross reactivity may be seen. Clinician must indicate to the laboratory which organism is being sought.
♦ Ehrlichial inclusion bodies (morulae) may be seen within buffy coat leukocytes or, rarely, CSF mononuclear cells with Wright stain.
♦ Ehrlichia may be isolated in culture but test is not widely available.

CSF may show increased lymphocytes and protein.

Varying combinations of anemia, thrombocytopenia, and leukopenia in 50–75% of cases.

Mild brief abnormalities in liver function tests.

Epidemic Typhus (Due to Rickettsia prowazekii), Brill-Zinsser Disease (Recrudescent Typhus Due to R. prowazekii), Murine Typhus (Due to R. typhi)

♦ Assay of paired sera for specific IgM and ≥ 4× rise in IgG (IFA, EIA) are best meth-ods and indicate recent infection. Single IFA titer of ≥ 1:128 is strongly suggestive. Specificity of these tests is close to 100%.

CF has insufficient sensitivity and specificity.

Presence of IgG generally indicates previous exposure and present immunity.

Q Fever

(Due to *Coxiella burnetii*)

♦ Single IgG titer of >1:128 or any IgM titer is diagnostically significant. ELISA is more sensitive (~95%) than IFA (~91%) and CF (~78%).

○ High specific IgM titer suggests hepatitis; high specific IgA titer is common in chronic Q fever and suggests endocarditis.

Rickettsialpox

(Due to *Rickettsia akari*)

♦ Paired early and later (2–3 wks) sera (showing 4× increase in titer) for CF and for IgM and total Ig (IFA) should be used. Should be absorbed with *R. rickettsii* and *R. akari* antigens to prove specificity of reaction.
♦ DFA reaction can be used on fixed tissue from presumed site of inoculation.

Rocky Mountain Spotted Fever

(Infectious vasculitis due to *Rickettsia rickettsii*)
♦ Direct immunofluorescence of skin biopsy specimen for antigen has sensitivity of ~70% and specificity of ~100%; is only specific test in early stages of disease.
♦ Culturing requires special conditions and is rarely performed.
♦ PCR has been used to detect *R. rickettsii* DNA in blood of patients with severe disease but is not yet available for clinical use.
♦ Paired sera showing ≥ 4× increase in IgG or total antibody by IFA or specific IgM is evidence of recent infection. IgM appears by day 3–8, peaks at 1 mo, may last 3–4 mos. IgG appears within 3 wks, peaks at 1–3 mos, and may last for 12 mos or more. Demonstrable IgG usually indicates previous exposure and immunity. Assay of paired sera for both IgG and IgM should always be done early and 10–14 days later.
CF is too insensitive to be used alone and appears too late (8–12 days) for early diagnosis and treatment. CF and IgG titers may be decreased by early treatment.
Infection may be life-threatening in patients with G-6-PD deficiency.

Scrub Typhus

(Due to *Rickettsia tsutsugamushi*)
♦ Presence of specific IgG and IgM (ELISA, IFA) strongly favors diagnosis.
○ Diagnostic Weil-Felix agglutination test shows ≥ 4× rise in titer to *Proteus vulgaris* OX-K and no reaction to *P. vulgaris* OX-2 or OX-19 (in 50–70% of patients); a single titer of ≥ 1:160 is also diagnostic; normal is ≤ 1:40. Better sensitivity and specificity than CF.

Fungi

See Table 15-11.

Actinomycosis

(Due to *Actinomyces israelii*)
♦ Recognition of organism in tissue or drainage material (e.g., fluid from sinus tracts or abscess cavities, empyema fluid; may be found normally in sputum) from sites of involvement (especially jaw, lung, cecum)
♦ Sulfur granules show radial gram-positive bacilli or filaments with central gram-negative zone.
♦ Histologic examination is suggestive; the diagnosis may be confirmed if a "ray fungus" is seen.
♦ Anaerobic culture methods (e.g., thioglycollate medium) are positive. Anaerobic growth on blood agar shows small colonies after 4–6 days. Hold 2–4 wks before considering negative.
No growth is seen on Sabouraud's medium.
Serologic tests are not useful.
Animal inoculation is negative.
WBC is normal or slightly increased (≤ 14,000/cu mm); high WBC indicates secondary infection.
ESR is usually increased.
Normocytic normochromic anemia is mild to moderate.

Aspergillosis

(Due to *Aspergillus fumigatus* and other species)
Clinical Types
- Invasive aspergillosis in immunocompromised individuals with invasion of bronchial wall. Serologic tests may be negative.
- Allergic bronchopulmonary aspergillosis occurs in 1–2% of patients with chronic asthma. EIA has ~90% sensitivity and specificity. Should be confirmed by immunoblotting. Can be monitored by changes in increased serum IgE.
- Fungus ball (pulmonary aspergilloma)—saprophytic aspergilloma superimposed on an anatomical abnormality. Serum IgG may be increased but IgE is not.
- Hypersensitivity pneumonitis (farmer's lung).
    Eosinophilia (>1000/cu mm; often >3000/cu mm)

Table 15-11. Summary of Laboratory Findings in Fungus Infections

Disease	Causative Organism	Source of Material												Diagnostic Methods					
		Blood	CSF	Stool	Urine	Nasopharynx, throat	Sputum, lung	Gastric washings	Vagina, cervix	Exudates, lesions, sinus tracts, etc.	Skin, nails, hair	Bone marrow	Lymph node	Fresh unstained material	Stained material	Culture	Animal inoculation	Serologic tests	Histologic examination
Cryptococcosis	*Cryptococcus neoformans*	+	+	+	+		+				+	+			+	+	+	+	+
Coccidioidomycosis	*Coccidioides immitis*	+	+	+			+	+			+	+	+	+		+	+	+	+
Histoplasmosis	*Histoplasma capsulatum*	+					+	+			+	+	+		+	+	+	+	+

Actinomycosis	*Actinomyces israelii*			+	+				+	+		+	+		+
Nocardiosis	*Nocardia asteroides*			+	+	+			+	+	+	+	+	+	+
North American blastomycosis	*Blastomyces dermatitidis*			+	+			+	+		+		+	+	+
South American blastomycosis	*Paracoccidioides brasiliensis*		+			+	+	+	+		+	+	+	+	+
Moniliasis	*Candida albicans*	+		+	+	+				+	+	+	+	+	
Aspergillosis	*Aspergillus fumigatus*, others			+			+		+	+	+	+	+	+	+
Geotrichosis	*Geotrichum candidum*			+					+	+	+				+
Chromoblastomycosis	*Fonsecaea pedrosoi, Phialophora verrucosa, compactum,* etc.				+			+	+	+	+				+
Sporotrichosis	*Sporotrichum schenckii*				+				+	+	+	+	+	+	+
Rhinosporidiosis	*Rhinosporidium seeberi*		+							+					+

Serum IgE antibody for *A. fumigatus* is markedly increased but not specific; significantly higher than in uncomplicated bronchial asthma.

Expectorated mucus plug contains eosinophils and mycelial elements.

♦ Recognition of organism in material (especially sputum) from sites of involvement (especially lung; also brain, sinuses, orbit, ear). *Organisms occur as saprophytes in sputum and mouth. Confirm by staining organisms in biopsy specimens.*

♦ Positive culture on most media at room temperature or 35°C.

♦ Serologic tests
  • CF has been used for detecting recent or active disease; has good specificity but less sensitive than immunodiffusion.
  • Immunodiffusion has high specificity but is often negative in invasive disease in immunocompromised patients, for whom EIA for IgG is best choice.
  • Antigen detection has good specificity but variable sensitivity.
  • Specific IgG levels (by ELISA) useful for early diagnosis and monitoring treatment. Precedes radiographic appearance of lung lesions and cytologic or microbiological identification by weeks.

Laboratory findings due to underlying or primary disease
  • Aspergilloma—superimposed on lung cavities caused by TB, bronchiectasis, carcinoma
  • Invasive aspergillosis—underlying condition (e.g., AIDS, malignant lymphoma, acute leukemia, other immunocompromising conditions, cystic fibrosis)

Blastomycosis

(North American blastomycosis due to *Blastomyces dermatitidis*; South American blastomycosis due to *Paracoccidioides brasiliensis*)
Clinical types
  • North American—involvement of skin and lungs.
  • South American—involvement of nasopharynx, lymph nodes, cecum.
  • Later, visceral involvement may occur in both types.

♦ Recognition of organism in material (e.g., pus, sputum, biopsied tissue) with special stains
  • Positive culture on Sabouraud's medium at room temperature and blood agar at 37°C; slow growth of *P. brasiliensis* on blood agar ≤ 1 mo. Culture of organism from tissue is the only certain diagnostic method. Observation of typical yeasts in tissue sections is less satisfactory.
  • Wet smear preparation in 20% potassium hydroxide.
  • Negative animal inoculation.

♦ Serologic tests for *B. dermatitidis*
  • Antibodies are usually detectable within 25 days of onset of illness; rise to peak at 51–75 days and then decrease. In chronic pulmonary disease, may peak within 25 days and then decrease.
  • EIA is most sensitive and specific, especially in early disease; is initial test of choice. Initial titers are often negative; therefore serial titers should be performed. Titer of ≥ 1:32 supports diagnosis and falling titers indicate improvement. Positive test should be confirmed with immunodiffusion assay.
  • RIA may be slightly less sensitive and specific.
  • Immunodiffusion assay for precipitin antibodies against antigen A is 17–65% sensitive and 95% specific; may be negative in early disease.
  • CF test is positive in high titer with systemic infection and high titer is correlated with poor prognosis, but test is not useful for diagnosis; sensitivity is <25%. CF shows 17% cross reaction with histoplasmosis.

WBC and ESR are increased.

Serum globulin is slightly increased.

Mild normochromic anemia is present.

Serum ALP may be increased with bone lesions.

Skin tests are positive in 40% of patients; false-positive results may occur in other fungal diseases (e.g., histoplasmosis) due to cross reactivity.

Chromoblastomycosis

(Due to *Phialophora pedrosi*, *Phialophora compactum*, etc.)
Usually skin; rarely brain abscess

♦ Recognition of organism from sites of involvement
  • Wet smear preparation in 10% potassium hydroxide
  • Positive culture on Sabouraud's medium (slow growth)
  • Biopsy of tissue
Hypersensitivity pneumonitis **(due to *Cladosporium carrionii*)**
♦ • Microscopy.
♦ • CIE and immunodiffusion assay show antibodies in sera in >85% of patients.

Coccidioidomycosis

(Due to *Coccidioides immitis*)
♦ Positive culture (e.g., sputum, BAL fluid) is diagnostic.
♦ Serologic tests are especially useful in this disease for both diagnosis and prognosis. Positive results are highly specific but false-negatives may occur, especially early in illness. Repeat testing during first 2 mos may be needed.
  • Determination of IgG and IgM by EIA has sensitivity and specificity of >92% for serum and CSF and is method of choice. Minimal cross reaction with other diseases and is rare. IgM occurs temporarily in 75% of cases of primary infection. IgG appears later and usually disappears in several months if infection resolves. Increased IgG titer indicates disseminated extrapulmonary disease but may not be found in meningitis.
  • Tube precipitin and immunodiffusion testing are used to detect IgM antibodies of early acute infection. Appear early, decrease after the third week, are uncommon after the fifth month. They occur at some stage of the disease in 75% of patients and usually indicate early infection. In primary infection, they are the only demonstrable antibodies in 40% of patients. If tests are negative, repeat three times at intervals of 1–2 wks. *Beware of occasional cross reaction with antibodies of primary histoplasmosis and cutaneous blastomycosis.*
  • CF is used to detect IgG antibodies that persist throughout disease course. Appear later (positive in 10% of patients in first week), and titer rises with increasing severity. Less than one-third of cases are positive in the first month; most positive reactions occur between the fourth and fifth weeks. Antibodies decrease after 4–8 mos but may remain positive in low titer for years. The titer parallels severity of infection and is useful for following the disease course. Low titers may be found early in disease and are significant; low titers may be seen in pulmonary, limited extrapulmonary, or inactive disease. Titers of 1:16–1:32 are highly suggestive of disease. Titers of >1:32 indicate active disease and suggest extensive, disseminated disease. Fall in titer suggests effective therapy but rising titer is diagnostic and denotes disease progression. High titer not always present in disseminated disease. May be found in other body fluids, usually 1–2 dilutions less than serum. In CSF, is diagnostic of meningitis (occurs in 75% of these cases). May cross-react with other mycoses, notably histoplasmosis.
  • EIA can detect antigen before appearance of antibodies.
♦ Wet preparation in 20% potassium hydroxide and culture on mycologic media of sputum, gastric contents, CSF, urine, blood, marrow biopsy specimen, liver biopsy specimen, exudate, skin scrapings, etc., or intraperitoneal injection of mice.
♦ Biopsy of skin lesions, affected lymph nodes, lung, etc., showing mature spherule with endospores is pathognomonic.
♦ DNA probe now commercially available allows confirmatory testing in hours.
CSF in meningitis shows 100–200 WBCs/cu mm (mostly mononuclear), increased protein, frequently decreased glucose.
♦ Positive IgG-specific antibody is diagnostic of meningitis in undiluted CSF; any titer is significant; is also used to indicate response to amphotericin B as well as relapse for 1–2 yrs after end of therapy. Serum titers are often negative or borderline in meningitis. CF antibodies are present in 75% of meningitis patients; latex agglutination results parallel CF results.
○Eosinophilia is ≤ 35%; >10% in 25% of patients.
WBC (with shift to the left) and ESR are increased.
Laboratory findings due to underlying immunosuppression (e.g., AIDS patients who may have concurrent disseminated and aggressive pulmonary disease; patients with Hodgkin's disease or those taking immunosuppressive drugs); also late stages of pregnancy and diabetes
○Skin test conversion strongly indicates recent infection; skin testing does not cause serological response.

Cryptococcosis

(Due to *Cryptococcus neoformans*. Usual manifestation is CNS although lung is usual portal of entry.)

♦ Serologic tests
  * Antibody detection (IFA, direct agglutination) is most useful in early disease when antigen production is small. Beware of false-positives due to the presence of IgM RF, other fungal infections, neurosyphilis, and bacterial meningitis, and false-negatives due to immune complexes, prozones, nonencapsulated variants, very early disease.
  * *Antibody* testing in serum and CSF is positive only in early CNS involvement or no CNS manifestations; may become positive only after institution of therapy. May be found in normal persons. Rising titer may be a favorable prognostic sign.
  * Antigen detection test is very useful. Latex slide agglutination on serum and CSF detects specific cryptococcal *antigen* (specificity = 100%). Measurement of cryptococcal antigen in serum and CSF is the most valuable test in meningitis. Use for screening of suspected cryptococcosis, because it is more sensitive (95%) than India ink smears of CSF; may be positive in 30% of cases without meningitis. Serum or CSF is positive in most cases; when negative, agglutination test may be positive. Antigen titers reflect extent of disease; are rarely positive with local involvement other than CNS (e.g., lung, skin); increasing titer suggests progressive disease and failure to decrease with treatment suggests insufficient therapy. EIA antigen detection has higher sensitivity and specificity.

♦ Cultures should always be done because false-positive antigen tests may occur due to presence of other fungi (e.g., *Trichosporon beigelii*). Culture of CSF for *C. neoformans* on Sabouraud's medium, which becomes positive in 1–2 wks (positive in 97% of cases), followed by mouse inoculation; 20% of cases require multiple cultures. Culture is commonly positive even without chemical changes in CSF. Repeated fungal cultures are often necessary; cisternal fluid is sometimes superior to lumbar CSF. Positive cultures may also be obtained from blood (25%), urine (37%), stool (20%), sputum (19%), and bone marrow (13%). Sputum cultures are most often positive when no radiographic evidence of pulmonary disease is found. Urine cultures are commonly positive with little kidney involvement. Positive blood culture indicates extensive disease and an extremely poor prognosis.

○ CSF
  Cell count is almost always increased to ≤ 800 cells (more lymphocytes than leukocytes). Protein is increased in 90% (<500 mg/dL). Glucose is moderately decreased in ~55% of patients. Relapse is less frequent when increase in protein and cells is marked rather than moderate. Poor prognosis is suggested if initial CSF examination shows positive results on India ink preparation, low glucose (<20 mg/dL), low WBC count (<20/cu mm). Positive serologic test without other CSF changes should be viewed with suspicion except in AIDS or other causes of serious immunosuppression. Low titer serology should always be confirmed with culture. Repeat CSF examination to evaluate therapy.

♦ India ink slide
  * CSF is positive in ~50% of meningitis patients (usually more acute onset); thus half of cases will be missed if India ink preparations are used as the sole criterion; rarely seen in other fungal types. Requires 10^5 organisms/cu mL.
  * India ink preparations are also used on sputum, pus, skin scrapings.

♦ In biopsy material, mucicarmine stain is positive; also positive results with intraperitoneal injection of white mice.

CBC and ESR usually remain normal.

Increased risk of failure of amphotericin B treatment if positive culture is obtained from sites other than CSF (e.g., blood, sputum, urine, etc.), anticryptococcal antibodies are absent, CSF or serum cryptococcal antigen titer initially is >1:32 or posttreatment titer is ≥ 1:8, and in immunosuppressed states.

Evidence of coexisting disease affecting T lymphocytes in ~50% of patients (e.g., those with AIDS, diabetes mellitus, Hodgkin's disease, lymphosarcoma, leukemia, those undergoing steroid therapy). Occurs in ≤ 9% of patients with AIDS. In AIDS, cryptococcal disease most commonly appears as meningitis but typical signs are seen in only ~50% of cases; dissemination to lungs, marrow, skin is common. In AIDS patients finding organisms in blood cultures and blood smear is more likely; CSF changes may be very slight and organisms may have smaller capsules, making recognition with India ink more difficult; although CSF antigen titer declines with treatment, serum antigen level often remains constant or increases.

Geotrichosis

(Due to *Geotrichum candidum*)
♦ Recognition of organisms in material from sites of involvement (respiratory tract; possibly colon)
  • Positive culture on Sabouraud's medium (room temperature). *Organisms occur as saprophytes in pharynx and colon.*
  • Microscopic visualization of organisms in biopsy material.

Histoplasmosis

(Due to *Histoplasma capsulatum*)
♦ Serologic tests
  • Antigen detection (by EIA and RIA)
    In urine in 90% of cases of disseminated disease, ~20% of cases of acute self-limited disease, <10% of cases of chronic pulmonary cavitary disease. Especially useful in disseminated disease in which patients may not show significant antibody response. Absent or low levels after amphotericin B therapy. Increase in serum or blood heralds relapse.
    In serum is less sensitive; found in 50% of cases of disseminated disease.
    In CSF in <50% of meningitis cases; may cross-react with coccidioidal meningitis (CSF antibodies may also cross-react).
    In BAL fluid, sensitivity = 70%.
  • CF titers
    A single serum titer of ≥ 1:32 or a 4× increase in titer is highly suggestive of active histoplasmosis; titer of <1:8 is considered negative. Rising CF titers occur in >95% of symptomatic primary infections. Increased titer is less common in disseminated primary infection. CSF titer of ≥ 1:8 is evidence for meningeal histoplasmosis. Appears during third to sixth week. Higher titers tend to be found in chronic pulmonary cavitary disease and lower titers in disseminated disease. Positive titers persist for months or years if disease remains active. Prognosis is not indicated by level of or changes in titers.
  • IgG and IgM detection by EIA and RIA is not clinically useful due to high false-positive rates (25–50%) caused by other infections and false-negative results in immunocompromised patients.
  • Skin testing can cause conversion of antibody titers within 1 wk. Skin tests are negative in 50% of cases of disseminated disease. Frequent cross reactivity with blastomycosis and coccidioidomycosis. Not helpful in clinical diagnosis but useful in epidemiologic studies.
♦ Culture of specimens from lung, skin, and mucosal lesions, sputum, bronchoalveolar washings, gastric washings, blood, or bone marrow may be difficult (Sabouraud's medium at room temperature; culture on blood agar at 37°C not specific). Blood and bone marrow cultures are positive in 50–70% of patients. Culture is positive in <10% of asymptomatic self-limiting cases, 65% of cavitary pulmonary cases, and 75% of cases with disseminated disease. Large volumes of CSF (30–40 mL) may be needed. Culture may require 2–6 wks. Mouse inoculation, especially from sputum, may give a positive subculture from spleen on Sabouraud's medium in 1 mo.
♦ Demonstration of *H. capsulatum* in stained smears of peripheral blood, buffy coat, bone marrow (25–60% positive), respiratory secretions is often the most rapid method of diagnosis but test is insensitive and should be performed with cultures.
♦ Biopsy (specially stained) of skin and mucosal lesions, bone marrow, and RE system specimens provides initial diagnosis in ~45% of cases.
Anemia, leukopenia, and thrombocytopenia are more common (60–80% of cases) in acute than in subacute or chronic disseminated types.
Laboratory findings due to involvement of various organ systems, e.g., meningitis, endocarditis, adrenal insufficiency, which are occasionally seen in subacute and less often in chronic disseminated histoplasmosis.

Because coinfection is common, specimens should be examined for other opportunistic organisms, especially mycobacteria. Underlying AIDS should be ruled out.

Moniliasis

(Due to *Candida albicans*)

♦ Definitive diagnosis by histopathology showing organisms invading tissue
♦ Positive culture on Sabouraud's medium and positive findings on direct microscopic examination of suspected material
♦ Serum antibody tests showing seroconversion, sharply rising titers, production of multiple precipitins usually indicate deep-seated infection in patients who are not immunosuppressed but may not distinguish transient candidemia. Precipitin titer of 1:8 or 4× increase in titer indicates invasive candidiasis rather than *Candida* colonization.
○ *In vaginitis, rule out underlying diabetes mellitus*; also pregnancy; use of antimicrobial drugs, oral contraceptives, corticosteroids, exogenous hormones; AIDS; local allergy due to perfumes, nylon underwear. Gram stain or 10% potassium hydroxide preparation confirms diagnosis but negative finding does not rule it out.
○ *In skin and nail involvement in children, rule out congenital hypoparathyroidism and Addison's disease.*
○ *In septicemia with endocarditis, rule out IV drug abuse, prosthetic heart valve. Persistent positive blood culture after removal of a central venous catheter indicates endocarditis rather than catheter contamination.*
○ *In myocarditis, rule out corticosteroid or intensive antibiotic therapy, or abdominal surgery.*
○ *In GI tract overgrowth, rule out AIDS or chemotherapy suppression of normal bacterial flora.*
○ *In positive blood culture, which is rare, rule out serious underlying disease (e.g., malignant lymphoma), use of multiple therapeutic antibiotics, and use of plastic IV catheters.*
♦ Ratio of serum D-arabinitol (in μmol/L) to creatinine (in mg/dL) of ≥ 4.0 in fungemia and deeply invasive tissue or mucosal candidiasis (sensitivity of 74% and specificity of >40%); highest values in persistent fungemia. Therapy that reduces tissue burden of *Candida* causes decline in ratio of D-arabinitol to creatinine.

Mucormycosis

(Due to *Zygomycetes* spp.)

Clinical types
- Cranial (acute diffuse cerebrovascular disease and ophthalmoplegia in uncontrolled diabetes mellitus with acidosis)
- Pulmonary (findings due to pulmonary infarction)
- In abdominal blood vessels (findings due to hemorrhagic infarction of ileum or colon)

♦ Histopathologic detection is the gold standard.
♦ Mycologic cultures from brain material and CSF are rarely positive; cultures of specimens from infected nasal sinuses or turbinate may be positive.

Serologic tests are mostly investigational.
- EIA for IgM and IgG gives best sensitivity and specificity.
- Immunodiffusion testing is positive in ~70% of patients.

Laboratory findings of underlying disease (e.g., diabetes mellitus with acidosis, leukemia, irradiation or use of cytotoxic drugs, uremic acidosis)
Laboratory findings due to complications (e.g., visceral infarcts)

Nocardiosis

(Due to *Nocardia asteroides*; now reclassified as bacterium [Mycobacteriaceae])

Clinical types
- Pulmonary disease (pneumonitis, abscess); metastatic brain abscesses in one-third of patients
- Maduromycosis

♦ Recognition of organism
- Sputum positive in only 30% of cases; bronchial washings, tracheal aspirate, or tissue biopsy material are preferred. Blood culture is rarely positive.
- Direct smear—gram positive and acid fast (*may be overdecolorized by Ziehl-Neelsen stain for tubercle bacilli*). Not significant in gastric washings as organism may be present in foods. *May be saprophytic in sputum.*

- Positive culture on Sabouraud's medium and blood agar. (*Beware of inactivation by concentration technique for tubercle bacillus.*)
- Positive guinea pig inoculation

♦ Serologic tests
- EIA is sensitive (titer >1:256) and specific.
- CF (titer = 1:16–1:32 3–4 wks after infection; sensitivity = 80%) and immunodiffusion (positive 2 wks after infection; sensitivity = 50–70%) are sometimes useful in diagnosis of systemic nocardiosis.

Laboratory findings due to predisposing immunocompromised conditions (e.g., AIDS, alcoholism, diabetes mellitus, lymphoma, organ transplant, long-term corticosteroid therapy) or underlying pulmonary disease (e.g., COPD)

Pneumocystis carinii *Infection*

(*P. carinii* recently classified as fungus closely related to yeasts)

♦ Diagnosis requires demonstration of organism.
- Transbronchial lung biopsy is very effective way to make a definite diagnosis. Also allows diagnosis of other infections or diseases (e.g., lymphoma), use of various stains, touch preparations. Open lung biopsy is rarely needed.
- BAL is equally successful in diagnosis (sensitivity ~95%).
- Analysis of induced sputum (nebulization with saline) is also effective for diagnosis, inexpensive, and can be performed on an outpatient basis. Use of immunofluorescent stain allows diagnosis in ~95% of cases.
- Organism is rarely found in routine sputum, bronchial washings or brushings.
- Organism can be found in postmortem histologic preparations.
- Immunologic stain with monoclonal antibodies is useful to diagnose extrapulmonary lesions.

♦ DNA hybridization and PCR have been used. PCR is very sensitive but may have high false-positive rate.

○ Morphology of the lung lesions suggests the diagnosis.

Organism does not stain with routine hematoxylin and eosin stains; requires immunofluorescence or special stains (e.g., Giemsa, Schiff).

Serologic tests are generally not useful at present. Do not distinguish old from new infections.
- Immunofluorescent tests have a reported sensitivity of 71% (titer = 1:16) in acute cases and 97% (titer = 1:16) in convalescent cases with overall sensitivity of 30–40%. High specificity with few cross reactions.
- CF is positive in <20% of patients.

No culture techniques are available.

○ Laboratory findings of associated diseases; found in >55% of sputum specimens from patients with various types of immunosuppression.
- Is the primary presenting opportunistic infection in 55–65% of AIDS cases; is twice as common in IV drug users as in homosexuals.
- Use of cytotoxic drugs and corticosteroids.
- Premature or debilitated infants.
- Underlying diseases (e.g., Ig defects; malignant lymphoma and leukemia patients more susceptible than those with other tumors).
- Other infections, especially CMV infection, systemic bacterial infections (especially with *Pseudomonas* or *Staphylococcus*), tuberculosis, cryptococcosis.
- 25% of patients who die after renal transplant.

Laboratory findings due to organ system involvement, e.g.,
Pulmonary disease
- Hypoxemia and hypercapnia.
- Increased serum LD.
- Pleural effusion may occur, but presence of a second condition (e.g., Kaposi's sarcoma, mycobacterial disease) should be considered.

May affect other organs (e.g., liver, spleen, marrow, eye, skin).

Leukopenia indicates a poor prognosis. Lymphopenia and anemia are common.

Rhinosporidiosis

(Due to *Rhinosporidium seeberi*)

♦ Recognition of organism in biopsy material from polypoid lesions of nasopharynx or eye (cannot be cultured)

Table 15-12. Serologic Tests in Diagnosis of Parasitic Diseases

Disease	Tests
Amebiasis	EIA, IHA
Babesiasis	IF
Chagas' disease	EIA, IF, CF, IHA
Cryptosporidiosis	EIA (Ag in stool)
Cysticercosis	IB, EIA
Echinococcosis	EIA, IHA, IB
Fascioliasis	EIA
Filariasis	EIA
Giardiasis	EIA, IF (Ag in stool)
Leishmaniasis	IF, CF
Malaria	IF
Paragonimiasis	EIA, IB
Pneumocystosis	Ag
Schistosomiasis	EIA, IB
Strongyloidiasis	EIA
Toxocariasis	EIA
Toxoplasmosis	EIA, IF, EIA-IgM
Trichinosis	BF, EIA
Trichomoniasis	Ag
Trypanosoma cruzi	EIA, IF, CF

Ag = antigen; BF = bentonite flocculation; CF = complement fixation; EIA = enzyme immunoassay; IB = immunoblot; IF = indirect immunofluorescence; IHA = indirect hemagglutination.
Source: Wilson M, Arrowood MJ. Diagnostic parasitology: direct detection methods and serodiagnosis. *Lab Med* 1993;24:145.

Sporotrichosis

(Due to *Sporothrix schenckii*)
♦ Recognition of organism in skin, pus, or biopsy material
  • Positive culture on Sabouraud's medium from unbroken pustule.
      Intraperitoneal mouse inoculation of these colonies or of fresh pus produces organism-containing lesions.
  • Direct microscopic examination is usually negative.
♦ Serologic tests
  • EIA is 100% sensitive at titer of ≥ 1:128. Titer much higher in extracutaneous disease than in cutaneous disease.
  • Tube and latex slide agglutination shows 94% sensitivity; persistent elevation or rising titer is common in pulmonary disease. Low titer (e.g., <1:16) in nonfungal disease (e.g., leishmaniasis). CSF titer of 1:32 in meningeal infection. CF is less sensitive (titer of ≥ 1:16); antibodies can be demonstrated in extracutaneous disease (e.g., pulmonary, disseminated). Cross reaction with other mycotic and bacterial infections.
  • Sera and CSF antibodies are present in meningeal disease (EIA of ≥ 1:8 is considered positive); titers decrease after onset of therapy. CSF may show oligoclonal IgG bands and elevated IgG index in meningeal infection.

Parasites

Diagnosis of Parasitic Diseases

See Tables 15-12 and 15-13.
♦ Diagnosis usually depends on demonstrating the causative organism in appropriate specimens concentrated and stained appropriately (e.g., sedimentation or flotation of stools; stained thick and thin smears of peripheral blood can detect parasites of malaria, babesiosis, lymphatic filariases, acute stage of trypanosomiasis).

Table 15-13. Identification of Parasites

Organism	Stool	Other Body Sites
Nematodes		
Ascaris lumbricoides	O, A	Rarely L in sputum early
Trichuris trichiura	O	
Enterobius vermicularis	Usually neg.; A after enema	Cellophane tape, perianal region—O and A
Strongyloides stercoralis	L	Occasionally L in sputum and duodenal contents
Ancylostoma duodenale	O, rarely L	
Necator americanus	O, rarely L	
Trichinella spiralis	Occasionally A and/or L	
Wuchereria bancrofti, W. malayi	None	Microfilariae in blood
Loa loa	None	Microfilariae in blood; A under conjunctiva
Onchocerca volvulus	None	A in subcutaneous nodules
Dracunculus medinensis	None	L in fluid from ulcer
Cestodes		
Taenia solium	G, O, S; A after treatment	
Taenia saginata	G, O, S	Cellophane tape, perianal region—O
Hymenolepis nana, H. diminuta	O	
Diphyllobothrium latum	O	
Echinococcus multilocularis	Not found	Histologic examination of biopsy specimen
Trematodes		
Schistosoma mansoni, S. japonicum,	O	See p. 868
S. haematobium	None	O in urine
Clonorchis sinensis	O	O in duodenal contents
Opisthorchis felineus	O	O in duodenal contents
Paragonimus westermani	O	O in sputum
Fasciola hepatica	O	
Fasciolopsis buski	O, occasionally A	

A = adult; G = gravid segments; L = larvae; O = ova; S = scolex; neg = negative.

Interferences
Foreign materials in stools, e.g., barium, bismuth, mineral oil, nonabsorbable antidiarrheal agents

Use of antimicrobial agents that may modify intestinal flora (e.g., tetracycline) within 1 wk before examination.

Serologic tests include IHA, CIE, EIA, ELISA, CF.
Use
Epidemiologic studies

Complementary when primary diagnostic method is negative.

Less expensive than direct microscopy

Negative test is useful to rule out certain diseases (e.g., invasive amebiasis).

Positive test in a traveler who has not previously been in an area where the disease is endemic can be helpful.

Disadvantages

May not distinguish between present and past infection.

Do not identify the causative species, which may be important for therapy (e.g., malaria).

Do not identify drug-resistant strains (e.g., malaria).

Not widely available in kit form or performed only in research or reference laboratories.

May require special equipment that is expensive to purchase and maintain and requires sophisticated operators (e.g., flow cytometry).

Newer technology (e.g., DNA probes, monoclonal antibodies for detection of antigen in stool) improves diagnostic utility when available, but genetic and molecular diversity of population of organisms (e.g., trypanosomes) makes it difficult to construct reliable serologic tests.

○Eosinophilia may be a clue to parasitic infection.

○Increased IgE in helminth infections

Ascariasis

(Due to *Ascaris lumbricoides*)

♦ Stools contain ova. Occasionally adult worms are spontaneously passed in stool.

○Eosinophils are increased during symptomatic phase.

Serologic tests are not useful.

Clonorchiasis

(Due to *Clonorchis sinensis*)

♦ Ova appear in stool or duodenal contents.

♦ EIA for antigen detection in stool has sensitivity, specificity, and positive predictive value of >90% when prevalence is 50%. Cross reactions may occur.

Clonorchiasis may cause laboratory findings due to biliary obstruction or recurrent cholecystitis.

Dirofilariasis (Pulmonary)

(Due to dog heartworm, *Dirofilaria immitis* [insect transmission, usually mosquito; rarely some species of fleas or ticks])

Filariform larvae transmitted by bite of intermediate host mosquito migrate to heart and die, resulting in pulmonary emboli and infarcts.

♦ Diagnosis is made by open lung biopsy.

Eosinophilia is not significant.

Cross reactions make EIA serologic tests difficult to interpret.

Fascioliasis

(Due to *Fasciola hepatica*)

♦ Ova appear in stool or duodenal contents.

♦ Serologic tests
  • Antibodies appear within 2–4 wks after infection (5–7 wks before eggs appear in stool).
  • Assay of antibodies by EIA and CIE has high sensitivity but may show cross reaction with schistosomiasis and trichinosis. CIE becomes negative with cure and thus is useful for monitoring therapy.
  • Indirect fluorescent antibody is positive in ~80% of cases; frequent cross reaction with infections due to other helminths, *C. sinensis* and *Opisthorchis* species.
  • EIA can detect antigen in serum.
  • CF is positive in only 14% of cases.

○Eosinophils are increased.

Liver function tests are abnormal.

Fasciolopsiasis

(Due to *Fasciolopsis buski*)

♦ Ova appear in stool.

Filariasis

Lymphatic Filariasis
(Due to *Wuchereria bancrofti* or *Brugia malayi*)

♦ Microfilariae are found in thick blood smear (Wright or Giemsa stain) or wet preparation; can be concentrated (e.g., centrifugation, membrane filtration). Collect blood after 8 p.m. *Persons with microfilariae in blood may be asymptomatic; circulating microfilariae may be absent in patients with this disease.*

○ Eosinophils are increased.

♦ Biopsy material from lymph node may contain adult worms.

Chyluria may occur.

Serologic tests
- Antibody detection lacks sensitivity and specificity.

♦ • Antigen detected in serum (50% of cases) and urine (100% of cases) in *W. bancrofti* infection. Can monitor treatment and relapse by measuring level in urine but not serum antibody levels.

Nonlymphatic Filariasis

Loaiasis
(Due to *Loa loa*)

○ Marked increase of eosinophils (50–80%) may occur.

♦ Identification of microfilariae in thick blood smears or concentrated filtrate of hemolyzed blood prepared with Giemsa stain; collect blood between 10 a.m. and 2 p.m.

♦ Identification of excised migrating subconjunctival adults.

♦ Identification of microfilariae in CSF in cases of meningoencephalitis.

Serologic tests—see previous Lymphatic Filariasis section.

Onchocerciasis (River Blindness)
(Due to *Onchocerca volvulus*)

♦ Identify microfilaria in skin

Tropical Pulmonary Eosinophilia
(Due to *Wuchereria bancrofti*)

○ Eosinophilia is extreme (usually >3000/cu mm) and persists for weeks.

○ Serum IgE levels are markedly elevated (usually >1000 U/mL).

♦ Microfilaria cannot be found in blood but may be found in enlarged lymph nodes when adenopathy is present.

Other laboratory abnormalities (e.g., increased ESR) are not diagnostically useful.

Hookworm Disease

(Due to *Necator americanus* or *Ancylostoma duodenale*)

○ WBC is normal or slightly increased, with 15–30% eosinophils; begins at 4 wks; peaks at ~50 days when ≤ 75% eosinophils are present.

Anemia due to blood loss is hypochromic microcytic. When anemia is more severe, eosinophilia is less prominent.

Hypoproteinemia may occur with heavy infection.

♦ Stools contain hookworm ova after ~5 wks.

Stools are usually positive for occult blood. Charcot-Leyden crystals are present in >50% of patients.

Serologic tests are not useful for diagnosis or monitoring of infection.

Laboratory findings due to frequently associated diseases (e.g., malaria, beriberi)

Larva Migrans, Cutaneous

(Due to *Ancylostoma caninum* and *Ancylostoma braziliense* from dogs, cats, other carnivores)

Serologic tests and biopsy are not useful.

Larva Migrans, Visceral

(Due to roundworms *Toxocara canis* or *Toxocara cati*; past exposure in humans is ~10%.)

○ WBC is increased; increased eosinophils (usually >30%) may be vacuolated and contain fewer than normal granules; persists for several months.

Serum gamma globulin, especially IgE, is often increased.

♦ Demonstration of larvae in tissue biopsy material is only definite way to make diagnosis; usually from liver, which shows granulomas.
♦ ELISA is 78% sensitive and 92% specific; positive test supports diagnosis. May be less sensitive in ocular than in visceral disease. IHA and bentonite flocculation tests are insensitive and nonspecific.
Increased anti-A and anti-B antibodies in most cases due to stimulation of isohemagglutinins
Laboratory findings due to organ system involvement (e.g., liver in 85% of cases and lung in 50% of cases—may cause Löffler's syndrome)

Opisthorchiasis

(Due to *Opisthorchis felineus*)
♦ Ova appear in stool or duodenal contents.
♦ EIA for IgG and IgE antibodies is useful.
♦ Antigen detection assay and DNA-based diagnosis should be useful.

Paragonimiasis

(Due to *Paragonimus westermani*)
○Eosinophilia is usual.
♦ Ova appear in stool or sputum, which may contain blood.
♦ Serologic tests
   • ELISA is method of choice; antibody levels decrease after treatment. Cross reactions may occur.
   • Antigen detection methods are under development.

Pinworm Infestation

(Due to *Enterobius vermicularis*)
♦ Ova and occasionally adults are found on cellophane tape swab of perianal region, which *should be taken on first arising early in morning*. Three tests will find 90% and five tests will find 95% of cases.
Stool is usually negative for ova and adults.
Eosinophil count is usually normal; may be slightly increased.
Serologic tests are not useful.

Schistosomiasis

(Due to *Schistosoma mansoni, Schistosoma japonicum, Schistosoma haematobium*)
Acute
○ • Eosinophilia occurs in 20–60% of cases.
   • ESR is increased.
   • Serum globulin is increased.
♦ Chronic
   • Diagnosis depends on detection of ova in stools or urine; only viable eggs indicate active infection. Quantification by egg count per gram of feces or per 10 mL of urine gives some indication of severity of infection. Species identification depends on egg morphology and is needed to determine drug dosage or select drugs.
   • Ova appear in urine sediment and in biopsy material from vesical mucosa in infection with *S. haematobium*. *S. haematobium* ova are sometimes found in stool and *S. mansoni* eggs are sometimes found in urine, especially in heavy infection.
   • Unstained rectal mucosa examined microscopically may show living or dead ova when stools are negative; granulomatous lesions may be present.
Changes secondary to clay pipestem fibrosis of liver with portal hypertension, esophageal varices, splenomegaly, etc. Liver function changes are quite minimal; increased serum bilirubin is rare, even with advanced cirrhosis. Increased serum globulin is frequent. Serum ALP is elevated in 50% of adult patients but is not useful measure in children.
♦ Ova may be found within granulomas.
Pulmonary involvement
♦ • Ova in sputum are very rare.
♦ • Lung biopsy may be positive in advanced cases.
   • Changes secondary to pulmonary hypertension.
Multiple granulomatous lesions may appear in uterine cervix.
♦ Serologic tests are particularly useful in chronic infections when stools contain no ova; they are not useful to assess chemotherapeutic cure. Do not determine activity

or intensity of current infection and may not distinguish new and old infections. Positive serology is most useful to support the diagnosis of acute schistosomiasis. Not useful for diagnosis in adults from endemic areas because specificity for active infection is too low. Cross reaction with other helminths may occur.
- IFA test is useful when IHA titer is <1:64; IHA titer is >1:256 in >90% of acute *S. mansoni* cases; cross reaction with other *Schistosoma* infections, filariasis, trichinosis.
- Screening of sera with ELISA and confirmation and speciation with enzyme-linked immunoelectro-transfer blot (Western blot) are most sensitive and specific methods.
- Antigen detection method is not yet available.

Strongyloidiasis

(Due to *Strongyloides stercoralis*; found in ~4% of rural Kentucky children)
♦ Stools contain larvae (sensitivity = 30–60% for direct examination, 70–80% after Baermann concentration). Larvae may also be found in duodenal washings (sensitivity = 60–70%). Sensitivity of string test (Entertest) is 60–80%. Presence of filariform larvae may suggest hyperinfection.
♦ Larvae appear in sputum with pulmonary involvement; eosinophils may also be present; presence indicates hyperinfection.
♦ Serologic tests (ELISA) for antibodies show sensitivity, specificity, and negative predictive value of >95%. Thus a positive test indicates need for examination of stool and duodenal contents, especially if a patient is to be treated with cytotoxic or immunosuppressive therapy, but may cross-react with *A. lumbricoides, L. loa,* or hookworm. A negative test without symptoms or other laboratory findings suggests no infection.
○ Leukocytosis is common. Increase in eosinophils is almost always present, but the number usually decreases in chronic disease; is most marked in patients with prominent skin manifestations; may be absent with immunosuppression. Leukopenia and absence of eosinophilia are poor prognostic signs. *Condition may be encountered in orphanages and mental institutions.*

Tapeworm Infestation

Due to *Taenia saginata* (Beef Tapeworm)
♦ In stool, ova cannot be distinguished from those of *Taenia solium*.
- Proglottids establish species diagnosis. Stool examination is positive in 50–75% of patients.
♦ Cellophane tape swab of perianal region is positive in ≤ 95% of patients.
Eosinophils may be slightly increased.

Due to *Taenia solium* (Pork Tapeworm)
♦ Stool (single specimen detects 50–75% of carriers) and cellophane tape swab of perianal region (may detect >75% of infections) are both used. Three to six specimens are examined over 1–2 wks.
○ Eosinophils may be increased (up to 10–15%).
Marked increase in ESR is unusual and suggests another diagnosis.
♦ With CNS involvement, CSF may show increased eosinophils (in 10–77% of cases), increased mononuclear cells (≤ 300/cu mm), slightly increased protein, normal or mildly decreased glucose; parasites are not found. Serologic tests are used in conjunction with CT scan or MRI. Older tests, e.g., IHA, IFA, CIE, immunoelectrophoresis, have sensitivity of ~80%. ELISA detects antibody in serum or CSF in 75–80% of patients with few or calcified cysts and 93% with severe CNS disease. Enzyme-linked immunoelectro-transfer blot test on serum or CSF has sensitivity and specificity of >94% in patients with multiple CNS lesions and of ~72% in those with single lesions. Change in titers is not reliable to judge cure. *Solitary CNS lesions may not produce antibodies consistently.* Status of antigen assays, ELISA, PCR, DNA probes, monoclonal antibody testing awaits future studies.
♦ Biopsy of solitary lesions may establish the diagnosis when serologic tests are negative.

Due to *Hymenolepis nana* (Dwarf Tapeworm)
♦ Stool shows ova, occasionally proglottids, etc.

Due to *Diphyllobothrium latum* (Fish Tapeworm)
♦ Stool shows ova.
○ Macrocytic anemia (see p. 365) may occur when worm is in proximal small intestine.
○ Increased eosinophils and leukocytes are found.

Due to *Echinococcus granulosus* (*Echinococcus multilocularis*) (Canine Tapeworm)

○Laboratory findings due to cystic lesion of liver in 65% of cases (see Space-Occupying Lesions of Liver, p. 248); cysts are widely scattered in 10% of cases; multiple in 20–40% of cases.

♦Identification of scolices and hooklets in cyst fluid and on histologic examination

♦Serologic tests
  • High titer (>1:256) on IHA has 90% sensitivity and ≤ 100% specificity in cases with hydatid cysts of liver or peritoneum; 60% sensitivity in cases of lung and bone involvement; 10% sensitivity in cases of calcified cysts. ≤ 10% false-positives (in cysticercosis, schistosomiasis, collagen disease, neoplasia); titers can persist for years after surgical removal.
  • EIA is method of choice. EIA but not IHA can differentiate *E. granulosus* from *E. multilocularis* in test for antigen on cyst fluid.

○Eosinophils are increased in 33% of cases; numbers rise dramatically if cyst leaks.
Stool examination is not helpful.

Trichinosis

(Due to *Trichinella spiralis*)

○Eosinophilia appears with values of ≤ 85% on differential count and 15,000/cu mm on absolute count. It occurs ~1 wk after the eating of infected meat and reaches maximum after third week. It usually subsides in 4–6 wks but may last up to 6 mos and occasionally for years. Occasionally it is absent; it is usually absent in fatal infections.

♦Stools do not contain adults or larvae.

♦Identification of larvae is made in suspected meat by acid-pepsin digestion followed by microscopic examination.

♦Muscle biopsy material may show the encysted larvae beginning 10 days after ingestion. Direct microscopic examination of compressed specimen is superior to routine histologic preparation.

♦Serologic tests become positive 1 wk after onset of symptoms in only 20–30% of patients and reach a peak in 80–90% of patients by fourth to fifth week. Rise in titer from acute- to convalescent-phase sera is diagnostic. Titers may remain negative in overwhelming infection. False-positive results may occur in polyarteritis nodosa, serum sickness, penicillin sensitivity, infectious mononucleosis, malignant lymphomas, and leukemia.
  • EIA is method of choice; peaks in 3 mos; may still be detected at 1 yr. Specificity >95%. IHA is also used. Previously used tests include CF, bentonite flocculation, precipitin, and latex fixation.
  • Antigen detection is said to be 100% specific but <50% sensitive.

Decrease in serum total protein and albumin occurs in severe cases between 2 and 4 wks and may last for years.

Increased (relative and absolute) gamma globulins parallel titer of serologic tests. The increase occurs between 5 and 8 wks and may last 6 mos or more.

ESR is normal or only slightly increased.

Decrease in serum cholinesterase often lasts 6 mos.

Serum muscle enzymes (e.g., CK) may be increased.

Urine may show albuminuria with hyaline and granular casts in severe cases.

With meningoencephalitis, CSF may be normal or ≤ 300 lymphocytes/cu mm with increased protein with higher antibody level in CSF than serum.

Trichostrongylosis

(Due to *Trichostrongylus* spp.)

♦Stools contain ova. Usually a concentration technique is required; *worm may be mistaken for hookworm.*

○Increase in WBC and eosinophils (≤ 75%) when patient is symptomatic.

Trichuriasis

(Due to whipworm, *Trichuris trichiura*)

♦Stools contain ova.

○Increased eosinophils (≤ 25%), leukocytosis, and microcytic hypochromic anemia may be present.

Serologic tests are not useful.

Protozoans

See Table 15-14.

Amebiasis

(Due to *Entamoeba histolytica*)

♦ Microscopic examination of stool for *E. histolytica*. Examination of six consecutive daily stools concentrated and stained identifies 90% of positive cases. Must be examined fresh or fixed immediately and stained. *(Beware of interfering substances in feces, e.g., bismuth, kaolin, barium sulfate, soap or hypertonic-salt enema solutions, antacids and laxatives, sulfonamides, and antibiotic, antiprotozoal, and antihelmintic agents.) Abundant RBCs but minimal WBCs on microscopic examination of stool helps to differentiate condition from bacillary dysentery.*

♦ Direct detection of *E. histolytica* antigen in stool by commercial kit

♦ Endoscopic biopsy (positive in 50% of cases) or smear of exudate of intestinal ulcers may show *E. histolytica*.

♦ Serologic tests
  • EIA is most sensitive and specific and is method of choice. IgG is present in all patients with invasive amebiasis and indicates current or previous infection; less sensitive in noninvasive disease. IgM is found in >90% of cases of liver abscess; usually disappears within 6 wks of successful treatment.
  • IHA test (>1:128) is sensitive and specific (~95% each) in patients with liver abscess or invasive intestinal disease but cannot distinguish these conditions from noninvasive intestinal infection, and positive results can persist for years after infection.
  • When severe diarrhea is due to *E. histolytica*, serologic tests are positive in >90%; when diarrhea has never been present, <50% of carriers have positive serologic tests.
Negative test results are unlikely with invasive disease if patient is not immunosuppressed and thus are useful for ruling out invasive amebiasis.
Liver abscess
♦ • Organism found in needle biopsy specimen of abscess in <20% of cases but absent in aspirate. *These tests should not be done.*
  • Stool is usually negative; bacterial culture is sterile.
  • Normochromic, normocytic anemia.
  • Leukocytosis (5000–33,000/cu mm).
  • Eosinophilia is not usually present.
  • ESR is markedly increased.
  • AST and ALT (2–6× normal) may be increased.
  • Increased serum ALP (usually 2–3× normal).
  • Serum albumin may be decreased and globulin increased.
  • Total bilirubin may be increased if complications occur.
  • Liver scanning.
  • See Space Occupying Lesions of Liver, p. 248.
  • Serologic tests—see previous paragraph.

Babesiosis

(Due to *Babesia microti* transmitted by bite of nymphal *Ixodes* tick; has been transmitted by blood transfusion.)

♦ Diagnosis is established by
  • Identification of parasite in RBCs on Wright- or Giemsa-stained thick or thin peripheral blood smears or by DFA staining.
  • Serologic studies—IFA of ≥ 1:64 is considered positive but is ≥ 1:1024 in most patients with acute illness; or 4× increase in serum titer between acute and convalescent phase. Increased titer may persist for months after resolution of symptoms. May cross-react with Colorado tick fever, malaria. Increased titer may occur in *R. rickettsii* infection.
  • PCR-based identification of *B. microti* DNA in blood is more sensitive than microscopy; parasitic DNA is rapidly cleared from blood after successful therapy and presence indicates active parasitemia. May be indicated to monitor course of infection; positive findings may persist for ≥ 6 mos along with symptoms.
  • Isolation in inoculated hamsters.
Hemolytic anemia may last days to months; most patients have thrombocytopenia.

Table 15-14. Summary of Laboratory Findings in Protozoan Diseases

Disease	Causative Organism	Blood	CSF	Stool	Urine	Vagina	Urethra	Exudates, ulcers, skin lesions	Bone marrow	Spleen	Lymph node aspirate
Malaria	*Plasmodium* species	+							+		
Babesiosis	*Babesia microti*	+									
Trypanosomiasis Acute sleeping sickness	*Trypanosoma rhodesiense*	+	+						+		+
Chronic sleeping sickness	*T. gambiense*	+	+						+		+
Chagas' disease	*T. cruzi*	+									+
Leishmaniasis Kala-azar	*Leishmania donovani*	+							+	+	+
American mucocutaneous	*L. brasiliensis*							+			
Oriental sore	*L. tropica*							+			
Toxoplasmosis	*Toxoplasma gondii*		+								+
Interstitial plasma cell pneumonia	*Pneumocystis carinii*										
Amebiasis	*Entamoeba histolytica*			+e							
Giardiasis	*Giardia lamblia*			+f							
Balantidiasis	*Balantidium coli*			+							
Coccidiosis	*Isospora hominis* or *belli*			+							
Trichomoniasis	*Trichomonas vaginalis*				+	+	+				

[a]Liver, lymph node.
[b]Hemagglutination, Sabin-Feldman dye test.
[c]Lymph node, muscle.
[d]Special stains.

Diagnostic Methods							Other Significant Laboratory Abnormalities									
Microscopic examination	Fresh unstained material	Stained material	Culture	Animal inoculation	Xenodiagnosis	Histologic examination	Anemia	WBC decreased	Monocytosis	Serum globulin increased	CSF abnormalities	Renal function abnormalities	Liver function abnormalities	Skeletal muscle abnormalities	Cardiac abnormalities	Other
		+					+	+	+	+	+	+	+			
		+		+		+	+					+	+			
	+	+	rare	+		+	+		+	+	+		+			
		+	rare	+		+	+		+	+	+		+			
		+	+	+	+	a				+				+	+	
		+	+				+	+		+		+				
		+	+	+		+	+	+								
		+	+			+										
		+		+		c				+						b
		+				+										d
		+				e							+			
		+														
		+														
+	+															

eIntestine.
fAlso duodenal washings.
Notes: Serologic tests can be performed at the Centers for Disease Control and Prevention (Atlanta, GA) on specimens submitted through state health department laboratories that do not perform such tests.
See Table 15-12.

Laboratory changes due to complications
* Renal failure
* Liver dysfunction (e.g., increased serum AST, LD)

~20% of patients have clinical and serologic evidence of concurrent Lyme disease. Ehrlichiosis may also be found.

Balantidiasis

(Due to *Balantidium coli*)

♦ Recognition of organisms in stool. *Intermittent appearance requires repeated examinations.*

No serologic tests are available.

Coccidiosis

(Due to obligate intracellular protozoans; includes *Cryptosporidium parvum*, *Isospora belli*, *Cyclospora cayetanensis*)

♦ Oocysts can be found in acid-fast stained smears of stool.

Coccidia—may cause acute, self-limited diarrhea in immunocompetent hosts; HIV-positive hosts with CD4 cell counts of >180/cu mm had self-limited disease but those with counts of <180/cu mm did not clear the parasite.

Cryptosporidiosis

(Cryptosporidium are small coccidian parasites, related to *I. belli*, that infect microvillus epithelial cells of GI tract.)

Transmitted via contaminated water supply (quality indicators are increase in 3–6 mm particles and turbidity) causing watery diarrhea. (Most U.S. surface water is contaminated.)

In immunocompetent persons, reported prevalence rates of 1–2% in Europe, <4.3% in North America, 3–20% in Asia, Africa, Latin America. Seroprevalence rates are higher. Probably a significant pathogen in diarrheal illness.

In HIV-infected persons, reported prevalence rates of >20%. Is one of the indicator diseases for AIDS (see p. 838) and can be a major factor leading to death.

♦ Identification of organism in stool or other body fluid that has been acid-fast stained is insensitive for diagnosis; requires 10,000–100,000 organisms for positive response.

♦ EIA for detection of antigen in stool has >98% sensitivity and specificity compared to acid-fast staining.

Immunofluorescent antibody assay is used to test water supply; presence of algae may cause false-positive result.

Giardiasis

(Due to *Giardia lamblia*)

♦ Recognition of organism in stools, or occasionally in material from small intestine, which have been concentrated and permanently stained. Sensitivity of ~50% for microscopic recognition of cysts in fecal smears.

♦ Serologic tests by CF, immunofluorescence, and ELISA are available. ELISA for IgG, IgM, IgA has negative predictive value of >98%, but presence of antibodies is not useful for diagnosis of recent infection.

♦ Detection of *Giardia* antigen in stool by ELISA has sensitivity and specificity >98% compared to microscopy. May use as complementary test when stool test is negative or as primary test that is cheaper and more efficient than microscopy.

Chronic infection may cause malabsorption syndrome.

Leishmaniasis

Kala-Azar
(Due to *Leishmania donovani*)

♦ Organism identified in stained smears from spleen, bone marrow, peripheral blood, liver biopsy material, lymph node aspirate

♦ Culture (incubated at 26°C) from same sources

♦ Serologic tests (ELISA, IFA, CIE, direct agglutination, IHA) may be done in immunosuppressed patients from areas of endemic disease who show appropriate clinical findings. Primarily for epidemiologic surveys. Tests are not generally available and require more study. May cross-react in trypanosomiasis, malaria, leprosy.

Anemia due to hypersplenism and decreased marrow production
Leukopenia
Thrombocytopenia
○Markedly increased serum globulin (IgG) with decreased albumin and reversed A/G ratio
Increased ESR, etc., due to increased serum globulin
Frequent urine changes (proteinuria, hematuria)
Laboratory findings due to amyloidosis in chronic cases

American Mucocutaneous Leishmaniasis
(Due to *Leishmania brasiliensis*)
♦ Organism identification by direct microscopy, culture, hamster inoculation, or histologic examination of scrapings or biopsy material from lesions occurs in 67% of cases. Results in literature vary widely.
Anemia sometimes present.

Oriental Sore (Cutaneous Leishmaniasis)
(Due to *Leishmania tropica*)
♦ Organisms identified by direct microscopy and culture of scrapings from lesion.

Malaria

(Due to *Plasmodium vivax, Plasmodium malariae, Plasmodium falciparum, Plasmodium ovale*)
♦ Organism is identified in thin or thick smears of peripheral blood or bone marrow. Thick smear method sensitive to 2 parasites/1,000,000 uninfected RBCs. Smears should be made every 6–12 hrs for 3 consecutive days.
♦ Serologic tests—useful when few parasites are found in blood, when smears are obtained after therapy, or to screen blood donors; not useful to determine species. Not useful in acute malaria because requires ≤ 3 wks to produce increase in titer.
  • IFA test (for IgG) shows high sensitivity (≤ 99%) and specificity and is useful for diagnostic purposes. Titer of >1:256 suggests recent infection (>1:64 where disease is not endemic). Titers rise ~1–2 wks after fever onset and remain increased for duration of infection. Titers fall ~6 mos after cure except in areas of endemic disease, where titer of 1:64 may be present with subclinical infection.
  • Monoclonal antibody testing to detect IgM and detection of antigen in serum have ≤ 100% sensitivity and specificity but do not distinguish past and present infection.
  • IHA test can detect antibody many years after infection and is useful for prevalence studies.
  • Nucleic acid probes using DNA can identify *P. falciparum* (50 parasites/μL of blood) and identify drug-resistant strains.
♦ Methods presently not generally available include
  • PCR-based assay, which is >90% sensitive and specific
  • Flow cytometry to detect infected RBCs
  • Centrifugal concentration of parasites in blood
Anemia (average 2.5 million RBCs/cu mm in chronic cases) is usually hypochromic; may be macrocytic in severe chronic disease. Reticulocyte count is increased.
Monocytes are increased in peripheral blood; pigment may occasionally be present in large mononuclear cells.
WBC is decreased.
Thrombocytopenia
Serum indirect bilirubin is increased, and other evidence of hemolysis is seen.
Bone marrow shows erythroid hyperplasia, RBCs containing organisms, and pigment in RE cells. Marrow hyperplasia may fail in chronic phase.
  • Agranulocytosis and purpura may occur late.
Serum globulin is increased (especially euglobulin fraction); albumin is decreased.
ESR is increased.
Biological false-positive test for syphilis is frequent.
Osmotic fragility of RBCs is normal.
P. malariae may cause acute hemorrhagic nephritis (albuminuria, hematuria); causes chronic renal disease in West Africa.
Blackwater fever (massive intravascular hemolysis) due to *P. falciparum*
  • Severe acute hemolytic anemia (1–2 million RBCs/cu mm) with increased bilirubin, hemoglobinuria, etc.

- May be associated with acute tubular necrosis with Hb casts, azotemia, oliguria to anuria, etc.
- Parasites absent from blood.

Laboratory findings due to involvement of organs
- Liver—vary from congestion to fatty changes to malarial hepatitis or central necrosis; malarial pigment in Kupffer's cells; moderate increase in AST, ALT, and ALP.
- Pigment stones in gallbladder.
- Cerebral malaria.

Persistence of parasite for years may cause contamination of donor blood.

Microsporidia

(*Encephalitozoon intestinalis* causes 10–20% of cases of intestinal microsporidiosis but should be distinguished from more common *Encephalitozoon bieneusi* because of propensity to cause disease in other organs and responsiveness to treatment. These are common opportunistic parasites of intestinal epithelium in AIDS patients with chronic diarrhea.)

Microsporidia may cause acute or chronic, life-threatening diarrhea in immunocompromised hosts; may also cause keratoconjunctivitis (Gram stain of sputum for spores), hepatitis, sclerosing cholangitis, peritonitis, respiratory tract infection, sinusitis, myositis, kidney disease.
- ♦ Identified by cytology, biopsy (light and electron microscopy) and touch preparations of intestinal mucosa.
- ♦ Microscopy of stool wet mounts or preparations using ultraviolet fluorescence or acid-fast or other special stains
- ♦ PCR testing limited to research setting.

Toxoplasmosis

(Due to *Toxoplasma gondii*)

- ♦ Presence of antibody is primary method of diagnosis because <10% of normal adults in the United States have evidence of past infection; causes 15% of unexplained lymphadenopathy. 30–80% of domestic cats have evidence of past infection.
  - Sabin-Feldman dye test detects primarily IgG antibodies; is benchmark for evaluating new tests but is superseded by other tests due to complexity and need for live organisms. Dye test detects antibodies 1–2 wks after onset of infection; level peaks to ≥ 1:1000 in 6–8 wks, then declines during months or years to low level (1:4–1:64) for life of patient; false-positive or false-negative tests are rare.
  - Testing for IgM and IgG by ELISA has fewer false-positives and false-negatives (major test currently in use).
  - IgG test (IFA, dye test, IHA, or CF) that shows a 2× rise in titer in samples taken at 3-wk interval indicates acute infection. IgG peak occurs within 1–2 mos, so initial specimen must be drawn early to demonstrate the rise in titer. Titers eventually reach 1:1000; IgG titer or dye test is rarely <1:1000 in acute toxoplasmosis. IgG antibodies may persist for many years.
  - IgM (IFA) appears in first week of infection, peaks within 1 mo, disappears in 2–3 mos (as early as 1 mo). Occurs in 75% of congenitally infected infants and 97% of adult with acute infections. A negative test rules out infection of <3 wks' duration but does not exclude infection of longer duration. A single titer (≥ 1:80) or serial rise in titer (>4×) indicates recent, new, or reactivated infection. (High titer is ≥ 1:16, low titer is <1:16, negative titer is <1:8; titers vary with laboratory.) ANA and RF may cause false-positive IgM IFA test. Not test of choice.
  - CF detects IgG later than IFA test, returns to normal earlier, is less sensitive than other tests, and is not widely used now.
  - IHA titer detects IgG antibodies; follows the same course as dye test but lags by a few days. Is useful for screening and population studies but not helpful in diagnosis of acute infection. Is less sensitive than IFA or CF tests.
  - Direct agglutination and latex agglutination tests are not available in United States.
  - Tests for specific antigen in serum, CSF, and urine are not commercially available.

In immunocompromised patients, IgM is usually absent and presence of IgG only confirms chronic infection. Serologic tests are often not helpful because IgM is usually negative and IgG is often moderately elevated and 4× rise is uncommon. Titer of 1:1024 strongly supports the diagnosis but is not usually found. Disease activity does not correlate with antibody titer or with changes in titer. Occurs in 5–10% of AIDS patients; absence of IgG in serum occurs in 3% of AIDS patients with toxoplasmic encephalitis. All AIDS patients with CNS symptoms should be tested for *T. gondii* antibodies.

♦ Determination of immune status

Acute infection is indicated by seroconversion or ≥ 4× increase in titer or dye test or IFA titer of ≥ 1:1024 or rising IgG in presence of compatible clinical illness.

Flat IgG titers in absence of IgM titers suggest infection more than 6 mos earlier.

High IgM and high IgG together indicate infection within past 3 mos.

Low to medium IgM and high IgG may indicate infection 3–6 mos earlier.

In organ transplantation, serology profile of both patient and donor are important; seronegative recipient should be monitored for disseminated toxoplasmosis if donor is seropositive.

♦ Mouse inoculation and tissue culture (e.g., from tissue, blood, or CSF) are most reliable methods.

♦ Only rarely is diagnosis made by recognition of trophozoite in appropriate material (CSF, lymph node, muscle) prepared with Wright or Giemsa stain. Confirmation by immunofluorescent antibody technique is often needed. May be aided by immunoperoxidase technique.

♦ Cysts may be incidental finding of chronic asymptomatic infection.

♦ PCR amplification of gene fragments is most sensitive for detection in both paraffin-embedded tissue and aqueous humor.

♦ Detection of DNA in amniotic fluid, CSF, or brain tissue

Adult Patients

WBC varies from leukopenia to leukemoid reaction; atypical lymphocytes may be found.

Anemia is present.

Serum gamma globulins are increased.

○ Heterophil agglutination test is negative, but hematologic picture may exactly mimic infectious mononucleosis; eosinophilia in 10–20% of patients.

Laboratory findings due to involvement of various organ systems

♦ • Lymph node shows distinctive marked hyperplasia; organism may be identified in histologic section.

♦ • CNS shows CSF changes (typically mild increase in number of mononuclear cells, normal glucose, moderate increase in protein; organism can be identified in smear of sediment). Occasionally biopsy of brain may be needed. Immunoperoxidase stain may be very valuable when histopathology is not definitive.

 • Coombs' test–negative hemolytic anemia.

 • Disseminated form (e.g., hepatitis, myositis, meningoencephalitis) is an important complication in the immunologically compromised patient but positive or changing titers may not be present.

 • Many patients in whom ocular findings are the only clinical disease show only very low titers that are not useful.

♦ Antibody titer may be greater in aqueous humor from anterior chamber tap than in serum.

Congenital Infection

Maternal infection rate of 1–5 in 1000 pregnancies. Occurs in 1 in 1000 live births in the United States. Infection rate = 11% in first trimester, 90% in late third trimester. With primary infection, risk varies from 25% in first trimester to 65% in third trimester. Severe disease is more likely with infection in first trimester. High mortality; 90% of infants have CNS sequelae. In mild infections, 80% have sequelae (e.g., chorioretinitis, CNS effects).

♦ Diagnosis by demonstration of *Toxoplasma* IgM in fetal serum but may be found in ~20% of cases, or by isolation of parasite from fetal WBCs or clotted blood inoculation into mice or tissue culture.

Screening has been performed by detection of IgM (ELISA) in neonatal blood on same filter paper used for detection of metabolic disorders.

Nonspecific changes may include increased WBC, eosinophil, and platelet counts, increased serum total IgM, GGT, and LD.

♦ Prenatal diagnosis

 • Tissue culture of chorionic villi (in first trimester).

 • Fetal cord blood, amniotic fluid at 2–22 wks' gestation by tissue culture.

 • PCR of amniotic fluid (sensitivity of >97%, negative predictive value of >99%).

Neonatal Infection
♦ Organism isolated in placenta from 95% of untreated mothers and 81% of treated mothers.
♦ Diagnosis can also be made by isolating *T. gondii* in blood, CSF, or histologic preparation of tissue.
♦ Persistent or increasing serum IgG titer in infant compared to mother; untreated newborn produces IgG by 3 mos; treatment delays production until 9 mos and sometimes prevents production.
♦ Demonstration of IgM antibody or of local production of IgG in CSF or eye fluid (body fluid titer/serum gamma globulin/body fluid gamma globulin).
♦ Demonstration of *Toxoplasma* antigen in blood, urine, or CSF
♦ Persistence of IgG in infant's serum after 1 yr indicates congenital infection.
Specific IgM is detected in <60% of cases. IgA may be detected more frequently.

Trypanosomiasis

Sleeping Sickness
(Acute Rhodesian due to *Trypanosoma rhodesiense*; chronic Gambian due to *Trypanosoma gambiense*)
♦ Identification of organism in appropriate material (blood, bone marrow, lymph node aspirate, CSF) by thick or thin smears or concentrations, wet mounts, animal inoculation, rarely culture. In Gambian type, lymph node aspirate is more likely to reveal organism than blood.
♦ Serologic tests are useful to establish suspicion of disease, but histologic confirmation of diagnosis is required because present drug therapy is not innocuous. Immunofluorescent antibody test or card agglutination test are particularly useful for early diagnosis of chronic infection. Other methods (e.g., IHA, ELISA, CIE) are not available commercially.
Hemolytic anemia, coagulation abnormalities (e.g., DIC), nonspecific liver function abnormalities may be present.
○ Increased serum globulin producing increased ESR, rouleaux formation, etc.
Increased monocytes in peripheral blood
CSF
♦ • Organisms may be identified by microscopic examination of CSF sediment. If organisms are not found, increased WBC and protein or increased IgM or presence of morula (Mott) cells is strongly suggestive.
 • Increased number of cells (mononuclear type)—≤ 30/cu mm during second month, later 100–400/cu mm.
 • Increased protein (use as index to severity of disease and to therapeutic response)—60–100 mg/dL with considerable increase in gamma globulin.
 • Latex agglutination or immunofluorescence tests of CSF give best results.

Chagas' Disease (American Trypanosomiasis)
(Due to *Trypanosoma cruzi*)
♦ Identification of organism
 • Definitive diagnosis is based on demonstration of parasite in blood, CSF, or lymph fluid, but presence is difficult to demonstrate in latent or chronic stages.
 • Blood concentration technique is useful only during acute stage; wet blood (buffy coat), not thin and thick smears, should be used.
 • Biopsy of lymph node or liver (shows leishmanial forms).
 • Culture on blood broth at 28°C from lymph node aspirate.
 • Intraperitoneal injection of mouse, which is killed after 1–2 wks.
 • Xenodiagnosis (laboratory-bred reduvid bug fed on patient develops trypanosomes in gut in 4 wks that are identified in feces) is only useful method during chronic stage; highly specific but sensitivity = 50%.
♦ Serologic tests—specific IgG increases soon after infection and usually remains increased for life.
 • IHA and direct agglutination tests at titers of >1:64 have good sensitivity (~100%) and specificity. IFA has poor specificity. Frequently cross-react in leishmaniasis, infection with other parasites, fungi, bacteria. Therefore, the recommendation is often made that serum test be positive by two different assays. In the United States, tests accepted by Food and Drug Administration for clinical testing but not for blood bank screening include EIA, ELISA.

- CF test is now considered less reliable.
- Gel tests (e.g., CIE) are most reliable but no commercial reagents are available.
- Newer methods (e.g., DNA probes) are being developed and may be available through the CDC or state laboratories or for research.
- Antigenuria can be detected in ~85% of chronic cases.

Laboratory findings due to organ involvement (e.g., heart, CNS, GI tract, skeletal muscle).

Transmission by natural insect vectors, contaminated food, blood transfusion, marrow and organ transplant, IV drug use; transmission through breast feeding and across placenta are possible.

Antenatal/Neonatal Infections[13]

Routine Screening

- Rubella
- Syphilis
- Viral hepatitis
- Group B *Streptococcus*
- HIV

Significant Prenatal Infections

- Varicella (chickenpox) (see p. 839)
- CMV (see p. 841)
- Toxoplasmosis (see p. 876)
- Listeriosis (see p. 807)
- Primary HSV (see p. 848)
- Syphilis (see p.816)

Opportunistic Infections

See Tables 15-15 through 15-17.

Laboratory findings due to underlying diseases (e.g., AIDS [see p. 828], malignant lymphoma and leukemia, diabetes mellitus, Ig defects, after renal transplant, uremia, hypoparathyroidism, hypoadrenalism)

Laboratory findings due to administration of drugs (antibiotics, corticosteroids, cytotoxic and immunosuppressive drugs)

Associated with other factors (e.g., plastic IV catheters, narcotic addiction)

Laboratory findings due to particular organism (see appropriate separate sections)

- *C. neoformans*
- *C. albicans*
- *Aspergillus*
- *Mucorales* fungi
- *S. aureus*
- *S. albus, Bacillus subtilis, Bacillus cereus*, and other saprophytes
- Enteric bacteria (*P. aeruginosa, E. coli, Klebsiella-Enterobacter, Proteus*)

For infectious diseases and pathogens that have been recognized in the past 25 yrs, see Table 15-18.

See Table 15-19 for a guide to human diseases that may be transmitted by or from animals.

See Table 15-20 for a list of biological warfare and terrorist agents.

[13]Gilbert GL. Diagnosis, prevention and management of infectious diseases in the fetus and neonate. In: Trent RJ, ed. *Handbook of prenatal diagnosis.* New York: Cambridge University Press, 1995.

Table 15-15. Commonly Associated Pathogens in Patients with Immunosuppression (e.g., Organ Transplantation, Treatment of Malignancies, AIDS)

Immune Response Depressed	Underlying Condition	Commonly Associated Pathogens
Humoral	Lymphatic leukemia Lymphosarcoma Multiple myeloma Congenital hypogammaglobulinemias Nephrotic syndrome Treatment with cytotoxic or anti-metabolite drugs	Pneumococci *Haemophilus influenzae* Streptococci *Pseudomonas aeruginosa* *Pneumocystis carinii* *Pneumocystis carinii*
Cellular	Terminal cancers Hodgkin's disease Sarcoidosis Uremia Treatment with cytotoxic or anti-metabolite drugs or corticosteroids	Tubercle bacillus *Listeria* *Candida* species *Toxoplasma* *Pneumocystis carinii*
Leukocyte bactericidal	Myelogenous leukemia Chronic granulomatous disease Acidosis Burns Treatment with corticosteroids Granulocytopenia due to drugs	Staphylococci *Serratia* *Pseudomonas* species *Candida* species *Aspergillus* *Nocardia*

Table 15-16. Commonly Associated Pathogens in Patients with Neoplasms

Neoplasm	Infection	Commonly Associated Pathogens
Acute nonlymphocytic leukemia	Sepsis with no apparent focus, pneumonia, skin, mouth, GU tract, hepatitis	Enterobacteriaceae, *Pseudomonas*, staphylococci, *Corynebacterium*, *Candida*, *Aspergillus*, *Mucor*, non-A, non-B hepatitis virus
Acute lymphocytic leukemia	Disseminated disease, pneumonia, pharyngitis, skin	Streptococci, *Pneumocystis carinii*, HSV, CMV, varicella-zoster virus
Lymphoma	Disseminated disease, sepsis, GU tract, pneumonia, skin	*Cryptococcus neoformans*, mucocutaneous *Candida*, HSV, herpes zoster virus, CMV, *Pneumocystis carinii*, *Toxoplasma gondii*, mycobacteria, *Nocardia*, *Strongyloides stercoralis*, *Listeria monocytogenes*, *Brucella*, *Salmonella*, staphylococci, Enterobacteriaceae, *Pseudomonas*
Multiple myeloma	Sepsis, pneumonia, skin	*Haemophilus influenzae*, *Streptococcus pneumoniae*, *Neisseria* meningitis, *Pseudomonas*, Enterobacteriaceae, herpes zoster virus, *Candida*, *Aspergillus*

Table 15-17. Pulmonary Infections

<30 days	30–120 days	>120 days
Following organ transplantation (continuing immunosuppressive therapy)		
Usually nosocomial gram-negative bacteria (e.g., *Pseudomonas aeruginosa, Klebsiella, Escherichia coli, Serratia*) Anaerobes Opportunistic organisms are uncommon	Opportunistic organisms (e.g., CMV, *Pneumocystis carinii, Nocardia, Aspergillus*, mycobacteria, HSV, varicella-zoster virus)	Routine bacterial and viral pathogens *P. carinii* *Cryptococcus neoformans* Nocardia Legionella
Following bone marrow transplantation (initial immunosuppressive therapy)		
(Prolonged neutropenia, progressive decrease in humoral and cell-mediated immunity)		(Delayed maturation of donor immune system leads to defective humoral immunity. Also graft-versus-host disease and use of chemotherapeutic drugs)
Gram-negative bacilli (*P. aeruginosa, Klebsiella, E. coli, Serratia*) Anaerobes *Candida* *Aspergillus* HSV	CMV, HSV, *P. carinii*, adenovirus	Encapsulated bacteria (*Streptococcus pneumoniae, Haemophilus influenzae, Staphylococcus aureus*) Varicella-zoster virus

INFECTIOUS

Table 15-18. Pathogens and Infectious Diseases Recognized in Past 25 Yrs

Viruses
Parvovirus B19 (aplastic crisis in chronic hemolytic anemia)
Rotavirus (infant diarrhea)
Hepatitis C, E
Human T-lymphotrophic virus 1 (T-cell lymphoma–leukemia)
Human T-lymphotrophic virus 2 (hairy cell leukemia)
Human immunodeficiency virus (acquired immunodeficiency syndrome [AIDS])
Herpesvirus 6 (roseola subitum)
Hemorrhagic fever viruses
    Ebola (Ebola hemorrhagic fever)
    Hantaan (hemorrhagic fever with renal syndrome)
    Guaranito (Venezuelan hemorrhagic fever)
    Sabia (Brazilian hemorrhagic fever)
Sin Nombre virus (adult respiratory syndrome)
Human herpesvirus 8 (associated with Kaposi's sarcoma in AIDS patients)
Bacteria
Campylobacter jejuni (enteric pathogen)
Toxin-producing strains of *Staphylococcus aureus* (toxic shock syndrome)
Legionella pneumophila (legionnaire's disease)
Escherichia coli O157:H7 (hemolytic-uremic syndrome; hemorrhagic colitis)
Borrelia burgdorferi (Lyme disease)
Helicobacter pylori (peptic ulcer)
Ehrlichia chaffeensis (ehrlichiosis)
Vibrio cholerae O139 (new strain; epidemic cholera)
Bartonella henselae (cat-scratch disease; bacillary angiomatosis)
Parasites
Cryptosporidium parvum (diarrhea)
Enterocytozoon bieneusi (persistent diarrhea)
Cyclospora cayatanensis (persistent diarrhea)
Encephalitozoon hellum (conjunctivitis; disseminated disease)
Encephalitozoon cuniculi (disseminated disease)
Babesia—new species (atypical babesiosis)

Table 15-19. Some Human Diseases that May Be Transmitted by or from Animals

Disease	Pathogen	Arthropod Vector[a]	Animal Reservoir[b]								
			D	C	B	F	P	R	M	X	H
Bacterial											
Campylobacter jejuni infections	C.jejuni		+	+	+	+	+	+	+		
Salmonella infections	Salmonella spp.	F, roaches	+	+	+	+	+	+	+		
Bacillary dysentery	Shigella spp.	F, roaches							+		
Yersinia infections	Y. enterocolitica		+	+		+	+	+			
Anthrax	Anthrax bacillus		+			+	+				
Brucellosis	Brucella spp.		+	+		+	+	+			
Tularemia	Francisella tularensis	T, biting flies	+	+		+	+	+			
Leptospirosis	Leptospira spp.		+	+			+	+			
Tuberculosis	Mycoplasma tuberculosis		+	+	+						
Lyme disease	Borrelia burgdorferi	T						+			
Relapsing fever	Borrelia hermsii, B. parkeri, B. turicatae, B. recurrentis	T, L						+		+	
Ehrlichiosis	Ehrlichia chaffeensis	T						+			
Plague	Yersinia pestis	Fl						+			+
Viral											
Rabies	Lyssavirus		+	+		+					
Cat-scratch disease	Bartonella spp.			+							
Psittacosis	Chlamydia psittaci				+			+			
Lymphocytic choriomeningitis			+					+			
St. Louis encephalitis	Flavivirus	M			+						
Western equine encephalitis	Alphavirus	M			+						
Eastern equine encephalitis	Alphavirus	M			+						
Venezuelan equine encephalitis	Alphavirus	M					+	+			
La Crosse encephalitis	Bunyavirus	M						+		3	
Dengue	Flavivirus	M									+
Yellow fever	Flavivirus	M						+	+		+
Colorado tick fever	Orbivirus	T						+			
Hemorrhagic fever with renal and pulmonary syndrome	Hantavirus						+	+			
California encephalitis	Arbovirus	M					+	+			

(continued)

Table 15-19. (continued)

Disease	Pathogen	Arthropod Vector[a]	D	C	B	F	P	R	M	X	H
Rickettsial											
Q fever	Coxiella burnetii	T								1	
Rocky Mountain spotted fever	Rickettsia rickettsii	T								2	
Rickettsialpox	R. akari	T						+			
Murine typhus	R. typhi	Fl						+			
Epidemic typhus	R. prowazekii	L								4	+
Fungal											
Ringworm	Microsporum, Tricophyton, Epidermophyton spp.			+			+	+			
Histoplasmosis	Histoplasma capsulatum				+					+	
Parasitic											
Leishmaniasis	Leishmania mexicana	F						+		6	
Roundworm infestation	Toxocara sp.		+	+							
Tapeworm infestation	Taenia spp.		+	+							
	Echinococcus		+	+		+					
Visceral larva migrans	Toxocara canis, T. cati		+	+							
Cutaneous larva migrans	Ancylostoma caninum, A. braziliense		+	+							
Dirofilariasis	Dirofilaria immitis	M	+	+							
Scabies	Sarcoptes scabiei		+	+							
Chagas' disease	Trypanosoma cruzi	O, kissing bugs (reduviids)						+		5	
Toxoplasmosis	Toxoplasmosis gondii		+	+							
Malaria	Plasmodium spp.	M									
Babesiosis	Babesia microti	T						+			+

Anisakiasis (nematode) from eating raw fish (e.g., sashimi).

Trichinosis from eating poorly prepared pork or exotic meats (e.g., bear, walrus, wild boar).

Capnocytophaga canimorsus (gram-negative bacteria) transmitted by dog bite or saliva causing acute overwhelming cellulitis, septicemia, meningitis, endocarditis; diagnosis by culture of blood, CSF, or tissue.

[a]Arthropod vector: F = fly; Fl = flea; L = louse; M = mosquito; O = other; T = tick or mite.

[b]Animal reservoir: B = birds; C = cat; D = dog; F = farm animals; H = human; P = poultry; M = monkeys; R = rodents; X = other; 1 = domestic livestock ticks; 2 = Dermacentor sp.; 3 = Aedes triseriatus mosquito; 4 = ?flying squirrels; 5 = opossums, raccoons, armadillos; 6 = opossums, cotton rats, ?armadillos.

Table 15-20. Biological Warfare and Terrorist Agents

Agent	See Page Number
Anthrax	794
Brucellosis	796
Plague	811
Q fever	854
Tularemia	825
Smallpox	852
Viral encephalitides	843
Viral hemorrhagic fevers	848
Botulinum toxin	796
Staphylococcal enterotoxin B	814

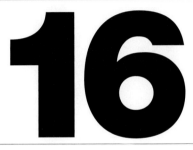

Miscellaneous Diseases

Laboratory Tests for Collagen/Vascular/Rheumatic Diseases

Antibodies, Antinuclear (ANA)

Use

Mainly to exclude SLE (see Table 16-1 and Table 16-2).

Interpretation

ANA is the most sensitive laboratory test for detecting SLE (detects up to 95% of cases); specificity is as low as 50% in rheumatic disease in general. May be present in healthy persons; the elderly; persons with other rheumatic diseases, infectious mononucleosis, or unrecognized chronic infections; persons using certain drugs (e.g., hydralazine, isoniazid, chlorpromazine); and family of SLE patients. Negative ANA finding in patient with active multisystem disease is strong (but not absolute) evidence against SLE; positive ANA finding without other manifestations is not diagnostic. High titers are most often associated with SLE; titers of <1:160 often have minimal clinical significance and may not be related to patient's symptoms. ANA may become negative during remission. Titers correlate poorly with remission and relapse; usually not useful to follow disease course or response to therapy. Persistently negative ANA tests occur in ~5% of SLE patients due to congenital deficiency of early complement component (usually C4 or C2); detected by absent total hemolytic complement (CH50). These patients tend to have prominent skin disease and low incidence of serious renal and CNS disease.

Pattern of ANA immunofluorescence is of limited value in discriminating SLE from other collagen vascular diseases but may suggest subsequent tests.
- Homogeneous (diffuse or solid) pattern is associated with antibodies to deoxyribonucleoprotein; high titers are more strongly associated with SLE than with other diseases and correlate with activity of SLE.
- Rim (peripheral) pattern is associated with anti-dsDNA (double-stranded DNA) and has the highest specificity for SLE.
- Speckled pattern detects numerous antigens (e.g., extractable nuclear antigen, Sm, nRNP, SS-A, SS-B); antibody tests for these antigens should be ordered when a speckled pattern is found.
- Nucleolar pattern is associated with anti-RNP; characteristic of scleroderma; rarely in other immune disorders.

Anti–extractable nuclear antigen (ENA) testing (by EIA or gel diffusion) detects only two extractable nuclear antigens: RNP and Sm.
- Anti-RNP is found in 25–30% of SLE patients, 10% of RA patients, 22% of scleroderma patients, and 100% of patients with mixed connective tissue disease.
- Anti-Sm (speckled immunofluorescence pattern) is found in 25–30% of SLE patients and *is the most specific diagnostic test for SLE*; occurs almost exclusively in SLE. Serum levels remain fairly constant and are not related to disease activity.

Anti-dsDNA is found in 40–80% of SLE patients and rarely in those with other diseases; *high specificity* is almost same as that of anti-Sm (rim or peripheral nodular

Table 16-1. Antinuclear Antibody Disease Profiles*

ANAs	SLE	Drug-Induced Lupus Erythematosus	Mixed Connective Tissue Disease	Scleroderma Syndrome	CREST Syndrome	Sjögren's Syndrome	Dermatomyositis and Polymyositis	RA
ANA screen	>95	>95	>95	70–90	70–90	75–90	40–60	R
Native DNA	**60**	R	R	R	R	R	R	40
Histones	30	**>95**	R	R	R	R	R	20
Sm	**30**	R	R	R	R	R	R	R
Nuclear RNP	40–50	R	**>95**	15	10	R	15	10
Scl-70	R	R	R	**30–70**	R	R	R	R
SS-A (Ro)	40–60		R	R	R	**≤90**	10	R
SS-B (La)	15		R	R	R	**≤60**	R	R
Centromere	R		R	30	**70–85**	R	R	R
Nucleolar	25	R	R	**40–70**	R	R	R	R
PM-Scl (PM-1) and Jo-1	R	R	R	~20	R	R	**10–50**	R

CREST = calcinosis, *R*aynaud's syndrome, *e*sophageal dysmotility, *s*clerodactyly, *t*elangiectasia; DNA = deoxyribonucleic acid; PM-Scl = polymyositis-scleroderma; R = rare; RNP = ribonucleoprotein; Scl = scleroderma; Sm = Smith; SS = Sjögren's syndrome.

*Reported frequency of ANAs in various diseases is given as a percentage. Boldface indicates significant correlation.

Source: Tan EM, Robinson CA, Nakamura RM. ANAs in systemic rheumatic disease: diagnostic significance. *Postgrad Med* 1985;78:141.

Table 16-2. Comparison of Idiopathic and Drug–Induced Lupus

	Idiopathic SLE	Drug–Induced Lupus
Renal, CNS involvement	Common	Rare
ANA pattern	Rim	Homogeneous
Immune complexes	Present	Rare
Low complement level	50–70%	5%
Antihistone antibodies	≤ 70% of patients	>95% of patients; if negative, drug–induced lupus is unlikely
Other antibodies (e.g., anti–dsDNA and anti–Sm)	Frequently present	Usually absent

dsDNA = double-stranded deoxyribonucleic acid.
Drug–induced ANA is histone dependent, but in idiopathic SLE, histone dependence is found in only 30% of patients and histone–dependent ANAs are never the only ones.

immunofluorescence pattern). Absence of anti-dsDNA throughout clinical course is associated with improved prognosis, and severe clinical disease frequently correlates with a high initial titer, which declines with clinical improvement; however, it may be present for prolonged periods without clinical activity. *High titers are characteristic of SLE and are found rarely in other conditions*; low titers (e.g., 1:10 to 1:20) are found in other rheumatic diseases. Anti–single-stranded DNA (ssDNA) is found in all other rheumatic diseases and many chronic inflammatory conditions; is not specific for SLE, but its presence in almost all SLE patients makes it a sensitive indicator. DNA-histone (deoxyribonucleoprotein) antibodies are found in drug-induced SLE, SLE, and many connective tissue diseases.

ANA Profile in SLE

♦ *Multiple (three or more) antibodies are characteristic of SLE.*
♦ *High titers of dsDNA are characteristic of SLE;* very specific for SLE; occur in 50–60% of patients. dsDNA may be present in chronic active hepatitis.
♦ *High titers of anti-Sm are very specific for SLE but not sensitive* (present in 30% of patients; 50–60% when measured by ELISA). Virtually absent in normal persons. May be found in absence of anti-dsDNA. Significance equal to that of dsDNA in identifying SLE patients. Titers remain constant. Does not correlate with disease activity.
ssDNA has low specificity; poor correlation with disease activity.
Deoxyribonucleoprotein in ≤ 70% of patients
Histones are found in ≤ 60% of patients.
SS-A is found in 25% of patients.
SS-B is found in 15% of patients.
RNP is found in ≤ 34% of patients, usually associated with anti-Sm.

ANA Profile in Drug-Induced Lupus

♦ *Antihistone antibodies are present in >95% of cases*; if negative, drug-induced lupus is unlikely. Other antibodies that are frequently seen in SLE (e.g., anti-dsDNA and anti-Sm) are usually absent.
Drug-induced ANA is histone dependent, but in idiopathic SLE, histone dependence is found in only 30% of patients and histone-dependent antibodies are never the only ANA.
Drugs that may cause positive tests for LE cells and/or ANA
Definite
  • High risk (e.g., procainamide, hydralazine)
  • Low risk (e.g., ethosuximide, hydantoins, isoniazid, lithium, quinidine, thiouracils, trimethadione)
Possible (rare) (e.g., D-penicillamine, chlorpromazine, reserpine)
Unlikely (e.g., allopurinol, gold salts, griseofulvin, methysergide, oral contraceptives, penicillin, streptomycin, sulfonamides, tetracycline)

MISC

ANA Profile in Sjögren's Syndrome

♦ Presence of SS-A (in 70% of patients) and SS-B (in 60% of patients) without other antibodies indicates probable Sjögren's syndrome; with other ANA probably indicates SLE. If SS-B is present, it usually accompanies SS-A. Virtually absent in normal persons.

ANA Profile in Mixed Connective Tissue Disease

(Combines clinical features of RA, polymyositis, SLE, and especially scleroderma; ~10% of SLE patients fulfill criteria for mixed connective tissue disease.)
♦ *High titer of anti-RNP in >95% of patients without anti-Sm and other antibodies is characteristic of mixed connective tissue disease.*
ANA positive with speckled pattern

ANA Profile in Progressive Systemic Sclerosis (Scleroderma) and CREST Syndrome

♦ Centromere is only antibody in 70–85% of patients with CREST (calcinosis, Raynaud's syndrome, esophageal dysmotility, sclerodactyly, telangiectasia) syndrome; moderate to high titers. Rare in other disorders.
♦ Finding of anti–Scl 70 in ~20% of patients is highly specific for scleroderma. More prevalent in severe scleroderma than in CREST syndrome.
High titer of nucleolar antibodies in 40–50% of patients
RNP, SS-A, SS-B at low titers

ANA Profile in Polymyositis and Dermatomyositis

♦ Anti–Jo 1 (PM-1) is found in 50% of polymyositis and 10% of dermatomyositis patients; strong association with interstitial lung disease. Rarely detected in other diseases. Syndrome may include pulmonary fibrosis, Raynaud's syndrome, dry cracked skin on hands ("mechanic's hands").

ANA Profile in Rheumatoid Arthritis

♦ RA nuclear antigen is found in 85–95% of patients.
Histones are found in 20% of patients.
♦ RF is present in ~80% of patients. Frequently present in Sjögren's syndrome; less often in other connective tissue diseases; occasionally in chronic infections (e.g., SBE, gammopathies).
ANAs are absent; low titer of anti–native DNA may be present.

Collagen/Vascular/Rheumatic Diseases and Miscellaneous Disorders

Amyloidosis[1]

♦ Diagnosis is established by demonstration of amyloid in tissue.
  • Congo red staining yields positive findings in one-third of patients with primary amyloidosis and approximately two-thirds of patients with secondary amyloidosis. *Congo red stain of tissue should be examined under polarized light (apple-green birefringence) as well as transmitted light.*
  • Findings of subcutaneous abdominal fat biopsy are positive in 85% of patients with light-chain (AL) amyloidosis.
  • Gingival biopsy findings are positive in one-half to two-thirds of patients.
  • Rectal biopsy findings are positive in one-half to two-thirds of patients.
  • Needle biopsy of kidney is useful when gingival and rectal biopsies are not helpful and there is a differential diagnosis of nephrosis.
  • Bone biopsy is positive in 30% of patients; also useful to identify multiple myeloma.

[1]Falk RH, Comenzo RL, Skinner M. The systemic amyloidoses. *N Engl J Med* 1997;337:898.

- Findings of needle biopsy of liver are often positive, but beware of intractable bleeding or rupture.
- Skin biopsy is taken from sites of plaque formation.
- Tissue from carpal-tunnel decompression is positive in 90% of amyloidosis cases.
- Other areas of involvement include GI tract, spleen, respiratory tract.
- Electron microscopy is the most specific diagnostic method.
- Immunohistochemical staining shows reaction of fibrils with kappa or lambda antisera.

Evans blue dye is retained in serum.

Classification

(AL) Light-Chain Amyloid (Primary)

(Paraprotein disorder characterized by monoclonal Ig light-chain deposits in tissues; Bence Jones proteinuria occurs; derived from malignant clone of plasma cells in neoplastic type or small nonproliferative population of plasma cells in nontumor type)

○One-third of cases show overt myeloma; occurs in ~15% of cases of multiple myeloma. Primary when no evidence of associated disease (e.g., myeloma) is present. May also be associated with Waldenström's macroglobulinemia, heavy-chain disease, etc.

○One organ usually shows predominant involvement.

- Cardiovascular system—involved in almost all cases; congestive failure in 25% of cases.
- Proteinuria and azotemia occur in most cases; nephrotic-range proteinuria (>3 gm/day) occurs in 45% of cases. Amyloidosis should always be ruled out in patients aged >30 yrs with unexplained nephrotic syndrome.
- Tongue is enlarged in 20% of cases.
- Peripheral neuropathy in 16% of cases; CNS is not involved.
- Carpal tunnel syndrome in 20% of cases.
- GI tract involvement—e.g., malabsorption.
- Bone marrow involved in 30%.
- Respiratory system is usually involved, but decreased pulmonary function is rare.
- Other (adrenal glands, thyroid, etc.).

○Serum protein electrophoresis shows hypogammaglobulinemia in 25% and an abnormal Ig (monoclonal spike) in another 45% of cases.

○Immunoelectrophoresis/immunofixation detects a monoclonal protein in 90% of cases. ~25% of patients have a free monoclonal light chain in serum (Bence Jones proteinemia). Lambda light chains (present in 65%) are more common than kappa light chains (present in 35%) in contrast to multiple myeloma.

○Urine contains free light chains in >75% of cases, two-thirds of these are lambda-type Bence Jones proteins; monoclonal peak is often hidden by nephrotic protein loss. Sensitivity for detection of free light chains is increased by concentration of urine (100–500×), and by immunoelectrophoresis and immunofixation. Low levels of urine monoclonal light chains (<200 mg/24 hrs) may indicate an immunocytic malignancy (multiple myeloma, CLL, or non-Hodgkin's lymphoma) even when serum is negative for M proteins, and thus occult malignancy should be ruled out. *Monoclonal proteins are not found in secondary, senile, familial, or localized amyloidosis.*

Serum creatinine level of >1.3 mg/dL is associated with a shorter survival time; some renal insufficiency in ~50% of cases.

Mild anemia in 50% of cases

Platelet count may be increased (>500,000/cu mm in ~10% of cases); may be due to functional hyposplenism.

WBC is frequently increased.

ESR is increased.

Bone marrow shows >5% plasma cells in 50% of cases.

See Multiple Myeloma (p. 420).

(ATTR) Familial Transthyretin Associated

(Autosomal dominant diseases; most commonly due to mutant transthyretin)

♦Many different types of abnormal transthyretin identified by isoelectric focusing of serum or DNA test for mutant transthyretin gene.

Renal disease less common than in AL type.

No tongue involvement

MISC

(AA) Reactive (Secondary) Systemic (Amyloid A Protein)
(Bence Jones proteinuria is absent.)
Due To
- RA
- Juvenile RA
- Ankylosing spondylitis
- Chronic infections (were most common cause before antibiotic era)
    Osteomyelitis, burns, decubital ulcers
    Leprosy
    TB
- Heroin use with chronic infection of skin injection sites
- Chronic inflammation (e.g., bowel disease)
- Neoplasms
    Hodgkin's disease
    Nonlymphoid solid tumors (e.g., renal and bladder adenocarcinoma)
- Heredofamilial systemic amyloidosis
    Familial Mediterranean fever (AA type)
    Neuropathic types (I, II, III, IV)—serum protein electrophoresis and immuno-
        electrophoresis are normal.

Increased concentration of serum amyloid A protein (an acute-phase protein)
  ♦ Immunohistochemical staining of tissue for AA protein

Local Amyloidosis Types
(Bence Jones proteinuria is absent.)
(SSA) Senile cardiac amyloid (formed from prealbumin)—found in 24% of patients >70
    yrs old; may cause heart failure.
(AF) Familial amyloid (formed from prealbumin)—occurs in autosomal dominant dis-
    ease with cardiac, renal, neuropathic involvement.
(CAA) Cerebral amyloid (subunit protein is called A4 or beta)—is found in cerebral ves-
    sels, plaques, and neurofibrillary tangles in Alzheimer's disease.
(A-beta$_2$-M) Systemic amyloid (from beta$_2$-microglobulin) due to dialysis
(IAPP) Amyloid of type II diabetes (from islet polypeptide)
(AE) Amyloid of medullary cancer of thyroid (from calcitonin)
Laboratory findings due to associated diseases (see previous)
Laboratory findings due to involvement of specific organs and systems (e.g., liver, kid-
    ney, GI system, endocrine system, skin, synovia and tendons in carpal-tunnel syn-
    drome, lung, bladder, skin, larynx; see appropriate separate sections)
Monoclonal Ig are not found in serum or urine.

Angioedema, Hereditary

**(Due to autosomal dominant congenital deficiency of inhibitor of first component
    of complement [C1 INH])**
Long history of clinical syndrome of episodes of upper airway obstruction, cramping
    abdominal pain, absence of urticaria, attacks precipitated by trauma, positive fam-
    ily history in 75–85% of cases
○ Serum C4 is the single most reliable screening test; is decreased even when patient
    is asymptomatic. If borderline, repeat at height of attack because C4 falls during
    episode.
♦ Low (0–30% of normal) C1 INH is necessary to confirm diagnosis. Do not use for
    screening.
RIA does not detect the 15% of cases of variant form in which C1 INH antigen is pres-
    ent but nonfunctioning; for these cases more difficult functional assay for C1 INH is
    needed. (Test is performed only at reference laboratories.)
CBC and ESR are usually normal when the manifestation is peripheral or facial
    angioedema, but they may be abnormal when the manifestation is diarrhea and
    abdominal pain.

Dermatomyositis

○ Increased serum CK and aldolase.
PM-1 antigen found in 10% of patients (see Table 16-1).
♦ Abnormal findings on biopsy of muscle.

Factitious Disorders

♦ Should always be suspected when significant discrepancy is seen between various laboratory data, laboratory results are impossible, or laboratory values are discordant with clinical picture.

Gastrointestinal [2–3]

Cause	Method of Detection
Self-induced vomiting	Hypochloremic metabolic alkalosis with increased serum bicarbonate, hyponatremia, and hypokalemia. Urine—increased potassium (>10 mEq/L) and decreased chloride.
Vomiting due to ipecac ingestion	Ipecac identified in stool as emetine by thin-layer chromatography; in stool and urine by HPLC (not by routine toxicology)
Diuretic abuse	Urine assay can detect thiazides, furosemide, ethacrynic acid, carbonic anhydrase inhibitors. Increased urine potassium (>10 mEq/L). *Any urine with potassium >30 mEq/L should be tested for diuretic agents.*
Diarrhea due to laxative abuse*	Hyperchloremic metabolic acidosis with decreased serum bicarbonate and potassium. Potassium is low in urine (<10 mEq/L) and increased in fecal fluid. Detection of laxative in urine (e.g., castor oil, phenolphthalein, bisacodyl, senna) and stool (e.g., phenolphthalein, mineral oil, anthraquinones, magnesium, sulfate, phosphate, bisacodyl [Dulcolax]) Alkalinization of stool causes color change due to phenolphthalein, some anthraquinones, bisacodyl. Detection of high concentration of sodium sulfate in stool when due to Glauber's salt (sodium sulfate) or high concentration of phosphate when due to Na_2PO_4. Sodium bicarbonate abuse causes hypokalemic metabolic alkalosis.
"Diarrhea" caused by dilution of stool with water (or another dilute fluid)*	Stool osmolality is very low (<250 mOsm/kg); is lower than plasma osmolality; is normal when defecation is supervised or colon contents are sampled endoscopically. Stool sodium, potassium, chloride, and magnesium concentrations are very low.
Vomiting and diarrhea due to salt poisoning	Very high sodium (>150 mEq/L) in serum and urine
Bleeding due to surreptitious ingestion of warfarin or brodifacoum (rodenticide) or trauma	Identification of anticoagulant in plasma, prolonged PT
Abdominal pain (pancreatitis)	Saliva was added to urine and is of salivary rather than pancreatic origin.

Hematologic

Hemorrhagic diathesis Ingestion of warfarin	Prolonged PT, which is restored to normal by administration of vitamin K. Warfarin can also be assayed in plasma. Prolonged PT due to "superwarfarin" (a rodenticide—brodifacoum) may not be controlled by standard doses of vitamin K. Warfarin assay is negative; requires a separate assay.

[2]Wallach J. Laboratory diagnosis of factitious disorders. *Arch Intern Med* 1994;154:1690.
[3]Phillips S, Donaldson BS, Geisler K, Pera A, Kochar R. Stool composition in factitial diarrhea: a 6-year experience with stool analysis. *Ann Intern Med* 1995;123:97.

Heparin injection	Prolonged aPTT but PT is normal; repeated aPTT rapidly becomes normal while patient is under observation. Prolonged TT and normal reptilase time. TT becomes normal on addition of protamine sulfate. Prolonged aPTT and TT are corrected after removal of heparin by an anion-exchange resin or heparinase. Assay can demonstrate heparin in plasma.
Anemia due to self–blood letting	Diagnosis by ^{59}Fe elimination rates and other erythrokinetic studies
Thrombocytopenia due to ingestion of drugs causing antiplatelet antibodies	Demonstration of antiplatelet antibodies
Pancytopenia due to ingestion of alkylating agents	

Endocrine

Hyperthyroidism (see Chapter 13)
Hypoglycemia (see Chapter 13)
Cushing's syndrome (see Chapter 13)

Genitourinary

Proteinuria	Waxing and waning proteinuria
	Unusual urine electrophoresis patterns
	Nonhuman protein is demonstrated by isoelectric focusing or immunofixation or immunodiffusion.
	Serum albumin remains normal.
Hematuria	RBC morphology is not of renal origin; no RBC or Hb casts.
Calculi	Analysis shows stones to be mineral (e.g., quartz, feldspar) or pepper grains.
Increased creatinine and potassium	Dilution of blood sample tube with urine.

Infectious

Bacteremia	May be polymicrobial. No evident source in obstruction of GI, GU, or biliary tracts.

Respiratory

Inhalation of talc simulating asthma	Analysis of crystals in lung biopsy specimen by electron microscopy and spectroscopy is identical to that of baby powder.

*Suspect if high daily stool volume (>500 mL/day), unexplained hypokalemia, or decreased serum bicarbonate with metabolic acidosis, melanosis coli on colonoscopy, cathartic colon on barium enema. See also Osmolal Gap, p. 68.

Fasciitis, Eosinophilic

(May be a scleroderma variant. Recent cases caused by L-tryptophan or Spanish toxic rapeseed oil. See Lyme Disease, p. 808.)
♦ Diagnosis is confirmed by characteristic findings in a deep biopsy of skin down to and including muscle.
Eosinophilia
Diffuse hypergammaglobulinemia

Lupus, Discoid

~10% of patients develop SLE.
Usually ANA negative
♦ Biopsy of skin lesions shows deposition of complement and Ig.
See Lupus Erythematosus, Systemic: Lupus Band Test, p. 897.

Lupus, Systemic Erythematosus (SLE)

Criteria for Classification of SLE

(American Rheumatism Association, 1982)
♦ Presence of four or more criteria at same or different times allows the diagnosis of
SLE and excludes other disorders.

	Sensitivity (%)	Specificity (%)
Malar rash	57	96
Discoid lupus	18	99
Oral/nasopharyngeal ulcers	27	96
Photosensitivity	43	96
Arthritis	86	37
Proteinuria (>0.5 gm/day or 3+ qualitative) or cellular casts	51	94
Seizures or psychosis not due to other causes	20	98
Pleuritis or pericarditis	56	86
Cytopenia (any of these four findings)	59	89
Autoimmune hemolytic anemia	15	
Neutropenia (<4000/cu mm on two or more occasions)		
Lymphopenia (<1500/cu mm on two or more occasions)		
Thrombocytopenia (<100,000/cu mm in absence of causative drugs)		
Immunologic findings (any of these four findings)	85	93
Anti–nuclear DNA antibodies		
Anti-Sm antibodies		
LE cells		
False-positive serologic test for syphilis of >6 mos' duration confirmed by FTA-ABS or *Treponema pallidum* immobilization test		
Positive ANA in the absence of known causative drugs	99	49
Overall	96	96

♦ *ANA is the most sensitive laboratory test for SLE* (detects up to 95% of cases). Most
patients with SLE have multiple (≥ 3) antibodies present, but those with drug-
induced lupus and other connective tissue diseases are likely to have fewer ANA present (see Table 16-1). *Combination of positive ANA test, positive dsDNA antibody test,
and hypocomplementemia has diagnostic specificity of virtually 100%.*
Traditional parameters of disease activity (Hb, WBC, ESR, CRP, urinalysis, serum creatinine) do not distinguish activity from superimposed infection or drug toxicity and
may not be sensitive enough to detect early exacerbation.
Current indicators of disease activity
  • Decrease in early complement components (C3, C4; C4 is most sensitive) and
    total hemolytic complement occurs in ~70% of patients with active SLE; is not
    specific for diagnosis but is helpful in managing patients who are at risk for renal
    and CNS involvement; C3 and/or C4 may be helpful in following response to
    therapy. Total hemolytic complement should be part of initial evaluation of SLE
    patients.
  ♦ Reduced C3, C4, and CH50 are rarely seen in those without immune complex dis-
    eases; therefore their reduction strongly supports diagnosis of SLE in patient with
    suggestive history and physical examination.
  • Increasing titers of anti-DNA; serial monitoring is probably not of value.
  • Presence of circulating immune complexes.
  • Presence of cryoglobulins (see p. 379) correlates well with disease activity.
  • Monoclonal RF assay.
  • C1q binding.
  • Raji cell assay is not recommended as indicator of SLE disease activity.
*These indicators do not predict which manifestations are likely to become active or the
time interval (may be weeks to months), and some patients with these laboratory*

abnormalities never manifest active disease. The strongest correlation is with active nephritis, but these tests may be normal in 10–25% of patients and in any case do not substitute for renal biopsy.

SLE may present as "idiopathic" thrombocytopenic purpura but serious thrombocytopenia occurs in <10% of patients.

Anemia is most commonly anemia of chronic disease or may be due to iron deficiency due to blood loss. Autoimmune hemolytic anemia occurs in ~15% of patients and correlates with disease activity.

ESR and CRP may be increased.

Abnormal serum proteins frequently occur.

- Biological false-positive test for syphilis is very common; occurs in ≤ 20% of patients. *This may be the first manifestation of SLE and may precede other features by many months; 7% of asymptomatic individuals with biological false-positive test for syphilis ultimately develop SLE.*
- Serum gamma globulin is increased in 50% of patients; a continuing rise may indicate poor prognosis. Alpha$_2$ globulin is increased; albumin is decreased. Ig's may be increased.

Tissue biopsy of skin, muscles, kidney, and lymph node may be useful.

Laboratory findings reflecting specific organ involvement

- Renal: Serologic changes may appear months before clinical renal involvement; urine findings are stronger indication to modify therapy. Urine findings indicate acute nephritis, nephrotic syndrome, chronic renal impairment, secondary pyelonephritis. Sediment is the same as in chronic active GN. Patients with azotemia and marked proteinuria usually die in 1–3 yrs. High antibody titer to native DNA associated with decreased serum complement indicates lupus nephritis. Disease activity often disappears when renal failure occurs. Recurrence in allograft is rare. Renal biopsy may not be indicated without significant proteinuria or urinary sediment abnormalities. (See p. 729.)
- CNS: Manifestations due to vascular changes causing occlusions, uremia, electrolyte imbalance, coagulopathy, hypertension, antineuronal antibodies, infection. (*Rule out complicating TB and cryptococcosis.*) CSF findings of aseptic meningitis (increased protein and pleocytosis are found in 50% of these patients).
- Cardiovascular: Bacterial and nonbacterial endocarditis; increased prevalence of coronary arteriosclerosis and valvular lesions.
- Pulmonary findings (acute or chronic disease) may be present. Pleural effusions are exudate in type.
- Joint involvement occurs in 90% of patients.
- Neonates of mothers with SLE may have discoid lupus, hematologic or serologic abnormalities due to transplacental passage of Ro antibodies.

Laboratory findings reflecting diseases due to autoantibodies

- Hashimoto's thyroiditis
- Sjögren's syndrome
- Myasthenia gravis
- Autoimmune thrombocytopenia in ≤ 25% of SLE patients
- Circulating lupus anticoagulants, antiphospholipid antibody syndrome (see p. 450)

Laboratory findings due to complications

- Various bacterial and viral opportunistic infections (e.g., herpes zoster) due to immunodeficiency (from SLE as well as therapy).
- Osteonecrosis.
- Malignancy—increased risk for lymphoma and soft tissue sarcomas.

Drug-induced lupus syndromes due to prolonged administration of drugs; most often associated with procainamide or hydralazine.

- Procainamide (15–100% develop ANA within 1 yr and 5–30% develop SLE; does not induce antibodies to dsDNA).
- Hydralazine (24–50% develop ANA and 8–13% develop SLE).
- Isoniazid and birth control pills may induce ANA without symptoms).
- Various anticonvulsants (e.g., phenytoin).
- Renal and CNS manifestations are very unusual.
- Usually high titer of ANA and absent dsDNA antibodies.
- See ANA profile in drug-induced lupus (p. 889 and Table 17-2).

○SLE should be ruled out in asymptomatic patients (especially women of child-bearing age) with false-positive VDRL, various unexplained conditions, e.g., thrombocytopenia, leukopenia, proteinuria or abnormal urine sediment, positive Coombs' test, prolonged aPTT.

LE cell test has been replaced by ANA tests.

Hematoxylin Bodies

(Homogeneous round extracellular material)
May be found in SLE, RA, multiple myeloma, cirrhosis. In SLE they may be found without LE cells in the same sample.

Lupus Band Test

Direct immunofluorescence on biopsy specimen from normal skin
Use
In patients without sufficient clinical manifestations of SLE (e.g., only renal or CNS findings)
In patients whose symptoms and other laboratory tests show remission due to steroid therapy
In differentiation of early SLE from RA
Interpretation
Is positive in 50% of all SLE patients and ≤ 80% of those with active multisystem (especially renal) disease; in discoid lupus findings are positive found only in skin lesions.
Specificity for SLE increases with the number of Ig's and complement components found.
May be positive in dermatomyositis, undifferentiated collagen vascular disease, and other nonrheumatic diseases but usually only one Ig is found.

Multiple Organ Dysfunction Syndrome

Sequela of certain severe conditions, especially in surgical intensive care unit (e.g., ruptured aneurysm, acute pancreatitis, septic shock, surgical complications, burns, trauma); four clinical stages with mortality ranging from 40% mortality in early stage to up to 90% in late stage.
• Episode of physiologic shock
• Active resuscitation lasting up to 24 hrs
• Stable hypermetabolism (hyperglycemia, hyperlactacidemia, polyuria, urine urea nitrogen >15 gm/day) lasting 7–10 days with appearance of acute lung injury and repeated septic episodes
• Onset of liver and kidney failure (serum bilirubin >3 mg/dL after 7–10 days with progressive rise followed by increase in serum creatinine); encephalopathy, consumption coagulopathy, GI bleeding, recurrent infection
Progressive increase in blood glucose, lactate, urine nitrogen excretion, and fall in serum albumin, transferrin, and other liver proteins.
Increasing consumption coagulopathy and thrombocytopenia.
Failure of immune system marked by bacteremia (especially due to gram-negative organisms) and positive cultures from urine, wounds, tracheal aspirate, invasive lines. *Candida* spp., viruses (especially HSV and CMV) can be cultured.
In one clinical variant no lung injury is clinically evident. In another clinical type (usually associated with a primary lung injury such as aspiration), liver and kidney failure does not manifest until a few days before death.
Poor prognostic findings are
• Initial ratio of mean pO_2 to fraction of inspired oxygen (FiO_2)of <250 (normal = 400)
• Serum lactate on day 2 of ≥ 3.4 mg/dL (normal <1.5 mg/dL)
• Liver failure by day 6 with mean serum bilirubin of 8.5 mg/dL and rising
• Kidney failure by day 12 with mean serum creatinine of 3.9 mg/dL and rising

Organ Transplantation

See sections on bone marrow transplantation (p. 415), liver transplantation (p. 248), heart transplantation (p. 130), kidney transplantation (p. 748).
Preoperative assessment (recipient and donor)
• Immunology and tissue typing
  ABO and Rh cross match

MISC

        HLA typing
        Panel of reactive antibodies
- Microbiology/virology
        HBV and HCV
        CMV
        HIV
        HTLV-I and HTLV-II
        HZV and VZV
        EBV
        Treponema pallidum
        Toxoplasma
        Blood and urine cultures (donor)

Organ function panels
    Liver
    Kidney
    Bone
    Nutrition
    Glucose
    Electrolyte/acid-base
    Hematology (coagulation, CBC)

Postoperative monitoring of recipient
- Graft function
- Rejection
- Nephrotoxicity
- Wound infection
- Opportunistic infection (e.g., CMV, *Pneumocystis*)
- Neoplasms (e.g., posttransplantation lymphoproliferative disorders)
- Bone demineralization
- Hypertension
- Recurrence of primary disease

♦ Most difficult distinction is between infection and rejection, for which organ biopsy is most diagnostic.

Sarcoidosis[4]

♦ Diagnosis is established by tissue biopsy that shows noncaseous granulomas at several sites for which a specific cause (e.g., fungal infection, acid-fast bacillus infection, or berylliosis) has been excluded. Kveim test may be used in place of another tissue biopsy.
- Results of needle biopsy of liver show granulomas in ≤ 75% of patients even if no impairment of liver function is noted.
- Lymph node biopsy findings are likely to be positive if lymph node is enlarged.
- Muscle biopsy findings are likely to be positive if arthralgia or muscle pain is present.
- Skin and transbronchial lung biopsies have higher yield, greater specificity, and less morbidity than liver and mediastinal lymph node biopsies.
- Other sites of biopsy are synovium, eye, lung, minor salivary glands of lower lip.
- Percentage of cases with involvement of given organ system.
    Pulmonary: >90%
    Peripheral lymph nodes: 50–75%
    Liver: 60–80%
    Skin: 35%
    Heart: 30%
    Bone: 1–35%
    Eye: ~25%
    Spleen: 15%
    Salivary glands: 5%
    CNS: 5%
    Joints

Kveim reaction (skin biopsy specimen 4–6 wks after injection of human sarcoid tissue shows a noncaseating granulomatous reaction at that site) has reported sensitivity of 35–88% and specificity of 75–99%. A positive reaction is less frequent if no lymph

[4]Newman LS, Rose CS, Maier LA. Sarcoidosis. *N Engl J Med* 1997;336:1224.

node involvement is present, if the disease is longstanding and inactive, and during steroid therapy.
- Positive Kveim tests may occur in other diseases in which lymph nodes are enlarged (e.g., TB, leukemia). Kveim test material is not available commercially; a few medical centers have limited quantities with variable specificities; not approved by FDA for general use.

○Serum Angiotensin-Converting Enzyme (ACE)

(Note: values vary between laboratories even with same method.)
Use
Monitor activity of disease and response to therapy
Little diagnostic value because of poor specificity
May Be Increased In
E.g.,
- Active pulmonary sarcoidosis (85% of patients but only 11% with inactive disease; increase is >35 U/mL by radioassay in adults and >50 U/mL for patients <19 yrs old)
- Gaucher's disease (100%)
- Diabetes mellitus (>24%)
- Hyperthyroidism (81%)
- Leprosy (53%)
- Chronic renal disease
- Cirrhosis (25%)
- Silicosis (>20%)
- Berylliosis (75%)
- Amyloidosis
- TB
- False-positive rate = 2–4%

Normal In
- Lymphoma
- Lung cancer

○Serum globulins are increased in 75% of patients, producing reduced A/G ratio and increased total protein (in 30% of patients). Is often the first clue to diagnosis.
○Serum protein electrophoresis shows decreased albumin and increased globulin (especially gamma) with characteristic "sarcoid-step" pattern.
WBC is decreased in 30% of patients.
Eosinophilia occurs in 15% of patients.
Mild normocytic, normochromic anemia occurs.
ESR is increased.
○Serum calcium may be mild to markedly increased in ~10% of patients; often transiently.
Increased urine calcium occurs twice as often as hypercalcemia. Increased frequency of renal calculi and of nephrocalcinosis in some patients.
Serum and urine calcium abnormalities are frequently corrected by cortisone administration; often within normal range in 1 wk.
Increased sensitivity to vitamin D is often present.
Increased serum 1,25-hydroxy-vitamin D, which is abnormally regulated.
Steroid administration rapidly lowers serum 1α, 25-hydroxy-vitamin D.
Serum phosphorus is normal.
Increased serum uric acid may occur even with normal renal function in ≤ 50% of patients.
Mumps CF test, which is positive in presence of negative mumps skin test (due to dissociation between normal circulating antibodies and defective cellular antibody response), supports the diagnosis but is not specific.
Serum lysozyme (muramidase) is increased in ~70% of cases but does not distinguish stable from progressive disease. Also increased with other chest diseases (e.g., TB, lung cancer).
Laboratory findings reflecting specific organ involvement
- Lung
- Diagnostic method of choice is transbronchial biopsy.
    Bronchoalveolar lavage (BAL) shows 3–5× increase in cells; T lymphocytes are increased to 36%; B lymphocytes = 4%; macrophages decreased to 55%; neutrophils and eosinophils are <5%.
^{67}Ga scan lacks specificity. Gas exchange is usually normal early in disease; later pO_2 is decreased with marked fall after exercise. BAL and ^{67}Ga scan have been used to assess disease activity.

- Kidney—renal function is decreased (because of hypercalcemia or increased uric acid with resultant nephrocalcinosis or renal calculi).
- Liver—cholestatic pattern in up to one-third of patients with increased serum ALP and relatively normal transaminases.
- Spleen—hypersplenism may occur (anemia, leukopenia, thrombocytopenia).
- CNS—CSF may be normal or may show no characteristic changes, e.g., moderate to marked increase in protein, and pleocytosis (chiefly lymphocytes). Glucose is sometimes decreased. In neurosarcoidosis, ACE is increased in serum or CSF in 50–70%, ESR in 40%, and serum calcium in 17% of cases. Oligoclonal bands may be present.
- Pituitary—diabetes insipidus, hypopituitarism, or hyperprolactinemia may occur.

Scleredema

WBC, ESR, and other laboratory tests are usually normal.

Sclerosis, Progressive Systemic (Scleroderma)

♦ Biopsy of skin, esophagus, intestine, synovia may establish diagnosis.

Laboratory tests are generally not diagnostic; no antibodies may be present.

ANA are found in low titers in 40–90% of patients. High titer of anti-nRNP alone may indicate risk of developing scleroderma.

♦ Antinucleolar pattern is most specific for scleroderma; is highly specific when no other antibody is present. Is rarely found in early scleroderma. May be found in 20% of other rheumatic diseases in association with other antibodies.

♦ Anticentromere antibody is sensitive and specific for CREST syndrome. May be present in early stage when only Raynaud's phenomenon is present.

♦ Anti–Scl 70 is found in 30–70% of patients with diffuse cutaneous scleroderma and is highly specific but occurs late in disease when diagnosis is obvious. Suggests a worse prognosis.

RF present in 30% of patients.

ESR is normal in one-third of patients, mildly increased in one-third of patients, markedly increased in one-third of patients.

Eosinophilia is described in all scleroderma syndromes.

Mild hypochromic microcytic anemia present in 10% of patients.

Serum gamma globulins are increased in 25% of patients (usually slight increase) and have no predictive value.

Abnormal serum proteins occasionally occur, as revealed by biological false-positive test for syphilis (5% of patients), positive RA test (35% of patients), cold agglutinins, cryoglobulins, etc.

Laboratory findings reflecting specific organ involvement, e.g.,

- Malabsorption syndrome due to small intestine involvement
- Abnormal urinary findings, renal function tests, and uremia due to renal involvement
- Myocarditis, pericarditis, secondary bacterial endocarditis
- Pulmonary fibrosis, secondary pneumonitis

Weber-Christian Disease (Relapsing Febrile Nodular Nonsuppurative Panniculitis)

♦ Biopsy of involved area of subcutaneous fat

WBC may be increased or decreased.

Mild anemia may occur.

Biochemical Changes in Cancer

Use

Prevention of misinterpretation of various findings in patients with cancer

Awareness of certain complications of cancers (e.g., anemia, hypercalcemia)

Decreased

Serum glucose
Serum protein and albumin (due to malnutrition, blood loss, etc.)
RBCs, Hct, Hb, or total volume (i.e., anemia) (due to hemorrhage, malnutrition, hemolysis, anemia of chronic disease, myelophthisis, etc.)

Increased

Serum uric acid
Serum calcium—occurs in ~20% of cancer patients, usually due to bone metastases, which sometimes cannot be detected. >14 mg/dL suggests cancer rather than hyperparathyroidism. (See Humoral Hypercalcemia of Malignancy, p. 598.)
Serum globulin (e.g., multiple myeloma), especially alpha$_2$ globulin
Serum lactic acid
Development of hemolytic anemia, autoantibodies (e.g., minimal change glomerular disease in Hodgkin's disease, membranous GN in solid tumors)
Occult blood in stool
ESR is often normal in patients with cancer and therefore is not a good test for screening and a normal value does not exclude metastases. In patients with known cancer, ESR >100 mm/hr is usually associated with metastases.
WBC may be increased due to tumor necrosis, secondary infection, etc.
Hypercoagulable state with recurrent thromboembolism
Laboratory findings due to metastatic tumor (e.g., liver, brain, bone)
Laboratory findings due to obstruction (e.g., ureters, bile ducts, intestine)
Laboratory findings due to metastases that interfere with endocrine secretion (e.g., adrenal, pituitary)
Laboratory findings due to fluid in body cavities (pleural, abdominal, CSF)
Laboratory findings due to myelophthisis (anemia, leukopenia, thrombocytopenia)
Laboratory findings due to complications of anticancer therapy
  • Blood dyscrasias including secondary leukemia
  • Bladder cancer after prolonged cyclophosphamide (Cytoxan) therapy
  • Cardiotoxicity (e.g., doxorubicin hydrochloride [Adriamycin])
  • Pulmonary fibrosis (e.g., methotrexate, bleomycin)
  • Sterility
  • Teratogenic effects
  • Diseases that occur with particular frequency in association with neoplasms (e.g., polymyositis, dermatomyositis)

Tumor Markers[5]

Use

Not generally useful to establish a definite diagnosis or for screening
May be useful to monitor effect of therapy or recurrence of lesion, to follow the clinical course, to pinpoint the tissue of origin.
May sometimes be useful to assess the extent of tumor and to estimate prognosis.
Contents may help to distinguish cystic lesions of pancreas.

Interpretation

Enzymes increased
  • Serum ALP and GGT in liver metastases; increase is predictive of positive liver scan but not of positive bone scan for metastases from breast cancer. Also in bone metastases, osteogenic sarcoma, myeloid leukemia. Placental isoenzyme of ALP increased in 30% of cases of ovarian cancer (especially serous cystadenocarcinoma), some cases of cancer of endometrium, lung, and breast, and 40% of cases of semi-

[5]Schwartz MK. Tumor markers in diagnostic endocrinology and metabolism. *Am Assoc Clin Chem* 1997;15:365.

noma (75% in metastatic seminoma); may also be increased in smokers. Intestinal isoenzyme is associated with hepatomas and malignant tumors of GI tract.
- 5'-NT in metastatic carcinoma of liver but not bone.
- Serum GGT in metastatic carcinoma of liver.
- Serum LD in metastatic carcinoma of liver, acute leukemia, lymphomas; less useful than GGT and 5'-NT in evaluating space-occupying lesions of liver.
- Serum LD total and LD-1 in testicular cancer; see LD isoenzymes (p. 65).
- Serum CK total and CK-BB in various cancers (e.g., prostate, breast, ovary, colon, small cell carcinoma of lung) in ~30% of early cases and ~45% with extensive cancer; rarely macromolecular forms of CK occur.
- Serum acid phosphatase in 80% of men with metastatic prostate cancer and 25% of those without metastases.
- Neuron-specific enolase in APUD (*a*mine *p*recursor *u*ptake and *d*ecarboxylation) tumors including small-cell carcinoma of lung, neuroblastoma, medullary carcinoma of thyroid. 32% accompanied by increased CK-BB.
- Serum amylase in 8–40% of cases of carcinoma of pancreas.
- Terminal deoxynucleotidyl transferase—large amounts in blast cells of ALL but little or none in nonlymphoid leukemia or nonleukemic cells; useful to differentiate acute lymphoid and acute myeloid leukemia.

Oncofetal antigens
- Serum AFP in hepatoma, teratoblastoma, yolk sac tumor; also increased in normal pregnancy
- Serum CEA in carcinoma of GI tract, breast, >40% of small-cell carcinoma of lung

Specific products of hormone-producing tumor of primary organ or ectopic, e.g.,
- Renin-producing tumor of kidney
- VMA, catecholamines in pheochromoblastoma, neuroblastoma by neural crest tumors, pheochromocytoma (see pp. 658–660)
- Urinary 17-KS in adrenal cortical carcinoma, androgenic arrhenoblastoma
- HIAA in carcinoid
- Erythropoietin in paraneoplastic erythrocytosis
- Thyroglobulin in patients with total thyroidectomy; detectable level indicates recurrent thyroid cancer (see p. 575)
- Prolactin (see p. 700)
- ACTH in Cushing's syndrome (e.g., due to adrenal tumor, due to oat cell carcinoma)
- Beta-hCG subunit (in blood or urine) (see p. 907)
- C-peptide in insulinoma
- Estrogen and progesterone receptors (see section Steroid Receptor Assays, p. 910)
- Parathormone-related protein produced by lung tumor, ovarian tumor, thymoma, carcinoid, islet cell tumor of pancreas, medullary carcinoma of thyroid
- ADH produced by small cell cancer of lung, carcinoid, Hodgkin's disease, bladder
- Calcitonin produced by medullary carcinoma of thyroid (see p. 569), breast, liver, kidney, lung carcinoid
- Gastrin in gastrinoma, gastric carcinoma; part of MEN type I syndrome, carcinoma of pancreas, parathyroid, pituitary
- Isoenzymes of ALP (Regan, Nagao)

Other proteins
- PSA (see p. 753).
- CA-125 (see p. 905).
- CA 19-9 (see p. 904).
- CA 15-3 (see p. 904).
- Ig's in multiple myeloma, lymphomas, Waldenström's macroglobulinemia. Beta$_2$-microglobulin is increased in multiple myeloma (currently used for research only).
- Interleukin-2 receptor may be increased in serum in adult T-cell leukemia.
- SCC (squamous cell carcinoma antigen; see p. 909).
- Plasma chromogranin A in pheochromocytoma (p. 662).
- Tumor-associated antigen (TA-90) in urine and sera of patients with metastatic melanoma (occult or clinical) with sensitivity, specificity, predictive values of ~75%.[6]

Ph[1] chromosome in chronic myeloid leukemia

---

[6]Kelley MC, et al. Tumor-associated antigen TA-90 immune complex assay predicts subclinical metastasis and survival for patients with early stage melanoma. *Cancer* 1998;83:1355.

Paraneoplastic syndromes
- One-third of these patients show ectopic hormone production (e.g., bronchogenic carcinoma).
- One-third show evidence of connective tissue (e.g., polymyositis, dermatomyositis) and dermatologic disorders (e.g., acanthosis nigricans).
- One-sixth show psychiatric and neurologic syndromes.
- Remainder show immunologic disorders, GI disorders (e.g., malabsorption), renal disorders (e.g., nephrotic syndrome), hematologic disorders (e.g., anemia of chronic disease, DIC), paraproteinemias (e.g., multiple myeloma), amyloidosis.

Alpha-Fetoprotein (AFP), Serum

(An alpha globulin found in fetal blood; originates in fetal liver, GI tract, yolk sac)

Use

Tumor marker for hepatoma
- Screening in high-prevalence areas (e.g., China, Eskimo lands).
- Patients with chronic active hepatitis or cirrhosis positive for HBsAg should be screened every 4–6 mos with serum AFP test and ultrasonography.
- Changes reflect the disease course.

Tumor marker for germ cell tumors of ovary and testis (see pp. 682–683, 684)
- Embryonal carcinoma (increased in 27% of cases)
- Malignant teratoma (increased in 60% of cases)
- *Should be used in conjunction with hCG and LD and LD-1; more often increased with advanced disease. These are useful to monitor chemotherapy; may predict relapse before clinical or radiographic evidence.*

To distinguish neonatal hepatitis (most patients have concentrations >40 ng/mL) from neonatal biliary atresia (most patients have concentrations <40 ng/mL).

Screening for fetal defects and placental disease during pregnancy (see p. 563)

Interpretation

(>50 ng/mL is essentially diagnostic of AFP-producing tumor.)

Primary cancer of liver (hepatoma)
- In 50% of whites and 75–90% of nonwhites; concentrations may be markedly elevated (>1000 ng/mL in ~50% of cases, which usually indicates tumor >3 cm in size). Increased in almost 100% of cases in children and young adults. In 90% of cases of hepatoma AFP is >200 and in 70% concentration is >400 ng/mL, but in benign liver diseases, AFP of >400 ng/mL is extremely rare. More likely to be increased in immature type of hepatoma compared to mature type.
- High initial concentrations indicate a poor prognosis.
- Failure to return to normal after surgery indicates incomplete resection or presence of metastases.
- Changes in concentrations can indicate effects of chemotherapy.
- Postoperative decreased concentration followed by an increase suggests recurrence. Short doubling time suggests occult metastases at time of surgery.

Increases associated with nonmalignant conditions are usually temporary and concentrations subsequently fall, but in malignant disease, concentrations continue to rise.

Increased In[7]

Other cancers
- Testicular teratocarcinomas (75%) (see p. 684)
- Pancreatic (23%)
- Gastric (18%)
- Bronchogenic (7%)
- Colon (5%)

Benign liver diseases
- Viral hepatitis (27%)
- Postnecrotic cirrhosis (24%)

[7]Aziz DC. Clinical use of tumor markers based on outcome analysis. *Lab Med* 1996;27:817.

- Laënnec's cirrhosis (15%)
- Primary biliary cirrhosis (5%)

Some patients with liver metastases from carcinoma of stomach or pancreas
Ataxia-telangiectasia
Hereditary tyrosinemia
Hereditary persistence of AFP

Absent In

Healthy persons after first weeks of life
Various types of cirrhosis and hepatitis in adults
Seminoma of testis
Choriocarcinoma, adenocarcinoma, and dermoid cyst of ovary

CA 15-3 and BR27.29

(Glycoproteins expressed on various adenocarcinomas, especially breast)

Use

FDA approval only to detect breast carcinoma recurrence before symptoms and to monitor response to treatment (clinical benefit is not established). Significant change is ±25%.

Not approved for screening although increased values may occur ≤ 9 mos before clinical evidence of disease.

Interpretation

Reported positive predictive value of 77% and negative predictive value of 90% at 49 U/mL.

Increases are directly related to stage of disease; increased in ~20% of patients with stage I or II disease and 70–80% of patients with metastatic or recurrent breast cancer.

Increases in 75% of patients with progressive disease and decreases in 38% of those responding to therapy.

Increased In

Benign breast and liver diseases, so that specificity is low.

CA 19-9, Serum

Use

To determine preoperative resectability of pancreatic cancer. Very high concentrations predict unresectable cancer—only 5% of patients with concentrations >1000 U/mL have surgically resectable disease; 50% of patients with concentrations <1000 U/mL have surgically resectable cancers. Postsurgical recurrence correlates with increased concentrations in 1–7 mos.

May be a useful adjunct to CEA for diagnosis and detection of early recurrence of certain cancers.

May indicate development of cholangiocarcinoma in patients with primary sclerosing cholangitis.

Increased (>37 U/mL) In

Carcinoma of pancreas (70–100%) (see p. 257)

Pancreatitis—concentrations are usually <75 U/mL but are much higher in pancreatic cancer.

Hepatobiliary cancer (22–51%)

Gastric cancer (42%)

Colon cancer (20%); is associated with very poor prognosis.

False-negative in 7% of U.S. population negative for Lewis[ab] blood group because CA 19-9 is an Le[ab] antigen.

CA 27-29, Serum

(Tumor marker similar to CA 15-3 antigen)

Use

Recently approved by FDA in conjunction with other procedures to monitor recurrence of stage II or III breast cancer.
Reported sensitivity is 58%; false-positive rate is 6%.

CA-125, Serum

(Glycoprotein derived from coelomic epithelium. Increased in benign or malignant conditions that stimulate peritoneal synthesis.)

Use

Monitor for persistent or recurrent *serous* carcinoma of ovary (see p. 681) after surgery or chemotherapy
Although may be increased ≤ 12 mos before clinical evidence of disease, is not recommended for screening women for serous carcinoma of ovary because it is not increased in 20% of cases at time of diagnosis and is found in <10% of patients with stage I or II disease (low sensitivity and specificity; high false-positive rate).
May be used for screening patients with a hereditary cancer syndrome or a family history of first-degree relative with ovarian cancer.
Not useful to distinguish benign from malignant pelvic masses even at high concentrations.
Little benefit to early detection of late-stage cancers.
Some authors have suggested that it be used to monitor therapy in patients with endometriosis.
Has also been used to predict survival in endometrial carcinoma (value of >35 U/mL predicts poor survival; value of >65 U/mL predicts extrauterine disease)[8]

Interpretation

Concentration of >35 U/mL indicates residual cancer in 95% of patients.
Prognosis may be better if
- 50% decline in concentration within 5 days after surgery.
- Ratio of postoperative/preoperative concentrations is 0.1 within 4 wks.
- Ratio of >0.1 but <0.5 indicates patient may benefit from chemotherapy but recurrence rate is high.
- Ratio of >0.8 indicates that alternative therapy (e.g., irradiation, different chemotherapy combinations) should be considered.

Remains increased in stable or progressive serous carcinoma of ovary. Rising concentrations may precede clinical recurrence by many months and may be indication for second-look operation, but lack of increased values does not indicate absence of persistent or recurrent tumor. Greater concentration is roughly related to poorer survival; value >35 U/mL is highly predictive of tumor recurrence.
90% of women with values >65 U/mL have cancer involving peritoneum.
Not helpful in early cases because related to tumor burden.
Normal concentration does not exclude tumor.

Increased In

(ULN is <35 U/mL.)
Malignant disease
- Nonmucinous epithelial ovarian carcinoma (85%)
- Fallopian tube tumors (100%)
- Cervical adenocarcinoma (83%)

---

[8]Sood AK, et al. Value of preoperative CA-125 level in the management of uterine cancer and the prediction of clinical outcome. *Obstet Gynecol* 1997;990:441.

- Endometrial adenocarcinoma (50%)
- Trophoblastic tumors (45%)
- Non-Hodgkin's lymphoma (40%), representing pleuropericardial or peritoneal involvement
- Squamous cell carcinomas of vulva or cervix (<15%)
- Cancers of pancreas, liver, lung

Conditions that affect the endometrium
- Pregnancy (27%)
- Menstruation
- Endometriosis

Pleural effusion or inflammation (see p. 148) (e.g., cancer, congestive heart failure)

Peritoneal effusion or inflammation (e.g., pelvic inflammatory disease, ovarian hyperstimulation syndrome, cirrhosis, other diseases of liver, pancreas, GI tract). *Especially increased in bacterial peritonitis in which ascitic concentration is higher than serum concentration.*

Some nonmalignant conditions
- Cirrhosis, severe liver necrosis (66%)
- Other disease of liver, pancreas, GI tract (5–8%)
- Renal failure

Healthy persons (1%)

Not increased in mucinous adenocarcinoma.

Interferences

Human antimouse or heterophile antibodies

Different assays do not produce equivalent values and should not be used interchangeably.

Carcinoembryonic Antigen (CEA), Serum

(High-molecular-weight glycoprotein)

Use

Monitoring for persistent, metastatic, or recurrent adenocarcinoma of colon after surgery; elevated in >30% of patients with breast, lung, liver, pancreas adenocarcinomas.

Determination of prognosis for patients with colon cancer

Not usually useful for diagnosis of local recurrence.

Not recommended for screening because of low sensitivity and specificity, especially in early stages of malignant disease, because CEA level reflects tumor bulk.

♦ Diagnosis of malignant pleural effusion (see p. 149)

Interpretation

♦ Monitoring of Disease Course

Same methodology should be used to monitor an individual patient. A significant change in plasma concentration is ±25%.

Failure to decline to normal concentrations postoperatively suggests incomplete resection. After complete removal of colon cancer, CEA should fall to normal in 6–12 wks. Immunohistochemistry of resected specimen is used to identify 20% of these cancers that do not express CEA for which monitoring is misleading.

Recurrence of colon cancer is indicated by progressive increase earlier than with other methods, but for most patients, this is not useful therapeutically although increasing concentrations may precede clinical evidence of recurrence by 2–6 mos. In ~50% of patients with advanced cancer, a latent phase of 4–6 wks may be seen from onset of therapy to change in CEA concentrations. Sensitivity is 97% for detecting recurrence of colon cancer in patients with preoperative elevation but only 66% in those with normal preoperative CEA. Specificity is >90%, positive predictive value is >70%. Increased concentrations indicates a poorer prognosis within a given stage. Levels are >3.0 ng/mL in ≤ 28% of patients with Dukes' stage A cancers, 45% of those with stage B cancers, and 70% of those with stage C cancers.

~30% of patients with metastatic colon cancer do not have increased CEA.

Undifferentiated or poorly differentiated tumors do not produce CEA.

♦ Prognosis

Is related to serum concentration at time of diagnosis (stage of disease and likelihood of recurrence). CEA concentration of <5 ng/mL before therapy suggests localized disease and a favorable prognosis, but a concentration of >10 ng/mL suggests extensive disease and a poor prognosis; >80% of colon carcinoma patients with values >20 ng/mL have recurrence within 14 mos after surgery. Plasma CEA levels of >20 ng/mL correlates with tumor volume in breast and colon cancer and are usually associated with metastatic disease or with a few types of cancer (e.g., cancer of the colon or pancreas); however, metastases may occur with concentrations <20 ng/mL. Values <2.5 ng/mL do not rule out primary, metastatic, or recurrent cancer. Increased values in node-negative colon cancer may identify poorer-risk patients who may benefit from chemotherapy.

Patterns of CEA change during chemotherapy.
* Uninterrupted increase indicates failure to respond.
* Decrease indicates response to therapy.
* Surge in CEA for weeks followed by a decrease indicates response.
* Immediate, sustained decrease followed by an increase indicates lack of response to therapy.
* Significant is a 25–35% change from baseline of larger or equal values during first 2 mos of therapy. Survival is significantly longer if titer decreases below this baseline.

Increased In

Cancer. A wide overlap in values is seen between benign and malignant disease. Increased concentrations are suggestive but not diagnostic of cancer.
* 75% of patients with carcinoma of entodermal origin (colon, stomach, pancreas, lung) have CEA titers of >2.5 ng/mL, and two-thirds of these titers are >5 ng/mL. Increased in approximately one-third of patients with small-cell carcinoma of lung and approximately two-thirds with non–small-cell carcinoma of lung.
* 50% of patients with carcinoma of nonentodermal origin (especially cancer of the breast, head and neck, ovary) have CEA titers of >2.5 ng/mL, and 50% of the titers are >5 ng/mL. Increased in >50% of breast cancer cases with metastases, 25% of cases without metastases, but not associated with benign lesions.
* 40% of patients with noncarcinomatous malignant disease have increased CEA concentrations, usually 2.5–5.0 ng/mL.
* Increased in 90% of all patients with solid-tissue tumors, especially with metastases to liver or lung, but only 50% of patients with local disease or only intraabdominal metastases.
* May be increased in effusion fluid due to these cancers (see p. 149).

Active nonmalignant inflammatory diseases (especially of the GI tract, e.g., ulcerative colitis, regional enteritis, diverticulitis, peptic ulcer, chronic pancreatitis) frequently show elevated concentrations that decline when the disease is in remission.

Liver disease (alcoholic, cirrhosis, chronic active hepatitis, obstructive jaundice)

Other disorders
* Renal failure
* Fibrocystic disease of breast

Smoking
* 97% of healthy nonsmokers have plasma CEA concentrations of <2.5 ng/mL.
* 19% of heavy smokers and 7% of former smokers have CEA concentrations of >2.5 ng/mL.

Interferences

Heparinized patients or plasma collected in heparinized tubes may interfere with accuracy of CEA assay.

Human antimouse antibodies may cause increased values.

Human Chorionic Gonadotropin (beta-hCG), Serum

(Glycoprotein produced by syncytiotrophoblast cell after trophoblast differentiation)

Use

Diagnosis, monitoring of course, and evaluation of prognosis of gestational trophoblastic tumors (with AFP)

Routine pregnancy test (see Pregnancy Test, p. 77); may also be used to gauge success of artificial insemination or in vitro fertilization.

Differentiation of ectopic pregnancy from other causes of acute abdominal pain. In ectopic pregnancy and in abortion, serial hCG levels usually decrease over 48 hrs (see pp. 761–762).

Prenatal screening for Down syndrome (see Chapter 12, p. 563)

Increased In

Gestational trophoblastic tumors, benign or malignant (see Germ Cell Tumors of Ovary and Testicle and Testicular Tumors, p. 684). Is valuable marker for management as changes in concentration reflect success or failure of therapy.
- Hydatidiform mole (sometimes markedly increased; after 12 wks of pregnancy, values of >500,000 U/24 hrs usually are associated with moles; values of >1,000,000 are almost always associated with moles).
- Choriocarcinoma (see pp. 681–683) in virtually 100% of cases, sometimes markedly. Elevated levels are most useful for monitoring remission after treatment; failure to fall to an undetectable level or a rise after an initial fall signals residual tumor or progression of disease and need for another form of therapy. Measure weekly during therapy; every 2 wks for 6 mos after therapy; then less frequently. After uterine evacuation, average disappearance times were 99 days for hydatidiform mole, 59 days for partial mole, 51 days for hydropic degeneration; therefore if levels show a steady fall, they may become negative by 100 days regardless of chemotherapy.
- Much poorer prognosis is indicated by failure of AFP to decline by 50% in 7 days and failure of beta-hCG to decline by 50% in 3 days.

Nonseminomatous germ cell tumors of testicle (found in 10% of patients with pure seminoma); should be used with AFP (see p. 684).

Some nontrophoblastic neoplasms (e.g., cancers of ovary, cervix, GI tract, lung, breast)

Normal pregnancy (secreted first by trophoblastic cells of conceptus and later by normal pregnancy. (See p. 77.)

Interferences

False-positive results have been found in
- Postorchiectomy patients (secondary to decreased testosterone)
- Marijuana smokers

Not Increased In

Endodermal sinus tumors
Nonpregnant state
Fetal death

Micrometastases, Detection of

Immunocytochemical analysis with manual microscopy can detect as few as 1 tumor cell in 1 million normal cells.

Flow cytometry has potential sensitivity of 1 cell in 10^6 or 10^7.

RT-PCR has theoretical detection sensitivity of 1 cell in 10^7 or 10^8.

Automated cell imaging with immunocytochemical staining may identify 1 cell in 10^8 normal bone marrow cells.

Neuron-Specific Enolase, Serum

Increased In

Neuroendocrine tumors
- Especially small-cell carcinoma of lung; found in 68% of patients with limited disease and 87% with extensive disease. Increased in 17% of cases of other lung cancers. Under investigation for use in assessing prognosis and monitoring treatment in small-cell lung cancer and neuroblastoma.
- Monitor patients with neuroblastoma, carcinoid, pancreatic islet cell tumor, pheochromocytoma, medullary carcinoma of thyroid.

Table 16-3. Comparison of Assays for Tumor Chemosensitivity Testing

Assay	Specimen	Specimens that Can Be Evaluated (%)	Accuracy in Determining Resistance (%)	Sensitivity (%)	Reporting Time (days)
Clonogenic	Single cell	40–60	90	70	10–21
Subrenal Capsule	Tumor fragments In vivo	80–90	80	80–90	7–10
Rotman fluorescent cytoprint	Tumor fragments	95–98	90	90–95	7–10

Source: Woltering EA. Tumor chemosensitivity testing: an evolving technique. *Lab Med* 1990;21(2):82.

Wilms' tumor, malignant lymphoma, seminoma; 20% of cancers of breast, GI tract, prostate
Occasional patients with benign liver diseases
Further studies are needed to define exact role.

Prostate-Specific Antigen (PSA) and Prostatic Acid Phosphatase (PAP), Serum

See Prostate Carcinoma, Chapter 14, p. 753.

SCC, SERUM

(Antigen purified from squamous cell carcinoma)

Use

Has been reported useful to monitor and detect recurrence of squamous cell carcinoma of uterine cervix, head and neck, esophagus, lung, skin, anus. In uterine cancer is reportedly increased in 29% of patients with stage I disease and 89% of those with stage IV disease.
Further studies are needed to define exact role.

Tumor Chemosensitivity Testing

(Assays to predict sensitivity/resistance of a tumor to specific chemotherapeutic agents)

See Table 16-3.
Requires sterile preparation transported on ice in cold tissue transport medium. Avoid freezing. Set up in tissue culture media within 24 hrs.
Clonogenic assay
- Minced solid tumor or fluids containing tumor (e.g., malignant effusions, urine, CSF).
- Incubated for 1 hr with test drug, then incubated on cell culture plates. Colonies are counted after 10–14 days and compared with count on control plates to determine percentage decrease in tumor colony–forming units.
Subrenal capsule assay
- Tumor fragments (not individual cells) are injected into immunocompetent mouse.
- Reported as percentage change in implantation weight.
Rotman in vitro chemosensitivity (fluorescent cytoprint) assay
- Measures ability of viable human tumor cells in culture to transport and hydrolyze fluorescein diacetate and retain fluorescein. Tumor is incubated with drug in media for 48 hrs. Sensitivity is defined as 100% cell death at lowest drug dose currently used.

Neoplastic Diseases

Basal Cell Nevus Syndrome

Rare disease that shows the following:
- Multiple basal cell tumors of skin
- Odontogenic cysts of jaw
- Bone anomalies (especially of ribs, vertebrae, and metacarpals) and defective dentition
- Neurologic abnormalities (calcification of dura, etc.)
- Ophthalmologic abnormalities (abnormal width between the eyes, lateral displacement of inner canthi, etc.)
- Sexual abnormalities (frequent ovarian fibromas; male hypogonadism, etc.)
- Normal karyotyping by chromosomal analysis
- Hyporesponsiveness to parathormone (Ellsworth-Howard test)

Rule out presence or development of occult neoplasms (e.g., ovarian fibroma, medulloblastoma).

Breast Cancer

♦Diagnosis is established by microscopic examination of tumor biopsy.
○Serum CEA increase becomes more likely with increasing stage and tumor burden. More frequent with bone and visceral involvement than with soft tissue involvement.
- An increasing concentration usually reflects disease progression and a decreasing concentration usually reflects remission.
- An increased or rising concentration may precede recurrence by 1–31 mos.
- May be increased in CSF in metastases to CNS, meninges, or spine but not in primary brain tumors.
- Not useful for screening or diagnosis of early breast cancer.
○Serum CA 15-3 (see p. 904)
Other markers (mucin-like carcinoma-associated antigen, MAM-6, mammary serum antigen) await further study of utility.

♦ Steroid Receptor Assays

Use

Determination of prognosis and treatment of breast carcinoma. Assay of both estrogen and progesterone receptors yields best information on response to hormone therapy.
Estrogen receptor (ER) is positive (>10 fmol/mg cytoplasmic protein) in ~50% of breast tumor specimens; levels are higher in post- than in premenopausal patients but this is not true for progesterone receptor (PgR).
When ER is negative, the chance of obtaining a favorable response to any endocrine therapy is <10%; thus chemotherapy would be the primary approach. The likelihood of visceral metastases is greater in patients with ER-negative tumors (>50%) than with those with ER-positive tumors (<6%).
When ER is positive, the chance of favorable response (i.e., tumor shrinkage and/or clinical improvement) is 55–60%.
When ER and PgR are both positive, response rate is 75–80%. No response to endocrine therapy in 10–15% of patients with ER/PgR-positive tumors.
Predictive value of assay is increased if ER and PgR levels are both high.
- ER titer of >100 fmol/mg protein.
- PgR titer is also positive, especially >100 fmol/mg.

Prognostic value
Recurrence rate is significantly greater for ER-negative tumors, both stage I (negative axillary lymph nodes) and stage II (positive axillary lymph nodes).
Overall response rate to endocrine therapy is ~50%.

	Response Rate to Endocrine Therapy
ER assay >100 fmol/mg protein	~75%
ER assay <100 fmol/mg protein	~40%
ER assay <3 fmol/mg protein	~12%
ER assay positive/PgR assay positive (60% of total group)	~80%

ER assay negative/PgR assay negative (31% of total group)   ~5%
ER assay positive/PgR assay negative   ~26%
ER assay negative/PgR assay positive (4% of total group;   ~50%
    this result may be due to inaccuracy in assay procedures)

Receptor assay should also be performed on recurrent carcinoma even when the original tumor has been previously assayed. Initially ER-positive tumors are later found to be ER negative in 19% and initially ER-negative tumors are later positive in 13%. Initially PgR-negative tumors are later positive in 8% and initially PgR-positive tumors are later reported negative in 28–44% of cases. These rates of discordance may be up to 75% in patients receiving antiestrogen tamoxifen within 2 mos.

Receptor assay may sometimes be useful in differential diagnosis of metastatic undifferentiated carcinoma in women.

Improved utility may result from newer technology using monoclonal antibody assays and immunocytochemical stains of tumor tissue.

Unfixed tissue specimen should be frozen immediately after removal.

Epidermal growth factor receptor (EGF-R) is an integral membrane protein. Elevated EGF-R correlates with poor prognosis and no detectable EGF-R is a good predictor of response to tamoxifen therapy.

HER2 (human epidermal growth factor receptor 2) overexpression (has partial homology with EGF-R). Measured by Southern blot, fluorescence in situ hybridization, immunohistochemistry (IHC), ELISA.

Genetic alteration of HER2 gene produces increased amount of HER2 identified by IHC staining of tumor cells in 25–30% of cases of metastatic breast cancer. These cancers show rapid tumor progression and metastasize at a faster rate. May show poor response to tamoxifen therapy alone, increased sensitivity to doxorubicin therapy, may respond to anti-HER antibody therapy, and may possibly benefit from change in chemotherapeutic agents.

DNA aneuploidy predicts shorter mean survival, independent of stage. 4-yr relapse-free rate is 72% for patients with DNA diploid tumors compared to 43% for those with DNA aneuploid tumors. ER and PgR negative tumors are more likely to be DNA aneuploid.

DNA ploidy strongly correlates with histopathologic grade—poorly differentiated tumors are more likely to be DNA aneuploid.

Mast Cell Disease (Mastocytosis)

(Rare condition with functional secretion or abnormal proliferation of tissue mast cells)

Localized
- Cutaneous (typically as urticaria pigmentosa[9])
- Solitary

Systemic
- Mast cell infiltration of bone marrow; may also show diffuse mast cell infiltration of multiple organs, especially skin, liver, spleen, lymph nodes, GI tract—10–30% of cases.

♦ Diagnosis by biopsy of tumor sites, e.g., skin (urticaria pigmentosa), lymph nodes, spleen, bone. Marrow biopsy is positive in ~90% of cases but marrow smears are less useful. Toluidine blue stains mast cell granules.

♦ Histamine is increased in blood, urine, and tissues. Increased levels of metabolites of histamine in random and 24-hr urine specimens; is more specific and sensitive than determination of histamine itself. Test is inadequate because histamine release is intermittent. Assay with mass spectroscopy is very accurate but not widely available. May also be increased in some patients with myeloproliferative disorders, carcinoid syndrome, insulinoma, medullary thyroid carcinoma, pheochromocytoma, vipoma, glucagonoma. False increase may occur from basophil degranulation during phlebotomy or if urine bacteria change histidine to histamine.

Serum tryptase has been reported to be a sensitive and specific marker of mast cell activation in systemic anaphylaxis and mastocytosis.

[9]Topar G, et al. Urticaria pigmentosa: a clinical, hematopathologic, and serologic study of 30 adults. *Am J Clin Pathol* 1997;109:279.

Transient increase of aPTT (restored to normal by addition of protamine) but normal
PT during severe episode

Gastric acid is increased; the incidence of peptic ulcer is higher; but hypochlorhydria
and achlorhydria have been reported.

Urinary 5-HIAA is normal.

Laboratory findings due to specific organ involvement
* Bone—abnormal hematologic findings in ≤ 70% of patients

May include:

Progressive anemia and thrombocytopenia

WBC may be increased or decreased.

Eosinophilia and occasionally basophilia may occur.

Mast cells are uncommon in peripheral blood, which may contain ≤ 10% mast cells.
Rarely, progresses to mast cell leukemia or other leukemias, lymphoma, or carcinoma
develop.
* Liver—fibrosis, portal hypertension, hypersplenism
* Spleen—myelofibrosis
* GI tract—malabsorption, diarrhea

Tumor Lysis Syndrome, Acute

Caused by effective induction chemotherapy of rapidly growing neoplasms (e.g., acute
leukemia, malignant, lymphoma, Burkitt's lymphoma), commonly 1–2 days after onset
of chemotherapy; persists for several days; unrelated to treatment in some patients.
Associated with higher WBC count in leukemias or cases of very large tumors, inade-
quate urine output, high pretreatment serum LD levels that rise further. Occurs in
one-third of nonazotemic and virtually all azotemic patients. Changes are greater in
those with preexisting azotemia and those who develop acute renal failure.
* Abrupt-onset oliguria (urine output of <400 mL/24 hrs).
* Hyperuricemia (often increases above elevation before therapy).
* Hyperkalemia begins within 12 hrs.
* Hypocalcemia as low as 2.8 mg/dL.
* Severe hyperphosphatemia—occurs only after chemotherapy; peaks in 48–96 hrs
(≤ 65 mg/dL); is criterion for instituting dialysis to avoid acute renal failure that
may occur. May cause rapid decrease in serum calcium. Pretreatment with allo-
purinol and diuresis may prevent syndrome unless concomitant renal failure is
present.
* Often acidosis and volume depletion.
* Changes due to urate nephropathy or renal calcification, which may cause or
worsen azotemia and further accentuate the above changes.

von Hippel–Lindau Disease

(Rare [1 in 36,000 live births] autosomal dominant trait with predisposition to develop the conditions listed below.)

Pheochromocytoma (see p. 658)
Islet cell carcinoma of pancreas (see p. 629)
Renal cell carcinoma (see p. 749)
Retinal angiomas
Hemangioblastomas of the brain and spinal cord
Cystadenomas of pancreas and epididymis
DNA polymorphism analysis can identify persons likely to carry this gene among
asymptomatic members of disease families; focus should be on those who should have
periodic screening.

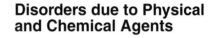
Disorders due to Physical and Chemical Agents

Acetaminophen Poisoning

♦ Blood levels
- 200 μg/mL within 4 hrs after ingestion or >50 μg/mL at 12 hrs predicts severe liver damage, and treatment with acetylcysteine should begin.
- <150 μg/mL at 4 hrs or <30–35 μg/mL at 12 hrs indicates no liver damage will occur.
- *Toxicity is dose dependent but is exaggerated by starvation and drugs, especially alcohol.*
- *Liver toxicity cannot be predicted from blood levels determined earlier than 4 hrs after ingestion.*
- *Exact time of ingestion is often difficult to ascertain.*
- *Patients taking other drugs or with concomitant cirrhosis may develop liver toxicity at different blood levels.*
- *Toxicity is less common in children <5 yrs old, and changes in liver function tests may be mild when serum drug levels are in toxic range.*

With hepatotoxicity (see Hepatic Failure, Acute, p. 221)
- During first 12–24 hrs, increased AST and ALT are found in only ~50% of patients and serum drug levels are the chief guide to therapy; this is the only stage at which treatment can prevent liver damage.
- During next 24–48 hrs, AST, ALT, serum bilirubin, PT are increased. AST and ALT are very high (typically >4000 U/L, often >10,000 U/L). AST/ALT ratio is <2 in ~90% of cases.
- On third to fourth day, liver function abnormalities peak; hypoglycemia, secondary renal failure may occur.

Addiction (Narcotics) and Chronic Usage; Drugs of Abuse (Usually Heroin)

See Table 17-1.

Persistent absolute and relative lymphocytosis occurs, with lymphocytes, often bizarre and atypical, that may resemble Downey cells.

Eosinophilia is seen in 25% of patients.

Liver function tests commonly show increased serum AST and ALT (increased in 75% of patients). Higher frequency of positive tests is evident on routine periodic repeat of these tests, which probably represents a mild, chronic viral hepatitis. Serum protein electrophoresis is usually normal.

HBsAg is found in 10% of patients.

Liver biopsy shows abnormal morphology in 25% of patients, and foreign particles are particularly suggestive.

Laboratory findings due to preexisting G-6-PD deficiency may be precipitated (by quinine, which is often used to adulterate heroin).

Laboratory findings due to malaria transmitted by common syringes. *(Malaria is not frequent; may be suppressed by quinine used for adulteration of heroin.)*

Laboratory findings due to active duodenal ulcer

Laboratory findings due to TB, which develops with increased frequency in narcotics addicts

Table 17-1. Drugs of Abuse

Drug	Street Names	Route	Usual Dose	Toxic Dose	Half-Life (hrs)	Duration of Effect (hrs)	% Not Changed in Urine
Stimulants							
Cocaine[a]	Coke, crack, snow	Nasal, smoke, IV, oral	1.5 mg/kg	>1.2 gm	2–5	1–2	<10
Amphetamine[b] (Benzedrine, Dexedrine)	Bennies, dexies, uppers	Oral, IV	10 mg	30–500 mg	4–24	2–4	~30
Methamphetamine (Desoxyn, Methedrine)	Speed, meth, crystal	Oral, IV	5–10 mg	>1 gm	9–24	2–4	10–20
Methylphenidate (Ritalin)		Oral, IV	5–20 mg	>2 gm	2–3	2–4	<1
Phenmetrazine (Preludin)		Oral, IV	75 mg		8	12	15–20
Cannabis							
Marijuana,[c] hashish	Grass, Mary Jane, pot, THC, hash	Smoke, oral, IV		50–200 µg/kg	14–38	2–4	<1
Narcotics							
Heroin[d]	Horse, smack, white lady, scag	IV, smoke, nasal	5–10 mg	100–250 mg	1–1.5	3–6	<1
Codeine[e] (e.g., with aspirin)		Oral, IV, IM	15–60 mg	500–1000 mg	2–4	3–6	5–20
Morphine[f] (morphine sulfate, Duramorph)	M, junk, morpho, white stuff	IV, IM, oral, smoke	5–10 mg	50–100 µg/kg	2–4	3–6	<10
Methadone[g] (Dolophine, Amidone)	Methadose	Oral, IV, IM	40–100 mg	100–200 mg	15–60	12–24	5–50
Meperidine (Demerol, Mepergan, Pethidine)		IV, IM, oral	25–100 mg	500–2000 mg	2–5	3–6	5
Propoxyphene[h] (Darvon, Darvocet, Dolene)	Yellow footballs	Oral	65–400 mg	500 mg	8–24	1–6	<1

Barbiturates[i]

Pentobarbital (Nembutal)	Yellow jackets, yellows	Oral, IV, IM	50–200 mg	2–10 gm	15–48	3–6	1
Amobarbital (Amytal, Tuinal)	Blues, bluebirds, rainbows	Oral, IV, IM	30–200 mg	1.5–10 gm	12–60	3–24	<1
Secobarbital (Seconal, Tuinal)	Reds, red devils, M & Ms	Oral, IV, IM	100–200 mg	2–5 gm	15–40	3–6	5
Butabarbital (Butisol)		Oral	15–100 mg	>2 gm	30–40	3–6	5–10
Butalbital (Fiorinal)		Oral	50–100 mg	>1 gm	30–40	3–6	5
Phenobarbital (Luminal)	Downers	Oral, IV, IM	50–200 mg	6–20 gm	48–120	10–20	20–35

Benzodiazepines[j]

Alprazolam (Xanax)		Oral	0.25–1 mg	>500 µg	7–13	4–8	20
Chlordiazepoxide (Librium)		Oral, IM	5–100 mg	>500 mg	6–27	4–8	<1
Diazepam (Valium)		Oral, IV, IM	5–30 mg	>250 mg	20–50	4–8	<1
Flurazepam (Dalmane)		Oral	15–30 mg	>500 mg	2–3	4–12	<1
Lorazepam (Ativan)		Oral, IV, IM	0.5–2 mg	25–100 mg	9–16	4–8	<1

Antidepressants

Tricyclics, e.g., imipramine (Tofranil, Janimine)		Oral, IM	100–500 mg	>1 gm	12–30		<1
Phenothiazines, e.g., chlorpromazine (Thorazine)		Oral, IV, IM, rectal	5–800 mg	>1 gm	7–120		<1

Sedatives, Depressants

Ethanol		Oral		100 gm	2–14	2–6	2–10
Methaqualone[k] (Quaalude)	'Ludes, soapers	Oral	150–500 mg	2 gm	20–60	4–8	<1
Meprobamate (Equanil, Miltown, Pathibamate)		Oral	400–1000 mg	2–5 gm	6–16	4–8	5
Glutethimide (Doriden)		Oral	150–500 mg	5 gm	5–22	4–8	<2
Chloral hydrate (Noctec)	Mickey Finn, joy juice	Oral, rectal	300–1000 mg	3 gm	<1	5–8	<1

(continued)

Table 17-1. (continued)

Drug	Street Names	Route	Usual Dose	Toxic Dose	Half-Life (hrs)	Duration of Effect (hrs)	% Not Changed in Urine
Hallucinogens							
Phencyclidine[l]	PCP, angel dust, killer weed	Oral, nasal, smoke, IV	0.25 mg/kg	10–20 mg	7–16	2–4 (psychosis may last weeks)	30–50
LSD	Acid, white lightning, microdots	Oral	1–2 μg/kg	100–200 μg	3–4	8–12	1
Amphetamine analogs	STP; DOM	Oral, IV	2 mg		4–8		20
Ketamine (Ketalar)		IV, IM	1–4.5 mg/kg	>500 mg	3–4	0.5–2	2–5
Mescaline	Peyote, mesc, buttons	Oral		200–700 mg	6	8–12	50–60

LSD = lysergic acid diethylamide.

Detection Times in Urine with EMIT Methods

[a]Cocaine   Up to 48 hrs after a single dose.
[b]Amphetamines   Detectable within 24–48 hrs after ingestion. Cold medicines that contain ephedrine, pseudoephedrine, or phenylpropanolamine may cause positive reaction.
[c]Marijuana   ≤ 5 days after occasional use; 21–32 days after last dose in habitual users.
[d]Heroin   One 10-mg dose detectable for up to 24 hrs. 4–5 days in habitual users.
[e]Codeine   Excreted as morphine. 120-mg dose detectable for up to 48 hrs.
[f]Morphine   Single 10-mg dose detectable for 24–48 hrs.
[g]Methadone   ~3 days. Interference from high levels of chlorpromazine, promethazine, and dextromethorphan may occur.
[h]Propoxyphene   Up to 48 hrs.
[i]Barbiturates   Up to 9 days after one 250-mg dose of phenobarbital; other common barbiturates can be detected for 1–2 days.
[j]Benzodiazepine   Not usually positive after one dose with normal renal function. Up to 5–7 days in habitual users.
[k]Methaqualone   ≥ 5 days after a typical dose.
[l]Phencyclidine   1 wk after a single dose. Up to 2 wks after last dose in habitual users.

Source: *Clin Chem News Laboratory Guide to Abused Drugs.* Compiled by Wilson J for Roche Diagnostic Systems.

Table 17-2. Lower Detectability Limits for Screening Urine for Drugs of Abuse

Drug Abuse Screen (Urine)	Lower Limit of Detectability
Alcohol	300 μg/mL
Amphetamines	500 ng/mL
Barbiturates	1000 ng/mL
Benzodiazepines	300 ng/mL
Benzoylecgonine	150 ng/mL
Cocaine	150 ng/mL
Opiates	300 ng/mL
Phencyclidine	25 ng/mL
Tetrahydrocannabinol carboxylic acid	15 ng/mL

Adapted from Leavelle DE, ed. *Mayo Medical Laboratories' Test Catalog.* Rochester, MN: Mayo Medical Laboratories, 1995.

Laboratory findings due to staphylococcal pneumonia or septic pulmonary emboli secondary to skin infections or bacterial endocarditis (conditions that are more frequent in narcotics addicts)

Laboratory findings due to endocarditis
- Right-sided—usually due to *Staphylococcus aureus* infection affecting previously normal tricuspid valve
- Left-sided—may be due to *Candida* infection superimposed on previously normal valve

Laboratory findings due to syphilis and other STDs, which occur with increased frequency in narcotics addicts. Biological false-positive tests for syphilis also occur with increased frequency.

Laboratory findings due to tetanus (which occurs with increased frequency in narcotics addicts because of "skin popping"). (*Tetanus causes 5–10% of addicts' deaths in New York City.*)

Laboratory findings due to other infections, e.g., pyelonephritis, phlebitis, abscesses

Laboratory findings due to concomitant use of sedatives, especially alcohol, barbiturates, and glutethimide (Doriden)

Oral and IV glucose tolerance curves are often flat (explanation for this finding is not known).

Urinalysis is usually normal unless renal failure due to endocarditis occurs.

Complications of drug addiction during pregnancy may also include premature rupture of membranes, abruptio placentae, stillbirth, meconium aspiration.

♦ Some drug testing thresholds (to report test as positive or negative)[1]

Drug	Screen (ng/mL)	Confirm (ng/mL)
Marijuana metabolites	100	15
Cocaine metabolites	300	150
Opiate metabolites	300	
Morphine		300
Codeine		300
6-Monoacetylmorphine		25
Phencyclidine (PCP)	25	25
Amphetamines	1000	
Amphetamine		500
Methamphetamine		500

Positive screening tests should always be confirmed by gas chromatography/mass spectrometry (Table 17-2).

♦ Blood level measurements only detect recent ingestion but do not predict toxicity. Have no clinical value but can be used to calculate when drug was used. Higher ratio of cocaine to benzoylecgonine (cocaine metabolite) indicates more recent use.

[1]Gerson B. *Drug monitoring and toxicology.* No. DM 91-4. ASCP Check Sample 1991:12.

PHYS/CHEM

- Chewing of coca leaves (practiced by Peruvian Indians)—usually 300–400 ng/mL.
- Snorting cocaine—600–800 ng/mL; snorting one line (~25 mg) produces level of ~50 ng/mL.
- IV cocaine—may reach 1200–1400 ng/mL.
- Considerable overlap between lethal and recreational levels; death is not usually dose related.

Urine screen detection time (approximate)

Alcohol: 6–12 hrs

Cocaine: 6–9 days in neonate; 2–4 days in adult

Amphetamines: 2–4 days

Cocaine and amphetamines are difficult to detect >48 hrs after use.

Opiates: 2–5 days

Marijuana: ≤ 30 days

PCP: ≤ 8 days

♦ Assay of hair permits estimate of cocaine use for previous several months and can indicate isolated or steady pattern (average hair growth = 1.3 cm [0.5 in] in 30 days). Thus 8 cm length of hair can detect cocaine user over a period of ~6 mos.

♦ RIA of hair for cocaine or heroin has 100% specificity for both, 97% sensitivity for cocaine, and 83% sensitivity for heroin.

Interferences

To detect adulteration[2] of urine specimen

- Temperature: Specimen should be within 1°C or 1.8°F of body temperature.
- Appearance: Dark color may be caused by goldenseal tea. Cloudy appearance may be due to liquid soap.
- pH: Range of 4.6–8.0 for preliminary screening. Acidification of urine may speed elimination of PCP or amphetamine before test. Alkalinization of urine may slow excretion during testing period.
- Creatinine level of <30 mg/dL or specific gravity of <1.003 may be due to external dilution of specimen, ingestion of large amounts of fluids, or use of diuretics. Creatinine of <10 mg/dL may indicate replacement by water. Specific gravity of >1.035 may be due to sodium chloride contamination.
- Nitrite is present in some commercial adulterants composed of KNO_3^-.
- Pyridinium chlorochromate ("urine luck") is an effective adulterant for urine drug testing for opiates and delta-9-tetrahydrocannabinol (THC). Suspect if abnormally low pH or orange tint to urine. Can be identified with a spot test for this oxidant but is not specific. Also produces a darker purple color with nitrate dipstick. Confirm by direct gas chromatography/mass spectrometry for pyridine and colorimetric assay for chromate.[3]
- Positive subject identification and chain of custody should be assured.

The clinician should be aware of which drugs are included in the screen, causes of false reactions, and detection levels for the particular methodology, e.g.,

False-negative immunoassay results may occur due to:

- Adulteration by addition to urine of various substances, e.g., Drano, bleach, acids, bases, Visine (benzalkonium), glutaraldehyde, soap, or table salt.
- Brief time after drug use.
- Ibuprofen may interfere with gas chromatography/mass spectrometry confirmation for marijuana.
- In urine testing for cannabinoids (marijuana metabolites), use of a lower level of 100 ng/mL for enzyme-multiplied immunoassay technique (EMIT) failed to detect 25–40% of cases identified by thin-layer chromatography (lower level of ~25 ng/mL).
- Traces of marijuana may be found by EMIT up to 1 wk after use or, in a heavy user, up to 4 wks; 15% false-positives by EMIT and 2% by HPLC.
- Screening tests not generally available for designer drugs, LSD, mescaline, psilocybin.

False-positive immunoassay results may occur due to:

- Barbiturates and benzodiazepines: ibuprofen ingestion.

---

[2]*The adulteration information booklet.* Tampa, FL: Chimera Research & Chemical, Inc.
[3]Wu AHB, et al. Adulteration of urine by "urine luck." *Clin Chem* 1999;45:1051.

- Opiates: ingestion of dextromethorphan, poppy seeds. Eating poppy seeds may cause a false-positive EMIT result for heroin confirmed by gas chromatography/mass spectrometry. Poppy seed ingestion as the only source of urinary morphine and codeine can be ruled out if: urine codeine is >300 ng/mL, urine morphine is >5000 ng/mL, morphine is >1000 ng/mL when no codeine is present, and morphine/codeine ratio is <2.
- Amphetamines: ingestion of ephedrine, other sympathomimetics.

Laboratory Findings due to Complications of Cocaine Abuse

(See appropriate separate sections.)

Catecholamine blood levels may reach several thousand ng/mL.

Sudden death due to AMI—may occur in relatively young persons (i.e., <40 yrs old) and without evidence of coronary artery obstruction, e.g., coronary artery spasm with arrhythmias.

Acute myocarditis, acute cardiomyopathy

Bacterial endocarditis

Aortic rupture

Pneumopericardium

Acute rhabdomyolysis that may cause acute renal failure and DIC, etc.

Cerebral vasculitis with cerebral and subarachnoid hemorrhage

Hyperthyroidism

Pulmonary hemorrhage and hemoptysis, pulmonary edema, "crack lung"

Laboratory Findings due to Phencyclidine (PCP) Abuse

Massive ingestion may cause
- Rhabdomyolysis
- Acute tubular necrosis
- Hypoglycemia

Alcohol (Isopropanol) Poisoning

♦ Increased blood levels of isopropanol. In absence of acetone, usually indicates an artifact.

Serum levels
- >400 mg/L—severe toxicity
- >1000 mg/L—coma

○ Presence of acetone in blood and urine, especially in high levels, suggests isopropanol poisoning.

Severe metabolic acidosis with increased AG is not a feature (as in ethanol poisoning but in contrast to methanol and ethylene glycol poisoning) unless lactic acid acidosis is present.

○ Osmolal gap increases 0.17 mOsm/L for every 1 mg of isopropanol; increase of 1 mOsm/L represents an isopropanol increase of 6 mg/dL.

Alcohol (Methyl) Poisoning

See Table 17-3.

Onset is 12–24 hrs after ingestion.

♦ Severe metabolic acidosis with increased AG and increased osmolar gap similar to that in ethanol intoxication (see Alcoholism) and ethylene glycol poisoning.

Frequent concomitant acute pancreatitis.

Treat with ethyl alcohol to achieve blood alcohol level of 100–150 mg/dL and maintain until methyl alcohol level is <10 mg/dL, formate level is <1.2 mg/dL, AG is normal, and acidosis resolves.

Institute hemodialysis if blood methyl alcohol is >50 mg/dL and severe resistant acidosis or renal failure is present. Lethal concentration = 80 mg/dL.

Alcoholism

See Tables 17-4 and 17-5.

PHYS/CHEM

Table 17-3. Comparison of Poisoning by Various Alcohols

Alcohol*	Metabolic Acidosis with I AG	Osmolal Gap	Serum Acetone	Urine Ketones	Urine Oxalate Crystals
Ethanol	V	I	V	V	–
Methanol	+	+	–	–	–
Isopropanol	–	I	+	+	–
Ethylene glycol	I	I	–	–	One-third of cases

+ = present; – = absent; AG = anion gap; I = increased; AG = anion gap; V = varies—findings depend on presence of lactic acidosis or alcoholic ketoacidosis.
*Measured by gas chromatography.

Table 17-4. Stages of Acute Alcoholic Intoxication

Ethanol Concentration (% Weight/Volume)		Stage of Alcohol Influence	Effects
Blood	Urine		
0.01–0.05	0.01–0.07	Sobriety	Little effect on most persons
0.04–0.12	0.03–0.16	Euphoria	Decreased inhibitions, decreased judgment, loss of fine control, increased reaction time ($\leq 20\%$)
0.09–0.20	0.07–0.30	Excitement	Uncoordination, loss of critical judgment, memory loss, increased reaction time ($\leq 100\%$)
0.15–0.30	0.12–0.40	Confusion	Disorientation Impaired emotional balance, slurred speech, disturbed sensation
0.25–0.40	0.20–0.50	Stupor	Paralysis, incontinence
0.30–0.50	0.25–0.60	Coma	Depressed reflexes, decreased respiration, possible death

Interference

False-positive values of ≤ 690 mg/L due to elevated lactate and LD concentrations can occur using EMIT but not protein-free ultrafiltrates or gas chromatography.
♦ Laboratory findings due to alcohol ingestion[4]
  • Blood alcohol level of >300 mg/dL at any time or >100 mg/dL in routine examination. (*Blood alcohol level of >150 mg/dL without gross evidence of intoxication suggests alcoholic patient's increased tolerance.*) In high-dose coma, blood alcohol should be >300 mg/dL; otherwise rule out other causes, especially diabetic acidosis and hypoglycemia (Table 17-4).
  • Rules of thumb to estimate blood alcohol level.
       Peak is reached 0.5–3 hrs after last drink.

[4]Laposata M. Assessment of ethanol intake. Current tests and new assays on the horizon. *Am J Clin Pathol* 1999;112:443.

Table 17-5. Diagnostic Efficiency of Some Markers for Alcoholism

Test	Sensitivity	Specificity	Predictive Value Positive	Negative
GGT (>50 U/L)	69	59	55	73
MCV	73	76	67	80
AST (>40 U/L)	69	68	55	74
ALT (>35 U/L)	58	57	49	66
AST/ALT (>1)	69	46	47	68

Source: Kwoh–Gain I, et al. Desialylated transferrin and mitochondrial aspartate aminotransferase compared as laboratory markers of excessive alcohol consumption. *Clin Chem* 1990;36:841.

Each ounce of whisky, glass of wine, or 12 oz of beer raises blood alcohol 15–25 mg/dL.

Women absorb alcohol much more rapidly than do men and show a 35–45% higher blood alcohol level. During premenstrual period, peak occurs more rapidly and reaches a higher level. Use of birth control pills causes a higher, more sustained level.

Elderly become intoxicated more quickly than young persons.

* Urine concentration is not well correlated with blood levels; cannot be used to determine level of intoxication or impairment.
* Breath test (Breathalyzer) has certain constraints and limitations.
* Alcohol content in saliva—determined by using cotton swab inserted into kit device. Method is used in drug abuse centers, hospital emergency and trauma units. Enzyme strip is colored in several minutes and is compared with a color scale to determine level of intoxication. One kit detects concentrations of >0.02%. Saliva to blood ratio = 1:1. Breath to blood ratio = 0.00048:1.
* Concentration in vitreous humor of refrigerated cadavers.
* Serum osmolality (reflects blood alcohol levels)—every 22.4 increment >200 mOsm/L reflects 50 mg/dL alcohol. Osmolar gap (difference between measured and calculated osmolality) is increased by >10. Absence of increased gap is evidence against elevated blood level of ethanol, methanol, or ethylene glycol.
* Laboratory findings due to other drugs of abuse may be present.
* Laboratory findings resulting from alcohol ingestion.
    Hypoglycemia
    Hypochloremic alkalosis
    Low magnesium level
    Increased lactic acid level (see Chapter 12, p. 496)
    Metabolic acidosis with increased AG (see Chapter 12, p. 497)
    Alcoholic ketoacidosis is preponderantly due to beta-hydroxybutyrate, and therefore increased ketone levels in blood and urine often yield negative or only weakly positive results because nitroprusside test detects acetoacetic but not beta-hydroxybutyric acid. As the patient improves, the ketone test may become more strongly positive (although total ketone level declines) because the improved liver function slows the conversion of acetoacetate to beta-hydroxybutyrate.
* Thrombocytopenia.
* Anemia most often due to folic acid deficiency; less frequently due to iron deficiency, hemorrhage, etc. (see appropriate separate sections).
* Alcohol is the most common cause of ring sideroblasts.
* Three types of hemolytic syndrome may occur (spur cell anemia, acquired stomatocytosis, Zieve syndrome).

Increase in the following blood values with no other known cause should arouse suspicion of alcoholism (Table 17-5).

* MCV (e.g., >97) (26% of cases) with round macrocytosis
* Serum GGT

PHYS/CHEM

- Uric acid (10% of cases)
- ALT, AST (48% of cases)
- ALP (16% of cases)
- Bilirubin (13% of cases)
- Triglycerides

After 4 wks of abstention, alcohol challenge in "moderate drinkers" causes increased AST and GGT in 24 hrs with slow decline thereafter. ALT, LD, ALP show little or no change.

Decrease of GGT after 1 wk of abstinence or decrease of MCV after 1–12 mos are markers of alcoholism in cirrhosis; persistent decrease of GGT to <2.5× ULN is marker of abstinence in alcoholic liver disease.

Declining serum potassium level to hypokalemia during alcohol withdrawal is said to be a reliable predictor of delirium tremens.

Laboratory findings due to major alcohol-associated illnesses (see the appropriate separate sections)
- Fatty liver (p. 216), alcoholic hepatitis (see p. 228), cirrhosis, esophageal varices, peptic ulcer, chronic gastritis, pancreatitis, malabsorption, vitamin deficiencies
- Head trauma, Korsakoff's syndrome, delirium tremens, peripheral neuropathy, myopathy
- Cardiac myopathy
- Various pneumonias, lung abscess, TB
- Associated addictions

Allergic Diseases

Increased serum total IgE is not a sensitive test and is of limited clinical value but extreme values may be helpful:
- Very low levels (<50 μg/L) help exclude atopic disease but not IgE sensitivity to special allergens such as penicillin or Hymenoptera venoms.
- If level is >900 μg/L, atopic disease is likely but tests for specific allergens are needed.
- Very high levels (2000 to >60,000 μg/L) are found in asthma associated with severe atopic dermatitis, allergic bronchopulmonary aspergillosis, Buckley's syndrome (staphylococcal infections with hyper-IgE), systemic parasitic infestations, IgE myeloma, immune deficiency.
- Principal value in infants is to alert the clinician to the possibility of allergic disease when this is not the presumptive diagnosis.

Radioallergosorbent test (serum IgE antibodies specific for various allergens) measures IgE specific for individual allergies. Useful when skin testing cannot be done (e.g., in children, those at risk for anaphylaxis) or when skin testing is unreliable (e.g., in cases of generalized dermatitis, severe dermographism). Less sensitive than skin and bronchial provocation tests.

Blood eosinophil count of >450/cu mm in adults and >750/cu mm in children suggest allergic disorders. Significant number of false-positive and false-negative results occur.

Nasal cytology smears stained with Wright's-Giemsa showing >5% eosinophils, >1% basophils, and/or >50% goblet/epithelial cells suggest allergic disease of respiratory tract. Does not correlate with blood eosinophilia. Large numbers of neutrophils suggest infection. Both eosinophils and neutrophils suggest chronic allergy with superimposed infection. Significant number of false-positive and false-negative results occur.

Measurement of serum complement is not useful.

Aluminum Toxicity

May occur in chronic renal failure patients on long-term dialysis treatment.
◆ • Serum aluminum should always be <200 μg/L (7.4 μmol/L); frequent monitoring and close observation for toxicity if serum level is >100 μg/L. Can be prevented by treatment of dialysate water (e.g., by reverse osmosis) so that final aluminum concentration in dialysate is <15 μg/L.

Microcytic hypochromic anemia (non–iron-deficient type)

Osteomalacic osteodystrophy is progressive, associated with a myopathy, resists treatment with vitamin D or its metabolites; may be associated with hypercalcemia. Metastatic calcification is common. Bone biopsy (special techniques) is most reliable test.

Dialysis encephalopathy

Chelation treatment with deferoxamine increases serum level with decrease in protein-bound fraction.

Apresoline (Hydralazine Hydrochloride) Reaction

(Occurs in hypertension therapy)
Anemia and pancytopenia occur infrequently.
○Prolonged use causes a syndrome resembling SLE (microscopic hematuria, leukopenia, increased ESR, presence of LE cells, altered serum proteins with increased gamma globulin). After cessation of drug, remission is aided by administration of ACTH.

Arsenic Poisoning

(From insecticides, rodenticides, herbicides, or therapeutic arsenic [e.g., Fowler's solution])
See Table 17-6.

Chronic

♦ Increased arsenic appears in urine (usually >0.1 mg/L; in acute cases may be >1.0 mg/L). Can be present for up to 10 days after a single exposure. With high industrial exposure, urine level may reach 1600 μg/L. After large seafood meal, level may reach 400 μg/L in 4 hrs.
♦ Increased arsenic appears in hair (normal = 0.05 mg/100 gm of hair; chronic toxicity = 0.1–0.5 mg/100 gm of hair; acute toxicity = 1–3 mg/100 gm of hair); may take several weeks to appear.
♦ Increased arsenic appears in nails 6–9 mos after exposure.
Moderate anemia is present; commonly normocytic, normochromic, basophilic stippling.
Moderate leukopenia occurs (2000–5000/cu mm), with mild eosinophilia.
Pancytopenia, aplastic anemia, and leukemia are associated with arsenic poisoning.
Liver function tests show mild abnormalities.
Abnormal renal function is frequent (oliguria, proteinuria, hematuria, casts).
Increased CSF protein (>100 mg/dL) is frequent; easily confused with Guillain-Barré syndrome.

Acute

(E.g., arsine gas [hydrogen arsenide])
Causes hemolysis with hemoglobinuria; may cause oliguric renal failure.
♦ Cleared from blood in 10 hrs; 40% is excreted in 48 hrs and 70% within 1 wk of ingestion; thus toxic blood levels may be missed. Urine levels are most useful to detect current poisoning (1–3 days previously).
Laboratory findings due to
  • Vomiting
  • Profuse watery or bloody diarrhea
  • Circulatory collapse
  • Renal damage (oliguria, proteinuria, hematuria)

Barbiturate Overdose

♦ Correlation between serum concentrations of barbiturates and state of intoxication in patients who have taken only a short-acting barbiturate, who are not habitual drug users, and who have no medical complications:

<6 μg/mL	Alert
6–10 μg/mL	Drowsy
11–17 μg/mL	Stuporous
16–20 μg/mL	Coma 1
20–24 μg/mL	Coma 2
24–28 μg/mL	Coma 3
28–40 μg/mL	Coma 4

If the serum drug level is less than expected for the state of intoxication, look for medical complications (e.g., aspiration pneumonia, head trauma) or presence of other drugs.

PHYS/CHEM

Table 17-6. Reported Reference Ranges of Some Common Toxic Substances and Trace Metals

Chemical	Specimen*	Normal Range	Toxic Concentration
Arsenic	Hair or nails	<1.0 μg/gm	
	Serum	<0.07 μg/mL	
	Urine	<25 μg/specimen	>150 μg/specimen
Cadmium	Blood	<5.0 ng/mL	
	Urine	<3 μg/24 hr	
Carbon monoxide	Blood	<7%	>20%
		<15% in heavy smokers	
Chromium	Serum	0.3–0.9 μg/L	
	Urine	<8.0 μg/specimen	
Copper	Serum	0.70–1.40 μg/mL (men)	
		0.80–1.55 μg/mL (women)	
		1.20–3.00 μg/mL (pregnancy)	
		0.80–1.90 μg/mL (children 6–12 yrs old)	
		0.20–0.70 μg/mL (infants)	
	Urine	15–60 μg/specimen	
	Liver tissue	10–35 μg/gm dry weight	
Ethanol	Blood		Toxic >2000 μg/mL
Ethylene glycol	Serum		Toxic >2 mmol/L, lethal >20 mmol/L
Lead	Blood	<0.2 μg/mL	
	Serum	0.8–2.5 ng/mL	
	Urine	<80 μg/specimen; abnormal, >400 μg/specimen; incon- clusive, 80–400 μg/ specimen	
	Hair or nails	<25 μg/gm	
Manganese	Serum or plasma	0.4–1.1 ng/mL	
	Whole blood	7.7–12.1 ng/mL	
	Urine	<0.3 μg/specimen	
Mercury	Blood	<0.005 μg/mL	>0.05 μg/mL
	Urine	<20 μg/specimen	>50 μg/specimen
	Hair or nails	<1.0 μg/gm	
Selenium	Serum	46–143 ng/mL	
	Whole blood	58–234 ng/mL	
	Urine	7–160 μg/L	
	Hair	0.2–1.4 μg/gm	
Silver	Serum	<0.2 μg/mL	
	Urine	<1.0 μg/specimen	
Thallium	Serum	<10 ng/mL	
	Urine	<10 μg/specimen	
Zinc	Plasma	0.70–120 μg/mL	
	Serum	5–15% higher than plasma	
	Urine	0.15–1.0 mg/day	

*Urine concentration is reported as per 7-mL aliquot of 24-hr urine collection.
Source: Some data from Jacob RA, Milne DB. Biochemical assessment of vitamins and trace metals. *Clin Lab Med* 1993;13:371.

Beta-Adrenergic Antagonist Overdose

(E.g., propranolol)
Drug levels are not useful for determining overdose.

Bromism

(Should always be ruled out in the presence of mental symptoms or psychosis.)
♦ Serum and urine bromide levels are increased.
CSF protein is increased in acute bromide psychosis.
○ False increase of serum "chloride" when measured by AutoAnalyzer. *If result of chloride determination with AutoAnalyzer is increased out of proportion to result with Cotlove coulometric titrator, bromism should be ruled out.* AG may be low or negative due to increased serum chloride.

Burns

Decreased plasma volume and blood volume. This decrease follows (and therefore is not due to) marked drop in cardiac output. Greatest fall in plasma volume occurs in the first 12 hrs and continues at a much slower rate for only 6–12 hrs more. In a 40% burn, plasma volume falls to 25% below preburn levels.
Infection—burn sepsis: gram-positive organisms predominate until the third day, when gram-negative organisms become dominant; reflects hospital's flora. By fifth day, untreated infection is active. *Fatal burn-wound sepsis shows no noteworthy spread of bacteria beyond wound in half the cases. Before antibiotic therapy, this caused 75% of deaths due to burns; it now causes 10–15% of deaths.*
♦ Diagnosis by quantitative biopsy of eschar showing $>10^5$ bacteria/gm of tissue and histologic evidence of bacterial invasion in underlying unburned tissue. Surface cultures do not accurately predict incipient burn wound sepsis. Local and systemic infection due to *Candida* and *Phycomycetes*.
Laboratory findings due to pneumonia, which now causes most deaths that result from infection. Two-thirds of pneumonia cases are airborne infections. One-third are hematogenous infections and are often due to septic phlebitis at sites of old cutdowns.
Laboratory findings due to inhalation injury
♦ • Carbonaceous sputum is pathognomonic; casts composed of mucin, fibrin, WBCs, cell debris may be present.
  • Hypoxemia.
  • Increased carboxyhemoglobin ($>15\%$).
Cyanide toxicity should be suspected if metabolic acidosis is present with apparently sufficient oxygen delivery.
Laboratory findings due to renal failure. Reported frequency varies from 1.3% of total admissions to 15% of patients with burns involving $>15\%$ of body surface.
Laboratory findings due to GI complications
  • Curling's ulcer. Occurs in 11% of burn patients. *Gastric ulcer is more frequent in general, but duodenal ulcer occurs twice as often in children as in adults. Gastric lesions are seen throughout the first month with equal frequency in all age groups, but duodenal ulcers are most frequent in adults during the first week and in children during the third and fourth weeks after the burns.*
  • Others include acute pancreatitis, superior mesenteric artery syndrome, adynamic ileus.
Laboratory findings due to complications of topical antibacterial therapy
  • Mafenide (Sulfamylon)—metabolic acidosis (carbonic anhydrase inhibition).
  • Silver nitrate—methemoglobinemia due to conversion of nitrate to nitrite by some strains of *Enterobacter cloacae*. Agyria does not occur.
  • Silver sulfadiazine (Silvadene)—hemolysis in patients with G-6-PD deficiency.
Blood viscosity rises acutely; remains elevated for 4–5 days although Hct has returned to normal.
Fibrin split products are increased for 3–5 days.
Other findings that may occur in all types of trauma
  • Platelet count rises slowly, with increase lasting for 3 wks.
  • Platelet adhesiveness is increased.
  • Fibrinogen falls during first 36 hrs, then rises steeply for up to 3 mos.
  • Factors V and VIII may be at 4–8× normal level for up to 3 mos.

PHYS/CHEM

Carbon Monoxide Poisoning, Acute

(Displaces oxyhemoglobin dissociation curve to left)
♦ Increased carboxyhemoglobin is diagnostic. Pulse oximetry cannot distinguish carboxyhemoglobin from oxyhemoglobin.

Symptoms are correlated with the percentage of carbon monoxide in Hb (% COHb):

% COHb	Symptoms
0–2%	Asymptomatic
2–5%	Found in moderate cigarette smokers; usually asymptomatic but may be slight impairment of intellect
5–10%	Found in heavy cigarette smokers; slight dyspnea with severe exertion
10–20%	Dyspnea with moderate exertion; mild headache
20–30%	Marked headache, irritability, disturbed judgment and memory, easy fatigability
30–40%	Severe headache, dimness of vision, confusion, weakness, nausea
40–50%	Headache, confusion, fainting, ataxia, collapse, hyperventilation
50–60%	Coma, intermittent convulsions
>60%	Respiratory failure and death if exposure is long continued
80%	Rapidly fatal

Blood pH is markedly decreased (metabolic acidosis due to tissue hypoxia).
Arterial pO_2 is normal, although O_2 is significantly decreased.
Arterial pCO_2 may be normal or slightly decreased.
♦ Increased carbon monoxide in patient's exhaled air or in ambient air at site of exposure can help confirm diagnosis if level of carbon monoxide in Hb has already fallen substantially.

Cigarette Smoking

♦ Cotinine increased in plasma or urine. Use to assess compliance in smoking cessation programs and to identify passively exposed nonsmokers. Has a longer half-life than nicotine, is more sensitive and specific than other markers to distinguish smokers from nonsmokers.

Reference ranges (HPLC)

	Plasma	Urine
Nonsmoker or passive exposure	0–8 μg/L	0.0–0.2 mg/L
Smoker	>8 μg/L	>0.2 mg/L

Increased blood carbon monoxide

Convulsive Therapy

(E.g., electroshock therapy)
Increased CSF AST and LD peak (at 3× normal) in 12 hrs; return to normal by 48 hrs.

Cyanide Poisoning

Potassium cyanide is in rodenticides, insecticides, laboratory reagents, film developer, amygdalin, silver polish, and acetonitrile used to remove artificial fingernails.

Hydrogen cyanide is in insecticides and fumigants and is released by the burning of plastics and synthetics.

pO_2 and oxygen saturation are normal except in severe cases when respiratory failure occurs.

Patient may first have respiratory alkalosis due to hyperventilation caused by tissue hypoxia.

Then severe lactic (metabolic) acidosis develops.

With respiratory depression, respiratory acidosis may occur.

Increased venous oxygen with decreased arteriovenous oxygen difference due to decreased tissue extraction of oxygen

♦ Blood cyanide is increased. Toxic concentration is >50 μg/dL.
Treat with nitrites to achieve methemoglobin level of >30%.

Drowning and Near-Drowning

Hypoxemia (decreased pO_2)
Metabolic acidosis (decreased blood pH)
In severe freshwater aspiration
- Decreased serum sodium and chloride
- Increased serum potassium
- Increased plasma Hb

In severe seawater aspiration
- Increased serum sodium and chloride
- Normal plasma Hb
- Hypovolemia

These changes follow aspiration of very large amounts of water. Electrolytes return toward normal within 1 hr after survival, even without therapy.
In near-drowning in freshwater, often
- Normal serum sodium and chloride.
- Variable serum potassium.
- Increased free plasma Hb; hemoglobinuria may occur.
- Oliguria with transient azotemia and proteinuria may develop.
- Fall in RBC, Hb, and Hct in 24 hrs.

In near-drowning in seawater, often
- Moderate increase in serum sodium and chloride
- Normal or decreased serum potassium
- Normal Hb, Hct, and plasma Hb

Blood Hb may appear normal even when considerable hemolysis is present because usual methodology does not distinguish between Hb within RBC and free Hb in serum. Decrease in Hb and Hct may be delayed 1–2 days.

Electric Current (Including Lightning), Injury due to

Increased WBC with large immature granulocytes
Albuminuria; hemoglobinuria in presence of severe burns
CSF sometimes bloody
Myoglobinuria and increased serum AST, CK, etc., indicate severe tissue damage.

Ethylene and Diethylene Glycol (Antifreeze) Poisoning

○Severe metabolic acidosis with increased AG and osmolal gap
◆Detection of ethylene glycol and its metabolite glycolic acid in serum
○Oxalate and hippurate crystals in urine
○Characteristic oxalate crystals in renal biopsy
○Urine may fluoresce under Wood's lamp due to fluorescein added to antifreeze.
Institute dialysis if glycol level is >50 mg/dL or renal failure or persistent severe acidosis is present.
Treat by IV administration of ethyl alcohol to achieve level >100 mg/dL.

Exercise, Severe

May occur with variable severity and in variable number of persons
- Increased serum enzyme concentrations due to skeletal muscle injury, e.g., CK total, CK-MB, LD, AST, aldolase, malate dehydrogenase
- Changes due to mechanical destruction of RBCs, e.g., increased serum and urine myoglobin, increased serum indirect bilirubin
- Increased serum uric acid, decreased serum phosphate

Heatstroke

Multiorgan dysfunction
Abnormal liver function and increased muscle-enzyme values
- Uniformly increased serum AST (mean is 20× normal), ALT (mean is 10× normal), and LD (mean is 5× normal) reach peak on third day and return to normal by 2

wks. Increased CK-MM. Lethal outcome is associated with significantly higher serum values that continued to increase in next 12–24 hrs. Consecutive normal values rule out diagnosis of heatstroke.

Hemoconcentration

Evidence of kidney damage may vary from mild proteinuria and slight abnormalities of urine sediment, to azotemia, to acute oliguric renal insufficiency.

Serum sodium is often decreased but may be high, especially in exertional heatstroke.

ARDS

Respiratory alkalosis occurs early and lactic acidosis and hyperkalemia later.

Hypoglycemia may occur.

Increased WBC count is usual.

DIC is common in severe cases.

Rhabdomyolysis, DIC, and acute renal failure are relatively uncommon in elderly because exertional heatstroke is less common in elderly.

CSF AST, ALT, and LD are normal.

Hypervitaminosis A

Acute intoxication after ingestion of 150–600 mg (500,000–2,000,000 U).

Chronic hypervitaminosis after ingestion of 7.5–90 mg/day (25,000–300,000 U) for minimum of 1 mo up to 2 yrs.

♦ Plasma vitamin A = 300–1000 μg/dL.

♦ Increased tissue levels of vitamin A and retinoic acid derivatives

May also show
* Increased ESR
* Increased serum ALP, GGT, bilirubin
* Decreased serum albumin
* Decreased Hb
* Slight proteinuria
* Slightly increased serum carotene
* Increased PT

Abnormal liver biopsy

Hypervitaminosis D

See p. 606.

Hypothermia, Accidental

Acid-base disturbances are very common.
* Initial hyperventilation causes respiratory alkalosis followed by respiratory acidosis due to carbon dioxide retention.
* Metabolic acidosis due to lactate accumulation. During rewarming, metabolic acidosis may become worse as lactic acid is mobilized from poorly perfused tissues.

Hemoconcentration is common.

WBC frequently falls, but differential is usually normal.

DIC may occur during rewarming.

"Cold diuresis," glycosuria, and natriuresis may occur; oliguria suggests complicating hypovolemia, acute tubular necrosis, rhabdomyolysis, or drug overdose.

Pancreatitis is a frequent complication.

Marked abnormalities in liver function tests are unusual.

Extreme hyperkalemia (>6.8 mEq/L) is a good indicator of death during acute hypothermia.

Insect Bite

(Due to ticks, lice, fleas, bugs, beetles, ants, flies, bees, wasps, etc.)

No specific laboratory findings without disease transmission or wound infection.

Iron Poisoning, Acute

(Occurs in children who have ingested medicinal iron preparations)

♦ Increased serum iron. Peak usually occurs 2–4 hrs after ingestion. Levels begin to fall after 6 hrs. If the first sample was taken 1–2 hrs after ingestion, a second sample should

Table 17-7. Centers for Disease Control and Prevention (CDC) Classification of Whole Blood Lead in Children 6–72 Mos Old for Prevention and Control

Level (μg/dL)	Classification
≤ 9	Not considered lead poisoning
$>10^*$	Rescreen; intervention; search for source
10–14	Need for more frequent screening of child and search for source
15–19	Rescreen; educational and nutritional intervention
20–44	Evidence of increased lead exposure; remedy environment; consider chelation
45–69	Chelation therapy; environmental intervention
>70	Emergency treatment should begin immediately

*CDC has recently lowered the intervention level from 25 to 10 μg/dL.
Source: Centers for Disease Control and Prevention. *Preventing lead poisoning in young children.* Washington, DC: U.S. Department of Health and Human Services, Public Health Service, 1994.

be obtained several hours later. Serum should be obtained after absorption is complete and before peak serum level falls due to protein-binding and tissue distribution.
- <350 μg/dL is rarely significant clinically; patient may have mild symptoms.
- 350–500 μg/dL: patient frequently has symptoms but risk of serious abnormality is mild; usually does not require prolonged chelation. 10% of patients develop coma or shock.
- >500 μg/dL within 6 hrs of ingestion with severe intoxication: patient needs urgent chelation treatment in hospital. 25% develop coma or shock.
- >1000 μg/dL may be lethal; patient may require hemodialysis or exchange transfusion. 70% develop coma or shock.

Increased TIBC itself is unreliable and not useful. Poor prognostic sign when serum iron greatly exceeds TIBC. Spuriously increased by deferoxamine chelation therapy.

Serum glucose of >150 mg/dL or WBC of $>15,000$/cu mm and radiopaque material noted on flat radiographic plate of abdomen correlate with increased serum iron level.

♦ In deferoxamine challenge (50 mg/kg up to 1 gm/kg administered IM) chelates free iron in circulation (100 mg binds 9 mg of iron, chiefly ferric); later appears in urine bound to iron, causing light orange to dark red-brown ("vin rose") color. Parenteral chelation should continue until serum iron is <100 μg/dL or urine loses vin rose color.

Renal changes may occur (e.g., acute renal failure, nephrotic syndrome, specific tubular defects).

Lead Poisoning (Plumbism)

See Tables 17-7 and 17-8, and Fig. 17-1.

Due To

- In adults, exposure is usually occupational (storage batteries, lead smelters) or environmental (improperly glazed earthenware, illicitly distilled whisky).
- In children, usually due to pica.
- In adolescents, may be due to gasoline sniffing.
- In all groups, epidemics may be due to contamination of water supply, use of contaminated pottery, etc.

♦ Measurements of zinc protoporphyrin (hematofluorometer) and FEP in blood using rapid micromethods are more sensitive indicators of lead poisoning than measurement of delta-ALA acid in urine. Especially useful for screening children. Zinc protoporphyrin appears only in new RBCs and remains for life of RBC; therefore zinc protoporphyrin does not increase until several weeks after onset of lead exposure and remains high long after lead exposure has ended; therefore is good indicator of total body burden of lead. FEP is sensitive measure of chronic exposure; increased whole blood level is sensitive measure of acute exposure. After therapy or removal of exposure, blood lead level becomes normal weeks to months before RBCs. CDC now recommends determination of whole blood lead in children because zinc protoporphyrin is not reliable below ~25 μg/dL.

Table 17-8. Screening for Lead Poisoning in High-Risk Children

Lead (μg/dL)	FEP (μg/dL)[a]			
	≤34	35–109	110–249	≥250
≤24	Retest in 1 yr	Rule out other causes of ↑ FEP[b]; retest in 3 mos	Rule out iron deficiency; retest in 3 mos	Rule out erythropoietic protoporphyria; retest in 3 mos
25–49	Retest next visit	Retest in 1–3 mos, then every 3–6 mos[c]	Rule out iron deficiency; retest in 2–4 wks[c]	
50–69	Usual pattern; retest to confirm	Retest in 2 wks, then every 1–3 mos[d]	Retest stat; rule out iron deficiency[d]	Retest stat; mobilization test or treat
≥70	Unusual pattern; retest to rule out contaminated specimen	Retest stat and treat	Retest stat and treat	Hospitalize stat

FEP = free erythrocyte protoporphyrin.
[a]Other causes of increased FEP are iron deficiency, anemia of chronic disease, sickle cell disease, and erythropoietic protoporphyria.
[b]Iron deficiency and thalassemia should be ruled out even if lead level is increased because iron deficiency and lead poisoning can occur together. Use blood lead and zinc protoporphyrin (ZPP) together for possible lead poisoning; blood ZPP with serum iron and ferritin for iron deficiency.
[c]Consider mobilization test if lead is ≥35 μg/dL.
[d]Consider mobilization test if lead = 35–55 μg/dL. Treat if lead = 56–69 μg/dL.
Source: Westchester County (N.Y.) Department of Health (Rev. 8.85).

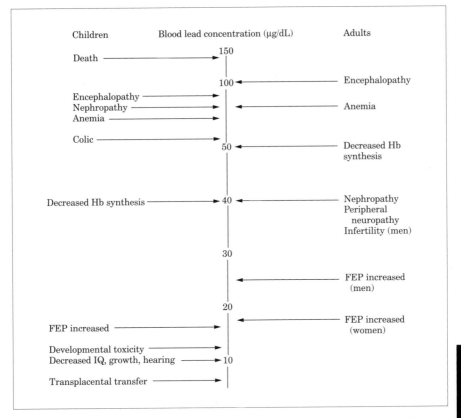

Fig. 17-1. Effects of lowest lead concentration on laboratory changes. (Data from Williams RH, Erickson T. Evaluating lead and iron intoxication in an emergency setting. *Lab Med* 1998;29:224.)

Other causes of increased FEP are iron deficiency, anemia of chronic disease, sickle cell disease, erythropoietic protoporphyria. FEP of ≥ 190 μg/dL is almost always due to lead intoxication. Iron deficiency and thalassemia should be ruled out even if lead level is increased because iron deficiency and lead poisoning can occur together. Use blood lead and zinc protoporphyrin together to evaluate for possible lead poisoning, blood zinc protoporphyrin with serum iron and ferritin to evaluate for iron deficiency.

♦ Delta-ALA is increased in urine. Because it is increased in 75% of asymptomatic lead workers who have normal coproporphyrin in urine, it can be used to detect early excess lead absorption. Is not increased until blood lead is >40 μg/dL.

♦ Confirm diagnosis with assay of blood lead—a single determination cannot distinguish chronic from acute exposure; reflects equilibrium between body compartments and therefore relatively recent exposure. *All blood and urine specimens for lead must be collected in special containers.*

Blood lead concentration in adults
• <10 μg/dL in most adults without occupational exposure.
• <20 μg/dL: considered normal.
• 25 μg/dL: report to state occupational health agency.
• >60 μg/dL: remove from occupational exposure; institute chelation therapy.

Urine lead level
• <150 μg/L is normal for adults.
• <80 μg/L is normal for children.
• >500 μg/24 hrs in children indicates excess mobile total body lead burden and suggests need for chelation therapy.

Lead mobilization test—administer 500 mg/sq m (up to 1000 mg) of edetate calcium disodium followed by measurement of 8-hr urine excretion of lead. Ratio of total urine lead (in μg) to edetate infused (in mgm) of >0.6 is considered positive. Difficulty in collecting urine usually makes test obsolete; begin chelation if blood lead is >45 μg/dL.

○Increased coproporphyrin in urine is a reliable sign of intoxication and is often demonstrable before basophilic stippling (but one should rule out a false-positive reaction due to drugs such as barbiturates and salicylates). This is a useful rapid screening test.

○Anemia is common, is usually mild (rarely <9 gm/dL). Is usually normochromic and normocytic but may be hypochromic and microcytic, especially in children. MCHC is reduced only moderately. Is often the first manifestation of chronic lead poisoning; due to decreased Hb production and increased hemolysis. In acute lead poisoning, hemolytic crisis may occur. Anemia may be seen at blood lead levels of 50–80 μg/dL in adults and 40–70 μg/dL in children.

Anisocytosis and poikilocytosis may be found, and a few nucleated RBCs may be seen. Some polychromasia is usual.

Stippled RBCs occur later in ~2% of cases (due to inhibition of 5'-pyramidine nucleotidase. Basophilic stippling is not pathognomonic of lead poisoning. Amount of stippling not correlated with severity of lead toxicity.

Bone marrow shows erythroid hyperplasia, and 65% of erythroid cells show stippling; some are ringed sideroblasts (thus this may be considered a secondary sideroblastic anemia).

Osmotic fragility is decreased, but mechanical fragility is increased.

Hematologic changes of lead poisoning are more marked in patients with iron deficiency.

Urine urobilinogen and uroporphyrin are increased.

Porphobilinogen is normal or only slightly increased in urine (unlike in acute intermittent porphyria).

Renal tubular damage occurs, with Fanconi's syndrome (hypophosphatemia, aminoaciduria, and glycosuria), usually in very severe or very chronic cases. Albuminuria, increased WBC, and transient rising BUN may occur. With chronic exposure interstitial nephritis develops with increased serum uric acid (saturnine gout); is most frequent renal finding.

CSF protein is increased, and frequently ≤ 100 mononuclear cells/cu mm are present in encephalopathy, which is rare with blood lead of <100 μg/dL.

In children, acute encephalopathy may be seen with blood lead of ≥ 80 μg/dL; abdominal and GI symptoms may occur with levels of 50 μg/dL but their presence usually indicate levels of ≥ 70 μg/dL.

Laboratory changes due to drug therapy using dimercaprol (BAL)
- Check daily for hematuria, proteinuria, cast formation.
- Check every other day for hypokalemia and hypercalcemia.
- Rule out G-6-PD deficiency and liver disease before starting therapy.

Lipid-Lowering Drugs, Side Effects

Nicotinic acid may cause
- Dramatic lowering (often) of blood triglyceride in hyperlipidemia types II and IV and probably also types III and V
- Increased blood sugar
- Increased blood uric acid
- Abnormal liver function tests
- Jaundice (rarely)

Cholestyramine in the form of a chloride salt may cause
- Lowering of cholesterol in familial type II hyperlipidemia
- Mild hyperchloremic acidosis

Mercury Poisoning

♦ Concentrations

Levels of mercury in serum, urine, and CSF are increased.

95% of asymptomatic normal people (not exposed to mercury) have a urine value of <20 μg/L and a blood level of <3 μg/L. Urine and blood levels are nondiagnostic, because they vary among patients with symptoms, and daily urine levels vary in the same patient. Thus, in one epidemic, urine levels of ≤ 1000 μg/L occurred in asymptomatic patients whereas other patients had symptoms at levels of 200 μg/L. The above values apply to mercury vapor and inorganic mercury salts.

Organic mercury (e.g., ethyl and methyl mercury) is more toxic; accumulates in RBCs and CNS. Most is slowly excreted in feces with half-life of 70 days. Only 10% is excreted in urine; urine levels may be normal even with significant exposure. Phenyl and methoxyethyl mercuries are less toxic and show higher urine levels.

Clinical correlation with organic mercury

	Whole Blood Total Mercury
	(μg/L or ng/mL or ppm)
Safe level	<100
Probably no symptoms	100–200
Symptoms occasionally present	>650
Symptoms usually present	>1000

Methemoglobinemia

See p. 416.

Milk Sickness ("Trembles")

(Poisoning from goldenrod, snakeroot, richweed, etc., or from eating poisoned animals)
Acidosis
Hypoglycemia
Increased nonprotein nitrogen (particularly guanidine)
Acetonuria

Mothball (Camphor, Paradichlorobenzene, Naphthalene) Poisoning

Paradichlorobenzene inhalation may cause liver damage.
Naphthalene ingestion may cause hemolytic anemia in patients with RBCs deficient in G-6-PD.

Oxalate Poisoning

(Due to ingestion of stain remover or ink eradicator containing oxalic acid)
Hypocalcemic tetany (due to formation of insoluble calcium oxalate)

Phenacetin, Long-Term Excessive Ingestion

Laboratory findings due to increased incidence of peptic ulceration, especially of stomach, often with bleeding, may be present.
○Laboratory findings associated with increased incidence of papillary necrosis and interstitial nephritis may be present.
• Proteinuria is slight or absent.
• Hematuria is often present in active papillary necrosis.
• WBC is increased in urine in absence of infection.
• Papillae are passed in urine.
• Creatinine clearance is decreased.
• Renal failure may occur.
Anemia is common and frequently precedes azotemia.

Phenol and Lysol Poisoning

Severe acidosis often occurs.
Acute tubular necrosis may develop.

Phenytoin Sodium (Dilantin) Therapy, Complications

Megaloblastic anemia may occur. It is completely responsive to folic acid (even when phenytoin sodium therapy is continued) but not always to vitamin B$_{12}$. Is the most common hematologic complication.
Rarely pancytopenia, thrombocytopenia alone, or leukopenia, including agranulocytosis may occur.

PHYS/CHEM

Laboratory findings of hepatitis may be present.

Laboratory findings resembling those of malignant lymphomas may be present.

Laboratory findings resembling those of infectious mononucleosis may occur, but heterophil agglutination is not increased.

Increased T_3 uptake, but RAIU, serum cholesterol level, etc., are normal (because of competition for binding sites of TBG).

Phenytoin sodium therapy may induce a lupus-like syndrome.

Phosphate (Organic) Poisoning (from Insecticides, e.g., Parathion, Malathion)

♦ RBC and serum cholinesterase decreased by $\geq 50\%$ due to inhibition of cholinesterase by organic phosphate pesticides (e.g., diazinon, malathion) and carbamates (e.g., carbaryl).
  • Decrease in serum of 40% when first symptoms of acute ingestion appear.
  • Decrease in serum of 80% when neuromuscular effects occur.
  • Patients with chronic low-level exposure may be asymptomatic even with decreased levels.
♦ RBC assay is a better reflection of cholinesterase activity in nerve tissue than is serum assay.

Worker experiencing industrial exposure should not return to work until these values rise to 75% of normal. RBC cholinesterase regenerates at rate of 1%/day and returns to baseline in 5–7 wks. Serum cholinesterase regenerates at rate of 25% in 7–10 days and returns to baseline in 4–6 wks.

Because of wide normal range, patient may lose 50% of their cholinesterase activity and still be within normal range. Therefore baseline levels should be determined for all workers at risk due to organophosphates or carbamates. A decrease of 30–50% from baseline indicates toxicity even if value is still within normal range.

When baseline levels are not available, retrospective diagnosis by serial measurements that increase after exposure.

Normal variation of $\pm 20\%$ in serum activity and $\pm 10\%$ in RBC activity prevents assessment of mild toxicity and recovery by only one or two assays.

Nonketotic hyperglycemia and glucosuria are common.

Serum amylase increase may reflect pancreatitis.

Serum cholinesterase may also be decreased in
  • Liver diseases.
      Especially hepatitis (30–50% decrease). Lowest level corresponds to peak of disease, and level becomes normal with recovery.
      Cirrhosis with ascites or jaundice (50–70% decrease). Persistent decrease may indicate a poor prognosis.
      Some patients with metastatic carcinoma (50–70% decrease), obstructive jaundice, congestive heart failure
  • Congenital inherited recessive decrease. Such patients are *particularly sensitive to administration of succinylcholine during anesthesia.*
  • Some conditions that may have decreased serum albumin (e.g., malnutrition, anemias, infections, dermatomyositis, AMI, pregnancy, recent surgery, liver diseases—see above).
  • Other drugs or chemicals (e.g., neostigmine methylsulfate [Prostigmin], quinine, fluoride, neostigmine, tetramethylammonium chloride, carbamate insecticides).

Phosphorus (Yellow) Poisoning

(Rat poison ingestion)
Acute yellow atrophy of liver occurs.
Vomitus may glow in the dark.

Potassium Chloride (Enteric-Coated) Poisoning

Laboratory findings due to small intestine ulceration, obstruction, or perforation.

Procainamide Therapy, Complications

Procainamide therapy may induce the findings of SLE.
○Positive serologic tests for SLE are very frequent, especially at dosage of ≥ 1.25 gm/day, and may precede clinical manifestations.

- LE cell tests become positive in 50% of patients.
- Anti-deoxyribonucleoprotein tests become positive in 65% of patients.
- Anti-DNA tests become positive in 35% of patients.
- One of these tests becomes positive in 75% of patients.

Perform serologic tests for SLE on all patients receiving procainamide.

Salicylate Intoxication

(Due to aspirin, sodium salicylate, oil of wintergreen, methylsalicylate)

♦ Increased serum salicylate (correlation does not apply to cases of chronic ingestion or ingestion of enteric-coated aspirin)
- >10 mg/dL when symptoms are present.
- 19–45 mg/dL when tinnitus is first noted.
- >40 mg/dL when hyperventilation is present.
- At ~50 mg/dL, severe toxicity with acid-base imbalance and ketosis occurs.
- At 45–70 mg/dL, death occurs.
- >100 mg/dL, hemodialysis is indicated.

Peak serum level is reached 2 hrs after therapeutic and at least 6 hrs after toxic dose. Serum levels drawn <6 hrs after ingestion cannot be used to predict severity of toxic reaction using Done's nomogram, although they confirm salicylate overdose. Done's nomogram cannot be used for ingestion of enteric-coated aspirin.
- 15–30 mg/dL for optimal antiinflammatory effect; 5–27 mg/dL in patients with RA on dose of 65 mg/kg/day.

When awaiting laboratory measurement, can estimate peak salicylate levels as follows:

$$\text{mg/dL of salicylate} = \frac{\text{(mg of salicylate ingested)}}{70\% \text{ of body weight (in gm)}^*} \times 100$$

* = Total body water.

In older children and adults, serum salicylate level corresponds well with severity; in younger children, correlation is more variable.

Gastric lavage may increase salicylate level by <10 mg/dL.

In early phase, serum electrolytes and carbon dioxide are normal.

Early respiratory alkalosis followed by metabolic acidosis; 20% of patients have either one alone.

Later, progressive decrease in serum sodium and pCO_2 occurs. 80% of patients have combined primary respiratory alkalosis and primary metabolic acidosis; change in blood pH reflects the net result. (*Infants may show immediate metabolic acidosis with the usual initial respiratory alkalosis. In older children and adults, the typical picture is respiratory alkalosis.*)

Hypokalemia accompanies the respiratory alkalosis. Dehydration occurs.

◯ Urine shows paradoxic acid pH despite the increased serum bicarbonate.
- Ferric chloride test is positive on boiled as well as unboiled urine (thus differentiating salicylate from ketone bodies); it may have a false-positive result because of phenacetin.
- Tests for glucose (e.g., Clinistix), reducing substances (e.g., Clinitest), or ketone bodies (e.g., Ketostix) are positive. All positive urine screening tests should be confirmed by serum sample.
- RBCs may be present.
- Number of renal tubular cells is increased because of renal irritation.

Hypoglycemia occurs, especially in infants on restricted diet and in diabetics.

Serum AST and ALT may be increased.

Hypoprothrombinemia after some days of intensive salicylate therapy is temporary and occasional; rarely causes hemorrhage.

Hydroxyproline is decreased in serum and urine.

Monitor patient by following blood glucose, potassium, pH.

Serum Sickness

Decreased WBC due to decreased polynuclear neutrophils; occasionally WBC is increased.

Eosinophils are usually normal.

ESR is normal.

Heterophil agglutination test is often positive and is decreased by guinea pig kidney absorption (see p. 844).

(see p. 844)

PHYS/CHEM

Snakebite

(Mortality is <1% in United States; 95% of cases are due to rattlesnakes.)

Pit Vipers

(Rattlesnake, copperhead, water moccasin; in United States all native snakes with elliptical pupils are poisonous.)

Increased WBC (20,000–30,000/cu mm)

Platelets decreased to ~10,000/cu mm within an hour; return to normal in ~4 hrs.

Burrs on almost all RBCs

Clotting caused by some venoms; normal coagulation prevented by others, which destroy fibrinogen so that fibrin split products are detected, fibrinogen levels are very low or absent, and PT and aPTT are very high. As a screening test, blood drawn into a modified Lee-White clotting tube that fails to clot within a few minutes of constant agitation is a reliable indication of envenomization.

Albuminuria

Elapidae

(Coral snakes, kraits, cobras)

Hemolytic manifestations

Monitor patients with CBC, platelet count, fibrinogen, PT, aPTT, BUN, bilirubin, electrolytes, bilirubin. Platelet count and fibrinogen are most sensitive.

80% of patients treated with antivenin develop serum sickness reaction.

Blood alcohol is >0.1% in 40% of people bitten.

Spider Bite

Black Widow Spider

(*Latrodectus mactans*)

Moderately increased WBC

Findings of acute nephritis

Brown Spider

(*Loxosceles reclusa*)

Hemolytic anemia with hemoglobinuria and hemoglobinemia

Increased WBC

Thrombocytopenia

Proteinuria

Steroids, Side Effects that Cause Laboratory Changes

Endocrine effects (e.g., adrenal insufficiency after prolonged use, suppression of pituitary or thyroid function, development of diabetes mellitus)

Increased susceptibility to infections

GI effects (e.g., peptic ulcer, perforation of bowel, infarction of bowel, pancreatitis)

Musculoskeletal effects (e.g., osteoporosis, pathologic fractures, arthropathy, myopathy)

Decreased serum potassium, increased WBC, glycosuria, ecchymoses, etc.

Vitamin D Intoxication

(See p. 606.)

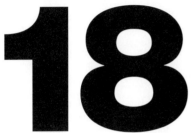

Therapeutic Drug Monitoring and Toxicology

The determination of toxic and effective therapeutic concentration of drugs has become one of the most important and widely used functions of the laboratory. In the past, drugs were measured by their effects (e.g., coumadins prolonged PT, antimicrobials inhibited growth of microorganisms). Newer methodologies now permit determinations of drug concentrations in the blood that were previously impossible or not generally available.

The clinician must be aware of the various influences on pharmacokinetics, factors such as half-life, time to peak and to steady state, protein binding, and excretion, that are not within the province of this book but are useful for the physician in prescribing these drugs appropriately.

The route of administration and sampling time after last dose of drug must be known for proper interpretation. For some drugs (e.g., quinidine), different assay methods produce different values, and the clinician must know the normal range for the test method used for the patient.

In general, peak concentrations alone are useful when testing for toxicity, and trough concentrations alone are useful for demonstrating a satisfactory therapeutic concentration. Trough concentrations are commonly used with such drugs as lithium, theophylline, phenytoin, carbamazepine, quinidine, tricyclic antidepressants, valproic acid, and digoxin. Specimens for measurement of trough concentrations can usually be drawn at the time the next dose is administered (*this does not apply to digoxin*). Both peak and trough concentrations are used to avoid toxicity but ensure bactericidal efficacy (e.g., gentamicin, tobramycin, vancomycin). With IV and IM administration, sample should usually be drawn 0.5 to 1 hr after administration is ended to determine peak concentration.

Concentrations given here are meant only as a general guide; the laboratory performing the test should supply its own values.

Blood should be drawn at a time specified by that laboratory, e.g., 1 hr before the next dose is due to be administered. This trough concentration should ideally be greater than the minimum effective serum concentration.

If a drug is administered by IV infusion, blood should be drawn from the opposite arm.

The drug should have been administered at a constant rate for at least 4–5 half-lives before blood samples are drawn.

See Table 18-1.

Indications for Therapeutic Drug Monitoring

Symptoms or signs of toxicity occur.

Therapeutic effect not obtained.

Noncompliance is suspected.

Drug has a narrow therapeutic range.

An optimal dosing schedule must be provided or confirmed.

Cause of organ toxicity (e.g., abnormal liver or kidney function tests) must be confirmed.

Other diseases or conditions exist that affect drug utilization.

Drug interactions that have altered desired or previously achieved therapeutic concentration are suspected.

Drug shows large variations in utilization or metabolism among individuals.

Table 18-1. Reported Reference Ranges of Some Common Therapeutic Drugs

Drug	Therapeutic Concentration	Toxic Concentration
Acetaminophen (e.g., Anacin, Dristan, Excedrin, Nyquil, Sinutab, Tylenol)	<50 μg/mL	>120 μg/mL
Amitriptyline + nortriptyline	75–225 ng/mL	>500 ng/mL
Nortriptyline (only)	50–150 ng/mL	>500 ng/mL
Bromide	1000–2000 μg/mL	$\geq$ 3000 μg/mL
Butabarbital	1–5 μg/mL	$\geq$ 10 μg/mL
Butalbital	10–20 μg/mL	$\geq$ 40 μg/mL
Caffeine	5–15 μg/mL	$\geq$ 30 μg/mL
Carbamazepine (P) (Tegretol for seizures)	2–10 μg/mL	$\geq$ 12 μg/mL
Carbamazepine-10-11-epoxide (P)	0.4–4.0 μg/mL	$\geq$ 8.0 μg/mL
Carotene (S)	48–200 μg/dL	
Chlordiazepoxide (S) (Librium)	5–10 μg/mL	$\geq$ 15 μg/mL
Chlorpromazine (S) (Thorazine)	>50 ng/mL	$\geq$ 1500 ng/mL
Clonazepam (for seizures)	10–50 ng/mL	$\geq$ 100 ng/mL
Cyclosporine (B)	100–300 mg/mL	$\geq$ 400 ng/mL
Diazepam	0.2–0.8 μg/mL	
Nordiazepam	0.2–1.0 μg/mL	
Total for both	0.4–1.8 μg/mL	$\geq$ 5.0 μg/mL
Dicumarol (P) (warfarin)	2–5 μg/mL	$\geq$ 10 μg/mL
Digitoxin	15–30 mg/mL	>30 ng/mL
Digoxin	0.5–2.0 ng/mL	$\geq$ 3.0 ng/mL
Disopyramide (P)	2.0–4.5 μg/mL	$\geq$ 8.0 μg/mL
Doxepin (combined with determination of metabolite desmethyldoxepin)	100–275 ng/mL	$\geq$ 500 ng/mL
Ethchlorvynol (S)	5–10 μg/mL	$\geq$ 20 μg/mL
Ethosuximide (P)	40–75 μg/mL	$\geq$ 100 μg/mL
Folate, RBC (B)		
$\geq$ 12 yrs old	150–800 ng/mL	
1–11 yrs old	96–362 ng/mL	
<1 yr old	74–995 ng/mL	
Folate (S)	$\geq$ 3.5 μg/L	
Fluoride (P)		$\geq$ 15 μmol/L
Glutethimide (S)	0.2–7.0 mg/mL	$\geq$ 10 μg/mL
Gold		
S	1.0–2.0 μg/mL	>5.0 μg/mL
24-hr urine	<1.0 μg/specimen	>5000 μg/specimen
Imipramine +		
Desipramine (P)	125–225 ng/mL	$\geq$ 500 ng/mL
Desipramine only	75–225 ng/mL	
Lidocaine (P) (Xylocaine)	2.0–5.0 μg/mL	$\geq$ 6.0 μg/mL
Lithium (S)	0.8–1.2 mEq/L	$\geq$ 1.5 mEq/L
Mephobarbital (P)	1–7 μg/mL	$\geq$ 15 μg/mL

Drug	Therapeutic Concentration	Toxic Concentration
(Phenobarbital should be determined on same sample)	See Phenobarbital	
Meprobamate (S)	<10 μg/mL	$\geq$ 100 μg/mL
Methaqualone (S)	1–5 μg/mL	$\geq$ 10 μg/mL
Methotrexate (S)	<0.1 μmol/L after 48 hrs	1.0×10^{-5} at 24 hrs 1.0×10^{-6} at 48 hrs 1.0×10^{-7} at 72 hrs
Methsuximide (S)	<1.0 μg/mL	>55 μg/mL
Normethsuximide (should be performed with methsuximide determination)	20–40 μg/mL	>55 μg/mL
Methyprylon (S)	<10 μg/mL	$\geq$ 30 μg/mL
Mexiletine (S or P)	0.75–2.0 μg/mL (trough)	$\geq$ 2.0 μg/mL (trough)
Pentobarbital (S)	1–5 μg/mL	$\geq$ 10 μg/mL
For reducing intracranial pressure	30–40 μg/mL	
Phenobarbital (P)		
Adults	20–40 μg/mL	$\geq$ 55 μg/mL
Infants and children	15–30 μg/mL	
Phenytoin		
Total (P)	10–20 μg/mL	$\geq$ 25 μg/mL
Free (P)	1–2 μg/mL	$\geq$ 2.5 μg/mL
Primidone (P) (should be performed with phenobarbital determination)	9–12.5 μg/mL (adults); 7–10 μg/mL (children <5 yrs old)	$\geq$ 15 μg/mL
Procainamide (P) (should be performed with NAPA determination)	4–8 μg/mL; <46 μg/mL (both)	$\geq$ 16 μg/mL; >46 μg/mL (both)
N-Acetylprocainamide (P) (NAPA)	$\leq$ 30 μg/mL	>30 μg/mL
Propoxyphene (S)	0.2–0.5 μg/mL	$\geq$ 2 μg/mL
Propranolol (P)	50–100 ng/mL	$\geq$ 1000 ng/mL
Quinidine (P)	2.0–5.0 μg/mL	$\geq$ 7.0 μg/mL
Salicylates (S)	2–20 mg/dL (adults)	$\geq$ 50 mg/dL
Secobarbital (S)	1.0–5.0 μg/mL	$\geq$ 7.0 μg/mL
Theophylline (P)	10–20 μg/mL (adults); 5–20 μg/mL (children)	$\geq$ 20 μg/mL
Thiocyanate (S)	4–20 μg/mL	$\geq$ 60 μg/mL
Thioridazine (S)	>50 ng/mL	$\geq$ 1500 ng/mL
Tocainide (S)	5–12 μg/mL	$\geq$ 15 μg/mL
Trazodone (S)	500–1100 ng/mL	$\geq$ 1500 ng/mL
Trifluoperazine (S)	<10 ng/mL	$\geq$ 50 ng/mL
	Note: Lower limit for detection is 20 ng/mL. Only useful to detect toxic concentration.	
Valproic acid (P)	40 μg/mL (trough); 100 μg/mL (peak)	$\geq$ 120 μg/mL

(*continued*)

TDM/TOXICOL

Table 18-1. (continued)

Antimicrobial Drug	Therapeutic Concentration (μg/mL)	High or Toxic Concentration (μg/mL)	Low Concentration (μg/mL)
Amikacin			
Peak	20–25	30	14
Trough	5–10	10	
Chloramphenicol			
Peak	15–25	30	15
Trough	8–10	15	8
5-Flucytosine			
Peak	100	125	50
Trough	50	125	30
Gentamicin			
Peak	4–8	8	3
Trough	1–2	2	
Netilmicin			
Peak	4–8	8	3
Trough	1–2	2	
Streptomycin			
Peak	5–20	40	
Trough	<5	40	
Sulfadiazine (S)	100–120	$\geq$ 300	
Sulfamethoxazole (S)	90–100	$\geq$ 300	
Sulfapyridine (S)	75–90	$\geq$ 300	
Sulfisoxazole (S)	90–100	$\geq$ 300	
Trimethoprim/sulfamethoxazole (TMP/SMX)			
Peak (trimethoprim)	$\geq$ 5		5
Peak (sulfamethoxazole)	$\geq$ 100		100
Tobramycin			
Peak	4–8	8	3
Trough	1–2	>2	
Vancomycin			
Peak	20–40	40	15
Trough	5–10	15	5

B = blood; P = plasma; S = serum.
Source: [1] Henry JB, ed. Symposium on therapeutic drug monitoring. *Clin Lab Med* 1981;1(3). [2] Gerson B, ed. Symposium on therapeutic drug monitoring. *Clin Lab Med* 1987;7(3). [3] Bakerman S. *ABCs of interpretive laboratory data*, 2nd ed. Greenville, NC: Interpretive Laboratory Data, 1984. [4] Leavelle DE, ed. *Mayo Medical Laboratories' interpretive handbook*. Rochester, MN: Mayo Medical Laboratories, 1995.

Medicolegal verification of treatment, cause of death or injury (e.g., suicide, homicide, accident investigation), or detection of use of forbidden drugs (e.g., steroids in athletes, narcotics) is needed.
Differential diagnosis of coma.

Criteria for Therapeutic Drug Monitoring

Available methodology must be specific and reliable.
Blood concentration must correlate with therapeutic and toxic effects.

Therapeutic window is narrow with danger of toxicity on therapeutic doses.
Correlation between blood concentration and dose is poor.
Clinical effect of drug is not easily determined.

Drugs for Which Therapeutic Drug Monitoring May Be Useful

Antiepileptic drugs (phenobarbital, phenytoin [Dilantin])
Theophylline
Antimicrobials (aminoglycosides [gentamicin, tobramycin, amikacin], chloramphenicol, vancomycin, flucytosine [5-fluorocytosine])
Antipsychotic drugs
Antianxiety drugs
Cyclic antidepressants
Lithium
Cardiac glycosides (digoxin)
Cardiac antiarrhythmics and antianginal drugs
Antihypertensive drugs
Antineoplastic drugs
Cannabinoids
Other drugs of abuse (cocaine, etc.)
Androgenic anabolic steroids
Immunosuppressant drugs (cyclosporine)
Antiinflammatory drugs
  • Nonsteroids (salicylates, propionic acids, oxicams, indoleacetic acids)
  • Steroids
TPN
At present, four drugs (digoxin, phenytoin, phenobarbital, theophylline) account for ~50% of drug monitoring

Antiarrhythmic Agents

(Data from refs. [2,4] in Table 18-1)

Amiodarone

(Used for supraventricular and some ventricular arrhythmias)
Therapeutic range: 1.5–2.5 μg/mL
Toxic concentration: ≥ 3.5 μg/mL
Effect on other laboratory test values:
  • Abnormal TSH and T_4 values are common and should be monitored during therapy.
  • Changes in laboratory results due to pulmonary fibrosis, which occurs in >2% of patients.
May increase the plasma concentration of digoxin, diltiazem, phenytoin, procainamide, quinidine.
Concentration may be increased by severe liver disease (amiodarone) or decreased renal function (dexethylamiodarone).

Diltiazem

(Calcium channel blocker used to treat angina pectoris and hypertension)
Therapeutic range: plasma concentration of 40–200 ng/mL
Effect of diltiazem on other laboratory tests: increased BT due to platelet dysfunction

Flecainide (Tambocor)

(Used for ventricular arrhythmias)
Therapeutic range: trough plasma concentration of 0.2–1.0 μg/mL
Toxic concentration: >1.0 μg/mL

Mexiletine (Mexitil)

(Used to treat many cardiac arrhythmias, e.g., ventricular arrhythmias)
Therapeutic range: plasma trough concentration of 0.75–2.0 μg/mL
Toxic concentration: >2.0 μg/mL

TDM/TOXICOL

Some drugs that may cause decreased plasma mexiletine concentration: phenobarbital, phenytoin, rifampin

Nifedipine

(Calcium channel blocker used to treat angina pectoris and hypertension)
Therapeutic range: serum concentration of 25–100 ng/mL
Effect on other laboratory tests: decreased glucose tolerance in normal and diabetic patients
Concentration of some drugs (e.g., digoxin) may be increased by nifedipine.

Procainamide

(Used to treat many cardiac arrhythmias)
Is measured along with its active metabolite N-acetylprocainamide
Therapeutic range: procainamide, 4–8 μg/mL; N-acetylprocainamide, $\leq$ 30 μg/mL; both, $\leq$ 30 μg/mL
Toxic concentration: procainamide, $\geq$ 16 μg/mL; N-acetylprocainamide, >30 μg/mL

Quinidine

(Used to treat many cardiac arrhythmias)
Therapeutic range: 2.0–5.0 μg/mL
Toxic concentration: $\geq$ 7.0 μg/mL

Tocainide (Tonocard)

(Used for long-term treatment of lidocaine-responsive ventricular arrhythmias)
Therapeutic range: plasma concentration of 5–12 μg/mL
Toxic concentration: $\geq$ 15 μg/mL (peak)
Effect on other laboratory test values:
- Presence of ANA antibodies or lupus syndrome is rare (in contrast to procainamide).
- Agranulocytosis is rare.
- Hepatitis.

Verapamil

(Calcium channel blocker used to treat supraventricular dysrhythmias, angina pectoris, hypertension)
Therapeutic range: serum concentration of 50–200 ng/mL (peak)
Toxic concentration: $\geq$ 400 ng/mL (peak)
Some drugs whose concentration may be increased by verapamil: carbamazepine, digoxin
Rifampin may decrease verapamil serum concentration.

Antidepressants, Cyclic

(Data from ref. [2] in Table 18-1)
Therapeutic drug monitoring is usually requested because of lack of clinical response.
Utility is decreased by the lack of objective monitoring criteria, poor correlation of plasma concentration with clinical response, and the presence of active metabolites.
Some conditions that may increase tricyclic antidepressant plasma concentration: aging, alcoholic liver disease, renal failure, use of chloramphenicol, cimetidine, haloperidol, methylphenidate
Some conditions that may decrease tricyclic antidepressant plasma concentration: barbiturate use, chloral hydrate use, smoking
Should maintain uniformity of collection (e.g., time related to last dose, serum versus plasma, type of container).

Antihypertensive Drugs

Little correlation is found between plasma concentration and clinical effect.

Antiinflammatory Drugs, Nonsteroidal

(Data from ref. [2] in Table 18-1)
Salicylates (aspirin, diflunisal)
Propionic acids (ibuprofen, diclofenac, naproxen, oxicams, piroxicam)

Indoleacetic acids (indomethacin, sulindac)

Except for salicylates, serum concentration does not correlate with drug effects, therapeutic ranges have not been established, and routine drug monitoring is not clinically useful.

Therapeutic drug monitoring of salicylates is indicated because of:

- Unreliability of clinical symptoms (e.g., tinnitus) as an indication of toxicity.
- Narrow anti-inflammatory therapeutic range: 2–20 mg/dL.
- Narrow anti-inflammatory toxic concentration: ≥ 50 mg/dL.
- Intraindividual variation of up to 300%.
- Drug interaction may significantly lower serum salicylate concentration (e.g., antacids, ACTH, prednisone).
- After 4 wks of therapy, serum salicylate concentrations decline to 65–80% of 1-wk concentration.

Antineoplastic Drug Monitoring

Despite the large number of classes and drugs available, monitoring is clinically useful only in the following instances and the clinical result is improved only with methotrexate:

5-Fluorouracil

To monitor systemic concentration with intrahepatic or intraperitoneal use

Melphalan

To monitor absorbance of oral drug

Doxorubicin

To determine kinetics in patients with liver dysfunction

Methotrexate

Therapeutic concentration: $\leq 1.0 \times 10^{-7}$ mol/L

Toxic concentration: 1.0×10^{-5}, 1.0×10^{-6}, 1.0×10^{-7} mol/L at 24, 48, and 72 hrs, respectively

Cannabinoids (Marijuana, Hashish)

(Data from ref. [4] in Table 18-1)

Testing (for THC) is done to detect drug abuse rather than for therapeutic monitoring. Lower limit of detectability is <15 ng/mL by definitive gas chromatography/mass spectrometry. Value of ≤ 25 mg/mL can be due to passive inhalation.

May be detected in plasma up to 6 days after smoking one marijuana cigarette.

In habitual marijuana users, cannabinoid metabolites have been detected in the urine up to 46 days after last use.

Urine adulterated with bleach, detergent, blood, salt, vinegar may produce negative test results with EMIT (enzyme immunoassay) methods.

Screening tests positive with one method (e.g., EMIT, RIA) should be confirmed with another method (e.g., gas chromatography/mass spectrometry). Qualitative EMIT screen has occasional false-positives.

Cyclosporine (Sandimmune)

(Used as immunosuppressant to prevent rejection of kidney, heart, liver, marrow, pancreas transplants; possible use in graft-versus-host disease and treatment of autoimmune diseases)

(Data from ref. [2] in Table 18-1)

Acts by selective inhibition of certain T lymphocytes; does not affect granulocytes. Often used in combination with corticosteroids.

Initial oral dose given 4–12 hrs before transplantation surgery. Oral dosage needs to be decreased (e.g., by 5%) during the following weeks or months to maintain constant blood concentration. Half-life = 4–6 hrs. Peak concentration occurs 2–6 hrs after oral dose. Trough concentration occurs 12–18 hrs after maintenance oral dose but longer after initial oral dose. Trough concentration occurs ~12 hrs after one IV dose.

Therapeutic range: 100–300 ng/mL (trough) in whole blood for kidney transplant patients. No immunosuppression with trough in whole blood of <100 ng/mL. For first weeks after transplantation, rejection occurs with trough values of <170 ng/mL; quiescence is usually maintained at values of ≥ 200 ng/mL; requirements diminish to 50–75 ng/mL by ~3 mos and dosage is maintained for rest of patient's life.

Monitoring: Draw blood just before next dose (trough concentration). Periodic monitoring (e.g., daily for liver transplant patients, three times/week for kidney transplant patients) should be performed, but this is not recommended as a stat procedure.

Threshold for renal toxicity is ≥ 400 ng/mL in whole blood. Nephrotoxicity occurs in up to one-half of renal transplant cases and approximately one-third of heart and liver transplant cases. Urine sediment unchanged.

- Nephrotoxicity includes four discrete syndromes:
  1. Delayed graft function in 10% of cases without cyclosporine therapy and 35% of cases with cyclosporine therapy; resolves when cyclosporine is withdrawn.
  2. Acute reversible functional impairment begins to occur at concentration of 200 ng/mL and is universal at >400 ng/mL. Serum creatinine begins to rise 3–7 days after rise in cyclosporine and falls 2–14 days after cyclosporine is reduced. Decreased GFR, hyperkalemia, acidosis.
  3. Hemolytic-uremic syndrome (see p. 480).
  4. Chronic nephropathy with interstitial fibrosis causes irreversible loss of renal function.
- Hepatotoxicity in 4–7% of cases is mild, transient, dose related; is monitored by testing for increased serum total bilirubin, AST, ALT, and ALP, by liver biopsy to look for hepatocyte damage.
- Lymphoma and epithelial malignancy are uncommon (0.1–0.4%); increase with combined immunosuppression.

Acute graft rejection occurs in 50% of patients after renal, heart, liver transplants. It may be difficult to differentiate from renal failure and renal biopsy may be indicated. Monitoring T-cell subsets is reported as not useful by some, whereas others have used rise in T_4 and decline in T_8 counts as indicator of graft rejection. Tests of complement-dependent cytotoxicity, antibody-dependent cell-mediated cytotoxicity, and lymphocyte-mediated cytotoxicity to donor spleen cells obtained at time of donor nephrectomy may help to distinguish nephrotoxicity from renal graft rejection. Also, in bacterial or viral infection, all target cells are destroyed, but in graft rejection, only donor cells are destroyed.

RIA measures parent compound and certain metabolites; HPLC measures only parent compound. Serum concentrations are ~60% lower than whole blood concentrations.

Some drugs that may cause increased serum cyclosporine concentrations: amphotericin B, cimetidine, corticosteroids, diltiazem, erythromycin, furosemide, ketoconazole, nicardipine.

Some drugs that may cause decreased serum cyclosporine concentrations: carbamazepine, glutethimide, phenobarbital, phenytoin, rifampin with isoniazid, sulfadimidine, trimethoprim/sulfamethoxazole.

Because cyclosporine contains ethanol, drug interactions may occur with: disulfiram (Antabuse), cefamandole, cefoperazone, chlorpropamide (Diabinese), metronidazole (Flagyl), moxalactam.

Digitoxin

Draw blood just before next dose or >6 hrs after last dose.
Therapeutic range: 15–30 ng/mL
Toxicity is common with concentration of >30 ng/mL.

Digoxin

(Data from refs. [2–4] in Table 18-1)
Draw blood 6–8 hrs (or 8–24 hrs, ref. [3]) after last oral dose after steady state has been achieved in 1–2 wks.
Therapeutic range: 0.5–2.0 ng/mL
Toxic range: ≥ 3.0 ng/mL, but 10% of patients may show toxicity at <2 ng/mL.

- Pediatric toxic concentration may be higher. Therapeutic index is very low, i.e., small difference between therapeutic and toxic blood concentration. However, ~10% of patients have serum concentration of 2–4 ng/mL without evidence of toxicity. On dose of 0.25 mg/day, mean serum concentration = 1.2±0.4 ng/mL; on dose of 0.5 mg/day, mean serum concentration = 1.5 ± 0.4 ng/mL. Digitalis leaf dose of 0.1 gm/day produces same serum concentration as 0.1 mg/day of crystalline digitoxin. ECG evidence of toxicity in one-third to two-thirds of patients with no symptoms or signs.

Toxicity may occur at lower blood concentration in presence of hypokalemia, hypercalcemia, hypomagnesemia, hypoxia, chronic heart disease.

Some drugs that may cause increased digoxin blood concentration: quinidine, verapamil, amiodarone, indomethacin, cyclosporine A.

Endogenous digoxin-like substances may give a positive test in persons who have not received the drug, especially in
- Uremia.
- Severe agonal states and postmortem. Thus, when concentration is high postmortem it may not have been high before death, and a normal postmortem concentration suggests that the antemortem concentration was not toxic. Therefore, only HPLC or mass spectrometry can definitely identify digoxin as a possible cause of death.

Because most methods measure both endogenous digoxin-like substances and inactive metabolites of digoxin, therapeutic monitoring should be used primarily to assess patient compliance and to confirm drug toxicity.

Ethanol

(Data from ref. [2] in Table 18-1)
Lower limit for detection = 100 μg/mL.
For treatment of methanol or ethylene glycol poisoning, desirable blood concentration = 100 mg/dL.
Criterion for driving an automobile while intoxicated = 100 mg/dL (= 0.1%; 1000 μg/mL).
♦ For diagnosis of alcoholism
- Major criterion:
    Blood concentration of >150 mg/dL without gross evidence of intoxication
- Minor criteria:
    Blood concentration of >300 mg/dL at any time
    Blood concentration of >100 mg/dL on routine examination
Toxic concentration: ≥ 200 mg/dL

Flucytosine (5-Fluorocytosine)

(Data from ref. [2] in Table 18-1)
(Used as antimycotic agent [e.g., *Cryptococcus neoformans, Candida*])
Therapeutic range: serum concentration of 50–100 mg/L. Most susceptible organisms are killed at 0.5–12.5 mg/L concentrations. Serum and CSF fungistatic concentration of 10–40 mg/L. Bone marrow toxicity becomes prominent at serum concentration of >125 mg/L or in presence of renal dysfunction.

In addition to drug monitoring, patients should be monitored for liver, kidney, and bone marrow toxicity.

Haloperidol

(Used for treatment of psychoses, Tourette's syndrome, unresponsive hyperexcitability in children)
Therapeutic drug monitoring is used to distinguish unresponsiveness from noncompliance or to detect high concentration in patients with abnormal liver function.
Therapeutic range: 5–16 ng/mL
Routine monitoring not indicated with good response to low-dose therapy.
Allow >1 wk for patient to reach steady state. Collect serum 12 hrs after last dose.

Lidocaine (Xylocaine)

(Used for prevention and treatment of ventricular arrhythmias)
(Data from refs. [3,4] in Table 18-1)
Draw blood 12 hrs after beginning therapy.
Indications for monitoring:
- Repeat every 12 hrs when drug clearance is altered by liver disease, heart failure, AMI.

- Toxicity is suspected.
- Ventricular arrhythmias occur despite therapy.

Therapeutic range: 2–5 μg/mL.

Toxic concentration: $\geq 6\ \mu$g/mL.

Concentration may be falsely low if blood is collected in some rubber-stoppered tubes.

Lithium

(Used for treatment of mania and as prophylaxis for manic and depressive episodes in bipolar disorders)

(Data from refs. [1,4] in Table 18-1)

Therapeutic concentration: 0.8–1.2 mEq/L based on serum trough concentration on sample drawn 12±0.5 hrs after evening dose; significant time differences can be misleading. Blood should be drawn after steady state has been achieved (3–10 days). ~25% of manic patients do not respond, and they can be tried at concentration of 1.5–2.0 mEq/L if closely monitored. Compliance is a major problem in these patients.

Toxic concentration: >1.5 mEq/L. >3.0 mEq/L can be lethal.

Thyroid and renal function should be monitored along with lithium concentration and clinical progress.

Peak concentration occurs 1–2 hrs after administration of lithium carbonate or citrate, 4 hrs after administration of slow-release preparations.

Recommended blood screening tests before beginning lithium therapy: sodium, potassium, calcium, phosphate, BUN, creatinine, TSH, T_4, CBC, urinalysis with specific gravity and osmolality

Some drugs that may cause increased serum lithium concentration: indomethacin, hydrochlorothiazide, diclofenac

Some drugs that may cause decreased serum lithium concentration: theophylline, aminophylline, acetazolamide, sodium bicarbonate, spironolactone, urea

Drug interactions may cause lithium toxicity at low lithium concentration (e.g., methyldopa, tetracycline).

Effect of lithium on other laboratory test values

- Increased TSH in 30% of patients (clinically euthyroid)
- Increased parathormone with resultant increased serum calcium and decreased phosphorus
- Decreased serum testosterone
- May affect TRH, GH, ADH

Serum lithium values may be increased by

- Decreased GFR (e.g., aging)
- Sodium deprivation and dehydration

Serum lithium values may be decreased

- By increased GFR (e.g., pregnancy, hemodialysis)
- In burn patients

Pentobarbital

(Data from ref. [4] in Table 18-1)

Therapeutic range: 1–5 μg/mL

Target for reducing intracranial pressure: 30–40 μg/mL

Toxic concentration: $\geq 10\ \mu$g/mL

Phenobarbital (Luminal)

(Used for treatment of seizure disorders)

Data from ref. [3] in Table 18-1)

Draw blood just before next oral dose, after steady state has been reached (11–25 days in adults; 8–15 days in children).

Therapeutic range: 20–40 μg/mL in adults; 15–30 μg/mL in children

Toxic concentration: >55 μg/mL

Monitoring is indicated when seizures are poorly controlled or patients have toxic symptoms, or 2–3 wks after change in dose or drug (e.g., primidone and mephobarbital, which are metabolized to phenobarbital).

Valproic acid may cause increased serum concentrations.

Phenytoin (Dilantin)

(Data from ref. [3] in Table 18-1)

(Testing is used to monitor therapeutic oral maintenance.)

Patient should be on stable dose for at least 1 wk; draw blood just before next dose. Draw trough sample 1 wk after beginning treatment and again in 3–5 wks. After IV administration, draw blood 2–4 hrs after loading dose.

Therapeutic drug monitoring is indicated when

- Medication or dosage has changed (allow 1 wk to reach steady state).
- Seizures are poorly controlled.
- Toxic symptoms occur.
- Patients are children (10–13 yrs old); monitor every 3–4 mos until stable concentration occurs.

Effect on other laboratory tests

Decreased serum free testosterone and increased total testosterone

May be artifactually increased in uremia when measured by various methods (e.g., immunoassay) compared to value obtained by HPLC.

Therapeutic or toxic effects may occur at a lower blood concentration in presence of decreased serum albumin, increased bilirubin, increased BUN.

Not altered by dialysis.

Some drugs that may cause increased phenytoin blood concentration (ref. [2] in Table 18-1): isoniazid, phenylbutazone, bishydroxycoumarin, diazepam, chlorpromazine

Some drugs that may cause decreased phenytoin blood concentration (ref. [2] in Table 18-1): ethanol, valproic acid, carbamazepine

Therapeutic range: total = 10–20 μg/mL; free = 1–2 μg/mL

Toxic concentration: total = $\geq$ 25 μg/mL; free = $\geq$ 2.5 μg/mL

Theophylline

(Data from ref. [4] in Table 18-1)

Therapeutic range: 10–20 μg/mL (adults), 5–20 μg/mL (children); <5 μg/mL is usually ineffective.

Toxic concentration: >20 μg/mL is toxic in 75% of persons.

Concentrations are usually measured at peak rather than trough.

Peak occurs 2 hrs after ingestion of oral standard form and ~5 hrs after ingestion of sustained-release form.

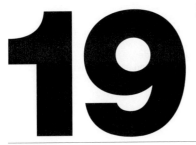

Body Substances

Amniotic Fluid

See Chapter 14.
Prenatal diagnosis of genetic disorders (see Chapter 13), e.g.,
   Hypophosphatemia
   Sickle cell disease, thalassemia
   Coagulopathies
Hemolytic disease of newborn (see p. 389)
Fetal/placental status
Fetal lung maturity
Prenatal/neonatal infection

Ascitic Fluid

See Chapter 7, p. 166.

Bile

See Chapter 8.
CEA (see p. 244)
Type of crystals (see Choledocholithiasis, p. 208)

Breath

Tests

Helicobacter pylori (see p. 804)
Lactase deficiency (see p. 108)
Fat malabsorption (see Chapter 7)
Alcohol—Breathalyzer (drunkometer) (see p. 921)

Odors[1]	Possible Toxic Substance or Condition
Acetone	Acetone, isopropyl alcohol
	Metabolic acidosis (e.g., salicylates, diabetic ketoacidosis)
Airplane glue	Ethchlorvynol, toluene
Alcohol	Ethanol (no odor with vodka or ethylene glycol)
Ammonia	Ammonia (e.g., uremia)
Bitter almonds	Cyanide (half of population cannot detect this odor)
Bleach	Hypochlorite
Carrots	Cicutoxin of water hemlock
Coal gas	Illuminating gas of gas stoves, heating units
Disinfectant	Creosote, phenol
Formaldehyde	Formaldehyde, methanol
Foul odor	Bromides, lithium
	Foreign body in orifices
	Lung abscess
Garlic	Arsenic, dimethylsulfoxide, malathion, parathion, yellow phosphorus, selenium, tellurium, zinc phosphide

[1]Viccellio P. *Handbook of medical toxicology*. Boston: Little, Brown, and Company, 1993.

Hemp	Marijuana
Mothballs	Camphor, naphthalene, paradichlorobenzene
Peanuts	Rodenticide (Vacor)
Pears	Chloral hydrate, paraldehyde
Rotten eggs	Sulfides (disulfiram, hydrogen sulfide), mercaptans, N-acetylcysteine
	Hepatic failure
Shoe polish	Nitrobenzene
Violets (urine)	Turpentine
Vinyl shower curtain	Ethchlorvynol
Wintergreen	Salicylate

Cerebrospinal Fluid

See Chapter 9.

Conjunctival Secretions

Smear (cytology)

Duodenal Contents

See pp. 185–188, 261.

Gastric Contents

See Chapter 7.

Hair

Disorder	Finding
Kwashiorkor	Pigmentary banding ("flag" sign)
Menkes' kinky-hair syndrome	Twisted hair
Argininosuccinicaciduria	Trichorrhexis nodosa
Ectodermal dysplasia	Misshapen hair
Irradiation and chemotherapy	Hair loss
Thallium poisoning	Specific changes in hair roots
Genetic mosaicism	Plucked hair roots
Low-sulfur hair syndrome	Polarizing light shows alternating light and dark zones (barber pole pattern), sharp cross breaks, low sulfur content, napkin-like folds
	Found in various conditions, e.g., dwarfism, ichthyosis, photosensitivity, complementation-positive xeroderma pigmentosum
Enzymatic heterozygosity	
Early deficiency of proteins or total calories	
Cystic fibrosis	Increased sodium and chloride

Not useful for assessing nutritional status of vitamins, minerals, other elements.

Drug Testing

Use (gas chromatography/mass spectrometry is method of choice)
- Drug screening (e.g., jails, workplaces, military environments)
- Investigate drug fatalities when other samples are not available (e.g., decayed or fragmented corpses)
- Screen neonate to detect drug abuse by mother during pregnancy
- Evaluate compliance in long-term drug therapy (e.g., antihypertensive, antipsychotic) or drug withdrawal in rehabilitation centers
- Detect doping (e.g., athletes, racehorses)

- Detection of
  - Heavy metals (e.g., lead, mercury, arsenic, aluminum, cadmium, uranium)
  - Drugs of abuse
    - Opiates (e.g., morphine, codeine)
    - Cocaine and metabolites, heroin
    - Amphetamine/methamphetamine
    - Hallucinogens (e.g., cannabis)
  - Hair analysis should not be used for forensic purposes without corroborative evidence because some substances (e.g., cocaine, benzoylecgonine) may also be incorporated from environmental exposure.[2]

Advantages for determination of drugs of abuse from hair samples include:
- Specimen easily obtained.
- Easy retesting of a second sample.
- Not affected by short periods of abstinence (in contrast to urinalysis) because hair grows at an average rate of 1.1 cm/mo (0.8–1.4 cm). Only the most recent 6 cms should be analyzed; telogen portion of hair may contain drug not used for more than 1 yr.
- Iron content has been described as a possible marker to monitor therapy in iron-deficient patients.[3]
- Not useful for assessment of zinc, copper, aluminum.

Interferences
Contamination due to selenium shampoo or lead-containing antigraying formulas.[4]

Meconium

See Cystic Fibrosis, p. 184, 256.

Milk

Infection: characterized by findings of $>10^6$ WBC/mL and $>10^3$ bacterial colonies/mL in contrast to cases of noninfectious inflammation or clogged duct. Usually due to *Staphylococcus aureus* or *Staphylococcus epidermidis* (penicillin resistant).
Infection develops in ~2.5% of nursing mothers, usually 2–5 wks postpartum.

Nails

See Table 19-1.
Heavy metal poisoning
Scrapings from under nails of victim in forensic cases

Nasal Secretions

Increased neutrophils in infection (see p. 139)
Increased eosinophils in allergy (Hansel's stain)
Increased eosinophils and neutrophils in infection superimposed on chronic allergy
Rapid antigen detection for RSV
Differentiate nasal secretions from CSF in possible skull fracture (See Trauma, Head, p. 291.)
Transferrin by immunoelectrophoresis
  CSF shows a double band
  Other body fluids (nasal secretions, tears, saliva, serum, lymph) show a single band
Glucose by test tape or tablets
  Positive in CSF
  Negative in nasal secretions (not reliable because may normally be positive in nasal secretions)

BODY SUBST

---

[2]Kintz P, ed. *Drug testing in hair*. New York: CRC Press, 1996.
[3]Bisse E, et al. Hair iron content: possible marker to complement monitoring therapy of iron deficiency in patients with chronic inflammatory bowel disease? *Clin Chem* 1996;42:1270.
[4]Crounse RG. The diagnostic value of microscopic examination of human hair. *Arch Pathol Lab Med* 1987;111:700.

Table 19-1. Nail Appearance and Associated Disorders

Nail Disorder	Nail Appearance	Associated Disorders	Drugs
Blue nails	Blue lunulae.	Wilson's disease	Minocycline
		Hemochromatosis	Silver nitrate
		Ochronosis	Antimalarials
Brown nails		Melanoma	Gold
		Addison's disease	
		Hemochromatosis	
Yellow nail syndrome	Diffuse yellow to green color; thickened; slow growth; increased side-to-side curvature.	Systemic disease (usually pulmonary effusion, bronchiectasis), cancer (e.g., lymphoma, melanoma)	
Half and half	Proximal half dull and white, obliterates lunula. Distal half is pink or brown.	Uremia (10% of patients)	
Terry's nails	Proximal two-thirds of nail is white; distal one-half is red.	Congestive heart failure Cirrhosis with decreased serum albumin	
Muehrcke's lines	Paired horizontal narrow white and normal color bands.	Nephrotic syndrome with decreased serum albumin	
Splinter hemorrhage		Multisystem disease (e.g., SBE) Trauma	
Koilonychia	Soft, thin nail plates causing concave or spoon-shaped nails.	Iron deficiency Raynaud's syndrome Hemochromatosis Trauma May be autosomal dominant trait	
Oncholysis (Plummer's) disease	Separation of nail plate from nail bed.	Hyperthyroidism Psoriasis Trauma	Chemicals
Nail fold telangiectasia		Dermatomyositis, SLE	

SBE = subacute bacterial endocarditis.

Pancreatic Secretions

See p. 185; Pancreatic Pseudocyst (p. 261).

Pleural/Pericardial Fluid

See p. 140.

Prostatic Fluid

WBC and Gram stain for infection/inflammation

Saliva[5-7]

Therapeutic drug monitoring (e.g., digoxin, phenytoin, lithium, theophylline, pheno-
    barbital, dexamethasone)
Testing for drugs of abuse (e.g., ethanol, amphetamines, barbiturates, benzodiazepines,
    cocaine, marijuana, heroin, codeine, PCP, nicotine [cotine]). Check winners of horse
    races for race fixing.
Diagnosis of infection in certain patients, e.g.,
    HIV—perinatal diagnosis
    Hepatitis A and B
    Rabies
Hormone assay, e.g.,
    Testosterone
    Androstenedione
    Estriol
    Radioactive iodine in hyperthyroidism, hypothyroidism (see Chapter 13)
Sjögren's syndrome (increased sodium, chloride; anti-Ro and anti-La antibodies)
Cystic fibrosis (see p. 256)

Saliva Test for Blood Alcohol

Use
Rapid identification of blood alcohol concentration of >0.02%
Saliva to blood ratio = 1:1.
Interferences
Alcohol vapors in air
Methyl and allyl alcohols
Peroxidases
Strong oxidizers
Ascorbic acid
Tannic acid
Pyrogallol
Mercaptans and tosylates
Oxalic acid
Uric acid
Bilirubin
L-Dopa
L-Methyldopa
Methampyrone

Semen

See pp. 678–681, 741, 764.

Skin

Fluid from pustule for cytology (inclusion bodies for various viral diseases), culture for
    some bacteremias (meningococcemia, Rocky Mountain spotted fever)
Fibroblasts for tissue culture for various genetic diseases

Sputum/Bronchoalveolar Lavage (BAL) Fluid

See Chapter 6.
See Cytology, Infection, Allergy
Pulmonary alveolar proteinosis (p. 154)

BODY SUBST

---

[5]Malamud D, Tabak L, eds. Saliva as a diagnostic fluid. *Ann N Y Acad Sci* 1993;694. New York. ASCP
Clinical Chemistry Check Sample CC 96-4.
[6]Read GF. Hormones in saliva. In: Tenovuo HFO, ed. *Human saliva. Clinical chemistry and microbiology.* Vol II. Boca Raton, FL: CRC Press, 1989:147–176.
[7]Millwe AM. Saliva: new interest in a nontraditional specimen. *Med Lab Observer* 1993;Apr:31–35.

Stool

See Chapter 7, p. 162.

Sweat

Color
    Brown: ochronosis
    Red: rifampin overdose
    Blue: occupational exposure to copper
    Blue-black: idiopathic chromhidrosis (in black persons, sweat of axillary chromhidro-
        sis may also be yellow, blue-green)
Electrolytes
    Cystic fibrosis (Chapter 8)
    Fucosidosis (Chapter 12)
Odor, e.g.,
    Maple syrup urine disease (Chapter 12)
    Organic acidemias (Chapter 12)

Synovial Fluid

See Chapter 10, pp. 307–317.

Tears

Decreased Volume In (Schirmer's test, Hamano thread test)

Sjögren's syndrome
Horner's syndrome
Decreased facial nerve function
Dehydration

Lysosomal Diseases that Can Be Identified by Enzyme Deficiency in Tears

See separate section for each disorder in Chapter 12.
Tay-Sachs disease
Sandhoff's disease
Fabry's disease
Fucosidosis
Mannosidosis
GM_1 gangliosidosis
Type II glycogenosis
Hurler-Scheie syndrome
Metachromatic leukodystrophy
Mucosulfatidosis

Urine

See Chapters 4 and 14.

Vaginal Secretions

See Chapter 14.
Forensic (e.g., rape/intercourse, p. 764)
Pap smear
    Hormone status
    Screening/monitoring gynecological atypias/cancers
Fern test
Fibronectin (see p. 772)
Infection (e.g., cultures, bacterial stains, wet mounts)
    Trichomonas/Candida

Vitreous Humor[8–10]

Postmortem glucose for diagnosis of hyperglycemia or diabetes mellitus, especially when ketones are also present and when blood is not available. Because glucose decreases after death, may not be useful to establish hypoglycemia.

Postmortem BUN for diagnosis of uremia when blood not available.

Sodium, chloride, carbon dioxide levels reflect antemortem values.

Increase in potassium of 12 mEq/L 100 hrs after death. Sometimes fluid is taken from both eyes at different times and the rate of change is used to establish the time of death.

Alcohol can be measured in vitreous humor even if body has been embalmed.

[8]Coe JI. Postmortem chemistries on human vitreous humor. *Am J Clin Pathol* 1969;51:741.
[9]Coe JI. Postmortem chemistry: practical considerations and a review of the literature. *J Forensic Sci* 1974;19:13.
[10]Burkhard M, Hensage C. Eye changes after death. In: Knight B, ed. *The estimation of the time since death in the early postmortem period*. London: Edward Arnold, 1995:106.

BODY SUBST

Bibliography

Baron EJ, Finegold SM. *Bailey & Scott's diagnostic microbiology*, 8th ed. St. Louis: Mosby, 1990.

Baum GL, Celli BR, Crapo JD, Karlinsky JB, eds. *Textbook of pulmonary diseases*, 6th ed. Philadelphia: Lippincott–Raven Publishers, 1997.

Becker KL, et al., eds. *Principles and practice of endocrinology and metabolism*, 2nd ed. Philadelphia: JB Lippincott, 1995.

Bennett JC, Plum F. *Cecil textbook of medicine*, 20th ed. Philadelphia: WB Saunders, 1996.

Black RM, Alfred HJ, Fan P, Stoff JS. *Rose & Black's clinical problems in nephrology*. Boston: Little, Brown and Company, 1996.

Carey CF, Lee HH, Woeltje KF. *The Washington manual of medical therapeutics*, 29th ed. Philadelphia: Lippincott–Raven Publishers, 1998.

Cotran RS, Kumar V, Robbins SL, Schoen FJ. *Robbins pathologic basis of disease*, 6th ed. Philadelphia: WB Saunders, 1998.

DeGroot LJ, et al., eds. *Endocrinology*. Philadelphia: WB Saunders, 1989.

Edelman CM, Bernstein J, Meadow SR, Spitzer A, Travis LB, eds. *Pediatric kidney disease*, 2nd ed. Boston: Little, Brown and Company, 1992.

Falk SA, ed. *Thyroid disease. Endocrinology, surgery, nuclear medicine, and radiotherapy*, 2nd ed. Philadelphia: Lippincott–Raven Publishers, 1997.

Frank MM, Austen KF, Claman HN, Unanue ER, eds. *Samter's immunologic diseases*, 5th ed. Boston: Little, Brown and Company, 1995.

Gantz NM, Brown RB, Berk SL, Esposito AL, Gleckman RA. *Manual of clinical problems in infectious diseases*, 4th ed. Philadelphia: Lippincott Williams & Wilkins, 1999.

Greene A, Morgan I. *Neonatal and clinical biochemistry*. London: ACB Venture Publications, 1993.

Greenfield LJ, Mulholland M, Oldham KT, Zelenock GB, Lillemoe KD, eds. *Surgery. Scientific principles and practice,* 2nd ed. Philadelphia: Lippincott–Raven Publishers, 1997.

Handin RI, Lux SE, Stossel TP, eds. *Blood. Principle & practice of hematology*. Philadelphia: JB Lippincott, 1994.

Hurst JW, ed. *Criteria for diagnosis*. Boston: Butterworth, 1989.

Jandl JH. *Blood: textbook of hematology*, 2nd ed. Boston: Little, Brown and Company, 1996.

Kelley WN, ed. *Textbook of internal medicine*, 3rd ed. Philadelphia: Lippincott–Raven Publishers, 1997.

Krisht AF, Tindall GT, eds. *Pituitary disorders. Comprehensive management*. Baltimore: Lippincott Williams & Wilkins, 1999.

Lawlor GL, Fischer TJ, Adelman DC, eds. *Manual of allergy and immunology*, 3rd ed. Boston: Little, Brown and Company, 1995.

Lee GR, Foerster J, Lukens J, Paraskevas F, Greer JP, Rodgers GM, eds. *Wintrobe's clinical hematology*, 10th ed. Philadelphia: Lippincott Williams & Wilkins, 1999.

Mazza JJ, ed. *Manual of clinical hematology*, 2nd ed. Boston: Little, Brown and Company, 1995.

McMillan JA, DeAngelis CD, Feigin RD, Warshaw JB, eds. *Oski's pediatrics: principles and practice*, 3rd ed. Philadelphia: Lippincott Williams & Wilkins, 1999.

Nyhan WL, Sakati NA. *Diagnostic recognition of genetic disease*. Philadelphia: Lea & Febiger, 1987.

Robinson SH, Reich PR, eds. *Hematology. Pathophysiologic basis for clinical practice*, 3rd ed. Boston: Little, Brown and Company, 1993.

Schiff ER, Sorrell MF, Maddrey WC, eds. *Schiff's diseases of the liver*, 8th ed. Philadelphia: Lippincott Williams & Wilkins, 1998.

Schrier RW, ed. *Renal and electrolyte disorders*, 5th ed. Philadelphia: Lippincott Williams & Wilkins, 1997.

Schrier RW, Gottschalk CW, eds. *Diseases of the kidney*, 6th ed. Boston: Little, Brown and Company, 1996.

Scott JR, DiSaia PJ, Hammond CB, Spellacy WN, eds. *Danforth's obstetrics and gynecology*, 8th ed. Philadelphia: Lippincott Williams & Wilkins, 1999.

Scriver CR, ed. *The metabolic and molecular basis of inherited disease*. New York: McGraw-Hill, 1989.

Stein JH, ed. *Internal medicine,* 4th ed. St. Louis: Mosby, 1994.

Tietz NW, et al., eds. *Clinical guide to laboratory tests*, 2nd ed. Philadelphia: WB Saunders, 1995.

Trent RJ, ed. *Handbook of prenatal diagnosis*. New York: Cambridge University Press, 1995.

Wallach J. *Interpretation of pediatric tests*. Boston: Little, Brown and Company, 1983.

Yamada T, Alpers DH, Laine L, Owyang C, Powell DW, eds. *Textbook of gastroenterology*, 3rd ed. Philadelphia: Lippincott Williams & Wilkins, 1999.

Appendices

Appendix A:
Abbreviations
and Acronyms

Ab	antibody
ACE	angiotensin-converting enzyme
ACh	acetylcholine
AChR	acetylcholine receptor
ACTH	adrenocorticotropic hormone
ADH	antidiuretic hormone
ADP	adenosine diphosphate
AFB	acid fast bacilli
AFP	alpha-fetoprotein
Ag	antigen
AG	anion gap
A/G	albumin/globulin ratio
AIDS	acquired immunodeficiency syndrome
ALA	aminolevulinic acid
ALL	acute lymphoblastic leukemia
ALP	alkaline phosphatase
ALT	alanine aminotransferase (SGPT)
AMI	acute myocardial infarction
AML	acute myelocytic, myeloid, nonlymphocytic, granulocytic, and myeloblastic leukemias
	acute myelogenous leukemia
ANA	antinuclear antibody
ANCA	antineutrophil cytoplasmic antibody
apo	apolipoprotein
aPTT	activated partial thromboplastic time
ARC	AIDS-related complex
ARDS	acute respiratory distress syndrome
ASO	antistreptolysin-O
ASOT	antistreptolysin-O titer
AST	aspartate aminotransferase (SGOT)
BAL	bronchoalveolar lavage
BCG	bacille Calmette-Guérin
BJ	Bence Jones (protein)
BT	bleeding time
BUN	blood urea nitrogen
CAD	coronary artery disease
CAH	congenital adrenal hyperplasia
cAMP	cyclic adenosine monophosphate
CAT	computerized axial tomography
CBC	complete blood cell count
CDC	Centers for Disease Control and Prevention
CEA	carcinoembryonic antigen
CF	complement fixation
CHD	coronary heart disease
CIE	counterimmunoelectrophoresis
CK	creatine kinase
CK-BB	creatine kinase isoenzyme BB
CK-MB	creatine kinase isoenzyme MB

CK-MM	creatine kinase isoenzyme MM
CLL	chronic lymphocytic leukemia
CML	chronic myelogenous leukemia
CMV	cytomegalovirus
CNS	central nervous system
CoA	coenzyme A
COPD	chronic obstructive pulmonary disease
CRH	corticotropin-releasing hormone
CRP	C-reactive protein
CSF	cerebrospinal fluid
CT	computed tomography
cTn	cardiac troponin
cTnI	cardiac troponin I
cTnT	cardiac troponin T
cu m	cubic meter
cu mm	cubic millimeter
DFA	direct fluorescent antibody
DHEA	dehydroepiandrosterone
DHEA-S	dehydroepiandrosterone sulfate
DIC	disseminated intravascular coagulation
DNA	deoxyribonucleic acid
DNase	deoxyribonuclease
dRVVT	dilute Russell viper venom time
dsDNA	double-stranded DNA
DST	dexamethasone suppression test
EBV	Epstein-Barr virus
ECG	electrocardiogram
EDTA	ethylenediaminetetraacetic acid
EGF-R	epidermal growth factor receptor
EIA	enzyme immunoassay
ELISA	enzyme-linked immunosorbent assay
EMIT	enzyme-multiplied immunoassay technique
ENA	extractable nuclear antigen
ER	estrogen receptor
ERCP	endoscopic retrograde cholangio-pancreatography
ESR	erythrocyte sedimentation rate
Fab	antigen-binding fragment of immunoglobulin
FAB	French-American-British classification for acute leukemias
Fc	crystallizable fragment of immunoglobulin
FDA	Food and Drug Administration
FDP	fibrinogen degradation products
FENa	fractional excretion of sodium
FEP	free erythrocyte protoporphyrin
FNA	fine needle aspiration
FSH	follicle-stimulating hormone
FTA-ABS	fluorescent treponemal antibody absorption test
FT_4	free T_4
FTI	free thyroxine index
G-6-PD	glucose-6-phosphate dehydrogenase
GFR	glomerular filtration rate
GGT	gamma-glutamyl transferase
GH	growth hormone
GI	gastrointestinal
gm	gram
GN	glomerulonephritis
GTT	glucose tolerance test
GU	genitourinary
HAI	hemagglutination inhibition
HATTS	hemagglutination treponemal test
HAV	hepatitis A virus
Hb	hemoglobin
HbA, HbC, etc.	hemoglobin A, hemoglobin C, etc.

HbA1c	glycosylated hemoglobin A, hemoglobin A1c
HBcAb	hepatitis B core antibody
HBcAg	hepatitis B core antigen
HBeAb	hepatitis B e antibody
HBeAg	hepatitis B e antigen
HBIg	hepatitis B immune globulin
HBsAb	hepatitis B surface antibody
HBsAg	hepatitis B surface antigen
HBV	hepatitis B virus
hCG	human chorionic gonadotropin
Hct	hematocrit
HCV	hepatitis C virus
HDAg	hepatitis D antigen
HDL	high-density lipoprotein
HDN	hemolytic disease of the newborn
HDV	hepatitis delta virus
HELLP	syndrome of hemolysis, elevated liver enzymes, low platelets
HER2	human epidermal growth factor receptor 2
HGPRT	hypoxanthine-guanine phosphoribosyltransferase
HGV	hepatitis G virus
HHM	humoral hypercalcemia of malignancy
HHV	human herpesvirus
5-HIAA	5-hydroxyindole acetic acid
HIV	human immunodeficiency virus
HLA	human leukocyte antigen
	histocompatibility antigen
HPF	high-power field
HPLC	high-pressure liquid chromatography
HPV	human papillomavirus
hr	hour
HSV	herpes simplex virus
HTLV	human T-cell leukemia virus
	human T-cell lymphotropic virus
HVA	homovanillic acid
HZV	herpes zoster virus
IEP	immunoelectrophoresis
IFA	indirect immunofluorescent assay
Ig	immunoglobulin
IgA, IgD, etc.	immunoglobulin A, immunoglobulin D, etc.
IHA	indirect hemagglutination
IM	infectious mononucleosis
	intramuscular
INH	isoniazid
INR	international normalized ratio
IRMA	immunoradiometric assay
ITP	idiopathic thrombocytopenic purpura
IV	intravenous
17-KGS	17-ketogenic steroids
17-KS	17-ketosteroids
L/S	lecithin/sphingomyelin
LA	latex agglutination
LAP	leucine aminopeptidase
LD	lactate dehydrogenase
LDL	low-density lipoprotein
LE	lupus erythematosus
LH	luteinizing hormone
LPD	low-power field
MAI	*Mycobacterium avium-intracellulare*
MAO	monoamine oxidase
MCH	mean corpuscular hemoglobin
MCHC	mean corpuscular hemoglobin concentration
MCV	mean corpuscular volume

ABBREV

MEN	multiple endocrine neoplasia (syndrome)
MHA-TP	microhemagglutination assay for *Treponema pallidum*
MI	myocardial infarction
min	minute
mo	month
MoM	multiples of the median. Unit used to express marker concentrations in maternal serum that allows for variations in concentration during gestation and between laboratories
MRI	magnetic resonance imaging
NANB	non-A, non-B hepatitis
NSAID	nonsteroidal anti-inflammatory drug
5'-NT	5'-nucleotidase
OGTT	oral glucose tolerance test
17-OHKS	17-hydroxyketosteroids
PA	pernicious anemia
Pap	Papanicolaou stain
PAP	prostatic acid phosphatase
PAS	p-aminosalicylic acid
pCO_2	partial pressure of carbon dioxide
PCP	phencyclidine
PCR	polymerase chain reaction
PDW	platelet distribution width
PgR	progesterone receptors
pH	hydrogen ion concentration
Ph^1	Philadelphia chromosome
PID	pelvic inflammatory disease
PKU	phenylketonuria
PMN	polymorphonuclear neutrophil
PO	per os
pO_2	partial pressure of oxygen
PRA	plasma renin activity
PSA	prostate-specific antigen
PSP	phenolsulfonphthalein
PT	prothrombin time
PTH	parathyroid hormone
PTHrP	parathyroid hormone–related protein
RA	rheumatoid arthritis
RAIU	thyroid uptake of radioactive iodine
RBC	red blood cell
RDS	respiratory distress syndrome
RDW	red cell distribution width
RE	reticuloendothelial
RF	rheumatoid factor
Rh	rhesus factor
RIA	radioimmunoassay
RIBA	recombinant immunoblot assay
RNA	ribonucleic acid
RNP	ribonucleoprotein
RPR	rapid plasma reagin
RSV	respiratory syncytial virus
RT-PCR	reverse transcriptase polymerase chain reaction
rT_3	reverse T_3
SBE	subacute bacterial endocarditis
SCID	severe combined immunodeficiency disorders
SD	standard deviation
sec	second
SGOT	serum glutamic oxaloacetic transaminase (aspartate aminotransferase, AST)
SGPT	serum glutamic pyruvic transaminase (alanine aminotransferase, ALT)
SI	Système International d'Unités
SIADH	syndrome of inappropriate ADH secretion

SLE	systemic lupus erythematosus
SMA	Sequential Multiple Analyzer
spp.	species
ssDNA	single-stranded DNA
STD	sexually transmitted disease
T_3	triiodothyronine
T_4	thyroxine
TB	tuberculosis
TBG	thyroxine-binding globulin
TDM	therapeutic drug monitoring
Tdt	terminal deoxynucleotidyl transferase
Tg	thyroglobulin
TGT	thromboplastic generation time
THC	delta-9-tetrahydrocannabinol (marijuana)
TIBC	total iron-binding capacity
TPN	total parenteral nutrition
TRH	thyrotropin-releasing hormone
TSH	thyroid-stimulating hormone
TSI	thyroid-stimulating immunoglobulin
TT	thrombin time
TTP	thrombotic thrombocytopenic purpura
ULN	upper limit of normal
URI	upper respiratory tract infection
UTI	urinary tract infection
VCA	viral capsid antigen
VDRL	Venereal Disease Research Laboratory (test for syphilis)
VIP	vasoactive intestinal polypeptide
VLDL	very-low-density lipoprotein
VMA	vanillylmandelic acid
vWF	von Willebrand's factor
VZV	varicella-zoster virus
WBC	white blood cell, white blood cell count
wk	week
yr	year
Z-E	Zollinger-Ellison (syndrome)

Symbols

$>$	greater than
$\geq$	equal to or greater than
$<$	less than
$\leq$	equal to or less than; up to
$\pm$	plus or minus
$\sim$	approximately
$\times$	times, e.g., $4\times$ increase = fourfold increase

ABBREV

Appendix B:
Conversion Factors between Conventional and Système International Units

This list is included to assist the reader in converting values between conventional units and the newer SI units (Système International d'Unités) that have been mandated by some journals. Only common analytes are included.

Data from:

Nichols Institute. *Endocrine interpretive guide*. Nichols Institute, 1995.

McQueen MJ. *SI unit pocket guide*. Chicago: ASCP Press, 1990.

Système International conversion factors for frequently used laboratory components. *JAMA* 1988;260:74.

Tietz NW, et al. *Clinical guide to laboratory tests*, 2nd ed. Philadelphia: WB Saunders, 1995.

Tietz NW, et al. *Textbook of clinical chemistry*. Philadelphia: WB Saunders, 1986.

Young DS. Implementation of SI units for clinical laboratory data. Style specification and conversion tables. *Ann Intern Med* 1987;106:114.

CONVERSIONS

Table B-1. Hematology

Analyte	Conventional Units	SI Units	Conversion Factors Conventional to SI Units	SI to Conventional Units
WBC count (leukocytes)				
(B)	/μL or /cu mm or /mm^3	cells $\times$ 10^9/L	0.001	1000
(CSF)	/cu mm or	10^6/L	1	1
	/cu μL	10^6/L	10^6	10^{-6}
(SF)	/μL	/L	10^6	10^{-6}
Platelet count	10^3/cu mm	10^9/L	1	1
Reticulocytes	/cu mm	10^9/L	0.001	1000
RBC count (erythrocytes)				
(B)	10^6/μL or /cu mm or /mm^3	10^{12}/L	1	1
(CSF)	/cu mm	10^6/L	1	1
Hct (packed cell volume [PCV])	%	Volume fraction	0.01	100
MCV (volume index)	μ^3 (cubic microns)	fL	1	1
MCH (color index)	pg (or $\mu\mu$g)	pg	1	1
	pg	fmol	0.06206	16.11
MCHC (saturation index)	gm/dL	gm/L	10	0.1
	gm/dL	mmol/L	0.6206	1.611
Hb	gm/dL	gm/L	10	0.1
(Whole blood)	gm/dL	mmol/L	0.155	6.45
(Plasma)	mg/dL	μmol/L	0.155	6.45
Fetal hemoglobin	%	mol/mol (may omit symbol)	0.01	100
Haptoglobin	mg/dL	mg/L	10	0.1
Fibrinogen	mg/dL	gm/L	0.01	100

For abbreviations, see Table B-2 footnotes.

Table B-2. Chemistry

Analyte	Conventional Units	SI Units	Conversion Factors Conventional to SI Units	SI to Conventional Units
ACTH	pg/mL	ng/L	1	1
	pg/mL	pmol/L	0.2202	4.541
Aldosterone				
(S)	ng/dL	nmol/L	0.0277	36.1
(U)	mEq/24 hrs	mmol/day	1	1
(U)	μg/24 hrs	nmol/day	2.77	0.36
Androstenedione	ng/dL	pmol/L	34.92	
Angiotensin II	ng/dL	ng/L	10	0.1
Angiotensin-converting enzyme (ACE)	nmol/min/mL	U/L	1	1
Antidiuretic hormone (ADH; vasopressin)	pg/mL	ng/L	1	1
Albumin				
(S)	gm/dL	gm/L	10	0.1
(CSF, AF)	mg/dL	mg/L	10	0.1
Alpha$_1$-antitrypsin	mg/dL	gm/L	0.01	100
AFP				
(S)	ng/mL	μg/L	1	1
	ng/dL	ng/L	10	0.1
	mg/dL	gm/L	0.01	100
	mg/dL	mg/L	10	0.1
	μg/dL	μg/L	10	0.1
Ammonia	μg/dL	μmol/L	0.714	1.4
(P)	μg/dL	μmol/L	0.5872	1.703
Anion gap	mEq/L	mmol/L	1	1
Base excess	mEq/L	mmol/L	1	1
Bicarbonate	mEq/L	mmol/L	1	1
Bilirubin	mg/dL	μmol/L	17.1	0.0584
Calcitonin	pg/mL	ng/L	1	1
Catecholamines (U)				
Norepinephrine	μg/24 hrs	nmol/day	5.91	0.169
	μg/mg creatinine	μmol/mol creatinine	669	0.00149
	pg/mL	pmol/L	5.91	0.169
	ng/mL	nmol/L	5.91	0.169
Epinephrine	μg/24 hrs	nmol/day	5.46	0.183
	μg/mg creatinine	μmol/mol creatinine	617	0.00162
	pg/mL	pmol/L	5.46	0.183
	ng/mL	nmol/L	5.46	0.183
Normetanephrine	ng/mL	nmol/L	5.46	0.183
	mg/gm creatinine	μmol/mmol creatinine		
Dopamine	μg/24 hrs	nmol/day	6.53	0.153
	μg/mg creatinine	μmol/mol creatinine	738	0.00136

(*continued*)

CONVERSIONS

Table B-2. (continued)

Analyte	Conventional Units	SI Units	Conversion Factors Conventional to SI Units	SI to Conventional Units
	pg/mL	pmol/L	6.53	0.153
	ng/mL	nmol/L	6.53	0.153
Metanephrines	mg/24 hrs	μmol/day	5.07	
	mg/gm creatinine	μmol/mol creatinine	0.5736	
Catecholamines (P)				
Epinephrine	pg/mL	pmol/L	5.458	
Norepinephrine	pg/mL	nmol/L	0.0059	
hCG, beta-subunit	mU/mL	U/L	1	1
	U/24 hrs	U/day	1	1
Calcium				
(S)	mg/dL	mmol/L	0.25	4.0
	mEq/L	mmol/L	0.5	2.0
(U)	mg/24 hrs	mmol/day	0.025	40
Carbon dioxide total (content CO_2 + bicarbonate)	mEq/L	mmol/L	1	1
CO_2 partial pressure, tension (pCO_2)	mm Hg	kPa	0.133	7.52
Standard bicarbonate (hydrogen carbonate)	mEq/L	mmol/L	1	1
Carotene	μg/dL	μmol/L	0.0186	
Chloride	mEq/L or mg/dL	mmol/L	1	1
CEA	ng/mL	μg/L	1	1
	μg/mL	mg/L	1	1
Ceruloplasmin	mg/dL	mg/L	10	0.1
Cholesterol	mg/dL	mmol/L	0.0259	38.61
HDL-cholesterol	mg/dL	mmol/L	0.0259	38.61
LDL-cholesterol	mg/dL	mmol/L	0.0259	38.61
Apolipoprotein A-I or B	mg/dL	mg/L	10	
Copper				
(S)	μg/dL	μmol/L	0.157	6.37
(U)	μg/24 hrs	μmol/day	0.0157	63.69
Coproporphyrins (I and III)	μg/dL	nmol/L	15	0.067
(U)	μg/24 hrs	nmol/day	1.5	0.67
(F)	μg/gm	nmol/gm	1.5	0.67
Cortisol (S)	μg/dL	μmol/L	0.028	35.7
	ng/mL	nmol/L	2.76	0.362
17-OHKS (cortisol) (U)	mg/24 hrs	μmol/day	2.759	0.3625
	μ/24 hrs	nmol/day	2.759	0.3625
Creatine (S)	mg/dL	μmol/L	76.3	0.0131
Creatinine				
(S, AF)	mg/dL	μmol/L	88.4	0.0113
(U)	gm/24 hrs	mmol/day	8.84	0.1131

(continued)

Table B-2. (continued)

Analyte	Conventional Units	SI Units	Conventional to SI Units	SI to Conventional Units
			Conversion Factors	
(U)	mg/24 hrs	mmol/day	0.00884	113.1
(U)	mg/kg/24 hrs	μmol/kg/day	8.84	0.113
(C)	mL/min/1.73 m^2	mL/s/m^2	0.00963	104
Cyclic adenosine monophosphate (cAMP)				
(S)	μg/L	nmol/L	3.04	0.329
(B)	ng/mL	nmol/L	3.04	0.329
(U)	mg/24 hrs	μmol/day	3.04	0.329
(U)	mg/gm creatinine	μmol/mol creatine	344	0.00291
DHEA-S				
(S)	μg/mL	μmol/L	2.6	0.38
(AF)	ng/mL	nmol/L	2.6	0.38
17-KS (as dehydro-epiandrosterone) (U)	mg/24 hrs	μmol/day	3.467	0.2904
17-KGS (as dehydroepian-drosterone) (U)	mg/24 hrs	μmol/day	3.467	0.2904
17-Hydroxycortico-steroids (17-OHCS) (U)	mg/gm creatinine	mg/mol creatinine	113.1	0.00884
11-Deoxycortico-sterone (DOC) (S)	pg/mL	pmol/L	3.03	0.33
Ferritin	ng/mL	μg/L	1	1
Gastrin	pg/mL	ng/L	1	1
Glucose	mg/dL	mmol/L	0.0555	18.02
Growth hormone	ng/mL	μg/L	1	1
HVA (U)	mg/24 hrs	μmol/day	5.49	0.182
	μg/24 hrs	μmol/day	0.00549	182
	μg/mg creatinine	mmol/mol creatinine	0.621	1.61
5-HIAA (U)	mg/24 hrs	μmol/day	5.2	0.19
Hormone receptors (T)				
Estrogen receptor assay	fmol/mg protein	nmol/kg protein	1	1
Progesterone receptor assay	fmol/mg protein	nmol/kg protein	1	1
Iron	μg/dL	μmol/L	0.179	5.587
Iron-binding capacity	μg/dL	μmol/L	0.179	5.587
Iron saturation	%	Fraction saturation	0.01	100
Lactate	mg/dL	mmol/L	0.111	9.01
Lead				
(S)	μg/dL	μmol/L	0.0483	20.72
(S)	mg/dL	μmol/L	48.26	
(U)	μg/24 hrs	μmol/day	0.00483	
Lipids (total)	mg/dL	gm/L	0.01	100

(*continued*)

CONVERSIONS

Table B-2. (continued)

Analyte	Conventional Units	SI Units	Conversion Factors Conventional to SI Units	SI to Conventional Units
Magnesium (S)	mEq/L	mmol/L	0.5	2
(S)	mg/dL	mmol/L	0.411	2.433
(U)	mg/24 hrs	mmol/day	0.411	2.433
Osmolality	mOsm/kg	mmol/kg		
Osteocalcin	ng/mL	μg/L	1	
O$_2$ partial pressure (pO$_2$)	mm Hg	kPa	0.133	7.5
PTH (S)	pg/mL	ng/L	1	1
(P)	μLEq/mL	mLEq/L	1	1
pH	nEq/L	nmol/L	1	1
Phosphate (inorganic phosphorus)				
(S)	mg/dL	mmol/L	0.323	3.10
(U)	gm/24 hrs	mmol/day	32.3	0.031
Porphobilinogen (U)	mg/24 hrs	μmol/day	4.42	0.226
Potassium				
(S)	mEq/L	mmol/L	1	1
(U)	mEq/24 hrs	mmol/day	1	1
(U)	mg/24 hrs	mmol/day	0.02558	39.1
Protein, total				
(S)	gm/dL	gm/L	10	0.1
(U)	mg/24 hrs	gm/day	0.001	1000
(CSF)	mg/dL	mg/L	10	0.1
Renin (PRA)	ng/mL/hr	μg/L/hr	1	1
Serotonin (S)	ng/mL	μmol/L	0.00568	176
Sodium				
(S)	mEq/L	mmol/L	1	1
(U)	mEq/24 hrs	mmol/day	1	1
(U)	mg/24 hrs	mmol/day	0.0435	22.99
Testosterone (total) (S)	ng/dL	nmol/L	0.0347	28.8
TBG	mg/dL	mg/L	10	0.1
	μg/dL	μg/dL	10	0.1
TSH	μU/mL	mIU/L	1	1
Thyroglobulin	ng/mL	μg/L	1	1
TRH	pg/mL	ng/L	1	1
	pg/mL	pmol/L	2.759	
T$_3$ total	ng/dL	nmol/L	0.0154	65.1
Free	pg/dL	nmol/L	15.4	
Reverse T$_3$ (rT$_3$)	ng/dL	nmol/L	0.0154	65.1
T$_4$ total	μg/dL	nmol/L	12.9	0.0775
Free	ng/dL	pmol/L	12.9	
Transferrin	mg/dL	gm/L	0.01	100
Triglycerides	mg/dL	mmol/L	0.0113	88.5

(*continued*)

Table B-2. (continued)

Analyte	Conventional Units	SI Units	Conversion Factors	
			Conventional to SI Units	SI to Conventional Units
Urea nitrogen				
(S)	mg/dL	mmol/L	0.357	2.8
(U)	gm/24 hrs	mol/day	0.0357	28
Uric acid				
(S)	mg/dL	mmol/L	0.05948	16.9
(U)	mg/24 hrs	mmol/day	0.0059	169
Uroporphyrin (U)	μg/24 hrs	nmol/day	1.204	
	μg/gm creatinine	nmol/mmol creatinine	1.1362	
VMA (U)	mg/24 hrs	μmol/day	5.05	0.198
	μg/gm creatinine	mmol/mol creatinine	0.571	1.75
Viscosity (S)	Centipoise	Same		
Vitamin B_6	ng/mL	nmol/L	5.982	
Folate	ng/mL	nmol/L	2.266	
Vitamin B_{12} (cyanocobalamin)	pg/mL	pmol/L	0.738	1.355
Unsaturated B_{12} binding capacity (S)	pg/mL	pmol/L	0.738	1.355
Vitamin C (ascorbic acid)	mg/dL	μmol/L	56.78	0.176
Vitamin A	μg/dL	μmol/L	0.0349	28.65
Vitamin D (calcitriol; 1,25-dihydroxy)	pg/mL	pmol/L	2.4	0.417
(25-hydroxy)	ng/mL	nmol/L	2.496	
Vitamin E (alpha-tocopherol)	ng/mL	nmol/L	23.22	
Xylose (U)	mg/dL	mmol/L	0.0666	15.01
	gm/5 hrs	mmol/5 hrs	6.66	0.15

AF = amniotic fluid; C = clearance; F = feces; S = serum; SF = synovial fluid; T = tissue; U = urine. All reference is to serum unless otherwise stated.

CONVERSIONS

Table B-3. Therapeutic and Toxic Drugs*

Analyte	Conventional Units	SI Units	Conventional to SI Units	SI to Conventional Units
			\multicolumn{2}{c}{Conversion Factors}	
Acetaminophen	μg/mL	μmol/L	6.62	0.151
Amikacin	μg/mL	μmol/L	1.71	0.585
Amitryptyline	ng/mL	nmol/L	3.61	0.277
Amobarbital	μg/mL	μmol/L	4.42	0.226
Amphetamine	ng/mL	nmol/L	7.4	0.135
	μg/mL	μmol/L	7.4	0.135
Bromide	μg/mL	mmol/L	0.0125	79.9
Caffeine	μg/mL	μmol/L	5.15	0.194
Carbamazepine (Tegretol, others)	μg/mL	μmol/L	4.23	0.236
Carbenicillin	μg/mL	μmol/L	2.64	0.378
Chloral hydrate	μg/mL	μmol/L	6.69	0.149
Chloramphenicol	μg/mL	μmol/L	3.09	0.323
Chlordiazepoxide (Librium, others)	ng/mL	μmol/L	0.00334	300
Chlorpromazine (Thorazine)	ng/mL	nmol/L	3.14	0.319
Chlorpropamide (Diabinese)	μg/mL	μmol/L	3.61	0.227
Cimetidine (Tagamet)	μg/mL	μmol/L	3.96	0.252
Clonazepam (Klonopin)	ng/mL	nmol/L	3.17	0.316
Clonidine (Catapres)	ng/mL	nmol/L	4.35	0.230
Cocaine	ng/mL	nmol/L	3.3	0.303
Codeine	ng/mL	nmol/L	3.34	0.299
Desipramine (Norpramin)	ng/mL	nmol/L	3.75	0.267
Diazepam (Valium)	ng/mL	μmol/L	0.0035	285
Digitoxin	ng/mL	nmol/L	1.31	0.765
Digoxin	ng/mL	nmol/L	1.28	0.781
Disulfiram	μg/mL	μmol/L	12.12	0.0761
Doxepin (Sinequan)	ng/mL	nmol/L	3.58	0.279
Ethanol	mg/mL	mmol/L	0.217	4.61
Ethchlorvynol (Placidyl)	μg/mL	μmol/L	6.92	0.145
Ethosuximide (Zarontin)	μg/mL	μmol/L	7.08	0.141
Gentamicin	μg/mL	μmol/L	2.09	0.478
Glutethimide	μg/mL	μmol/L	4.60	0.217
Haloperidol (Haldol)	ng/mL	nmol/L	2.66	0.376
Hydromorphone (Dilaudid)	ng/mL	nmol/L	4.85	0.206
Ibuprofen	μg/mL	μmol/L	4.85	0.206
Imipramine (Tofranil)	ng/mL	nmol/L	3.57	0.28
Isoniazid	μg/mL	μmol/L	7.29	0.137
Kanamycin (Kantrex)	μg/mL	μmol/L	2.06	0.485
Lidocaine (Xylocaine)	μg/mL	μmol/L	4.27	0.234
Lithium	mEq/L	mmol/L	1	1
Lorazepam	ng/mL	nmol/L	3.11	0.321
LSD (lysergic acid diethylamide)	μg/mL	μmol/L	3.09	0.323

(continued)

Table B-3. (continued)

Analyte	Conventional Units	SI Units	Conversion Factors	
			Conventional to SI Units	SI to Conventional Units
Meperidine (Demerol)	ng/mL	nmol/L	4.04	0.247
Meprobamate	mg/L	μmol/L	4.58	0.218
Methadone	ng/mL	μmol/L	0.00323	309
Methotrexate	ng/mL	nmol/L	2.2	0.454
Methsuximide	μg/mL	μmol/L	5.29	0.189
Methyldopa (Aldomet)	μg/mL	μmol/L	4.73	0.211
Morphine	ng/mL	nmol/L	3.5	0.285
	ng/mL	μmol/L	0.0035	285
Nortriptyline	ng/mL	nmol/L	3.8	0.263
Oxazepam	μg/mL	μmol/L	3.49	0.287
Oxycodone (Percodan, others)	ng/mL	nmol/L	3.17	0.315
Paraldehyde	μg/mL	μmol/L	7.57	0.132
Pentobarbital (Nembutal)	μg/mL	μmol/L	4.42	0.179
Phenacetin	μg/mL	μmol/L	5.58	0.179
Phenobarbital (Luminal)	μg/mL	μmol/L	4.31	0.232
Phenytoin (Dilantin)	μg/mL	μmol/L	3.96	0.253
Primidone	μg/mL	μmol/L	4.58	0.218
Procainamide (Pronestyl),	μg/mL	μmol/L	4.23	0.236
Propoxyphene (Darvon)	μg/mL	μmol/L	3.07	0.326
Propranolol	ng/mL	nmol/L	3.86	0.259
Quinidine	μg/mL	μmol/L	3.08	0.324
Quinine	μg/mL	μmol/L	3.08	0.324
Salicylic acid	μg/mL	μmol/L	7.24	0.138
Secobarbital (Seconal)	μg/mL	μmol/L	4.2	0.238
Theophylline (aminophylline, others)	μg/mL	μmol/L	5.55	0.180
Tobramycin	μg/mL	μmol/L	2.14	0.467
Valproic acid	μg/mL	μmol/L	6.93	0.144
Vancomycin	μg/mL	mg/L	1	1
Warfarin (Dicumarol, others)	μg/mL	μmol/L	3.24	0.308

*Only some of the more common or better known drugs are included.

CONVERSIONS

Table B-4. Measurements

Factor	Fraction	Decimal	Name	Prefix	Symbol
10^{-1}	1/10	0.1	One tenth	deci	d
10^{-2}	1/100	0.01	One hundredth	centi	c
10^{-3}	1/1,000	0.001	One thousandth	milli	m
10^{-4}	1/10,000	0.000 1			
10^{-5}	1/100,000	0.000 01			
10^{-6}	1/1,000,000	0.000 001	One millionth	micro	μ
10^{-7}	1/10,000,000	0.000 000 1			
10^{-8}	1/100,000,000	0.000 000 01			
10^{-9}	1/1,000,000,000	0.000 000 001	One billionth	nano	n
10^{-10}	1/10,000,000,000	0.000 000 000 1			
10^{-12}	1/1,000,000,000,000	0.000 000 000 001	One trillionth	pico	p
10^{-15}	1/1,000,000,000,000,000	0.000 000 000 000 001	One quadrillionth	femto	f
10^{-18}	1/1,000,000,000,000,000,000	0.000 000 000 000 000 001	One quintillionth	atto	a
10^{-21}	1/1,000,000,000,000,000,000,000	0.000 000 000 000 000 000 001	One sextillionth	zepto	z
10^{-24}	1/1,000,000,000,000,000,000,000,000	0.000 000 000 000 000 000 000 001	One septillionth	yocto	y

Factor	Fraction	Name	Prefix	Symbol
10^{0}	1	standard unit	none	
10^{1}	10	ten	deka	da/dk
10^{2}	100	hundred	hecto	h
10^{3}	1,000	thousand	kilo	k
10^{4}	10,000	ten thousand	myria	my
10^{5}	100,000			
10^{6}	1,000,000	million	mega	M
10^{7}	10,000,000			
10^{8}	100,000,000			
10^{9}	1,000,000,000	billion	giga	G
10^{10}	10,000,000,000			
10^{12}	1,000,000,000,000	trillion	tera	T
10^{15}	1,000,000,000,000,000	quadrillion	peta	P
10^{18}	1,000,000,000,000,000,000	quintillion	exa	E
10^{21}	1,000,000,000,000,000,000,000	sextillion	zetta	Z
10^{24}	1,000,000,000,000,000,000,000,000	septillion	yotta	Y

Appendix C:
Summary of Causes of and Diagnostic Tests for Spurious Laboratory Results

Effect of Artifacts on Laboratory Test Values

See Table C-1, p. 980.

Spurious values are false results due to various interferences in laboratory analysis but not due to clerical error, improper performance of tests, instrument failure, or poor reagents. They are sufficiently frequent that the clinician and laboratorian should be aware of them, especially in the face of discrepant laboratory results. Particular methodologies, reagents, and instruments are all important in determining these occurrences, and opposite results may derive from different technologies. Only those spurious results of greatest clinical significance and frequency are noted here. This section does not include discussion of the effect of drugs on laboratory test values that are even more numerous, factitious disorders (Munchausen syndrome), or technician or clerical errors.

Common causes of spurious chemical values are hemolysis and lipemia.

- Hemolysis releases RBC analytes and enzymes into serum (characteristically increasing serum LI), potassium, acid phosphatase and prostatic acid phosphatase, cholesterol [if hemolysis is marked]; AST, ALT, creatine kinase, iron, and magnesium may be affected to a lesser extent).
- Lipemia may cause hyponatremia, hypokalemia, hyperchloremia, and negative ion gap by means of three mechanisms

    Turbidity due to light scattering caused by lipid particles interfering with photometry.

    Partitioning errors that cause the analyte to enter the lipid, nonpolar phase, making it inaccessible for the chemical reaction.

    Fat replacing serum water and altering the distribution and concentration of electrolytes in the total volume of the specimen. This does not become a problem until triglycerides are >1500 mg/dL at which time serum is milky rather than just cloudy. Serum sodium decreases 1.5 mEq/L for every 1000-mg/dL increase in triglycerides. Serum iron may decreased.

In addition to spurious blood cell counts, histograms are often abnormal and may vary from one instrument to another. All histograms must be carefully scrutinized when spurious blood counts are suspected.

Table C-1. Summary of Causes of and Diagnostic Tests for Spurious Laboratory Results

Spurious Manifestation	Cause	Diagnostic Clue or Confirmation
Decreased platelet count	(a) Temperature-dependent agglutinins	(a) Accurate platelet count when sample is maintained at 37°C
	(b) EDTA-dependent agglutinins	(b) Associated low WBC, high Hb or Hct. Accurate platelet count using citrate- or heparin-anticoagulated blood
		(a,b) Histograms may be abnormal. Blood smear shows normal number of platelets; may show clumping. Normal blood smear from finger stick.
	(c) Overfilling of faulty vacuum blood collection tubes	(c) Use different lot of vacuum tubes
Increased platelet count	(a) Platelet clumping due to EDTA in patient with rheumatoid arthritis. Particles counted as platelets on automated blood cell counters.	(a) Rheumatoid factor present.
	(b) Bacteremia	(b) Bacteria on blood smear
	(c) Leukemic blast cell fragments	(c) Low MPV; leukemic cells present
	(d) RBC fragmentation	(d) High MPV
	(e) Small RBCs	(e) Blood smear, manual RBC count
	(f) Cryoglobulinemia due to globulin crystals being counted	(f) Normal manual platelet count or with warming; cryoglobulin deposits seen on blood smear; abnormal histogram
Increased WBC	Particles counted as WBCs on automated blood cell counters	
	(a) Clumped platelets	(a) Blood smear does not show increased WBCs; clumped platelets seen
	(b) Incomplete RBC lysis	(b) Abnormal hemoglobins or severe liver disease present
	(c) Cryoglobulinemia due to globulin crystals being counted in automated blood cell counters	(c) Normal manual WBC or with warming; cryoglobulin deposits seen on blood smear; abnormal histogram
	(d) Platelet satellitosis	(d) Satellitosis seen on blood smear of EDTA specimen but not on heparinized sample
Decreased neutrophils	(a) Cold-induced clumping (cold agglutinins, cryofibrinogenemia)	(a) Clumped WBCs on blood smear; abnormal WBC histogram. Corrected by count at 37°C.
	(b) Lymphocyte fragility in lymphocytic leukemia. Occurs with automated cell counters	(b) Corrected by manual count
	(c) Overfilled blood tubes causing inadequate mixing	(c) Associated low platelet count, high Hb and Hct

Finding	Cause	Comment/Action
High reticulocyte count		
Increased hemoglobin	Massive *Plasmodium* infection (a) Turbidity due to high WBC (b) Markedly increased serum bilirubin	*Plasmodium* seen on blood smear (a) Normal manual WBC and blood smear (b) Interference with Hb determination may occur at > 30 mg/dL of bilirubin; MCHC and MCH may also be increased
Increased MCH and MCHC; Hb may be disproportionately high	Hyperlipidemia interferes with Hb determination, especially with triglycerides > 1000 mg/dL	Normal count after replacing patient plasma with diluent; abnormal WBC histograms
Increased RBC count, decreased WBC and platelet counts	Inadequate mixing of blood tube before testing	Compare counts on properly and improperly prepared specimens
Increased MCV	(a) Increased blood glucose (600–2000 mg/dL) (b) Delayed testing for 24–48 hours, stored at 25°C (c) Fibrin strands	(a) Repeat CBC when glucose is normal (b) Compare with prompt testing or storage at 5°C (c) Repeat CBC using properly drawn specimen; fibrin strands may be seen on blood smear; falsely increased WBC and decreased platelet counts may be present with normal RBC count and histogram
Increased MCV with decreased MCHC	(d) Increased WBC > 50,000/cu mm	(d) Manual WBC
Increased MCV, anisocytosis	(e) Reticulocytosis > 50%	(e) Reticulocyte count
Decreased automated RBC count, increased MCV, decreased Hct	Cold agglutination of RBCs	Perform CBC at 37°C
	Cold agglutination of RBCs	Perform CBC at 37°C
Decreased RBC, WBC, platelet counts	Collection through catheter, diluting blood	Compare with correctly collected specimen
Decreased ESR	(a) Polycythemia (b) Abnormal RBC shapes (c) Very high WBC (d) Hypofibrinogenemia	(a) Hct, RBC count (b) Smear for sickle cells, spherocytes, acanthocytes (c) WBC (d) Evidence of DIC, massive hepatic necrosis
Decreased serum glucose	In vitro utilization of glucose by WBCs, platelets, or organisms	Increased number of cells (e.g., leukemic WBCs, nucleated RBCs, reticulocytes) or organisms (e.g., trypanosomiasis)[d]

(continued)

Table C-1. (continued)

Spurious Manifestation	Cause	Diagnostic Clue or Confirmation
Decreased serum sodium	(a) Specimen drawn distal to IV infusion of hypotonic fluid (b) Hyperlipidemia interferes with flame photometry but not with ion-specific electrode methods[a] (c) Hyperproteinemia[b] (d) Hyperglycemia[c]	(a) Measure glucose in same specimen; draw repeat specimen from another site (b) Repeat analysis with ion-specific electrode instrument
Increased serum sodium	Umbilical blood sample drawn through catheter coated with cationic benzalkonium chloride, which causes increased sodium and potassium with some ion-selective electrodes	Serum potassium also increased. Draw blood from other sites or without catheter or do not use ion-selective electrode methodology
Decreased serum potassium	Gross lipemia [see "Decreased serum sodium" (a)]	
Increased serum potassium	(a) Hemolytic anemia (b) In vitro cell lysis of markedly increased platelets or WBCs (c) Tight or prolonged tourniquet use (d) In vitro lysis of RBCs due to improper specimen collection or handling (e) Umbilical blood sample drawn through catheter coated with cationic benzalkonium chloride, which causes increased sodium and potassium with some ion-selective electrodes	(a) Evidence of hemolytic process (b) Very high WBC or platelet count (e.g., > 1 million/cu mm; serum level higher than simultaneously drawn plasma potassium level) (c) Compare with specimen drawn without tourniquet (d) Repeat analysis of appropriately collected specimen (e) Serum sodium also increased. Draw blood from other sites or without catheter or do not use ion-selective electrode methodology.
Increased serum chloride, negative anion gap	Hyperlipidemia causes light scattering in colorimetric assay	Hyponatremia also present; remove lipid before to assay
Increased serum chloride	Bromide in serum	Test for serum bromide
Decreased serum chloride	Same as for "Decreased serum sodium"	
Increased serum phosphate	Multiple myeloma	Evidence of multiple myeloma. May have normal serum calcium and renal function; normal value if serum is first deproteinized
Increased or decreased serum calcium	Increased or decreased serum albumin[e]	Increased or decreased serum albumin or total protein

Finding	Explanation	Corrective Action
Decreased blood CO_2 and bicarbonate, increased anion gap	(a) Dilutional effect of sodium heparin solution in blood sample (b) Loss of CO_2 by evaporation from sampling curvette may be up to 8.8 in 2 hours (c) Underfilling of blood collection tubes	(a) Different blood collection system (b) Prompt analysis of simultaneously drawn samples (c) Repeat with properly filled tubes
Decreased serum creatinine	Extreme hyperbilirubinemia interferes with creatinine measurement on certain instruments	Use different instrument (e.g., Astra-8 instead of Dupont ACA or Abbot-VP). BUN not affected
Increased serum creatinine	Acetoacetate as in diabetic ketoacidosis interferes with Jaffé method	BUN not affected
Increased PO_2	Exposure of blood to air bubbles, especially with microsampling	Repeat after proper collection and transport
Hypoxemia shown by pulse oximetry	Very increased WBCs (500,000/cu mm) or platelets, which utilize oxygen	Higher oxygen saturation shown by pulse oximetry
Spurious O_2 and CO_2 shown by pulse oximetry	Abnormal hemoglobins (carboxyhemoglobin, methemoglobin); IV administration of methylene blue	Arterial blood gases; demonstrate abnormal hemoglobins
Increased serum TSH, CEA, hCG, or CA-125	Patient's sera contains antimouse antibodies (or those of other animal such as rabbit) used in test kit	No other evidence of causative disease (e.g., hypothyroidism). Adding mouse serum or IgG produces normal TSH results.
Increased antibody titer for infectious agents	Treatment with IV immunoglobulins	Measure titers on suspected lots of IgG and on patient's serum obtained before treatment
Positive infectious mononucleosis rapid slide test	Very high levels of horse RBC agglutinins in patient sera	Minimal absorption with test guinea pig kidney or beef RBC suspensions
Stool-positive guiac test for blood	Toilet sanitizers present in toilet bowl	Compare with test of stool not collected from toilet bowl
Stool-negative test for blood	Blood leached from fecal surface into water	Compare with test of blood not collected from toilet bowl
Decreased urine creatinine	Cotton or rayon sponges in diapers or diaper material selectively absorb creatinine	Use alternate urine collection methods

[a]DIC = disseminated intravascular coagulation; CEA = carcinoembryonic antigen; hCG = human chorionic gonadotropin.
[b]Same mechanism as for hyperlipidemia and cationic effect of paraproteins, which displace sodium, decreasing sodium 0.7 mEq/L for each 1 gm/dL of monoclonal protein.
[c]Osmotic effect of hyperglycemia decreases sodium 1.6 mEq/L for each 100-mg/dL increase in serum glucose.
[d]Even with a normal blood count, glucose decreases at a rate of 7 mg/dL/hour at room temperature if blood cells are not separated from serum.
[e]0.8 mg of calcium is bound to 1.0 gm of albumin in serum, allowing for correction of serum calcium values. Binding to globulin only affects total calcium if globulin is > 6 gm/dL. Serum albumin and total protein should always be measured simultaneously with calcium determinations.
Source: Data from D Yucel and K Dalva, Effect of in vitro hemolysis on 25 common biochemical tests, *Clin Chem* 38:575, 1992. MH Kroll and RJ Elin, Interference with clinical laboratory analysis. *Clin Chem* 40:1996, 1994.

SPUR LAB

983

Index

Note: Page numbers followed by *f* indicate figures; page numbers followed by *t* indicate tables.

INDEX

INDEX